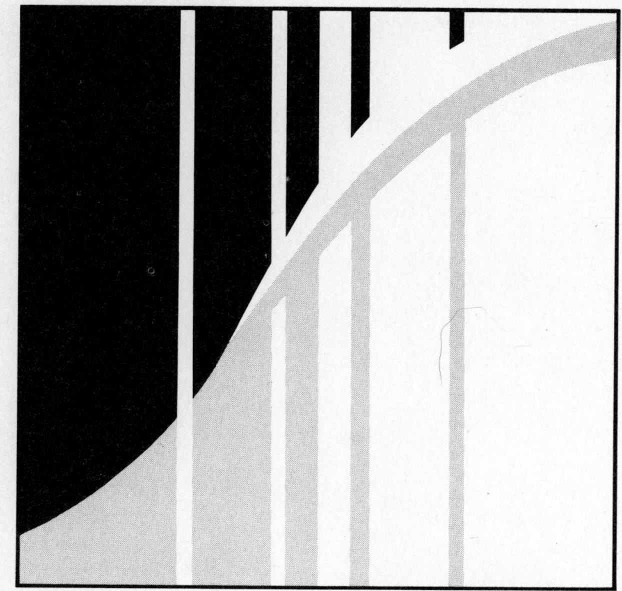

Pharmacological basis of nursing practice

JULIA B. CLARK, Ph.D.

Associate Professor of Pharmacology,
Indiana University School of Medicine,
Indianapolis, Indiana

SHERRY F. QUEENER, Ph.D.

Associate Professor of Pharmacology,
Indiana University School of Medicine,
Indianapolis, Indiana

VIRGINIA BURKE KARB, R.N., M.S.N.

Assistant Professor of Nursing,
School of Nursing,
University of North Carolina at Greensboro,
Greensboro, North Carolina

with 51 illustrations

The C. V. Mosby Company

ST. LOUIS • TORONTO • LONDON 1982

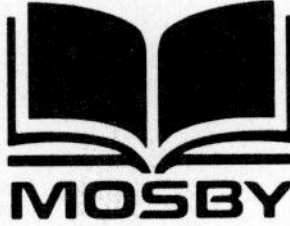

A TRADITION OF PUBLISHING EXCELLENCE

Editorial director: Thomas Allen Manning
Manuscript editors: Mary Dolan, Kathy Howell, Elaine Steinborn
Design: Diane Beasley
Production: Margaret B. Bridenbaugh

Great care has been used in compiling and checking the information in this book to ensure its accuracy. However, because of changing technology, recent discoveries, research, and individualization of prescriptions according to patient needs, the uses, effects, and dosages of drugs may vary from those given here. Neither the publisher nor the authors shall be responsible for such variations or other inaccuracies. We urge that before you administer any drug you check the manufacturer's dosage recommendations as given in the package insert provided with each product.

Printed in the United States of America

The C.V. Mosby Company
11830 Westline Industrial Drive, St. Louis, Missouri 63141

Library of Congress Cataloging in Publication Data

Clark, Julia B., 1940-
Pharmacological basis of nursing practice.

Bibliography: p.
Includes index.
1. Pharmacology. 2. Nursing. I. Queener, Sherry F., 1943- . II. Karb, Virginia Burke. III. Title. [DNLM: 1. Pharmacology—Nursing texts. QV 4 C593p]
RM300.C5 615'.1'024613 81-14192
ISBN 0-8016-4061-X AACR2

GW/VH/VH 9 8 7 6 5 4 3 2 01/C/068

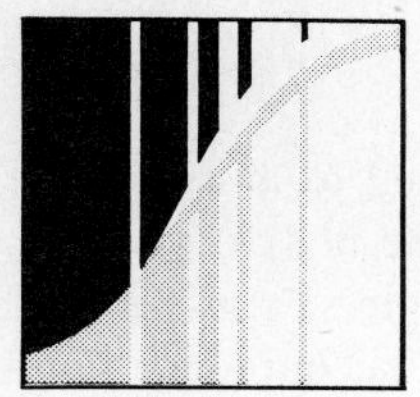

Preface

Having taught pharmacology since 1971 to more than 2000 nursing students in the baccalaureate program at Indiana University School of Nursing, we have been constantly dismayed with the pharmacology textbooks available for our students. We perceived a need for an up-to-date, scientifically based textbook in pharmacology that fulfilled the three basic requirements of the nursing student studying pharmacology: (1) a clear presentation of the concepts of pharmacology that guide all drug use, (2) a thorough treatment of major classes of drugs, emphasizing mechanisms of action, and (3) a clear and easily accessible reference on the patient care implications that grow out of an understanding of the pharmacology of specific drugs. With the help of another experienced teacher of nursing students, Virginia Karb, and with the guidance of the editorial staff in nursing at The C.V. Mosby Company, we have tried to produce a pharmacology textbook that meets these needs.

The book is divided into ten sections that represent the grouping we have found to be most effective with our curriculum. However, each chapter within the book is restricted to discrete topics, thereby allowing flexibility for instructors who wish to adapt the textbook to their own curriculum. This organization not only allows the instructor to rearrange the order in which material is presented but also gives the students succinct sections to master.

Students of nursing look forward to pharmacology as one of the important background courses for their professional education but often express frustration at trying to remember the large number of drugs they are called on to learn. We have minimized that difficulty for our students by dealing with drug classes first and then by emphasizing the similarities between members of a single drug class. This pedagogical technique of grouping drugs according to mechanism of action is reinforced by our chapter divisions, which are narrower than those of most textbooks in pharmacology for nursing students.

In this textbook we have emphasized the rational quality of pharmacology by relating the physiology of disease processes to drug mechanisms. Although we are more thorough than most textbooks for nursing students in describing the scientific basis of drug action, we do not neglect to review carefully the pertinent physiology so that students can readily see how drugs modify physiological processes. We do not present drug structures and we do not present biochemical reactions in molecular detail, choosing rather to discuss the physiological importance of chemistry and biochemistry when appropriate.

The first eight chapters that make up Sections I and II contain introductory material. The goal of these chapters is to provide the background information necessary for discussing drug action. These are the only chapters that are biased toward the science of pharmacology rather than the pharmacology of nursing practice. These sections form a necessary introduction to the concepts of pharmacology. We have written these materials so that students can see how this information can be applied to each drug or group of drugs to be studied. These concepts can be used as a guide for study of the drug classes presented later in the text. It is our experience as teachers that basic concepts need to be reinforced throughout the study of pharmacology or students fall out of the habit of organizing material according to these logical precepts. We have, therefore, systematically referred students back to these early chapters at logical points throughout the text.

The chapters in Sections III through X are organized in a consistent manner. The student is first presented with the physiology and cell biology required as background. When appropriate, disease processes are discussed briefly with reference to what is known about the aberrant physiological processes involved. However, we do not pretend to present clinical pharmacology in detail. Drug classes are presented, dealing first with the mechanisms of action of the class followed by the pharmacokinetics, side effects, toxicity, drug interactions if appropriate, and special comments on the clinical use of the drugs when necessary for clarity. To promote conciseness, we rarely discuss fixed dosage combination drugs, choosing rather to deal with individual agents. Following the basic material, the appropriate nursing assessment and management are reviewed in a section called *The Nursing Process*. A chapter summary follows in which the main points of the chapter are reviewed. A special chapter section called *Patient Care Implications* is then presented in which the specialized information required by a nurse for the appropriate administration of the drug and for the proper care, evaluation, and education of the patient is given in a straightforward manner. At the end of the chapter, study questions and suggested readings are provided for the student. The suggested readings offer readable discussions on the clinical uses of the drug and generally supplement and expand the information in the text.

The section in each chapter called *The Nursing Process* is meant to serve as a guide, particularly to the nursing student, in relating knowledge of medications with the overall plan of care for the patient. This section is not meant to supplant the use of additional textbooks of nursing and current literature. The focus is almost exclusively on the pharmacology rather than on the disease process itself. *The Nursing Process* section is divided into three parts. The first is patient assessment, in which some of the more frequent types of patients requiring the use of the drugs discussed in the chapter are identified. In addition, the assessment section identifies specific areas to be assessed that are particularly relevant to the type of patient usually receiving the drugs under consideration. The second section of *The Nursing Process* is management. This section encompasses the planning and implementation phase of the nursing process. This section identifies the type of data that should be monitored throughout therapy and some of the nursing activities needed to promote the drug activity or to promote patient well-being. Management also contains information on teaching the patient material required for self-management. The third section of *The Nursing Process* is evaluation, in which the usual desired outcome following administration of the selected category of drugs is described. We anticipate that the beginning practitioner and the nursing student may have difficulty in translating knowledge of a drug action into appropriate nursing interventions. *The Nursing Process* section leads the student into this translation process; the *Patient Care Implications* section carries this process on to the level of defining concrete clinical activities.

The specific clinical details of drug use and patient care are purposefully separated from the body of the text in the *Patient Care Implications* section. We believe that this method of presentation enables the student to use the book more efficiently at two levels. First, the student can master the scientific basis of the action of a particular drug. General comments on nursing assessment and management of patients are made in the text and are summarized and brought into focus in *The Nursing Process* section of the chapter. However, when students enter the clinical setting, they require much more specific information than can be effectively included in the body of the text. We have therefore gathered this information in the *Patient Care Implications* section, where it is easily accessible and where it does not interrupt the flow of the discussion on basic principles of drug action. The *Patient Care Implications* presuppose that the student is familiar with the drug being discussed. Therefore a person using this section for reference on a completely unfamiliar drug would be well advised to first read the appropriate material on the drug in the body of the text.

The specific organization of chapters is as follows. Section I begins with two chapters that introduce pharmacology and the principles of pharmacodynamics and pharmacokinetics. A chapter on drug administration that includes dosage calculations is then included. We have developed this material on drug calculation to introduce our students to this quantitative area of pharmacology. The chapter on the regulation of the manufacture, sale, and use of drugs is intended to give the student an understanding of the legal status concerning all aspects of drug manufacture, sale, and use. The chapter on over-the-counter drugs provides an overview of this often neglected section of pharmacology. Common combination over-the-counter products are considered in depth at this point, since with few exceptions combination products are not described in the remainder of the textbook.

Section II is an introduction to neuropharmacology. The principles of neuropharmacology are central to so many areas of pharmacology that three short chapters are used to present these basic principles. These chapters are written to provide an introduction on first reading and a review at a later reading. Drugs stemming from autonomic pharmacology have developed into so many clinical areas that we have found that the most successful approach in our own teaching is to present autonomic pharmacology first on a theoretical level and later on a systems level.

Section III is designed to cover those areas of pharmacology that are hard to define other than that they are systems under cholinergic control. In this section drugs affecting muscle tone, the eye, and the gastrointestinal tract are discussed.

Section IV presents those drug classes affecting the cardiovascular and renal systems. The drugs affecting the sympathetic nervous system appear primarily in Chapters 12 and 13, in which circulation and blood pressure are described. We are convinced from our teaching that it is more rational to present a systems approach to these areas of pharmacology than to describe all of cardiovascular pharmacology as variations of adrenergic pharmacology. However, within each chapter, we have taken an adrenergic mechanisms approach to the discussion of the cardiovascular disease processes. One chapter is devoted to drug classes affecting the kidney, two chapters to drug classes affecting the heart, and three chapters to drug classes affecting the blood.

Section V presents drug classes that affect the local mediators, prostaglandins and histamine. This area of pharmacology is rapidly expanding, with several new agents of this type recently appearing on the market. The mechanism of action of aspirin, from its role in pain and fever to its antiinflammatory activity, is first presented and used to introduce the other nonsteroidal, antiinflammatory drugs and drugs used to treat rheumatoid arthritis and gout. The antihistamines are next presented, followed by a chapter on bronchodilators and drugs used to treat asthma. This latter chapter and the following chapter on drugs controlling bronchial secretions contain the remaining sympathomimetic drugs not described in detail in the cardiovascular and renal sections.

Section VI presents drugs used for treating mental and emotional disorders. Drug abuse is not treated in a separate chapter in this textbook, but the pharmacological basis of drug abuse and its pharmacological treatment are carefully described for each class of drugs. The chapter on sedative-hypnotic and antianxiety drugs also includes a section on alcohol and the treatment of alcoholism. The antipsychotic and antidepressant drugs are presented as separate chapters, since psychoses and depression no longer are held to be the two ends of the same molecular seesaw. We have not emphasized neuroanatomy in discussing any central nervous system processes, having found that this approach does little beyond confusing the student. Instead we have presented central nervous system pharmacology in terms of neurotransmitter mechanisms, another reason for having reviewed the principles of neuropharmacology in an introductory chapter.

Section VII presents drugs used to control severe pain. The chapter on the narcotic analgesics highlights the recent explosion in the understanding of how these drugs mimic endogenous substances. The chapter on general anesthetics includes inhalation agents, intravenous agents, and the combinations now used for balanced anesthesia and neuroleptanesthesia. Local anesthetics are discussed with special reference to the routes of administration.

Section VIII covers those drugs used for disorders of central muscle control. The spectrum of anticonvulsant drugs is first presented, followed by a chapter that covers the antiparkinsonian drugs and drugs used to treat muscle spasms and spasticity.

Section IX presents drugs that affect the endocrine system. The first chapter in the section describes basic principles that may be applied to all of the endocrine organs. Subsequent chapters deal with the pharmacology associated with a particular endocrine organ. Sufficient information about endocrine disease states is presented so that students may understand the nursing assessment of these patients. Unlike most texts in pharmacology, this text includes enough information about endocrine testing methods to allow a student to understand the diagnostic procedures patients with many endocrine conditions must undergo. This information again facilitates and complements the material on patient management and teaching.

Section X presents antimicrobial agents and chemotherapeutic agents. The first chapter of this section introduces the general principles of antimicrobial therapy and explains how these drugs differ from the other agents discussed up to this point. Thereafter, each chapter describes the pharmacology of a major family of antibiotics. Enough microbiology is presented to make the clinical uses of each family of drugs obvious. Antifungal, antiviral, and antiparasitic agents are each considered separately, appropriately prefaced by information explaining why these organisms present more therapeutic difficulties than bacteria. The last chapter of the book deals with the many selective poisons used to treat neoplastic diseases. Again, mechanism of drug action is emphasized because an understanding of mechanisms allows the clinical properties of these drugs to be more easily appreciated and puts the nursing procedures into perspective.

The planning of this textbook has stretched over several years and has involved many people to whom we would like to give credit. In the early phases of preparation, we were assisted most ably by Nancy Evans, an experienced editor with The C.V. Mosby Company. Through Ms. Evans we established the collaborative arrangement that has worked so well throughout this project. In the latter phases of preparation, Mr. Tom Manning of the editorial staff of The C.V. Mosby Company contributed to the design of the book. Both of these editors strongly influenced the final form of the textbook.

Many of our professional colleagues at Indiana University have generously contributed time and expertise in reviewing materials for this book. We especially wish to thank the following people, many of whom critiqued large sections of material for us: Marlene A. Aldo-Benson, M.D., Associate Professor of Medicine; Grace Boxer, M.D., Assistant Professor of Medicine; Richard N. Dexter, M.D., Professor of Medicine; Joseph A. DiMicco, Ph.D., Assistant Professor of Pharmacology and Medicine; William C. Duckworth, M.D., Professor of Medicine; Joseph R. Holtman, Ph.D., Research Assistant in Pharmacology; Bonnie Klank, Pharm. D., Drug Information Specialist; Friederich C. Luft, M.D., Associate Professor of Medicine; Sandi Mazorati, R.N., Research Assistant in Neurobiology; Donald Niederpruem, Ph.D., Professor of Microbiology and Immunology; Raymond R. Paradise, Ph.D., Professor of Pharmacology and Anesthesia; Richard Powell, M.D., Professor of Medicine and Biochemistry; Judith A. Richter, Ph.D., Associate Professor of Pharmacology; Robert Strawbridge, M.D., Assistant Professor of Medicine; Robert Tight, M.D., Chief of Infectious Diseases, Veterans Administration Hospital, Fargo, North Dakota; Frank N. Vinicor, M.D., Associate Professor of Medicine; August M. Watanabe, M.D., Professor of Pharmacology and Medicine; Lynn R. Willis, Ph.D., Pharm. D., Associate Professor of Pharmacology and Medicine; and Thomas M. Wolfe, M.D., Assistant Professor of Anesthesia. Dr. H.R. Besch, Chairman of the Department of Pharmacology at Indiana University School of Medicine, deserves special mention for the support and help he has given us during the course of this endeavor.

Three professional colleagues deserve special credit, since they not only read and reviewed materials but also lived with the book as we did. These are our husbands: Dr. Charles M. Clark, Jr., Professor of Medicine and Director of the Diabetes Research and Training Center, Indiana University School of Medicine; Dr. Stephen W. Queener, Research Scientist, Department of Antibiotic Culture Development, Eli Lilly and Company; and Dr. Kenneth S. Karb, Clinical Oncologist, Greensboro, North Carolina.

Actual typing and preparation of the manuscript was ably performed by Ms. Julie Metcalf, Ms. Naomi Wilson, Ms. Brenda Heady, Ms. Vicki Lester, and Ms. Debbie Jubenville. Mrs. Janie Siccardi guided and organized the typing of the manuscript through some of the critical last phases of the project. Illustrations were rendered by Phil Wilson Artcraft.

Julia B. Clark
Sherry F. Queener
Virginia Burke Karb

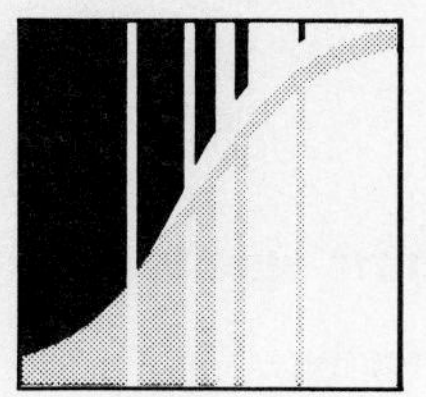

Contents

IX
Drugs affecting the endocrine systems

X
Antiinfective and chemotherapeutic agents

Pharmacological basis of nursing practice

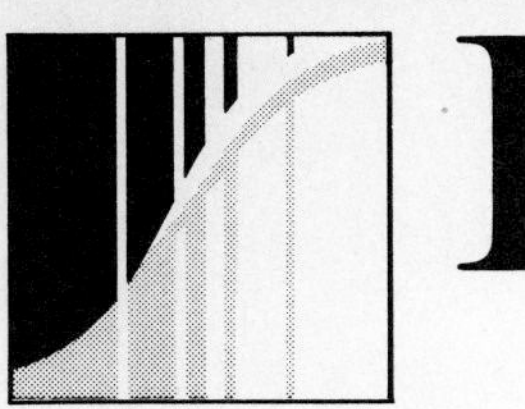

I GENERAL PRINCIPLES OF PHARMACOLOGY

The first two chapters of this textbook cover the principles that govern the action of all drugs in the body. These basic concepts and the terms defined in these first two chapters recur repeatedly throughout the study of pharmacology. By studying these concepts initially the student is made aware of how to approach the study of individual drugs and how to rationalize the manner in which an individual drug is used clinically.

Drug administration and dosage calculations are covered in Chapter 3 **(Drug Administration).** We have tried not to usurp the role of the clinical instructor in this area but rather have attempted to support clinical instruction with a basic presentation of the pharmacological considerations in drug administration. Drug dosage calculations are presented as a guide to the level of proficiency expected of practicing nurses. Whereas students with good arithmetic skills can readily acquire the ability to solve problems of the level presented in this chapter, our experience has been that many students initially experience difficulty because they have forgotten basic rules of arithmetic and algebra. Such students should seek to repair these gaps before attempting the drug dosage calculations.

Chapter 4, **Regulation of the Manufacture, Sale, and Use of Medications,** is intended to place the legal status of modern drugs into perspective. This chapter also introduces the Schedule of Controlled Substances and the D.E.S.I. rating, topics which recur at appropriate places throughout the text.

Chapter 5, **Over-the-Counter Drugs,** is included to emphasize the importance of these agents in nursing practice. The legal status of these agents, their properties, and drug interactions are discussed. The material presented in this chapter is a ready reference for the nurse in assessing the use of nonprescription medications.

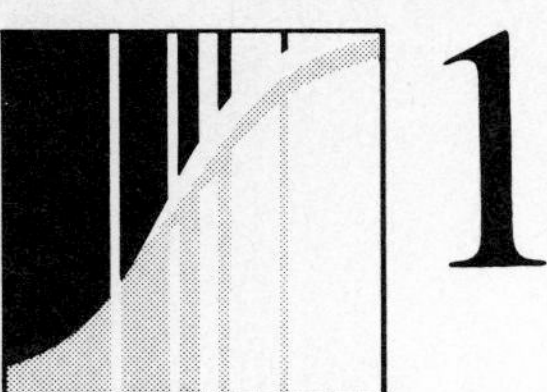

1 General principles of drug action

Pharmacology is the study of the interaction of chemicals with living organisms to produce biological effects. In this text are presented those chemicals that produce therapeutically useful effects, chemicals referred to as *drugs*. This chapter reviews the general principles of drug action that form the basis for understanding the action of specific drugs.

■ PRINCIPLE 1: DRUGS DO NOT CREATE FUNCTIONS, BUT MODIFY EXISTING FUNCTIONS WITHIN THE BODY

This principle explains the necessity for understanding the physiology of normal humans and the changes wrought by disease as a background for pharmacology. Drugs must always be considered in terms of the physiological functions they alter in the body. In no case do drugs *create* a function in a tissue or organ. For example, digitalis is a drug used to strengthen the action of the heart. Digitalis has this action because the drug alters the existing pattern of ion flow into and out of heart cells; it does not create a new way for the heart to contract. The drug simply alters the natural process.

■ PRINCIPLE 2: NO DRUG HAS A SINGLE ACTION

The *desired action* of a drug is an expected, predictable response. Ideally, each drug would have the desired effect on one physiological process and produce no other effect. However, all drugs have the potential for altering more than one function in the body. The desired action of the drug is distinguished from all other actions by referring to these unwanted actions as *side effects* or *drug reactions*. Again, digitalis is an example. Digitalis strengthens the failing heart; this is the desired clinical effect of the drug. At the same time, however, digitalis may cause erratic heartbeats. This action of digitalis is an undesirable side effect.

Predictable reactions arising from the known pharmacological action of a drug account for between 70% and 80% of all drug reactions. For example, barbiturates put a patient to sleep because the drugs depress the central nervous system. However, excessive depression of the central nervous system is lethal, since the brain centers controlling breathing will be depressed. Respiratory depression would therefore be an expected toxic reaction when barbiturates are used at doses that allow the drug to accumulate in the body. This type of toxic reaction to excessive amounts of the drug may be distinguished from predictable side effects seen at normal doses of the drug. These predictable side effects are related to the secondary actions of the drug. For example, barbiturates increase the drug-metabolizing activity of the liver at normal therapeutic doses. This ability of the barbiturates is unrelated to the therapeutically desired activity of these drugs and, in fact, is the mechanism by which barbiturates cause a number of reactions with other drugs.

Unpredictable reactions to drugs account for between 20% and 30% of all drug reactions. Although experience shows that a certain percent of the population may be expected to react to a drug in an unusual manner, it is not usually possible to predict which individual patient will show the reaction. The unpredictable drug reactions are of two types: idiosyncratic reactions and allergic reactions.

Idiosyncratic reactions are unusual, unexpected reactions to a drug that are usually explained by a genetic difference between the patient and the normal population. For example, a certain small percentage of the population lacks an enzyme called pseudocholinesterase, which is usually found in the bloodstream. Persons lacking this enzyme show no signs of this abnormality until they are exposed to drugs such as succinylcholine. Succinylcholine is a paralyzing agent used before surgery to relax the muscles and allow easy tracheal intubation. In normal persons the drug is very short acting, since it is destroyed by pseudocholinesterase. In persons lacking this enzyme, succinylcholine stays in the bloodstream and the drug is very long acting. These patients require artificial ventilation until the paralyzing effects of succinylcholine wear off, whereas a normal person recovers within a minute or so and requires no assistance. This prolonged reaction to succinylcholine is one example of an idiosyncratic reaction.

Allergic reactions to drugs account for between 6% and 10% of all drug reactions. The allergic reaction may be triggered by the drug in its original form or by a metabolite of the drug formed in the body. Most drugs are not very allergenic, but others are very efficient at stim-

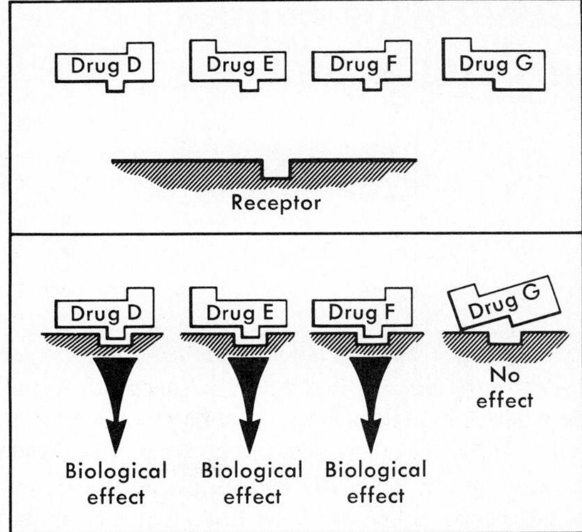

FIG. 1-1

Lock-and-key fit between drugs and receptors through which they act. Site on the receptor that interacts with a drug has a definite shape. Those drugs that conform to that shape can bind and produce a biological response. In this example, only the shape along lower surface of drug molecule is important in determining whether or not the drug will bind to receptor.

ulating antibody reactions from the immune system of the body. The exact symptoms of allergic reactions may vary from patient to patient and, to a certain extent, from drug to drug. The most common reactions involve the skin. One form of allergic reaction is *urticaria,* also called *hives*. These raised, irregular-shaped patches on the skin are frequently accompanied by severe itching. Other skin reactions include simple rashes (eczema) or contact dermatitis, which may occur when drugs are applied directly to the skin.

Although allergic reactions involving the skin are annoying, they are not usually serious, although extreme reactions can certainly occur. In contrast, allergic reactions involving the cardiovascular and respiratory systems are life threatening. This type of severe acute allergic reaction is called *anaphylaxis* or *anaphylactic shock*. Anaphylaxis is marked by sudden contraction of the bronchiolar muscles and frequently by edema of the mouth and throat. These reactions may completely cut off air flow to the lungs. In addition, blood pressure falls and the patient may go into shock. These violent reactions may occur within a very short time, and aggressive therapy is required to save the patient's life. Few people react to drugs in this way.

Allergic reactions may also involve other internal organ systems, and the symptoms may include fever, enlarged glands, joint pains, as well as others. For example, some drugs cause cholestatic hepatitis, which is an allergic reaction with symptoms resembling viral hepatitis. Other drugs cause allergic reactions that interfere with bone marrow function, lowering the production of one or more types of blood cells. The exact mechanism by which these reactions occur is not fully understood. However, since certain drugs are specifically linked to these reactions, patients receiving these drugs can be tested to detect early signs of these allergic responses and thereby be protected from extensive injury.

Allergic reactions do not occur during the first exposure to a drug, since time is required for the immune system to develop the antibodies that cause these reactions. In theory this fact should aid in predicting which patients are at risk of an allergic reaction; however, documenting prior exposure to a drug is not always easy. Neither do patients always know the names of drugs they have received, nor are patients always reliable sources of information on prior reactions to drugs. Moreover, persons may be exposed unknowingly to penicillins and certain other antibiotics through food or milk, since these drugs are sometimes used in animal medicine.

■ PRINCIPLE 3: DRUG ACTION IS DETERMINED BY HOW THE DRUG INTERACTS WITH THE BODY

■ Drugs chemically altering body fluids

Drugs produce their actions in one of three ways. First, some drugs alter the chemical properties of a body fluid. Examples of drugs that work in this way are antacids, which enter the stomach and neutralize excess stomach acid. Alteration of the pH of stomach fluid is the only intended action of these drugs. Other examples are drugs that accumulate in the urine and alter the pH of that fluid. By acidifying the urine with ammonium chloride or alkalinizing the urine with sodium bicarbonate, the ion flow in the kidney is altered and drug excretion patterns are changed.

■ Drugs chemically altering cell membranes

The second way drugs may act is by nonspecifically interacting with cell membranes. The interaction of the drugs with the cell membrane involves a chemical attraction and is usually based on the lipid nature of the cell membrane and the lipid attraction of the drugs. General anesthetic gases act in this way (Chapter 29). These agents dissolve in lipid-containing membranes and thereby alter the properties of the cells involved.

■ Drugs acting through specific receptors

The third and most common mechanism by which drugs act is through specific *receptors*. The biological activity of many drugs is determined by the ability of the drug to bind to a specific receptor, and in turn the ability to bind to the receptor is determined by the chemical structure of the drug. The interaction of a drug with a specific receptor may be thought of as being analogous to a lock-and-key fit (Fig. 1-1). Only drugs and naturally occurring compounds that have a similar shape, that is, chemical structure, may bind to the receptor and produce the biological response (Drugs D and F in Fig. 1-1). Only a certain critical portion of the drug is usually involved in binding, not the entire molecule. Therefore drugs that are alike in the critical region but different in other parts of the molecule might also be expected to have biological activity (Drug E in Fig. 1-1). In general, the better the drug fits at the receptor site, the higher the affinity (attraction) between the drug and the receptor and the more biologically active the drug will be.

When receptors are highly specific and have high affinities for the compounds that bind to them, very low concentrations of these compounds may show biological activity. For example, hormones naturally found in the body act through specific receptors. Some of these hormones are found at concentrations in the bloodstream of less than 1 picomolar, or less than one part per trillion. Nevertheless, these tiny amounts are biologically effective because the hormone is detected and bound by the specific receptor.

Receptors also allow for localization of drug effects to certain tissues. Each tissue or cell type will possess its own unique array of specific receptors. For example, certain cells in the kidney possess specific receptors for antidiuretic hormone. These cells therefore have the capacity to respond to this hormone. Cells in other tissues that lack these receptors are unable to respond to antidiuretic hormone.

Pharmacologists frequently speak of drug receptors. The concept of drug receptors is one of the major concepts in pharmacology. The specific receptors called *drug receptors* are actually natural components of the body intended to respond to some chemical normally present in blood or tissues. For example, there are specific receptors within the brain that respond to morphine and related compounds from the opium poppy, but until 1975 the natural function of these receptors was not known. It is now known that the brain and other tissues contain compounds called enkephalins and endorphins. These natural compounds bind to the so-called morphine receptor and are more potent than morphine in producing analgesia (Chapter 28).

Any compound, either natural or man-made, which binds to a specific receptor and produces a biological effect by stimulating that receptor is called an *agonist*. For example, the hormone norepinephrine binds to specific sites in the heart called beta-1 adrenergic receptors. Stimulation of these receptors causes the heart to beat faster. A synthetic drug called *isoproterenol* acts on the same receptors in the heart and produces the same effects. Both norepinephrine and isoproterenol are therefore called agonists for the beta-1 adrenergic receptor (Chapter 8).

Some drugs produce their action not by stimulating receptors but by preventing natural substances from stimulating receptors. These drugs are called *antagonists*. For example, the drug propranolol blocks beta-1 adrenergic receptors and prevents agonists such as norepinephrine from stimulating the receptor normally. Propranolol is therefore classed as an antagonist of the action of norepinephrine. Another example of a drug that acts by antagonizing the action of the normal agonist at the receptor is tubocurarine. Tubocurarine blocks the acetylcholine receptors at the neuromuscular junction that are required to maintain muscle tone. In the presence of tubocurarine, the natural agonist acetylcholine cannot stimulate the receptors and muscular paralysis results (Chapter 9).

• • •

The material presented in this chapter forms the framework on which subsequent specific information about drugs may be placed. For example, as each drug class is studied, the student should first seek to understand the mechanism of action of the drug. Does this drug operate through specific receptors? Does it alter a body fluid or cell membranes? Second the student should consider what side effects are likely to occur as a result of the action of the drug in tissues. For example, does the drug affect receptors in more than one organ or tissue? The student should note whether experience has indicated that allergies or idiosyncratic reactions are common with the drug. Finally, the student should consider the balance between the positive effects of the drug and the negative reactions to understand what place the particular drug may have in clinical practice. For example, some very effective drugs have limited clinical use because the side effects are unacceptable for most patients.

With this framework for study, understanding the pharmacology of individual drugs becomes a more rational process and is much more easily accomplished.

■ THE NURSING PROCESS

The concepts presented in this chapter translate logically and directly into the actions required in the nursing process.

■ Assessment

Assessment is that process through which information is obtained about and from the patient relative to the patient's medical condition. Assessment involves collecting both subjective and objective data. Subjective data are the information the patient reports to the nurse about present or past complaints. For example, when a patient reports being recently exposed to an infection and currently complains of specific symptoms such as fever, these bits of information would constitute subjective data. Objective data are obtained directly by the nurse or physician through observation, auscultation, percussion, and palpation. Laboratory data such as blood counts, x ray films, electrocardiograms, and other tests would also fall under the heading of objective data.

Assessment of a patient requires understanding what physiological systems are altered by the patient's disease. Assessment at this level allows the nurse to put the pharmacological therapy of the disease into the proper perspective.

■ Management

Management is a two-step process involving planning and implementation. Management of a patient arises naturally as a result of understanding the physiological basis of the patient's disease and the physiological processes altered by the drugs prescribed for this patient. Since drugs do not have single actions, this understanding also leads directly to an appreciation of expected side effects of the drug and explains the nursing actions that may be required to aid the effectiveness of the drug. Management also includes a teaching component. Nurses are expected to be able to prepare the patient for the use of the drug on an outpatient basis if necessary.

■ Evaluation

Evaluation involves determining whether the therapy has achieved the goals established in the planning stage of patient management. For example, knowing the mechanism of action of a drug and the expected effects on various body systems, the nurse may, by continuing assessment, determine if the expected effects are being observed. Evaluation also involves determining that the patient can explain how to take the medication prescribed, why it is being given, and what side effects may be necessary sequelae of drug administration and what side effects may require notifying the nurse or the physician. This phase of evaluation is obviously different for hospitalizied patients than for outpatients.

■ SUMMARY

Pharmacology is the study of how chemicals interact with living organisms to produce biological effects in that organism. The chemicals used as drugs do not create functions, but modify existing functions within the body. All drugs have multiple effects. Drugs may produce predictable side effects or may produce unpredictable reactions such as allergies or idiosyncratic responses.

Drugs alter the properties of body fluids, nonspecifically affect cell membrane function, or produce biological effects by interacting with receptors in various tissues. Drugs that bind to receptors and produce the natural response expected from that receptor are called agonists. Drugs that prevent the binding of agonists to receptors are called antagonists.

Understanding drug effects in the body in terms of basic, generalized mechanisms allows the health care provider to remember details of drug reactions and toxicity as part of a predictable pattern. This rational approach eliminates the need for rote memorization of repetitious material, since the same information may be common to many drugs of a class.

■ STUDY QUESTIONS

1. Why is an understanding of physiology basic to an understanding of pharmacology?
2. What is the difference between a drug action and a side effect?
3. What are two major types of unpredictable reactions drugs may produce?
4. Give three examples of types of allergic reactions drugs may produce.
5. What are the three general mechanisms by which drugs interact with the living organism to produce a biological effect?
6. What is an agonist?
7. What is a drug antagonist?

■ SUGGESTED READINGS

Bungaard, H.: Drug allergy: chemical and pharmaceutical aspects, Pharmacy International **1**(5):100, 1980.

Goth, A.: Drug-receptor interactions. In Goth, A., editor: Medical pharmacology, ed. 10, St. Louis, 1981, The C.V. Mosby Co.

Goth, A.: Medical pharmacology, ed. 10, St. Louis, 1981, The C.V. Mosby Co., p. 46.

Handwerger, R.L., and Hambrick, G.W.: Recognizing and managing drug eruptions, Postgraduate Medicine **52**(5):119, 1972.

Levine, R.R.: How drugs act on the living organism. In Pharmacology: drug actions and reactions, ed. 2, Boston, 1978, Little, Brown & Co.

Levine, R.R.: The scope of pharmacology—definitions. In Pharmacology: drug actions and reactions, ed. 2, Boston, 1978, Little, Brown & Co.

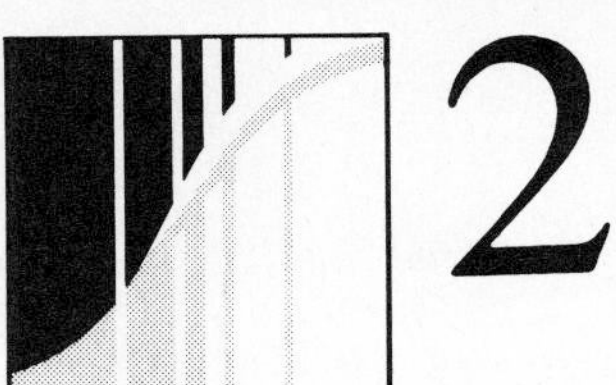

2 Principles relating drug dose to drug action

Most drugs produce biological effects by interacting with specific receptors at the site of action of the drug. The magnitude of the biological effect produced by a drug is related to the amount of the drug present at the site of action. Drugs differ not only in their intrinsic ability to produce an effect but also in their ability to penetrate to the site of action and in their rates of removal from that site. *Pharmacokinetics* is the study of how drugs enter the body, reach their site of action, and are removed from the body. *Pharmacodynamics* is the study of drug action at the biochemical and physiological level. Both the pharmacokinetics and the pharmacodynamics of a drug determine how a drug will be administered, how often it will be given and at what dose.

■ PHARMACOKINETICS

■ Factors controlling drug absorption by enteral routes

Drug dissolution. About 80% of the drugs used in clinical practice are administered orally, primarily because of the ease and convenience of administration by this route. The drug may be given in liquid form, but most often the drug will be given in a solid form such as a pill, tablet, or capsule (Table 2-1). To achieve this solid form, the drug is usually mixed with other compounds that serve various functions. Starches and other compounds may be added as inert fillers, especially when the actual amount of drug required per dose is too small to be conveniently handled. Adhesive substances called binders may also be added to allow the tablet to hold together after it is compressed in manufacture. Other compounds called disintegrators may be required to allow the tablet to absorb water and to break apart. Lubricants are frequently added to prevent the tablet from sticking to machinery during manufacture. These other additions to the dosage form may make up the bulk of the tablet. The formulation shown in Table 2-2 for tablets containing 100,000 units of potassium penicillin illustrates the use of these agents. In the formulation the active ingredient, potassium penicillin, makes up only 11% of the tablet mass. Stearic acid acts as a lubricant and acacia is a commonly used binder. The other compounds act as fillers and disintegrators.

Bioavailability. Bioavailability refers to the ability of the drug to be released from its dosage form, dissolved, and absorbed. To be effective the solid dose of the drug must break apart in the gastrointestinal tract and allow the drug to go into solution. Only the dissolved drug is absorbed from the gastrointestinal tract into the blood. Since breakdown of the solid dosage form is the required first step in absorption of the drug, any variability in this process can affect how rapidly and completely the drug is absorbed. The formulation of a tablet or capsule is one important factor that obviously affects dissolution rates. Tablets from different manufacturers that contain the same amount of active ingredient but different types and amounts of inert ingredients may not be identical in clinical action, since each formulation may have different dissolution properties. Tablets may also change with age and conditions of storage. In general, older tablets tend to dry out and become more difficult to disintegrate; hence bioavailability of the drug may be reduced.

Contents of the gastrointestinal tract. The presence of food may interfere with dissolution and absorption of certain drugs. However, some drugs are so irritating to the stomach that food may be useful to dilute high local concentrations of the drug. There is considerable variation from person to person in gastric emptying times and, therefore, in the length of time the drug spends in the acid environment of the stomach. In addition, the amount of acid in the stomach varies with the individual and the time of day. The very young and the elderly have less stomach acid than middle-aged persons. Lower acidity may mean less drug is degraded and more is available for absorption.

Chemical properties of the drug. In addition to the physical state of the drug, the chemical nature of the drug determines how satisfactory oral administration will be. First, to pass through the membrane lining the gastrointestinal tract, a drug must be relatively *lipid soluble,* since the membranes themselves contain a high concentration of lipid. Ionic (charged) forms of drugs do not easily pass through these membranes. Many drugs can exist in an ionic state or in an uncharged lipid-soluble state, depending on the chemical environment (pH) in

TABLE 2-1. Forms of medications

Form	Description
Capsules	Solid dosage forms for oral use in which medication is enclosed in a gelatin shell that dissolves in the stomach or intestine. The gelatin of the capsules is colored to aid in product identification. Various manufacturers have distinctive shapes distinguishing their capsules from those of other companies.
Douche	Aqueous solution used as cleansing or antiseptic agent for a part of the body or a body cavity. Douches are usually sold as a powder or liquid concentrate to be dissolved or diluted before use.
Elixirs	Clear fluids designed for oral use and containing primarily water and alcohol with glycerin and sorbitol or another sweetener sometimes added. The alcohol content of these preparations varies.
Glycerites	Solutions of drugs in glycerin that are primarily for external use. The solution must be at least 50% glycerin.
Pills	Solid dosage forms for oral use in which drug and various vehicles are formed into small globules, ovoids, or oblong shapes. True pills are rarely used, having been replaced by compressed tablets.
Solution	Liquid preparations, usually in water, containing one or more dissolved compounds. Solutions for oral use may contain flavoring and coloring agents. Solutions for injection intravenously must be sterile and particle free. Other injectable solutions must be sterile. Solutions of certain drugs may also be used externally.
Suppositories	Solid dosage forms to be inserted into a body cavity where the medication is released as the solid melts or dissolves. Suppositories frequently contain cocoa butter (cacao butter or theobroma oil), which is solid at room temperature but liquid at body temperature, or glycerin, polyethylene glycol, or gelatin, which dissolves in secretions from mucous membranes.
Suspension	Finely divided drug particles that are suspended in a suitable liquid medium before being injected or taken orally. Suspensions must not be injected intravenously.
Sustained action	Form of medication that is altered so that dissolution is slow and continuous for an extended period. Total dosage in sustained action medication is greater than for regular formulations, since the drug is not all released at once but over an extended period.
Syrups	Medication dissolved in a concentrated solution of a sugar such as sucrose. Flavors may be added to mask the unpleasant taste of certain medications.
Tablets	Solid dosage forms frequently shaped like disks or cylinders which contain drug in addition to the drug, one of the following ingredients: binder (adhesive substance that allows tablet to stick together), disintegrators (substances promoting tablet dissolution in body fluids), lubricants (required for efficient manufacturing), and fillers (inert ingredients to make the tablet size convenient).
Enteric-coated tablets	Solid dosage forms intended for oral use. Medication in tablet form is coated with materials designed not to dissolve in the stomach. The coatings do dissolve in the intestine, where the medication may be dissolved.
Press-coated or layered tablets	Preformed tablet has another layer of material pressed on or around it. This practice allows incompatible ingredients to be separated and causes them to be dissolved at slightly different rates.
Tincture	Alcoholic or water-alcohol solutions of drugs.
Troches (also called lozenges or pastilles)	Solid dosage forms shaped frequently like disks or cylinders which contain drug, flavor, sugar, and mucilage. Troches dissolve or disintegrate in the mouth, releasing medication such as antiseptic or anesthetic for action in the mouth or throat. Troches dissolve more slowly than tablets.

TABLE 2-2. Sample pharmaceutical formulation for penicillin (potassium) tablets

Ingredient	Amount contained in each tablet (mg)
Potassium penicillin (1595 units/mg)	69
Calcium carbonate	362
Starch	85
Sugar	25
Acacia	78
Stearic acid	3

which the drug is found. This environment changes along the gastrointestinal tract as illustrated in Fig. 2-1. The stomach fluid is highly acidic. A drug such as aspirin, which is a weak acid, will be converted from a charged to an uncharged form by the strong acid in the stomach. Since the uncharged form of the drug can readily diffuse through the lipid membranes of the stomach cells, the drug is rapidly absorbed. In contrast, drugs such as penicillins are not stable in the acid of the stomach, and part of the dose will be destroyed rather than absorbed.

Some drugs that are sensitive to the acid in the stomach may be protected by using *enteric coatings* on the tablets or capsules (Table 2-1). These coatings are designed to be inert at low (acidic) pH but soluble at higher (alkaline) pH. Therefore the drug passes through the stomach and is released in the intestine. Enteric coatings are also used for drugs that are highly irritating to the gastric mucosa.

The fluids in the small intestine are slightly alkaline. This higher pH favors the absorption of weakly basic drugs, since at this pH range weak bases are uncharged (Fig. 2-1). The small intestine also has an enormous surface area for drug absorption, making it a major site of absorption. However, some drugs, particularly proteins such as insulin or growth hormone, are destroyed in the small intestine by the action of digestive enzymes from the pancreas.

Drugs that are absorbed from the small intestine are transported by the portal circulation directly to the liver before entering the circulation to the rest of the body as illustrated in Fig. 2-2. The liver metabolizes a significant proportion of certain types of drugs before the drug can enter the general circulation. This process of absorption into the portal circulation with metabolism of the drug in the liver before the drug reaches systemic circulation is called the *first pass phenomenon*. The first pass phenomenon explains why oral doses of drugs that are readily metabolized by the liver must be much larger than would be given by other routes. The larger oral doses compensate for the drug lost through liver metabolism. The first pass phenomenon may be avoided by using

FIG. 2-1

Effect of pH on ability of drugs to cross gastrointestinal membranes. Strongly acidic environment of the stomach (pH 1 to 3) maintains weak acids in an uncharged form, which is more easily absorbed. Weak bases remain charged in the stomach, but are converted to uncharged forms as the pH approaches neutrality (pH 7) or becomes slightly alkaline (pH 7 to 8).

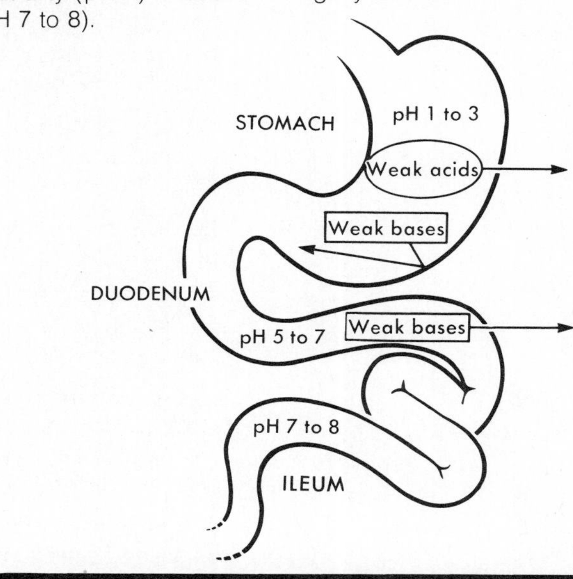

FIG. 2-2

Two circulatory pathways for materials absorbed from the gastrointestinal tract. Materials absorbed from stomach, small intestine, or colon enter portal circulation, which perfuses the liver before returning to heart. Materials absorbed from these sites are therefore exposed first to the action of liver microsomal enzymes and then are circulated to the rest of the body. In contrast, absorption through membranes lining mouth or rectum deliver the material directly to systemic circulation.

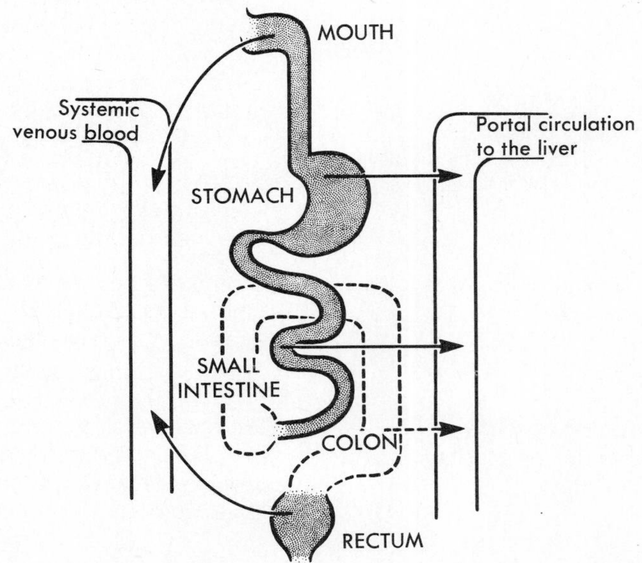

TABLE 2-3. Summary of major routes for systemic administration of drugs

Route	Description	Advantages	Disadvantages
Oral	Drug swallowed; absorbed from stomach and/or small intestine	1. Convenient. 2. Nonsterile procedure. 3. Economical.	1. Unpleasant taste may cause patient to discontinue medication. 2. Irritation to gastric mucosa may induce nausea and vomiting. 3. Patient must be conscious. 4. Drug may be partly or completely destroyed by digestive juices. 5. Absorbed drug enters portal circulation to liver where drug may be destroyed.
Sublingual	Drug dissolved under tongue; absorbed across mucous membranes of the mouth	1. Convenient. 2. Nonsterile procedure. 3. Drug enters general circulation before passing through liver.	1. Route is not useful for drugs that taste bad. 2. Irritation to oral mucosa could occur. 3. Patient must be conscious. 4. Only very lipid-soluble drugs are absorbed rapidly enough to be administered by this route.
Buccal	Drug dissolved between cheek and gum; absorbed across mucous membrane of the mouth	As for sublingual.	As for sublingual.
Rectal	Drug inserted into rectum; absorbed through mucous membranes of the rectum	1. May be used in unconscious or vomiting patient. 2. Drug enters general circulation before passing through liver.	1. Route is inconvenient. 2. Drug may irritate rectal mucosa. 3. Drug must be made up into a suppository.
Lung	Drug inhaled as a gas or aerosol	1. Useful for drugs intended to act directly on the lung. 2. Useful for drugs that are gases at room temperature and are very lipid-soluble (i.e., inhalation anesthetics).	1. Absorption across the membranes of the lung is too slow to be useful for most drugs.
Subcutaneous	Drug injected under the skin	1. Useful for drugs in soluble or relatively insoluble forms. 2. May be used in unconscious or uncooperative patients.	1. Sterile procedures are necessary. 2. Route produces a relatively painful site, and patient may suffer irritation from the drug.
Intramuscular	Drug injected into muscle mass	1. Relatively rapid absorption, since blood supply is good. 2. Useful for drugs in soluble or relatively insoluble forms. 3. May be used in unconscious or uncooperative patients.	1. Sterile procedures are necessary. 2. Minor pain is present on injection for most drugs, but irritation and local reactions may occur.
Intravenous	Drug injected directly into vein	1. Allows direct control of blood concentration of drug. 2. Most rapid attainment of effective blood levels.	1. Sterile procedures are necessary. 2. Too rapid injection may produce transient, dangerously high blood concentrations of drug.

other routes of administration, such as sublingual (drug dissolved under the tongue), buccal (drug dissolved between the cheek and gum), and rectal routes (Fig. 2-2). Drugs administered by these routes are absorbed directly across the mucous membranes and rapidly enter the systemic circulation. The sublingual and buccal routes are useful when a palatable, very lipid-soluble drug is involved. The rectal route is useful, especially when a patient is unconscious. The best physical form for a drug intended for rectal use is a suppository that will melt in the rectum and release the drug for absorption (Table 2-3).

■ Factors controlling drug absorption by parenteral routes

The parenteral routes of drug administration are primarily those which require injection of the drug into the skin, muscle, or blood. Injection necessarily involves breaking the skin, and sterile technique must be used to prevent bacteria from gaining entry (Table 2-3). Special precautions must often be taken to avoid producing undue tissue damage with irritating drugs. Sometimes these precautions involve preventing the drug from contacting the skin; other drugs require dilution before administration.

Subcutaneous injection (under the skin) is appropriate for drugs that will be used in small volumes and drugs for which slow absorption is desirable. Insulin is an example of such a drug.

Intramuscular injection (into a muscle) is appropriate when larger volumes of a drug must be injected. An example is streptomycin. Absorption from intramuscular sites is faster than from subcutaneous sites, since the muscles are better supplied with blood vessels than is the skin. Absorption from either subcutaneous or intramuscular sites can be speeded somewhat by applying heat or massage to the site to accelerate blood flow to the area. Absorption can be slowed by decreasing blood flow to the injection site by applying ice packs or by the simultaneous injection of a drug such as epinephrine, which constricts blood vessels.

Drugs intended for intramuscular or subcutaneous injection may be in relatively insoluble forms. Indeed, some drugs are formulated to dissolve slowly and therefore to be absorbed slowly from injection sites. These dosage forms are called *depot* injections.

Intravenous injection (directly into a vein) requires special precautions. Drugs that are to be used intravenously must always be in solution and can contain no particulate matter. Some drugs irritate the veins and cause thrombophlebitis if administered at too high a concentration. Other drugs must be injected slowly to avoid toxic concentrations of the drug reaching the heart or other vital organs. The intravenous route is valuable when drug concentrations must be maintained continuously, but it has the disadvantage that potential harm to the patient is greater by this route than by other routes discussed so far.

Special injection routes may be employed in certain circumstances. For example, local anesthetics may be injected into the spinal column to produce certain types of anesthesia. In other circumstances, drugs may be injected directly into body cavities or joints. These specific routes are employed when conventional routes of injection do not allow high enough drug concentrations to be achieved at the desired site of drug action.

■ Factors controlling drug persistence in the blood

Once a drug has entered the blood, its ultimate fate is determined by the chemical properties of the drug and how it is affected by the blood and tissues it contacts. Some drugs are metabolized by enzymes in the blood. An example is succinylcholine, already mentioned in Chapter 1. Drugs that persist for any length of time in the blood are usually bound to proteins in the blood rather than being simply dissolved directly in plasma. The most important carrier protein is albumin, a protein formed in the liver and released into the blood. Drugs bound to albumin or other carrier proteins remain in the blood, since these proteins as a rule do not diffuse through capillary walls. Drug binding to albumin is a reversible process, and in the blood an equilibrium is established between drug bound to the protein and drug that is free in solution. Only free drug is able to diffuse into tissues, interact with receptors, and produce biological effects. The same proportion of bound and free drug is maintained in the blood at all times. Thus, when free drug leaves the blood, some drug is released from protein binding to reestablish the proper ratio between bound and free drug.

An example of a drug that binds to plasma protein is the anticoagulant bishydroxycoumarin. In the blood, 99% of this drug is bound to plasma albumin. Therefore only 1% of the blood content of this coumarin is free to diffuse to its site of action or to its sites of elimination. The net effect of binding to albumin is to create a reservoir of the drug that is released to replenish free drug removed to other sites. In general, drugs that do not bind to plasma albumin remain in the body for shorter periods than drugs that are tightly bound. A drug such as bishydroxycoumarin, which is very strongly bound to albumin, remains in the body for up to 3 days. A longer duration of action is thus one characteristic of drugs that are bound to plasma proteins.

■ Factors controlling drug distribution throughout the body

Two of the factors that influence drug distribution have already been mentioned: lipid solubility of the drug and protein binding. A small molecular weight also favors diffusion of the drug through membranes. In general, the smaller and more lipid-soluble a drug, the better able it is to penetrate tissues. This consideration is especially important for drugs that act on organs with a high lipid content, such as the brain. All transport from the blood, however, involves passing through lipid-containing membranes. High concentrations of free drug in the blood and high lipid solubility favor this process.

■ Factors controlling drug metabolism in the body

Biotransformation. Biotransformation is the ability of living organisms to modify the chemical structure of drugs. Most drugs are metabolized in the body by the liver, specifically by the *microsomal enzyme* system. These enzymes allow the body to metabolize potentially toxic compounds. Many types of chemical transformations are carried out, but in general these reactions create water-soluble compounds that are more easily eliminated from the body by the kidney. These enzymes have two important properties. First, the enzymes are relatively nonspecific. Therefore many drugs may be metabolized by the same enzyme system. Second, the liver has the capacity to synthesize more enzyme in response to being exposed to higher than normal concentrations of certain drugs. This property means that the liver can increase its capacity to destroy a drug over a period of a few days. This increase in microsomal enzyme content in the liver is called *enzyme induction*.

The liver is by far the most important site for biotransformation of drugs, but it is not the only site. For example, systemically administered prostaglandins are destroyed almost instantaneously in the lung. Therefore prostaglandins, which might have use in stimulating uterine contractions, cannot be administered systemically for this purpose. The kidney is another important site for biotransformation of certain types of drugs.

Biotransformation may be carried out by bacteria within the colon. This process may limit absorption of the drug from the bowel following oral administration or it may be a mechanism by which the drug is eliminated from the blood after administration by parenteral routes.

■ Factors controlling drug elimination from the body

There are three main routes by which drugs may be eliminated from the body. These routes involve the liver, kidney, and bowel.

Elimination in the feces. The first of these routes involves uptake of the drug by the liver, release into bile, and elimination in the feces. For some drugs such as erythromycin and certain penicillins, the concentration of drug in the bile may be much higher than the concentration in the blood. Since between 600 and 1000 ml of bile is formed each day, this route of elimination may dispose of significant amounts of drug. However, drugs in the bile enter the small intestine where they may be reabsorbed into the blood, returned to the liver, and again secreted into bile. This secretion and reabsorption process is called *enterohepatic circulation*. Drugs that are extensively reabsorbed from the intestinal tract after biliary secretion obviously persist in the body much longer than drugs that remain in the lumen of the intestine and pass out with the feces. If the reabsorbed drug is in an active form, the duration of action of the drug is prolonged.

Elimination in the urine after metabolism by the liver. The second route of elimination involves the liver and the kidney. Common biotransformations of drug by the liver include formation of glucuronides, hydroxylations, and acetylations. The kidney is also capable of forming glucuronides and sulfates. All of these reactions tend to form more polar compounds, which can be more efficiently excreted by the kidney. For example, a drug such as the antibiotic chloramphenicol normally enters glomerular fluid by passive diffusion but is reabsorbed from the tubules and reenters the blood. In the liver, however, chloramphenicol is transformed into chloramphenicol glucuronide. In this form the drug enters glomerular fluid, cannot be reabsorbed from the tubules, and hence is excreted in the urine.

Various factors may influence the ability of the liver to metabolize drugs. For example, premature infants and neonates have immature livers that are incapable of carrying out certain biotransformations. Therefore these patients may accumulate those drugs that must be metabolized in the liver before they can be excreted by the kidney. Another group of patients who may accumulate drugs normally excreted by this route are patients who have suffered hepatic damage, such as that frequently seen in chronic alcoholics.

Elimination in the urine without metabolism by the liver. Some drugs are not extensively metabolized anywhere in the body and are excreted unchanged in the urine. This excretion may take place in one of two ways. Some drugs are excreted by passive diffusion into glomerular fluid and are not extensively reabsorbed; hence these drugs enter the urine. Other drugs are actively secreted by specific systems in the renal tubule. These active processes lead to more rapid drug elimination and allow much higher urinary concentrations of drug to be achieved. The antibiotic penicillin G is a good example of a drug that is actively secreted by the renal tubule. One-half of an intravenous dose of penicillin G can be eliminated in about 20 minutes by active tubular secretion. In contrast, an antibiotic such as tetracycline that is eliminated primarily by passive diffusion in the kidney persists in the body for several hours.

Those drugs which are normally eliminated unchanged in the urine will accumulate in the body when there is a loss of kidney function. Patients with kidney disease must frequently have drug dosages lowered to compensate for the reduced ability of the kidney to excrete various substances. Kidney function declines with age even in healthy persons, and elderly patients may show a reduced ability to excrete drugs in their urine. Certain drugs such as aminoglycoside antibiotics are themselves nephrotoxic and may directly damage the kidneys and thereby interfere with their own excretion.

■ PHARMACODYNAMICS

■ The dose-response curve

The relationship between the dose of drug administered and the response produced is an S-shaped (sigmoid) curve called the *dose-response curve* as shown in Fig. 2-3. This curve is obtained by plotting the observed response (on a linear scale) against the dose of the drug used to elicit that response (on a logarithmic scale). This curve illustrates several important quantitative properties about drugs. First, there is a threshold for each drug-induced response. Doses of drug below that threshold will produce no observable effect. Second, the drug-induced response will reach a plateau rather than increase indefinitely. For example, the drug shown in Fig. 2-3 produces its maximal response at a dose of about 512 units. Doubling the dose produces no detectable further effect. Even beginning at lower drug concentrations, doubling the dose still does not double the effect. In this example, the 50% maximal response to this drug is produced by a dose of 16 units, but at double that dose (32 units) only about 70%, not 100%, of the maximal response is produced. In summary, the dose-response curve demonstrates that a finite dose is required to see a response and that the intensity of the response produced is not linearly related to the dose.

The dose-response curve in Fig. 2-3 shows the effect of a drug on an individual (or average responses from several individuals). The same type of curve is produced when the drug response is instead defined as an all-or-none phenomenon (such as asleep versus awake) and the logarithm of the drug dose is plotted against the percentage of patients who show the drug effect at that given dose. The plateau for this curve will be the drug dose at which all patients respond and the threshold will be the drug dose below which no patients respond. The recommended therapeutic dose of the drug will be a dose at which most patients respond to the drug.

Drugs produce multiple predictable biological effects, and for each of these effects a dose-response curve may be drawn. For example, the drug digitalis, although increasing the force of contraction of the failing heart, also produces nausea, causes neurological symptoms such as headaches and visual disturbances, induces cardiac arrhythmias, and ultimately triggers ventricular fibrillation. Each of these responses can be plotted as a dose-response curve as illustrated in Fig. 2-4. Comparing the dose-response curves for these other reactions to the curve for the principal therapeutic effect, nausea is seen as an effect observed in a significant number of patients receiving therapeutic doses of digitalis. With increasing doses of the drug, more and more patients will suffer visual disturbances and arrhythmias. At drug concentrations well above normal therapeutic doses, ventricular fibrillation will occur. These predictable drug reactions become an important part of patient care. For digitalis, the visual disturbances are a warning that the concentration of digitalis in the patient is approaching concentrations that can cause cardiac arrhythmias and ventricular fibrillation.

Each drug may be described as relatively safe or relatively dangerous, based on consideration of dose-response curves such as those in Fig. 2-4. For example, nausea is frequently associated with the use of digitalis because the doses that produce nausea are only slightly greater than those which increase the force of contraction of the heart. Doses of digitalis that produce more serious reactions are only slightly higher than those which cause nausea. Digitalis, therefore, is a drug with a narrow margin of safety, and doses must be rigorously controlled and great care must be taken to keep blood levels of the drug within a very narrow range. In contrast, a drug with a wide margin of safety, such as penicillin G, may be given in doses greatly exceeding normal therapeutic doses without much danger of producing direct toxic effects.

Therapeutic index. The relative safety of drugs is also sometimes expressed as the therapeutic index. The therapeutic index (TI) is defined as the ratio of the dose of the drug that is lethal in 50% of the tested population (LD_{50}) to the dose of the drug that is therapeutically effective in 50% of the tested population (ED_{50}), or TI = LD_{50}/ED_{50}. Obviously, these figures come from tests conducted in animals. A drug with a high therapeutic index has a wide safety margin; the lethal dose is greatly in excess of the therapeutic dose. A drug with a low therapeutic index is more dangerous for the patient, because small increases over normal doses may be sufficient to induce toxic reactions.

■ Time course of drug action

Drugs may enter the body by a number of routes, but except for the intravenous route, some time will be required for the drug to enter the blood after administration. There is also a delay between the time the drug enters the blood and the time the drug reaches its site of action. If the response to a single dose of a drug is mea-

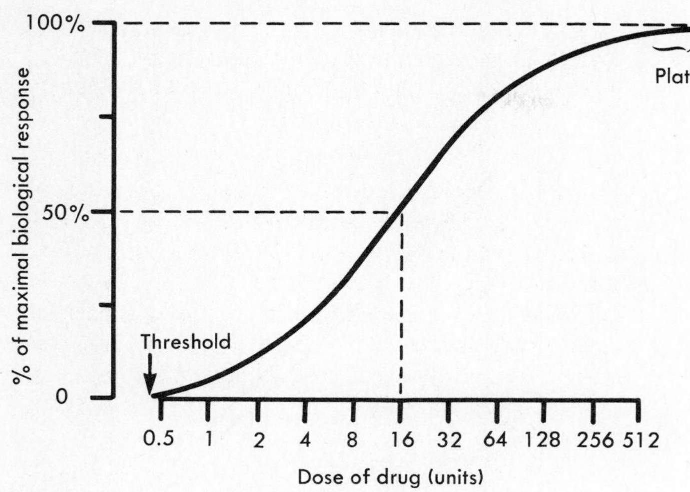

FIG. 2-3

A log dose-response curve. Percent of maximal biological response is plotted on a linear scale on vertical axis. Dose of the drug is plotted on a logarithmic scale on horizontal axis. The threshold is the dose of drug required to cause a measurable response. The plateau is region of curve where increasing drug dose does not increase the biological response.

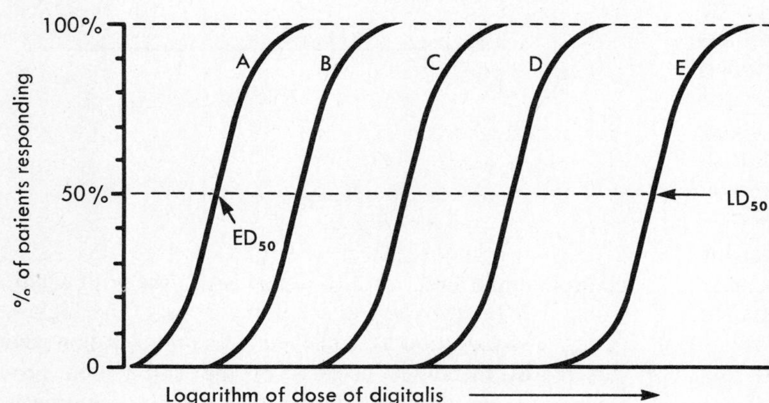

FIG. 2-4

Log dose-response curves for effects of digitalis. In this example, percent of patients responding to digitalis is plotted on vertical axis and dose of digitalis is plotted on logarithmic scale on horizontal axis. *Curve A* represents strengthened force of contraction of the heart produced by digitalis; *curve B* measures nausea; *curve C* measures visual disturbances; *curve D* measures cardiac arrhythmias; and *curve E* measures ventricular fibrillation and death. These undesirable effects are all dose-related responses to digitalis.

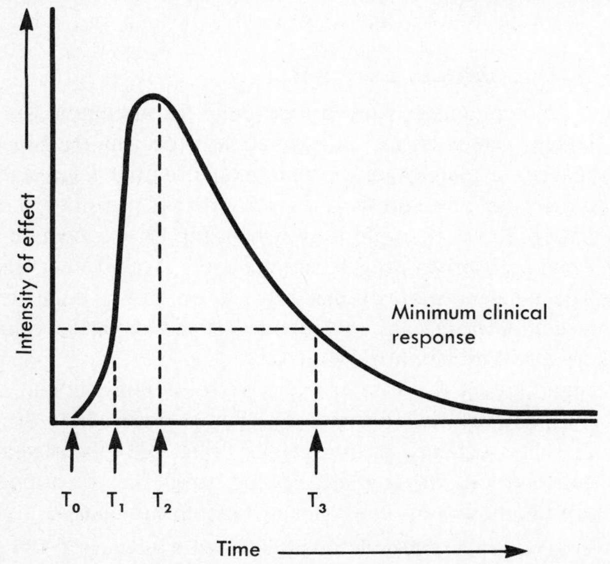

FIG. 2-5

Time course of action of a single dose of a drug. Drug is administered at T_0. Time interval between T_0 and T_1 represents time of onset of action of the drug. Peak action occurs at T_2. Time interval between T_0 and T_2 represents the time for peak action. At T_3 drug response falls below that required for minimal clinical effectiveness. Time interval between T_1 and T_3 represents duration of action of the drug.

sured as a function of time, the pattern shown in Fig. 2-5 is observed. The time for the *onset of drug action* is the time it takes after the drug is administered to reach a concentration that produces a response. As drug continues to be absorbed, higher concentrations of the drug reach the site of action, and the response increases. As the drug is being absorbed, it is also subject to the influences that tend to eliminate the drug from the body. Ultimately elimination will dominate, and the actual concentration of the drug in the body will begin to fall. As a result, the response will also begin to diminish. The *time to peak effect* is the time it takes for the drug to reach its highest effective concentration. The *duration of action* of a drug is the time during which the drug is present in a concentration large enough to produce a response and is determined by the rate of absorption and the rate of elimination.

The insulins are a good example of drugs for which an understanding of onset and duration of action is critical to the success of drug therapy. Insulin lowers blood sugar levels, and the peak drug action must be planned to coincide with the absorptive period after meals when blood sugar levels will rise rapidly if no insulin is present. If insulin is injected at the proper dose but at the wrong time, a serious hypoglycemic (low blood sugar) reaction may endanger the patient.

FIG. 2-6

Absorption and elimination rates for drug administered by oral or intravenous route. Plasma concentration of drug is plotted on a logarithmic scale on the vertical axis.

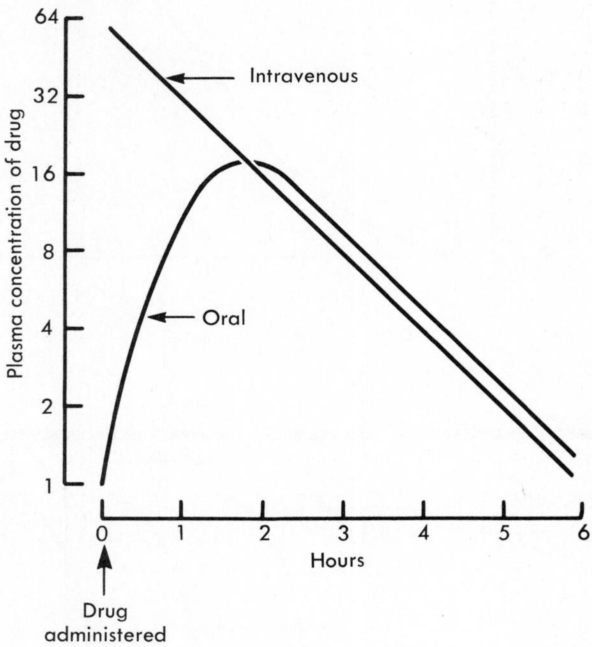

■ The half-life of a drug

The concepts of onset and duration of drug action are also important for understanding the proper timing of administration of drugs that are given repeatedly for a course of therapy. The *drug half-life* or *elimination half-time* is simply how long it takes for elimination processes to reduce the blood concentration of the drug by half. For example, consider a drug like penicillin G. The peak concentration of penicillin in the blood would occur a few moments after the drug is administered intravenously. Thereafter penicillin would be rapidly excreted by the kidney and would disappear from the blood. The length of time required for these processes to decrease the blood concentration of penicillin by 50% is the drug half-life or elimination half-time, which for penicillin G is around 20 minutes. Therefore 20 minutes after the intravenous dose of penicillin, only one half of the initial concentration of the drug would remain in the blood. After 40 minutes, only one quarter of the initial concentration would remain, and after 60 minutes, only one eighth would remain. During each succeeding 20-minute period the remaining concentration decreases by one half.

For a drug administered by a route where drug absorption is not instantaneous, the elimination processes compete with the absorptive processes, delaying the appearance of peak blood concentrations of the drug. The example shown in Fig. 2-6 is for a drug with a half-life of 1 hour. When given intravenously, the highest drug concentration is achieved on administration and decreases thereafter because of the elimination processes. When the same dose is given orally, the drug is absorbed relatively slowly so that drug elimination is responsible for lowering the peak drug concentration that can be achieved. Once in general circulation, however, the drug is eliminated in the same way, no matter what the initial route of administration.

■ The plateau principle

When a drug is given repeatedly for therapy at fixed dosage intervals, the concentration of drug in the blood reaches a plateau and is maintained at that level until either the dose or the frequency of administration is changed. An example is shown in Fig. 2-7, in which a rapidly absorbed drug is administered at fixed intervals. The concentration of the drug in the blood fluctuates around a mean value, which approaches a plateau value after 4 elimination half-times have passed; this happens regardless of the dose or frequency of administration, as long as they are constant. The actual dose of the drug and the frequency of dosage determine what the plateau concentration of drug in the blood is, but they do not determine how long it will take to reach that plateau.

As an example of this plateau principle, consider a

FIG. 2-7

Plateau principle. In this example, drug is administered once every elimination half-time for the drug. The plasma concentration of drug rises and falls as drug doses are rapidly absorbed and slowly eliminated. Drug accumulates over a period of time so that after 4 elimination half-times the average plasma concentration of the drug has reached a steady state. By adjusting the dose, average plasma concentration of drug may be adjusted.

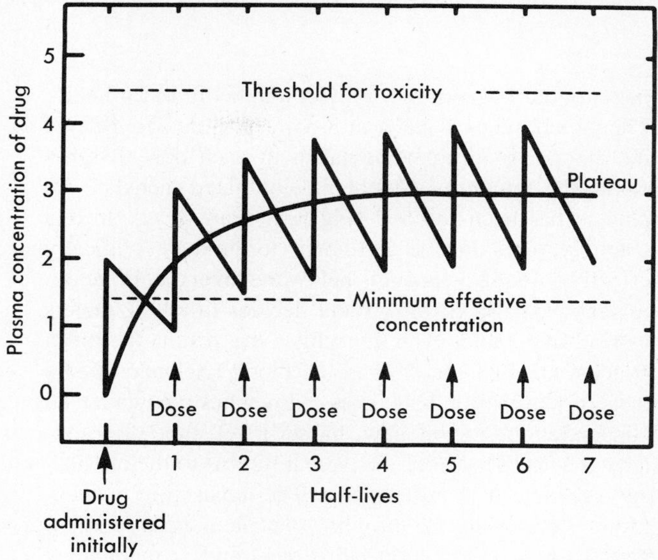

FIG. 2-8

Plateau principle in practice. *Patient A* receives a drug with half-time of 24 hours. Increasing dose of the drug from 1 to 2 tablets in a single daily dose increases plateau concentration of the drug. In contrast, *patient B* illustrates that by dividing the dose (taking ½ tablet every 12 hours rather than 1 tablet once daily) fluctuations in drug concentration are minimized but average concentration is unchanged.

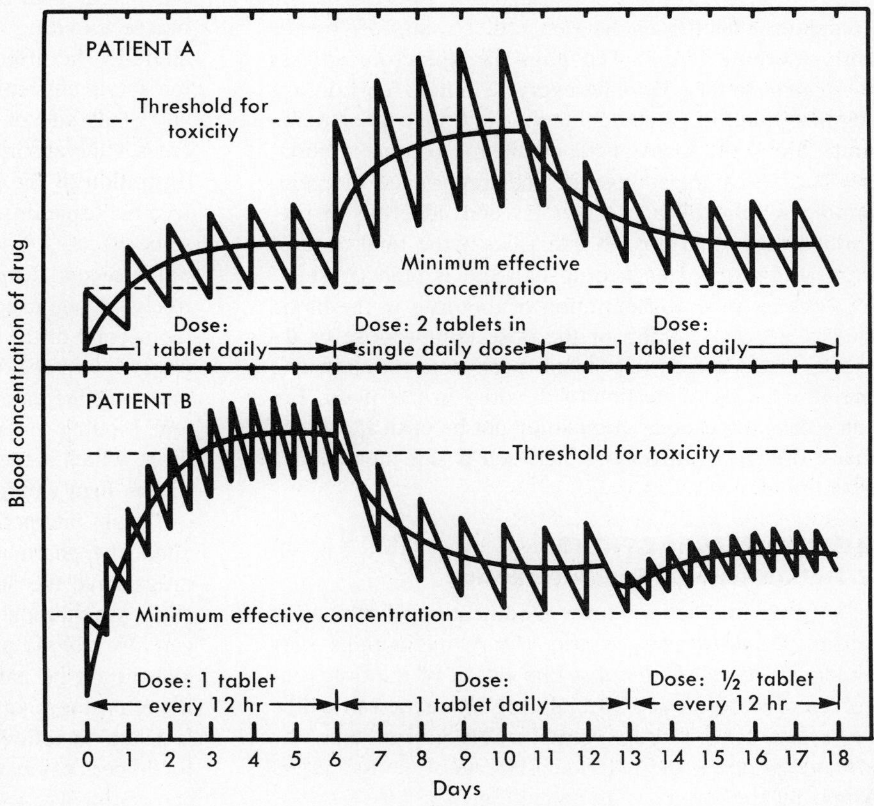

patient who is given a drug with a half-life of 24 hours. The patient takes 1 tablet at 8 AM every day. In 4 days, the amount of drug being taken in each dose roughly equals the amount of drug being eliminated each day; the plateau has been reached (Fig. 2-8, Patient A). In this example, this dose is sufficient to produce clinically effective blood levels but is below the level that produces toxicity. On day 6, the patient decides to take 2 tablets instead of 1 tablet each morning. As a result, the mean concentration of the drug in the blood rises and after 4 days (4 elimination half-times), it reaches a new plateau concentration. At this new, higher level some drug toxicity is seen. Therefore the patient returns to the old dosage schedule of 1 tablet daily. The mean drug concentration returns to the original plateau concentration 4 days later (4 elimination half-times) and is maintained until the dosage amount or intervals change.

Patient B in Fig. 2-8 receives the same drug as patient A, but patient B takes 1 tablet every 12 hours instead of once daily. As a result, the plateau concentration of drug in the blood is higher than for patient A. Note, however, that it still takes 4 days (4 elimination half-times) to reach the plateau concentration. After 3 days of therapy, patient B mentions some unusual symptoms, which the nurse recognizes as toxic reactions to the drug. On the basis of this report, the physician reduces the frequency of drug administration to 1 tablet daily. After 5 days on this dosage schedule the patient complains that the medication effect wears off by the early morning hours. The physician therefore advises the patient to take ½ tablet every 12 hours. This dosage regimen minimizes the fluctuations in drug concentration in the blood but does not change the mean concentration.

These examples illustrate the importance of maintaining regular dosage schedules and adhering to prescribed doses and dosage intervals. If the total dose of drug administered each drug half-life is held constant, then the average concentration of the drug in the blood stays constant. Timing of the dose (single dose or divided doses) affects the actual peak concentration and the minimal concentration of the drug in the blood. For some drugs, these variations may not be critical, but for many drugs the difference between a safe dose and a toxic dose is not very great.

■ DRUG INTERACTIONS

■ Definition of a drug interaction

A drug interaction is any modification of the action of one drug by another drug. Drug interactions may either *potentiate* or *diminish* the action of the drugs involved. *Synergism* is a special drug interaction in which the effect of two drugs combined is greater than the effect expected if the individual effects of the two drugs acting independently were added together.

Drug interactions are commonly encountered in clinical practice and are sometimes actively sought as part of a therapeutic program. An excellent example is the treatment of chronic moderate hypertension, which frequently employs several drugs, each amplifying the action of the others to lower the blood pressure.

The negative side of drug interaction is that the therapeutic result expected from a drug can be greatly distorted by the presence of other drugs. This negative side can be diminished when health care personnel are aware of the major drug interactions; are thorough in determining which drugs a patient is taking, including over-the-counter drugs, alcohol, and tobacco; and give careful instruction to the patients about which drugs will interact with their prescribed medication.

Comprehensive lists of drug interactions have been published and may be referred to if necessary when information about rare or unlikely interactions is sought. Clinically important common interactions are discussed with each drug class in this text.

■ Origin of drug interactions

Drug interactions may arise when one drug alters the pharmacokinetics of another drug. For example, one drug may alter the dissolution, absorption, protein binding, metabolism, or elimination of another drug. Drug interactions of the pharmacokinetic type are generally one sided, with one drug altering the pharmacokinetics of a second drug without its own pharmacokinetics being altered. The effect of the drug interaction is to change the actual concentration of the second drug in the blood and at its site of action. For instance, if one drug decreases the absorption of a second drug, the actual concentration of the second drug is diminished, and therefore the usual dose will not give the expected result. The same effect is produced if the metabolism or elimination of the second drug is increased by the first drug. Alternatively, if one drug increases the actual concentration of the second drug, the result is potentiation of the second drug. Pharmacokinetic potentiation may arise because one drug increases the absorption or decreases the protein binding, metabolism, or elimination of a second drug, which is therefore present in higher actual concentration than would be anticipated at that dose.

Drug interactions may also arise when one drug alters the pharmacodynamics of a second drug. If two drugs have the same action, drug potentiation will result. An example is seen with the vasodilators, which can lower blood pressure. A vasodilator such as hydralazine might be part of a therapeutic program to control hypertension. Nitroglycerin is another vasodilator that is taken to relieve angina. Patients taking hydralazine for hypertension who also take nitroglycerin for angina can anticipate a severe hypotensive response to nitroglycerin, and they may have to lie down when taking nitroglycerin to avoid fainting.

An example of drug interaction of the pharmacodynamic type that diminishes the response of both drugs at the usual therapeutic doses are drugs that are antagonists. An example would be the beta receptor antagonist propranolol, which might be prescribed for a patient with hypertension. If that patient developed asthma, a beta receptor agonist such as isoproterenol would be indicated. Although in this example the therapeutic target for propranolol is the heart and for isoproterenol the therapeutic target is the bronchioles, these drugs would antagonize each other at all organs with beta-adrenergic receptors and neither drug would give the desired therapeutic effect. (In fact, propranolol on its own would make the asthma worse and could not be used.)

Alcohol is a frequent cause of pharmacodynamic drug interactions. As a central nervous system depressant, alcohol acts synergistically with the other drug classes that depress the central nervous system: antihistamines, sedative-hypnotics, antianxiety drugs, antidepressants, antipsychotics, general anesthetics, and the narcotic analgesics. At low doses the drowsiness characteristic of these drug classes is exaggerated by alcohol, although at higher doses respiration can be dangerously depressed.

■ BIOLOGICAL VARIATION

Not all patients respond to a set drug dosage in the same way. Moreover, it is not possible to predict in most cases which patients will be more or less sensitive to a drug than normal. The term *normal* in this context really means average for the population.

Biological variability is based on subtle differences in physiological functions that exist among people. For example, absorption of oral drug doses can be greatly influenced by stomach acidity, gastrointestinal motility, pancreatic function, and gastrointestinal microbiological flora. Yet these parameters vary greatly in normal people. Likewise, people vary in the sensitivity of certain tissue to drugs. This variability may be the result of differences in the numbers of drug receptors, differences in permeability barriers, or many other factors. These factors are all hard to assess and yet greatly influence the magnitude of drug effects in patients.

In the clinical setting, the causes of biological variation are not usually known with any degree of certainty. Patients are observed for the proper response to a drug, and dosages are usually adjusted on the basis of clinical assessment of progress. Although the exact causes of biological variation are not known for an individual patient, some general factors can be delineated that may influence patient responses to medications. These factors include age, sex of the patient, overall health status, and genetic background.

■ THE NURSING PROCESS

An understanding of pharmacokinetics and pharmacodynamics is involved in the treatment of every patient. Specific drugs may involve consideration of difference aspects of pharmacokinetics and pharmacodynamics, but the following presentation outlines in general how these principles may be applied.

■ Assessment

In the course of assessing the patient, the nurse should ascertain whether any route of administration is inappropriate for the patient. For example, a patient with stomach ulcers might not receive some oral medications. The nurse might also assess which routes of elimination are available in a given patient. For example, the nurse might determine whether the patient has compromised kidney function that would prevent the safe use of many drugs eliminated by the kidney. The nurse might also consider the desired site of action of the drug and consider which drugs would not be able to penetrate to this site because of their distribution properties in the body.

■ Management

In identifying goals of therapy, the nurse should consider the problem of getting the drug to its site of action at the proper concentration. This consideration would include a knowledge of the proper timing of dosages as well as a knowledge of ways to improve the effectiveness of the drug. For example, the excretion rates of some drugs may be influenced by the pH of the urine. Thus changing the pH of the urine may change the duration of action of a drug and improve the therapeutic effect in the patient. To teach the patient, the nurse should emphasize the appropriate actions the patient might take to maintain drug effectiveness. For example, a patient might be cautioned to avoid antacids with medications if they were known to lower bioavailability of an orally administered drug. Proper timing of doses might be especially emphasized for drugs with short half-lives, whereas the dangers of changing the drug dose without the knowledge of the physician might be emphasized for a drug with a low therapeutic index. Drug interactions might be anticipated and avoided by good patient teaching.

■ Evaluation

If therapy has not achieved the desired goals, the pharmacokinetics and pharmacodynamics of the drugs being used should be examined as possible causes for the therapeutic failure. Drug interactions may also be involved and should be considered.

■ SUMMARY

The activity of a drug is related to its ability to reach its site of action and its rate of removal from that site. Enteral administration introduces the drug into the gastrointestinal tract and requires that the drug dissolve and pass through the lipid membranes of cells lining the gastrointestinal tract to enter the blood. Therefore small, lipid-soluble drugs are absorbed better than highly ionic (charged) drugs, which are very water soluble. Drugs adsorbed from the stomach or intestine enter the portal circulation, which exposes a drug to the microsomal enzymes in the liver before the drug enters systemic circulation. In contrast, drugs administered by sublingual, buccal, or rectal routes of administration enter the systemic circulation before reaching the liver. Parenteral routes of administration require injection of the drug into a fluid or tissue. Subcutaneous injection produces slower absorption rates and is suitable for smaller volumes of drug than intramuscular injections.

Drugs are eliminated from the body by three major mechanisms: (1) excretion into the bile, (2) biotransformation of the drug by the liver followed by excretion by the kidney, or (3) excretion of unchanged drug by the kidney. The persistence of a drug in the body is influenced by these elimination processes and by the ability of the drug to enter tissues or be bound by plasma proteins.

The magnitude of the biological effect produced by a drug is related to the amount of drug administered. This relationship is expressed by the dose-response curve. The threshold dose of a drug is the minimum dose required to produce an observable biological effect. Higher doses produce increasing effects until the maximal response is achieved. Doses above those required for maximal drug effects are at best wasteful and increase the incidence of side effects.

When drugs are given repeatedly at fixed dosage intervals, the concentration of drug in the blood reaches a plateau and is maintained at that level until the dose or frequency of dosage is changed. The actual concentration of drug in the blood fluctuates around some mean value. This mean value, or plateau concentration, is achieved after about 4 elimination half-times for the drug. The elimination half-time or drug half-life is the time required for the concentration of drug in the blood to be decreased by half. The dose of a drug influences the plateau concentration of the drug in the blood but does not influence how long it takes for that plateau concentration to be reached. The frequency of drug dosage influences the degree of fluctuation around the mean concentration of that drug in the blood.

When patients receive more than one drug at the same time, the drugs may interact, either diminishing or potentiating the drug response. Drug interactions may arise when one drug alters the dissolution, absorption, protein binding, metabolism, or elimination of another drug. Drug interactions may also occur when drugs either enhance or block the action of other drugs in tissues containing the receptors. Drug interactions frequently involve nonprescription medications and alcohol.

Not all patients respond to a set drug dosage in the same way, primarily because of the biological variability among people. Subtle physiological differences as well as differences in age, sex, health status, and genetic background strongly influence the response to many drugs.

■ STUDY QUESTIONS

1. Why are pharmacodynamics and pharmacokinetics helpful in understanding the clinical uses of drugs?
2. Describe how a drug in tablet form enters the blood after oral administration. What factors may influence the absorption of this drug?
3. What is the first pass phenomenon? Does the first pass phenomenon affect all routes of administration?
4. What are the advantages and disadvantages to subcutaneous, intramuscular, and intravenous routes of drug administration?
5. How does the binding of drugs to proteins in the blood influence the effect of the drug?
6. What are the microsomal enzymes of the liver and how do they influence the biological activity of drugs?
7. What is biotransformation?
8. What is enterohepatic circulation?
9. How does glomerular excretion of a drug differ from tubular secretion of a drug in the kidney?
10. What information is expressed in a log dose-response curve?
11. What is the therapeutic index of a drug?
12. What is the onset time for a drug and how does it differ from the duration of action of a drug?
13. What is the elimination half-time of a drug?
14. What is the plateau principle?
15. How long does it take for a constant, average concentration of drug to be achieved if the drug is given at a constant dose and at fixed intervals?
16. What is a drug interaction?
17. Do drug interactions increase or decrease the action of the drugs involved?
18. What are the two major mechanisms by which drug interactions can occur?
19. Which type of drug interaction may actually change the concentration of one of the drugs involved?
20. Which type of drug interaction does not change drug concentrations but does change observed drug responses?
21. Why must biological variability be considered in drug therapy?
22. What are some of the possible reasons for the observed differences in drug response seen among patients?

■ SUGGESTED READINGS

Alvares, A.P., Pantuck, E.J., Anderson, K.E., Kappas, A., and Conney, A.H.: Regulation of drug metabolism in man by environmental factors, Drug Metabolism Reviews **9**(2):185, 1979.

Baker, C.: Reference chart for drug interactions, American Family Physician **12**(4):127, 1975.

Bauwens, E., and Clemmons, C.: Foods that foil drugs, RN **41:**79, 1978.

Black, C.D., Popovich, N.G., and Black, G.: Drug interactions in the GI tract, American Journal of Nursing **77:**1426, 1977.

Brater, D.C.: The pharmacological role of the kidney, Drugs **19**(1): 31, 1980.

Cadwallader, D.E.: Biopharmaceutics and drug interactions, ed. 2, Nutley, N.J., 1974, Roche Scientific Monograph, Roche Laboratories, Rocom Press.

Carruthers, S.G.: Duration of drug action, American Family Physician **21**(2):119, 1980.

DiPalma, J.R.: Pharmacogenetics, American Family Physician **9**(4): 148, 1974.

Dollery, C.T., Fraser, H.S., Mucklow, J.C., and Bulpitt, C.J.: Contribution of environmental factors to variability in human drug metabolism, Drug Metabolism Reviews **9**(2):207, 1979.

Editors: Pharmcokinetics, Emergency Medicine **4**(10):106, 1972.

Foerst, H.: Drug-prescribing patterns in skilled nursing facilities, American Journal of Nursing **79:**2002, 1979.

Garrett, E.R.: Biological responses and pharmacokinetics. Part 1, Pharmacy International **1**(6):121, 1980.

Garrett, E.R.: Biological responses and pharmacokinetics. Part 2, Pharmacy International **1**(7):133, 1980.

Gibaldi, M.: Biopharmaceutics and clinical pharmacokinetics, ed. 2, Philadelphia, 1977, Lea & Febiger.

Gotz, B.E., and Gotz, V.P.: Drugs and the elderly, American Journal of Nursing **78:**1347, 1978.

Greenblatt, D.J., and Allen, M.D.: Intramuscular injection-site complications, Journal of the American Medical Association **240:**542, 1978.

Hansten, P.D.: Drug interactions, ed. 4, Philadelphia, 1979, Lea & Febiger.

Jusko, W.J.: Influence of cigarette smoking on drug metabolism in man, Drug Metabolism Reviews **9**(2):221, 1979.

Lamy, P.P.: How your patient's diet can affect drug response, Drug Therapy **10**(8):82, 1980.

Lamy, P.P., Reichel, W., and Wag, R.: Make age a factor in the drug equation, Patient Care **9**(14):136, 1975.

Libert, I.: Pediatric drug use, Nurses' Drug Alert **1**(19):165, 1977.

Mayersohn, M.: Clinical pharmacokinetics: applying basic principles to therapy, Drug Therapy **10**(9):79, 1980.

Mennear, J.H.: Familial pharmacology, American Family Physician **15**(6):100, 1977.

Palmer, H.A., and Fraser, G.L.: Crushing tablets, opening capsules: when is it safe? RN **41:**53, 1978.

Reidenberg, M.M., and Drayer, D.E.: Drug therapy in renal failure, Annual Review of Pharmacology and Toxicology **20:**45, 1980.

Robinson, L.A., and Fischer, R.G.: Pediatric drug information, Pediatric Nursing **4:**36, 1978.

Strauss, S.: Patient dosage instructions: a guide for nurses, Ambler, Pa., 1976, Medical Business Services.

Tatro, D.S.: Adverse drug reactions in children, Drug Intelligence and Clinical Pharmacy **7:**109, 1973.

Toothaker, R.D., and Welling, P.G.: Effect of food on drug bioavailability, Annual Review of Pharmacology and Toxicology **20:**173, 1980.

Ward, M., and Baltman, M.: Drug therapy in the elderly, American Family Physician **19**(2):143, 1979.

Weintraub, M.: Drugs in the elderly, Nurses' Drug Alert **1**(17):149, 1977.

Weintraub, M.: The therapeutic window: when more is much, much less, Drug Therapy **9**(10):163, 1979.

Welling, P.G.: How food and fluid affect drug absorption, Postgraduate Medicine **62**(1):73, 1977.

3 Drug administration

In Chapter 2 we discussed the various routes by which a drug may be administered and we illustrated the importance of careful control of drug levels in the body. Administering the proper drug dose by the appropriate route is the obvious first step in assuring that the desired drug concentration will appear in the bloodstream. In this chapter we consider the principles of drug administration. Teaching the mechanics of drug administration we leave to its proper place in the clinic.

■ THE ROLE OF THE NURSE

The nurse shares moral and legal responsibility with the physician and pharmacist in administering drugs. In many hospitals, the pharmacist calculates and prepares the drug for administration to the patient, based on the physician's order. This practice does not remove legal responsibility from the nurse who actually administers the drug to the patient. It is the nurse who must verify that the correct drug at the proper dose has been prepared. For this reason, the nurse should be familiar with the forms of drugs and be able to recognize common medications.

The nurse's proper role in the clinic may also include questioning a physician's order for a drug when that order seems inappropriate. For example, a drug dose well outside normal clinical dosage ranges might be questioned. It may also be appropriate to question an order for a drug producing toxic reactions to which a particular patient might be more susceptible than normal. For example, the patient may have complained of stomach distress during hospitalization. That fact might influence the physician to select an enteric-coated drug form that would be less irritating to the stomach than normal tablets. For this reason, it is appropriate for the nurse to call attention to the patient's complaint.

The nurse has access to several sources of information about specific drugs. Manufacturers include specific information related to dosage and toxicity as a package insert with medication. The same information can be found in the *Physician's Desk Reference* (PDR), which also contains a series of color plates showing the dosage forms of specific drugs. The PDR is organized according to drug manufacturer. Other books of similar content are organized according to drug class. One such publication is *Facts and Comparisons*. Either the PDR or *Facts and Comparisons* might be found in the nursing unit. Another source of information more likely to be found in a library is the *AMA Drug Evaluations*. This publication not only lists available drugs but also comments on clinical use and toxic reactions. Another useful book is the *Nurse's Guide to Drugs*. In addition to these publications, numerous drug handbooks or handbooks of therapy are available from several publishers. Some publications such as the PDR are published annually, whereas others are published less frequently. Since medical opinion on such subjects as drug toxicity or efficacy can change with increased clinical experience with a drug, it is wise to consult the most recent reference available when questions arise.

■ READING DRUG ORDERS

Physicians and pharmacists sometimes employ a system of abbreviations in writing orders or prescriptions. These abbreviations are derived from Latin phrases and, although Latin is no longer used in medical communication, these abbreviations persist through custom. For this reason the nurse must be familiar with the more common abbreviations listed in Table 3-1. Many of the abbreviations designate how the drug is to be administered. For example, a physician's order might read "Penicillin G 100,000 U q. 3h., p.o." This order would be translated to "100,000 units (U) of penicillin G are to be administered every 3 hours (q. 3h.) by mouth (p.o.)."

Some confusion can be generated by the use of these abbreviations, and the nurse must be certain that the physician's intent is clearly understood. Among the most troublesome are the abbreviations ad lib. and p.r.n. A drug given p.r.n. should be taken at the prescribed interval if the patient requires the drug. For example, a post-surgery patient might have the following order on the chart: "Morphine 10 mg q. 4h., p.r.n.". Every 4 hours the nurse should assess whether the patient requires the morphine for pain relief. If the patient is sleeping or is comfortable, the dosage may be postponed. According to the drug order, the morphine may be given less fre-

TABLE 3-1. Abbreviations encountered in physicians' orders and prescriptions

Abbreviation	**Latin phrase**	**Translation**
ad lib.	ad libitum	Freely; as much or as often as wanted
aa. (or $\overline{aa}$)	ana	of each
a.c.	ante cibum	before meals
b.i.d.	bis in die	twice daily
$\bar{c}$	cum	with
gtt.	guttae	drops
h.s.	hora somni	at bedtime
non rep.	non repetatur	do not repeat
o.d.	oculus dexter	right eye
o.s.	oculus sinister	left eye
o.u.	oculus uterque	both eyes
p.c.	post cibum	after meals
p.o.	per os	by mouth
p.r.	per rectum	by rectal route
p.r.n.	pro re nata	according to circumstances
q.s.	quantum sufficit	as much as is necessary
q.d.	quaque die	every day
q.h. q. 4 h	quaque hora	every hour every 4 hours
q.i.d.	quarter in die	four times daily
ss. (or $\overline{ss}$)	semis	one half
stat.	statim	immediately
t.i.d.	ter in die	three times daily

quently than every 4 hours but not more frequently. In contrast a medication prescribed "ad lib." is given whenever the patient needs it.

The abbreviations we have discussed are used as a medical shorthand to save time in communicating between medical personnel. If the use of an abbreviation creates any uncertainty in the mind of the nurse administering the medication, the physician or pharmacist should be consulted for clarification.

■ UNITS OF DRUG DOSAGE

In clinical practice, nurses will encounter situations in which they will be called on to translate a physician's order for a certain drug dosage into the proper number of tablets or the proper volume of drug for an individual patient. This section is to prepare the student of nursing to handle these problems with skill and confidence.

TABLE 3-2. Systems of units in common use in the United States

System	**Unit of mass**	**Unit of volume**
Metric	Gram (Gm)	Liter (L)
Apothecaries'	Grain (gr)	Minims (m)
Household	Pound (lb)	Pint (pt)

TABLE 3-3. Table of equivalents within systems

System	**Equivalents**
Metric	1.0 Gm = 0.001 kg 1.0 Gm = 1000 mg 1.0 L = 1000 ml
Apothecaries'	1.0 gr = 1/60 dram (dr or ʒ) = 1/480 oz 60 gr = 1 dr 8 dr = 1 oz (or ℥) 1.0 minim (m) = 1/60 f dr = 1/480 f oz 60 m = 1 f dr (or f ʒ) 8 f dr = 1 f oz (or f ℥)
Household	1.0 lb = 16 oz 1.0 pt = ½ quart (qt) = ⅛ gallon (gal) 1.0 pt = 16 f oz = 32 tablespoonsful (T) 1.0 T = 3 teaspoonsful (t)

Before turning to the rather simple arithmetical principles required to solve dosage problems, we must familiarize ourselves with the three systems of units in common use in the United States today. These are the metric system, the apothecaries' system, and the common, or household, system (Table 3-2). Within each of these systems we are concerned with the primary units of mass and volume, since all of the problems we will be called on to solve will be expressed in some unit of drug mass and some unit of drug volume.

The primary unit of mass within the metric system is the *gram* (Gm). With prefixes, this unit can be adjusted to express thousan*ds* of grams (1 *kilo*gram = 1000 grams) or thousan*dths* of grams (1 *milli*gram = 0.001 grams). In less common usage are the prefixes *deci* and *centi,* meaning 1/10 and 1/100, respectively. The primary unit of volume within the metric system is the liter (L). With prefixes, the liter is commonly divided into thousandths (1 L = 1000 *milli*liters), and less commonly into millionths (1 L = 1,000,000 *micro*liters), or hundredths (1 L = 10 *deci*liters).

TABLE 3-4. Conversion of units between systems

Apothecaries'	Metric
15 gr	= 1 Gm*
1 dr	= 4 Gm
1 oz	= 32 Gm
15 m	= 1 ml
1 f dr	= 4 ml
1 f oz	= 30 ml†

Household	Metric
1 t	= 5 ml
1 T	= 14 ml
1 pt	= 480 ml (or 500 ml)
1 qt	= 960 ml (or 1000 ml)
1 gal	= 3.84 L (or 4 L)
1 lb (avoirdupois)	= 0.46 kg or 1 kg = 2.2 lb

*Two factors have been used for converting grains to milligrams. The older conversion factor is 65 mg = 1 gr. This factor is the basis for aspirin and acetaminophen formulations (i.e., a 5-gr aspirin tablet contains 325 mg of aspirin). The newer conversion factor agreed on is 60 mg = 1 gr. This new conversion factor is easier to use for drugs such as morphine which are frequently administered in small doses that are fractions of grains. For example, ¼ gr of morphine equals 15 mg, using the new conversion factor. The student should remember that these factors are simply agreed on for ease of calculation. All the problems presented in this book use the conversion 15 gr = 1000 mg.

†30 ml has been agreed on as the equivalent for 1 f oz, rather than the more exact approximation of 32 ml, since 30 ml is more conveniently and accurately estimated in most clinical glassware.

The milliliter (ml) is the metric unit equivalent to the unit of gas volume commonly encountered in the clinic, the cubic centimeter (cc).

The primary unit of mass in the apothecaries' system is the grain (gr). It must be remembered that 60 gr constitutes 1 dram and that 8 drams is equivalent to 1 ounce. The primary unit of volume in the apothecaries' system is the minim. The equivalent of 60 minims is 1 fluid dram (f dr); 8 f dr = 1 f oz.

Equivalents within the household system may be familiar from domestic experience. Table 3-3 will refresh your memory on those points that may have become unclear.

Any of the three systems of units may be used by a physician in ordering drugs. The metric system possesses many advantages in terms of ease of calculation and convenience of units, but despite this fact the older systems still persist in some situations. A nurse may be called on to convert drug doses from one system to another. Unfortunately, the exact equivalents result in awkward and unwieldy values. For example, 1 L = 0.26418 gallons; 1 quart = 0.9643 L; 1 grain = 0.0648 Gm; 1 f oz = 29.57 ml; 1 oz (apothecary) = 31.1 Gm. Obviously these numbers are not convenient in calculations. For this reason certain approximations have been agreed on and are used in ordinary circumstances for converting between systems. These conversions are listed in Table 3-4.

TABLE 3-5. Abbreviations for various units

Unit	Abbreviation used in this text	Other acceptable abbreviations
Gram	Gm	gm, g
Milligram	mg	mgm
Microgram	μg	mcg
Liter	L	l
Milliliter	ml	cc*

*Used for gases only.

Abbreviations for the various units are not entirely standardized in the medical literature. For example, gram may be abbreviated Gm, gm, or g. One set of abbreviations has been adopted for use throughout this book. Table 3-5 summarizes the abbreviations in use for various units.

The apothecaries' system also has some unusual expressions that require explanation. Unlike any other system, apothecaries' units are frequently used with small Roman numerals rather than Arabic numerals. Moreover, in the apothecaries' system the units precede the numeral. For example, 5 gr may be written gr v, gr being the abbreviation for grain and v the Roman numeral for 5. In this system the abbreviation *ss* designates one half. For example, gr iss is translated 1½ gr. Smaller fractions of grains are written out in Arabic numerals. For example, a quarter grain would be written gr ¼.

The nurse in practice deals daily with solutions of drugs. A solution is defined as a given mass of solid substance dissolved in a known volume of fluid (w/v; weight/volume) or as a given volume of a liquid substance dissolved in a known volume of another fluid (v/v; volume/volume). The concentration of a w/v solution is always expressed as units of mass per units of volume. Common concentration units are Gm/ml, Gm/L, mg/ml, gr/m, and dr/f oz. Concentrations are also commonly expressed as percentages, based on the definition of a 1% solution as 1 Gm of solid/100 ml of solution. Proportions are also used as expressions of concentrations. For example, 1:1000 designates a solution containing 1 Gm/1000 ml of solution. Blood levels of certain metabolites are frequently expressed as mg% (mg/100 ml) of solution. Mg/100 ml is equivalent to mg/deciliter, that is, a 1 mg% solution is the same as a 1 mg/deciliter solution.

The relationship between the various expressions of concentration is illustrated in Table 3-6.

TABLE 3-6. Equivalents of concentration expressions

%	Ratio	Gm/L	mg/ml	mg/dl	μg/ml
10.0	1:10	100	100	10,000	100,000
1.0	1:100	10	10	1,000	10,000
0.1	1:1000	1.0	1.0	100	1,000
0.01	1:10,000	0.1	0.1	10	100
0.001	1:100,000	0.01	0.01	1.0	10
0.0001	1:1,000,000	0.001	0.001	0.1	1.0

■ CALCULATIONS

■ Calculating the strength of drug solutions

Calculating the concentration of a drug solution utilizes the following equation:

Concentration = Mass of drug/volume of solution

If you know any two of these quantities, you may solve directly for the third, provided all the quantities are expressed in the same system of units. Therefore as a first step in the solution of any problem it is frequently necessary to convert units from one system to another, as we see in example 1.

EXAMPLE 1: *Prepare 1 L of a 5% solution.*

You know:

1. Volume of solution (1 L)
2. Concentration (5%)

To solve:

1. Convert all quantities to the same system of units:

   5% = 5 Gm/100 ml; 1 L = 1000 ml

2. Substitute the known quantities into the equation:

   5 Gm/100 ml = Mass of drug/1000 ml

3. Solve for mass of drug:

$$\text{Mass} = \frac{1000 \text{ ml} \times 5 \text{ Gm}}{100 \text{ ml}} = 50 \text{ Gm}$$

EXAMPLE 2: *What is the strength of a 2 L solution containing 10 Gm of drug?*

You know:

1. Mass of drug (10 Gm)
2. Volume of solution (2 L)

To solve:

Substitute the known quantities into the equation:

$$\text{Concentration} = \frac{10 \text{ Gm}}{2 \text{ L}} = \frac{5 \text{ Gm}}{\text{L}} = \frac{0.5 \text{ Gm}}{100 \text{ ml}} = 0.5\% = 1{:}200$$

EXAMPLE 3: *How much of a 2% solution can be prepared with 6 Gm of drug?*

You know:

1. Concentration (2%)
2. Mass of drug (6 Gm)

To solve:

1. Convert all quantities to the same system of units:

$$2\% = \frac{2 \text{ Gm}}{100 \text{ ml}}$$

2. Substitute the known quantities into the equation:

   2 Gm/100 ml = 6 Gm/Volume of solution

3. Solve for volume of solution:

$$\text{Volume} = \frac{6 \text{ Gm} \times 100 \text{ ml}}{2 \text{ Gm}} = 300 \text{ ml}$$

EXAMPLE 4: *Prepare 4 oz of a 0.5% solution from tablets gr v each.*

You know:

1. Volume of solution required (4 oz)
2. Concentration of solution (0.5%)

To solve:

1. Convert all quantities to the same system of units:

   0.5% = 0.5 Gm/100 ml
   4 oz = 4 × 32 ml = 128 ml
   gr v = 5 gr = 0.333 Gm

2. Substitute the known quantities into the equation:

   0.5 Gm/100 ml = Mass of drug/128 ml

3. Solve for mass of drug:

$$\text{Mass} = \frac{128 \text{ ml} \times 0.5 \text{ Gm}}{100 \text{ ml}} = 0.64 \text{ Gm}$$

4. Determine the number of tablets required to total 0.64 Gm:

$$\frac{0.64 \text{ Gm}}{0.33 \text{ Gm/tablet}} = 2 \text{ tablets}$$

Therefore two tablets would be dissolved in 4 oz to prepare the desired solution. Note that the conversion was not exact but was very close to a value of 2 and was rounded off. In dealing with scored tablets, one may calculate to the nearest half tablet.

Self-test for proficiency in drug calculations

After thorough study of the previous section the student should be able to work the following problems. You may check your answers and see the calculations worked out in the answers at the end of this chapter.

SET 1: *Conversions of units and expressions of concentration*

1. A solution is $^1/_{50}$ gr/m. Express this concentration in the following units:
   a. Gm/L ____________
   b. mg/ml ____________
   c. % ____________

d. mg% ____________
e. ratio ____________
f. μg/ml ____________

SET 2: *Conversion of units used in calculations*

1. The tablets on hand are 0.9 mg each. The order is for gr 1/150. How many tablets should you give?
2. A drug in liquid form contains gr iiss in 1 t. What is the drug concentration in Gm/L?
3. Prepare 3 f oz of a 0.1% solution from tablets gr iss each.
4. How would you prepare 15 gallons of a 1:6000 solution from a powder?
5. The tablets on hand are marked 0.1 mg each. The order is for gr 1/300. How should the nurse proceed?
6. What is the strength of 100 ml of solvent containing gr v?

■ Calculating the strength of diluted solutions

The examples just given have all dealt with weight/volume problems. In examining volume/volume problems we may modify our basic equation slightly and solve problems in much the same way as before. Our equation becomes:

(Concentration of solution) × (Volume of solution) = (Concentration of stock) × (Volume of stock).

When we say stock or stock solution we refer to a concentrated, storage form of a drug, which must ordinarily be diluted before use. Using this equation, calculations are performed much as before, as shown in the following examples.

EXAMPLE 5: *Prepare 1 quart of a 1:5000 solution from a 10% solution.*

You know:

1. Volume of solution (1 qt)
2. Concentration of solution (1:5000)
3. Concentration of stock (10%)

To solve:

1. Convert all quantities to the same system of units:

$$1 \text{ qt} \simeq 1 \text{ L} \simeq 1000 \text{ ml}$$
$$1{:}5000 = 1 \text{ Gm}/5000 \text{ ml}$$
$$10\% = 10 \text{ Gm}/100 \text{ ml}$$

2. Substitute into the equation:

$$1 \text{ Gm}/5000 \text{ ml} \times 1000 \text{ ml} = 10 \text{ Gm}/100 \text{ ml} \times \text{Volume of stock}$$

3. Solve for the unknown:

$$\text{Volume of stock} = \frac{1 \text{ Gm} \times 1000 \text{ ml}}{5000 \text{ ml}} \times \frac{100 \text{ ml}}{10 \text{ Gm}} = 2 \text{ ml}$$

EXAMPLE 6: *Prepare 500 ml of a 1% solution from a 1:25 stock.*

You know:

1. Volume of solution (500 ml)
2. Concentration of solution (1%)
3. Concentration of stock (1:25)

To solve:

1. Convert all quantities into the same system of units:

$$1\% = 1 \text{ Gm}/100 \text{ ml}$$
$$1{:}25 = 4 \text{ Gm}/100 \text{ ml}$$

2. Substitute into the equation:

$$\frac{500 \text{ ml} \times 1 \text{ Gm}}{100 \text{ ml}} = \frac{4 \text{ Gm}}{100 \text{ ml}} \times \text{Volume of stock}$$

3. Solve for the unknown:

$$\text{Volume of stock} = 500 \text{ ml} \times \frac{1 \text{ Gm}}{100 \text{ ml}} \times \frac{100 \text{ ml}}{4 \text{ Gm}} = 125 \text{ ml}$$

EXAMPLE 7: *How much of a 0.5% solution will 10 ml of a 20% solution prepare?*

You know:

1. Concentration of solution (0.5%)
2. Volume of stock (10 ml)
3. Concentration of stock (20%)

To solve:

1. Convert all quantities into the same system of units:

$$0.5\% = 0.5 \text{ Gm}/100 \text{ ml}$$
$$20\% = 20 \text{ Gm}/100 \text{ ml}$$

2. Substitute into the equation:

$$0.5 \text{ Gm}/100 \text{ ml} \times \text{Volume of solution} = 20 \text{ Gm}/100 \text{ ml} \times 10 \text{ ml}$$

3. Solve for the unknown:

$$\text{Volume of solution} = \frac{20 \text{ Gm}}{100 \text{ ml}} \times 10 \text{ ml} \times \frac{100 \text{ ml}}{0.5 \text{ Gm}} = 400 \text{ ml}$$

Self-test for proficiency in drug calculations

After thorough study of the previous section, the student should be able to work the following problems. You may check your answers and see the calculations worked out in the answers at the end of this chapter.

SET 3: *Dilution of stock solutions*

1. A stock solution of a drug contains 10,000 units/ml.
   a. Calculate the amount of stock needed to include in 500 ml of infusion fluid if a 150 lb patient is to receive 20,000 units of drug in this volume.
   b. Calculate the concentration of the diluted drug.
2. Prepare 1 qt of a 2% solution from a 1:10 stock.
3. How would you prepare 1 gal of a 5% solution from a 50% solution?
4. The attending physician has left orders to infuse a patient with 25,000 units of a drug in 0.5 L of normal saline solution. The drug is supplied as 50,000 units/ml stock solution. What volume of the drug stock would you use to make up the 0.5 L drug solution for administration?

■ Calculating drug dosage

All of the examples thus far have dealt with the preparation of the drug for administration. We now turn to the next step: the use of those materials to fulfill the physician's drug order for a patient. Our equation is:

Body weight × Dosage = Volume of drug × Drug concentration

A drug dosage is expressed as units or mass of drug per body weight of patient. For example, 0.1 Gm of drug/kg body weight is a drug dosage expression, but 0.1 Gm of drug is not. Occasionally a physician may order a dose of, for example, 500 mg of an antibiotic to be taken every 4 hours. Technically this form does not constitute a drug dosage, but in practice it is understood that 500 mg is the appropriate dose for an average-size patient, that is, the intended dosage is 500 mg/70 kg body weight. More accurate dosages must of course be calculated for persons who deviate greatly from the normal weight range or when highly toxic drugs are involved. Common types of problems in drug dosage are presented in the following examples.

EXAMPLE 8: *A 100 kg patient is to receive a dose of 4 units/kg body weight. How many ml of the supplied drug at 100 units/ml will be required?*

You know:

1. Drug dosage (4 units/kg body weight)
2. Patient body weight (100 kg)
3. Concentration of the drug to be administered (100 units/ml)

To solve:

1. Substitute into the equation:

$$100 \text{ kg} \times \frac{4 \text{ units}}{\text{kg}} = \text{Volume of drug} \times 100 \text{ units/ml}$$

2. Solve for volume of drug:

$$\text{Volume of drug} = 100 \text{ kg} \times \frac{4 \text{ units}}{\text{kg}} \times \frac{\text{ml}}{100 \text{ units}} = 4 \text{ ml}$$

EXAMPLE 9: *The physician orders 0.2 Gm of drug for a patient. How many capsules at gr iss each will you administer?*

To solve:

1. Convert 0.2 Gm to 3 gr.
2. Convert gr iss to 1.5 gr.

Therefore

$$\frac{3 \text{ gr}}{1.5 \text{ gr/capsule}} = 2 \text{ capsules}$$

Self-test for proficiency in drug calculations

After thorough study of the previous section, the student should be able to work the following problems. You may check your answers and see the calculations worked out in the answers at the end of this chapter.

SET 4: *Drug dosages*

1. A 70 kg patient is to receive 1.2 Gm of a drug administered in a 3.0 ml volume. What is the concentration of the drug solution administered to the patient, and what is the drug dosage?
2. A 60 kg patient is to receive 600 mg of a drug administered in a 2 ml volume. What is the drug dosage?
3. A certain drug is dispensed in tablets marked 250 mg. The drug package insert says that the dose of the drug is not to exceed 10 mg/kg. If a 60 kg adult patient receives 2 tablets, will the dosage exceed that which the manufacturer considers safe?
4. A certain patient is to receive a drug at a dose of 5 mg/kg. The drug is supplied in a vial marked 500 mg/ml. What volume of drug from the vial should be administered to a 70 kg patient?
5. A certain drug is known to cause thrombophlebitis when given intravenously at high concentrations. For this reason the package insert says the drug must be infused at a concentration of less than 10 mg/ml. A 50 kg patient is to receive 500 mg of the drug by intravenous infusion. What is the drug dosage, and what volume will have to be infused?

■ Calculating infusion rates

Many drugs must be administered intravenously by slow infusion rather than as a rapid bolus injection. Large volumes of fluids of various types are also given by intravenous infusion. Disposable infusion sets are available from several manufacturers. These sets are commonly calibrated to deliver 10, 12, 15, 20, 50, or 60 drops/ml of fluid. The nurse in practice can find the calibration, or drop factor, for any particular infusion set by examining the package in which it is supplied. Usually a hospital will only have two sizes available to minimize confusion: one regular, or macrodrip, set of 10, 12, 15 drops/ml (abbreviated gtt/ml), and one pediatric, or microdrip, set of 50 or 60 gtt/ml.

Calculations of infusion rates can be carried out with the following equation:

$$\text{gtt/minute} = \frac{\text{gtt/ml calibration}}{60 \text{ minute/hour}} \times \frac{\text{Total ml to be administered}}{\text{Total hours of infusion}}$$

The use of this formula can be illustrated with the following examples:

EXAMPLE 10: *A physician's order reads "3500 ml %5 dextrose in water IV in 24 hours." What is the correct infusion rate if the infusion set delivers 60 gtt/ml?*

You know:

1. gtt/ml calibration = 60 gtt/ml
2. Total ml to be administered = 3500
3. Total hours of infusion = 24

To solve:

Substitute into the equation:

$$\text{gtt/minute} = \frac{60 \text{ gtt/ml}}{60 \text{ minute/hour}} \times \frac{3500 \text{ ml}}{24 \text{ hours}} = 145 \text{ to } 146 \text{ gtt/minute}$$

EXAMPLE 11: *To give 50 ml of antibiotic solution IV in 30 minutes, what should the infusion rate be in drops per minute? The infusion set is calibrated for 60 gtt/ml.*

You know:

1. gtt/ml calibration = 60 gtt/ml
2. Total ml to be administered = 50 ml
3. Total hours of infusion = 0.5

To solve:

Substitute into the formula:

$$\text{gtt/minute} = \frac{60 \text{ gtt/ml}}{60 \text{ minute/hour}} \times \frac{50 \text{ ml}}{0.5 \text{ hour}} = 100 \text{ gtt/minute}$$

EXAMPLE 12: *If an infusion set calibrated for 15 gtt/ml is running at a rate of 45 gtt/minute, how long will be required to infuse 1 L of fluid?*

You know:

1. gtt/ml calibration = 15 gtt/ml
2. Total ml to be administered = 1000 ml (1 L)
3. Flow rate = 45 gtt/minute

To solve:

Substitute into the equation:

$$45 \text{ gtt/minute} = \frac{15 \text{ gtt/ml}}{60 \text{ minute/hour}} \times \frac{1000 \text{ ml}}{\text{Hours of infusion}}$$

We rearrange the formula to solve for the number of hours:

$$\text{Hours of infusion} = \frac{15 \text{ gtt/ml}}{60 \text{ minute/hour}} \times \frac{1000 \text{ ml}}{45 \text{ gtt/minute}} = 5.55 \text{ hours}$$

Self-test for proficiency in drug calculations

After thorough study of the previous section, the student should be able to work the following problems. You may check your answers and see the calculations worked out in the answers at the end of this chapter.

SET 5: *Calculating IV infusion rates*

1. The physician's order reads "1000 ml of D5W IV in 8 hours." What is the correct infusion rate if the administration set delivers 10 gtt/ml?
2. To give 50 ml of antibiotic solution IV in 30 minutes, what should the infusion rate be in drops per minute if the infusion set is calibrated to deliver 10 gtt/ml?
3. One-half liter of normal saline solution is to be infused over a 5-hour period. The infusion set delivers 20 gtt/ml. What should the rate of infusion be?
4. The physician's order reads "1000 ml D5W in 24 hours." If the infusion set calibration is 60 gtt/ml, how many drops per minute should be administered?
5. An infusion of 500 ml of IV fluid is to be carried out over 3 hours. What infusion rate must be used with an infusion set delivering 10 gtt/ml?

■ Calculating pediatric dosages

Calculation of pediatric dosages requires special knowledge of each drug and how it interacts with the unique metabolism of the infant. Some drugs may be given to children and infants in doses that are in the same proportion to body weight as the doses used in adults. Other drugs must be given in greatly reduced doses because the infant is more sensitive or is incapable of metabolizing the drug as rapidly as an adult. These considerations are taken into account in determining recommended pediatric doses. For many drugs the pediatric doses listed in various drug reference publications will include a statement that the dosage may be calculated for children according to body weight, for example, but should not exceed a stated upper limit.

Several methods for calculating pediatric dosages exist. We will present three of the more common methods. The first method, called *Young's rule,* is based on the age of the child and applies to children between 1 and 12 years of age. The equation is:

$$\text{Child's dose} = \frac{\text{Age of the child in years}}{\text{Age of child in years} + 12} \times \text{Adult dose}$$

The use of Young's rule is illustrated in the following example.

EXAMPLE 13: *What is the appropriate dose of aspirin for a 3-year-old child? A normal adult dose is gr v.*

You know:

1. The age of the child = 3 years
2. The adult dose = gr v

To solve:

Substitute the known quantities into the equation:

$$\text{Child's dose} = \frac{3 \text{ years}}{3 + 12} \times 5 \text{ gr}$$

$$= \frac{1}{5} \times 5 \text{ gr} = 1 \text{ gr, or gr i}$$

A second method for calculating pediatric dosages is based on a comparison of the child's weight to the average weight of an adult. This formula, which applies to all ages of children, is called *Clark's rule*. The equation is:

$$\text{Child's dose} = \frac{\text{Weight of child in pounds}}{150 \text{ lb}} \times \text{Adult dose}$$

The use of Clark's rule is illustrated in the following example.

EXAMPLE 14: *What is the appropriate dose of aspirin for a 30 lb child, if the normal adult dose is gr v?*

You know:

1. The weight of the child = 30 lbs.
2. The adult dose = 5 gr.

To solve:

Substitute the known quantities into the equation:

$$\text{Child's dose} = \frac{30 \text{ lb}}{150 \text{ lb}} \times 5 \text{ gr} = 1 \text{ gr}$$

Note that Clark's rule and Young's rule give the same answer when the child is not greatly lighter or heavier than the normal weight for his or her age. The 3-year-old child used in examples 14 and 15, at 30 lbs, is near the normal weight for his or her age. Clark's rule

TABLE 3-7. Body surface area as a function of weight

Weight kg	Weight lb	Surface area (M^2)	Approximate age of patient	Weight kg	Weight lb	Surface area (M^2)	Approximate age of patient
4.0	8.8	0.25	3 weeks	19	41	0.73	5 years
5.7	12.5	0.29	3 months	21	47	0.82	6 years
7.4	16	0.36	6 months	24	53	0.90	7 years
10	22	0.46	1 year	27	59	0.97	8 years
12	27	0.54	2 years	32	71	1.12	10 years
14	31	0.60	3 years	39	86	1.28	12 years
16	36	0.68	4 years	70	150	1.7	Adult

is considered the more accurate of the two rules, since it will adjust dosage for a child who does deviate from normal weight.

The most accurate method of calculating pediatric dosage is based on the surface area of the child's body relative to that of an adult. Surface area is obviously more difficult to measure than age or weight. Measurements under laboratory conditions have allowed us to take 1.7 square meters (M^2) as the average body surface area for an adult. Measurements under similar conditions with children have enabled us to construct charts and nomograms that relate the child's body weight to surface area. An example of such a chart is shown in Table 3-7. The equation used for the drug dose calculation is:

$$\text{Child's dose} = \frac{\text{Surface area of child in M}^2}{1.7\ \text{M}^2} \times \text{Adult dose}$$

The use of the formula is illustrated in the following example:

EXAMPLE 15: *What dose of Demerol does a child weighing 10 kg require? The adult dose for Demerol is 50 mg.*

To calculate the dosage on the basis of body surface area, we must first determine from Table 3-7 the surface area that corresponds to a body weight of 10 kg. That value is 0.46 M^2. We may now proceed.

You know:

1. Surface area of child = 0.46 M^2
2. Adult dose = 50 mg

To solve:

Substitute these values into the equation:

$$\text{Child's dose} = \frac{0.46\ \text{M}^2}{1.7\ \text{M}^2} \times 50\ \text{mg} = 13.5\ \text{mg}$$

Self-test for proficiency in drug calculations

After thorough study of the previous section, the student should be able to work the following problems. You may check your answers and see the calculations worked out in the answers at the end of this chapter.

SET 6: *Calculating pediatric doses.*

1. A physician orders the antibiotic cephalexin for a 25 lb child. The normal adult dose for this drug is 250 mg q.i.d. Using Clark's rule, calculate the appropriate dose for this child. Does the prescribed dose fall within the recommended dose of 6 to 12 mg/kg listed in the package insert?
2. A 5-year-old child is to be given phenobarbital. The adult dose is 60 mg. Using Young's rule, calculate the appropriate dose for the child.
3. A 10-year-old child requires codeine sulfate. The normal adult dose is 30 mg. Using body surface area, calculate the appropriate dose for this child.
4. A 4-year-old child is to be given aspirin. Adults take either 5 or 10 gr of aspirin, depending on the severity of the pain to be relieved. Using Young's rule, calculate the appropriate dose for the child, based on the maximum adult dose.
5. A 9 kg infant is to receive atropine. The normal adult dose is gr $\frac{1}{150}$. What is the appropriate dose for this infant, based on body surface area?
6. Penicillin G is being given to a child weighing 40 lb. The adult dose is 300,000 units. Using Clark's rule, calculate the child's dose.

■ THE NURSING PROCESS

In this chapter, drug administration has been emphasized. Drug therapy is, in fact, only a part of the total patient care, but for drug therapy to be successful it must be properly carried out. The patient has the right to expect to receive the right drug, in the right dose, at the right time, via the right route of administration.

■ Assessment

In assessing a patient the nurse should be answering the question of why this patient might need a particular type of drug. Identifying the reason for medication being prescribed helps the nurse to detect inadvertent errors in which the wrong drug is in danger of being administered to a patient.

■ Management

Implementing the therapeutic plan involves proper administration of the prescribed medication. The nurse may seek information on specific drugs from a variety of sources, such as those mentioned in this chapter. For a student nurse, the prospect of learning about all the medications to be administered is overwhelming. Once the nurse is in practice, however, repeated administration of medications will facilitate developing a basic understanding of many of the categories of drugs frequently used.

Not only must the nurse be knowledgeable about the prescribed medication, but caution must be exercised that the prescribed medication is actually what the patient receives. Thus medications should remain in labelled packages or containers until the drug is administered. The increasing use of unit-dose packaging is helpful in allowing the nurse to remove the drug form only at the bedside of the patient.

The patient has a right to receive the medication in the correct dose. Currently many hospital pharmacies are preparing medications in the pharmacy and supplying them to the floor in the desired dose. Regardless of how drugs are supplied, however, the nurse has the responsibility to check labels carefully and to double-check all calculations that must be done. Some nurses have difficulty with the mathematical calculations necessary for dosage calculation; these nurses should get into the habit of having a colleague verify dosage calculations rather than possibly subjecting the patient to an incorrect dose of medication. The pharmacy may also be of assistance in dosage calculation.

Successful drug therapy may depend on the proper timing of drug doses, as discussed in Chapter 2. This requirement may involve close control of the intervals between doses. For example, many antibiotics must be administered at regular intervals around the clock to maintain continuous therapeutic blood levels. For other drugs, the most important time factor may be the time of day and time of meals. For example, certain medications should not be administered with meals. Therefore scheduling should be done to ensure that those medications are administered between meals.

To ensure that the patient receives each drug via the right route of administration, the nurse must know what routes are appropriate for a specific drug and must know how to administer drugs via that route. This textbook makes no attempt to teach techniques of drug administration. The student should refer to other fundamental nursing textbooks and use all available opportunities during laboratory and clinical instruction to develop facility in using all equipment for all routes of administration.

It is not possible in this book to list all possible sources of error in medication administration. There are, however, a few principles that should be followed in administering any medication. Regardless of what administration system an institution uses, the nurse should alway check the working tools of drug administration with the original written physician's order. Thus medication Kardexes or medication cards should always be checked against

■ THE NURSING PROCESS—cont'd

■ Management—cont'd

the original written medication order to ensure that transcription was correct. If there is any question because of difficulty in reading the physician's handwriting, the physician should be consulted. When the nurse reaches the patient's bedside, the patient should be clearly identified before any medication is administered. This involves asking patients to identify themselves as well as checking the patient's wristband.

The nurse must develop a sense of suspicion whenever a medication order seems to be out of the ordinary. For example, a dose of medication that seems unusually large or unusually small should be double-checked. If at the bedside the patient seems hesitant to take the medication, stating that the medication is new or that it is not what is usually taken, this should suggest to the nurse a need to double-check the physician's orders before insisting that a patient take a medication. Recording that a patient has received a medication should be done as soon as possible after the medication is administered to avoid inadvertent duplicate medication administration by other members of the health care team.

Local practices regarding safety checks for drug administration should be followed; they usually have been developed in response to a problem related to drug administration. Thus in many hospitals insulin doses are double-checked by two professional nurses before insulin is administered. The same procedure is used for administering doses of heparin, intravenous cardiotonics, and certain other dangerous medications. Some pediatric units require that all intramuscular and intravenous medications be checked by two professional nurses before the drugs are administered. Other units require that dosage calculations be double-checked by another professional before a dose is prepared and administered. Many hospitals have standing orders regarding automatic expiration dates for narcotics, antibiotics, anticoagulants, and other medications. These policies should be observed by the nurse.

■ Evaluation

In the process of evaluating a patient, the nurse may discover that a medication error has been made. When this occurs, the procedure within the institution should be followed for reporting the error. The usual procedure involves immediately reassessing the patient and observing the effects resulting from the incorrect medication or incorrect dose, notifying the physician, and recording the error on appropriate forms, which are usually provided by the institution. The nurse should not be afraid to report an error; the professional acknowledges when mistakes have been made, placing the well-being of the patient above false pride. The nurse should seek to learn from the error and modify practice to help ensure that the error will not occur again.

■ SUMMARY

The nurse bears moral and legal responsibility for seeing that each patient receives the prescribed drug at the proper dosage. If the physician's order for a drug creates any uncertainty as to intended dose or method of administration, the physician should be asked to clarify the written or verbal order. The nurse should refer to the package insert or to standard reference works to seek specific information about the dose, side effects, or special properties of a drug in question.

■ ANSWERS TO SELF-TESTS FOR PROFICIENCY IN DRUG CALCULATIONS

The correct answer for each question is given first, followed by the calculation.

Solution to Set 1

1/50 gr/m = 0.02 grains per minim (1 ÷ 50). We remember 15 gr = 1 Gm and 15 m = 1 ml. We know therefore that 1 gr/m = 1 Gm/ml $\left(\frac{15 \text{ gr}}{15 \text{ m}} = \frac{1 \text{ Gm}}{1 \text{ ml}}\right)$.

Hence 0.02 gr/m = 0.02 Gm/ml. We have now converted our expression of concentration from the apothecaries' system to the metric. We may now readily carry out the other conversions required. The answers are given first, followed by the calculation.

a. *20 Gm/L:* 1 ml = 0.001 L. Therefore 0.02 Gm/ml = 0.02 Gm/0.001 L or 20 Gm/L.
b. *20 mg/ml:* 1 Gm = 1000 mg. Therefore 0.02 Gm = 20 mg and 0.02 Gm/ml = 20 mg/ml.
c. *2%:* % is defined as Gm/100 ml. Solving by proportion, $\frac{0.02 \text{ Gm}}{1 \text{ ml}} = \frac{? \text{ Gm}}{100 \text{ ml}}$, ? Gm = $\frac{(0.02 \text{ Gm})(100 \text{ ml})}{1 \text{ ml}}$ = 2 Gm. Therefore 0.02 Gm/ml = 2 Gm/100 ml, or 2%.
d. *2000 mg%:* mg% is defined as mg/100 ml. 0.02 Gm = 20 mg; therefore 0.02 Gm/ml = 20 mg/ml, 20 mg/ml = ? mg/100 ml, ? = 2000 mg; therefore 20 mg/ml = 2000 mg%.
e. *1:50:* Ratio is defined as Gm:ml with both usually expressed as whole numbers. $\frac{0.02 \text{ Gm}}{1 \text{ ml}} = \frac{1 \text{ Gm}}{? \text{ ml}}$, ? = $\frac{1 \text{ Gm}}{0.02 \text{ Gm/ml}}$ = 50 ml. Therefore 0.02 Gm/ml = 1 Gm/50 ml, or 1:50.
f. *20,000 μg/ml:* 1 Gm = 1,000,000 μg. Therefore 0.02 Gm = 0.02 (1,000,000) = 20,000 μg.

Solution to Set 2

1. *0.5 tablet:* 15 gr = 1 Gm = 1000 mg. 1 gr = $\frac{1000 \text{ mg}}{15}$ and $\frac{1}{150}$ gr = $\frac{1000 \text{ mg}}{(150)(15)}$ = 0.44 mg. $\frac{0.44 \text{ mg}}{0.9 \text{ mg/tablet}}$ = 0.5 tablet.
2. *33.3 Gm/L:* gr iss = 2½ (ii = 2; ss = ½) gr. Solving by proportion, $\frac{15 \text{ gr}}{1 \text{ Gm}} = \frac{2.5 \text{ gr}}{? \text{ Gm}}$ and ? (Gm) = $\frac{(1 \text{ Gm})(2.5 \text{ gr})}{15 \text{ gr}}$ = 0.167 Gm. 1 t = 5 ml = 0.005 L, so the drug concentration is $\frac{0.167 \text{ Gm}}{0.005 \text{ L}}$ = 3.33 Gm/L.
3. *Add 1 tablet to 90 ml of water:* gr iss = 1.5. Solving by proportion, $\frac{15 \text{ gr}}{1 \text{ Gm}} = \frac{1.5 \text{ gr}}{? \text{ Gm}}$. ? Gm = $\frac{(1 \text{ Gm})(1.5 \text{ gr})}{15 \text{ gr}}$ = 0.1 Gm. 1 f oz = 30 ml, so 3 f oz = 90 ml. 0.1% = $\frac{0.1 \text{ Gm}}{100 \text{ ml}}$, and since we want 90 ml, solving by proportion, $\frac{0.1 \text{ Gm}}{100 \text{ ml}} = \frac{? \text{ Gm}}{90 \text{ ml}}$ and ? Gm = 0.09 Gm. Each tablet is 0.1 Gm: $\frac{0.09 \text{ Gm}}{0.1 \text{ Gm/tablet}}$ = 0.9 tablet, rounding off to 1 tablet.
4. *10 Gm of drug is added to 15 gal of water:* 15 gal = 60 L, and a 1:6000 solution = 1 Gm/6 L = 10 Gm.
5. *The nurse should administer 2 tablets:* gr 1/300 = 0.0033 gr, and 0.1 mg = 0.0015 gr; therefore the number of tablets required = gr 0.0033/(gr 0.0015/tablet) = 2 tablets.
6. *0.33%:* gr v = 0.33 Gm; therefore strength = 0.33 Gm/100 ml = 0.33%.

Solution to Set 3

1. a. *2 ml:* Calculate the *amount of stock* that contains 20,000 units. Solving by proportion, $\frac{10{,}000 \text{ units}}{1 \text{ ml}} = \frac{20{,}000 \text{ units}}{? \text{ ml}}$. ? ml = $\frac{(1 \text{ ml})(20{,}000 \text{ units})}{10{,}000 \text{ units}}$ = 2 ml.
   b. *40 units/ml:* Diluted drug is 20,000 units in 500 ml, so $\frac{20{,}000 \text{ units}}{500 \text{ ml}}$ = 40 units/ml.
2. *Dilute 200 ml of 1:10 stock to 1 qt (1000 ml):* 1:10 stock = $\frac{1 \text{ Gm}}{10 \text{ ml}}$; 1 qt = 1000 ml; 2% solution = $\frac{2 \text{ Gm}}{100 \text{ ml}}$. To make 1 qt of 2% would require: $\frac{2 \text{ Gm}}{100 \text{ ml}} = \frac{? \text{ Gm}}{1000 \text{ ml}}$. ? Gm = $\frac{(3 \text{ Gm})(1000 \text{ ml})}{100 \text{ ml}}$ = 20 Gm. To get 20 Gm from the 1:10 stock: $\frac{1 \text{ Gm}}{10 \text{ ml}} = \frac{20 \text{ Gm}}{\times \text{ ml}}$. ? ml = $\frac{(20 \text{ Gm})(10 \text{ ml})}{1 \text{ Gm}}$ = 200 ml.
3. *Add 400 ml of the 50% stock solution to 3600 μl of water:* 1 gal = 4000 ml, a 5% solution = 5 Gm/100 ml, and a 50% solution = 50 Gm/100 ml; therefore the volume of stock solution to be added = $\frac{(5 \text{ Gm/100 ml}) \times 4000 \text{ ml}}{(50 \text{ Gm/100 ml})}$ = 400 ml. Note that this volume is to be mixed with 3600 ml of water for the final volume of the solution to be 1 gal.
4. *0.5 ml:* You require 25,000 units from a stock solution of 50,000 units/ml; therefore the volume to be used = 25,000 × units/(50,000 units/ml) = 0.5 ml.

Solution to Set 4

1. *The concentration is 0.4 Gm/ml and the dosage is 17 mg/kg:* Concentration = $\frac{1.2 \text{ Gm}}{3 \text{ ml}}$ = 0.4 Gm/ml = 0.4 Gm/ml. Dosage = $\frac{1.2 \text{ Gm}}{70 \text{ kg}} = \frac{0.017 \text{ Gm}}{\text{kg}}$ = 17 mg/kg.

2. *Dosage is 10 mg/kg:* Dosage $= \frac{600 \text{ mg}}{60 \text{ kg}} = 10$ mg/kg.
3. *So:* $\frac{2 \text{ tablets}}{\text{Dose}} \times \frac{250 \text{ mg}}{\text{Tablet}} = \frac{500 \text{ mg}}{\text{Dose}}$

   Dosage $= \frac{500 \text{ mg}}{60 \text{ kg}} = 8.33$ mg/kg. Therefore the dose as prescribed should be within the accepted safety limits.
4. *0.7 ml:* $\frac{5 \text{ mg}}{\text{kg}} \times 70$ kg $= 350$ mg drug in each dose. $\frac{350 \text{ mg}}{500 \text{ mg/ml}} = 0.7$ ml volume from the vial.
5. *Dosage = 10 mg/kg and the minimum infusion volume is 50 ml:* Dosage $= \frac{500 \text{ mg}}{50 \text{ kg}} = 10$ mg/kg. Minimum infusion volume $= \frac{500 \text{ mg}}{10 \text{ mg/ml}} = 50$ ml.

Solution to Set 5

1. *20 to 21 gtt/minute:* gtt/minute $= \frac{10 \text{ gtt/ml}}{60 \text{ minute/hour}} \times \frac{1000 \text{ ml}}{8 \text{ hours}} = 20$ to 21 gtt/minute.
2. *16 to 17 gtt/minute:* gtt/minute $= \frac{10 \text{ gtt/ml}}{60 \text{ minute/hour}} \times \frac{50 \text{ ml}}{0.5 \text{ hours}} = 16$ to 17 gtt/minute.
3. *33 to 34 gtt/minute:* gtt/minute $= \frac{20 \text{ gtt/ml}}{60 \text{ minute/hour}} \times \frac{500 \text{ ml}}{5 \text{ hours}} = 33$ to 34 gtt/minute.
4. *41 to 42 gtt/minute:* gtt/minute $= \frac{60 \text{ gtt/ml}}{60 \text{ minute/hour}} \times \frac{1000 \text{ ml}}{24 \text{ hours}} = 41$ to 42 gtt/minute.
5. *27 to 28 gtt/minute:* gtt/minute $= \frac{10 \text{ gtt/ml}}{60 \text{ minute/hour}} \times \frac{500 \text{ ml}}{3 \text{ hours}} = 27$ to 28 gtt/minute.

Solution for Set 6

1. *Dosage prescribed = 3.8 mg/kg, which is less than the suggested lower limit of 6 mg/kg:* Child's dose $= \frac{25 \text{ lb}}{150 \text{ lb}} \times 250$ mg $= 42$ mg. 25 lb = 11 kg. Dosage = 42 mg/11 kg = 3.8 mg/kg.
2. *17.6 mg:* Child's dose $= \frac{5 \text{ years}}{5 + 12} \times 60$ mg $= 17.6$ mg.
3. *19.8 mg:* Body surface area of 10-year-old child from Table 3-7 = 1.12 M^2. Child's dose $= \frac{1.12 \text{ M}^2}{1.7 \text{ M}^2} \times 30$ mg $= 19.8$ mg.
4. *2.5 gr:* Child's dose $= \frac{4 \text{ years}}{4 + 12} \times 10$ gr $= 2.5$ gr.
5. *0.11 mg:* Body surface area of 9 kg infant from Table 3-7 = 0.41 M^2. Child's dose $= \frac{0.41 \text{ M}^2}{1.7 \text{ M}^2} \times$ (1/150 gr) = 0.24 (0.44 mg) = 0.11 mg.
6. *80,000 units:* Child's dose $= \frac{40 \text{ lb}}{150 \text{ lb}} \times 300{,}000 = 80{,}000$ units.

■ SUGGESTED READINGS

Specific information about individual drugs

AMA drug evaluations, ed. 4, New York, 1980, The American Medical Association and John Wiley & Sons, Inc.

Facts and comparisons, 1979, St. Louis, 1979, Facts and Comparisons, Inc.

Gilman, A.G., Goodman, L.S., and Gilman, A., editors: The pharmacological basis of therapeutics, ed. 6, New York, 1980, Macmillan, Inc.

Goth, A.: Medical pharmacology: principles and concepts, ed. 10, St. Louis, 1981, The C.V. Mosby Co.

Loebl, S., Spratto, G., and Heckheimer, E.: The nurse's drug handbook, ed. 2, New York, 1980, John Wiley & Sons, Inc.

Modell, W., editor: Drugs of choice 1980-1981, St. Louis, 1980, The C.V. Mosby Co.

Nurse's guide to drugs, Horsham, Pa., 1980, Intermed Communications, Inc.

Physicians' desk reference, Oradell, N.J., 1981, Medical Economics Co.

Dosage calculations

Blume, D.M.: Dosages and solutions, ed. 3, Philadelphia, 1980, F.A. Davis.

Campbell, J.: The BSA method of calculating pediatric drug dosages, MCN **3**:357, 1978.

Carr, J.J., McElroy, N.L., and Carr, B.L.: How to solve dosage problems in one easy lesson, American Journal of Nursing **76**:1934, 1976.

Eisenbach, R.: Calculating and administering medications, Philadelphia, 1977, F.A. Davis Co.

Engram, B.: Computing I.V. flow rates, Nursing '81 **11**:89, 1981.

Hart, L.K.: The arithmetic of dosages and solutions: a programmed presentation, ed. 5, St. Louis, 1981, The C.V. Mosby Co.

Jessee, R.W., and McHenry, R.W.: Self-teaching tests in arithmetic for nurses, ed. 9, St. Louis, 1975, The C.V. Mosby Co.

Keane, C.B., and Fletcher, S.M.: Drugs and solutions: a programmed introduction for nurses, ed. 2, Philadelphia, 1970, W.B. Saunders Co.

Medici, G.A.: Drug dosage calculations: a guide for current clinical practice, Englewood Cliffs, N.J., 1980, Prentice-Hall, Inc.

Radcliff, R.K., and Ogden, S.J.: Calculation of drug dosages: a workbook, ed. 2, St. Louis, 1980, The C.V. Mosby Co.

Richardson, L.I., and Richardson, J.K.: The mathematics of drugs and solutions with clinical applications, ed. 2, New York, 1980, McGraw-Hill, Inc.

Sackheim, G.I., and Robins, L.: Programmed mathematics for nurses, ed. 4, New York, 1979, Macmillan, Inc.

Tso, Y.: Drug dosing for pediatric patients, Nurse Practitioner **2**:35, 1977.

Whisler, B.: Mathematics for health professionals, North Scituate, Mass., 1979, Duxbury Press.

Techniques of drug administration

Bjeletich, J., and Hickman, R.O.: The Hickman indwelling catheter, American Journal of Nursing **80**(1):62, 1980.

Brill, E.L., and Kilts, D.F.: Foundations of nursing, New York, 1980, Appleton-Century-Crofts.

Burgess, A.W.: Nursing: levels of health interventions, Englewood Cliffs, N.J., 1978, Prentice-Hall, Inc.

Du Gas, B.W.: Introduction to patient care, ed. 3, Philadelphia, 1977, W.B. Saunders Co.

Feeley, E.M., Shine, M.S., and Sloboda, S.B.: Fundamentals of nursing care, New York, 1980, D. Van Nostrand Co.

Giving medications, Horsham, Pa., 1980, Intermed Communications, Inc.

Giving medications through a nasogastric tube, Nursing '80 **10**(5): 71, 1980.

Kozier, B., and Erb, G.L.: Fundamentals of nursing. Concepts and procedures, Reading, Mass., 1979, Addison-Wesley Publishing Co., Inc.

Lewis, L.V.W.: Fundamental skills in patient care, ed. 2, Philadelphia, 1980, J.B. Lippincott Co.

Murray, M.: Fundamentals of nursing, ed. 2, Englewood Cliffs, N.J., 1980, Prentice-Hall, Inc.

Newton, D.W., and Newton, M.: Route, site and technique: three key decisions in giving parenteral medication, Nursing '79 **9**(7):18, 1979.

Newton, M., and Newton, D.W.: Guidelines for handling drug errors, Nursing '77 **7**(9):62, 1977.

Saperstein, A.B., and Frazier, M.A.: Introduction to nursing practice, Philadelphia, 1980, F.A. Davis Co.

Sorensen, K.C., and Luckmann, J.: Basic nursing. A psychophysiologic approach, Philadelphia, 1979, W.B. Saunders Co.

Uretsky, S.: Drug information sources, a valuable resource, Nurses' Drug Alert, Special Report **3**:69, 1979.

Wolff, L.V., Weitzel, M.H., and Fuerst, E.V.: Fundamentals of nursing, ed. 6, Philadelphia, 1979, J.B. Lippincott Co.

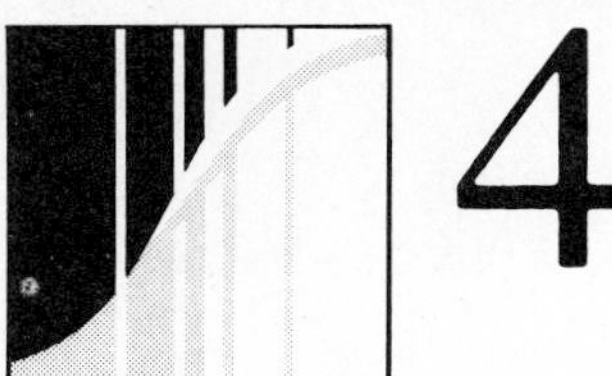

4 Regulation of the manufacture, sale, and use of medications

Patients receiving medications have always faced certain risks, which include the possibility that (1) the medication will not produce the beneficial effect claimed by those who make and sell the drug, (2) the medication may be directly harmful, and/or (3) the medication may be improperly administered. Modern drug legislation is designed to reduce or to eliminate these risks to patients.

■ ESTABLISHING THE SAFETY AND EFFICACY OF DRUGS

■ History of materia medica

The earliest form of medical practice involved the use of various natural products that were discovered by trial and error to have certain effects on the body. For example, parts of the poppy plant were known by the ancient Egyptians to relieve pain. This remedy was already ancient when it was recorded in the Papyrus of Ebers in 1500 BC. Equally ancient is the use of parts of the Ephedra shrub by the Chinese, who called the preparation *ma huang*. In the New World, South American Indians used the bark of the cinchona tree to relieve the symptoms of malaria. Even in more recent times, natural products have been introduced into medical practice. For example, in 1785 a British physician named Withering described the use of the leaf of the foxglove plant to relieve edema of a certain type, which had previously resisted all therapy.

Until very recently, natural products such as those just listed were the only medicinal agents, or *materia medica,* available. The most common medications were made from plants or parts of plants, and were therefore called botanicals. Some botanicals continue to be used in medical practice, but most have been replaced as chemists have analyzed these crude products and identified active ingredients. The active ingredients are the chemicals found in the crude preparation, which are responsible for producing the biological effect of the medicinal agent. For example, the poppy plant relieves pain because the plant contains opium. *Ma huang* produces its effects on the heart, lungs, and other organs because it contains ephedrine, an agent that stimulates the sympathetic nervous system. Similarly, it is the quinine in cinchona bark that relieves the symptoms of malaria, and it is the digitalis in foxglove leaves that relieves the edema associated with heart failure.

Identification of the active ingredient in a crude medicinal agent has two benefits. First, the active ingredient may be measured (or assayed) in the crude preparation and the dose adjusted for the content of the active ingredient. For example, the digitalis content of the foxglove leaf may vary from plant to plant. Therefore a dosage based on the amount of the leaf administered may actually contain a variable amount of digitalis and may therefore have variable biological effects. Since the biological activity of a drug is related to the actual dose of the active ingredient, dosages based on the weight of pure digitalis should have a more predictable biological effect.

The second benefit of identifying the active ingredient of a medicinal agent is that the chemical structure and properties of the active drug are revealed. This knowledge can lead to better ways to isolate the active material from natural sources. Digitalis is an example of a drug that is still prepared by extracting the drug from its plant source. Alternatively, once the structure of an active agent is known, chemists may be able to synthesize the material. Ephedrine is an example of a drug now chemically synthesized in a simple, economic process, which has replaced the procedure of isolating the drug from plant materials.

■ Standardization of medicinal agents

Recognizing the relationship between drug dose and biological effect produced, most nations of the world have attempted to adopt codes to standardize the content of medicinal agents. Drugs sold in the United States must comply with the standards established in *The United States Pharmacopeia and National Formulary,* or the *United States Homeopathic Pharmacopeia*.

The United States Pharmacopeia and National Formulary, abbreviated USP, contains chemical, physical, and biological information on all active ingredients used in medications. To qualify as a standard, or official, medication, the preparation must conform to the information listed in this source. The *National Formulary,* abbreviated NF, was originally independent of the USP and contained information on medications that were

TABLE 4-1. Chronological listing of federal drug legislation in the United States

Date	Title of Law	Major provisions
1906	Food and Drug Act	1. Established the USP and NF as official standards 2. Set standards for proper drug labelling
1912	Sherley Amendment	1. Prohibited fradulent claims for therapeutic effects of drugs
1914	Harrison Narcotic Act	1. Legally defined the term *narcotic* 2. Regulated and restricted the importation, manufacture, sale, or use of opium, cocaine, marihuana, and other drugs likely to produce dependence
1938	Federal Food, Drug, and Cosmetic Act	1. Maintained major provisions of previous laws 2. Required that a drug be demonstrated to be safe before it was marketed 3. Added the Homeopathic Pharmacopoeia of the United States as a third standard for drugs.
1945	Amendment to the Food and Drug Act	1. Required that biological products used as drugs (e.g., insulin or antibiotics) be certified on a batch by batch basis by a government agency
1952	Durham-Humphrey Amendment	1. Designated certain drugs as *legend drugs* (must be marked "Caution: Federal Law prohibits dispensing without prescription") 2. Restricted the right of the pharmacist to distribute legend drugs
1962	Kefauver-Harris Amendment	1. Required proof of efficacy for a drug to remain on the market 2. Authorized the FDA to establish official names for drugs
1970	Comprehensive Drug Abuse Prevention and Control Act (or the Controlled Substances Act)	1. Defined drug dependency and drug addiction 2. Classified drugs according to abuse potential and medical usefulness 3. Established methods for regulating manufacture, distribution, and sale of controlled substances 4. Established education and treatment programs for drug abuse

compounded from several different ingredients and on materials which had been dropped from the USP as standard medications. However, the distinctions between the NF and the USP became blurred in the last few editions. Therefore the fourteenth edition of the NF, published in 1975, was the last to be published separately. The new edition, USP XX and NF XV, was published as a single volume, which became official July 1, 1980.

As an example of the type of information found in the USP we may consider aspirin. The USP classifies aspirin as an antipyretic (fever-reducing), analgesic (pain-reducing) agent. In the USP, aspirin powder is listed separately from aspirin tablets. A variety of tablet sizes are described, containing amounts of aspirin ranging from 65 to 650 mg (approximately 1 to 10 gr). To meet USP standards, tablets must actually contain between 95% and 105% of the amount of aspirin on the label. For example, an aspirin tablet labeled 500 mg must contain between 475 and 525 mg of aspirin by actual assay. The aspirin used in these tablets must meet the chemical and physical standards listed for that compound in the USP. Although drug doses for adults and children are listed, the USP is less useful for clinical personnel than for persons in pharmaceutical manufacture or pharmacy.

Some drugs in use in the clinic cannot be standardized easily by chemical analysis, since the drug preparations are relatively complex mixtures of compounds. Standardization of these products may be obtained by measuring a biological effect. For example, insulin isolated from porcine or bovine pancreas glands is standardized on the basis of the amount of the preparation required to reduce the blood sugar of a test animal a certain amount. Antibiotics may be standardized on the basis of the amount of the preparation required to kill 99.9% of a certain sensitive strain of bacteria in a rigidly controlled laboratory test. Other complex pharmaceutical preparations, such as serums, vaccines, and human blood products, are tested and licensed by the National Institutes of Health, Division of Biological Standards (Table 4-1).

■ Government regulations concerning medicinal agents

Drug manufacturing and sale are regulated by both state and federal agencies. For federal laws to apply, a drug must enter interstate commerce. A drug totally manufactured within a single state and sold only in that state would not be subject to the federal drug laws. Very few drugs fall into this category.

The first effective federal law concerning drugs in the United States was passed in 1906 (Table 4-1). This law was intended to protect citizens from adulterated medicines and from medicines that contained harmful ingredients but failed to list these ingredients on the label. Each new law passed since that time has been intended to overcome specific problems that have arisen. For example, in the early 1900's a certain patent medicine was advertised as a cure for cancer. The federal government sought to force this company to halt the false advertisement. However, the drug label as it appeared on the bottle was accurate in naming the contents of the medicine. Under the 1906 law, accurate labelling of the contents was all the government could require. When the Sherley amendment was added in 1912, the federal government gained the ability to control advertising claims as well as the contents of the drug label.

The next major piece of drug legislation, passed in 1938, added the requirement that a drug sold in the United States had to be shown to be safe before it could be marketed. Prior to this law, a pharmaceutical company was not responsible for the safety of the drugs it manufactured and sold. For example, in 1937 over 100 people died from taking a product that was sold as "elixir of sulfanilamide." Investigations revealed that the cause of death was not the sulfanilamide, but the propylene glycol used to dissolve the drug. Amazingly, no one had tested the toxicity of propylene glycol before using it in this medication. Under the laws in 1937, however, the company responsible for this disaster could be charged only with mislabelling the drug, since an elixir is by definition an alcohol solution.

One of the major provisions of the legislation currently controlling drug marketing and use in the United States is that drugs must be efficacious in treating the medical condition for which the drug is recommended (Table 4-1). The requirement for proving efficacy as well as safety has greatly increased the amount of drug testing done by private companies who develop new drugs. As a result, the number of new drugs entering the market has been sharply reduced, and the time and money required to get a drug on the market have increased. On the other hand, drugs that do enter the market are much more reliable medications than newly introduced drugs have been in the past.

Another current provision of drug legislation is that pharmaceuticals be produced by what are termed "good manufacturing practices." Under this provision of the Food and Drug Act, the Food and Drug Administration inspects manufacturing facilities and oversees the general production of medications. Good manufacturing practices are general procedures, not specific processes. Indeed, the methods employed to produce the same medication can vary widely from company to company. Such variation is perfectly acceptable, as long as both procedures are in accordance with good manufacturing practices.

A number of federal agencies are involved in regulating drug trade, under the existing drug laws. In addition to the official government agencies, there are a number of private organizations that contribute advice or expertise to the government on matters concerning medicines. These organizations are listed and described in Table 4-2.

■ Assessing the safety of drugs

All medications intended for human use must undergo extensive toxicity testing in at least two species of animals. These toxicity tests must include both acute and chronic studies. Acute toxicity tests assess the short-term effects of extreme doses of the drug. The intent of these tests is to identify organs or tissues that may be sensitive to an action of the drug. These acute tests also allow researchers to determine how dangerous the drug might be in cases of overdose in human beings.

Chronic toxicity tests assess the effects of prolonged dosage with the experimental agent. Several exposure levels are usually tested, with at least one group of animals receiving doses far in excess of those expected to be received by human patients. After prolonged exposure to the test drug, the animals are sacrificed and extensive pathological and histological examinations are performed. Again, any pathological effects on organs or tissues, if present, must be noted. Significant toxicity observed in animals is usually sufficient cause for abandoning development of a drug.

Chronic toxicity tests are carried out in both males and females, since the sensitivity of the reproductive systems may differ. Certain other organs may differ between the sexes as well. Bladder cancer, for example, is more easily induced in males than in females with many chemicals.

TABLE 4-2. Organizations involved in regulating the manufacture and sale of drugs in the United States

Name	Common abbreviation	Function
Department of Health and Human Services (formerly Department of Health, Education, and Welfare)	HHS	The secretary of HHS is a cabinet-level officer whose duties include designating the official names for drugs sold in the United States and overseeing the Public Health Service.
Drug Enforcement Administration	DEA	This agency within the Department of Justice is the sole drug enforcement arm of the U.S. government, under the Controlled Substances Act of 1970.
Federal Trade Commission	FTC	This federal agency regulates the advertisement of medications aimed at the general public (not medical personnel).
Food and Drug Administration	FDA	This federal agency is responsible for guaranteeing the safety, purity, effectiveness, and reliability of drugs sold in the United States. In addition, this agency regulates the advertising of medications to medical personnel.
National Academy of Sciences–National Research Council	NAS–NRC	The NAS is a private organization composed of outstanding scientists in the United States. The NRC is the research arm of the NAS and was involved in evaluating the efficacy of drugs for the FDA in the Drug Efficacy Study Implementation.
Public Health Service	PHS	This federal agency not only funds extensive clinical research but also is responsible for maintaining basic research programs under the National Institutes of Health. Biologicals used as drugs are also certified by this agency.
Pharmaceutical Manufacturers Association	PMA	This private organization represents the pharmaceutical houses where most drugs are developed. This group functions as an advisory group to the FDA on occasion and as a lobbying group to Congress.
United States Adopted Names Council	USAN	This private group contains members from government, private industry, the medical profession, and research institutions whose function is to advise the Secretary of HHS as to the appropriate official name for each new drug introduced.

Chronic toxicity tests are also the point at which a drug is usually tested for carcinogenic (cancer-inducing) effects. The carcinogenic effects of compounds may also be assessed by the Ames test, which is based on the fact that mutagenic chemicals (chemicals that induce genetic mutations) accelerate the rate at which mutant bacteria revert to normal. Since many chemicals that are mutagens are also carcinogens, this test can help predict which drugs may be carcinogenic. This bacterial test is both less expensive and faster than chronic toxicity tests in animals, which may run months or years.

Drugs are also tested for their effects on pregnant animals and on fetuses. Drugs that cause fetal abnormalities are called *teratogens*. Some drugs are very dangerous to fetuses at certain stages in embryonic development but relatively harmless to adult animals or more mature fetuses. The stage of fetal development most sensitive to drugs or toxins is approximately the first one third of fetal life. A tragic example of this principle occurred with the drug thalidomide. Thalidomide is a sleeping medication that was widely marketed in Europe during the 1960's. The drug was not dangerous to adults, but when used by women in the early stages of pregnancy, the drug inhibited the proper development of fetal limb buds. The result was a number of babies born with tiny, nonfunctional limbs—a tragedy that could have been prevented by more extensive drug testing. Thalidomide was, in fact, never marketed in the United States because insufficient information was available to satisfy the Food and Drug Administration (FDA) guidelines for new drugs.

■ Assessing the efficacy of drugs

The clinical trial. Once an experimental drug has been thoroughly tested for toxicity in animals, the manufacturer may be ready to file with the FDA a "Notice of Claimed Investigational Exemption for a New Drug (IND)." Included in this notice must be information on the chemical structure of the new drug, partly to aid in establishing that the drug is, in fact, new. All the toxicity data in animals, data on drug absorption and metabolism, and data on the expected biological activity of the drug must be included. The manufacturer or licenser must outline in great detail the tests that will be run in human subjects.

The first testing of a drug in human beings is done in normal volunteers to establish how well the animal studies correlate with the results in humans. For example, drug absorption in humans may be quite different from that observed in certain animal species. It may therefore be necessary to repeat certain studies in humans. Occasionally, an unexpected side effect may show up at this stage of testing. For example, alterations of mood may not be easily recognized in experimental animals and yet may be severe enough in humans to prevent further development of an experimental drug.

The second stage of testing in human beings is properly called the *clinical trial*. Clinical trials may take many forms, but all are designed to answer the question, "Is this drug an effective treatment for a defined medical condition?" To answer this question, a relatively large number of patients must be studied, and the results must be analyzed in an objective manner, usually with statistical methods.

The *double-blind* design is one very effective format for a clinical trial. In this type of study, patients are randomly assigned to treatment groups or are assigned so that groups have the same average age, the same proportion of men and women, or some other desired characteristic. One group will receive the drug to be tested. Another group may receive a *placebo* (a dosage form containing no pharmacologically active ingredient). The drug and the placebo should be in the same form so that they are indistinguishable by sight or by taste. The placebo-treated group of patients serves as a control and allows the researcher to assess what percentage of patients would improve without therapy. The term *double-blind,* used to describe this experimental design, refers to the fact that during the experiment neither the patient nor the medical personnel dispensing medication know which patients are receiving the test drug and which are receiving placebo. In some studies, the control group receives the therapy that is currently accepted as the best available for the condition being tested, rather than placebo. This type of control allows the researchers to compare the efficacy of the new drug to existing therapy.

Patients who receive placebo in clinical trials and who show clinical improvement may be of two types. The first type includes patients whose disease has gone into spontaneous remission during the course of the clinical trial. For example, spontaneous remission is commonly observed in certain types of depressive diseases and in certain types of arthritis. The second type of patient who improves while receiving placebo is the patient who improves simply as a result of receiving medical attention rather than an effective drug. For example, as many as 30% of a group of patients suffering mild pain will report significant pain relief when they are given a placebo. With drugs affecting mood, the response to placebo will be observed in an even higher percentage of patients.

The *placebo effect* (clinical improvement in response to placebo) is a complication in clinical trials and makes the task of clearly evaluating the role of a particular drug in therapy more difficult. The existence of such an effect, however, emphasizes the importance of sympathetic human contact in relieving the suffering of a patient. A patient who responds to a placebo should by no means be considered to have originally been suffering from an imaginary complaint. We are now beginning to understand the normal mechanisms by which the body produces analgesia (endogenous morphine-like compounds, or endorphins, Chapter 28) and to realize that these internal mechanisms may be regulated by the central nervous system and affected by emotional states. Therefore the attention and support given to patients may alter the emotional state of the patient and allow the natural mechanisms of the body to improve their clinical condition.

Once a drug has been proven effective in controlled clinical trials, the manufacturer may file a request with the FDA to release the drug into limited circulation so that the drug can be tested in several medical centers on large numbers of patients. During the first round of clinical trials, the total number of patients tested may only

■ THE NURSING PROCESS IN DRUG TESTING

State laws differ in the provisions regulating the role of the nurse in drug testing. Therefore the nurse should examine the nurse practice act that is applicable and determine whether nurses are allowed to participate in drug testing studies and to what extent.

■ Assessment

Patient assessment should be performed on patients involved in drug testing programs just as for patients receiving normal therapy.

■ Management

Patient management in a drug testing study may be different than in a normal clinical setting. For example, the nurse should be certain that the institution where the study is taking place permits the nurse to administer investigational drugs. Many institutions require that the person conducting the experiment actually administer experimental drugs. The nurse should also find out whether a nurse is legally allowed to obtain informed consent. Some institutions in some states do not permit anyone but the principal investigator to obtain informed consent from the patient.

■ Evaluation

Evaluation of the patients receiving experimental drugs may be a major portion of the research aspect of drug testing programs. In many cases, detailed evaluation is carried out by the physician/researcher. Nevertheless, the nurse should continue to evaluate these patients in a manner consistent with good nursing practice. The extent to which the nursing evaluations become part of the permanent record of the experiment will depend on the institution and the protocol established by the investigator.

---

be a few hundred. When the drug is released into limited circulation, it may be tested in a few thousand patients. This larger number of patients allows assessment of rare complications of drug therapy that could not be predicted from more limited trials. Before a tested drug is finally released for interstate marketing, its developer must file with the FDA a New Drug Application (NDA). The NDA includes all information available on toxicity of the new drug, its use in patients, and the results of the clinical trials. If the FDA rules that the drug has been proven safe and efficacious, and that the claims made for the drug in the package insert and other professional advertising are supported by the results of the clinical trials, then the drug may be released for sale in interstate commerce.

■ The rights of the patient in drug testing

Anyone involved in assessing the clinical usefulness of a new drug is bound by certain moral and legal constraints. No one may be coerced into receiving an investigational drug. All drug studies must be done on volunteers who have read, understood, and signed "informed consent" forms. The law requires that all potential hazards associated with the use of the drug be clearly explained to the patient. The patient or volunteer must not be promised unrealistic benefits from therapy. The patient must also be free to withdraw from the study at any time without fear that the level of medical care received will be compromised.

Although compliance with the constraints just mentioned seems a simple matter, there are complications in practice. For example, some people believe that experimental drugs are always better than currently used drugs. These people may not have realistic expectations, in spite of having been told the properties of the drug being tested. Another problem concerns patients who are intimidated by medical personnel and who are afraid to refuse to participate in a drug study. These patients may confide their fears to an accessible and sympathetic nurse. It is the duty of the nurse to assist such patients in making their true feelings known.

■ Drug Efficacy Study Implementation (DESI)

All drugs introduced after the Harris-Kefauver amendment in 1962 are required to go through the extensive testing just described and must be proven efficacious and safe before they can be marketed. However, the drugs that were already on the market in 1962

TABLE 4-3. DESI rating system for drugs

Rating	Description
Effective	Substantial evidence exists to demonstrate the drug is effective treatment for the defined medical condition.
Probably effective	Some evidence exists but more will be required to prove the drug effective.
Possibly effective	Minimal evidence exists to suggest the drug may be effective.
Ineffective	Controlled trials have failed to show the drug to be more effective than placebo.
Ineffective as a fixed combination	Individual components of the medication might be effective alone at appropriate doses, but no evidence suggests all components of the medication are necessary to the effect.
Effective but	A qualification to the use of the drug is made, which must be added to the labelling.

posed a special problem, since they had been tested primarily for safety and not efficacy. To bring all drugs up to the same standard, the FDA contracted the National Research Council of the National Academy of Sciences to evaluate all medications being sold in the United States. This project was called the Drug Efficacy Study Implementation (DESI).

To carry out this project, scientific and clinical experts were called to study data from clinical trials. Based on this information, drugs were rated according to the scale shown in Table 4-3. Drugs that were rated as ineffective were removed from the market. Those drugs listed as possibly effective or probably effective required reformulation and/or retesting to stay on the market. This drug testing program begin in 1967 with prescription drugs and was later extended to over-the-counter medications (Chapter 5).

■ CONTROLLED SUBSTANCES

■ Properties of controlled substances

Certain substances can alter the normal function of the human body so profoundly that the body becomes dependent on that substance and will suffer physical harm if the substance is withdrawn. This condition is called *physical addiction* or *physical dependence*. Other substances, although not producing clear evidence of physical addiction, nevertheless produce profound changes in the psychological makeup of the user and produce what is called *psychological addiction*. Examples of types of compounds producing each of these types of addiction are listed in Table 4-4.

Because the substances that produce physical or psychological addiction clearly have the capacity to harm their users, these substances have been regulated extensively in the United States as well as elsewhere throughout the world. The original legislation in the United States was the Harrison Narcotics Act of 1914. This law restricted the importation of many of these addictive substances. One of the major aims of the Food and Drug Act of 1906 and the Harrison Act was to prevent the sale of patent medicines that contained no active ingredient except one of these addicting agents.

The Harrison Act did not eliminate the problem of illicit drug use and drug addiction. The existing law was also clearly limited in dealing with certain synthetic agents that were useful clinically but were also highly addicting. This legislation was replaced by a more comprehensive law in 1970, called the Controlled Substances Act. In addition to supplying guidelines on what constitutes drug dependency and establishing education and treatment programs, this law clearly classifies drugs based on abuse potential and clinical usefulness and specifies the restrictions that apply to each type of controlled drug. The drug schedules are described in Table 4-5.

■ Regulation of controlled substances in the clinic

Drugs in each of the schedules defined by the Controlled Substances Act are regulated by a defined set of rules appropriate to those drugs. For example, Schedule I substances have no approved medical uses and are therefore simply banned. Schedule II drugs are controlled at every stage from initial manufacture through distribution and final use. By law, no prescription for a Schedule II drug may be refilled. Physicians must be licensed to prescribe these medications and must keep accurate records to ensure that drugs are used strictly for legitimate purposes. Likewise, pharmacies must be specially licensed and keep accurate records for Schedule II drugs.

Drugs in Schedules III, IV, and V are considered less dangerous than those in Schedule II. For the most part this greater safety is a result of the inherent properties of the chemicals that appear in these schedules. However, some chemicals appear in more than one schedule. For example, codeine used alone as an antitussive is a Schedule II drug. However, medications containing codeine compounded with aspirin, acetaminophen, or other agents are Schedule III drugs, even when the total dose of codeine is the same as that used in the Schedule II preparations. One reason these compounded

TABLE 4-4. Compounds that produce dependence with continued use

Type of dependence	Drug category	Specific drugs
Physical and psychological	Narcotic analgesics	Morphine, heroin, codeine, paregoric, methadone
Physical and psychological	General depressants	Ethanol, barbiturates, glutethimide, methaqualone
Psychological*	Psychomotor stimulants	Amphetamines, cocaine, methylphenidate
Psychological	Hallucinogens	LSD, mescaline (peyote), *NN*-dimethyl-tryptamine (DMT), 2,5-dimethoxy-4-methyl amphetamine (STP), phencyclidine
Psychological	Cannabis	Marihuana, hashish

*Physical dependence has been suggested for certain of these drugs, but remains controversial.

TABLE 4-5. Classification of controlled substances according to the Controlled Substances Act of 1970

Classification	Description	Specific substances
Schedule I	Drugs that have high potential for abuse and no accepted medical use. The containers are marked C-I.	Heroin, LSD, peyote, marihuana, *NN*-dimethyltryptamine
Schedule II	Drugs that have a high potential for abuse but have an accepted medical use. Dependence may include strong physical and psychological dependence. The containers are marked C-II.	Amobarbital, amphetamine, benzedrine, codeine, dextroamphetamine, meperidine, methadone, hydromorphone, methaqualone, morphine, opium, pentobarbital, phenazocine, methylphenidate, secobarbital
Schedule III	Medically accepted drugs that may cause dependence, but are less prone to abuse than drugs in Schedules I and II. The containers are marked C-III.	Codeine-containing medications, butabarbital, hexobarbital, paregoric, nalorphine
Schedule IV	Medically accepted drugs that may cause mild physical or psychological dependence. The containers are marked C-IV.	Chloral hydrate, chlordiazepoxide, diazepam, meprobamate, phenobarbital
Schedule V	Medically accepted drugs with very limited potential for causing mild physical or psychological dependence. The containers are marked C-V.	Drug mixtures containing small quantities of narcotics, such as over-the-counter cough syrups containing codeine

forms of codeine are considered less likely to be abused is that adverse symptoms from overdoses of the other ingredients in the compounds discourage abuse of these forms of codeine. Codeine also appears in several cough syrups that are Schedule V drugs. The recommended single dose of codeine for adults in these Schedule V medications is 5 or 10 mg, whereas the doses found in Schedule II or III forms are 15 to 60 mg. This lower dosage in the cough medications is responsible for the Schedule V classification.

■ THE NURSING PROCESS INVOLVED WITH CONTROLLED SUBSTANCES

Because of the addictive potential of many controlled substances, legal restraints have been placed on the use of these drugs in medical practice. These regulations as well as the special nature of the drugs add a special burden and responsibility to the nurse.

■ Assessment

The nurse should take special care to observe whether an individual patient displays signs and symptoms that make the use of the controlled substance appropriate. Nurses should be alert to signs of drug abuse in patients. Patients may have obtained prescriptions from several physicians in order to acquire excessive amounts of controlled substances. The nurse should be alert not only to physical signs of excessive drug use but also to the psychological signs pointing to this problem. For example, a patient who is dependent on drugs obtained under false pretenses may be reluctant to enter the hospital even for the most routine testing, fearing that the drug dependency will be discovered in the closely regulated hospital environment.

■ Management

In dealing with controlled substances, the nurse has both legal and medical responsibilities. The legal responsibilities include ensuring that controlled substances (Schedules II through V) are kept under lock and key. These substances must be available only to authorized personnel. Records on the use of these substances must be kept so that all of the material is accounted for. Any unauthorized use of controlled substances must be reported to the proper authorities.

The nurse should be aware of the institutional policy on standing orders for controlled substances. For Schedule II drugs, the physician's order may require renewal every 48 hours. A nurse who administers the drug after the 48-hour period without obtaining a renewal order is in violation of the law.

Patients receiving controlled substances may express concern about possible drug dependence. The use of the medication should be explained in terms of the patient's own condition, and the patient may be appropriately reassured.

■ Evaluation

Patient evaluation is at two levels for controlled substances. First, the medical evaluation should be performed as for any other type of drug. The nurse should ascertain if the medication is successfully controlling the signs and symptoms for which it was given. For example, the nurse might evaluate the patient to determine if pain is being adequately relieved in a postsurgery patient receiving morphine. Second, the patient should be evaluated for psychological responses to the addictive drugs. Signs of drug dependence should be noted, as well as excessive fears of addiction. These observations may dictate changes in the therapeutic program.

■ SUMMARY

The earliest medicinal agents were natural products discovered by trial and error to have certain effects on the body. Most of these crude natural products have now been replaced by preparations containing known amounts of active ingredients. The United States Pharmacopeia and National Formulary and the United States Homeopathic Pharmacopeia serve as the reference works establishing the chemical properties, physical properties, and content of medications sold in the United States. Legislation in effect in the United States requires that medicinal agents be accurately labelled and advertised and be safe as well as effective when used as directed. The safety and efficacy of drugs in humans is determined in controlled clinical trials carried out before the drug is released into trade. Drugs may not enter clinical trials until extensive toxicity tests in animals have shown the drug is likely to be safe in human beings.

Drugs that can cause psychological or physical addiction are regulated according to the provisions of the Controlled Substances Act of 1970. Substances are assigned to Schedules I through V according to their clinical uses and potential for abuse. Substances assigned to Schedule I have a high abuse potential and no accepted clinical uses. At the other extreme, substances assigned to Schedule V are medically accepted drugs that have a very limited potential for causing mild physical or psychological dependence. Substances listed in Schedule I are illegal to sell or possess in the United States. Those substances in Schedule II that do have accepted medical uses are closely regulated throughout manufacture and sale. The appropriate distribution and use of drugs in Schedules II through V must be documented by accurately kept records.

■ STUDY QUESTIONS

1. What is the "active ingredient" of a medicinal preparation?
2. What advantages are gained by identifying the active ingredient in a crude medicinal preparation?
3. What is the function of The United States Pharmacopeia and National Formulary?
4. Outline the steps involved in getting a new drug approved for the United States market.
5. What is a clinical trial?
6. Describe a clinical trial following the *double-blind* design.
7. What is the placebo effect?
8. Suggest two explanations for the placebo effect observed in drug trials.
9. What is the purpose of the informed consent form?
10. What was the purpose of the Drug Efficacy Study Implementation?
11. What are controlled substances?
12. What special precautions are required in handling controlled substances?

■ SUGGESTED READINGS

Annas, G.J.: Informed consent, Annual Review of Medicine **29:**9, 1978.

Bok, S.: The ethics of giving placebos, Scientific American **231**(5): 17, 1974.

Cazalas, M.W.: Nursing and the law, ed. 3, Germantown, Md., 1978, Aspen Systems Corporation.

Creighton, H.: Law every nurse should know, ed. 3, Philadelphia, 1975, W.B. Saunders Co.

Editors: The curious case of therapeutic failures, Emergency Medicine **6**(11):81, 1974.

Goth, A.: Drug safety and effectiveness. In Goth, A.: Medical pharmacology, ed. 10, St. Louis, 1978, The C.V. Mosby Co.

Lawson, D.H.: Detection of drug-induced disease, British Journal of Clinical Pharmacology **7**(1):13, 1979.

Lowry, W.T., and Garriott, J.C.: Forensic toxicology; controlled substances and dangerous drugs, New York, 1979, Plenum Press.

Seligman, J., Hager, M., and Shapiro, D.: Drug test creates a doctor's dilemma, Newsweek, p. 52D, July 14, 1980.

U.S. Department of Justice: Regulations implementing the Comprehensive Drug Abuse Prevention and Control Act of 1970, Federal Register **36**(No. 80): 1, Apr. 24, 1971.

Vogel, A.V., Goodwin, J.S., and Goodwin, J.M.: The therapeutics of placebo, American Family Physician **22**(7):105, 1980.

Wertheimer, A.I.: The placebo effect, Pharmacy International **1:**12, 1980.

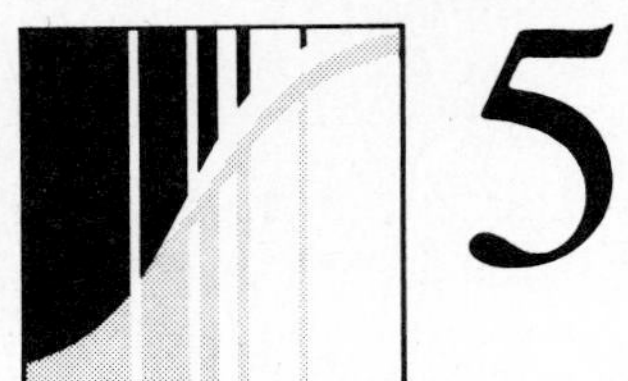

5 Over-the-counter drugs

■ THE LEGISLATIVE ORIGIN OF OVER-THE-COUNTER (OTC) DRUGS

Products intended for the self-medication of a variety of illnesses have been sold in the United States for more than 250 years. Until the early 20th century, there were no restrictions that governed the contents, potency, purity, safety, efficacy, sale, or advertising of these products, which came to be known as "patent medicines." Consequently, some were of marginal safety and most provided no therapeutic benefit. Although most of the patent medicines were essentially harmless as well as ineffective, many contained alcohol, narcotics, or other dangerous drugs in unspecified quantities.

Some element of control of the patent medicine industry was achieved with passage of the first Pure Food and Drug Act of 1906 (Chapter 2). The new law required that product labels accurately list the ingredients of the medicine. Any substance present but not listed was deemed an adulterant. A later amendment to the law, the Sherley Amendment (1912), forbade false and fradulent labelling claims. In 1938, a new Food and Drug Law was enacted that required that all marketed medicinal products be of proven safety; in 1951, the Durham-Humphrey amendment specified two categories of drugs, those safe enough for sale without a prescription (over-the-counter, or OTC), and those deemed sufficiently dangerous to require sale only by prescription.

Present control of OTC drugs stems from the Kefauver-Harris amendment requiring medicinal products to be proven safe and effective and to be tested for teratogenicity. While the proof of efficacy has been limited largely to prescription drugs, OTC products have recently come under scrutiny. Federal Drug Administration OTC Review Panels are continuing to review the various classes of OTC drugs, judging them as follows:

Category I: Recognized as safe and effective for the claimed therapeutic indication
Category II: Not recognized as safe and effective
Category III: Additional data needed to decide safety and/or effectiveness

□ This chapter was contributed by Lynn Roger Willis, Ph.D., Associate Professor of Pharmacology and Medicine, Indiana University School of Medicine.

■ COMMON PROPERTIES OF OTC MEDICATIONS

■ Low doses

A principal concern of today's manufacturers of OTC products is safety. Drug toxicity is dose related, and its risk is reduced when drug dosage is low. Thus most OTC products are provided with low, and sometimes far less than therapeutic, amounts of active ingredient. Such preparations may serve as little more than placebos, especially for such subjective minor complaints as pain, itch, and sleeplessness. For such indications, proof of product efficacy may be difficult, even when adequate drug dosage is provided.

■ Combination of ingredients

Most OTC products contain several drugs. The drugs may be totally different from each other, or they may be of the same or similar classification. When drugs are taken in combination, there is a risk of adverse interactions occurring between two or more of the drugs. Although the risk of interactions occurring with the drugs in a given product may be low, it is not so low when other drugs are taken simultaneously.

OTC medications containing several ingredients are examples of *fixed combination* medications. This term means that the dosages of the various components of the medication are fixed and cannot be altered according to need by the user because the dosage of an ingredient of a combination OTC product cannot be adjusted without altering the dosage of all the other ingredients. For example, if a tablet contains 4 mg of antihistamine and 60 mg of decongestant, a patient who wished to increase the antihistamine dosage would also have to take more of the decongestant, which might not be needed or even safe. On the other hand, many single-entity OTC drugs are available. Examples include analgesic-antipyretics, decongestants, cough suppressants, antihistamines, and antifungal agents. Often single entity drugs can be purchased less expensively than can the advertised combination products, and control of dosage is optimal with a single entity product. By understanding the pharmacology of OTC drugs and the specific requirements of a patient, the nurse can advise a rational product selection.

■ MAJOR CLASSES OF OTC DRUGS

The classes of OTC drugs chosen for discussion in this chapter include cold and cough remedies, weight control products, and sleeping aids; component drugs are discussed in other chapters. This chapter emphasizes the combination of drugs in each type of OTC product and the rationale for OTC combination drugs. Also chosen for discussion are vitamin C, ophthalmic products, acne treatments, topical antiinfectives, and hemorrhoidal products that are not discussed elsewhere in this text. Finally, several classes of OTC drugs are discussed in detail in Chapter 11 and are not included in this chapter: antacids, antidiarrheals, laxatives, and antiemetics. For an exhaustive review of all OTC drugs, the reader is referred to the American Pharmaceutical Association's *Handbook of Nonprescription Drugs*.

■ Cold remedies

Most of the available OTC cold remedies contain one or more of the following classes of drugs: a *sympathomimetic*, an *antihistaminic*, and/or an *analgesic* drug. Some products may also contain *caffeine, ascorbic acid,* and/or *belladonna alkaloids*. A few products are sold singly, but the vast majority are sold as combination products.

Drugs of the sympathomimetic class that are commonly available in OTC products as *decongestants* are *phenylephrine, phenylpropanolamine, ephedrine,* and *pseudoephedrine*. Only phenylephrine, phenylpropanolamine, and pseudoephedrine are efficacious as orally administered decongestants. The pharmacology of these drugs is discussed in Chapter 32.

Phenylephrine hydrochloride (10 mg every 4 hours) can reduce nasal congestion, although its bioavailability is not predictable owing to its rapid hydrolysis in the gastrointestinal tract. Phenylpropanolamine hydrochloride is effective in doses of 25 to 50 mg three times per day. Pseudoephedrine promotes decongestion in doses of 60 mg every 4 hours. Administered systemically, these drugs have a relatively long onset of peak action (3 to 4 hours). They may produce generalized vasoconstriction that ordinarily is not sufficient to elevate blood pressure; nevertheless, hypertension may occur in some individuals.

The rationale for including an antihistamine in a product intended to treat the symptoms of the common cold is questionable. Unless the cold is associated with conditions of increased histamine release such as allergic rhinitis, the blocking action of the drug at the histamine receptor will be of no use. (See chapter 21 for a detailed discussion of antihistamine pharmacology.) Antihistamines also possess some degree of anticholinergic action, which reduces somewhat the production of mucus by the nasal and bronchial mucosa. This action likely provides the principal justification for inclusion of the drugs in OTC cold remedies. Although some "drying" effect may actually occur with antihistamines, their drying efficacy is low, especially at recommended OTC doses. On the other hand, the therapeutic index of antihistamines is relatively high, and there is little risk of serious toxicity in adults. Thus the antihistamines have some potential for producing relief of mild rhinorrhea (runny nose) with little risk, especially those patients who are subject to allergic rhinitis. Aside from the antihistaminic properties, the most dominant action is the production of sedation and drowsiness. Although this action is of no therapeutic value in treating a cold, it does serve as the basis for the inclusion of antihistamines in OTC sleep aids (see section on sleeping aids). Patients seeking relief of rhinitis with an antihistamine may find the drug-induced drowsiness to be highly undesirable and, in some hazardous occupations, dangerous.

The analgesic-antipyretic ingredients most often found in OTC cold remedies are *aspirin, acetaminophen,* and *salicylamide*. Salicylamide is the amide of salicylic acid. It is inferior to aspirin as an analgesic and antipyretic and is no longer listed in the United States Pharmacopeia. It occurs in OTC products in subeffective doses. The therapeutic value of aspirin and acetaminophen in OTC cold remedies lies in their effectiveness for relief of the aches and pains that commonly accompany a cold, since fever in the absence of bacterial infection is rare. However, one need never purchase a cold remedy that contains an analgesic drug. If analgesia is desired, cut-rate (but good quality) aspirin can be obtained at considerable savings. Indeed the complicated pharmacology of aspirin and acetaminophen (Chapter 20) requires that they be administered separately and only as needed.

There is no rationale for the inclusion of *caffeine* or *ascorbic acid* (vitamin C) in OTC cold remedies. In those products that contain caffeine, it is present in doses far below those that produce central nervous system stimulation. If ascorbic acid is to be effective at all, it must be used in doses far in excess of those in the cold remedies and before the onset of a cold to reduce its severity or to prevent it altogether (see section on vitamin C). The *belladonna alkaloids* have marked anticholinergic properties, but are present in generally subeffective doses in the few OTC products that currently contain these agents.

■ Vitamin C

Vitamin C *(ascorbic acid)* is necessary for a number of important biochemical reactions in the body such as synthesis of collagen and adrenal steroids. Collagen provides the supporting framework for tooth, bone, and capillary structures. Vitamin C deficiency manifests itself in several ways, with scurvy and its attendant breakdown of the gums, loss of teeth, and diminished rate of wound healing as the most notable effects.

Ascorbic acid is found in a variety of foods but especially in citrus fruits and vegetables. It is readily absorbed from the intestine, and, when taken in minimum daily amounts (60 mg daily in adults), little ascorbate appears in the urine. Metabolic conversion of ascorbate to oxalate with subsequent urinary excretion occurs in humans. However, when the daily intake of ascorbic acid exceeds 100 mg, and the plasma ascorbate level exceeds 1.5 mg/dl, ascorbate is excreted in the urine.

Some years ago, the Nobel laureate Dr. Linus Pauling proposed that vitamin C might be effective in treating and preventing the common cold. To date, that proposal remains controversial. Proponents of the vitamin C theory assert that, to be effective, large doses (termed *megadoses*) of ascorbic acid must be taken (1 to 5 Gm daily to prevent a cold and as much as 15 Gm daily to treat a cold). A number of investigators have conducted clinical trials of megadose therapy with vitamin C. While none have been totally negative, likewise none have shown unequivocal evidence that the vitamin is effective in altering the severity, occurrence, or duration of the common cold. On the other hand, there are several known disadvantages to megadose therapy with vitamin C. Diarrhea is a common, though not serious, side effect of high-dose ascorbic acid treatment. The precipitation of urate, oxalate, or cystine stones resulting from metabolic conversion of large amounts of ascorbic acid is a dose-related risk, although it is low at doses below 1 Gm per day. Increased urinary excretion of ascorbic acid and resulting acidification of the urine can alter the rate of excretion of other drugs such as amphetamines and salicylates. Finally, one must consider the major financial burden that a person assumes when he begins a prophylactic course of megadose vitamin C therapy. At present, for many patients this negative factor may outweigh the dubious and as yet unsubstantiated benefit of vitamin C in relationship to the common cold.

■ Cough remedies

The cough that may accompany the common cold may be *productive* or *nonproductive*. The productive cough serves to remove phlegm from the lower respiratory tract and, unless it becomes nonproductive and excessive, should not be suppressed. Generally, but not always, colds with accompanying chest congestion will be associated with a productive cough. The dry, "hacking," nonproductive cough can be excessive, discomforting, and, because of local irritation caused by the rapid movement of air, self-perpetuating. Such coughs can safely be suppressed and relieved with available OTC medications. Two classes of antitussive agents can be purchased without a prescription: *expectorants* and *cough suppressants* (antitussives). The detailed pharmacology of these drugs is discussed in Chapter 23.

Expectorants. The use of *expectorants* in clinical medicine is controversial. The generally available expectorants have not been shown to be more effective than placebo, and their place in any aspect of clinical medicine has been criticized. In part, the controversy stems from the lack of objective methods for assessing the efficacy of expectorant drugs. At present, the FDA OTC Panel on Cold, Cough, Allergy, Bronchodilator, and Antiasthmatic Products must rely on subjective evidence in support of these drugs. They have concluded that the available information is insufficient to provide proof of efficacy (category III). The commonly available expectorants are *ammonium chloride* (300 mg every 2 to 4 hrs), *guaifenesin* (200 to 400 mg every 4 hours), *ipecac syrup* (0.5 to 1.0 ml 3 or 4 times a day), and *terpin hydrate* (200 mg every 4 hours). Ammonium chloride, guaifenesin, and ipecac are thought to stimulate the reflex production of bronchial secretion by irritation of the gastric mucosa. In higher dosage, they can produce emesis. Terpin hydrate is believed to directly stimulate secretory glands in the lower respiratory tract. Recommended dosages for ammonium chloride, guaifenesin, and terpin hydrate in children from 6 to 12 years of age are ½ the adult dosage, and ¼ the adult dosage for children from 2 to 6 years of age. Ipecac syrup is not recommended for children younger than 6 years.

Cough suppressants (antitussives). The commonly available cough suppressants, *codeine* and *dextromethorphan,* have been designated safe and effective (category I).

Codeine (Chapter 28) is an opium alkaloid and a narcotic. It has a liability for psychological and physical dependence. This liability is less than that for morphine and is virtually nonexistent when the drug is used in recommended dosage for short periods of time (10 to 20 mg every 4 to 6 hours). In excess of recommended dosage, codeine may cause nausea, drowsiness, and constipation. Abuse of codeine-containing OTC cough preparations has been a problem in the United States, and varying restrictions on the OTC sale of such products have been enacted by state legislatures. These restrictions range from limiting the quantity that can be sold to complete prohibition of sale without a prescription.

Dextromethorphan is a nonnarcotic cough suppressant with approximately the same antitussive potency as codeine. Unlike codeine, however, dextromethorphan does not depress respiration or have addiction liability. Side effects caused by recommended doses of dextromethorphan are mild and uncommon, consisting largely of drowsiness and gastrointestinal upset. In doses of 10 to 20 mg every 4 hours, the drug suppresses coughs through direct inhibition of the medullary cough reflex center.

In children 6 to 12 years of age, one half of the recommended adult dose may be given. One quarter of the adult dose is recommended for children between the ages of 2 and 6 years.

Noscapine is an opium alkaloid, which, like codeine, suppresses the cough reflex center in the medulla of the brain. Unlike codeine, however, noscapine has no central nervous system or respiratory depressant action, and is devoid of addiction liability. Noscapine exerts its antitussive effect at doses of 15 to 30 mg every 4 to 6 hours. Only a few of the many OTC antitussive products contain noscapine, but this is more a reflection of the more extensive sales promotion and wider acceptance of codeine and dextromethorphan than of the effectiveness of noscapine.

The incidence of side effects with noscapine use is low. Constipation and gastrointestinal upset have not been widely reported. Although the evidence for the antitussive, nonnarcotic properties of noscapine goes back many years, it is not as convincing as is that for codeine and dextromethorphan. Consequently, the FDA Review Panel has classified noscapine as category III, and awaits additional proof of efficacy, although it allows its OTC sale.

Combination of an expectorant and an antitussive. Some cough suppressant products consist only of the antitussive drug in a flavored base. Others include an expectorant. Either is suitable, although preparations containing only an expectorant in a flavored base are of unproven value. If a cough suppressant and a decongestant are desired, the pharmacologically rational approach would be to purchase two separate products, one for cough suppression and one for decongestion. One or the other (or both) can then be taken to achieve the desired result. More importantly, individual preparations provide optimum control of dosage. In some cases, the nurse may find a patient who will insist on "needing" the full combination of ingredients for cough and cold. The recommended choices should be those that deliver optimal, or nearly optimal, doses of the active ingredients, and contain only essential ingredients.

Other drugs in cough preparations. Many OTC cough preparations, especially liquids, contain a decongestant and an antihistamine in combination with a cough suppressant and/or an expectorant. If the cough is the result of postnasal drip due to rhinitis or allergy, preventing the drip should alleviate the cough, thus eliminating the need for an antitussive drug. On the other hand, if the cough is due to irritation, low humidity, or "smoker's cough," a decongestant and/or antihistamine will be of no value and a cough suppressant alone would be sufficient.

■ Weight control products

Obesity is most frequently defined as a body weight more than 20% greater than the ideal body weight. Obesity is a complex problem that requires complex treatment. Drug treatment of obesity is of limited value at best. Amphetamines (Chapter 27) have been prescribed for weight control for a number of years. Amphetamine and related drugs suppress appetite via a central mechanism, but the appetite remains suppressed only as long as sufficient levels of the drug are present in the brain. Unless the overweight person willfully resists the temptation to overeat when hungry, the amphetamines will be of no value. Moreover, tolerance develops to the anorectic action of the amphetamines, and they may produce dependence. They are not available without prescription.

The OTC armamentarium for the treatment of obesity and weight control consists of *phenylpropanolamine, bulk-producing agents,* and *benzocaine*. Weight loss will occur if caloric utilization exceeds intake. No available product will enhance the rate at which calories are expended. The OTC products can only serve to reduce caloric intake. To that end, it matters little if a dietary aid possesses true pharmacological activity; a placebo can be totally effective in some persons if, while taking the medication, they consume fewer calories.

Phenylpropanolamine, discussed as an OTC nasal decongestant, is structurally related to ephedrine and amphetamine and is used in OTC weight control products. It is an indirect acting sympathomimetic drug (Chapters 8 and 27). Phenylpropanolamine differs from amphetamine principally in having lower central nervous system potency than does amphetamine. Amphetamine-like appetite suppression requires an action in the central nervous system; thus phenylpropanolamine does enter the brain, but milligram for milligram, its central effects are less. The drug is clearly effective as an appetite suppressant in experimental animals, but its effect in human subjects is controversial. As a result, not all authorities recognize its usefulness as a weight control drug. Nevertheless, an FDA advisory panel has classified the drug as safe and effective (category I) for aid in diet control when used for up to about 12 weeks as an adjunct in weight reduction.

The effects of phenylpropanolamine on the cardiovascular system and the central nervous system are less than those of the amphetamines, but amphetamine-like side effects can occur, especially if recommended dosages are exceeded (Chapter 27). The label on products containing phenylpropanolamine warns against an intake exceeding 75 mg per day, although the FDA considers a dose of 25 to 30 mg every 4 hours, not to exceed 150 mg per day, to be safe.

Common side effects of phenylpropanolamine include nervousness, insomnia, restlessness, headache, nausea, and hypertension. Because phenylpropanolamine is an alpha adrenergic agonist and may elevate blood glucose concentration and produce tachycardia, persons with diabetes mellitus, heart disease, hypertension, or thyroid disease should not take the medication unless on the advice of a physician. Persons taking phenylpropanolamine should know of its potential for interaction with other adrenergic drugs (Chapter 8).

Amphetamines are widely known as "diet pills" and are abused as "pep pills." Unscrupulous producers and advertisers have capitalized on this level of public awareness by promoting phenylpropanolamine as an "energy booster" or the "strongest diet medication available without prescription," and by linking product nomenclature to established trade names for amphetamines. In recommending a dietary aid containing phenylpropanolamine, the nurse should emphasize the importance of the desired short-term drug therapy with phenylpropanolamine, and the fact that the drug will be useless as a weight reduction aid if caloric intake is not permanently reduced.

A variety of bulk-producers are sold as aids to weight reduction. The rationale behind their use stems from the tendency, when taken with one or two glasses of water, to expand and swell in the stomach, thereby producing a feeling of fullness and suppression of appetite. Examples of OTC bulk producers are *methylcellulose, carboxmethylcellulose, agar, psyllium hydrophilic mucilloid,* and *karaya gum*. The problem with these agents is that the swollen bulk spends little time in the stomach, moving rapidly into the intestine. There is stimulates peristalsis and exerts a laxative effect. Indeed, some bulk-producers are also marketed as laxatives and stool softeners (Chapter 11). From a pharmacological standpoint, bulk-producers are probably no more effective at suppressing appetite and caloric intake than is drinking 2 or 3 glassfuls of water before each meal. Nevertheless, the FDA has approved bulk producers for dietary use.

Several OTC weight control products incorporate the local anesthetic drug *benzocaine* into their formulations. The products are intended either for internal administration or for local application (i.e., chewing gum) to the lips and mucous membranes. Presumably, benzocaine exerts a local anesthetic effect on the gastric mucosa to suppress appetite, but there is no evidence to support this possibility. Similarly, studies of the value of producing local anesthesia in the mouth as an aid to diet suppression are inconclusive.

In selecting or recommending an OTC weight control product, the importance of a diet plan, preferably supervised by a family member, friend, nurse, or physician, cannot be too strongly emphasized. The OTC products will not themselves produce weight loss. Caloric intake must be reduced, and the success of a weight loss program will depend on the maintenance of diminished caloric intake.

■ Sleeping aids

From time to time, insomnia in one form or another disrupts the restful nights of nearly everyone. Some persons may find it difficult to fall asleep, others may awake in the middle of the night and be unable to go back to sleep. The cause of sleep difficulties may be physiological or psychological. In most cases sleep difficulties are temporary. A wide variety of common remedies for sleeplessness exist, including warm soaking baths, a dull book, or a glass of warm milk or wine. In severe cases of insomnia, the assistance of a physician may be sought who may prescribe one of several powerful sedative-hypnotic drugs (Chapter 24). Many people fear the addictive properties of these drugs, but find little or no relief from simple home remedies. Between these extremes lies the OTC sleep aid. The FDA has greatly simplified the job of selecting such a product by severely restricting the number of drugs that may be sold as sleeping aids without a prescription. Since 1979, OTC sleep aids must consist of an antihistamine alone or in combination with analgesic drugs (aspirin and/or acetaminophen). Earlier preparations contained bromides, scopolamine, vitamins, and/or combinations of antihistamines, but recent FDA Review Panels have ruled the bromides and scopolamine unsafe at therapeutic doses and vitamins and antihistamine combinations as irrational.

The rationale for inclusion of an antihistamine in OTC sleep preparations stems from their tendency to promote drowsiness. This tendency, plus their wide margin of safety, lends credence to marketing claims for their use in the short-term treatment of insomnia. Some sleeping aids contain analgesic drugs as well, on the basis that mild nighttime pain may be the cause of the sleeplessness. Clinical comparisons of antihistamines with placebo in sleep laboratories have tended to support the notion that they may be effective; nevertheless, some authorities remain doubtful. *Pyrilamine maleate* (25 to 50 mg at bedtime) and *doxylamine succinate* (25 mg at bedtime) are the only presently approved antihistamines in OTC sleeping aid products.

Product selection in this category of drugs is relatively simple owing to the limited number of available active ingredients. Of perhaps more importance from the nursing standpoint is assessment of the cause of the sleeplessness and the actual need for a sleeping aid. If mild pain is keeping someone awake, relief of the pain with aspirin or acetaminophen will often be sufficient to allow sleep to occur. If anxiety is the cause, antihistamine-induced drowsiness may be helpful, but it also may be no more effective than a glass of warm milk or a warm bath, although more expensive. Wise nursing counsel may be the most effective remedy for mildly insomniac patients.

■ Ophthalmic products

OTC ophthalmic products are intended only for the symptomatic relief of mild, self-limiting conditions such as "eye fatigue," tearing, "redness," itching, or stinging associated with allergic or chemical conjunctivitis. Conditions associated with marked eye pain or blurred vision require attention by a physician. Selection and use of an OTC ophthalmic preparation should be guided by several factors. The available products are effective for the designated applications; however, they are designed solely for symptomatic relief and short-term use, usually not to exceed 48 hours. Decongestant products constrict blood vessels in "bloodshot" eyes, but the extent to which that action provides more than cosmetic effects has not been clearly established. Simple, inexpensive eye washes may provide the same relief from itching or stinging eyes as do the more expensive decongestant preparations.

OTC ophthalmic products must be initially sterile and must contain preservatives to maintain sterility. They must be clear solutions that contain no agents for color or odor, and they should have a tonicity and pH approximating that of natural tears. OTC ophthalmic products are sold as *eye washes, artificial tears, or decongestants*. *Eye washes* are merely sterile, isotonic buffer solutions. *Artificial tears* have a viscosity-increasing agent added to the buffer solution, and *decongestant* products contain a vasoconstrictor drug in buffer solution, with or without a viscosity-increasing agent. All ophthalmic preparations carry the risk of becoming contaminated, and thereby transferring the contamination to the eye. Thus cloudy or discolored solutions should be discarded. All products carry an expiration date for the unopened package and a warning on the label that they should be discarded within 3 months of the date of opening.

Nonmedicinal ingredients. OTC ophthalmic products contain a variety of nonmedicinal ingredients, all of which have been reviewed by the FDA OTC Panel on Ophthalmic Drugs. *Tonicity adjusters* (dextran, glycerin and others) are added to render the solutions isotonic or nearly so. Adjustment of tonicity prevents excessive tearing and subsequent dilution and washout of active ingredients. *Antioxidants* and *stabilizers* such as edetic acid (0.01% to 0.1%), sodium bisulfite or metabisulfite (0.1%), or thiourea (0.1%) prevent the chemical alteration of the product and its active ingredient. *Buffers* (boric acid, potassium bicarbonate, sodium acetate, and others) maintain product pH within a range of 6.0 to 8.0. Products with a pH outside this range may be irritating. *Wetting agents* (such as Polysorbate 80, [1.0%] or poloxamer 282 [0.025%]) reduce surface tension. *Preservatives* are added to prevent bacterial growth. Benzalkonium chloride (0.013%), benzethonium chloride (0.010%), chlorobutanol (0.5%) edetic acid with benzalkonium chloride (0.1% to 0.01%), phenylmercuric nitrate (0.004%), and thimerosal (0.01%) have all been classified as safe and effective (category I) preservatives by the FDA. *Viscosity-increasing agents* such as gelatin (1%), glycerin, lanolin, or polyethylene glycol are used to increase the tendency of the ophthalmic liquid to spread over the eye.

Decongestants (vasoconstrictors). The principal medicinal agent contained in OTC ophthalmic preparations intended as a decongestant is a vasoconstrictor drug. Drugs that are used for this purpose include *ephedrine hydrochloride* (0.12%), *naphazoline hydrochloride* (0.03%), *phenylephrine* (0.08% to 0.2%), and *tetrahydrozoline* (0.05% to 0.1%). These drugs are also found in nasal decongestants (Chapter 23). All have been classified as safe and effective for use (category I) by the FDA Panel. Local application of one of those drugs to the eye promptly relieves the symptoms of allergic conjunctivitis. The drugs constrict dilated blood vessels, thereby relieving the "bloodshot" appearance and returning the normal color to the whites of the eyes. These drugs can also stimulate the receptors affecting pupillary size, causing mydriasis. For this reason they are contraindicated in narrow-angle glaucoma.

Although effective in controlling redness of the eyes, the OTC ophthalmic decongestant products are intended only for occasional use and for purely cosmetic purposes.

Ephedrine provides the shortest duration of action, and naphazoline and tetrahydrozoline the longest. Phenylephrine is the most commonly used decongestant in the OTC preparations, but owing to its instability in solution, it is the most variable in effectiveness.

Several problems can occur in association with the use of ophthalmic decongestant preparations. Rebound congestion may occur after prolonged use of the drugs. It is manifest as a return of the original symptoms, only more intensely; if the preparation is used to treat the renewed symptoms, it results in a worsening and self-perpetuating condition. In addition, the products are ineffective if the symptoms are the result of a problem occurring within the eyeball itself, and, in the case of bacterial infection, the product may mask its presence.

Antipruritics and astringents. Other medicinal agents that are found in some decongestant and other OTC ophthalmic preparations include antipruritics such as *antipyrine* (0.01% to 0.14%), *camphor, menthol,* and astringents (*zinc sulfate,* 0.25%). Antipruritics produce mild local anesthesia and a cooling sensation. They are considered unsafe because they can mask the presence of foreign, abrasive substances in the eye that can damage the cornea. Zinc sulfate is the only acceptable astringent in ophthalmic preparations.

■ Acne treatments

Acne vulgaris is the curse of adolescence, a time when individuals are highly sensitive to alterations of their physical appearance and to peer influences. For this age-group, the prevention and treatment of even mild cases of acne assume a high priority. Virtually everyone has experienced an attack of acne at some time in their life, most often during adolescence, but the disease can occur in adults. In most cases the disease is not serious, although severe cases can produce scarring of the face, back, and chest.

Origin of acne. The pimples and skin eruptions of acne are termed *comedones*. They consist of a mixture of sebum that is produced by the sebaceous glands of the hair follicles and epithelial cells shed from the infundibulum of the follicle. In acne, excessive sebum production occurs. In adolescents, increased sebum production has been attributed to elevated androgen levels as puberty approaches. The oily sebaceous fluid impairs the normal washout of shed infundibular cells. The cells become compacted and plug the follicle, which then becomes distended with accumulated sebum and cells. The condition is relieved by removal of the plug either by lancing of the comedone or by the natural growth of the hair that brings the plug to the surface of the skin. Scarring can occur with this noninflammatory form of acne, although it is more likely to occur with the inflammatory form of the disease. Inflammatory acne is characterized by pustule formation and local inflammation. It occurs when comedones do not open at the skin surface to relieve the pressure within the hair follicle. An inflamed follicle may rupture beneath the skin surface, thereby spreading sebum, cells, and any bacteria present to surrounding tissues and initiating local inflammation. Whereas noninflammatory acne can be treated with OTC products, cases of inflammatory acne should be directed to a physician for treatment.

Nonmedicinal treatment. The widespread incidence and variable severity of acne has spawned speculation that external factors may contribute to its development. These factors include diet, personal cleanliness, and self-image, and they remain controversial. Certainly personal hygiene is important in combating excessive skin oiliness, but there is no evidence that compulsive and vigorous cleansing of the skin is any more effective in preventing acne than is normal washing. Since bacterial infection is not ordinarily associated with acne, the use of antibacterial soaps and antiseptic solutions is neither necessary nor recommended.

The role of diet in acne is controversial. Chocolate has long been condemned as a causative factor in the development of acne, but evidence of the cause-and-effect relationship is lacking. Similarly, the evidence does not support the presumed need for dietary restriction of other sweets, nuts, and greasy foods. On the other hand, until a clearer understanding of acne and its cause emerges, individual trial-and-error with diet, hygiene, and other factors should certainly not be excluded.

Noninflammatory acne is treated symptomatically. It cannot be cured. Treatment consists of removing excess sebum from the skin by washing, and promoting the production and turnover of new skin to prevent closure of the pilosebaceous orifices of the hair follicles. Washing should involve warm water, mild soap, and a soft washcloth, and the face should be washed no more than three times daily. The washing and rubbing will produce some drying and peeling of the skin. Medicated or abrasive soaps are not necessary. Closure of the pilosebaceous orifices is prevented by the topical application of mildly irritating agents that promote desquamation (peeling). These agents stimulate growth of new skin cells.

Medicinal treatment. The agents that are most widely used to promote desquamation are *sulfur* (2% to 10%), *resorcinol* (1% to 4%), and *salicylic acid* (0.5% to 2%). All three are generally accepted as effective. Resorcinol and salicylic acid often appear in alcoholic solutions. They dry quickly and do not leave a visible film. Some products contain all three desquamating ingredients. Dosage forms of these drugs primarily include creams, lotions, gels, and liquids. Ointment bases tend to be greasy and messy. Some soaps include desquamating agents. Their presence in this formulation is irrational, since they will be removed from the skin by rinsing and drying. (Salicylic acid is also the principle active ingredient of OTC products for the treatment of bunions, calluses, and warts).

Benzoyl peroxide is a stronger irritant and desquamating agent than sulfur, resorcinol, and salicylic acid. It is used in concentrations of 5% to 10% and generally produces sensations of mild stinging and warmth. It is probably no more effective than the milder agents for most acne problems. Benzoyl peroxide is highly irritating. It should not come in contact with the eyelids, neck, or lips, and its use should be discontinued if it produces severe and prolonged stinging or irritation.

OTC products are effective only against noninflammatory acne. Initially only the milder irritants should be utilized in combination with faithful adherence to a regular schedule of skin washing. Only if the milder agents are ineffective should benzoyl peroxide be tried and only then when adequate precautions against its very irritating properties are observed.

■ Topical antiinfectives

Antifungal products

Several common tineal (fungal) infections of the skin generally respond to self-medication with OTC products, although responsiveness is dependent on several factors. These factors include the strain of fungus involved and the site, severity, and duration of the infection. The microorganisms most often causing superficial tinea infections in man include: *Trichophyton, Microsporum, Epidermophyton,* and *Candida*. All but *Candida* can be treated with OTC antifungal products (Chapter 47). Moreover, the products are effective only for superficial, acute infections. Chronic and extensive infections will respond slowly, if at all, and will often require the attention of a physician. Fungal infections of the toenails, fingernails, or those that have penetrated the hair shafts will generally respond poorly to OTC antifungal products. The nurse should exercise care in selecting or recommending OTC antifungal medication. If the condition involves an apparent tinea infection of the foot (athlete's foot), groin (jock itch), or scalp, for example, reasonably rapid results can be expected from OTC products. Suspected fungal infections of other body regions should be referred to a physician.

OTC antifungal products include *keratolytic agents, fungistatic agents,* and *fungicides*.

Keratolytic preparations include *selenium sulfide* and *Whitfield's ointment (benzoic acid,* 6%, and *salicylic acid,* 3%). These agents irritate the skin and cause peeling of the superficial layers, thereby exposing deeper sites of infection to other antifungal compounds. Selenium sulfide stops cellular growth when applied in concentrations of 1% to 2%. It is a common and effective ingredient in antidandruff preparations.

Fungistatic agents include *fatty acids* and *salicylanilide* (5%). *Sodium propionate* and *undecylenic acid* are fungistatic fatty acids. Sodium propionate is effective in solution (1%) and ointment (5%) forms. Undecylenate is effective as the acid (5%) and as the zinc salt (20%). It is commonly employed as an ointment, powder, or spray for the relief of tinea pedis.

The *fungicidal* drug *tolnaftate* is effective against the majority of superficial fungal infections except those caused by *Candida* species. Tolnaftate is sold in powder, liquid, cream, spray, or gel forms (all 1%). Relief of itching occurs within several days, but complete resolution of the infection generally requires 2 to 3 weeks. If the skin is rough and scaly, prior treatment with a keratolytic agent to remove the scale will improve the effectiveness of tolnaftate.

Tinea pedis is probably the most common of fungal infections. For antifungal therapy to be optimally effective, the affected area must be kept clean and dry. In advanced cases, which are characterized by macerated, soggy tissue, appropriate drying or astringent agents (e.g., aluminum chloride compresses) should be used to dry the tissue. Tolnaftate is most effective when used on dry skin.

Antibacterial products

OTC antibacterial preparations have been the subject of controversy and repeated review by the FDA. At present, the antibiotic drugs that are available without a prescription include *bacitracin, neomycin, polymyxin B sulfate, tetracycline hydrochloride, chlortetracycline hydrochloride,* and *oxytetracycline hydrochloride*. The FDA OTC Panel on Antimicrobial Drugs recognizes two classifications of product: skin wound antibiotics and skin wound protectants. The former includes products for the treatment of overt skin infections, and the latter refers to products with antibiotics added to prevent the subsequent infection of a wound and to prevent the growth of organisms in the product. As of 1979, all OTC antibiotics sold as skin wound antibiotics were classified in category III (i.e., insufficient data to enable determination of safety and/or efficacy). All but neomycin sulfate were classified as safe and effective (category I) for use as skin wound protectants. (These antibiotics are discussed in detail in Chapters 43 and 44.)

The OTC topical antibiotics are generally safe when used as directed. However, their low concentration in the available products makes questionable their effectiveness against skin wound infections. Bacitracin, neomycin, and polymyxin B sulfate are nephrotoxic if absorbed systemically. With ordinary topical use, such toxicity is rare. Nevertheless, the risk is real, and, in view of the questionable topical efficacy of the drugs and of their allergenicity, their use is not recommended.

■ Hemorrhoidal products

As the result of environment, heredity, and posture, human beings suffer from a number of painful anorectal disorders, the most prevalent of which is hemorrhoids. Hemorrhoids (varicosities) are caused by increased pressure in the hemorrhoidal veins. In addition to upright posture itself, among the factors that can elevate pressure in the hemorrhoidal veins and lead to the formation of varicosities are hypertension, coughing, pregnancy and labor, physical exertion, straining during defecation, and rectal carcinoma. Hemorrhoids can occur external or internal to the anorectal line and are associated with a variety of symptoms that include itching, burning, inflammation, and swelling. Mild pain and discomfort are common, but bleeding, prolapse of an internal hemorrhoid, and severe chronic pain are symptoms that require the attention of a physician.

OTC products for the treatment of anorectal disorders are intended for the symptomatic relief of pain, itching, and burning. They contain a variety of pharmacological agents including *local anesthetics, vasoconstrictors, antiseptics, astringents, emollients/lubricants, keratolytics, anticholinergics,* and a variety of miscellaneous agents including *counterirritants* and *"wound-healing" agents*. The FDA OTC Review Panel on Hemorrhoidal Drug Products has ruled on the efficacy of these agents in relieving hemorrhoid symptoms. Antiseptics, "wound healers," and anticholinergics have all been classified as ineffective (category II) in hemorrhoidal products, and the purchase of products containing them is not recommended.

Local anesthetics have been judged effective for the relief of the itching and burning of hemorrhoids. Of the many local anesthetics available, only two have been shown to be both safe and effective, *benzocaine* (5% to 20%) and *pramoxine hydrochloride* (1%). Diperodon has been shown to be ineffective, and phenacaine may produce systemic toxicity. Other local anesthetics, including dibucaine, tetracaine, and lidocaine, for example, remain to be proven effective.

The *vasoconstrictor drugs, ephedrine sulfate, epinephrine hydrochloride,* and *phenylephrine hydrochloride,* have been judged effective for the symptomatic relief of hemorrhoidal itching and swelling, although conclusive evidence of effectiveness on swollen hemorrhoidal tissue itself is lacking. Presumably, the vasoconstrictor drugs directly constrict the vascular smooth muscle in the anorectal area.

A variety of *emollients-lubricants (protectants)* have been recommended for use in hemorrhoidal preparations. These include such compounds as *calamine, cocoa butter, cod liver oil, glycerin, mineral oil, petrolatum, shark liver oil,* and *zinc oxide*. All can be administered externally and internally to the rectum except glycerin, which is intended for external use only. Petrolatum may be the most effective of these agents. To be effective, the total protectant concentration of an OTC hemorrhoidal product should be 50%.

Mildly *keratolytic agents* may have some value in relieving the itching and burning of hemorrhoids. *Aluminum chlorhydroxy allantoinate* is one such compound. The usefulness of keratolytic agents is confined to the external anal tissues, but stronger agents such as resorcinal and sulfur are not recommended.

Astringents coagulate skin cell protein, thereby protecting underlying skin cells from dehydration and irritation. *Calamine, zinc oxide,* and *Hamamelis water* (witch hazel) have been judged effective for the relief of hemorrhoidal itching, irritation, and pain. Calamine and zinc oxide may be applied externally and internally to anorectal tissue, whereas hamamelis water is intended for external use.

Antiseptics are considered to be no more effective than washing with soap and water for the prevention of anorectal infections. Indeed, they may adversely alter the normal bacterial flora in that region.

Anticholinergic drugs (e.g., atropine) are of dubious value in OTC hemorrhoidal preparations. The drugs are not absorbed through the skin and, if applied to the external anal tissues, do not relieve itching or pain. Anticholinergic drugs can be absorbed across the rectal mucosa and, in sufficient dosage, can interfere with autonomic nerve function in the gut and elsewhere in the body. There is no evidence, however, that a local or systemic anticholinergic effect is of any value in the treatment of hemorrhoids.

A *counterirritant drug* distracts from the discomfort of itching, irritation, and pain by stimulating local nerve endings to provide a sensation of warmth, tingling, or coolness. Counterirritation is the basis for the OTC products that are available for the relief of minor muscular aches and pains, providing "deep-heating" and "penetrating" warmth. In reality, these "muscle ache" preparations do not directly affect the musculature. Rather their effects are localized to the skin. To be effective in relieving pain, a counterirritant must stimulate local sensory nerve endings. Since no sensory nerves occur in the rectal mucosa, there is no rational basis for including a counterirritant in an internal hemorrhoidal preparation. However, counterirritants can provide temporary relief of pain and itching if applied externally to the anorectal region. At present, *menthol* is the only recommended counterirritant for external hemorrhoidal preparations. Camphor, oil of turpentine, and hydrastis have been included in various products in the past, but they are considered to be either too toxic even for external use or of unproven efficacy against the symptoms of hemorrhoids.

"Wound-healing agents" include an extract of Brewer's yeast, skin respiratory factor (SRF), cod liver oil, vitamins A and D, and others. No convincing evidence of their effectiveness as wound healers has been demonstrated, and, until such evidence emerges, their value is questionable.

Dosage forms. OTC products for the treatment of hemorrhoids and other mild anorectal disorders are pro-

■ THE NURSING PROCESS

Over-the-counter, or nonprescription, drugs will not form a major part of the clinical responsibilities of the practicing nurse. Nevertheless, the nurse is frequently sought as a source of information on these agents. The following presentation is one suggestion for a method of patient counseling about nonprescription medications.

■ Assessment

Since the patient is involved in self-care, the nurse might assist the individual to clearly state what condition or symptoms are to be treated. For example, if the individual is seeking a medication to treat the symptoms of a cold, the nurse might lead that person to consider exactly what symptoms require treatment. For some persons, a cough might be the most outstanding symptom, whereas for others it might be nasal congestion or headache.

■ Management

After leading the patient to define exactly what symptoms are to be treated, the nurse might appropriately teach the patient what types of medications are available to treat these symptoms. The nurse might suggest that fixed combinations of ingredients are more difficult to use, since dosages are impossible to regulate for each component of the combination. More control may be gained by using single agents at appropriate doses as necessary for defined symptoms. The nurse should also suggest other sources of information about nonprescription drugs, one of the most valuable being the pharmacist.

■ Evaluation

Evaluation would be expected to be carried out by the patient involved in self-care. If the patient seeks advice because therapy is unsuccessful, the nurse might lead the patient to consider if the proper medication was administered for the symptom to be controlled and if the right dose was given.

---

vided in a variety of dosage forms. These forms include ointments, creams, suppositories, pads, and foams.

Ointments (oil base), *creams* (water base), and *gels* are equally effective in delivering active ingredients to the affected areas. Devices such as the ''pile pipe,'' a tube with lateral exit ports, are useful for applying the medication directly into the rectum.

Suppositories are not particularly useful for the treatment of hemorrhoids. They may slip beyond the affected site, releasing their active ingredients in contact with healthy mucosa. In addition, the degree of coverage of the affected area may be erratic with suppositories and cannot be controlled. Finally, because they must melt to release their active ingredients, relief of painful symptoms by suppositories is delayed.

Foams provide no advantages over ointments and creams. Moreover, they tend to be unnecessarily messy.

Other hemorrhoidal treatments. Personal hygiene and normal bowel habits are important in the successful treatment of hemorrhoids. Many physicians recommend regular sitz baths or soaks with astringent solutions as an adjunct to the use of OTC products for the relief of mild itching and burning symptoms. In addition, the diet should be adjusted to avoid either excessively loose or excessively compact stools.

■ SUMMARY

Over-the-counter (OTC) medications are medicinal agents deemed safe enough for sale without a prescription. The distinction between prescription and OTC drugs was created by the Durham-Humphrey amendment in 1951. OTC medications are being evaluated by the FDA and assigned to one of three categories:

Category I: Recognized as safe and effective for the claimed therapeutic indication

Category II: Not recognized as safe and effective

Category III: Additional data required to establish safety and/or effectiveness

Many OTC products contain low doses of active ingredients, sometimes less than therapeutic doses. Many OTC drugs contain several ingredients in fixed combination. These combinations increase the risk of drug interactions and prevent the adjustment of dosage of a single component of the medication.

Cold remedies may contain decongestants, antihistamines, analgesics, caffeine, vitamin C, and/or belladonna alkaloids. The decongestants commonly used are sympathomimetics (Chapter 32). Antihistamines are more appropriate for allergic conditions than for colds. Analgesics are often present in cold remedies in doses too low to be effective. Caffeine and vitamin C inclusion has no rational basis. Belladonna alkaloids are not recommended.

Cough remedies are appropriate only for the nonproductive cough associated with colds. Expectorants increase respiratory secretions. Cough suppressants (antitussives) block the cough reflex in the central nervous system. Coughs due to postnasal drip may be treated directly by eliminating rhinitis with a decongestant or allergy with an antihistamine.

Weight control products available without prescription are phenylpropanolamine, bulk-producing agents, and benzocaine. Phenylpropanolamine suppresses appetite by effects on the central nervous system. Tolerance may develop, and the agent is of limited use for short-term control. Bulk-forming agents produce a feeling of fullness and may briefly suppress appetite if taken before meals. Benzocaine is a local anesthetic of unproven effectiveness in weight control.

Sleeping aids contain antihistamines alone or in combination with an analgesic. These drugs may be effective for mild insomnia, since a side effect of antihistamines is drowsiness. Analgesics relieve minor aches and pains that can interfere with sleep.

Ophthalmic products include eye washes, artificial tears, and decongestants. Eye washes are isotonic buffers. Artificial tears have, in addition, a viscosity-increasing agent. Decongestants are intended to reduce the redness in the white of the eye by constricting blood vessels.

Acne medications are primarily intended to promote desquamation (peeling), thereby preventing closure of pilosebaceous orifices. This action decreases the formation of comedones (pimples and inflamed, plugged follicles). Antibacterial or antiseptic agents are not recommended.

Antifungal agents for use against tinea (fungal) infections of the skin include keratolytic agents, fungistatic agents, and fungicides. Keratolytic agents promote peeling and allow infected lower layers of skin to be penetrated by fungistatic or fungicidal medications.

Topical antibiotics have limited usefulness in treating skin wound infections or preventing infections.

Hemorrhoidal products may contain local anesthetics, vasoconstrictors, antiseptics, astringents, emollients-lubricants, keratolytics, anticholinergics, counterirritants, and/or wound-healing agents. Wound-healing agents are ineffective. Antiseptics and anticholinergic agents are not recommended. Local anesthetics can relieve local itching and burning, as can vasoconstrictors, astringents, emollients, and counterirritants.

■ STUDY QUESTIONS

1. The present laws that regulate the OTC drug industry have evolved from which law?
2. The Durham-Humphrey Amendments to the 1938 law created two classes of drugs. What are they?
3. What does the Kefauver-Harris amendment to the 1938 law require?
4. The present-day FDA OTC review panels classify OTC drugs into three distinct categories. List them.
5. List the advantages and disadvantages of fixed-ratio combination OTC products.
6. List the ingredients of OTC cold remedies.
7. What are the major side effects of antihistaminic drugs?
8. List the OTC expectorant drugs.
9. List the available OTC cough suppressants.
10. Which drugs are used in OTC products for the treatment of obesity and for weight control?
11. Phenylpropranolamine is related to which drugs? What are its side effects?
12. What is the rationale for the use of a bulk-producing agent in a weight control product?
13. What drugs are available in OTC sleeping aids?
14. List the medicinal and nonmedicinal ingredients of OTC ophthalmic products.
15. How should OTC ophthalmic products be used?
16. List the commonly available OTC drugs for treatment of acne.
17. OTC antifungal products include which drugs?
18. Distinguish between keratolytic agents, fungistatic agents, and fungicides.
19. Which antibiotics are currently available in OTC preparations?
20. List the ingredients and their actions in OTC hemorrhoidal products.

■ SUGGESTED READINGS

Benowicz, R.J.: Non-prescription drugs and their side effects, New York, 1977, Grosset and Dunlop.

DiCyan, E., and Hessman, L.: Without prescription, New York, 1972, Simon and Schuster.

Handbook of non-prescription drugs, ed. 6, Washington, D.C., 1979, American Pharmaceutical Association.

Physician's desk reference for non-prescription drugs, New York, 1981, Litton Educational Publishing, Inc.

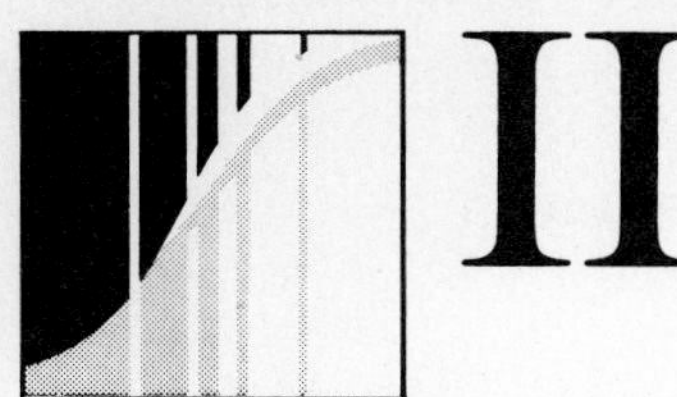

II GENERAL PRINCIPLES OF NEUROPHARMACOLOGY

A separate introductory section on neuropharmacology is unique in pharmacology texts for nursing students. We have chosen this format to introduce the student to key concepts in neuropharmacology and to ask the student to concentrate first on mechanisms and effects before moving to drugs and therapeutics.

The autonomic and motor nervous systems provide the prototypes for our knowledge of neuropharmacology. Chapter 6 reviews these systems and the function and regulation of the neurotransmitters acetylcholine and norepinephrine. Chapter 7 reviews mechanisms of cholinergic drugs, and Chapter 8 reviews mechanisms of adrenergic drugs. The purpose of these latter two chapters is to introduce the student to the spectrum of mechanisms and therapeutic uses for drugs that affect these two neurotransmitters. The student is cautioned not to be concerned initially with actual drugs listed because these drugs, their therapeutic uses, and the implications for nursing are all discussed in detail in the appropriate following chapters. However, the student will find the detailed classification of drugs by mechanism useful as a review later in the course of study.

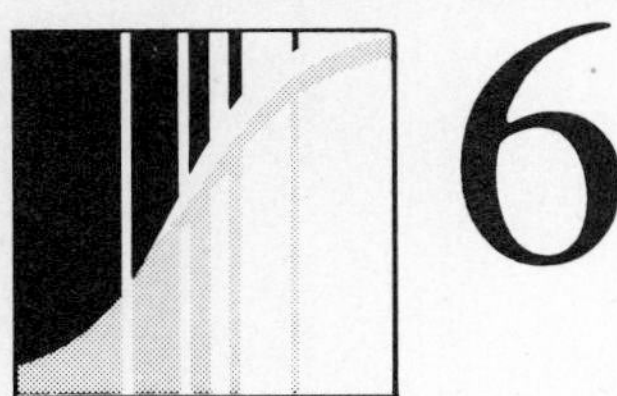

6 Introduction to neuropharmacology

■ OVERVIEW

Many different classes of drugs, used for a variety of therapeutic purposes, affect the nervous system at some level. Some of these drugs are designed to alter the function of some portion of the nervous system, whereas others alter functions of the nervous system as a side effect. A review of the anatomy and biochemical function of the nervous system is necessary to understand the mechanisms of these drugs and the array of side effects they produce. The purpose of this chapter is to present that review.

The central nervous system includes the brain and spinal cord. The functions of these structures are twofold: first, to monitor, convey, and process signals from sensory receptors throughout the body by way of ascending neuronal pathways; and, second, to sequence information and to convey signals to initiate or to modify body actions.

The neurons that relay information from the central nervous system to the rest of the body are called *efferent neurons*. The ascending sensory neurons and the efferent neurons form the *peripheral nervous system*. The peripheral nervous system is subdivided into the *motor nervous system* and the *autonomic nervous system*.

■ NEUROTRANSMITTERS

■ Neurotransmitters and receptors

All neurons use neurotransmitters to contact neurons and other cells. A neurotransmitter is a chemical that is synthesized in the nerve cell and stored inside vesicles (sacs) in the terminal. Most neurons appear to make only one kind of neurotransmitter. When the neuron is stimulated, some of the vesicles merge with the nerve terminal membrane and quantities of neurotransmitter are released. There is a space between the neuron and the cell with which the neuron is communicating. This space is the *synaptic cleft*. The neurotransmitter molecules diffuse across the synapse and occupy specific *receptors* on the next cell. The function of the receptor is to recognize only one specific neurotransmitter and to initiate a cellular response to that neurotransmitter. The binding of the neurotransmitter to its receptor is reversible. When the neurotransmitter diffuses away from the receptor, the stimulation of the cell is terminated.

Two neurotransmitters, acetylcholine and norepinephrine, are used in the peripheral nervous system. A given class of neurons, however, will use only one of these neurotransmitters. The synthesis and degradation of each neurotransmitter will first be discussed. A description of where each neurotransmitter is found in the peripheral nervous system and the responses produced will follow.

■ The neurotransmitter acetylcholine (Fig. 6-1)

Acetylcholine is synthesized in the nerve terminal by the enzyme choline acetylase from choline and an acetate molecule activated by coenzyme A. This acetylcholine is packaged in vesicles. On stimulation of the nerve, some of the vesicles release acetylcholine into the synapse where the acetylcholine diffuses to the opposing membrane and binds at the specific receptors for acetylcholine. In addition, the membrane contains the enzyme acetylcholinesterase, which degrades acetylcholine to acetate and choline. The acetylcholinesterase is very active, and the half-life of the acetylcholine released is only a few milliseconds. Any acetylcholine that diffuses from the synapse into the blood is degraded by nonspecific cholinesterases in the blood or tissues. Thus, when released, acetylcholine produces a response in the next cell by way of the acetylcholine receptor and/or is rapidly degraded by the membrane-bound enzyme acetylcholinesterase or by nonspecific cholinesterases in the blood plasma.

■ The neurotransmitter norepinephrine and the neurohormone epinephrine (Fig. 6-1)

Norepinephrine is synthesized in the nerve terminal from the amino acid tyrosine. Norepinephrine is a neurotransmitter because it is released from a neuron to act on an adjacent cell. The chromaffin cells of the adrenal medulla also synthesize norepinephrine but convert 80% to 85% of the norepinephrine to epinephrine. These adrenal stores of epinephrine and norepinephrine are released into the blood on stimulation of the adrenal medulla in response to stress. Epinephrine is called a neurohormone because it is released into the blood to produce effects at distant sites.

FIG. 6-1

A, Acetylcholine. *(1)* Choline is taken up by the neuron, and *(2)* used to synthesize acetylcholine, which *(3)* is stored in vesicles. On stimulation of the neuron *(4)*, some vesicles merge with the membrane to discharge acetylcholine into the synapse, where acetylcholine diffuses to *(5)* its receptor to activate the cell, or to *(6)* acetylcholinesterase, the enzyme that degrades acetylcholine. Plasma cholinesterases can also degrade acetylcholine.

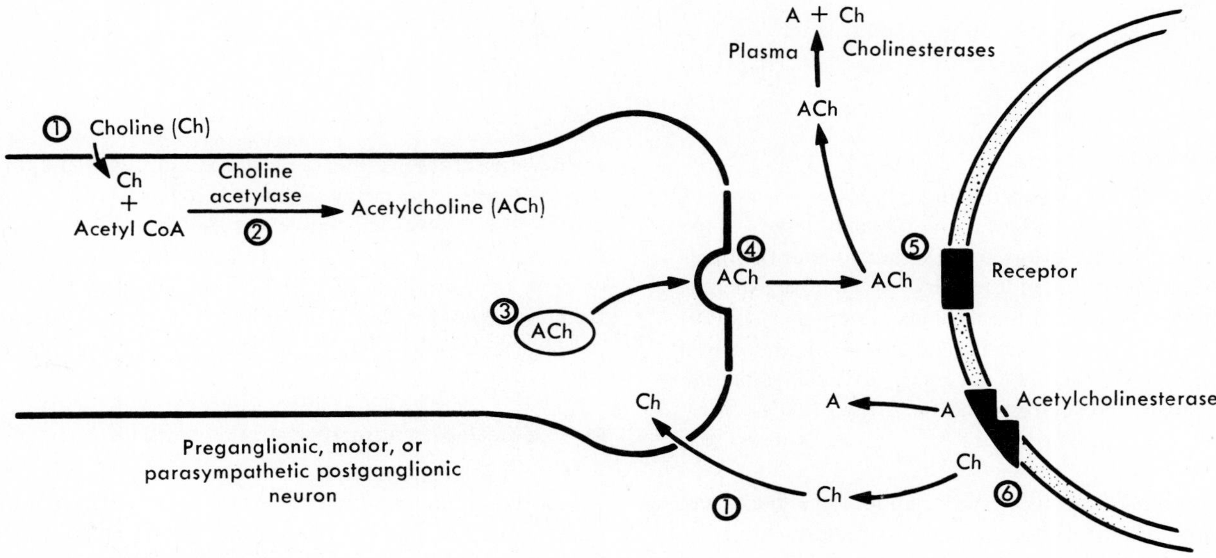

B, Norepinephrine. *(1)* Tyrosine is taken into the neuron and in three reactions is modified to norepinephrine, which is *(2)* stored in vesicles. On stimulation of the neuron *(3)*, some vesicles merge with the membrane to discharge norepinephrine into the synapse, where it diffuses to *(4)* its receptor to activate the cell. Most of the norepinephrine is *(5)* taken up by the neuron and reused. Some norepinephrine is degraded by *(6)* the mitochondrial enzyme monoamine oxidase (MAO) or *(7)* the enzyme catechol-O-methyl transferase (COMT) found in most body tissues.

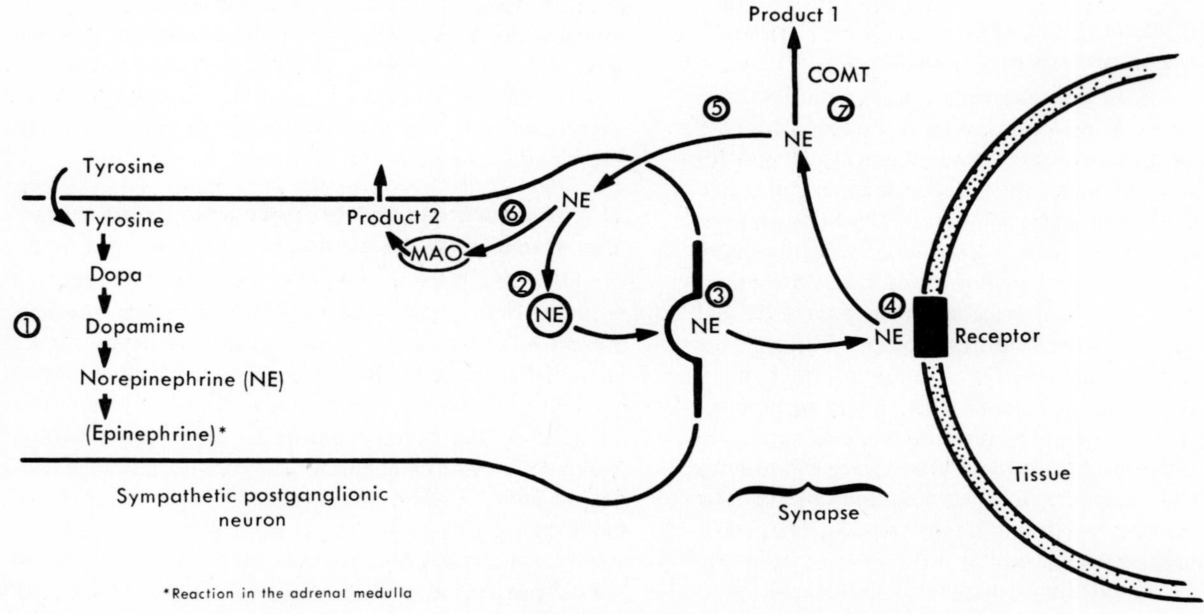

*Reaction in the adrenal medulla

FIG. 6-2

Neurotransmitters of the autonomic nervous system. Sites of release. Acetylcholine and norepinephrine are released from neurons as indicated on adjacent cells. Epinephrine is released from adrenal medulla into blood to act throughout the body.

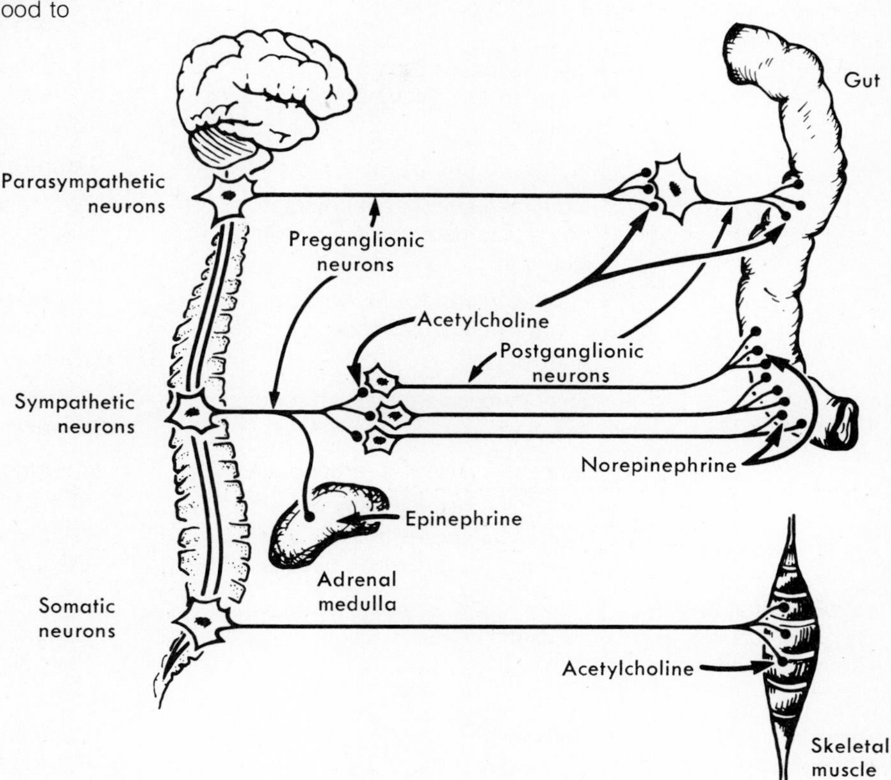

Most norepinephrine is *not* degraded after release. Instead norepinephrine is taken back up into the neuron from which it was released and stored again in granules. This process is called *reuptake*. There are two enzymes that can degrade norepinephrine and epinephrine. Monoamine oxidase (MAO) is located in the mitochondria of most cells, including nerve terminals that release norepinephrine. Catechol-O-methyltransferase (COMT) is found in the cytoplasm of most cells. Both MAO and COMT are found in large concentrations in the liver and kidney. Any norepinephrine that diffuses into the blood or any epinephrine in the blood is quickly degraded by the liver and/or kidney. No drugs are used that interfere with COMT, but in later chapters we shall see that drugs which inhibit MAO are used as antidepressant drugs, as an antihypertensive drug, and in the treatment of parkinsonism.

The main features of the peripheral nervous system and its neurotransmitters acetylcholine and norepinephrine will be reviewed as a preparation for discussing drugs that act by modifying neurotransmitter action within the peripheral nervous system. We shall start first with the motor nervous system, and then discuss the more complex autonomic nervous system.

■ MOTOR (SOMATIC) NERVOUS SYSTEM (Fig. 6-2)

The motor or somatic nervous system is under both conscious and unconscious control to initiate muscle contraction. A motor neuron has a cell body in the spinal cord and contacts a striated muscle at a specialized region, the neuromuscular junction. Motor neurons are found in several cranial nerves and in all spinal nerves. Stimulation of a motor neuron releases acetylcholine at the neuromuscular junction, and the muscle cell reacts to acetylcholine by contracting. Stimulation of a motor neuron may arise as a result of a willed impulse originating in the brain and transmitted to the appropriate neuron in the spinal cord or, unconsciously, as a reflex. A reflex is initiated by sensory input (i.e., heat, touch, pressure, pain), which is transmitted to the spinal cord, then out to the motor neurons without processing by the brain.

■ AUTONOMIC NERVOUS SYSTEM (Fig. 6-2)

■ Divisions of the autonomic nervous system

The role of the autonomic nervous system is to monitor and to control internal body functions such as

TABLE 6-1. Actions of the autonomic nervous system

Tissue	Sympathetic (adrenergic) response	Parasympathetic (cholinergic or muscarinic) response
Eye	Dilation (mydriasis)	Constriction (miosis) Accommodation (focus on near objects)
Glands	Increased sweating* Increased salivation (thick, contains proteins)	Increased salivation (copious, watery) Increased tears and secretions of respiratory and gastrointestinal tract
Heart	Increased rate (positive chronotropy)	Decreased rate (negative chronotropy)
	Increased strength of contraction (increased contractility or positive inotropy)	Decreased strength of contraction (negative inotropy)
	Increased conduction velocity through the atrioventricular node (positive dromotropy)	Decreased conduction velocity through the atrioventricular node (negative dromotropy)
Bronchioles	Smooth muscle relaxation (opens airways)	Smooth muscle constriction (restricts airways)
Blood vessels	Dilates vessels in heart and skeletal muscle	Constricts vessels in heart (not a prominent effect in humans)
	Constricts vessels in skin, viscera, salivary gland, erectile tissues, kidney	Dilates vessels in salivary gland and erectile tissues
Gastrointestinal tract		
Smooth muscle	Relaxation	Contraction
Sphincters	Contraction	Relaxation
Urinary bladder		
Fundus	Relaxation	Contraction
Trigone and sphincter	Contraction	Relaxation
Uterus	Contraction	
Liver	Glycogenolysis	

*Acetylcholine is the neurotransmitter for this sympathetic response. This is the exception to the rule that norepinephrine is the postganglionic neurotransmitter.

cardiac output, blood volume, blood composition, blood pressure, and digestive processes, primarily by modifying the tone of tissue smooth muscle and the quantity of tissue secretions. The autonomic nervous system has two distinct efferent divisions, the *parasympathetic (cholinergic) nervous system* and the *sympathetic (adrenergic) nervous system*. Both divisions commonly act on a given organ, but produce opposite responses. This is highlighted in Table 6-1, in which the prominent effects of the two divisions on key tissues are summarized. For example, the parasympathetic division slows the heart rate, whereas the sympathetic division increases the heart rate. This *dual antagonistic innervation* is a hallmark of the autonomic nervous system, allowing full control of organ function according to bodily requirements. This antagonism is a result of two distinct kinds of receptors, adrenergic receptors and cholinergic receptors, coexisting on the same organ. Activation of the cholinergic receptor, in general, produces the opposite cellular response from activation of the adrenergic receptor.

■ Autonomic tone

The concept of autonomic tone is also important. Although a minimal but constant release of each neurotransmitter affects each tissue, one branch of the autonomic nervous system is dominant and sets the tone of that tissue to coordinate with other tissues. The sympathetic nervous system provides the dominant tone for the cardiovascular system, so that the magnitude of cardiac and blood pressure responses reflects predominantly the degree of sympathetic tone, which is itself determined and coordinated within the central nervous system. Parasympathetic control of the cardiovascular system is primarily that of a reflex decelerator system to protect against rapid rises in cardiovascular function. On the other hand, parasympathetic tone is coordinated within certain brain centers to dominate visual, digestive, and eliminatory functions and to determine the intensity of these responses. The role of the sympathetic nervous system is primarily that of an override system to depress these functions in times of stress.

■ Preganglionic and postganglionic neurons

Each efferent division of the autonomic nervous system is a two-neuron system. The first neuron *(preganglionic neuron)* has its cell body in the brain stem or spinal cord and terminates outside the spinal cord in a special nervous tissue, a ganglion (Fig. 6-2). The first neuron sends a projection out of the spinal cord *(preganglionic fiber),* which contacts a second neuron *(postganglionic neuron)* within the ganglion. The neurotransmitter for the synapse in the ganglion is acetylcholine. The second neuron has its cell body in a ganglion and by means of a *postganglionic fiber* innervates an internal organ, usually modifying the action of involuntary muscle such as smooth muscle or cardiac muscle.

■ Role of acetylcholine, norepinephrine, and epinephrine

The most important pharmacological difference between the parasympathetic and sympathetic nervous system is that the final postganglionic transmitter is different for the two divisions. The preganglionic neurotransmitter at the synapses within the ganglia for both divisions is acetylcholine. However, the parasympathetic nervous system also uses acetylcholine as a postganglionic neurotransmitter. It is for this reason that the parasympathetic nervous system is often called the *cholinergic nervous system*. The sympathetic nervous system uses norepinephrine as the postganglionic transmitter. The sympathetic nervous system has another component, the neurohormone epinephrine. Epinephrine is released from the adrenal medulla as a reaction to stress. The adrenal medulla acts like a postganglionic neuron because it is innervated by a preganglionic fiber and on stimulation releases epinephrine. Epinephrine is carried by the blood throughout the body where epinephrine not only activates tissue receptors for norepinephrine but also activates additional receptors more specific for epinephrine itself as well. The synonym for the sympathetic nervous system is the *adrenergic nervous system*. The term *adrenergic* comes from the British word for epinephrine, *adrenaline*. (Norepinephrine is called noradrenaline.) The identity of the neurotransmitter at the various sites of the peripheral nervous system is diagrammed in Fig. 6-2.

■ Functional and anatomical characteristics of the autonomic nervous system

Functional characteristics. Certain characteristics readily distinguish the parasympathetic and sympathetic nervous systems functionally. These characteristic functions are listed in Table 6-1. The parasympathetic nervous system has dominant control over "regulatory" processes of the body, whereas the sympathetic nervous system provides immediate adaptation for "fight or flight." Indeed, the easiest way to remember the actions of the sympathetic nervous system (and by contrast the parasympathetic nervous system) is to review the "fight or flight" adaptations: the eyes dilate so that vision is improved even in dim light, the bronchioles dilate to let air flow to and from the lungs more readily, the heart beats faster and with greater strength to get blood to muscle, the visceral blood vessels are constricted but muscle blood vessels are dilated so that the increased blood flow can meet demands of cardiac and skeletal muscle for oxygen and nutrients, digestive and excretory processes are slowed, and the liver breaks down stored glycogen to provide glucose for fuel. All of these actions represent actions of the sympathetic nervous system.

Anatomical characteristics. The parasympathetic and the sympathetic nervous system also differ in their anatomy. The postganglionic neurons of the two systems derive from distinct areas of the spinal cord. The efferent neurons for part of the parasympathetic nervous system arise in the lower area of the brain. These parasympathetic cell bodies include the respiratory and circulatory centers of the medulla, which control cardiovascular and gastrointestinal processes. The remainder of the preganglionic neurons of the parasympathetic nervous system arise from the sacral portion of the spinal cord and allow parasympathetic control of digestive, excretory, and reproductive processes. In contrast, the preganglionic neurons of the sympathetic nervous system all arise in the thoracic and lumbar regions of the spinal cord. Also the number of postganglionic to preganglionic neurons is highly characteristic of each division. In the parasympathetic nervous system each preganglionic neuron contacts one or two postganglionic neurons so that there is discrete neuronal control over organ function. In contrast, the sympathetic nervous system may have 20 or more postganglionic neurons in contact with each preganglionic neuron so that the action on stimulation of preganglionic neurons is diffuse, in keeping with the "alarm" nature of the sympathetic nervous system.

■ COMMENTS ON THE CENTRAL NERVOUS SYSTEM

The brain and spinal cord are more complex in their neuronal organization than is the peripheral nervous system. This is because information must be processed rather than just transmitted. This processing is accomplished in two ways. First, a given neuron may send out many axonal projections and thereby form synaptic junctions with many different neurons. This serves to send a flow of information to several areas for further processing. Second, a given neuron can receive information from more than one neuron. Thus dendrites from a given neuron may have synaptic junctions with axons from many neurons. This serves to collect information from different sources.

■ Neurotransmitters of the central nervous system

An important difference between the central nervous system and the peripheral nervous system is the number of neurotransmitters believed to exist. In addition to acetylcholine and norepinephrine, the probable central neurotransmitters that will be encountered in discussing central nervous system pharmacology in later chapters include dopamine, serotonin, epinephrine, histamine, gamma aminobutyric acid (GABA), glycine, and enkephalins. Some neurotransmitters, in particular GABA and glycine, are inhibitory rather than excitatory. The neuronal response to these neurotransmitters is to develop a more negative resting potential with a decreased likelihood of firing rather than to depolarize more readily and fire.

■ Correlations of function with neurotransmitters in the central nervous system

In the past few years, nerve tracts have been described in the brain and characterized by their neurotransmitter content. These nerve tracts have cell bodies in different areas of the brain to collect information, but the neurons will then converge and form synaptic junctions with many neurons in other regions of the brain. Through surgery or chemical destruction of specific nerve tracts it has been possible to associate control of mental and motor behavior with some of the nerve tracts and their neurotransmitters. Examples include a role for acetylcholine and dopamine in the central coordination of muscle movement (Chapter 32, Central motor control: drugs for parkinsonism and centrally acting skeletal muscle relaxants), a role for dopamine in psychosis (Chapter 25, Antipsychotic drugs), a role for dopamine and serotonin in depression (Chapter 26, Antidepressant drugs), and the role of enkephalins in analgesia (Chapter 28, Narcotic analgesics [opioids]). A current goal in neuropharmacology is to identify how drugs modify behavior through their modification of neurotransmitter synthesis, storage, release, action, and inactivation.

■ SUMMARY

The actions of the nervous system depend on the release of neurotransmitters to act on specific receptors of the next cell. In the peripheral nervous system the preganglionic neurons of both the sympathetic and parasympathetic nervous system release acetylcholine. Motor neurons also release acetylcholine to stimulate skeletal muscle. The identity of the neurotransmitter differs in the postganglionic neurons: acetylcholine is the neurotransmitter of the parasympathetic or cholinergic nervous system, and norepinephrine is the neurotransmitter of the sympathetic or adrenergic nervous system. In reaction to stress, epinephrine is released by the adrenal medulla to augment and expand the role of the sympathetic nervous system, producing the "fight or flight" adaptations of the body organs.

Body tissues contain distinct receptors for acetylcholine and for norepinephrine. The two neurotransmitters produce opposite tissue responses, and the relative activity of a tissue is controlled by the degree of sympathetic versus parasympathetic activity. The following chapters discuss mechanisms by which drugs either mimic or inhibit the action of the neurotransmitters acetylcholine and norepinephrine. Emphasis will be placed on the receptor populations on which drugs act. This chapter has discussed how each neurotransmitter can potentially act at many tissues. Relatively specific actions, for example, stimulation of the bladder or heart, may be achieved by appropriate doses of selected drugs. However, because it is usually difficult to administer the drug to a single tissue, many predictable side effects are seen resulting from actions in other tissues.

■ STUDY QUESTIONS

1. What are neurotransmitters?
2. Describe the synthesis, storage, release, and termination of action of acetylcholine and norepinephrine.
3. What are the two divisions of the autonomic nervous system? How are they involved in dual antagonistic innervation and in determining autonomic tone?
4. Describe the neurons of the autonomic nervous system and of the motor nervous system with respect to anatomy and identity of the neurotransmitter used.
5. Describe the "flight or fight" adaptations of the sympathetic nervous system.

■ SUGGESTED READINGS

Axelrod, J.: Neurotransmitters, Scientific American **230:**59, 1974.

Cooper, J.R., Bloom, F.E., and Roth, R.H.: The biochemical basis of neuropharmacology, ed. 3, New York, 1978, Oxford University Press, Inc.

De Robertis, E.: Molecular biology of synaptic receptors, Science **171:**963, 1971.

Hall, Z.W.: Release of neurotransmitters and their interaction with receptors, Annual Reviews of Biochemistry **41:**925, 1972.

Kolata, G.B.: New drugs and the brain, Science **205:**774, 1979.

Langer, S.Z.: Presynaptic receptors and their role in the regulation of transmitter release, British Journal of Pharmacology **60:**481, 1977.

7 Mechanisms of cholinergic control

This chapter is intended to be read at two different times during a course in pharmacology. The beginning student should read the chapter for the mechanisms and therapeutic applications and should not be overly concerned with the drugs given as examples. Later in a course in pharmacology, the student can return to this chapter to review the drugs learned by their mechanism of action. The exception is the drug atropine, which is presented in detail in this chapter but not elsewhere.

■ POPULATIONS OF CHOLINERGIC RECEPTORS AS DEFINED BY DRUG ACTION

In the preceding chapter, three distinct populations of receptors for acetylcholine in the peripheral nervous system were presented: receptors on striated muscle at the neuromuscular junction, receptors on postganglionic neurons within the ganglia, and receptors on other innervated tissues.

■ Muscarinic receptors

This distinction among acetylcholine receptors is not just anatomical. Chemical differentiation is made with muscarine, a chemical found in certain mushrooms, which mimics the effects of acetylcholine by slowing the heart rate or stimulating smooth muscle when applied to those tissues. Muscarine produces no effect when applied to skeletal muscles or to ganglia. Muscarine only mimics acetylcholine at the postganglionic receptors. The parasympathetic postganglionic receptors are therefore called *muscarinic* receptors.

Muscarine is a laboratory tool and is encountered clinically only as the agent responsible for acute mushroom poisoning. (There is another kind of mushroom poisoning in which symptoms take several hours to appear.) The symptoms of acute mushroom poisoning appear within an hour or so of ingestion and consist of generalized parasympathetic overstimulation that includes glandular stimulation (sweating, tearing, salivation), an overactive gastrointestinal system (nausea, cramps, diarrhea), cardiovascular symptoms (flushed skin and slow heart rate), constricted pupils, and excessive urination.

■ Nicotinic receptors

Nicotine, found in tobacco, is the laboratory agent that mimics the effects of acetylcholine at the skeletal muscle and ganglionic receptors. Therefore the "nicotinic" receptors are the ganglionic and neuromuscular receptors for acetylcholine.

■ DIRECT- AND INDIRECT-ACTING CHOLINOMIMETIC DRUGS

Drugs that mimic the action of acetylcholine act by one of two mechanisms: *directly,* by mimicking acetylcholine (these drugs are chemically related to acetylcholine) or *indirectly,* by inhibiting acetylcholinesterase (these drugs allow acetylcholine to remain intact longer because its degradation is inhibited).

Acetylcholine itself is not commonly used as a therapeutic agent because it produces too many responses and because it is too rapidly degraded in the blood. Rarely, acetylcholine is used topically in eye surgery. Carbachol (Carbacel) and pilocarpine (Pilocar) are examples of direct-acting cholinomimetic drugs used principally in ophthalmology. Bethanechol (Urecholine) is the only direct-acting cholinomimetic drug used systemically.

■ Reversible and irreversible acetylcholinesterase inhibitors

The acetylcholinesterase inhibitors can be subdivided into the reversible inhibitors and the irreversible inhibitors. The reversible inhibitors, as the name implies, bind to the enzyme reversibly, and therefore the drug effect wears off as the drug is eliminated from the body, usually in a few hours. Examples of reversible inhibitors of acetylcholinesterase include physostigmine (Eserine), pyridostigmine (Mestinon), and neostigmine (Prostigmin).

The irreversible inhibitors form a permanent covalent bond with acetylcholinesterase, and the enzyme must be completely replaced before the drug effect wears off, a process requiring days to weeks. The most common examples of irreversible acetylcholinesterase inhibitors are the organophosphate compounds, which include potent

TABLE 7-1. Receptor selectivity of cholinomimetic drugs at therapeutic doses

Generic and trade names	Muscarinic receptor*	Nicotinic† (neuromuscular) receptor	Therapeutic uses
DIRECT-ACTING			
Bethanechol (Urecholine)	+	0	To stimulate an atonic bladder or intestine
Carbachol (Carbacel and others)	+ [topical]		Miotic (constricts pupil)
Pilocarpine (Pilocar and others)	+ [topical] + [topical]		Miotic (constricts pupil)
INDIRECT-ACTING: REVERSIBLE INHIBITORS OF ACETYLCHOLINESTERASE			
Ambenonium (Mytelase)	(+)	+	To restore muscle strength in myasthenia gravis
Edrophonium (Tensilon)	(+)	+	To diagnose myasthenia gravis; to differentiate a myasthenic crisis from a cholinergic crisis
Neostigmine (Prostigmin)	+	+	To restore muscle strength in myasthenia gravis To stimulate an atonic bladder or intestine
Physostigmine (Eserine)	+ [topical]		Miotic (constricts pupil)
Pyridostigmine (Mestinon)	(+)	+	To restore muscle strength in myasthenia gravis
INDIRECT-ACTING: IRREVERSIBLE INHIBITORS OF ACETYLCHOLINESTERASE			
Demecarium (Humorsol)	+ [topical]	(+) near eye	Miotic (constricts pupil)
Echothiophate (Phospholine)	+ [topical]	(+) near eye	Miotic (constricts pupil)
Isoflurophate (Floropryl)	+ [topical]	(+) near eye	Miotic (constricts pupil)
Pralidoxime (Protopam)	+	+	Reactivate acetylcholinesterase

*+, Stimulation. (+), Stimulation, at high concentrations, of muscles near the eye. 0, No stimulation.
†No drugs are used therapeutically that primarily stimulate nicotinic-ganglionic receptors. Stimulation of nicotinic-ganglionic receptors is a toxic effect of cholinomimetic drugs.

drugs for constricting the pupil (miotics): demecarium (Humorsol), echothiophate (Phospholine), and isoflurophate (Floropryl); the insecticides parathion and malathion; and several agents developed for chemical warfare. Interestingly, the antidote for poisoning by an irreversible acetylcholinesterase inhibitor is pralidoxime (PAM), which is itself an acetylcholinesterase inhibitor. Pralidoxime, however, is able to compete with the enzyme for the phosphate group of the inhibitor, thereby eliminating itself and the inhibitor from the enzyme, reversing the ''irreversible'' inhibition.

■ THERAPEUTIC USES OF CHOLINOMIMETIC DRUGS

Cholinomimetic drugs are used clinically for three effects in the peripheral nervous system:

1. To restore muscle tone in patients with myasthenia gravis or in surgical patients treated with tubocurarine. This is a nicotinic effect at the neuromuscular junction. The drugs used to increase muscle strength are all acetylcholinesterase inhibitors. Cholinomimetic drugs acting at the neuromuscular junction are discussed in Chapter 9.
2. To constrict the pupil (miosis), a muscarinic effect that is used in ophthalmology. Cholinomimetic drugs administered to act in the eye are described in Chapter 10.
3. To stimulate an atonic bladder or intestine. This is a muscarinic effect. Cholinomimetic drugs affecting the gastrointestinal system are discussed in Chapter 11.

Table 7-1 reviews the receptor selectivity of cholinomimetic drugs discussed in detail in other chapters. Note that no clinical use is made of drugs stimulating the nicotinic receptors of the ganglia. The ganglia are involved

FIG. 7-1

Acetylcholine is the peripheral neurotransmitter at three receptor populations. Each receptor population is characterized by an agonist and an antagonist as pictured. Muscarine and atropine are the agonist and antagonist of parasympathetic postganglionic (muscarinic) receptors. Nicotine and hexamethonium are the agonist and antagonist of parasympathetic preganglionic (nicotinic) receptors. Nicotine and tubocurarine are the agonist and antagonist of neuromuscular junction (nicotinic) receptors.

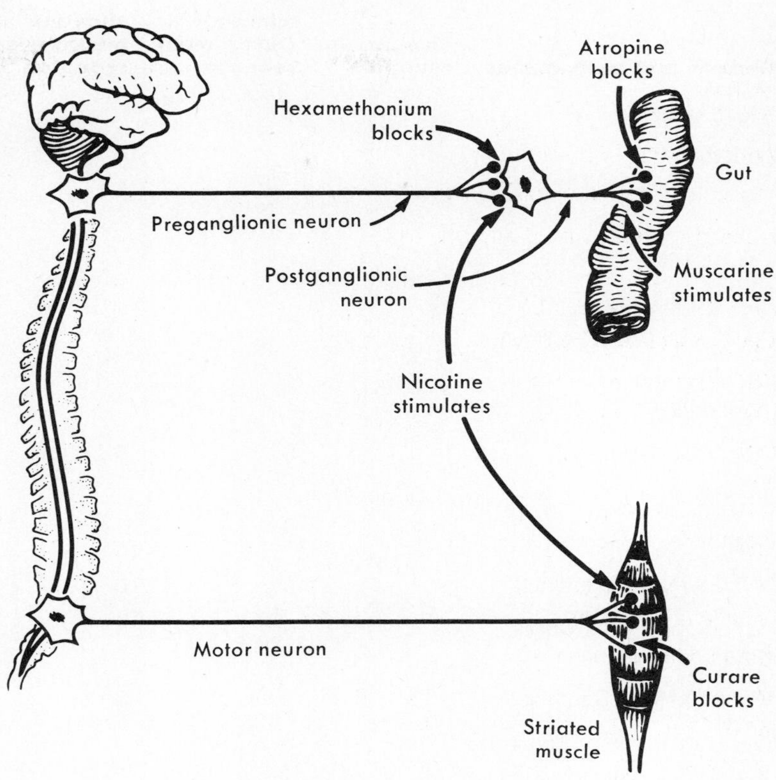

in so many responses as to make their stimulation by drugs clinically useless.

■ CHOLINERGIC ANTAGONISTS

As illustrated in Fig. 7-1, each of the three groups of receptors for acetylcholine is characterized by a drug that blocks the action of acetylcholine at that type of receptor by occupying the receptor and preventing cholinergic action. Since each class of acetylcholine antagonist acts on a discrete receptor population, the clinical use of each class of antagonist differs greatly. Table 7-2 reviews the receptor selectivity of cholinergic receptor antagonists discussed in detail in other chapters.

■ Neuromuscular receptor antagonists

Tubocurarine primarily blocks the receptors for acetylcholine at the neuromuscular junction and thereby causes muscular relaxation or paralysis. Antagonists of the neuromuscular cholinergic receptor are used chiefly as an adjunct to anesthetics and will be discussed in Chapter 9 (Drugs to control muscle tone).

■ Ganglionic receptor antagonists

The receptors for acetylcholine in the ganglia are blocked by *hexamethonium,* thus blocking transmission for both parasympathetic and sympathetic impulses. Antagonists like hexamethonium lack much specificity in the response produced. Limited use of drugs antagonizing the action of acetylcholine in the ganglia is made in treating severe cases of hypertension. One such drug, trimethaphan, will be discussed in Chapter 13 along with the other antihypertensive drugs.

■ Muscarinic receptor antagonists

Atropine and *scopolamine* are the prototypes of drugs that block acetylcholine at the muscarinic receptors. These are the parasympathetic, postganglionic receptors for acetylcholine on the heart, smooth muscle, and exocrine glands.

Atropine is an alkaloid originally derived from the leaves of the plant "deadly nightshade" or *Atropa belladonna,* which belongs to the potato family. Several other plants also contain atropine and a related drug, scopolamine. These two drugs are often referred to as *belladonna alkaloids*. References to the use of these plants as medicinal agents are found in all ancient medical literature. To this day, atropine remains the most useful and widely versatile of the antimuscarinic drugs.

■ THERAPEUTIC USES OF MUSCARINIC RECEPTOR ANTAGONISTS

1. To block secretions. Salivation is readily blocked by atropine. Indeed one classic side effect of atropine is a dry mouth (xerostomia). Secretions in the respiratory tract are also inhibited by atropine. This inhibition of bronchial and salivary secretions is the desired effect

TABLE 7-2. Receptor selectivity of cholinergic receptor antagonists at therapeutic doses*

Generic and trade names	Muscarinic receptor	Nicotinic (ganglionic) receptor	Nicotinic (neuromuscular) receptor	Therapeutic uses
Anisotropine	–	0	0	Same as homatropine
Atropine	–	0	0	Topical to the eye for mydriasis (dilated pupil) and cycloplegia (paralysis of accommodation); systemic, reduces gastric acid secretion and reduces gastrointestinal motility and tone of the bladder and ureter
Cyclopentolate (Cyclogyl)	– [topical]			Mydriasis and cycloplegia
Decamethonium (Syncurine)	0	0	–	Same as succinylcholine
Diphemanil (Prantal)	–	0	0	To control gastric acid
Eucatropine	– [topical]			Mydriasis and cycloplegia
Gallamine (Flaxedil)	(–)	0	–	Same as tubocurarine
Glycopyrrolate (Robinul)	–	0	0	Same as homatropine methylbromide
Homatropine methylbromide (Homopin)	–	0	0	To reduce gastrointestinal hypermotility and gastric acidity
Methantheline (Banthine)	–	0	0	Same as homatropine methylbromide
Methscopolamine (Pamine)	–	0	0	Same as homatropine methylbromide
Metocurine (Metubine)	0	0	–	Same as tubocurarine
Oxyphencyclimine (Daricon)	–	0	0	To control gastrointestinal hypermotility, gastric acidity, and hypermotility of the genitourinary and biliary tracts
Pancuronium (Pavulon)	0	0	–	Same as tubocurarine
Propantheline (Pro-Banthine)	–	0	0	Same as oxyphencyclimine
Scopolamine	–	0	0	Same as atropine
Succinylcholine (Anectine)	0	0	–	Depolarizing skeletal muscle relaxant
Trimethaphan (Arfonad)	0	–	0	To lower blood pressure in selected cases of hypertensive crisis
Tropicamide (Mydriacyl)	– [topical]			Mydriasis and cycloplegia
Tubocurarine (Tubarine)	0	(–)	–	Nondepolarizing skeletal muscle relaxant

*–, Inhibition. (–), Inhibition at high concentrations. 0, No inhibition.

when atropine is administered as a preanesthetic agent before surgery. The "drying" effect of atropine reduces secretions that may be involuntarily aspirated when the patient is drowsy or unconscious.

Atropine and related drugs are moderately effective in depressing gastric acid secretion in patients with peptic ulcers. The role of cholinergic antagonists in treating gastrointestinal disorders is discussed in Chapter 11.

Large doses of atropine and scopolamine dilate the blood vessels in the skin, especially around the face and particularly in children, thus producing a pronounced blushing. The mechanism for this vasodilation is not clear, but since sweating is inhibited by atropine, this flush may represent a mechanism to dissipate heat and a fever may be noted.

2. To depress an overactive gastrointestinal tract. A prominent antimuscarinic effect of atropine is to inhibit the tone and motility of smooth muscle. The gastrointestinal smooth muscle is very sensitive to atropine. Drugs affecting gastrointestinal motility are discussed in Chapter 11.

3. To dilate the eye (mydriasis) and to paralyze accommodation (cycloplegia). Atropine is applied by drops to the eye to block the actions of acetylcholine. The result of this antagonism is dilation of the pupil, since the circular muscles of the iris are relaxed, and blurred vision, since there is paralysis of accommodation. This mydriasis and cycloplegia allow measurements of lens refraction, examination of the retina, and aid in the healing of some infections. Drugs affecting the eye are discussed further in Chapter 10.

Atropine taken orally will also reach the eye. Photophobia (sensitivity to light) as a result of the dilation and blurring of vision (caused by the cycloplegia) are frequent side effects of oral administration of atropine.

4. To increase the heart rate. Atropine is administered to increase the heart rate by antagonizing the acetylcholine released by the vagus nerve at the atrioventricular node of the heart (Chapter 16).

5. To treat toxicity of cholinergic agents. The most frequent cause of cholinergic toxicity is overexposure to insecticides such as malathion and parathion, which are organic phosphate acetylcholinesterase inhibitors. Atropine will reverse the muscarinic effects (i.e., salivation, tearing, diarrhea, bradycardia) but will not reverse the neuromuscular paralysis. Pralidoxime (PAM), which regenerates acetylcholinesterase at all sites, is therefore the drug of choice.

■ Other uses of drugs blocking muscarinic receptors

Drugs that are muscarinic receptor antagonists have other uses unrelated to peripheral muscarinic receptors. Many anticholinergic drugs also have effects in the central nervous system. Some drugs have antitremor activity and are used to relieve certain tremors called *extrapyramidal motor effects* caused by Parkinson's disease, other diseases, and some drugs. Anticholinergic drugs used in the treatment of parkinsonism are discussed in Chapter 32.

■ Differences in the central nervous system effects of atropine and scopolamine

Atropine, particularly in an overdose, produces generalized excitement, which, in the toxic state, may result in hallucinations. In contrast, while scopolamine can produce hallucinations, scopolamine also produces sleepiness, sedation, and amnesia. Scopolamine, unlike atropine, is effective in preventing motion sickness.

■ SUMMARY

There are three types of receptors for acetylcholine outside the central nervous system. These receptor populations, defined by the drugs muscarine, nicotine, atropine, hexamethonium, and tubocurarine, are as follows:

1. Postganglionic receptors are stimulated by muscarine and blocked by atropine.
2. Ganglionic receptors are stimulated by nicotine and blocked by hexamethonium.
3. Neuromuscular receptors are stimulated by nicotine and blocked by tubocurarine.

The physiological activities associated with these receptor populations are

Muscarinic: Increased glandular secretion, stimulation of the gastrointestinal smooth muscle, vasodilation and slowing of the heart rate, increased urge for urination, and constriction of the pupils.

Nicotinic (ganglionic): Nonspecific activation of both the sympathetic and parasympathetic nervous systems.

Nicotinic (skeletal muscle): Increased muscle tone and, in excess, fasciculations (rapid, small contractions).

Cholinomimetic drugs may act *directly,* by stimulating receptors for acetylcholine, or *indirectly,* by slowing the degradation of acetylcholine released. This is accomplished by inhibiting the enzyme acetylcholinesterase, which degrades acetylcholine after it is released from the nerve terminal. The indirect-acting cholinomimetic drugs may be subdivided into reversible and irreversible inhibitors.

Therapeutic uses of cholinomimetic drugs are to restore muscle tone (increase muscle strength), to constrict the pupil, and to stimulate an atonic bladder or intestine.

Cholinergic antagonists act by blocking a receptor from occupation and activation by acetylcholine.

1. Tubocurarine is the prototype of an antagonist of the neuromuscular nicotinic receptor. The blockade produces muscular relaxation.
2. Hexamethonium is the prototype antagonist of the ganglionic nicotinic receptor. The effects of ganglionic receptor blockage are complex and clinically useful only in reversing severe hypertension.
3. Atropine is the prototype antagonist of the muscarinic receptor. Therapeutic uses of atropine-like drugs (muscarinic antagonists) include
   a. Blocking secretions

b. Depressing the tone of the gastrointestinal tract
c. Dilating the pupil and paralyzing accommodation
d. Raising the heart rate
e. Counteracting toxicity of cholinergic agents

The classic atropine-like (anticholinergic) effects are dry mouth, blurred vision, photophobia (from dilated pupils), flushed, dry skin, increased heart rate, mental confusion and excitement, constipation, and urinary retention.

Many drug classes other than the anticholinergic drugs have atropine-like side effects. Examples of these drug classes are the antihistamines, the antipsychotic drugs, the monoamine oxidase inhibitors, and the tricyclic antidepressants.

■ STUDY QUESTIONS

1. What are muscarine and nicotine and how do they relate to receptors for acetylcholine?
2. Contrast the mechanisms of a direct- and an indirect-acting cholinomimetic drug.
3. What three therapeutic uses are made of cholinomimetic drugs?
4. What are the three prototype antagonists and with which receptor population is each associated?
5. List the five actions of atropine that are useful therapeutically.
6. What are "atropine-like" or anticholinergic side effects? List them.

■ SUGGESTED READINGS

Bebbington, A., and Brimblecombe, R.W.: Muscarinic receptors in the peripheral and central nervous systems, Advances in Drug Research **2:**143, 1965.

Birdsall, N.J.M., and Hume, E.C.: Biochemical studies on muscarinic acetylcholine receptors, Journal of Neurochemistry **27:**7, 1976.

Ketchum, J.S., Sidell, F.R., Crowell, E.B., Jr., Aghajanian, G.K., and Hayes, A.H., Jr.: Atropine, scopolamine, and ditran: comparative pharmacology and antagonists in man, Psychopharmacologia **28:**121, 1973.

Krnjevic, K.: Central cholinergic pathways, Federation Proceedings **28:**113, 1969.

Rumack, B.H.: Anticholinergic poisoning: treatment with physostigmine, Pediatrics **52:**449, 1973.

Snyder, S.H., Chang, K.J., Kuhar, M.J., and Yamamura, H.I.: Biochemical identification of the mammalian muscarinic cholinergic receptor, Federation Proceedings **34:**1915, 1974.

Unna, K.R., Glaser, K., Lipton, E., and Patterson, P.R.: Dosage of drugs in infants and children. I. Atropine, Pediatrics **6:**197, 1950.

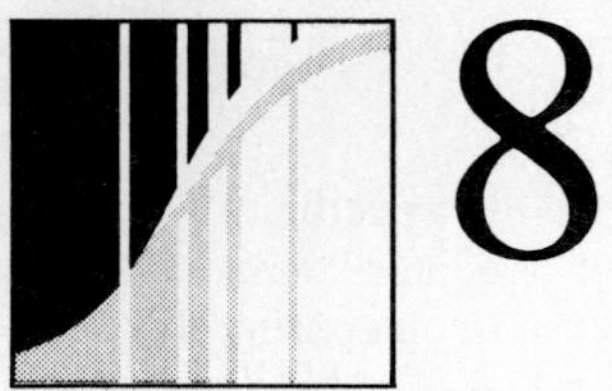

8 Mechanisms of adrenergic control

As in Chapter 7, this chapter is intended to be read at the beginning of a course in pharmacology as an introduction and at a later time as a review. When read as an introduction, the student should read for the mechanisms and the effects associated with these mechanisms. The drugs given as examples and their classification by mechanism will be of interest when the chapter is read at a later time for review.

■ CATECHOLAMINES AND THEIR RECEPTORS

■ The naturally occurring catecholamines

Dopamine, norepinephrine, and epinephrine are the naturally occurring *catecholamines,* which function as neurotransmitters and neurohormones. Dopamine is derived from the amino acid tyrosine and is the chemical precursor of norepinephrine:

Tyrosine →→ Dopamine → Norepinephrine → Epinephrine

All three catecholamines are important neurotransmitters in the central nervous system. In the autonomic nervous system, norepinephrine is the sympathetic, postganglionic neurotransmitter, and epinephrine is the neurohormone released from the adrenal medulla in reaction to stress. Dopamine plays a role in the autonomic nervous system that, at present, is not completely understood.

■ Classes of adrenergic receptors and adrenergic responses

The first synthetic catecholamine to be studied was isoproterenol. The existence of two classes of adrenergic receptors was proposed in the late 1940's to explain the different physiological effects elicited by norepinephrine, epinephrine, and isoproterenol. *Alpha receptors* are those receptors for which norepinephrine and epinephrine are equally potent but isoproterenol is less potent. *Beta receptors* are those receptors for which isoproterenol is more potent or as potent as epinephrine or norepinephrine. Subsequent studies over the years have expanded this classification to include two subtypes in each class: alpha-1, alpha-2, beta-1, and beta-2.

Alpha-1 adrenergic receptors. Alpha-1 receptors account for the primary responses elicited by norepinephrine released from sympathetic postganglionic neurons. Epinephrine is as potent as norepinephrine in stimulating alpha-1 receptors. Physiological effects resulting from stimulation of alpha-1 receptors include the following:

1. Contraction of the radial muscles of the iris. The radial muscles are arranged like the spokes of a wheel so that contraction causes dilation of the pupil (mydriasis). Adrenergic drugs used therapeutically for this effect are discussed in Chapter 10.
2. Constriction of arterioles and veins, which causes an increase in blood pressure. Adrenergic drugs that are used to raise the blood pressure are discussed in Chapter 13.
3. Contraction of smooth muscle sphincters in the stomach, intestine, and bladder.
4. Contraction of the uterus (female) and stimulation of ejaculation (male).
5. Decreased secretions from the pancreas.
6. Breakdown of glycogen in the liver (glycogenolysis) and synthesis of glucose (gluconeogenesis).

No therapeutic use is made of drugs mimicking the adrenergic effects listed in items 3 through 6.

Systemic effect of alpha-1 receptor activation. The general role of the alpha-1 receptor is to stimulate contraction of smooth muscle. The most prominent effect systemically is an increase in blood pressure resulting from the constriction of blood vessels, mainly arterioles. The blood vessels controlled by alpha-1 receptors are those servicing the internal organs, mucosal surfaces, and the skin. Blood pressure is in part a reflection of the degree of constriction of these blood vessels, since blood pressure is determined by the cardiac output and the peripheral resistance to blood flow in blood vessels.

Local vasoconstriction. Therapeutic use is made of local vasoconstriction by epinephrine and some other alpha-1 adrenergic receptor agonists (stimulants). Nasal decongestion may be achieved by local application of a vasoconstrictive drug (Chapter 23). Drug absorption from parenteral sites is slowed when a drug is injected with a vasoconstricting agent. Local anesthetics in particular will have a longer duration of action when injected with epinephrine to slow systemic absorption.

Alpha-2 adrenergic receptors. The concept of and experimental proof for a second class of alpha receptors, the alpha-2 receptors, was developed in the 1970's. Alpha-2 receptors are presynaptic receptors that when stimulated inhibit further release of norepinephrine. Therefore the two important distinctions between alpha-1 and alpha-2 receptors are their location and their function. Alpha-1 receptors are part of the tissue innervated by the sympathetic postganglionic neurons and are frequently referred to as *postsynaptic alpha receptors,* whereas the alpha-2 receptors are called *presynaptic alpha receptors* to reflect their location on the nerve terminal of those same postganglionic sympathetic neurons. As with the alpha-1 receptors, both norepinephrine and epinephrine are equally potent agonists (stimulants) of the alpha-2 receptor. However, stimulation of the presynaptic (alpha-2) receptors acts as a negative feedback system to limit the amount of norepinephrine released by the neuron. Therefore the norepinephrine released from the sympathetic postganglionic nerve terminal performs two functions: activation of the alpha-1 receptors on the tissue (usually to elicit smooth muscle contraction) and activation of alpha-2 receptors on the nerve terminal, which inhibits further release of norepinephrine. A drug with specificity for the alpha-2 receptor over alpha-1 receptors will have the apparent effect of inhibiting norepinephrine because less norepinephrine will be released. The therapeutic potential of drugs acting at alpha-2 receptors remains to be developed. The antihypertensive drugs clonidine and methyldopa have been found to stimulate the alpha-2 receptor. This action does not account for their antihypertensive effect, which has been shown to be a result of their activity in the central nervous system.

Beta-1 adrenergic receptor. The beta-1 receptor is stimulated by norepinephrine and by epinephrine but isoproterenol is a more potent stimulant than either. Physiological responses to activation of beta-1 receptors include the following:

1. Stimulation of the heart. There are three cardiac effects. Activation of the beta-1 receptor in the conducting tissue of the heart speeds the repolarization of the cells. An increase in heart rate (positive chronotropic effect) and an increase in impulse conduction speed (positive dromotropic effect) are the two consequences. Stimulation of the beta-1 receptors in the ventricular muscle increases the force of contraction (positive inotropic response). In Chapter 12 drugs acting on beta-1 receptors that are used for stimulating the heart under certain restricted conditions are presented.

2. Stimulation of the beta-1 receptor of fat tissue stimulates lipolysis, the breakdown of stored fat. The

TABLE 8-1. Receptor selectivity of adrenergic drugs*

Generic and trade names	Alpha receptor	Beta-1 receptor	Beta-2 receptor	CNS	Main therapeutic uses
CATECHOLAMINES					
Dobutamine (Dobutrex)	0	+D	0	0	Fairly specific in increasing cardiac contractility with little increase in heart rate or conductivity
Dopamine (Intropin)	(+) I	(+) I	0	0	At low doses dilates renal arteries by activating dopamine receptors and preventing kidney shutdown in shock
Epinephrine	+D	+D	+	(+)	To treat anaphylactic shock To treat acute asthma attacks To limit systemic absorption of drugs applied for local action

*+I, Indirectly acting (releases norepinephrine). +D, Directly acts on the receptor. (+), Effect is modest except at high concentrations. 0, No effect.

TABLE 8-1. Receptor selectivity of adrenergic drugs—cont'd

Generic and trade names	Alpha receptor	Beta-1 receptor	Beta-2 receptor	CNS	Main therapeutic uses
Isoproterenol (Isuprel)	0	+D	+	(+)	Bronchodilator (asthma)
Norepinephrine, levarterenol (Levophed)	+D	+D	0	(+)	To counteract the hypotension of spinal anesthesia
NONCATECHOLAMINES					
Albuterol (Ventolin, Proventil)	0	0	+	0	Bronchodilator
Amphetamine	+I	+I	0	+	To depress appetite To stimulate respiration To counteract narcolepsy
Ephedrine	+I,D	+I,D	+	+	Bronchodilator (asthma) Nasal decongestant To dilate the pupil (mydriasis)
Hydroxyamphetamine (Paredrine)	+I	+I	0	0	To dilate the pupil (mydriasis)
Isoetharine (Bronkosol)	0	0	+	0	Bronchodilator
Mephentermine (Wyamine)	+I,D	+I,D	0	+	To counteract the hypotension of spinal anesthesia To depress appetite
Metaproterenol (Alupent, Metaprel)	0	(+)	+	0	Bronchodilator
Metaraminol (Aramine)	+I,D	+I,D	0	0	To counteract the hypotension of spinal anesthesia
Methoxamine (Vasoxyl)	+D	0	0	0	To counteract the hypotension of spinal anesthesia To terminate paroxysmal atrial tachycardia
Naphazoline (Privine)	+	0	0	0	Nasal decongestant
Nylidrin (Arlidin)	0	0	+	0	To stimulate blood flow to heart, brain, and muscles
Oxymetazoline (Afrin)	+	0	0	0	Nasal decongestant
Phenylephrine	+D	0	0	0	Nasal decongestant To terminate paroxysmal atrial tachycardia
Phenylpropanolamine	+I,D	+I,D	+	(+)	Nasal decongestant
Propylhexedrine (Benzedrex)	+	0	0	0	Nasal decongestant
Terbutaline (Brethine, Bricanyl)	0	0	+	0	Bronchodilator
Tetrahydrozoline (Tyzine)	+	0	0	0	Nasal decongestant
Tuaminoheptane (Tuamine)	+	0	0	0	Nasal decongestant
Xylometazoline (Otrivin)	+	0	0	0	Nasal decongestant

fatty acids that are released can then be used as energy sources by the heart and liver. No therapeutic use is made of drugs mimicking this adrenergic effect.

Beta-2 adrenergic receptor. In contrast to their relative activities on the beta-1 receptors, epinephrine and isoproterenol are equipotent in stimulating beta-2 receptors, whereas norepinephrine is a weak stimulant. Physiological responses to activation of *beta-2 receptors* include the following:

1. Dilation of the bronchioles. The relaxation of bronchial smooth muscle decreases airway resistance and makes it easier to breathe. Drugs acting through activation of beta-2 receptors are used to treat patients with restricted airways, primarily caused by asthma or chronic obstructive lung disease. These drugs will be discussed in Chapter 22.

2. Dilation of the blood vessels in the skeletal muscle, brain, and heart. Activation of these beta-2 receptors causes vasodilation and shunts blood to the skeletal muscle, brain, and heart. The drug nylidrin (Arlidin) is used to increase blood flow to these organs (Chapter 12).

Systemic effects of beta-adrenergic receptor activation. The value of the responses to two classes of beta receptors can be appreciated by recalling the "fight or flight" nature of the sympathetic nervous system discussed in Chapter 6. The heart rate and cardiac output go up because epinephrine reinforces the action of norepinephrine on the beta-1 receptors. Blood is shunted to the muscle, brain, and heart, where stimulation of beta-2 receptors results in vasodilation, and from the skin and abdominal organs, where stimulation of alpha-1 receptors causes vasoconstriction. Epinephrine also stimulates the liver to break down glycogen to glucose and stimulates the fat cells to break down lipid to fatty acids to provide readily used energy sources for the body.

Table 8-1 reviews the receptor selectivity of these sympathomimetic drugs discussed in detail in other chapters.

■ The second messenger concept and the beta receptor

In the 1950's Earl Sutherland began his work to elucidate how epinephrine caused glycogenolysis (breakdown of glycogen to glucose) in the dog liver. He and his colleagues subsequently showed that epinephrine acts by binding to what we now recognize as the beta-2 receptor on the liver cell membrane. When the beta-2 receptor is occupied, there is a structural change that activates the membrane-bound enzyme, adenylate cyclase. The active portion of adenylate cyclase is inside the cell. The enzyme catalyzes the conversion of adenosine triphosphate (ATP) to pyrophosphate (PP) and cyclic adenosine 3′,5′-monophosphate (cyclic AMP). Cyclic AMP is the key to the intracellular action of epinephrine. Epinephrine is the hormone released to signal the cell to act. Cyclic AMP is the "second messenger" that translates the presence of epinephrine at the cell surface to the internal machinery of the cell. Many cyclic AMP molecules are formed as a result of each receptor occupation, amplifying the epinephrine signal. Cyclic AMP produces cellular effects by stimulating other enzymes. The enzymes present in the cell that can be stimulated by cyclic AMP determine what the cellular response will be. In the case of the liver, the response is the breakdown of glycogen. In the heart, the response is an increase in heart rate, force of contraction, and conduction speed. In smooth muscle, the response is relaxation. This second messenger concept is illustrated in Fig. 8-1. The cyclic AMP system mediates the response of the beta-1 and beta-2 receptors but not those of the alpha receptors. The intracellular mechanisms for the alpha receptors are unknown but are believed to involve the movement of calcium.

Two more features of the cyclic AMP system need to be pointed out. First, epinephrine is not the only hormone that stimulates the formation of cyclic AMP. Most polypeptide hormones discussed in Chapter 33 are known to work through cyclic AMP. The exceptions are insulin, growth hormone, and prolactin. Each hormone has its specific receptor on its target tissues. This is why each hormone can have tissue specific actions while using the same second messenger system. Second, cyclic AMP is rapidly degraded by the enzyme phosphodiesterase to 5′-adenosine monophosphate (AMP). A few drugs have been identified that inhibit phosphodiesterase and thereby produce elevated cyclic AMP concentrations. The main drug is theophylline and its dimer, aminophylline. These drugs are used to produce vasodilation in cerebral ischemia and, more importantly, in treating asthma by promoting bronchial dilation (Chapter 22).

■ Therapeutic uses and features of adrenergic drugs

The therapeutic use of an adrenergic drug depends on whether it acts on alpha-1, beta-1, or beta-2 receptors. A variety of drugs have been synthesized that are relatively specific for activating a given receptor type and thereby *directly mimic* some portion of norepinephrine or epinephrine action. Other adrenergic drugs act by a second mechanism of action. These are *indirect-acting* adrenergic drugs, which act by causing the sympathetic, postganglionic neurons to release norepinephrine. This increased amount of norepinephrine activates alpha-1, alpha-2, and beta-1 receptors. Drugs such as amphetamine, ephedrine, and mephentermine also act in the central nervous system, which determines as well

FIG. 8-1

Second messenger concept is illustrated. Binding of the hormone at the cell surface initiates a series of reactions that modify activity through phosphorylation of key enzymes and thereby modify cellular responses. Cyclic AMP is the *second messenger* because it carries the message that the hormone is at cell surface and translates this message into action by stimulating a phosphorylating enzyme (cyclic AMP dependent protein kinase). Cellular responses to epinephrine characteristic for a given organ are given as examples of biological responses mediated through cyclic AMP.

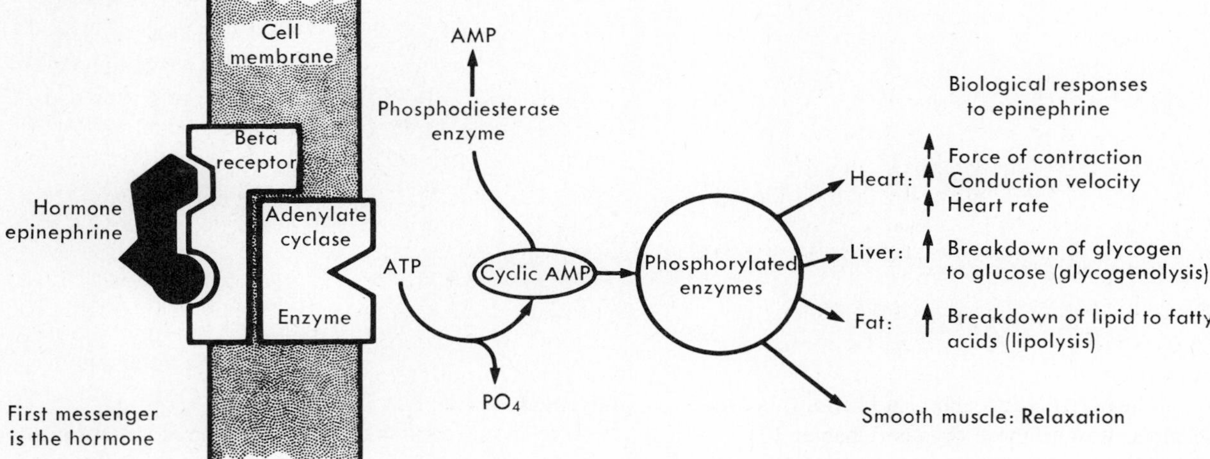

as limits their use. The catecholamines are relatively or completely ineffective when taken orally because they are rapidly destroyed in the gastrointestinal tract or by the liver, whereas many noncatecholamines can be taken orally.

■ DRUGS INHIBITING ADRENERGIC ACTIVITY

Table 8-2 lists the drugs interfering with peripheral adrenergic activity and the therapeutic use of these drugs. Several different drug mechanisms interfere with adrenergic activity. These mechanisms include

1. Blockade of alpha adrenergic receptors
2. Blockade of beta adrenergic receptors
3. Depletion of peripheral neuronal stores of norepinephrine
4. Inhibition of peripheral sympathetic activity through an action in the central nervous system

Each of these mechanisms will be discussed further as to the spectrum of physiological effects produced.

■ Blockade of alpha adrenergic receptors

Each of the drugs phenoxybenzamine, phentolamine, and prazosin acts selectively to antagonize norepinephrine at the alpha-1 receptors. Infusion of one of these drugs into a person with normal blood pressure produces little change in blood pressure as long as the person is lying down. However, any sudden shift to the upright position causes orthostatic (postural) hypotension because the blockade of the alpha-1 receptors prevents the vasoconstriction necessary to redistribute blood flow. Therefore in orthostatic (postural) hypotension the blood pools in the legs and drains from the head to cause fainting.

Other effects characteristic of blockade of the alpha-1 receptors include a pinpoint pupil (miosis), nasal stuffiness, or, in males, inhibition of ejaculation.

The uses and pharmacokinetics of the alpha-1 receptor antagonists in the treatment of hypertension are discussed in Chapter 13.

■ Blockade of beta adrenergic receptors

Nonselective antagonists. The physiological effects of beta-receptor antagonists can be anticipated by considering the functions of the beta receptors. Blockade of the beta-1 receptors in the heart causes little change in the normal person at rest but limits the increase in cardiac functions normally elicited by exercise and hypertension. Conditions improved by beta-1 receptor blockade include angina and some cardiac arrhythmias. Beta-receptor antagonists are also effective in treating hypertension, although the mechanism responsible for this improvement is not clear. However, when a beta-receptor antagonist is given with a vasodilator drug, the beta-receptor antagonist inhibits the reflex activation of the heart caused by the drop in blood pressure. For this reason, a beta-receptor antagonist combined with a vasodilator drug is especially effective in treating hyperten-

TABLE 8-2. Drugs inhibiting adrenergic receptor activity*

Generic and trade names	Alpha receptor	Beta-1 receptor	Beta-2 receptor	CNS	Main therapeutic uses
ALPHA-ADRENERGIC RECEPTOR ANTAGONISTS					
Phenoxybenzamine (Dibenzyline)	–	0	0	0	To treat hypertension secondary to pheochromocytoma To treat vasospastic disorders of the digits (Raynaud's syndrome)
Phentolamine (Regitine)	–	0	0	0	To treat hypertension secondary to pheochromocytoma
Prazosin (Minipress)	–	0	0	0	To treat chronic hypertension
BETA-ADRENERGIC RECEPTOR ANTAGONISTS					
Metoprolol (Lopressor)	0	–	0	–	To treat chronic hypertension Prophylactic treatment of angina
Naldolol (Corgard)	0	–	–	–	To treat chronic hypertension Prophylactic treatment of angina
Propranolol (Inderal)	0	–	–	–	To treat chronic hypertension Prophylactic treatment of angina To treat cardiac arrhythmias Prophylactic treatment for migraine
Timolol (Timoptic)	0	–	–	0	Ophthalmic, to treat glaucoma
DRUGS DEPLETING NEURONAL STORES OF NOREPINEPHRINE					
Guanethidine (Ismelin)	–I	–I	–I	0	To treat severe chronic hypertension
Reserpine (Serpasil)	–I	–I	–I	–	To treat chronic hypertension
DRUGS INHIBITING SYMPATHETIC ACTIVITY THROUGH AN ACTION IN THE CNS					
Alpha methyldopa (Aldomet)	–CNS	0	0	–	To treat chronic hypertension
Clonidine (Catapres)	–CNS	0	0	–	To treat chronic hypertension

*– denotes inhibition, 0 denotes no effect, –I denotes indirect inhibition resulting from depletion of norepinephrine stores, –CNS denotes a decrease in peripheral sympathetic tone through an action in the CNS.

sion. The use of beta-receptor antagonists in the therapy of hypertension is discussed in Chapter 13.

Blockade of beta-2 receptors will limit bronchiole dilation and therefore can severely compromise the pulmonary function in patients with asthma. This fact has led to the search for beta-1 selective antagonists (cardioselective antagonists) such as metoprolol (Lopressor).

Propranolol (Inderal) was the first beta-receptor antagonist approved for clinical use in the United States. Propranolol blocks both beta-1 and beta-2 receptors and is used to treat hypertension, angina, and cardiac arrhythmias. In addition, propranolol is an effective prophylactic in the treatment of migraine headaches, although the mechanisms involved are not clear.

Naldolol (Corgard) was introduced in 1980 as a nonselective beta-receptor antagonist for use in treating angina and hypertension. Additional nonselective beta receptor antagonists that may be released for clinical use in the United States include pindolol and oxprenolol. Acebutolol is a cardioselective beta-receptor antagonist that may be released.

Timolol (Timoptic) is a nonselective beta-receptor antagonist used to treat glaucoma. Timolol reduces the production of aqueous humor in the eye and is discussed with other ophthalmic drugs in Chapter 10.

■ Depletion of peripheral neuronal stores of norepinephrine

Guanethidine (Ismelin) and reserpine (Serpasil) are antihypertensive drugs that deplete norepinephrine from peripheral neurons.

Guanethidine is taken up into the postganglionic sympathetic nerve terminals, where it then prevents the release of norepinephrine. After several days the neuronal content of norepinephrine is depleted.

Reserpine also causes a depletion of norepinephrine stores not only in the periphery but also in the brain. The central action of reserpine is believed to contribute in a major way to the depression of sympathetic tone with this agent.

Reserpine and guanethidine are useful in treating chronic hypertension (Chapter 13) and Raynaud's disease (Chapter 12).

■ Inhibition of peripheral sympathetic activity through an action in the central nervous system

The central nervous system controls sympathetic activity, although the mechanism of this control is not understood. The preceding section indicated that part of the effect of reserpine is believed to be mediated through an action in the central nervous system. It is now recognized that two other antihypertensive drugs, clonidine (Catapres) and methyldopa (Aldomet), decrease sympathetic tone mainly through an action in the central nervous system. The role of these drugs in the treatment of hypertension is described in Chapter 13.

■ SUMMARY

Effects of adrenergic receptor agonists (stimulants) depend on how selective the drug is for the four classes of adrenergic receptors.

Activation of the alpha-1 receptors causes vasoconstriction, which is seen systemically as a rise in blood pressure. In the eye, pupil dilation (mydriasis) is mediated by activation of alpha-1 receptors. Activation of alpha-2 receptors will appear as a diminution of sympathetic activity because activation of these presynaptic receptors inhibits the further release of norepinephrine. The characterization of the alpha-2 receptor is recent, and the clinical implications are not yet developed.

Activation of the beta-1 adrenergic receptors increases cardiac activity, whereas activation of beta-2 receptors relaxes the bronchioles. Selective beta-2 adrenergic receptor agonists (stimulants) have been developed for use in treating asthma and other types of reversible bronchiole constriction. The intracellular pathway activated by stimulation of beta receptors is the production of cyclic AMP, a compound that alters the activity of key enzymes. A drug that inhibits the degradation of cyclic AMP will produce the effects characteristic of a beta-adrenergic receptor agonist.

Four mechanisms are described for the inhibition of adrenergic activity. All four mechanisms can be related to drugs effective in treating chronic hypertension. Drugs inhibiting alpha-1 adrenergic receptors would appear to offer the most direct means of lowering blood pressure, but in practice drugs inhibiting the beta-1 adrenergic receptors are clinically more efficacious. In addition to blockade of alpha-1 and beta-1 adrenergic receptors, adrenergic activity can be inhibited by drugs that deplete the norepinephrine stores in the sympathetic postganglionic nerve terminals and by drugs that act in the central nervous system to depress sympathetic activity. These latter two classes of drugs also find primary use as drugs to treat chronic hypertension.

Beta-1 adrenergic receptor antagonists (blockers) are also effective in treating angina and some types of cardiac arrhythmias. Beta-receptor antagonists also limit the production of aqueous humor in the treatment of chronic glaucoma.

■ STUDY QUESTIONS

1. Which are the three naturally occurring catecholamines and where are they found?
2. What actions are associated with stimulation of the alpha-1 adrenergic receptor? With the stimulation of the alpha-2 adrenergic receptor? With the stimulation of the beta-1 adrenergic receptor? With the stimulation of the beta-2 adrenergic receptor?
3. What does the "second messenger" (cyclic AMP) do?
4. Contrast the mechanism of action of direct-acting and indirect-acting sympathomimetic drugs.
5. What are the four major drug mechanisms that inhibit adrenergic activity? What therapeutic use is made of each of these actions?

■ SUGGESTED READINGS

Axelrod, J.: Noradrenaline: fate and control of its biosynthesis, Science **173:**598, 1971.

Axelrod, J., and Weinshilboum, R.: Catecholamines, The New England Journal of Medicine **287:**237, 1972.

Christensen, N.J.: The role of catecholamines in clinical medicine, Acta Medica Scandinavia, Supplement **624:**9, 1979.

Von Euler, U.S.: Adrenergic neurotransmitter functions, Science **173:** 202, 1971.

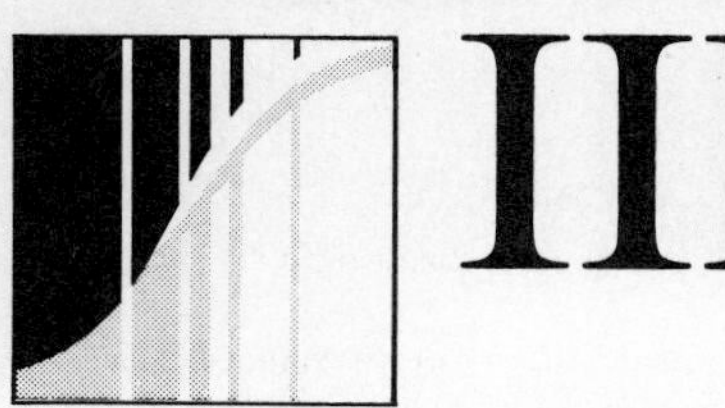

III DRUGS AFFECTING SYSTEMS UNDER CHOLINERGIC CONTROL

In this section the cholinergic drug classes are presented within the framework of their major therapeutic targets: the skeletal muscle, the eye, and the gastrointestinal system. The goal of this section is to present the traditional cholinergic drug classes but within a systems setting to allow assessment of the therapeutic role of drugs affecting cholinergic mechanisms relative to drugs acting by other mechanisms.

The drug classes in Chapter 9, **Drugs to Control Muscle Tone,** are the acetylcholinesterase inhibitors and the neuromuscular blocking drugs, so that only cholinergic mechanisms are discussed. The drug classes in Chapter 10, **Drugs Affecting the Eye,** are more diverse. The anticholinergic drugs of the atropine type are supplemented with the adrenergic drugs for pupillary dilation. The discussion of cholinomimetic drugs in treating glaucoma is supplemented by reference to the role of additional drug classes: the adrenergics, carbonic anhydrase inhibitors, and osmotic diuretics.

The final chapter in this section, Chapter 11, **Drugs Affecting the Gastrointestinal Tract,** considers several drug classes in addition to the cholinergic classes. The role of the cholinergic system is emphasized initially by discussing cholinomimetics to increase and anticholinergics to decrease small intestinal motility. Next the role of anticholinergic drugs in inhibiting stomach acid secretion is discussed, and the more important roles of antacids to neutralize stomach acid and the H_2 receptor antagonist cimetidine to inhibit stomach acid secretion are presented. Nausea and vomiting, which can be considered hyperactivity of the upper gastrointestinal tract, are then considered. Central mechanisms rather than cholinergic mechanisms are cited as the target for drug therapy of nausea and vomiting. The different roles of antihistamines and the dopamine antagonists are only briefly reviewed here because they are discussed fully in Chapters 21 and 25. Finally, the two major drug classes affecting the large intestine, laxatives and antidiarrheals, are discussed. Cholinergic mechanisms play no role in these drug classes. Antidiarrheals rely chiefly on opiate mechanisms to halt hyperactivity, whereas laxatives basically provide bulk by one means or another to stimulate activity.

9 Drugs to control muscle tone

■ OVERVIEW

Motor neurons are single neurons originating in the spinal cord and terminating on the muscle. In this chapter, two classes of drugs affecting skeletal muscle that act at the neuromuscular junction to affect the neurotransmitter acetylcholine or its receptor will be discussed. The first class of drugs is the *acetylcholinesterase inhibitors,* which are indirect-acting cholinomimetic drugs. These drugs are used to diagnose and to treat myasthenia gravis, a disease of muscular weakness, by increasing the quantity of acetylcholine at the neuromuscular junction to restore muscle contraction. The second class of drugs is the *neuromuscular blocking* drugs that occupy the receptors for acetylcholine on muscles and thereby prevent muscle contraction. These drugs are used to produce muscular relaxation for intubation and surgical procedures.

■ DESCRIPTION OF MYASTHENIA GRAVIS

Myasthenia gravis is a disease in which the skeletal muscles quickly show weakness and become fatigued. The muscles most commonly involved are those controlling facial movements, and one early sign of myasthenia gravis is drooping eyelids (ptosis). As the disease progresses, chewing and swallowing become increasingly difficult, and the voice becomes less distinct. Death can result if the intercostal muscles and the diaphragm, muscles essential for breathing, become affected.

The basic defect in myasthenia gravis is a reduction by 70% to 90% in the available receptors for acetylcholine at the neuromuscular junction. This reduction in the number of available receptors appears to be an autoimmune disease brought about by antibodies produced against the receptors. These antibodies block the active site for acetylcholine on the muscle (nicotinic) receptor and also increase the rate at which the receptors are degraded by the cell. A number of drugs are contraindicated for the patient with myasthenia gravis and are listed here. These drugs block the neuromuscular receptor to a degree that is not noticeable in a normal person but can dangerously weaken the patient with myasthenia gravis.

- ACTH and glucocorticoids
- Anesthetics
  - Diethyl ether
  - Halothane (Fluothane)
  - Lidocaine IV (Xylocaine)
- Antiarrhythmics
  - Procainamide (Pronestyl)
  - Propranolol (Inderal)
  - Quinidine
- Antibiotics
  - Bacitracin (Bacitracin)
  - Colistimethate (Coly-Mycin M)
  - Colistin (Coly-Mycin S)
  - Gentamicin (Garamycin)
  - Kanamycin (Kantrex)
  - Lincomycin (Lincocin)
  - Neomycin (Mycifradin, Neobiotic)
  - Paromomycin (Humatin)
  - Polymyxin B (Aerosporin, Polymyxin B)
  - Streptomycin (Streptomycin)
  - Viomycin (Viocin)
- Anticonvulsants
  - Magnesium sulfate
- Antimalarials
  - Quinine
- Diuretics and other drugs or circumstances promoting hypokalemia (low blood potassium concentration)
- Muscle relaxants
  - Gallamine (Flaxedil)
  - Metocurine (Metubine)
  - Pancuronium (Pavulon)
  - Succinylcholine (Anectine)
  - Tubocurarine
- Sedatives, especially those with respiratory depressant effects, such as barbiturates, narcotics, and tranquilizers
- Thyroid compound

■ ACETYLCHOLINESTERASE INHIBITORS FOR MYASTHENIA GRAVIS (Table 9-1)

■ Mechanism of action

Drugs that inhibit the degradation of acetylcholine, acetylcholinesterase inhibitors (anticholinesterases), are

TABLE 9-1. Cholinomimetic drugs for the diagnosis and treatment of myasthenia gravis

Generic name	Trade name	Dosage and administration	Comments
Ambenonium chloride	Mytelase	ORAL: *Adults*—5 mg 3 or 4 times daily increased every 1 to 2 days as required. *Children*—0.3 mg/kg body weight daily in divided doses, increased gradually if necessary to a maximum of 1.5 mg/kg daily.	Acetylcholinesterase inhibitor. Rapidly absorbed.
Edrophonium chloride	Tensilon	For diagnosis of myasthenia gravis: INTRAVENOUS: *Adults*—2 mg injected over 15 to 30 sec. If no response, 8 mg is given. May repeat test after 1 hr. *Children:* 2 mg initially as above followed by 5 mg (under 75 lb) or up to 10 mg (over 75 lb).	Very short acting acetylcholinesterase inhibitor. Diagnosis is positive if muscle strength increases within 3 min (duration, 5 to 10 min).
		To differentiate a myasthenic from a cholinergic crisis: 1 to 2 mg.	A cholinergic crisis if muscle strength decreases (lower medication dose). A patient in cholinergic crisis may require ventilatory assistance after edrophonium injection.
Neostigmine bromide	Prostigmin Bromide	ORAL: *Adults*—15 mg every 3 to 4 hr initially, then adjust upward as required. *Children*—begin with 2 mg/kg body weight daily in divided doses.	Acetylcholinesterase inhibitor. High incidence of side effects.
Neostigmine methylsulfate	Prostigmin Methylsulfate	INTRAMUSCULAR: *Adults*—0.022 mg/kg body weight (atropine, IM, 0.011 mg/kg may be given to control muscarinic side effects). *Children*—1.5 mg (with 0.6 mg atropine, IM).	Injectable form for diagnosis of myasthenia gravis
Pyridostigmine bromide	Mestinon	ORAL: *Adults*—60 to 120 mg every 3 or 4 hr initially, increased as necessary. *Children*—7 mg/kg in divided doses as required.	Acetylcholinesterase inhibitor; drug of choice for controlling muscular weakness of myasthenia gravis.
	Regonol	INTRAMUSCULAR, INTRAVENOUS: *Adults*—1/30 of oral dose. *Newborn infants of myasthenic mothers*—0.05 to 0.15 mg/kg body weight.	

the first line of treatment for myasthenia gravis. Acetylcholinesterase inhibitors allow the accumulation of acetylcholine at the neuromuscular junction, and this increase in the concentration of acetylcholine at the neuromuscular junction ensures that available receptors are activated.

The acetylcholinesterase inhibitors used to treat myasthenia gravis are also used to reverse the effects of the competitive neuromuscular blocking drugs used in surgery. This use is discussed in the section on neuromuscular blocking drugs.

■ Side effects

Side effects arising from overstimulation of neuromuscular (nicotinic) receptors include muscle cramps, rapid, small contractions (fasciculations), and weakness. Acetylcholinesterase inhibitors can also act at sites other than neuromuscular sites. These inhibitors act at muscarinic sites and produce side effects classic for parasympathetic stimulation: excessive salivation, perspiration, abdominal distress, and nausea and vomiting.

■ Specific drugs

Neostigmine

Neostigmine (Prostigmin) can be used for the diagnosis and treatment of myasthenia gravis. As a diagnostic tool, an intramuscular injection of neostigmine should improve the patient's muscular strength in 10 minutes, and this improvement should last 3 to 4 hours. Neostigmine is also prescribed to relieve the symptoms of

■ THE NURSING PROCESS FOR DRUGS USED IN MYASTHENIA GRAVIS

■ Assessment

Patients requiring acetylcholinesterase inhibitors are those in whom the diagnosis of myasthenia gravis is either confirmed or suspected. The patient may come to the hospital with a wide range of symptoms from mild ptosis (drooping eyelids) and easy fatigability to acute muscular weakness. A total body assessment should be done. The nurse should monitor not only the temperature, pulse, respiration, and blood pressure but also vital capacity, ability to swallow, muscle strength (all of which are impaired in myasthenia gravis), and the degree of ptosis. The nurse should assess the patient's condition for any additional medical problems that may coexist and influence treatment.

■ Management

The treatment of the patient with myasthenia gravis can be complex and sometimes tricky. It is beyond the scope of this book to discuss all aspects of treatment; consult an appropriate textbook of nursing. The nurse should continue to monitor signs of myasthenia gravis including the ptosis, ability to swallow, vital capacity, and overall muscle strength as well as the vital signs. Medications should be administered exactly on time. A suction machine should be at the bedside if the patient displays any signs of being unable to swallow secretions adequately. Drugs that should be at the bedside include edrophonium, pyridostigmine, atropine, and neostigmine, along with syringes. In addition, equipment for intubation should be readily available if the patient's condition warrants it. The nurse should begin teaching the patient and family about the management of myasthenia gravis in the home setting. If appropriate, the patient can be referred to other members of the health care team for physical therapy or social service, or to the local visiting nurse association.

■ Evaluation

It is not possible to cure or halt the progression of myasthenia gravis. Successful drug therapy aids the patient to maintain as normal a life-style as possible. With this disease, perhaps more than with many other diseases, patient compliance and understanding are essential to good control of the symptoms. Before discharge the patient should be able to explain how and why the medication should be taken, the signs and symptoms that indicate overdose and underdose with medications, the symptoms that would require notification of the physician, other measures that should be employed to assist in managing the disease (such as the use of a nonelectric alarm clock to awaken the patient for nighttime doses of medication), and medications that should be avoided. For more specific information, see the patient care implications section at the end of this chapter.

---

myasthenia gravis. Because neostigmine is irregularly absorbed from the gastrointestinal tract, effective drug levels can be difficult to establish with oral administration. Muscarinic side effects, particularly salivation, cramps, and diarrhea, are common enough to limit the long-term use of neostigmine. If neostigmine is used, atropine may also be prescribed to block the muscarinic effects.

Pyridostigmine

Pyridostigmine (Mestinon) is the drug of choice for the treatment of myasthenia gravis. Compared to neostigmine, pyridostigmine is better absorbed from the gastrointestinal tract and longer acting. Adverse effects such as miosis, sweating, salivation, gastrointestinal distress, and slow heart rate are less common with pyridostigmine than with neostigmine.

Ambenonium

Ambenonium (Mytelase) is slightly longer acting than pyridostigmine or neostigmine. Occasionally, patients experience side effects such as jitteriness, headaches, confusion, and dizziness, which are not seen with pyridostigmine or neostigmine. An advantage of ambenonium is that it is not a bromide salt, whereas pyridostigmine and neostigmine are bromide salts. Ambenonium is thus the drug of choice for patients with an allergy to bromides.

Edrophonium

Edrophonium (Tensilon) is a very short-acting acetylcholinesterase inhibitor used as a diagnostic agent. When a new patient with suspected myasthenia gravis is given 2 mg of edrophonium IV, an increase in muscle strength should be seen in 1 to 3 minutes. If no response is seen, another 4 to 10 mg of edrophonium is given over the next 2 minutes and muscle strength is again tested. If no increase in muscle strength is seen with this higher dose, the muscle weakness is caused by something other than myasthenia gravis. Patients receiving injections of edrophonium commonly show a drop in blood pressure and feel faint, dizzy, and flushed.

A second diagnostic use for edrophonium is to aid in diagnosing what to do when a patient under treatment for myasthenia gravis becomes weaker. The problem is to identify whether the patient is suffering from an overdose of medication (cholinergic crisis) or increasing severity of the disease (myasthenic crisis). An injection of edrophonium will make the patient in the cholinergic crisis temporarily worse but will temporarily improve the patient in a myasthenic crisis.

■ NEUROMUSCULAR BLOCKING DRUGS

(Table 9-2)

■ Mechanism of action

Neuromuscular blocking drugs produce complete muscle relaxation by binding to the receptor for acetylcholine at the neuromuscular junction. The nondepolarizing or competitive blockers bind to the receptor without initiating depolarization of the muscle membrane. The depolarizing drugs also bind to the receptor for acetylcholine but do cause depolarization of the muscle membrane. Since the depolarizing drugs do not readily dissociate from the receptor, the depolarization persists. Larger doses of a depolarizing drug also desensitize the receptor to restimulation. Both types of blockade, nondepolarizing and depolarizing, result in muscle paralysis. The two types of neuromuscular blocking drugs can be differentiated by the response to an injection of a drug such as edrophonium, which inhibits the degradation of acetylcholine by acetylcholinesterase. As the concentration of acetylcholine rises in the neuromuscular junction, a nondepolarizing drug will be displaced and muscle tone will be regained. The depolarizing drug will not be displaced.

■ Therapeutic uses

Because neuromuscular blockers can produce complete paralysis, they are administered only to an anesthetized patient. Assisted ventilation should be available for the short-acting succinylcholine and is mandatory when administering the longer acting neuromuscular blockers. The skeletal muscle relaxants do not inhibit pain in any way. The major use of the neuromuscular blocking drugs is to provide muscle relaxation during surgery, particularly relaxation of the abdominal muscles, without using deep general anesthesia, which would relax abdominal muscles by depressing the spinal cord. The neuromuscular blockers are also used with light anesthesia to allow a tube to be passed down easily to the trachea (endotracheal intubation), to relieve spasm of the larynx, to prevent convulsive muscle spasms during electroconvulsive therapy for depression, and to allow breathing to be controlled totally by a respirator (controlled ventilation) during surgery.

■ Nondepolarizing drugs

Tubocurarine (curare)

Tubocurarine was originally isolated as the active principle of the South American arrow poison. An animal hit with an arrow containing curare would fall paralyzed a short time later.

Uses. The main uses of tubocurarine are to produce muscle relaxation during surgery or electroconvulsive shock therapy, to reduce muscle spasm in tetanus, and to allow controlled ventilation. Administration is by slow (60 to 90 seconds) intravenous injection. Maximal paralysis occurs within 5 minutes and persists for 60 minutes (range: 25 to 90 minutes). The progression of paralysis begins with the eyelids, then the face, the extremities, and finally the diaphragm, resulting in the cessation of spontaneous breathing. The recovery from neuromuscular blockade can be assisted by injecting edrophonium, neostigmine, or pyridostigmine to increase the amount of acetylcholine at the neuromuscular junction.

Excretion. About 40% of tubocurarine is excreted unchanged in the urine. Patients with renal failure or acidosis will excrete tubocurarine less rapidly and require a smaller dose.

Side effects. Tubocurarine can cause the release of histamine, which in turn causes hypotension or bronchospasm (Chapter 21). Hypotension can also arise from ganglionic blockade by tubocurarine. Tubocurarine does not cross the placenta or the blood-brain barrier.

Drug interactions. Many drugs potentiate the action of tubocurarine, including the anesthetics halothane, ether, methoxyflurane, and enflurane. Other drugs that can markedly potentiate the action of tubocurarine include the aminoglycoside antibiotics and the antiarrhythmic quinidine. Since patients with myasthenia gravis have an exaggerated response to tubocurarine, very small doses of tubocurarine can be used to diagnose

TABLE 9-2. Neuromuscular blocking drugs

Generic name	Trade name	Dosage and administration	Comments
NONDEPOLARIZING (COMPETITIVE) DRUGS			
Gallamine triethiodide	Flaxedil Triethiodide	INTRAVENOUS: *Adults*—1 to 1.5 mg/kg body weight. Supplemental doses, 0.3 to 1.2 mg/kg. *Children*—2.5 mg/kg initially with 0.3 to 1.2 mg/kg supplemental doses. *Newborns*—to 1 ml, 1.5 mg/kg initially, with 1 mg/kg supplemental doses.	May cause increased heart rate. Not for use in patients in renal failure. Doses given are for use with nitrous oxide. Other inhalation anesthetics may require smaller doses.
Metocurine	Metubine Iodide	INTRAVENOUS: *Adults*—0.1 to 0.3 mg/kg body weight. Supplemental doses, 0.02 to 0.03 mg/kg.	See tubocurarine chloride. Doses given are for use with nitrous oxide, Other inhalation anesthetics may require smaller doses.
Pancuronium bromide	Pavulon	INTRAVENOUS:*Adults and children*—0.04 to 0.1 mg/kg body weight initially with 0.01 to 0.02 mg/kg supplemental doses. Newborns may be very sensitive; use a test dose of 0.02 mg.	Does not cause hypotension. May stimulate heart rate and cardiac output. Doses given are for use with nitrous oxide. Other inhalation anesthetics may require smaller doses.
Tubocurarine chloride (curare)		INTRAVENOUS: *Adults and children*—0.2 to 0.4 mg/kg body weight initially. Supplemental doses, 0.04 to 0.2 mg/kg. Diagnosis of myasthenia gravis: $^1/_{15}$ to $^1/_5$ of above dose.	Intravenous injection should be slow (1 to 1½ min). Do not combine with the alkaline intravenous barbiturate solutions. Doses are for use with nitrous oxide. Other inhalation anesthetics may require smaller doses.
DEPOLARIZING DRUGS			
Succinylcholine chloride	Anectine Quelicin Sucostrin Sux-Cert	INTRAVENOUS: *Adults*—0.6 to 1.1 mg/kg body weight initially. Continuous infusion, 0.1% or 0.2% solution at a rate of 0.5 to 10 mg/min. *Children*—1.1 mg/kg body weight initially with 0.3 to 0.6 mg/kg supplemental doses. *Newborns*—2 mg/kg. Continuous infusion is not recommended for children and newborns.	Duration is only 5 min because of hydrolysis by plasma cholinesterase. This enzyme is missing genetically in some patients, and a prolonged action is seen. May cause cardiac arrhythmias. Doses given are for use with nitrous oxide. Other inhalation anesthetics require smaller doses.
Decamethonium bromide	Syncurine	INTRAVENOUS: *Adults*—0.03 to 0.06 mg/kg body weight.	Duration of action is about 20 min. Excreted unchanged in the urine.

myasthenia gravis if tests with edrophonium or neostigmine are inconclusive.

Metocurine (dimethyl tubocurarine) iodide (Metubine)

Metocurine iodide, a semisynthetic derivative of tubocurarine, is 2 to 3 times as potent as tubocurarine but otherwise similar.

Gallamine triethiodide (Flaxedil)

Gallamine triethiodide is a synthetic drug similar in action to tubocurarine but with a shorter duration of action. Gallamine does not cause histamine release or ganglionic blockade. The major side effect of gallamine is an increase in heart rate (tachycardia), which is seen a few minutes after injection and then declines. Gallamine is excreted unchanged in the urine and should not be used in patients with kidney failure.

Pancuronium bromide (Pavulon)

Pancuronium bromide has a faster onset of action than tubocurarine, although the duration of action is similar. Pancuronium does not cause the histamine release or ganglionic blockade characteristic of tubocurarine. Heart rate, cardiac output, and atrial pressure are increased by pancuronium, effects that may be desired in cardiac surgery. Pancuronium is partially excreted unchanged in the urine, and doses must be decreased for patients with renal failure.

■ THE NURSING PROCESS FOR NEUROMUSCULAR BLOCKING AGENTS

■ Assessment

Patients receiving neuromuscular blocking drugs will be those undergoing anesthesia, patients having certain diagnostic studies in which brief muscle relaxation is necessary for the completion of the study, some patients who are "bucking" ventilators, and patients undergoing electroconvulsive therapy. The nurse should determine the pulse, respiratory rate, and blood pressure of these patients. A thorough patient assessment should be done, focussing on the major problems being treated and what diagnostic or therapeutic procedure is to be carried out. The neuromuscular blocking agents usually are used for such a brief period of time that under normal circumstances there are no appropriate laboratory tests that should be monitored.

■ Management

Because neuromuscular blocking agents paralyze the patient completely, management includes rapid assessment of the respiratory system and assisted ventilation for the patient when necessary. Before using a neuromuscular blocking agent, equipment for intubation and suctioning should be at the bedside. The nurse should observe the rate, quality, and depth of respirations and ventilate the patient as needed. If the drugs are being administered by constant infusion, an infusion monitoring device should be used. Remember that neuromuscular blockade agents, when used alone, do not produce anesthesia; medicate the patient for pain if necessary. The nurse should position the patient carefully and check to see that instruments and bed linens are not causing unnecessary pressure on any areas of the patient's body. After the drug has been used, it may take minutes to hours for the effect of the neuromuscular blocking agents to wear off. During this period of time it is important to assess the ability of the patient to breathe unassisted, to cough, and to handle secretions. Patients should be positioned on their sides and the side rails should be kept up. Patients should not be left unattended until it is certain that the patient can adequately cough, handle secretions, and call for help.

■ Evaluation

These agents are considered successful if they produce sufficient muscle relaxation to allow the procedure or activity to proceed. These are all short-acting drugs, and they are not appropriately prescribed for use outside of a hospital setting. For additional specific information, see the patient care implications section at the end of the chapter.

■ Depolarizing neuromuscular blocking drugs

Succinylcholine chloride (Anectine and others)

Succinylcholine chloride has the briefest duration of action (5 minutes) of the neuromuscular blocking drugs because plasma cholinesterases readily degrade succinylcholine. Longer action requires continuous infusion of succinylcholine, but care must then be taken to avoid desensitizing the muscle. The duration of action is increased by drugs that inhibit cholinesterases. Some patients have abnormal plasma cholinesterases that do not readily degrade succinylcholine. In these patients, the action of succinylcholine will be very prolonged. Conditions that elevate the plasma potassium concentration (hyperkalemia), such as burns, tetanus, massive trauma, or brain or spinal cord injury will prolong the action of succinylcholine.

Uses. The short duration of action makes succinylcholine a drug of choice for such procedures as endoscopy, terminating laryngospasm, endotracheal intubation, orthopedic procedures, and electroconvulsive shock therapy.

Side effects. Children are not as sensitive to succinylcholine on a weight basis as adults and require higher doses. Children are more apt to show side effects of succinylcholine resulting from parasympathetic stimulation: slow heart rate (bradycardia) and cardiac arrhythmias. Succinylcholine does not cross the blood-brain barrier or the placenta.

Succinylcholine initially causes rapid but small contractions of the muscles (fasciculations) before the muscles are paralyzed. This is believed to be the cause of the stiffness and soreness experienced by many patients 12 to 24 hours after receiving succinylcholine. Succinylcholine will also transiently raise intraocular pressure and must be administered before surgery to the eye begins.

Decamethonium bromide (Syncurine)

Decamethonium bromide produces a neuromuscular blockade that lasts for 20 minutes by a mechanism like that of succinylcholine. Decamethonium is excreted unchanged in the urine.

■ PATIENT CARE IMPLICATIONS

Drugs for the diagnosis and treatment of myasthenia gravis

1. Health care professionals should be well-versed in the difference between a myasthenic crisis and a cholinergic crisis before attempting to care for the patient with myasthenia gravis. Overdose with an acetylcholinesterase inhibitor can produce a cholinergic crisis.
2. Edrophonium (Tensilon), pyridostigmine (Mestinon), atropine, neostigmine, and syringes should be kept at the patient's bedside or together in a convenient place on the hospital unit for rapid treatment of a myasthenic or cholinergic crisis.
3. Assess the ability of the myasthenic patient to swallow before preparing an ordered dose of oral anticholinesterase. If the ability to swallow is deteriorating, it may be necessary to administer a parenteral dose of medication rather than an oral dose. Ideally, the physician will have written orders for both oral and parenteral doses of anticholinesterases so that valuable time is not lost in trying to call the physician for a medication order if the patient is slipping into a myasthenic crisis.
4. In the hospital setting, careful scheduling of diagnostic studies and x-ray studies should be done for the patient with myasthenia because the administration of anticholinesterase medications cannot be delayed while waiting for the patient to return to the unit. If the patient is not on the unit when a medication is due, the medication should be taken to the patient.
5. Appropriate parameters to assess in managing the patient with myasthenia include blood pressure, pulse, vital capacity, the presence or degree of ptosis, muscle strength, and ability to swallow. These assessments should be made before each dose of medication is given and whenever the patient's condition seems to be changing.
6. In planning for discharge of a patient with myasthenia gravis, it is important to emphasize the following points to the patient:
   a. Anticholinesterases must be taken as ordered. In all but the mildest cases of the disease, forgetting a dose of medication, taking a dose too early or too late, or omitting an inconvenient dose may cause the disease to go out of control.
   b. No medications, whether prescription or over-the-counter, should ever be taken without first checking with the physician.
   c. Patient should also be taught about and given a list of drugs known to cause weakness.
7. Patients with myasthenia gravis may find it helpful to plan their medication schedule in such a way that they take their anticholinesterase 30 to 60 minutes before meals to increase strength for chewing and swallowing.
8. Taking anticholinesterases with milk or crackers will help to reduce gastric irritation.
9. If the patient at home is ordered to take a dose of medication during the night, a reliable, nonelectric alarm clock should be used to awaken the patient.
10. The patient should be reminded to keep a careful watch on the supply of medication on hand and to refill prescriptions before they run out.
11. Family members need to be taught about the disease and signs and symptoms of myasthenic and cholinergic crises. If the family feels that a patient is not responding appropriately, the patient should be brought to the emergency room.
12. Patients with myasthenia gravis should be encouraged to wear a medical identification tag or bracelet and to carry with them the names and doses of medications being taken.
13. For additional information about the treatment and care of the patient with myasthenia gravis, see appropriate textbooks of medicine or nursing, or the suggested readings listed at the end of this chapter. In addition, patient and health care professionals will find many additional readings by contacting the Myasthenia Gravis Foundation, Inc., New York Academy of Medicine Building, 2 East 103rd Street, New York, New York 10029.
14. If neostigmine is being used, the prior or concomitant use of atropine sulfate may be appropriate to decrease muscarinic side effects. Neostigmine and atropine should never be mixed in the same syringe.
15. When used as an antidote for tubocurarine, neostigmine is administered via slow intravenous push. Appropriate ventilatory support should be continued until the patient is breathing well unassisted. If the pulse is less than 80 beats/minute, atropine should be administered prior to the neostigmine.

16. In any situation in which an anticholinesterase is being administered via continuous infusion, a volume control device and an infusion monitoring device are recommended to control the dilution and rate of administration. Monitor carefully and frequently the respiratory and cardiovascular status.
17. Patients should be reminded to keep these and all medications out of the reach of children.

Neuromuscular blocking agents

1. Monitor the blood pressure, pulse, respirations, and overall respiratory status at regular intervals.
2. Neuromuscular blocking agents should only be used in settings where personnel and equipment are available to provide immediate endotracheal intubation of the patient. There should also be available a suction machine, oxygen, a mechanical ventilator or resuscitation bag, and resuscitation equipment and drugs.
3. Neuromuscular blocking agents are not anesthetics. Patients, unless also anesthetized, can still hear, feel sensations, and see if the eyelids are opened. Health care personnel should be careful not to permit inappropriate discussions in the presence of the patient. Because the patient can still experience pain, it may be appropriate to medicate the patient with analgesics at regular intervals. Careful positioning of the patient should be done, and care should be taken that equipment, instruments, or linens are not placed in an uncomfortable way or against the patient, who would be unable to communicate discomfort.
4. When therapy with a neuromuscular blocking agent is being discontinued, the patient should not be left unattended until enough muscle tone has returned that the patient can breathe, handle secretions, and if not intubated, call for assistance if needed.
5. Patients receiving a depolarizing agent may complain of pain or discomfort in the back, neck, trunk, lower intercostal region, or abdominal wall when first ambulating.
6. Quinidine administered in the immediate postoperative period after tubocurarine has been used may enhance the action of tubocurarine, resulting in respiratory paralysis. Appropriate personnel and equipment should be available (see item 2).
7. Neostigmine is the antidote for tubocurarine; see the patient care implications section for drugs to treat myasthenia gravis.
8. When these drugs are administered via continuous infusion, an infusion monitoring device should be used to control the rate of infusion.
9. Consult the manufacturer's literature for specific guidelines regarding calculation of dosage.

■ SUMMARY

Acetylcholine is the neurotransmitter at the neuromuscular junction. Acetylcholinesterase inhibitors increase the amount of acetylcholine in the neuromuscular junction. This effect is used therapeutically to restore muscle strength in patients with myasthenia gravis or to terminate the action of nondepolarizing neuromuscular blocking drugs after surgery.

Neuromuscular blocking drugs produce muscle relaxation by preventing acetylcholine from stimulating the neuromuscular receptor. These drugs may themselves cause an initial stimulation with subsequent paralysis (depolarizing drugs), as shown by succinylcholine, or the drug may cause paralysis only (nondepolarizing drugs), as shown by tubocurarine.

Neuromuscular blockers are used to produce muscle relaxation during surgery, intubation, or electroconvulsive shock therapy.

■ STUDY QUESTIONS

1. Contrast the mechanisms by which the acetylcholinesterase inhibitors (anticholinesterases) increase activation of the neuromuscular junction and the neuromuscular blockers inhibit activation at the neuromuscular junction.
2. List the muscarinic side effects of neostigmine and pyridostigmine. Which drug may be used as an antidote for neostigmine?
3. Describe two diagnostic uses of edrophonium.
4. Contrast the mechanism of the depolarizing and the nondepolarizing neuromuscular blocking drugs. How does edrophonium distinguish between these actions?
5. List the nondepolarizing neuromuscular blocking drugs.
6. List the depolarizing neuromuscular blocking drugs.
7. List the uses of tubocurarine.
8. What genetic alteration do some patients have that prolongs the action of succinylcholine?

■ SUGGESTED READINGS

Dahl, D.S.: The management of myasthenia gravis, Drug Therapy **6**(10):21, 1976.

DiPalma, J.R.: Pharmacology of myasthenia gravis, American Family Physician **22**(4):158, 1980.

Kao, I., and Drachman, D.B.: Myasthenic immunoglobulin accelerates acetylcholine receptor degradation, Science **196:**527, 1977.

Kinney, A.B., and Blount, M.: Systems approach to myasthenia gravis, Nursing Clinics of North America **6:**435, Sept., 1971.

Winkler, L.H., and Winkler, G.F.: Myasthenia gravis, pathogenesis, diagnosis, and therapy, Postgraduate Medicine **66**(8):50, 1979.

10 Drugs affecting the eye

■ ROLE OF THE AUTONOMIC NERVOUS SYSTEM

The autonomic nervous system plays a major role in controlling the amount of light entering the eye and in focussing images. The amount of light penetrating the eye is controlled by the size of the pigmented iris, which contains two sets of muscles: the sphincter muscles and the dilator muscles. The sphincter muscles are circular muscles with muscarinic receptors innervated by the parasympathetic nervous system. As diagrammed in Fig. 10-1, the pupil is constricted when the sphincter muscles contract so that only a small surface on the eye passes light. The dilator muscles contain alpha receptors innervated by the sympathetic nervous system. *Miosis* is the term that refers to a constricted pupil and is achieved primarily by stimulating the muscarinic receptors of the sphincter muscles. *Mydriasis* is the term that refers to a dilated pupil and is achieved either by blocking the muscarinic receptors of the sphincter muscles or by stimulating the alpha receptors of the dilator muscles.

The cornea and the lens determine the focus of images onto the retina. The cornea accomplishes the coarse focussing, but the fine focussing for sharp images and near vision is accomplished by the lens. The shape of the lens is controlled by muscarinic receptors of the parasympathetic nervous system. As diagrammed in Fig. 10-1, the accommodation for near vision requires the contraction of ciliary muscles to change the shape of the lens. Ligaments normally pull the lens to keep it relatively flat. The contraction of the ciliary muscles relaxes the ligaments so that the lens becomes rounder as required for near vision. *Cycloplegia* refers to the paralysis of the ciliary muscles by drugs that block muscarinic receptors. Cycloplegia causes blurred vision because the shape of the lens can no longer be adjusted for near vision.

■ ANTICHOLINERGIC DRUGS FOR MYDRIASIS AND CYCLOPLEGIA

(Table 10-1)

■ Actions

Classic anticholinergic actions include dilated pupils (mydriasis) and blurred vision (cycloplegia). Accurate measurement of lens refraction requires both of these anticholinergic actions. The relaxation of sphincter and ciliary muscles when anticholinergic drugs are instilled into the eye hastens healing of inflammatory conditions, especially after surgery of the eye. Atropine, scopolamine, and homatropine are used for this type of treatment.

■ Side effects

Anticholinergic drugs used ophthalmically are applied directly to the eye. Systemic reactions may nevertheless occur when the drug is absorbed into the body, particularly with atropine. These systemic reactions are those associated with anticholinergic effects: a dry mouth and dry skin, fever, thirst, confusion, and hyperactivity. Children are the most prone to systemic toxicity from ophthalmic drugs.

■ Specific drugs

Atropine

Atropine is the drug of choice for use in children because atropine is potent and long-acting and children have a very active accommodation. Mydriasis may last 12 days, although accommodation usually returns in 6 days. Since atropine is applied for 3 days, children should be carefully watched for systemic reactions and application discontinued if any reactions appear. Atropine has been reported to cause a contact dermatitis of the eyelids.

Scopolamine

Scopolamine is used like atropine, but cycloplegia lasts for only 3 days instead of 6 days.

Homatropine

Homatropine is applied 2 or 3 times at 10-minute intervals to produce mydriasis and cycloplegia, which are achieved in 60 minutes. Recovery may take 2 days.

Cyclopentolate (Cyclogyl) and tropicamide (Mydricyl)

Cyclopentolate and tropicamide are rapidly acting mydriatic and cycloplegic drugs. Cyclopentolate is ef-

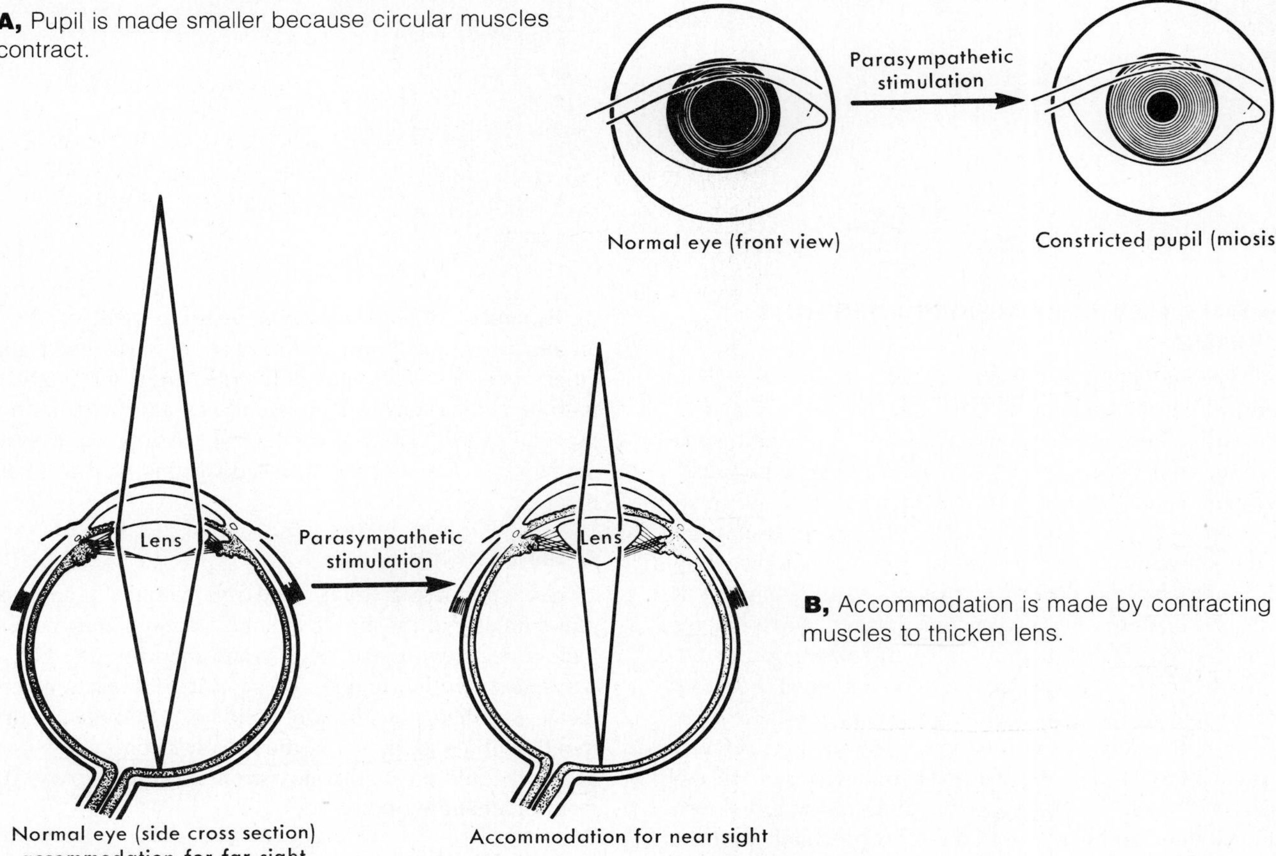

FIG. 10-1

Effects of the parasympathetic nervous system on the eye are shown. These are mediated through muscarinic receptors.

A, Pupil is made smaller because circular muscles contract.

B, Accommodation is made by contracting muscles to thicken lens.

fective in 25 to 75 minutes and accommodation returns in 6 to 24 hours. Tropicamide is effective in 20 to 35 minutes, and accommodation returns in 2 to 6 hours. Systemic reactions have been reported with cyclopentolate but not with tropicamide.

Eucatropine

Eucatropine is a weak anticholinergic drug that causes mydriasis with little cycloplegia and is used when only dilation is desired to examine the interior of the eye.

■ ADRENERGIC DRUGS FOR MYDRIASIS

(Table 10-1)

The adrenergic drugs phenylephrine and hydroxyamphetamine are used as mydriatics when only the interior structures of the eye are to be examined and cycloplegia is not required.

Phenylephrine (Neo-Synephrine and others)

Phenylephrine acts on the alpha receptors of the dilator muscles to produce mydriasis. Dilation is maximal in 60 to 90 minutes, and recovery is in 6 hours. Cyclomydril is a combination of cyclopentolate and phenylephrine used when maximal dilation is required.

Hydroxyamphetamine (Paredrine)

Hydroxyamphetamine is an indirect-acting alpha adrenergic drug that acts by releasing neuronal stores of norepinephrine. Dilation is maximal in 45 to 60 minutes, and recovery is in 6 hours.

■ GLAUCOMA AND DRUG THERAPY

■ Description of glaucoma

Glaucoma is the increase in intraocular pressure as a result of fluid accumulation between the lens and the cornea. The space between the lens and cornea is filled with *aqueous humor*. Aqueous humor is a protein-poor fluid formed by the ciliary body. As indicated in Fig. 10-2, this fluid is normally reabsorbed through the trabecular spaces into Schlemm's canal in a special region of the cornea called the *anterior chamber*. If the aqueous humor cannot be reabsorbed through the anterior chamber, the fluid accumulates and intraocular pressure increases. If the intraocular pressure is not re-

TABLE 10-1. Drugs for mydriasis and cycloplegia

Drug	Trade name	Dosage and administration	Comments
ANTICHOLINERGIC DRUGS FOR MYDRIASIS AND CYCLOPLEGIA			
Atropine sulfate	Atropine Sulfate Atropisol Bufopto Atropine Isopto Atropine	Topical solutions, 0.5% to 3%. *Adults*—1 drop of 1% to 3% solution to each eye. Frequency of administration depends on the condition being treated. *Children*—1 drop of 0.125 to 0.5% solution (under 8 yr) or 0.25 to 1% solution (over 8 yr) 3 times daily for 3 days before and once on the morning of the day refraction is measured. Duration: 6 days.	*Children*—refraction measurements. *Adults*—to relax eye muscles during surgery or treatment of eye inflammation. For adults, to aid in eye surgery or treatment of eye inflammation.
Cyclopentolate hydrochloride	Cyclogyl	Topical solutions, 0.5%, 1%, and 2%. *Adults*—1 drop of solution in each eye, repeated after 5 min. Darker irises or children require the stronger solutions. *Children*—1 drop of solution in each eye, repeated after 10 min. Onset: 25 to 75 min. Duration: 6 to 24 hr.	To aid in measuring refraction.
Homatropine hydrobromide	Isopto Homatropine Homatrocel Homatropine Hydrobromide	Topical solutions, 2% and 5%. *Adults*—for refraction 1 drop of 5% solution every 10 min 2 or 3 times. Duration: 2 days.	To aid in refraction measurements in adults. To aid in treating mild eye inflammation.
Scopolamine hydrobromide	Isopto Hyoscine Hydrobromide	Topical solutions, 0.2% to 0.3%. *Adults*—1 drop of solution or ointment to each eye, 1 or more times daily depending on the condition being treated. *Children*—1 drop of 0.2% to 0.25% solution or ointment twice daily for 2 days before refraction measurement. Duration: 3 days.	For children, to measure refraction. For adults, to treat eye inflammation.
Tropicamide	Mydriacyl	Topical solutions, 0.5% and 1%. 1 drop in each eye, repeated in 5 min. Onset: 20 to 35 min. Duration: 2 to 6 hr	To aid in measuring refraction.
ANTICHOLINERGIC DRUGS FOR MYDRIASIS ONLY			
Eucatropine hydrochloride	Eucatropine Hydrochloride	Topical solutions, 5% and 10%. 1 drop in each eye repeated in 10 to 15 min for dilation. 2 drops in one eye to test for acute glaucoma. Onset: 30 min. Duration: 2 to 4 hr.	To dilate the eye for examination with little cycloplegia. To test for intraocular pressure rise when acute glaucoma is suspected.
ADRENERGIC DRUGS FOR MYDRIASIS ONLY			
Hydroxyamphetamine hydrobromide	Paredrine	Topical use, 1 drop of a 1% solution.	Maximal mydriasis in 45 to 60 min. Recovery in 6 hr.
Phenylephrine hydrochloride	Efricel Mydfrin Neo-Synephrine Hydrochloride	Topical use, 1 drop of a 2.5% solution.	Maximal mydriasis in 60 to 90 min. Recovery in 6 hr.

FIG. 10-2

A, Normal eye or eye with chronic glaucoma. Flow of aqueous humor is shown from the ciliary body and around iris. Aqueous humor is normally absorbed into the body through trabecular network into Schlemm's canal. In chronic glaucoma, aqueous humor accumulates because trabecular network degenerates.

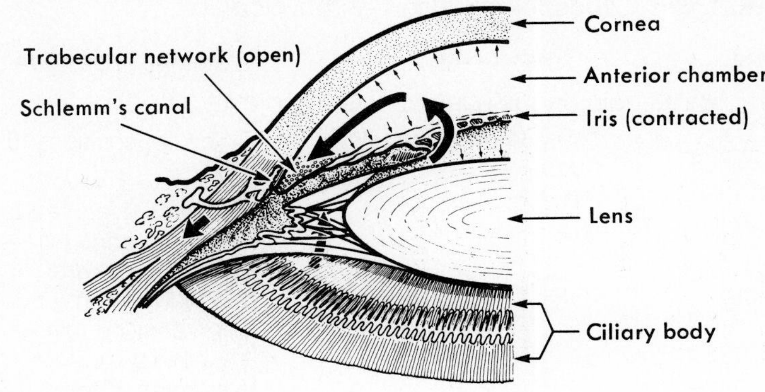

B, Eye in acute glaucoma. Flow of aqueous humor is stopped because iris has blocked trabecular network and Schlemm's canal. Aqueous humor can accumulate quickly to cause a marked rise in ocular pressure that may damage optic nerve.

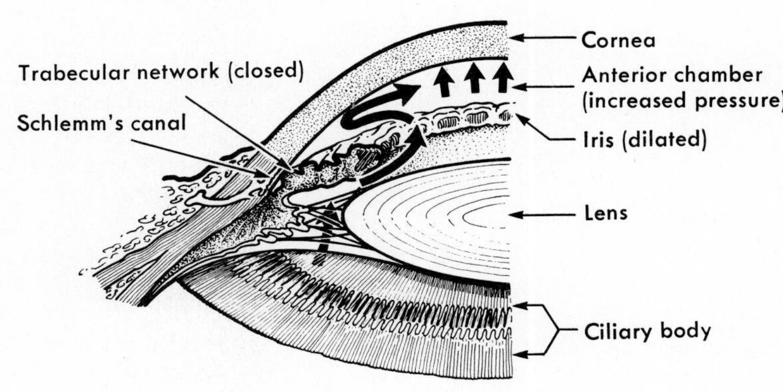

lieved, the optic nerve will become damaged, resulting in blindness.

Chronic (open-angle) glaucoma is the more common form of glaucoma and is very gradual in its onset. The defect is a slow degeneration of the anterior chamber so that the uptake of aqueous humor is impaired (Fig. 10-2).

The initial treatment for chronic glaucoma is usually the application of a weak cholinomimetic drug to cause constriction of the pupil (miosis). The therapeutic effectiveness is a result of the spread of the trabecular spaces of the anterior chamber when the sphincter muscles contract. The larger area allows improved uptake of the aqueous humor, which relieves intraocular pressure.

The adrenergic drug epinephrine is the alternate drug to initiate therapy or the next drug added when the miotic drug alone is inadequate. Epinephrine stimulates both alpha and beta receptors, and in the eye, stimulation of alpha receptors reduces resistance to the outflow of aqueous humor, whereas stimulation of the beta receptors decreases production of aqueous humor.

The new adrenergic beta-blocking drug timolol may also be used initially to treat chronic glaucoma or may be applied in addition to the miotic and epinephrine. The mechanism by which blockade of the beta receptors of the eye decreases intraocular pressure is not clear, particularly since stimulation of the beta receptor also causes reduction of intraocular pressure.

The drugs discussed so far are all applied directly to the eye. In resistant cases of glaucoma, systemic drugs are added. A carbonic anhydrase inhibitor is the next drug added because aside from being weak diuretics, carbonic anhydrase inhibitors are also effective in decreasing the production of aqueous humor.

Osmotic agents such as glycerin, isosorbide, urea, or mannitol provide an immediate but short-term reduction in intraocular pressure by drawing fluid from the eyeball to the hyperosmotic blood.

Acute (closed-angle) glaucoma is characterized by the iris bulging up to shut off access of the aqueous humor to the anterior chamber, as shown in Fig. 10-2. This creates an emergency because the build-up of intraocular pressure may become severe rapidly, damaging the optic nerve and causing blindness. Emergency treatment consists of a cholinomimetic drug, a carbonic anhydrase inhibitor, epinephrine, and an osmotic diuretic. This drug regimen is transient treatment while the patient is being prepared for eye surgery in which the iris is cut to allow fluid access to the anterior chamber again.

■ Cholinomimetic (miotic) drugs to treat glaucoma (Table 10-2)

Pilocarpine (Pilocar and others)

Pilocarpine is the drug of choice for chronic and acute glaucoma. It is a direct-acting cholinomimetic that is active 15 to 30 minutes after application and which

TABLE 10-2. Drugs to treat glaucoma

Generic name	Trade name	Dosage and administration	Comments
CHOLINOMIMETIC DRUGS (WEAK MIOTICS)			
Carbachol	Carbacel Isopto Carbachol Mistura-C	TOPICAL: 1 drop 0.75% to 3% solution every 8 hr. Onset: 15 to 30 min.	Direct-acting cholinomimetic; miotic, for treating chronic glaucoma.
Physostigmine sulfate	Eserine Sulfate	TOPICAL: 1 drop of 0.25% to 1% every 4 to 6 hr. Ointment at night. Onset: 30 min.	Acetylcholinesterase inhibitor; miotic for chronic glaucoma; conjunctivitis and allergic reactions common if use is prolonged.
Physostigmine salicylate	Isopto Eserine		
Pilocarpine hydrochloride	Isopto Carpine Pilocar Various others	TOPICAL: 1 drop, 1% to 2% every 6 to 8 hr. Onset: 15 to 30 min.	Direct-acting cholinomimetic; miotic; drug of choice for treating glaucoma, acute and chronic.
Pilocarpine nitrate	P.V. Carpine Liquifilm	TOPICAL: 1 drop, 1% to 2% every 6 to 8 hr. Onset: 15 to 30 min.	Direct-acting cholinomimetic; miotic; drug of choice for treating glaucoma, acute and chronic.
CHOLINOMIMETIC DRUGS (STRONG MIOTICS)			
Demecarium bromide	Humorsol	TOPICAL: 1 drop 0.125% to 0.25% solution every 12 to 48 hr. Onset: 12 hr.	Irreversible acetylcholinesterase inhibitor; potent miotic for resistant chronic glaucoma. Cataracts can develop with long-term administration.
Echothiophate iodide	Phospholine Iodide	TOPICAL: 1 drop 0.03% to 0.06% every 12 to 48 hr. Onset: 12 hr.	Same as for demecarium.
Isoflurophate	Floropryl	¼ in strip of 0.025% ointment every 12 to 72 hr. Onset: 12 hr.	Same as for demecarium.
ADRENERGIC DRUGS			
Epinephrine bitartrate	Epitrate Murocel Mytrate	TOPICAL: 1 drop of a 0.25% to 2.0% solution one or two times daily.	Persons with darkly pigmented irises may require a higher concentration of solution.
Epinephrine borate	Epinal Eppy	Same.	
Epinephrine hydrochloride	Epifrin Glaucon	Same.	
Timolol maleate	Timoptic	TOPICAL: 1 drop of 0.25% solution twice daily. If not sufficient, a 0.5% solution is used.	A beta-adrenergic receptor antagonist.
CARBONIC ANHYDRASE INHIBITORS			
Acetazolamide	Diamox	ORAL: *Adults*—250 mg every 6 hr. *Children*—10 to 15 mg/kg body weight daily in divided doses. Timed-release capsules are taken every 12 to 24 hr but may not be as effective.	A weak diuretic.
Acetazolamide sodium	Diamox, Parenteral	INTRAVENOUS, INTRAMUSCULAR: *Adults*—500 mg repeated in 2 to 4 hr if necessary. *Children:* 5 to 10 mg/kg body weight every 6 hr.	

Continued.

TABLE 10-2. Drugs to treat glaucoma—cont'd

Generic name	Trade name	Dosage and administration	Comments
Dichlorphenamide	Daranide Oratrol	ORAL: *Adults*—50 to 200 mg every 6 to 8 hr.	
Ethoxzolamide	Cardrase Ethamide	ORAL: *Adults*—125 mg every 6 to 8 hr.	
Methazolamide	Neptazane	ORAL: *Adults*—25 to 100 mg every 8 hr.	
OSMOTIC AGENTS			
Glycerin	Glyrol Osmoglyn	ORAL: *Adults and children*—1 to 1.5 Gm/kg body weight as a 50% or 75% solution once or twice daily.	May flavor with instant coffee or lemon juice to increase palatability. May chill with chipped ice. May cause hyperglycemia in diabetic patients.
Isosorbide	Ismotic	ORAL: *Adults*—1.5 Gm/kg body weight up to 4 times daily.	May chill with chipped ice.
Mannitol	Osmitrol	INTRAVENOUS: *Adults and children*—0.5 to 2 Gm/kg body weight as a 20% solution infused over 30 to 60 min.	May discontinue when intraocular pressure is decreased even though the full dose has not been given.
Urea	Ureaphil Urevert	INTRAVENOUS: *Adults*—0.5 to 2 Gm/kg body weight as a 30% solution infused at 60 drops/min. *Children*—0.5 to 1.5 Gm/kg body weight of a 30% solution infused over 30 min.	Infuse carefully. Patients with hereditary fructose intolerance should not be given urea made up in invert sugar.

lasts 4 to 8 hours. Since pilocarpine is the weakest of the cholinomimetic drugs used, it is the least likely to produce side effects, although it must be applied more frequently. The Ocusert system has been devised to overcome the need for frequent application of pilocarpine. The system is placed in the upper or lower cul-de-sac of the eye. Pilocarpine is contained in a reservoir between two membranes and is released over a period of 1 week. The drawbacks include the occasional sudden leakage of pilocarpine, the migration of the system over the cornea, and the unrealized loss of the system from the eye.

Carbachol (Carbacel and others)

Carbachol is also a direct-acting cholinomimetic agent. It is more potent and slightly longer acting than pilocarpine.

Physostigmine (Eserine)

Physostigmine is a short-acting acetylcholinesterase inhibitor that is occasionally used in place of pilocarpine or carbachol in the treatment of chronic glaucoma.

Demecarium (Humorsol), echothiophate (Phosphaline), and isoflurophate (Floropryl)

These three potent acetylcholinesterase inhibitors are used to treat chronic glaucoma not responsive to the combination of a weak miotic, epinephrine, and timolol. The effect of these acetylcholinesterase inhibitors is not seen for about 24 hours, but a single application is effective for 12 to 72 hours. Unfortunately, side effects are frequent with these potent miotics. They can cause congestion in the blood vessels of the ciliary body, resulting in a rise in the intraocular pressure. For this reason, they are seldom used to treat acute glaucoma. Spasms may be produced in the muscles of the eyelid as well as the eye itself, resulting in twitching of the eyelids or eyebrows, ocular pain, and headaches.

■ Additional drugs to treat glaucoma

(Table 10-2)

Epinephrine (Glaucon and others)

Epinephrine stimulates both alpha and beta adrenergic receptors to increase uptake of aqueous humor and to decrease production of aqueous humor, respectively. When applied directly to the eye in the treatment of chronic glaucoma, epinephrine produces a fall in intraocular pressure that lasts 12 to 24 hours. Mydriasis is transient. Epinephrine may be used as the initial therapy for glaucoma in young patients, who may suffer spasms of the ciliary muscles controlling accommodation if a miotic is used, and in elderly patients with cataracts, whose vision is compromised by small pupils. Highly pigmented eyes are more resistant to epinephrine than lightly pigmented eyes.

Side effects. Epinephrine can cause a browache and can irritate the eyes. With prolonged use, epinephrine can cause swelling of the eyelids and bloodshot eyes. Symptoms of systemic absorption of epinephrine include a fast heart rate (tachycardia), high blood pressure, headache, sweating, and tremors.

Timolol (Timoptic)

Timolol is a beta adrenergic antagonist that blocks both beta-1 and beta-2 receptors. Since timolol is a new drug, its role and long-term effectiveness in treating glaucoma is still being established. The major advantage of timolol is that neither pupil size nor reactivity to light is altered. There may be some irritation and blurred vision at the start of therapy, but these effects usually disappear.

Timolol lowers intraocular pressure within 20 minutes after administration in eyes with normal or elevated pressure and requires application only twice a day. Other beta adrenergic antagonists have proved unsatisfactory because they have a local anesthetic effect, produce systemic effects, or have some activity as beta adrenergic agonists. Tolerance may develop to timolol so that in long-term therapy intraocular pressure is no longer reduced.

Side effects. Timolol may also produce systemic effects after absorption into the circulation. The most common effects are a decrease in heart rate (bradycardia) and a fall in blood pressure, effects expected with a drug that blocks beta-1 adrenergic receptors. Bronchospasm resulting from blockade of the beta-2 adrenergic receptors has also been reported. Because of these systemic effects, timolol should be used cautiously with patients who have asthma, heart block, or heart failure.

Carbonic anhydrase inhibitors

Carbonic anhydrase inhibitors to treat glaucoma include *acetazolamide (Diamox), dichlorphenamide (Daranide, Oratrol), ethoxzolamide (Cardrase, ethamide),* and *methazolamide (Neptazane).* Although carbonic anhydrase inhibitors are weak diuretics, the effective action in treating glaucoma is to decrease the formation of aqueous humor. A fall in intraocular pressure is seen only in those individuals with elevated ocular pressure (glaucoma). The fall in intraocular pressure is negligible in individuals with normal ocular pressure.

The carbonic anhydrase inhibitors are taken orally and are maximally effective in 2 hours. The duration of action is 6 to 12 hours. Carbonic anhydrase inhibitors may be added to glaucoma therapy when the combination of a weak miotic, epinephrine, and timolol does not adequately lower the intraocular pressure of chronic glaucoma. Carbonic anhydrase inhibitors are also used with a miotic and epinephrine to lower intraocular pressure in acute (closed-angle) gluacoma.

Side effects. Carbonic anhydrase inhibitors have a number of unpleasant side effects including a loss of appetite, gastrointestinal upset, and a general feeling of lethargy and depression. A tingling sensation (paresthesia) in the fingers, toes, and face is common. Carbonic anhydrase inhibitors commonly produce a slight hypokalemia early in treatment; thus caution should be used in treating patients who are receiving digitalis.

Osmotic agents

Osmotic agents include glycerin (Glyrol, Osmoglyn), isosorbide (Ismotic), mannitol (Osmitrol), and urea (Ureaphil, Urevert). These are used for the short-term treatment only to lower the intraocular pressure of glaucoma prior to surgery or as an emergency treatment of acute (closed-angle) glaucoma. Glycerin and isosorbide are administered orally, whereas mannitol and urea are administered intravenously.

Glycerin. Glycerin is effective in lowering intraocular pressure 60 minutes after ingestion, and the effect lasts 5 hours. Since glycerin is metabolized, it does not cause a diuresis, but glycerin can cause hyperglycemia in a patient with diabetes. A headache and nausea and vomiting are other side effects of glycerin.

Isosorbide. Isosorbide is sometimes used in the emergency treatment of acute (closed-angle) glaucoma. Isosorbide does produce a diuresis but otherwise has few side effects.

Mannitol. Mannitol is effective in lowering intraocular pressure in 30 to 60 minutes, and the effect lasts for 6 to 8 hours. Mannitol produces a pronounced diuresis and will often cause a headache, nausea and vomiting, and dehydration.

Urea. Urea is less satisfactory than mannitol because urea can penetrate the eye and cause a rebound increase in intraocular pressure when the systemic osmotic effect is over, 8 to 12 hours after administration. Urea is also highly irritating on injection.

■ THE NURSING PROCESS

■ Assessment

Patients requiring treatment of eye conditions often have no externally visible signs of their condition. A thorough patient assessment should be done, especially of symptoms related to the eye. The nurse should check peripheral vision and test visual acuity using a Snellen chart or asking the patient to read something during the examination process. The patient should be questioned about recent difficulties in driving or ambulating in the home setting; such difficulties might include tripping or bumping into objects. The nurse should examine the eyes closely for any signs of infection, exudate, excessive tearing or dryness, or any other deviation from normal.

■ Management

The drugs discussed in this chapter are used for purposes of assisting in further evaluation of eye problems or in treating glaucoma. Before receiving these eye medications for the first time, the patient should be warned about effects that will occur, particularly those related to vision. Blurred vision, photophobia, and other eye symptoms can be frightening to a patient when they occur without warning. In addition, the nurse should teach the patient about possible systemic side effects that may occur.

■ Evaluation

Drugs used to assist in diagnostic evaluation of the eye are considered successful if they aid in the examination desired without producing local or systemic side effects. Drugs used to treat glaucoma are considered successful if the intraocular pressure is lowered to within safe limits. Before discharging any patient taking eye medications, it is important that the patient be able to explain why the drug is being used, to demonstrate how to administer the drug correctly, to explain the local and systemic side effects that might occur as a result of drug therapy, to explain what signs and symptoms should prompt the patient to contact the physician, and, particularly in the case of glaucoma, to explain the need for continuing therapy as ordered. For additional specific information, see the patient care implications section at the end of the chapter.

■ PATIENT CARE IMPLICATIONS

General guidelines for use of eye drops

1. Patients receiving any topical eye medications should be taught to apply or instill them properly. Medications should be placed in the lower conjunctival sac and never directly on the cornea. The patient should avoid touching any part of the eye with the applicator or dropper. Each patient should have a separate bottle of medication; patients at home should be instructed to avoid sharing a bottle of eye medications. Finally, patients should be instructed to avoid putting anything in the eye that is not clearly marked for ophthalmic use only. For additional information on administration of eye medications, see the suggested readings at the end of the chapter or any fundamental nursing textbook.
2. Though eye drops may seem to be less harmful than other medications, they should be kept out of the reach of children.
3. Some eye preparations are available in a variety of concentrations. Review with patients the prescribed concentration, and caution patients to read labels carefully, especially when prescriptions are refilled, to ensure the correct dose is being used.
4. To prevent overflow of medications into the nasal and pharyngeal passages and to reduce the incidence of systemic side effects with some preparations, the patient may be instructed to occlude the nasolacrimal duct with one finger for 1 to 2 minutes after the medication has been applied and before the patient closes the eyelid. Check with the physician.

Drugs for mydriasis and cycloplegia

1. Atropine and the belladonna alkaloids may precipitate an attack of acute glaucoma in elderly patients or those predisposed to angle closure; thus they should be given cautiously to these patients.

2. Patients receiving mydriatics should be warned that their vision will be temporarily impaired. Wearing sunglasses may lessen the photophobia.
3. Review with patients and parents of children receiving atropine the possible systemic side effects that can occur (Chapter 7). Instruct patients to report any unusual signs or symptoms.
4. Patients receiving drugs causing cycloplegia should be cautioned to avoid activities requiring visual acuity, such as driving or operating machinery, until the paralysis of the ciliary muscles disappears and visual acuity returns to normal. Patients being treated in an outpatient setting should not be permitted to drive home alone.
5. Review with patients the anticipated duration of action of the specific eye medication being used so that the patient can anticipate how long vision may be reduced.

Drugs used to treat glaucoma

1. Patients receiving miotic drugs should be warned not to drive immediately after administration of the drug.
2. The pain and blurred vision commonly experienced at the beginning of treatment will usually diminish with repeated usage. Painful eye spasms can be relieved by application of cold compresses.
3. Patients with glaucoma should be instructed that their eye medications are as important to their well-being as any other medications and should not be discontinued without prior consultation with the physician.
4. One drop of a 1% to 2% epinephrine solution reverses the redness caused by the potent acetylcholinesterase inhibitors.
5. Pralidoxime (PAM), 0.1 to 0.2 ml of a 5% solution, reverses the action of the irreversible acetylcholinesterase inhibitors. PAM must be injected subconjunctivally to be effective in the eye.
6. Acetylcholinesterase inhibitors should be discontinued 2 weeks before surgery because of possible interactions with anesthetic agents.
7. Systemic side effects to epinephrine are rare and usually only occur if there is damage to the eye or the epithelium that comes in contact with the drug.
8. The carbonic anhydrase inhibitors and osmotic agents are discussed in chapter 14.
9. Monitor the pulse of patients receiving timolol and teach the patients to check their pulse regularly, if appropriate. Because this drug causes bradycardia, it should not be administered if the pulse is below 50 or 60 beats/minute; check with the physician.

■ SUMMARY

Miosis refers to constricted pupils and is achieved with instillation of certain cholinomimetic drugs.

Mydriasis refers to a dilated pupil and is achieved with instillation of certain anticholinergic drugs that also paralyze the muscles of accommodation (cycloplegia). Mydriasis is produced without cycloplegia by sympathomimetic drugs acting at alpha adrenergic receptors.

Glaucoma refers to a condition in which there is a build-up of aqueous humor behind the cornea such that the pressure may damage the optic nerve if not relieved. Drainage of aqueous humor is achieved by instillation of drugs that decrease the production of aqueous humor and/or increase the uptake of aqueous humor.

■ STUDY QUESTIONS

1. Define miosis, mydriasis, and cycloplegia.
2. What are the anticholinergic actions in the eye? How are these actions medically useful?
3. Which anticholinergic drugs are used in the eye?
4. What action is mediated by the alpha adrenergic receptor in the eye? Which drugs are used for this effect?
5. Describe glaucoma and the role of aqueous humor.
6. Differentiate between chronic and acute glaucoma.
7. What role do cholinomimetic drugs play in the treatment of glaucoma? Which drugs are used?
8. What role do drugs acting at adrenergic receptors play in the treatment of glaucoma? Describe the actions of epinephrine and timolol.
9. What role do carbonic anhydrase inhibitors and osmotic agents play in the treatment of glaucoma?

■ SUGGESTED READINGS

Boyd-Monk, H.: Screening for glaucoma, Nursing '79 **9**(8):42, 1979.

Editors: When the eyes get it, Emergency Medicine **7**(8):35, 1975.

Giving medication, Horsham, Pa., 1980, Intermed Communications, Inc.

Katz, I.M., and Soll, D.B.: Beta blockers and glaucoma, American Family Physician **21**(4):150, 1980.

Kosman, M.: Trends in therapy, Department of Drugs: timolol in the treatment of open angle glaucoma, J.A.M.A. **241:**2301, 1977.

Quail, C., and Waddleton, C.: Treating the glaucomas, Nurses' Drug Alert **4**(9):93, 1980.

Soll, D.B., and Philips, A.: Update on glaucoma management, Drug Therapy **9**(10):88, 1979.

Waddleton, C.: Eye openers: uses and precautions, Nurses' Drug Alert **2:**132, Nov., 1978.

Wong, E.K., Wang, S., and Leopold, I.H.: How ophthalmic drugs can fool you, RN **43:**36, March, 1980.

11 Drugs affecting the gastrointestinal tract

■ OVERVIEW

The gastrointestinal system processes food and water and eliminates undigestible material. The parasympathetic (cholinergic) nervous system acts as a major stimulant of the digestive processes by increasing both digestive secretions and the tone and motility of the smooth muscle of the stomach and intestines. The sympathetic (adrenergic) nervous system plays a minor role in the digestive processes. Although the parasympathetic nervous system acts on all parts of the digestive tract, current research is uncovering a complex system in which activities in each section of the digestive tract are further regulated by a variety of peptide hormones, prostaglandins, and the biogenic amines histamine and serotonin. At the present time the roles of only a few of these factors are well characterized. This chapter focuses on specific conditions affecting the gastrointestinal tract for which there are pharmacological interventions.

Tone and motility of the small intestine

Drugs affecting the activity of the parasympathetic nervous system in the gastrointestinal tract are presently used mainly to modify the tone and motility of the smooth muscle layers of the intestinal tract.

■ CHOLINOMIMETIC DRUGS TO INCREASE TONE AND MOTILITY (Table 11-1)

Cholinomimetic drugs play a minor role in the treatment of gastrointestinal disorders. Occasionally, bethanecol or neostigmine is administered to stimulate an atonic intestine or bladder.

Bethanechol (Urecholine)

Bethanechol is the only direct-acting cholinomimetic drug with sufficient tissue specificity to be administered systemically. At therapeutic doses, bethanechol is relatively specific for the urinary and gastrointestinal tracts. This stimulation is useful for situations in which the bladder or intestine has lost its tone, such as after childbirth, surgery, or other abdominal trauma.

Side effects of bethanechol are those expected from muscarinic stimulation: salivation, flushing of the skin, sweating, diarrhea, nausea and belching, and abdominal cramps.

Bethanechol should never be administered if there is any mechanical obstruction of the gastrointestinal or urinary tract, such as stones or adhesions, because the hypermotility caused by the drug could lead to rupture of the tissue in the presence of an obstruction. Also bethanechol is never administered intravenously or intramuscularly because the rate of absorption is so fast that toxic plasma concentrations of the drug are reached, resulting in possible heart block or a severe drop in blood pressure. Bethanechol may be administered subcutaneously if the oral route is not effective.

Neostigmine (Prostigmin)

Neostigmine is a reversible acetylcholinesterase inhibitor that is prescribed for its muscarinic as well as

TABLE 11-1. Cholinergic drugs affecting gastrointestinal motility and secretion

Generic name	Trade name	Dosage and administration	Comments
CHOLINOMIMETIC DRUGS: TO INCREASE TONE AND MOTILITY			
Bethanechol chloride	Urecholine Duvoid Myotonachol	ORAL: *Adults*—10 to 30 mg every 6 to 8 hr. SUBCUTANEOUS: *Adults*—2.5 to 5 mg every 6 to 8 hr; maximum, 10 mg/day. Never give IV or IM Onset: 30 min.	Direct-acting cholinomimetic; stimulates atonic bladder, gastrointestinal tract.
Neostigmine methylsulfate	Prostigmin Methylsulfate	SUBCUTANEOUS, INTRAMUSCULAR: *Adults*—0.25 to 0.5 mg every 3 to 4 hr to stimulate bladder or gastrointestinal tract. Onset: 10 to 20 min.	Acetylcholinesterase inhibitor; stimulates atonic bladder, gastrointestinal tract.
ANTICHOLINERGIC DRUGS—ANTISPASMODIC DRUGS: TO DECREASE TONE AND MOTILITY			
Belladonna alkaloids (uncharged)			
Atropine sulfate		ORAL, SUBCUTANEOUS: *Adults*—0.3 to 1.2 mg every 4 to 6 hr. SUBCUTANEOUS: *Children*—0.01 mg/kg every 4 to 6 hr.	Reduces gastrointestinal motility and gastric acid secretion. Also reduces the tone of the bladder and ureter.
Belladonna extract		ORAL: *Adults*—15 mg every 8 hr.	As above. Atropine is the active ingredient.
Belladonna fluid extract		ORAL: *Adults*—0.06 ml every 8 hr.	As above. Atropine is the active ingredient.
Belladonna leaf		ORAL: *Adults*—30 to 200 mg.	As above. Atropine is the active ingredient.
Belladonna tincture		ORAL: *Adults*—0.6 to 1 ml every 6 to 8 hr. *Children*—0.03 ml/kg in 3 or 4 divided doses.	As above. Atropine is the active ingredient.
Hyoscyamine hydrobromide (L-isomer of atropine)		ORAL, INTRAMUSCULAR, SUBCUTANEOUS, INTRAVENOUS: *Adults*—0.25 mg every 6 to 8 hr.	As above. Atropine is the active ingredient.
Hyoscyamine sulfate	Anaspaz Levsin	ORAL: *Adults*—0.125 to 0.25 mg every 4 to 6 hr. *Children*—2 to 10 yr, ½ adult dosage; under 2 yr, ¼ adult dosage. INTRAMUSCULAR, SUBCUTANEOUS, INTRAVENOUS: *Adults*—0.25 to 0.5 mg every 4 to 6 hr.	As above. Atropine is the active ingredient.
Charged derivatives of atropine			
Homatropine methylbromide	Homapin Mesopin-PB	ORAL: *Adults*—2.5 to 10 mg every 6 hr. *Children*—3 to 6 mg every 6 hr. *Infants*—0.3 mg dissolved in water every 4 hr.	To reduce gastrointestinal hypermotility and gastric acidity.
Methscopolamine bromide	Pamine	ORAL: *Adults*—2.5 to 5 mg every 6 hr. *Children*—0.2 mg/kg every 6 hr. INTRAMUSCULAR, SUBCUTANEOUS: *Adults*—0.25 to 1 mg every 6 to 8 hr. Onset: 1 hr.	To reduce gastrointestinal hypermotility and gastric acidity.
Synthetic substitutes for atropine			
Anisotropine methylbromide	Valpin	ORAL: *Adults*—50 mg 3 times daily. Onset: 1 hr.	To treat gastrointestinal spasms and to control gastric acid secretion.

Continued.

TABLE 11-1. Cholinergic drugs affecting gastrointestinal motility and secretion—cont'd

Generic name	Trade name	Dosage and administration	Comments
ANTICHOLINERGIC DRUGS—ANTISPASMODIC DRUGS: TO DECREASE TONE AND MOTILITY—cont'd			
Synthetic substitutes for atropine—cont'd			
Diphemanil methylsulfate	Prantal	ORAL: 100 to 200 mg every 4 to 6 hr initially, then 50 to 100 mg every 4 to 6 hr for maintenance. Onset: 1 to 2 hr. Timed-release, 100 to 200 mg every 8 hr.	Aid in control of gastric acid or excessive sweating.
Glycopyrrolate	Robinul-PH	ORAL: 1 to 2 mg 3 times daily initially, then 1 to 2 mg 2 times daily for maintenance. Onset: 1 hr. INTRAMUSCULAR, SUBCUTANEOUS, INTRAVENOUS: 0.1 to 0.2 mg every 4 hr. Onset: 10 min.	To treat gastrointestinal hypermotility and control gastric acidity.
Mepenzolate bromide	Cantil	ORAL: *Adults*—25 mg 4 times daily. Increase to 50 mg if necessary.	
Methantheline bromide	Banthine	ORAL: *Adults*—50 to 100 mg every 6 hr initially; reduce by ½ for maintenance. *Children*—6 mg/kg daily in 4 doses. Onset: 30 min. INTRAMUSCULAR: *Adults*—50 mg every 6 hr. *Children*—6 mg/kg daily in 4 doses. Onset: 30 min.	Used like atropine.
Oxyphen-cyclimine hydrochloride	Daricon	ORAL: 10 mg 2 times daily; can be increased to 50 mg if tolerated.	To treat gastric acidity or hypermotility of the gastrointestinal, genitourinary, or biliary tract.
Propantheline bromide	Pro-Banthine	ORAL: *Adults*—15 mg 3 times daily plus 30 mg at bedtime or 30 mg timed-release every 8 to 12 hr. *Children*—1.5 mg/kg daily every 6 hr. INTRAMUSCULAR OR INTRAVENOUS: *Adults*—30 mg every 6 hr.	To control gastric acidity and hypermotility of gastrointestinal, genitourinary, and biliary tracts.
Antispasmodic drugs			
Dicyclomine hydrochloride	Bentyl Dyspas	ORAL OR INTRAMUSCULAR: *Adults*—10 to 20 mg 3 or 4 times daily. *Children*—10 mg 3 or 4 times daily. *Infants*—5 mg 3 or 4 times daily.	To control hypermotility of the colon.
Methixene hydrochloride	Trest	ORAL: 1 mg 2 to 3 times daily.	To control hypermotility of the gastrointestinal tract.
Thiphenamil hydrochloride	Trocinate	ORAL: *Adults*—400 mg every 4 hr. *Children*—over 6 yr, 200 mg every 4 hr.	To control hypermotility of the gastrointestinal tract.
Tridihexethyl-chloride	Pathilon	ORAL: 25 mg 3 times daily before meals and 50 mg at bedtime. Timed-release, 75 mg every 6 to 12 hr. INTRAMUSCULAR, SUBCUTANEOUS, INTRAVENOUS: *Adults*—10 to 20 mg every 6 hr.	To control gastric acidity and hypermotility of the gastrointestinal tract.

■ THE NURSING PROCESS WITH CHOLINOMIMETIC DRUGS USED TO INCREASE TONE AND MOTILITY

■ Assessment

Patients requiring cholinomimetic drugs to increase tone and motility are patients who have had recent trauma or surgery and have resultant atonic intestines or bladder. A thorough patient assessment should be done, especially to rule out any obstruction of the bladder or intestine. The nurse should assess the vital signs, check for the presence of bowel sounds, check the fluid intake and output, and palpate the bladder for distention. If a urinary catheter is in place, the nurse should ascertain that it is patent.

■ Management

Because both bethanechol and neostigmine are potent, the nurse should anticipate remaining at the bedside for at least 15 minutes after the drug is administered to observe the patient for side effects. Side effects will usually occur with bethanechol, especially if given via the subcutaneous route. The known drug antidote, atropine, should be readily available before the drug is administered. After the drug is administered, the nurse should monitor the vital signs and measure any fluid or solid output that results from the administration of the medication. If side effects become serious, the nurse should notify the physician and/or consider administering atropine (0.6 mg).

■ Evaluation

These drugs are considered effective if they increase intestinal tone and/or bladder tone, enhancing the patient's ability to defecate or urinate. In some patients only one or two doses are necessary, after which the patient's body is able to maintain motility unaided. Other patients will require continuous use of these drugs on an outpatient basis. Before discharging a patient for self-management, the patient should be able to explain how to take the drug correctly, the anticipated effects of the drug, the side effects that may occur and what to do about them, and which symptoms should prompt the patient to seek medical attention. For additional specific information, see the patient care implications section at the end of this chapter.

---

its neuromuscular effects (Chapter 9). Neostigmine may be given subcutaneously or intramuscularly in place of bethanechol to restore bladder or intestinal tone. If urination does not occur within 1 hour, the patient should be catheterized.

■ ANTICHOLINERGIC AND ANTISPASMODIC DRUGS TO DECREASE TONE AND MOTILITY

(Table 11-1)

Anticholinergic drugs (drugs that block muscarinic receptors) inhibit gastric acid secretion and depress gastrointestinal motility. These actions are useful in treating a peptic ulcer or in treating hyperactive bowel disorders.

Table 11-1 lists atropine and its derivatives as well as the synthetic anticholinergic drugs that are used to depress gastric acid secretion in treating peptic ulcers. Homatropine and the synthetic drugs are charged compounds that do not cross the blood-brain barrier to act in the central nervous system. Oxyphencyclimine is an uncharged synthetic compound and is the exception.

Common side effects of anticholinergic drugs are the classic anticholinergic effects described for atropine: dry mouth, photophobia from dilated pupils (mydriasis), blurred vision (cycloplegia), fast heart rate (tachycardia), constipation, and acute urinary retention. In fact, patients are not getting a dose large enough to suppress acid secretion if they do not have a dry mouth.

Toxic doses of the uncharged anticholinergic drugs atropine (and its L-isomer, hyoscyamine) and oxyphencyclimine reach the central nervous system and produce central nervous system stimulation: restlessness, tremor, irritability, delirium, or hallucinations. Toxic doses of the charged anticholinergic drugs that do not reach the central nervous system cause ganglionic blockade (usually seen as orthostatic hypotension) or neuromuscular blockade. Death can result from respiratory arrest secondary to neuromuscular blockade.

Table 11-1 also lists drugs that were found to have antispasmodic but not anticholinergic effects. These

■ THE NURSING PROCESS WITH ANTICHOLINERGIC AND ANTISPASMODIC DRUGS TO DECREASE TONE AND MOTILITY

■ Assessment

The drugs in this section are used for selected patients who have problems related to excessive intestinal motility or peptic ulcer. A generalized patient assessment should be done with attention to the following points: the vital signs, any subjective patient complaints, the frequency and character of stools, and a check for the presence of occult blood in the stools.

■ Management

These drugs are usually used in conjunction with dietary management and other therapies to decrease gastric acid or the symptoms associated with hyperactive bowel disease. The nurse should continue to monitor the patient's subjective complaints and vital signs and to observe the patient for the presence of side effects. The anticholinergic drugs and related compounds should produce side effects if administered in effective dosages. The nurse should assist the patient in finding ways to deal with unpleasant side effects, for instance, sucking on hard candy for treatment of dry mouth. The intake and output of solids and liquids should be checked and the patient questioned about constipation. The nurse should look for central nervous system effects such as restlessness, tremor, or irritability, since these symptoms may indicate a need to reduce the drug dose.

■ Evaluation

These drugs are effective if the patient complains of fewer symptoms and/or the signs of ulcer disease disappear. Before discharge, patients should be able to explain why and how to take the medications ordered, which side effects will probably occur, possible ways to treat these side effects, which symptoms would warrant notification of the physician, and how to perform any related therapies that have been prescribed, such as dietary manipulation for treatment of ulcer disease. For additional specific information, see the patient care implications section at the end of this chapter.

drugs relax the smooth muscle of the gastrointestinal tract and are used to treat hyperactivity or spasm of the intestine. Side effects of these drugs are not as prominent as those reported for the anticholinergic drugs. Side effects reported include constipation or diarrhea, rash, euphoria, dizziness, drowsiness, headache, nausea, and weakness.

Activity of the upper gastrointestinal tract

■ STOMACH ACID: DRUGS TO TREAT ULCERS (Table 11-2)

■ Ulcers and stomach acid

An ulcer is the loss of the skin or mucosal tissue that provides the protective layer of cells normally surrounding an organ. In the gastrointestinal system, an ulcer (peptic ulcer) occurs in the esophagus, the stomach, or the duodenum as a consequence of the destruction of the mucosal barrier to expose the underlying tissue to stomach acid and to the enzyme pepsin. The cause of an ulcer is a defect in the anatomy of the stomach or in the regulation of stomach secretions. The goal in treating an ulcer is to depress or to neutralize stomach acid to allow the ulcer to heal and to prevent the recurrence of the ulcer.

It is important for patients with esophageal or duodenal ulcers to learn that the conditions causing the ulcer

TABLE 11-2. Drugs to treat an ulcer*

Generic name	Trade name	Dosage and administration	Comments
ANTACIDS			
Aluminum hydroxide gel	ALterna GEL Amphojel	ORAL: *Adults*—5 to 30 ml up to 40 ml every 30 min if pain is severe.	Constipating. Long-term use may cause hypophosphatemia. Complexes with tetracycline and can interfere with the absorption of warfarin, digoxin, quinine, and quinidine.
Dihydroxyaluminum aminoacetate	Robalate	ORAL: *Adults*—0.5 to 2 Gm 4 times daily.	Constipating.
Dihydroxyaluminum sodium carbonate	Rolaids	ORAL: *Adults*—1 to 2 tablets 4 times daily.	Constipating in large doses.
Calcium carbonate	Dicarbosil Titralac Tums	ORAL: *Adults*—1 to 4 Gm 1 and 3 hr after meals and at bedtime. Tablets should be chewed before swallowing.	Can be used hourly to keep acid neutralized but some patients will become hypercalcemic. Constipating.
Magnesium carbonate Magnesium hydroxide Magnesium oxide Magnesium phosphate Magnesium trisilicate	Milk of Magnesia		These magnesium salts are laxatives. Must be taken with an aluminum or calcium antacid to maintain normal stool consistency.
H_2 RECEPTOR ANTAGONIST			
Cimetidine	Tagamet	ORAL: *Adults*—300 mg with meals and at bedtime until ulcer is healed (3 to 6 wk); then 300 mg at bedtime to inhibit nocturnal secretion.	Long-term safety in human beings not established. May cause gynomastia (breast development) in men and breast tenderness in women. May suppress white cells.
Cimetidine hydrochloride	Tagamet Hydrochloride	INTRAVENOUS: *Adults*—1 to 4 mg/kg/hr or 300 mg diluted and infused over 15 to 20 min. INTRAMUSCULAR: *Adults*—300 mg every 6 hr. ORAL, INTRAVENOUS: *Children*—20 to 40 mg/kg in divided doses.	Switch to oral doses when ulcer bleeding has stopped.

*See also Table 11-1, anticholinergic-antispasmodic drugs.

will always be present and only preventive therapy will decrease the incidence of recurrence. An esophageal ulcer results when there is reflux of stomach acid up into the esophagus because of a defective esophageal sphincter. An ulcer in the duodenum results from an overactive secretion of acid in the stomach to the point that the stomach contents cannot be neutralized in the duodenum. The acidic contents then damage the duodenal mucosa. Stomach ulcers are most frequently caused by a tumor, but a nonmalignant cause of stomach ulcers is the reflux of duodenal contents back into the stomach because of a faulty pyloric sphincter. The duodenal contents contain bile acids that disrupt the mucosal barrier normally protecting the stomach from acid and pepsin.

The factors controlling the secretion of hydrochloric acid by the parietal cells of the stomach are diagrammed in Fig. 11-1. The neurotransmitter acetylcholine (released from a branch of the vagus nerve), the hormone gastrin, and histamine all stimulate the secretion of acid. The role of the hydrochloric acid is to aid in the breakdown of connective tissue in food, to activate pepsinogen to pepsin (which degrades protein), and to kill any bacteria ingested in the food. The acidic digest leaves the stomach to enter the duodenum. This movement of

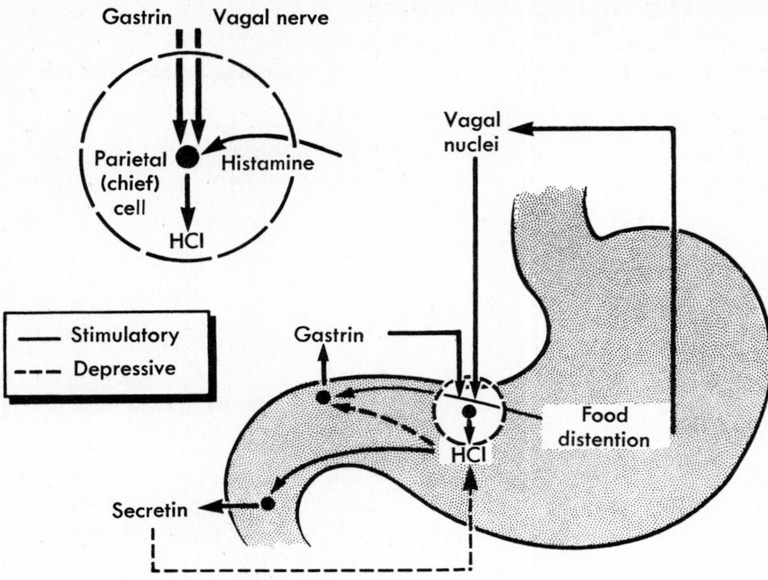

FIG. 11-1

Secretion of acid by parietal cells of the stomach is under control of the duodenally released hormone, gastrin; the parasympathetic nervous system, via the neurotransmitter acetylcholine; and histamine. Histamine is the most effective stimulant of gastric acid secretion. Note that acid secretion is discontinued when food reaches duodenum, where hydrochloride *(HCl)* inhibits gastrin release and stimulates secretin release, and distention of the stomach is lessened, decreasing vagal stimulation.

digested food lessens stomach distention and thereby removes a stimulus for the release of gastrin and for vagal activity. In response to acidity, the duodenum releases secretin, a hormone that stimulates the release of bicarbonate and digestive enzymes from the pancreas. Secretin also depresses the release of hydrochloric acid by the parietal cells and depresses the motility of the stomach. The bicarbonate released by the pancreas neutralizes the acidity of the partially digested food as it enters the duodenum. This neutralization is also necessary for the digestive enzymes in the intestine to be active.

■ Drug treatment of ulcers

Three classes of drugs are used to treat an ulcer: antacids, anticholinergic drugs, and an antihistamine.

Antacids

Antacids (Table 11-2) are weak bases that can be ingested to neutralize the hydrochloric acid secreted by the stomach.

Sodium bicarbonate (baking soda) reacts with hydrochloric acid to yield water and carbon dioxide. Carbon dioxide is a gas and causes the belching frequently associated with the ingestion of sodium bicarbonate. Sodium bicarbonate is the only antacid commonly used that is readily absorbed from the gastrointestinal tract. Taken in excess, sodium bicarbonate also makes the blood slightly alkaline, and in turn the urine becomes alkaline. Excess bicarbonate will stimulate the stomach to secrete more acid (rebound hypersecretion). This hypersecretion can persist after the bicarbonate has been absorbed. For these reasons, sodium bicarbonate is not an antacid of choice when prolonged therapy is required.

Nonsystemic antacids include *alkaline salts of aluminum, magnesium,* and *calcium,* which neutralize acid but are not readily absorbed into the bloodstream. The aluminum and calcium salts tend to cause constipation, whereas magnesium salts tend to have a laxative effect. For this reason, most antacids are a combination of a magnesium salt or hydroxide and an aluminum or calcium salt or hydroxide. Nonsystemic antacids are most effective when taken on an hourly basis. This regimen neutralizes acid without causing the rebound secretion of acid.

The nonsystemic antacids are available as liquids or chewable tablets. The most common side effect is diarrhea or constipation even with a combination antacid. The patient must then add additional antacid: more aluminum or calcium antacid to correct diarrhea or more magnesium antacid to correct constipation. Antacids can impede the absorption of drugs, most notably tetracyclines (an antibiotic), digoxin (a cardiac glycoside), and quinidine (a cardiac antiarrhythmic drug).

Anticholinergic drugs

Anticholinergic drugs used to treat an ulcer are those already discussed with antispasmodic drugs (Table 11-1).

Anticholinergic drugs are taken before meals so they can then depress the secretion of acid that occurs on eating. Anticholinergic drugs should not be taken with antacids because the antacids will slow the absorption of the anticholinergic drugs. Moreover, the administration of an antacid with an anticholinergic drug is not rational: the acid will have already been released in response to the meal and neutralized by the antacid, making the anticholinergic drugs useless.

■ THE NURSING PROCESS WITH ANTACIDS AND ANTIHISTAMINES IN THE TREATMENT OF ULCER DISEASE

■ Assessment

Patients with diagnosed or suspected ulcer disease may come to the hospital with a wide variety of symptoms. The presenting picture may range from the patient who is asymptomatic to the patient who is critically ill from excessive blood loss from a large gastric ulcer. The presenting condition of the patient will guide the examiner in the focus of the assessment. In addition to a baseline total patient assessment, the nurse should assess the vital signs, the level of consciousness, and the character or quality of any emesis or stool, including the presence of occult blood. Fluid balance is monitored by the fluid intake and output. The nurse should question the patient about possible relevant history, such as recent alcohol intake or previous ulcer disease. Appropriate laboratory tests include a hematocrit and hemoglobin determination.

■ Management

The goal of treating an ulcer is to stop blood loss and to promote the healing of the ulcerated area. The management will in part be based on the severity of the presenting picture. Nursing care includes continued monitoring of the vital signs, the fluid intake and output, the level of consciousness, and the character of any emesis or stool. Appropriate laboratory work such as the hematocrit, hemoglobin, and serum electrolyte measurements are continually monitored. When the patient's condition is stable, appropriate diagnostic studies, such as upper gastrointestinal x-ray films or endoscopy, may be done. Dietary restrictions to limit the amount of such irritants as coffee, alcohol, and spices ingested by the patient may be imposed, and the frequency of meals may be increased with an emphasis on inclusion of milk and milk-related products. Antacids and/or cimetidine are often ordered prophylactically for patients falling into categories associated with frequent ulceration. Examples of such patients include those with head injury, those requiring intensive care treatment for any major surgical or medical problem, and patients on high-dose glucocorticoid therapy.

■ Evaluation

These drugs are considered successful if they promote the healing of the ulcer without the patient experiencing side effects resulting from the drug therapy. Before discharge, the patient should be able to explain why the drugs have been ordered; how to take them correctly; how to treat side effects that may occur, such as constipation or diarrhea associated with antacid therapy; which side effects should be reported to the physician; and how to implement dietary or other restrictions prescribed by the physician.

For additional specific information, see the patient care implications section at the end of this chapter.

Antihistamine

Cimetidine (Tagamet) (Table 11-2) is a drug introduced in the 1970's. Cimetidine acts specifically to block the H_2 histamine receptors that control the basal and stimulated secretion of hydrochloric acid by the parietal cells (Fig. 11-1). (The H_1 receptors are blocked by the classic antihistamines and are discussed in Chapter 21.) Many investigators believe that both gastrin and acetylcholine act through histamine to cause the release of hydrochloric acid because cimetidine is effective in decreasing acid secretion stimulated by pentagastrin (an active analog of gastrin) or bethanechol (an agonist of acetylcholine), as well as by food, insulin, and caffeine.

Cimetidine is effective in blocking acid secretion by 70% for at least 4 hours after administration. Much of the drug (50% to 70%) is excreted unchanged in the urine so that a decrease in dose is required for patients with renal insufficiency. Side effects are mild and infrequent but include headache, dizziness, fatigue, muscle pain, and diarrhea or constipation. Elderly patients may become confused.

Duodenal ulcers heal within 8 weeks of therapy with cimetidine. The safety of cimetidine for long-term therapy to prevent the recurrence of duodenal ulcers is being examined. Cimetidine is also being tested for its effectiveness in alleviating a variety of conditions in which stomach acid impedes therapy. These include

1. The Zollinger-Ellison syndrome. A tumor secretes excessive gastrin that stimulates excessive acid production.
2. Benign gastric ulcers.
3. Esophageal ulcers.
4. Pancreatic insufficiency. Digestive enzymes must be administered orally. Without cimetidine, stomach acid inactivates most of the administered enzymes.
5. Gastrointestinal hemorrhage. Stomach acid intensifies the inflammation of the stomach, worsening the hemorrhaging.

■ CENTRAL CONTROL: DRUGS AFFECTING VOMITING (EMESIS) (Table 11-3)

■ Origin of nausea and vomiting

Vomiting (emesis) is an involuntary act regurgitating the contents of the stomach and is coordinated by an area in the medulla called the *vomiting center*. Nausea is the unpleasant sensation that usually precedes vomiting. Input from three major neural sites can stimulate the vomiting center. The first input is that controlled by the higher central nervous system functions, with vomiting being secondary to emotion, pain, or disequilibrium (motion sickness). The second pathway is that arising from peripheral stimuli, with vomiting being secondary to injury or disease of a body tissue or organ. In particular, irritation of the mucosa of the gastrointestinal tract or bowel or biliary distention stimulates the vomiting center by way of the autonomic neurons carrying information to the central nervous system (afferent neurons). The third pathway is that from the chemoreceptor trigger zone, a medullary center sensitive to stimulation by circulating drugs and toxins.

■ Nonmedicinal treatments of nausea and vomiting

Nausea and vomiting are not necessarily treated with drugs. For instance, the nausea and vomiting of pregnancy is best treated by having the patient sip water or tea and eat small meals because antiemetic drugs have been shown to cause fetal abnormalities in experimental animals. Many drugs cause nausea and vomiting as side effects because they act directly on the chemoreceptor trigger zone. Examples of such drugs include levodopa, digitalis, opiates (narcotic analgesics), and aminophylline. The effective treatment is to lower the dose of the offending drug or to increase the dose slowly.

Drugs may also irritate the gastric mucosa to cause a reflex stimulation of nausea and vomiting. Aspirin is an example of an irritant drug. The effective treatment is to take the drug with a large volume of liquid or with a meal to dilute the drug.

■ Drug therapy for nausea and vomiting

Drugs currently used to prevent nausea and vomiting are listed by drug class in Table 11-3. These drugs include antagonists of histamine, acetylcholine, and dopamine, as well as drugs with actions not yet determined. The choice of an antiemetic is determined by the cause of the nausea and vomiting. Drugs for treating nausea and vomiting are most effective when administered before nausea and vomiting have begun rather than after. For instance, the drugs effective in treating motion sickness or vertigo are effective when taken about 30 minutes before travelling is begun, but are relatively ineffective if taken after motion sickness has started. The drugs for treating the nausea and vomiting of chemotherapy or radiation therapy are most effective when taken 30 to 60 minutes before the therapy is begun.

Motion sickness and vertigo are most effectively treated prophylactically with certain of the antihistamines or the anticholinergic drug scopolamine. The action of these drugs is not clear. Presumbly they reduce the stimulation of receptors in the labyrinth from which signals governing the sense of equilibrium arise.

The effective drugs for reducing the vomiting from the chemotherapy and radiation therapy of cancer are those which act at the chemoreceptor trigger zone and are antagonists of dopamine, the major neurotransmitter of the chemoreceptor trigger zone. Most of these dopamine antagonists are drugs that are used as antipsychotic drugs (Chapter 25). These drugs include chlorpromazine (Thorazine), fluphenazine (Prolixin), haloperidol (Haldol), perphenazine (Trilafon), prochlorperazine (Compazine), promazine (Sparine), thiethylperazine (Torecan), and triflupromazine (Vesprin). These drugs are also effective in controlling postoperative vomiting, although they are not effective in preventing motion sickness.

In addition to the anticholinergic, antihistaminergic, and antidopaminergic drugs, there are a few additional drugs that have antiemetic action: benzquinamide (Emete-Con), diphenidol (Vontrol), and trimethobenzamide (Tigan). The active compound in marijuana, Δ^9-tetrahydrocannabinol (THC), and a related drug, nabilone, are being tested for their reputed superior antiemetic effect in cancer chemotherapy.

TABLE 11-3. Drugs to control vomiting

Generic name	Trade name	Dosage and administration	Comments
ANTICHOLINERGIC DRUGS			
Scopolamine hydrobromide		ORAL, SUBCUTANEOUS: *Adults*—0.6 to 1.0 mg. *Children*—0.006 mg/kg body weight.	One of the most effective drugs in preventing motion sickness, but side effects (dry mouth, drowsiness) limit its use.
ANTIHISTAMINIC DRUGS			
Buclizine hydrochloride	Bucladin-S	ORAL: *Adults*—50 mg 30 min before traveling and 4 to 6 hr later. For vertigo, 50 mg 2 times daily.	Effective for preventing motion sickness.
Cyclizine hydrochloride; cyclizine lactate	Marezine	ORAL: *Adults*—50 mg 30 min before traveling and 4 to 6 hr later; maximum, 200 mg daily. *Children*—6 to 10 yr, 3 mg/kg body weight divided into 3 doses daily.	Effective for preventing motion sickness and vertigo.
Dimenhydrinate	Dramamine	INTRAMUSCULAR: *Adults*—50 mg as needed. *Children*—5 mg/kg body weight divided into 4 doses daily; maximum, 300 mg daily. INTRAVENOUS: *Adults*—50 mg diluted in 10 mg saline solution, injected over 2 min. ORAL: *Adults*—50 to 100 mg every 4 hr. *Children*—5 mg/kg body weight divided into 4 doses; maximum, 150 mg daily. RECTAL: *Adults*—100 mg 1 to 2 times daily.	Effective for preventing vertigo, motion sickness, and the nausea and vomiting of pregnancy. Also causes drowsiness.
Diphenhydramine hydrochloride	Benadryl hydrochloride	DEEP INTRAMUSCULAR: *Adults*—10 mg, increased to 20 to 50 mg every 2 to 3 hr if needed; maximum, 400 mg daily. *Children*—5 mg/kg body weight divided into 4 doses; maximum, 300 mg daily. INTRAVENOUS: *Adults*—same as deep intramuscular. ORAL: *Adults*—50 mg 30 min before traveling, then 50 mg before each meal. *Children*—5 mg/kg body weight divided into 4 doses; maximum, 300 mg daily.	Causes sedation. Effective for preventing vertigo motion sickness and the nausea and vomiting of pregnancy.
Hydroxyzine hydrochloride	Isaject Vistaril	INTRAMUSCULAR: *Adults*—25 to 100 mg. *Children*—1 mg/kg body weight.	An antianxiety drug. Effective for preventing motion sickness and postoperative nausea and vomiting.
Hydroxyzine pamoate	Vistaril	ORAL: *Adults*—25 to 100 mg 3 to 4 times daily. *Children*—over 6 yr, 50 to 100 mg daily divided into 4 doses; under 6 yr, 50 mg daily divided into 4 doses.	
Meclizine hydrochloride	Antivert Bonine	ORAL: *Adults*—25 to 50 mg once daily, taken 60 min or longer before traveling; 25 to 100 mg daily in divided doses for vertigo or radiation sickness.	Effective for preventing motion sickness, vertigo, and the nausea and vomiting of radiation therapy. Longer acting than most antihistamines.

Continued.

TABLE 11-3. Drugs to control vomiting—cont'd

Generic name	Trade name	Dosage and administration	Comments
Promethazine hydrochloride	Phenergan Remsed	INTRAMUSCULAR, RECTAL: *Adults*—25 mg, then 12.5 to 25 mg as needed every 4 to 6 hr. *Children*—under 12 yr, no more than half the adult dose. ORAL: *Adults*—25 mg 2 times daily. *Children*—12.5 to 25 mg twice daily.	Effective for preventing motion sickness and vertigo and postoperative nausea and vomiting.
ANTIDOPAMINERGIC DRUGS			
Chlorpromazine hydrochloride	Thorazine	RECTAL: *Adults*—50 to 100 mg every 6 to 8 hr. *Children*—1 mg/kg body weight every 6 to 8 hr. INTRAMUSCULAR: *Adults*—25 mg, then 25 to 50 mg every 3 to 4 hours to stop vomiting. *Children*—0.5 mg/kg body weight every 6 to 8 hr; maximum, 40 mg (up to 5 yr or 50 lb), 75 mg (5 to 12 yr or 50 to 100 lb) daily. ORAL: *Adults*—10 to 25 mg every 4 to 6 hr. *Children*—0.5 mg/kg body weight every 4 to 6 hr.	Watch for hypotension with initial injection. Effective for postoperative nausea and vomiting and that caused by toxins, radiation therapy, or chemotherapy. May cause considerable drowsiness.
Fluphenazine hydrochloride	Prolixin	INTRAMUSCULAR: *Adults*—1.25 mg every 6 to 8 hr as needed.	Effective for postoperative nausea and vomiting and that caused by toxins, radiation, therapy, or chemotherapy.
Haloperidol	Haldol	INTRAMUSCULAR, ORAL: *Adult*—1, 2, or 5 mg every 12 hr as needed.	Effective for postoperative nausea and vomiting and that caused by toxins, radiation therapy, or chemotherapy.
Perphenazine	Trilafon	ORAL: *Adults*—8 to 24 mg daily in 2 or more divided doses. INTRAMUSCULAR: *Adults*—5 mg daily.	Effective for postoperative nausea and vomiting and that caused by toxins, radiation therapy, or chemotherapy.
Prochlorperazine	Compazine	RECTAL: *Adults*—25 mg 2 times daily. *Children*—over 10 kg, 0.4 mg/kg body weight daily divided into 3 to 4 doses.	Effective for postoperative nausea and vomiting and that caused by toxins, radiation therapy, or chemotherapy.
Prochlorperazine edisylate	Compazine	DEEP INTRAMUSCULAR: *Adults*—5 to 10 mg every 3 to 4 hr; maximum, 40 mg daily. *Children*—over 10 kg, 0.2 mg/kg body weight daily.	
Prochlorperazine maleate	Compazine	ORAL: *Adults*—5 to 10 mg every 3 to 4 hr; maximum, 40 mg daily. *Children*—over 10 kg, 0.2 mg/kg body weight daily.	

TABLE 11-3. Drugs to control vomiting—cont'd

Generic name	Trade name	Dosage and administration	Comments
Promazine hydrochloride	Sparine	ORAL: *Adults*—25 to 50 mg every 4 to 6 hr as needed. INTRAMUSCULAR: *Adults*—50 mg.	Effective for postoperative nausea and vomiting and that caused by toxins, radiation therapy, or chemotherapy. Watch for hypotension after intramuscular injection. Sedation and anticholinergic effects common.
Thiethylperazine maleate	Torecan	ORAL, INTRAMUSCULAR, RECTAL: *Adults*—10 to 30 mg daily.	Effective for postoperative nausea and vomiting and that caused by toxins, radiation therapy, or chemotherapy. May cause some hypotension and anticholinergic effects.
Triflupromazine hydrochloride	Vesprin	ORAL: *Adults*—20 to 30 mg daily. *Children*—0.2 mg/kg body weight divided into 3 doses; maximum daily dose, 10 mg. INTRAMUSCULAR: *Adults*—5 to 15 mg every 4 hr as needed; maximum daily dose, 60 mg. *Elderly*—2.5 to 15 mg daily. *Children*—0.2 to 0.25 mg/kg body weight; maximum daily dose, 10 mg.	Effective for postoperative nausea and vomiting and that caused by toxins, radiation therapy, or chemotherapy.
MISCELLANEOUS DRUGS			
Benzquinamide hydrochloride	Emete-Con	INTRAMUSCULAR: *Adults*—0.5 to 1 mg/kg body weight at least 15 min before chemotherapy or emergence from anesthesia. Repeat in 1 hr, then every 3 to 4 hr as required. INTRAVENOUS: *Adults*—0.2 to 0.4 mg/kg body weight diluted in 5% dextrose, sodium chloride injection, or lactated Ringer's injection and administered over 1 to 3 min. Additional doses are given IM.	A new rapidly acting antiemetic with a short duration of action. Effective in controlling postoperative nausea and vomiting. Acts by inhibiting the chemoreceptor trigger zone.
Diphenidol hydrochloride	Vontrol	ORAL: *Adults*—25 to 50 mg 4 times daily. *Children*—over 6 mo and 12 kg, 5 mg/kg body weight daily divided into 4 doses. INTRAMUSCULAR: *Adults*—20 to 40 mg 4 times daily. *Children*—3 mg/kg body weight divided into 4 daily doses. INTRAVENOUS: *Adults*—20 mg; repeat once at 1 hr if necessary.	Acts on vestibular apparatus to prevent vertigo after surgery on the middle ear. Effective for postoperative nausea and vomiting caused by toxins, radiation therapy, or chemotherapy.
Trimethobenzamide hydrochloride	Tigan	INTRAMUSCULAR: *Adults*—200 mg 3 to 4 times daily. For preventing postoperative nausea and vomiting, give 1 dose before or during surgery and another 3 hr after surgery. ORAL: *Adults*—250 mg 3 to 4 times daily. *Children*—15 mg/kg body weight divided into 3 to 4 doses.	Relieves nausea and vomiting of radiation therapy, in the immediate postoperative period, and with gastroenteritis.

■ THE NURSING PROCESS WITH DRUGS TO TREAT NAUSEA AND VOMITING

■ Assessment

Patients may develop nausea with associated vomiting as a result of a variety of causes, including reaction to general anesthesia, reaction to other drugs, motion sickness, viral and bacterial infections, or other medical problems such as intestinal obstruction. After doing a total patient assessment, the nurse should focus on the patient's vital signs, assess the character and quantity of any emesis, listen for the presence of bowel sounds, obtain a brief neurological examination, and measure the fluid intake and output. Relevant history to be obtained from the patient might include such things as precipitating factors, exposure to recent infectious processes, and recent changes in diet or recent medications that have been taken.

■ Management

Drugs used to treat nausea and vomiting only provide symptomatic relief; they do not treat the actual cause of the nausea. During the management phase, attempts will be made to treat the underlying condition and/or diagnose causative agents. Antiemetics will be used for relief of symptoms. The nurse should continue to monitor the vital signs and the fluid intake and output and should assess the subjective complaints of the patient related to nausea and vomiting. The patient should be observed for side effects, although these are usually not severe when these drugs are used in their usual doses. Central nervous system depression, hypotension, and dry mouth are seen frequently. Reducing odors of food and other substances from the patient's environment, limiting intake to clear liquids, and providing back rubs or cool washcloths applied to the forehead are measures that may aid patient comfort.

■ Evaluation

Because these drugs only treat symptoms, their success is measured by a reduction in the subjective complaint of nausea and by less vomiting. Often the condition causing the nausea and vomiting is self-limiting, and with time the need for antiemetics will decrease. When discharged with an antiemetic drug, the patient should be able to explain why and how to take the drug, what the frequency of drug administration should be, the anticipated side effects of the medication, and what should be done if nausea and vomiting are unrelieved by the medication.

For additional specific information, see the patient care implications section at the end of the chapter.

■ Side effects and drug interactions of antiemetic drugs

The side effects of antiemetic drugs are those characteristic of the drug class. All of the drugs used as antiemetics cause drowsiness. Scopolamine also causes the classic anticholinergic side effects of blurred vision, dilated pupils, and dry mouth. Because of these anticholinergic effects, antihistamines are more frequently prescribed to prevent motion sickness than is scopolamine in spite of the superior effectiveness of scopolamine.

Occasionally extrapyramidal symptoms are seen with the dopamine antagonists. Extrapyramidal symptoms are disorders of motor control associated with too little dopamine in a certain area of the brain. The side effects of the dopamine antagonists are more fully discussed in Chapter 25.

The major drug interactions of antiemetics is a synergistic depression with drugs depressing the central nervous system, particularly when respiratory depression is involved. For instance, vomiting secondary to alcohol intoxication or ingestion of narcotic analgesics can be relieved with a dopamine antagonist, but the resultant respiratory depression makes this treatment undesirable.

TABLE 11-4. Drugs to control diarrhea

Generic name	Trade name	Dosage and administration	Comments
OPIOIDS AND RELATED DRUGS			
Codeine phosphate; codeine sulfate		ORAL: *Adults and children over 12 yr*—15 to 60 mg every 4 to 8 hr as needed. INTRAMUSCULAR: *Adults and children over 12 yr*—15 to 30 mg every 2 to 4 hr.	A Schedule II drug.
Diphenoxylate hydrochloride with atropine	Colonil Lomotil Lofene Various others	ORAL: *Adults*—5 mg 3 to 4 times daily. *Children*—8 to 12 yr; 10 mg daily in 5 divided doses; 5 to 8 yr, 8 mg daily in 4 divided doses; 2 to 5 yr, 6 mg daily in 3 divided doses.	A Schedule V drug.
Loperamide	Imodium	ORAL: *Adults*—4 mg initially, then 2 mg with each diarrheal episode, up to 16 mg daily.	A Schedule V drug.
BISMUTH SALTS			
Bismuth subsalicylate	Pepto-Bismol	ORAL: *Adults*—30 ml. *Children*—10 to 14 yr, 20 ml; 6 to 10 yr, 10 ml; 3 to 6 yr, 5 ml.	A nonprescription drug. Effective for "traveler's" diarrhea. May turn stools gray-black.

Activity of the large intestine

■ DRUGS TO CONTROL DIARRHEA

(Table 11-4)

About 8 liters of fluid travel through the intestines of the average adult in 24 hours. Water ingested in food or drink accounts for about 2 liters, and secretions (salivary, gastric, biliary, and pancreatic) account for about 6 liters. Since only 100 to 200 ml of water is normally excreted daily in the feces, the intestines are very efficient in reabsorbing water and electrolytes.

■ Definition

Diarrhea has no precise definition but rather refers to bowel movements that are frequent (more than three per day), fluid (unformed stools), or large (greater than 200 Gm per day). Acute diarrhea lasts for hours or days, whereas chronic diarrhea lasts more than 3 to 4 weeks. Chronic diarrhea requires a thorough examination to establish a cause, which can then be specifically treated. Acute diarrhea rarely requires treatment beyond the avoidance of food and adequate intake of liquids.

■ Replacement therapy for diarrhea

The primary treatment of diarrhea is to replace lost fluids and electrolytes. The presence of glucose is required for the intestinal absorption of water and electrolytes, so mild dehydration can be treated with carbonated drinks (which add glucose and bicarbonate) and broths or clear soups (which add sodium and chloride). Infants and the elderly can become seriously dehydrated if an adequate intake of glucose and salts is not maintained to replace the fluid and electrolytes lost. Commercially available drinks for replacement of glucose and electrolytes include Gatorade and Lytren. A similar drink can be made at home with ½ teaspoon of corn syrup or honey and a pinch of table salt added to 1 cup (8 oz) of fruit juice (to provide potassium), alternating with a drink made by adding ¼ teaspoon of baking soda (sodium bicarbonate) to 1 cup (8 oz) of water. A simpler drink is made with following recipe: 1 teaspoon table salt, 1 teaspoon baking soda, and 4 teaspoons of sugar in a quart of boiled water. This latter recipe does not provide needed potassium, however, and if possible ½ teaspoon of potassium chloride should be added to a quart of the solution.

■ Drug therapy for diarrhea (Table 11-4)

The most effective nonspecific antidiarrheal agents are the opioids, which decrease the tone of the small and large intestines in a manner that slows the transit of material. The longitudinal contractions propelling the contents (peristalsis) are inhibited by the opioids, but the circular contractions which cause the segmental activity that mixes the intestinal contents are stimulated by the opioids. The treatment of diarrhea with opioids is nonspecific, and when diarrhea is caused by poisons, infec-

■ THE NURSING PROCESS WITH DRUGS USED TO CONTROL DIARRHEA

■ Assessment

Diarrhea may have a variety of causes, including viral and bacterial infections, response to various medications, and physiological diseases of the colon. The nurse should do a thorough patient assessment. Specific points include monitoring the vital signs and the intake and output of solids and liquids, auscultating bowel sounds, and checking the character and quantity of diarrhea. Appropriate laboratory studies related to diarrhea include culturing a stool specimen and testing stools for ova and parasites and the presence of occult blood. The nurse should question the patient about recent exposure to new water or dietary sources, recent exposure to infectious agents, and any new medications that have been started recently.

■ Management

The treatment of diarrhea is directed at providing symptomatic relief for the patient and at identifying the cause of the diarrhea and treating the cause. The nurse should continue to monitor the vital signs and the intake and output of liquid, and should observe the frequency and character of any additional stools. If laboratory work has indicated a possible specific cause for diarrhea, treatment of this causative agent should be started. Limiting the diet to clear fluids may help to limit diarrhea. In cases in which diarrhea is the result of milk intolerance or other dietary causes, the patient is referred to the dietician for appropriate teaching about prescribed dietary restrictions. The nurse should observe the patient for side effects resulting from the medications, in particular, constipation and sedation. If diarrhea is severe or persists, the serum electrolyte concentrations should be monitored and replacement fluids provided as necessary.

■ Evaluation

These drugs are considered effective if the frequency of bowel movements is decreased to the patient's normal range. In addition, there should be no side effects such as constipation resulting from drug therapy. Before discharge the patient should be able to explain when and how to take the medication prescribed, symptoms that may indicate too high a dose, and what to do if the drugs do not relieve the symptoms.

For more specific information, see the patient care implications section at the end of the chapter.

---

tions, or bacterial toxins, opioids can make the condition worse by delaying the elimination of these agents. Opioids that are used to control diarrhea include *opium tincture, paregoric, codeine,* and *diphenoxylate (Lomotil).* The effective antidiarrheal dose is lower than that which can cause euphoria or analgesia. Toxic doses produce respiratory depression, which can be reversed with a narcotic antagonist.

Opium tincture

Opium tincture is a 10% solution of opium containing 10 mg/ml morphine. The antidiarrheal dose of opium tincture is measured in drops (usually 6 to 20), and this dose does not usually produce euphoria or analgesia.

Paregoric

Paregoric (camphorated opium tincture) contains only 0.4 mg/ml morphine and is administered by the teaspoonful. Paregoric has an unpleasant taste.

Codeine

Codeine can be given orally or intramuscularly.

Diphenoxylate (Colonil, Lomotil)

Diphenoxylate is an opioid that has a lower potential than codeine or opium tincture for causing drug dependence. Diphenoxylate is combined with atropine to diminish abdominal cramping while reducing the loss of water and electrolytes.

Loperamide (Imodium)

Loperamide is a relatively new antidiarrheal drug that acts to depress both longitudinal and circular contractions of the intestinal smooth muscle and to decrease the release of acetylcholine. This is a broader spectrum of actions on the intestine than is seen with opioids. Loperamide is listed as a Schedule V drug and is structurally related to diphenoxylate, although loperamide has no effects on the central nervous system and does not appear to produce physical dependence. Loperamide is concentrated by the liver and excreted into the bile. Use of loperamide is contraindicated in the presence of liver disease.

Bismuth salts

In addition to the opioids that depress intestinal motility, many agents have been used as antidiarrheal drugs with the belief that they absorb toxins and thereby remove the cause of diarrhea. Of these drugs, only the bismuth salts have been proven effective.

Bismuth subsalicylate (Pepto-Bismol) is effective in controlling "traveler's" diarrhea, apparently by binding the bacterial toxins. Bismuth causes the feces to become black, which should not be taken as an indication of blood in the feces. Use in infants or the elderly may produce feces that cannot be expelled (impacted feces).

■ DRUGS TO RELIEVE CONSTIPATION: LAXATIVES

■ Origin of constipation

The major muscular activity of the large intestine is a contraction of circular smooth muscle, which decreases the diameter to segment and knead the fecal mass without moving it along. About 2 liters of water are removed from the fecal mass in the large intestine. Bulk in the large intestines stimulates stretch receptors to cause a reflex peristalsis, which moves the fecal mass forward. Periodically, usually 3 to 4 times daily, strong propulsive contractions occur spontaneously to move the fecal mass through the large intestine. The strongest movements usually occur after the first meal of the day, and the perception of the need to defecate follows the filling of the rectum. The relaxation of the external anal sphincter is a voluntary act, as are the straining movements to expel the feces. The pattern of defecation described implies that defecation is a regular morning event, but the timing of defecation is highly individual and may occur more or less frequently. A normal bowel movement refers to whatever pattern of defecation results in readily passed feces for a given individual. Constipation arises when the frequency of bowel movements decreases and defecation yields hard stools that are difficult to pass.

■ Classes of laxatives (Table 11-5)

Laxative, cathartic, and *purgative* are all terms describing agents that act on the large intestine (colon, bowel) to promote defecation, but these terms have evolved to represent different degrees of action. A laxative produces soft stools with a minimal incidence of abdominal cramping. A cathartic produces a soft to fluid stool and may also cause abdominal cramping. A purgative produces a watery stool and violent cramping to such an extent that shock and hemorrhaging may result. Purgatives are no longer used in medical practice, and only some cathartics, also called stimulant cathartics, are commonly used.

Table 11-5 lists the drugs used as laxatives. Traditionally, laxatives are classified as (1) bulk-forming, (2) stimulant (irritant) cathartic, (3) saline (osmotic) cathartic, (4) wetting agent (softener), and (5) lubricant. Laxatives are indicated for those with true constipation. Causes of constipation include poor bowel habits, narcotic analgesics, drugs with anticholinergic side effects, and the loss of intestinal muscle tone because of surgery, bed rest, or age. Laxatives are also indicated when straining is painful or risky, such as in women with episiotomies and patients with hemorrhoids, hernias, or aneurysms. Laxatives are also used to clean out the large intestine before surgery or examination. With the exception of mineral oil, laxatives act by providing a greater bulk to the fecal mass, primarily by keeping water in the large intestine. The large, hydrated fecal mass can fill the rectum to stimulate defecation, and defecation is accomplished with minimal irritation or strain.

Bulk-forming laxatives

This class of laxatives includes bran, methylcellulose, polycarbophil, and psyllium hydrophilic mucilloid. These laxatives act by retaining water so that the stool remains large and soft. Bulk-forming laxatives provide what should be a part of good nutrition. It is generally felt that people in the developed countries eat a diet that contains too little fiber and favors the formation of small, hard stools. The inclusion of bran, whole grain products, and fibrous fruits and vegetables in the diet promotes the formation of large, soft stools that readily stimulate the large intestine and the rectum.

In a person who does not regularly use laxatives, bulk-forming laxatives will be effective in 12 to 24 hours. Bulk-forming laxatives can also relieve a mild watery diarrhea by absorbing water to produce a soft stool.

TABLE 11-5. Drugs to relieve constipation

Generic name	Trade name	Dosage and administration	Comments
BULK-FORMING AGENTS			
Karaya gum		ORAL: 5 to 10 Gm daily, taken with water.	Nonprescription.
Methylcellulose; carboxymethyl cellulose	Cologel Hydrolose	ORAL: *Adults*—4 to 6 Gm daily. *Children*—over 6 yr, 1 to 1.5 Gm daily.	Nonprescription.
Plantago (psyllium) seed		ORAL: *Adults*—2.5 to 30 Gm daily. *Children*—over 6 yr, 1.25-15 Gm daily. Add to water and drink rapidly.	Nonprescription.
Polycarbophil		ORAL: *Adults*—4 to 6 Gm daily. *Children*—6 to 12 yr, 1.5 to 3 Gm daily; 2 to 5 yr, 1 to 1.5 Gm daily; to 2 yr, 0.5 to 1 Gm daily.	Nonprescription.
Psyllium hydrocolloid Psyllium hydrophilic mucilloid	Effersyllium Konsyl L.A. Formula Metamucil Modane Bulk	ORAL: *Adults*—1 round teaspoonful (7 Gm) or 1 packet. Add to a glass of water and drink rapidly and then follow with a second glass of water. Repeat 1 to 2 times daily if necessary.	Nonprescription.
STIMULANT (IRRITANT) CATHARTICS			
Bisacodyl	Biscolax Dulcolax Various others	ORAL: *Adults*—10 mg. Up to 30 mg may be given to clear gastrointestinal tract. *Children*—over 6 yr, 5 mg. RECTAL: *Adults and children over 2 yr*—10 mg. *Children under 2 yr*—5 mg.	Initial response in 6 to 12 hr. Nonprescription. Do not take within 60 min of milk or antacids. Rectal administration effective in 15 min.
Cascara sagrada	Bileo-Secrin Cas-Evac	ORAL: *Adults*—200 to 400 mg of extract, 0.5 to 1.5 ml of fluid extract, or 5 ml of aromatic extract.	Nonprescription. One of the mildest of the stimulant cathartics.
Castor oil		ORAL: *Adults*—15 to 60 ml. *Children*—over 2 yr, 5 to 15 ml; under 2 yr, 1 to 5 ml.	Castor oil is degraded to ricinoleic acid, which is the active drug. Nonprescription.
Castor oil, emulsified	Neoloid	ORAL: *Adults*—30 to 60 ml. *Children*—over 2 yr, 7.5 to 30 ml; under 2 yr, 2.5 to 7.5 ml.	Nonprescription. This emulsion is mint flavored. Turns alkaline urine pink.
Danthron	Anavac Danivac Dorbane Modane Weslax	ORAL: *Adults*—75 to 150 mg. *Children*—6 to 12 yr, 37 to 75 mg; 1 to 6 yr, 10 to 15 mg.	Nonprescription. Turns alkaline urine pink.
Glycerin suppositories		RECTAL: *Adults*—3 Gm. *Children*—under 6 yr, 1 to 1.5 Gm.	Nonprescription. Effective in 15 to 30 min.
Phenolphthalein	Chocolax Ex-lax Feen-A-Mint Phenolax Various others	ORAL: *Adults*—30 to 270 mg daily. *Children*—over 6 yr, 30 to 60 mg daily; 2 to 6 yr, 15 to 20 mg daily.	Nonprescription. Turns alkaline urine pink.
Senna concentrate	Senokot suppositories	RECTAL: *Adults*—1 suppository. *Children*—over 60 lb, ½ suppository.	
Senna pod	Senokot Various others	ORAL: *Adults*—twice daily give 1 to 2 teaspoonfuls (granules), 2 to 3 teaspoonfuls (syrup), or 2 to 4 tablets. *Children, pregnant or postpartum women, or geriatric patients*—½ adult dose. *Children*—1 mo to 1 yr, 1.25 to 2.5 ml (syrup).	Nonprescription. Not all preparations are recommended for children.

TABLE 11-5. Drugs to relieve constipation—cont'd

Generic name	Trade name	Dosage and administration	Comments
Senna, whole leaf		ORAL: *Adults*—0.5 to 2 Gm or 2 ml of senna fluidextract. *Children*—6 to 12 yr, ½ adult dose; 2 to 5 yr, ¼ adult dose; under 2 yr, ⅛ adult dose.	Nonprescription.
Sennosides A & B	Glysennid	ORAL: *Adults*—12 to 24 mg at bedtime. *Children*—over 10 yr, same as adult; 6 to 10 yr, 12 mg at bedtime.	Nonprescription.
SALINE CATHARTICS			
Magnesium hydroxide	Milk of Magnesia	ORAL: *Adult*—10 to 15 ml (concentrated) or 15 to 30 ml (regular).	Nonprescription.
Magnesium sulfate	Epsom salt	ORAL: *Adults*—15 Gm in a glass of water.	Nonprescription.
Monosodium phosphate	Sal Hepatica	ORAL: *Adult*—5 to 20 ml with water.	Nonprescription.
Sodium phosphate		ORAL: *Adults*—4 Gm in a glass of warm water.	Nonprescription.
Sodium phosphate with sodium biphosphate	Phospho-Soda	ORAL: *Adult*—20 to 40 ml in a glass of cold water.	Nonprescription.
LUBRICANTS			
Mineral oil	Agoral, Plain Kondremul Plain Neo-Cultol Petrogalar Plain	ORAL: *Adults*—15 to 30 ml at bedtime. *Children*—5 to 15 ml at bedtime.	Nonprescription. To ease strain of passing hard stools. Should not be used regularly because the fat-soluble vitamins (A, D, E, and K) are not absorbed.
FECAL SOFTENERS			Response in 1 to 3 days.
Dioctyl calcium sulfosuccinate	Surfak	ORAL: *Adults*—50 to 360 mg daily. *Children*—50 to 150 mg daily.	Nonprescription.
Dioctyl sodium sulfosuccinate	Colace Comfolax D-S-S Various others	ORAL: *Adults*—50 to 360 mg. *Children*—6 to 12 yr, 40 to 120 mg; 3 to 6 yr, 20 to 60 mg; under 3 yr, 10 to 40 mg.	Nonprescription.

Stimulant (irritant) cathartics

Stimulant cathartics include cascara, danthron, senna, phenolphthalein, bisacodyl, castor oil, and glycerin. These drugs usually form a soft to fluid stool in 6 to 12 hours. Stimulant cathartics were believed to act only by directly stimulating the motility of the large intestine, but recent research indicates that these drugs also inhibit the reabsorption of water in the large intestine.

The stimulant cathartics are the most abused laxatives. When a stimulant cathartic is used for more than a week, the large intestine loses its tone and becomes less responsive to any stimulation. Continued use of a stimulant cathartic can produce a diarrhea severe enough to cause dehydration and to lower blood concentrations of sodium and potassium.

Cascara and *senna* are extracted from plants while *danthron* is a chemically related synthetic compound. Cascara is the mildest and senna is the most potent of these three laxatives. They should not be used by mothers breast-feeding infants, since these laxatives are excreted in the milk. Senna and cascara color an acid urine yellow-brown and an alkaline urine red. Danthron imparts a pink color to an alkaline urine.

Phenolphthalein is found in many over-the-counter laxative preparations. Phenophthalein enters the enterohepatic circulation and may be effective for several days. In an alkaline urine, phenolphthalein is pink.

Bisacodyl is a synthetic compound that is available both as a suppository and as a tablet. As a suppository, bisacodyl is effective in 15 minutes. As a tablet, bi-

■ THE NURSING PROCESS WITH DRUGS TO RELIEVE CONSTIPATION

■ Assessment

Constipation may occur for various reasons, including enforced bed rest, concomitant use of medications such as narcotic analgesics or drugs with anticholinergic action, recent surgery, dehydration, and improper use of drugs used to treat diarrhea. The nurse should do a thorough patient assessment with attention to the vital signs, the fluid intake and output, and the presence of bowel sounds. A digital rectal examination is performed if appropriate to determine the presence of impacted stools. Additional helpful data might include any previous history of constipation and its treatment, the patient's perception of what constipation is, and any recent change in life-style, diet, or medications that might promote constipation.

■ Management

The actual treatment of constipation is usually relatively simple. If the problem is a persistent one, it is important to rule out serious causes such as cancer. In addition to stimulating the intestine to produce a bowel movement, it is important to begin teaching the patient about other factors that influence the frequency of stools. The patient can be taught the importance of adequate fluid intake and adequate activity. The patient should also be instructed that certain foods and juices tend to cause bulk in the stool and produce gastrointestinal stimulation. The treatment of a complaint of constipation may be different from the final drug program prescribed for the patient for management of chronic constipation at home.

■ Evaluation

These drugs,are considered effective if they either produce a bowel movement within 12 to 24 hours or allow the patient to have bowel movements unaided on a regular basis. Before discharging a patient to home, it is important that the patient be able to explain how to take the medications ordered and what the desired effects of the medications are, since some cause a laxative effect whereas others keep the stool soft; the patient should also know what to do if the prescribed therapy is no longer effective for treatment of constipation.

For further specific information, see the patient care implications section at the end of this chapter.

---

sacodyl is effective in 6 hours. Since bisacodyl irritates the stomach, the tablet is coated to dissolve only in the intestine. This enteric-coated tablet should not be taken within an hour of ingestion of such things as milk or antacids, which neutralize stomach acid. Bisacodyl is often used to clear the large intestine for proctoscopic or coloscopic examination.

Castor oil is an old remedy for constipation and is still used medically. Castor oil is the most potent of the stimulant cathartics, producing a watery stool in 2 to 6 hours, which thoroughly removes gas and feces from the intestine. Castor oil has an unpleasant taste that is best disguised by chilling it and giving it with fruit juice.

Glycerin is used only as a suppository. It acts by stimulating the rectum as well as by attracting water to increase bulk and is effective in 15 to 30 minutes.

Saline (osmotic) cathartics

Saline cathartics are poorly absorbed salts of magnesium or sodium: magnesium carbonate, oxide, citrate, hydroxide, or sulfate; sodium phosphate or sulfate; and potassium, sodium tartrate. The concentrated solutions of these salts attract water osmotically into the lumen of the large intestine, and the resulting bulk stimulates peristalsis. Saline cathartics empty the bowel in 2 to 6 hours.

Patients with poor kidney function should not use saline cathartics because these patients cannot excrete the extra salt load from the small fraction of the salt that is absorbed systemically.

Wetting agents (stool softeners)

Wetting agents are detergents that inhibit the absorption of water so that the fecal mass remains large and soft. This class of laxatives is indicated when the objective is to avoid straining to pass the stools. The wetting agent laxatives include dioctyl sodium sulfosuccinate (docusate sodium) and dioctyl calcium sulfosuccinate (docusate calcium).

Lubricant

The only lubricant laxative still used is *mineral oil,* which is indigestible and acts to soften the feces, thus easing the strain of passing the stools and lessening the irritation to hemorrhoids. Long-term use of mineral oil interferes with the absorption of the fat-soluble vitamins A, D, E, and K. Mineral oil can cause a lipid pneumonia if accidentally aspirated. The wetting agents are regarded as superior to mineral oil in softening the stools for easy passage.

■ PATIENT CARE IMPLICATIONS

Cholinomimetics: Bethanechol and neostigmine

1. Atropine sulfate (0.5 to 1.0 mg) should be on hand to counteract excessive cholinergic side effects in patients receiving bethanechol or neostigmine subcutaneously for an atonic bladder or gastrointestinal tract.
2. Check dosages carefully. The oral dose of bethanechol may be as high as 50 mg, whereas the subcutaneous dose should not exceed 5 mg.
3. Use either of these drugs with caution in patients with epilepsy, Parkinson's disease, bradycardia, ulcer, heart disease, or pregnancy.
4. Oral doses of bethanechol should be taken when the stomach is empty; if taken with meals or just after eating, nausea and vomiting may occur.
5. Patients receiving subcutaneous bethanechol, especially the first dose, should not be left unattended for the first 10 minutes. The drug acts very rapidly, with results apparent in 5 to 15 minutes and if serious side effects are going to occur, they usually will do so within minutes.
6. In selected situations, the physician may order a test dose of one-half or less of the desired dose to monitor the patient's response. Monitor the blood pressure and pulse.
7. Check the pulse before administering neostigmine. Notify the physician if the rate is below 80, and withhold the dose pending physician approval.
8. For additional information about neostigmine, see Chapter 9.
9. Remind patients to keep these and all medications out of the reach of children.

Anticholinergic and antispasmodic drugs

1. Anticholinergic drugs may precipitate an attack of acute angle-closure glaucoma, although this is more common with parenteral forms. Patients with open-angle glaucoma who have their glaucoma under control with miotics can safely take anticholinergics.
2. These drugs are usually taken before meals and at bedtime unless a timed-release form is being used. These medications should not be taken at the same time antacids are taken, because the antacid will slow absorption of the other drug.
3. These medications should be used cautiously in patients with prostatic hypertrophy, pyloric obstruction, obstruction of the bladder neck, or severe cardiac disease. They are contraindicated in patients with myasthenia gravis.
4. Urinary retention can occur occasionally, although this is more common in men with preexisting prostatic hypertrophy. Instruct the patient to report inability to void, increasing difficulty in initiating urination, or feelings of incomplete bladder emptying. It may help to instruct the patient to void at the time a dose is taken. In the hospital, monitor the fluid intake and output.
5. Constipation often occurs, especially with long-term use. Instruct the patient to increase the daily fluid intake to at least 3000 ml and to add to the diet more roughage and fiber, if allowed. Increasing the level of activity may also help. If diarrhea occurs, it may indicate incomplete obstruction of the gastrointestinal tract and should be investigated. Instruct the patient to keep a record of bowel movements so that constipation, if it occurs, can be treated before becoming too severe. The patient should consult the physician if a bowel movement has not occurred in 3 days. Instruct the patient not to take cathartics or other aids to defecation without consulting the physician, since these drugs may be contraindicated in diseases that require anticholinergic therapy.
6. Because tachycardia is a side effect of these drugs, they should not be used in patients with an existing tachycardia (pulse over 90 to 100) or with a history of heart disease associated with tachycardia. Monitor the pulse.
7. Both drowsiness and blurred vision have been reported with these drugs. Caution the patient to avoid engaging in activities requiring mental alertness and/or visual acuity (e.g., driving, operating machinery) until the effects of the medication can be evaluated.
8. These drugs inhibit the ability of the body to perspire and may predispose patients to heatstroke or heat exhaustion if patients work in a setting with a high environmental temperature. Caution patients about this possible hazard, and encourage them to take occasional periods to cool off. Atropine may

produce a fever, especially in children, because of the decreased ability to perspire.

9. Chewing gum or sucking on hard candies may help relieve a dry mouth. There are also available commercially prepared saliva substitutes that some patients may wish to use; consult the physician.
10. Because side effects almost always occur at therapeutic doses, patient compliance may be poor. Review with patients the need for the medication at regular intervals. Try to be accepting of the patient's complaints about side effects, yet reinforcing of the need to continue the medication in the dose and frequency prescribed.
11. Keep these and all medications out of the reach of children.
12. These drugs should be used during pregnancy and by nursing mothers only if the benefit outweighs the risk; consult the physician.
13. Many anticholinergics are manufactured in combination with other drugs, including barbiturate and antianxiety agents. If a combination drug has been prescribed for the patient, review the side effects of each of the component parts of the combination with the patient.
14. Neostigmine is used to treat overdose with any of these medications.
15. Tincture of belladonna may be prescribed by the number of drops. Dilute the dose in 15 to 30 ml of water before administering to ensure that the patient receives the entire dose.

Drugs to treat peptic ulcers

1. *Antacids*
   a. As indicated in the text, antacids should not be taken with tetracyclines, digoxin, or quinidine.
   b. Most patients will find it necessary to alternate aluminum and calcium salts with magnesium salts to regulate bowel movements. Even combinations tend to cause either constipation or diarrhea in many individuals.
   c. Read labels carefully and instruct patients to do the same. Many antacids are now available in several forms (e.g., double strength or with simethicone), and the names are almost identical. If in doubt, consult the pharmacist.
   d. Many antacids are high in sodium and should be used judiciously in patients with cardiac disease, hypertension, or renal disease. The following is a partial list of some antacid liquids, both single entity and mixtures, and their sodium concentration per 5 ml. Note that the acid-neutralizing ability, which is not included on the table, varies from product to product. Note also that some products listed also contain simethicone, an antiflatulent agent, or other ingredients.

Drug	Sodium content
AlternaGEL	less than 2.0 mg sodium
Amphojel	6.9 mg sodium
Basaljel	2.4 mg sodium
Gaviscon*	26.8 mg sodium
Gelusil*	0.7 mg sodium
Kudrox*	15.0 mg sodium
Maalox	2.5 mg sodium
Mylanta*	0.7 mg sodium
Riopan†	0.3 mg sodium

   e. Antacid tablets should be chewed and not swallowed whole.
   f. Liquid and tablet preparations should be followed by enough water to ensure that the dose reaches the stomach.
   g. Since antacids may interfere with the absorption of other drugs the patient may be taking, review the dosage schedules of all the prescribed medications, and rearrange the schedules as needed to prevent this problem. Remind patients to keep health care providers informed of all medications that are being taken, including antacids.
2. *Cimetidine*
   a. Cimetidine may potentiate the action of coumarin anticoagulants, particularly warfarin. Monitor the prothrombin time. Instruct the patient to report any signs of bruising or bleeding. Monitor the stools for occult blood.
   b. Cimetidine is not recommended for use in pregnancy or by nursing mothers unless the benefits outweigh the risks. If in doubt, consult the physician.
   c. Cimetidine may be given orally, in tablet or liquid forms. It may be given undiluted intramuscularly. For intravenous "push" infusion, dilute 300 mg with sodium chloride solution or other diluent (see manufacturer's instructions) to make a total volume of 20 mg; inject over 1 to 2 minutes. For intermittent infusion, dilute in an appropriate solution to a volume of 100 ml, and infuse over 15 to 20 minutes.
   d. Oral doses are best administered with or just before meals.

Antiemetics

1. Drowsiness is a side effect of all of these drugs. Caution patients to avoid activities requiring mental alertness, such as driving or operating machinery, until the effects of the drug have worn off.

*Contains simethicone
†This drug (magaldrate) is a chemical entity, not a combination of antacids.

2. Individuals who suffer from motion sickness may find that riding in the front seat of the car is less nauseating than the back seat.
3. Sucking on hard candy or chewing gum may help to relieve the dry mouth associated with some of these drugs. If the patient has vomited, assisting the patient to rinse the mouth out with water or mouthwash will help to decrease the unpleasant taste. The postoperative patient who still may not eat may find relief by sucking on ice chips; check with the physician.
4. If possible, measure the emesis as a part of the fluid intake and output record.
5. Keeping the environment neat and free of odors may ease the discomfort of the nauseated patient somewhat. The nauseated person may not tolerate the sight of food; keep the door closed or the curtains drawn during meal times if appropriate. Begin feeding the person who has been experiencing nausea with small amounts of clear liquids before progressing to a more complete diet.
6. Intramuscularly administered antiemetics may cause pain or burning at the injection site.
7. Antiemetics should be used with caution in children who may be suffering from Reye's syndrome. This syndrome is characterized by an abrupt onset of persistent severe vomiting, lethargy, irrational behavior, progressive encephalopathy, convulsions, coma, and death.
8. The use of these agents in pregnant women is contraindicated unless the benefits clearly outweigh the risks. Consult the physician.
9. Keep these and all medications out of the reach of children.
10. The antihistamines are discussed in detail in Chapter 21. Bendectin is a combination of the antihistamine doxylamine and pyridoxine hydrochloride (vitamin B_6) and is frequently prescribed for morning sickness.
    a. In addition to drowsiness, this drug may cause vertigo, nervousness, epigastric pain, headache, diarrhea, disorientation, or irritability.
    b. The patient should be instructed to take 2 tablets at bedtime to relieve morning sickness. If nausea continues during the day, the dose may be increased or changed; check with the physician.
    c. The use of Bendectin in pregnancy is being reevaluated because the antihistamine has been alleged to cause birth defects.
11. The antidopaminergic drugs are discussed in detail in Chapter 25.
12. *Benzquinamide*
    a. Intravenous administration has been associated with an increase in blood pressure and transient cardiac arrhythmias, including premature ventricular contractions (PVCs). The intramuscular route is preferred.
    b. Monitor the blood pressure and pulse.
13. *Diphenidol*
    a. This drug may cause hallucinations, disorientation, or confusion. If these symptoms occur, notify the physician. Assess whether the patient can be left unattended.
    b. Monitor the blood pressure and pulse every 4 hours.
    c. This drug may be given undiluted via the intramuscular or intravenous route.
14. *Trimethobenzamide*
    This drug is not recommended for intravenous use.
15. *THC (Δ^9 tetrahydrocannabinol)*
    a. Some patients may have difficulty taking or may be unwilling to take this drug because it has been illegal to possess or use. Discussion with the patient of the possible benefits anticipated may help to convince the patient to take the drug, but the patient's psychological objection to the drug may predispose to an increased number of side effects that are reported or to complaints that the drug does not work.
    b. Frequently reported side effects include tachycardia, reddened conjunctiva, decreased lacrimation (dry eyes), and dry mouth. Monitor the pulse. The use of artificial tears may be helpful. If dry mouth is a problem, chewing gum or sucking on hard candy may bring some relief. There are also available commercially prepared artificial saliva preparations that some patients may find helpful.
    c. Psychological side effects are often dose related and are those effects seen when marijuana is taken for its mind-altering effects. These sensations include euphoria, sense of well-being, giddiness, illusions, and distorted time sense. Some patients experience anxiety or paranoia. Hallucinations are rare. Keeping the environment quiet and remaining with the patient may help when psychological side effects are prominent. Encourage patients to discuss their feelings.
    d. The side effects of therapeutic THC are still being investigated. For additional information, consult the references or current studies about the use of THC.

Drugs to control diarrhea

1. Keep a record of the frequency of bowel movements. Often after several days of treatment with

antidiarrheal agents, the patient may become constipated from the effects of the drug.
2. As indicated in the text, fluid and electrolyte loss can be severe. Encourage patients with diarrhea to switch to a clear liquid diet. Total fluid intake should be at least 3000 ml per day, although in cases of severe diarrhea, up to 5000 to 6000 ml per day may be necessary.
3. Most cases of short-term diarrhea are self-limiting, especially if a result of a viral infection. Instruct the patient to consult the physician if any of the following occur: diarrhea persists longer than 3 to 5 days; the medications are not bringing relief; the stools are particularly foul-smelling or contain flecks of blood or large amounts of mucus; or the patient is unable to take in sufficient replacement fluids. Symptoms of hypokalemia are muscle weakness, fatigue, anorexia, vomiting, drowsiness, irritability, and eventually coma and death. Symptoms of hypochloremia include hypertonic muscles, tetany, and depressed respirations.
4. Question the patient carefully about recent activities that might have caused diarrhea. Examples include recent travel, especially international; recent antibiotic use; or recent cancer chemotherapy.
5. The use of these agents during pregnancy and by nursing mothers without prior clearance by the physician is not recommended.
6. Keep these and all medications out of the reach of children.
7. Opium tincture is not used frequently now. Dilute the ordered number of drops in 15 to 30 ml of water to ensure that the patient receives the entire dose.
8. Paregoric is very unpleasant to the taste. Many patients find combination drugs such as Parepectolin much more palatable. (Parepectolin, 30 ml, contains 3.7 ml equivalents of paregoric, 162 mg pectin, and 5.5 Gm kaolin. Note that combination drugs subject the patient to additional ingredients that may or may not be helpful or needed.)
9. Codeine, used primarily as a narcotic analgesic, is discussed in more detail in Chapter 28.
10. Diphenoxylate hydrochloride, which is related to meperidine, can cause similar side effects if given in high enough doses. Caution the patient that these preparations can cause decreased mental alertness; therefore the patient should avoid dangerous activities, such as driving or operating machinery, until the effects of the drug can be evaluated. If patients are taking other drugs that depress the central nervous system (e.g., barbiturates, antianxiety drugs, alcohol) the drowsiness may be more pronounced.
11. Theoretically, addiction to diphenoxylate is possible. Overdose with this drug resembles an overdose by a narcotic analgesic and is treated the same way (Chapter 28).
12. Diphenoxylate preparations contain a small amount of atropine. A single dose of these preparations would cause few if any side effects as a result of the atropine, but the accumulated dose following a day of treatment might cause problems. Review the side effects of and contraindications to atropine use.
13. Side effects of loperamide are rare in prescribed doses, but may include abdominal pain or distention, constipation, drowsiness, nausea and vomiting, and tiredness.

Agents to relieve constipation

1. When used in the correct dosage and at recommended frequency, there are few side effects associated with these drugs other than an increasing dependence on them.
2. In many cases of constipation, long-term cure could better be achieved by the patient through modification of dietary habits. Instruct the patient to increase dietary intake of foods known to be bulk-producing or stimulating to the gastrointestinal tract. Such foods are bran cereals, fresh fruits and vegetables, fruit juices, or foods known by that patient to be stimulating to defecation, such as coffee or hot chocolate.
3. Advise the patient to increase the fluid intake to at least 2500 to 300 ml per day. Specific directions may be more helpful to patients who do not know how much fluid they consume in a day. For example, the patient might be instructed to drink a full glass of water at each meal (in addition to the other beverages that might be ordinarily consumed with that meal) and to have a glass of water at midmorning and midafternoon.
4. Increasing the level of activity may assist in decreasing constipation.
5. Abuse of drugs to relieve constipation sometimes occurs with individuals who feel that a daily bowel movement is necessary. Try to teach patients that it may be normal to defecate only every 2 or 3 days.
6. If these drugs have been used for a long time, it may be difficult to establish a normal pattern after discontinuing the drugs.
7. Many of these drugs are sold over-the-counter. Remind patients to follow the directions on the package in terms of dose and frequency. These and all medications should be kept out of the reach of children.
8. These drugs should not be used if the patient is vomiting or has diarrhea, severe abdominal pain, suspected intestinal obstruction, suspected appendicitis, or other possible acute abdominal process.

9. Read the physician's order carefully. Many of these drugs have similar names. Many of these drugs are manufactured as combination products containing two or more kinds of agents.
10. The stimulant cathartics and saline cathartics may cause some mild abdominal cramping. If cramping is excessive, it may indicate that the dose of medication was too high or that there may be some additional pathological condition present such as obstruction. In the elderly, smaller doses of these drugs may be sufficient to stimulate defecation.
11. When one or more of these drugs is prescribed to prepare the patient for a diagnostic procedure, it is important to review the instructions with the patient and to emphasize the necessity of following the directions carefully. The major reason that many studies of the gastrointestinal tract are poor in quality or need to be repeated is that the preparations of the gut or colon were inadequate.
12. Pregnant women should consult their physicians before self-dosing to relieve constipation. Women who are nursing should use only preparations cleared with the physician to prevent the possibility of the infant consuming one of these drugs in the breast milk.
13. Changes in bowel habits, especially when no easily explainable cause can be found, should be investigated with a thorough medical examination.
14. Keep a record of bowel movements on all immobilized, incapacitated, or institutionalized patients. Early detection and treatment of constipation, followed by preventive treatment and change in diet, are much easier and less time-consuming than treatment of severe constipation or impaction.
15. *Bulk-forming laxatives*
    a. The prescribed dose should be stirred into an 8 oz glass of fluid and consumed while still suspended in solution. For best results, the dose should be followed by another full glass of water. These drugs should never be taken dry because they could cause obstruction. If taken in pill form, the pill should be swallowed whole and not chewed first.
    b. Regular use of these agents (1 to 3 times daily) is usually needed to promote regular defecation.
16. *Stimulant (irritant) cathartics*
    a. Because most of these medications, when taken orally, require about 6 hours to stimulate defecation, they are often better taken at bedtime, allowing the patient to have a bowel movement the next morning.
    b. Enteric-coated tablets, such as bisacodyl preparations, should be swallowed whole and not chewed.
    c. Bisacodyl oral preparations, as noted in the text, should not be given within 60 minutes of milk or antacids. Do not administer bisacodyl suppositories before eating or at any time in which the stimulation of defecation 15 to 20 minutes later will interfere with other activities in the patient's day.
    d. Before administering castor oil preparations, check with the patient to see which juice the patient prefers as a diluent. Some patients may even prefer to take the medication "straight" with the juice as a follow-up liquid so that the taste of the juice is not ruined by the medication.
    e. Regular castor oil will not mix with a water-based diluent and sits on the top of the juice. The addition of a small amount of baking soda (less than ¼ teaspoon) immediately before administering to the patient will cause the mixture to fizz, and the castor oil will be partially suspended in the juice for a minute or two; the patient may find it easier to drink this way. In an institution, the routine use of baking soda for this purpose should be cleared by the pharmacy or physician.
    f. Review with patients the anticipated changes in the color of urine and/or feces (see text and Table 11-5).
    g. Suppositories should be kept in the refrigerator if they are to be kept for long periods of time. The cold suppository, especially the glycerin suppository, may be easier to insert than one at room temperature, which may be too soft.
17. *Saline cathartics*
    a. Magnesium citrate is usually better tolerated if chilled first. The entire dose should be consumed at one time.
18. *Mineral oil*
    a. When mineral oil is used on a regular basis, there may be leakage of the oil and/or fecal material from the anus. Warn patients of this. The oil will stain clothing. It may be necessary for patients to wear a perianal pad to protect clothing and sheets.
    b. The regular use of mineral oil has been associated with an increased incidence of lipid pneumonia, especially in the elderly. Caution the patient to always sit upright when taking this medication. If the patient will be using an agent on a long-term basis to relieve constipation, a medication other than mineral oil might be a better choice.
    c. Mineral oil, or any oil-based substance, should never be used to lubricate around the nose because of the possibility of inhaling minute quan-

tities that might contribute at a later time to lipid pneumonia.

19. *Fecal softeners*
    a. Explain to the patient the action of fecal softeners. Many patients misunderstand their function, and expect defecation to occur a few hours following a dose of a fecal softener, just as it might after a stimulant-type drug.
    b. To be effective, fecal softeners need to be used on a daily basis or more often to keep the stools at a softer consistency regularly. If used once or twice a week or on an "as needed" basis, they will be much less effective.

■ SUMMARY

Tone and motility of the small intestine are stimulated by cholinomimetic drugs and inhibited by anticholinergic and antispasmodic drugs.

Stomach acid is neutralized by antacids and its secretion is inhibited by anticholinergic drugs and cimetidine, the H_2-histamine receptor antagonist.

Vomiting is best controlled prophylactically. Antihistamines and scopolamine are most effective for preventing motion sickness. Antidopaminergic drugs are most effective for preventing vomiting from chemotherapy and radiation therapy.

Diarrhea refers to bowel movements that are frequent, watery, and/or large. Lost fluids must be replaced, and, if appropriate, certain drugs can be given. Opioids act to decrease tone and motility of the intestine. Bismuth salts can absorb toxins and other irritants that cause diarrhea.

Constipation refers to bowel movements that are infrequent and difficult to pass. Laxatives promote defecation and are used to relieve constipation or to clean out the large intestine for examination. Classes of laxatives include bulk-forming, stimulant (irritant), saline (osmotic), wetting agent (softener), and lubricant. Chronic use of stimulant or saline laxatives can irritate the large intestine to the point that it becomes inactive. Chronic use of the lubricant mineral oil can create a deficiency of the fat-soluble vitamins A, D, E, and K.

■ STUDY QUESTIONS

1. What actions do cholinomimetic drugs have on the gastrointestinal tract? Name two cholinomimetic drugs that are used for their activity on the gastrointestinal tract.
2. What actions do anticholinergic drugs have on the gastrointestinal tract?
3. What three factors stimulate the secretion of stomach acid?
4. How do ulcers arise? What does the location of the ulcer indicate?
5. What do antacids do?
6. Name the major side effects of sodium bicarbonate, aluminum and calcium alkaline salts, and magnesium alkaline salts.
7. Why does cimetidine inhibit gastric acid secretion, whereas other commonly used antihistamines do not?
8. What are the three major pathways stimulating vomiting?
9. What are some nonmedicinal treatments of nausea and vomiting?
10. Describe the major differences in the effectiveness of the antihistamines versus the antidopaminergic drugs for types of nausea and vomiting.
11. What is diarrhea? Why is fluid and electrolyte replacement important?
12. What drugs are effective in treating diarrhea? What is their mechanism of action?
13. List the five classes of laxatives. How do they differ in the time for a laxative effect to be produced and in the type of stool produced?
14. Why is the continued use of the stimulant (irritant) cathartics of little help in establishing regular bowel habits?

■ SUGGESTED READINGS

Aman, R.A.: Treating the patient, not the constipation, American Journal of Nursing **80:**1634, 1980.

Andrysiak, T., Carroll, R.M., and Ungerleider, J.T.: Marijuana for the oncology patient, American Journal of Nursing **79:**1396, 1979.

Bertholf, C.B.: Protocol: acute diarrhea, Nurse Practitioner **3:**8, Feb., 1980.

Black, F.O., Correia, M.J., and Stucker, F.J.: Easing proneness to motion sickness, Patient Care **14**(6):114, 1980.

Burkle, W.S.: What you should know about Tagamet. New drug therapy for peptic ulcers, Nursing '80 **10:**86, April, 1980.

Derezin, M.: Laxatives and fecal modifiers, American Family Physician **10**(1):126, 1974.

Dhar, G., and Soergel, K.: Principles of diarrhea therapy, American Family Physician **19**(1):165, 1979.

Dretchen, K., Hollander, D., and Kirsner, J.B.: Roundup on antacids and anticholinergics, Patient Care **9**(6):94, 1975.

Finkelstein, W., and Isselbacher, K.: Medical intelligence: drug therapy, New England Journal of Medicine **299:**992, 1978.

Hendrix, T.: Antacids, American Family Practice **9**(3):184, 1974.

Lucas, V., and Laszlo, J.: Delta ^{9}-tetrahydrocannabinol for refractory vomiting induced by cancer chemotherapy, Journal of the American Medical Association **243:**1241, 1980.

Marshall, J.B., and Settles, R.H.: Zollinger-Ellison syndrome, Postgraduate Medicine **68**(1):38, 1980.

Rodman, M.J.: The drug interactions we all overlook, RN **43:**46, Oct., 1980.

Samborsky, V.: Drug therapy for peptic ulcer, American Journal of Nursing **78:**2064, 1978.

Sause, R.B.: Antacid therapy, Journal of Nursing Care **12:**8, Sept., 1979.

Sause, R.B.: Cimetidine treatment for peptic ulcer disease, Journal of Nursing Care **13:**8, Feb., 1980.

Schlipper, W.: Cimetidine: H_2-receptor blockade in gastrointestinal disease, Archives of Internal Medicine **138:**1257, 1978.

Shambaugh, G.E., III, and Major, N.D.: When your patient asks about enemas, Patient Care **14**(6):129, 1980.

Summers, R., and Christensen, J.: Acute and chronic diarrheas: diagnostic and therapeutic considerations, Drug Therapy **8**(11):31, 1978.

Texter, E., Jr., Smart, D., and Butler, R.: Antacids, American Family Physician **11**(4):111, 1975.

Tollison, J., and Graffin, J., Jr.: High-fiber diet and colorectal disease, American Family Physician **22**(7):121, 1980.

Wyman, J., and Wick, M.: The vomiting patient, American Family Physician **21**(2):139, 1980.

IV DRUGS AFFECTING THE CARDIOVASCULAR AND RENAL SYSTEMS

This section can be divided into three groups: drugs affecting circulation and blood pressure (Chapters 12, 13, and 14), drugs affecting the heart (Chapters 15 and 16), and drugs affecting the blood (Chapters 17, 18, and 19).

In Chapters 12 and 13, which cover the pharmacology of circulation and blood pressure, the student will find drugs with the adrenergic mechanisms discussed in Chapter 8 as well as direct-acting vasodilators. Chapter 12 covers the sympathomimetic amines and their use as acute agents to maintain circulation and/or blood pressure. The vasodilators used principally to treat angina and those used principally to treat impaired peripheral vascular circulation are discussed. Antihypertensive drugs are presented in Chapter 13 according to their mechanism of action. The importance of planned drug interaction in the treatment of chronic hypertension is reviewed in the chapter summary.

Chapters 14 through 19 are each devoted to a given area of therapeutics for which the pharmacology is rather distinctly focused on a physiological process. Here the chapter titles indicate the traditional scheme of presentation: diuretics, cardiac glycosides, antiarrhythmic drugs, drugs affecting blood clotting, drugs to lower blood lipids, and drugs to treat nutritional anemias.

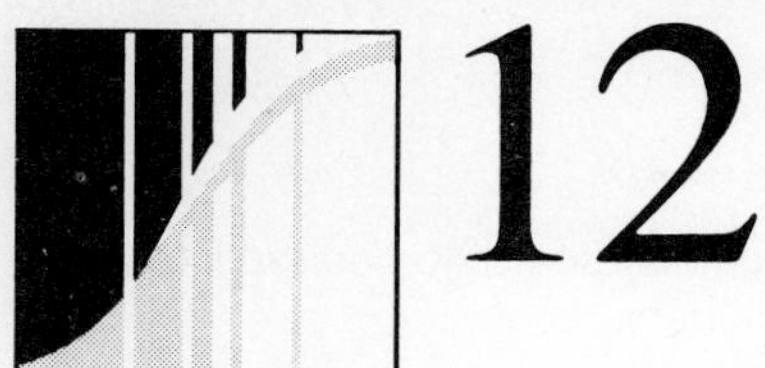

12 Drugs to improve circulation: sympathomimetics and vasodilators for angina and peripheral vascular disease

This chapter covers drugs used primarily to improve circulation: sympathomimetic drugs and selected vasodilators.

Sympathomimetic drugs restore functions mediated through adrenergic receptors. These drugs are used primarily in the treatment of shock, a condition of poor tissue perfusion in which selective adjustment of cardiac or vascular function may prevent shock from progressing to death.

Vasodilators improve blood flow by increasing the size of the blood vessels. Vasodilation has been used in treating angina and peripheral vascular disease. Although some of the activity of vasodilators may be related to alpha or beta adrenergic receptors, most vasodilators work by a mechanism not well understood. As an understanding of these diseases progresses, the role of vasodilators is being reevaluated. Vasodilators used primarily as antihypertensive agents are discussed in Chapter 13.

Sympathomimetic amines

■ DIRECT-ACTING SYMPATHOMIMETIC AMINES

■ Cardiovascular actions

The rate of blood flow through a tissue is determined by the size of the blood vessels and the atrial-venous blood pressure differential across the tissue. The systemic blood pressure reflects the cardiac output, whereas the diastolic blood pressure reflects the resistance of the tissue vessels to flow. As discussed in Chapter 8, the sympathetic nervous system plays a major role in controlling cardiovascular function. Stimulation of the alpha adrenergic receptors of blood vessels causes vasoconstriction. On a systemic level, this vasoconstriction shows up as a higher blood pressure. Stimulation of the cardiac beta-1 receptors increases heart rate and force of contraction, resulting in an increased cardiac output. Stimulation of the beta-2 receptors, found primarily in the blood vessels of the skeletal muscle, causes vasodilation. Only in unusual circumstances, however, does systemic stimulation of the beta-2 receptors decrease blood pressure.

The net change in cardiovascular function produced by direct-acting sympathomimetic drugs depends on the degree of activity at the three adrenergic receptor subtypes.

■ Uses in shock

Shock is a disruption of circulation. Frequently, the blood pressure is too low to force blood through vital tissues. Poor perfusion of the brain results in confusion or coma; poor perfusion of the kidney results in low urine output (less than 30 ml per hour); and poor perfusion of the skin makes the skin cold and clammy. In shock, the body has already activated the sympathetic nervous system to increase blood pressure. Fluid replacement or fluid addition is often the first choice in treating shock to overcome the decrease in the circulating volume caused by the constriction of the peripheral blood vessels. Selected use of direct-acting sympathomimetic amines is made in treating certain types of shock, raising blood pressure by increasing peripheral resistance (activation of alpha-1 adrenergic receptors) and/or by increasing cardiac output (activation of beta-1 adrenergic receptors).

■ Specific drugs (Table 12-1)

Levarterenol (Norepinephrine, Levophed)

Mechanism of action. Norepinephrine, the neurotransmitter of the sympathetic nervous system, is a potent agonist of the alpha-1 and beta-1 adrenergic receptors when administered as the drug levarterenol. Levarterenol has relatively little effect on the beta-2 adrenergic receptors.

Levarterenol produces a potent peripheral vasoconstriction and inotropic response. Blood flow is shifted from the skin and visceral and renal vessels (where blood vessels are constricted) to the heart and brain (where blood vessels do not have alpha receptors). On administration, levarterenol initially raises blood pressure dramatically. The increase is quickly great enough to stimulate the baroreceptors in the aorta, thereby triggering reflex stimulation of the vagus nerve, a physiological

TABLE 12-1. Sympathomimetic drugs used to treat hypotension and shock

Generic name	Trade name	Dosage and administration	Comments
Dobutamine hydrochloride	Dobutrex	INTRAVENOUS: *Adults*—2.5 to 10 μg/kg/min. A 12.5 to 25 mg/ml solution is made up and used.	To stimulate cardiac contractility in cardiogenic shock.
Dopamine hydrochloride	Intropin	INTRAVENOUS: *Adults*—1 ampule (40 mg of the chloride salt in 5 ml) is diluted in 250 ml (800 μg/ml) or 500 ml (400 μg/ml) of solution. Initial intravenous infusion is 2 to 5 μg/kg/min. Onset: 5 min. Duration: 10 min.	To maintain renal blood flow in shock with mild cardiac stimulation.
Epinephrine hydrochloride	Adrenalin Chloride	INTRAMUSCULAR, SUBCUTANEOUS, INTRAVENOUS: *Adults*—0.5 ml of a 1:1000 solution IM or SC followed by 0.25 to 0.5 ml of a 1:10,000 solution IV every 5 to 15 min. *Children*—0.3 ml of a 1:1000 solution IM. May be repeated every 15 min for 1 hr if necessary. Onset: minutes. Duration: 1 to 4 hr.	To treat anaphylactic shock.
Isoproterenol hydrochloride	Isuprel Hydrochloride	INTRAVENOUS: *Adults*—1 to 2 mg (5 to 10 ml) diluted in 5% dextrose and infused at a rate of 1 to 10 μg/min. Onset: minutes. Duration: 1 to 2 hr.	To stimulate cardiac contractility.
Levarterenol (norepinephrine) bitartrate	Levophed Bitartrate	INTRAVENOUS: *Adults*—2 to 8 ml of a 0.2% solution in 500 ml 5% dextrose and given by continuous infusion for desired response. Onset: immediate. Duration: minutes.	To maintain blood pressure in life-threatening situations.

process called *reflex bradycardia* (slow heart rate). This results because stimulation of the vagus nerve releases acetylcholine. Since acetylcholine slows the heart, this vagal stimulation counteracts the direct stimulation of the heart by levarterenol. The net result of administering levarterenol is therefore an increase in blood pressure with a modest and variable change in heart rate but very strong contractions of the heart.

Administration and fate. Levarterenol is ineffective when taken orally, being rapidly degraded in the stomach. Levarterenol is administered intravenously, and if it does infiltrate the infusion site, the alpha adrenergic receptor antagonist phentolamine must be infiltrated in the area to counteract the profound vasoconstriction that may lead to tissue ischemia.

Levarterenol is rapidly inactivated by the liver. Some of the drug is taken up and stored in sympathetic neurons identical to the native norepinephrine.

Side effects. Anxiety and a slow forceful heartbeat are common side effects on administration of levarterenol. Some patients may develop a transient hypertension that presents as a severe headache.

Uses and contraindications. Levarterenol is used to restore blood pressure in acute hypotensive states but only after blood volume has been restored. In the absence of adequate blood volume, tissue perfusion is inadequate after vasoconstriction by levarterenol in spite of increased blood pressure. Kidney perfusion in particular is poor. Levarterenol provides a temporary treatment when the brain or heart is compromised in shock. Levarterenol may be used immediately after cardiac arrest has been terminated to restore and maintain blood pressure.

Levarterenol is contraindicated for patients who have vascular thrombosis because the resulting vasoconstriction could cause tissue death. Levarterenol should not be used to raise blood pressure in patients anesthetized

TABLE 12-1. Sympathomimetic drugs used to treat hypotension and shock—cont'd

Generic name	Trade name	Dosage and administration	Comments
Mephentermine sulfate	Wyamine Sulfate	INTRAVENOUS: *Adults*—600 mg to 1 Gm is diluted in 1 L 5% dextrose and given by continuous infusion to maintain pressure. Onset: immediate. Duration: 30 to 45 min.	To maintain arterial blood pressure during spinal, epidural, or general anesthesia.
Metaraminol bitartrate	Aramine	INTRAMUSCULAR, INTRAVENOUS: *Adults*—2 to 5 mg as a single intravenous injection or 200 to 500 mg diluted in 1 L 5% dextrose given by continuous infusion to maintain pressure. Alternatively, 5 to 10 mg given IM. Onset: 1 to 2 min. Duration: 20 to 60 min.	To maintain pressure during spinal, epidural, or general anesthesia.
Methoxamine hydrochloride	Vasoxyl	INTRAMUSCULAR, INTRAVENOUS: *Adults*—5 to 20 mg in a single intramuscular dose or 2 to 5 mg given slowly IV. Onset: immediate. Duration: 60 min.	To maintain pressure during spinal and general anesthesia. To control hypotension after ganglionic blockade.
Phenylephrine hydrochloride	Neo-Synephrine Hydrochloride Isophrin	ORAL, INTRAMUSCULAR, SUBCUTANEOUS, INTRAVENOUS: *Adults*—1 to 10 mg IM or SC; 0.25 to 0.5 mg given IV or 10 mg in 500 ml 5% dextrose infused slowly; 20 mg 3 times per day orally for orthostatic hypotension. Onset: minutes. Duration: 1 to 2 hr.	To maintain pressure during general and spinal anesthesia. To treat orthostatic hypotension and paroxysmal atrial tachycardia.

with a drug that sensitizes the heart to catecholamine-induced arrhythmias (Chapter 29).

Drug interactions. Administration of levarterenol to a patient taking an antidepressant drug (either a monoamine oxidase inhibitor or a tricyclic antidepressant) may cause a severe hypertensive response, since these drugs interfere with the degradation and reuptake, respectively, of norepinephrine. A persistent hypertensive response may be elicited if levarterenol is administered after an oxytocic drug during labor.

Epinephrine

Mechanism of action. Epinephrine is a potent agonist of the beta-1 receptors of the heart, increasing heart rate and force of contraction. This cardiac stimulation is achieved with an increase in the oxygen demand of the heart, which may not be tolerable in cardiac disease. Epinephrine also stimulates alpha receptors to cause vasoconstriction, particularly of the vessels in the skin, mucosa, kidney, and visceral organs. Epinephrine also stimulates beta-2 receptors, which alters blood flow because beta-2 receptors mediate vasodilation in the blood vessels in skeletal muscle. The overall response to intravenous administration of epinephrine is a marked increase in heart rate and force of contraction with little or no increase in blood pressure.

Administration and fate. Epinephrine is not active when given orally because it is rapidly inactivated by the gastric mucosa. Epinephrine is administered intramuscularly or subcutaneously. Epinephrine may be inhaled from a nebulizer for relief of bronchospasm. Intravenous administration of epinephrine must be done very slowly and cannot be made using one of the epinephrine suspensions. Intracardiac injection of epinephrine is a last step in attempting cardiac resuscitation when other measures have failed.

Epinephrine is rapidly degraded by the monoamine oxidase and catechol-*O*-methyltransferase of the liver and kidney. Epinephrine is unstable in alkaline solutions and when exposed to light or air. Pink or brown solutions should not be used.

Side effects. Fear and anxiety are side effects of epinephrine arising from stimulation of the central nervous system. Other side effects include a throbbing headache, dizziness, and pallor caused by vasoconstriction. Stimulation of skeletal smooth muscle causes tremor and weakness and stimulation of the heart causes palpitation. These effects are usually transient. Hyperthyroid and hypertensive patients are prone to an exaggerated hypertensive response to epinephrine. Cerebral hemorrhage and cardiac arrhythmias are serious reactions to epinephrine.

Uses and contraindications. Epinephrine, administered as soon as possible, is the drug of choice for treating anaphylactic shock. Anaphylactic shock is the result of massive histamine release caused by an allergic reaction and must be promptly treated. Histamine causes profound vasodilation and bronchial constriction. Epinephrine opposes the actions of histamine: epinephrine produces vasoconstriction, raising the blood pressure, and relaxes the bronchioles, restoring breathing. Epinephrine quickly reverses the edema of the larynx and the bronchospasm of anaphylactic shock.

Epinephrine may be administered systemically or by inhalation for relief of bronchospasm resulting from asthma or allergic reactions. Because epinephrine causes vasoconstriction, it is applied topically as a hemostatic agent. Epinephrine injection prolongs the action of local anesthetics by slowing their systemic absorption.

Epinephrine is contraindicated for patients under a general anesthetic that sensitizes the heart to catecholamines. Neither should patients with narrow-angle glaucoma receive epinephrine nor should women in labor. Epinephrine must be used with extreme care in patients with cardiac arrhythmias, cardiovascular disease, hypertension, or hyperthyroidism. The hyperglycemic, hypoinsulinemic effects of epinephrine will interrupt control of diabetes mellitus.

Drug interactions. Epinephrine should not be administered simultaneously with isoproterenol because the combination can cause cardiac arrhythmias. Cardiac effects of epinephrine are also potentiated by tricyclic antidepressants, antihistamines, thyroxine, digitalis, and mercurial diuretics. A hypertensive response to epinephrine may be seen in patients receiving a monoamine oxidase inhibitor or oxytocin.

Isoproterenol (Isuprel)

Mechanism of action. Isoproterenol is a synthetic catecholamine that stimulates beta-1 and beta-2 adrenergic receptors but has little activity on alpha adrenergic receptors. Isoproterenol will therefore stimulate heart rate and cardiac output. At sufficient doses of isoproterenol, blood pressure will fall because activation of the beta-2 receptors of the blood vessels in skeletal muscle will shunt blood to the muscles and lower peripheral resistance. Smooth muscle, particularly the bronchial and gastrointestinal smooth muscle, is stimulated by isoproterenol. Isoproterenol is effective in treating bronchospasm.

Administration and fate. Isoproterenol is not very effective orally. Absorption from a sublingual site is unreliable. Isoproterenol may be given effectively subcutaneously, intramuscularly, or intravenously. The catechol-*O*-methyltransferase of the liver and other tissues is the major enzyme for degrading isoproterenol.

Side effects. Side effects of isoproterenol include palpitation, tachycardia (fast heart rate), headache, and flushing of the face. Sweating and mild tremors, nervousness, dizziness, and nausea may be experienced.

Uses. The principal use of isoproterenol is as a bronchodilator, and this use is discussed in Chapter 22. Isoproterenol is infrequently used as a cardiac stimulant in heart block and in cardiogenic shock secondary to a myocardial infarction or septicemia.

Contraindications and drug interactions. Patients taking digitalis or otherwise disposed toward cardiac arrhythmias should not receive isoproterenol. Isoproterenol should not be administered with epinephrine because together they can induce severe cardiac arrhythmias.

Dopamine (Intropin)

Mechanism of action. Dopamine is a naturally occurring catecholamine capable of acting at alpha and beta adrenergic receptors as well as at its own specific dopaminergic receptors. Appropriate doses of this catecholamine can be selected such that cardiac output is increased while heart rate and mean blood pressure remain unchanged. The unusual and highly desirable property of dopamine is that renal blood flow is directly stimulated at these same doses. Renal function may therefore be maintained in patients being treated for shock as long as supportive therapy maintains adequate blood volume.

Administration and fate. Dopamine must be administered by constant intravenous infusion. Dopamine is rapidly taken up and stored or destroyed by tissues. The infusion rate must be meticulously adjusted to achieve the desired therapeutic results.

Side effects. Dopamine can cause tachycardia (fast heart rate), palpitation, nausea and vomiting, angina, headache, hypertension, and vasoconstriction. A reduction or discontinuance of dopamine infusion is usually sufficient to reverse side effects because dopamine has such a short plasma half-life. Leakage of dopamine around the infusion site must be avoided, but if extravasation does occur, the alpha adrenergic receptor antagonist phentolamine should be infused into the area to reverse vasoconstriction. Untreated extravasation can cause tissue death and sloughing.

Uses. Dopamine is the most widely used sympathomimetic amine for treating shock. The action of dopamine may be controlled by the rate of infusion. Dopamine is primarily used as a renal vasodilator to prevent renal failure in shock and is secondarily used to increase cardiac output. At low doses (0.5 to 2 μg/kg/min), dopamine acts exclusively on dopamine receptors in the renal arterioles to cause vasodilation. At higher doses (1 to 10 μg/kg/min), dopamine acts at cardiac beta-1 receptors to stimulate cardiac contractility. The beta-1 receptors controlling heart rate and the alpha receptors on blood pressure are not activated. At doses above these, dopamine causes the release of norepinephrine, thereby increasing heart rate and blood pressure.

Contraindications and drug interactions. Like the other sympathomimetic amines, dopamine is contraindicated for patients predisposed to cardiac arrhythmias. Dopamine is not stable in alkaline solutions and should not be made up in a sodium bicarbonate solution. Patients medicated with a monoamine oxidase inhibitor require a reduced dosage of dopamine. Tricyclic antidepressants potentiate the hypertensive action of dopamine. Dopamine should not be administered to women in labor receiving an oxytocic drug because a severe persistent hypertension may be produced. Patients receiving one of the general anesthetics that sensitize the heart to catecholamines may develop arrhythmias if dopamine is administered. Since dopamine dilates renal arteries, the action of diuretic drugs is potentiated.

Dobutamine (Dobutrex)

Mechanisms of action. Dobutamine is a new drug, which, like dopamine, will at low doses selectively increase the contractility of the heart without increasing the heart rate. Dobutamine neither stimulates the dopamine receptors of the kidney blood vessels nor releases norepinephrine. At high doses, dobutamine does increase heart rate and conduction velocity (beta-1 adrenergic receptor) and stimulates beta-2 adrenergic receptors.

Administration and fate. Dobutamine has a plasma half-life of about 2 minutes and must be administered by continuous intravenous infusion. Dobutamine is rapidly metabolized to inactive compounds in the liver.

Side effects. An increase in heart rate and blood pressure are the most frequent side effects and can be reversed by lowering the infusion rate. Palpitations, shortness of breath, angina, nausea, and headache are infrequent side effects of dobutamine.

Uses. Dobutamine improves cardiac output in patients with congestive heart failure with little effect on heart rate or systolic blood pressure.

Contraindications and drug interactions. Dobutamine is a relatively new drug, and contraindications and drug interactions are not extensively characterized. Since the actions of dobutamine are similar to dopamine and isoproterenol, similar contraindications and drug interactions should be anticipated.

Methoxamine (Vasoxyl)

Methoxamine acts selectively to stimulate alpha adrenergic receptors. Methoxamine is administered intravenously or intramuscularly and increases blood pressure for 60 to 90 minutes. This vasopressor action is used to treat the hypotension of anesthesia during surgery, primarily for spinal anesthesia when the patient is conscious and aware of the unpleasant effects of hypotension. The increased blood pressure in a patient with normal blood pressure will cause a reflex slowing of the heart rate (reflex bradycardia). Use of this action is made in terminating episodes of paroxysmal supraventricular tachycardia.

Side effects of methoxamine include sustained hypertension with a severe headache. Goose flesh (pilomotor erection), desire to urinate, and vomiting are occasional side effects.

Like the other sympathomimetic vasopressors, methoxamine should be used with caution in patients with heart disease or hypertension and is potentiated in patients receiving oxytocic drugs, monoamine oxidase inhibitors, tricyclic antidepressants, or those patients under general anesthesia of the type that sensitizes the heart to catecholamines.

Phenylephrine (Isophrin, Neo-Synephrine)

Phenylephrine acts selectively to stimulate alpha adrenergic receptors. Phenylephrine is shorter in duration (20 to 50 minutes) than methoxamine, but otherwise the description of methoxamine and its uses, side effects, and drug interactions can be applied to phenylephrine.

Phenylephrine is used mainly as a nasal decongestant (Chapter 23) and is also used to dilate the pupil (Chapter 10). These actions result from stimulation of alpha adrenergic receptors.

■ INDIRECT-ACTING SYMPATHOMIMETIC AMINES

■ Mechanism and uses

Indirect-acting sympathomimetic drugs cause the release of norepinephrine from sympathetic neurons. The norepinephrine so released accounts for the activity of the drug. Like methoxamine, the selective alpha

■ THE NURSING PROCESS FOR SYMPATHOMIMETIC DRUGS

■ Assessment

Sympathomimetics are used primarily to treat shock. There may be many causes for shock, including trauma, blood loss, burns, overwhelming sepsis, cardiac failure (cardiogenic shock), anaphylaxis, and extreme reactions to some drugs. The patient in shock appears pale, with clammy skin. The blood pressure is usually low or may even be absent: the pulse rate may be increased and thready. If alert, the patient may complain of fear of impending doom and may be anxious. The respiratory rate may be increased. Assessment should begin with a thorough patient examination. If the shock is of acute onset, the assessment needs to be rapid, and needs to focus on the most important areas quickly. The nurse should assess the pulse, respirations, blood pressure, and level of consciousness. The patient should be observed and examined for obvious causes of the shock. The nurse should obtain and assess appropriate laboratory work, examples of which might be arterial blood gas concentrations, serum electrolyte concentrations, hematocrit and hemoglobin values, additional blood counts, and blood sugar concentrations.

■ Management

The treatment of shock usually begins while data collection continues. Vasopressors used to increase and maintain the blood pressure may be ordered immediately. An infusion control device and a microdrip infusion set should be used if possible for intravenous administration. The nurse should monitor the vital signs frequently, as often as every 5 minutes. Replacement fluids and blood are given if ordered. The fluid intake and output are checked and a Foley catheter inserted if needed. The level of consciousness is monitored and the patient attached to a cardiac monitor if necessary. Appropriate emergency care equipment such as a suction machine and resuscitation equipment should be readily available. The nurse should remain with the patient and maintain a calm external appearance. Additional data that might identify the underlying process causing the shock should be obtained and the patient observed for side effects, whether the result of shock or the medications being administered. For example, decreased perfusion of the kidneys resulting in decreased urinary output may be the result of shock itself or may be the result of side effects of the drugs being used. In addition to the physiological side effects of the medications, the nurse should look for symptoms such as fear and anxiety that may result from either the shock process or the drugs being administered. The patient and family should be kept informed of what is being done. Finally, the patient should be moved to an acute care setting as soon as the patient is stable. For further information about the treatment of shock and its causes, see appropriate textbooks of nursing.

■ Evaluation

Drugs to treat shock are considered successful if the blood pressure is maintained to provide adequate tissue perfusion. However, successful treatment of shock involves more than maintenance of blood pressure; there should also be successful treatment of the underlying condition and prevention of side effects resulting from the shock process or from the drugs that were used to treat the patient. Only a few vasopressors are used in self-management situations; most are used only in the acute care setting for the patient in shock. An example of a situation in which a patient would be prescribed a vasopressor for home use might be that of a patient with a long history of serious allergic reactions for whom the physician might prescribe epinephrine to be used in certain emergency situations. Before discharging any patient on a vasopressor, the patient should be able to explain when the medication should be used and how to use it, to demonstrate the correct administration of the medication, and to explain the side effects that occur resulting from the medication; the patient should also know when emergency assistance should be sought. For further specific guidelines, see the patient care implications section at the end of the chapter.

adrenergic receptor agonist, the indirect-acting sympathomimetic amines find primary use in treating the hypotension of spinal anesthesia. During spinal anesthesia, the sympathetic ganglia lying near the spinal cord may be affected, thereby disrupting sympathetic control of blood pressure. This is usually not to a degree that is life-threatening, but the sensation is unpleasant to the conscious patient. The indirect-acting sympathomimetic amines act directly on the postganglionic nerve terminals to release norepinephrine and restore blood pressure.

■ Specific drugs (Table 12-1)

Ephedrine

Mechanism of action. Ephedrine is the prototype of the indirect-acting sympathomimetic amines, although ephedrine can be shown to have direct sympathomimetic actions at alpha and beta adrenergic receptors. Ephedrine has been isolated from several plants and has been used in Chinese medicine for 2000 years. The major uses of ephedrine are as a bronchodilator (Chapter 22) and to dilate the pupil (mydriasis) (Chapter 10). Ephedrine is seldom used as a vasopressor and is not included in Table 12-1. The vasopressor response to ephedrine is primarily a result of cardiac stimulation, increasing blood pressure through an increase in cardiac output.

Administration. Ephedrine is active administered orally, subcutaneously, intramuscularly, or intravenously for 4 to 6 hours.

Side effects. Ephedrine is a potent stimulant of the central nervous system, and this stimulation is the major side effect. Insomnia, agitation, euphoria, and confusion may be noted. Delirium and hallucinations can occur at high doses. As with other sympathomimetic drugs, headache, palpitation, nausea and vomiting, and difficulty in voiding may be side effects. Repeated administration of ephedrine decreases the effectiveness of the drug. This rapidly developing tolerance (tachyphylaxis) results from the depletion of stored norepinephrine.

Contraindications and drug interactions. Ephedrine should be used cautiously in patients with hypertension, hyperthyroidism, diabetes mellitus, or in males with prostate obstruction. The vasopressor response to ephedrine is potentiated by monoamine oxidase inhibitors, tricyclic antidepressants, and oxytocic drugs. Cardiac arrhythmias may be precipitated by ephedrine in the presence of digitalis or one of the general anesthetics that sensitize the heart to catecholamines.

Metaraminol (Aramine)

Metaraminol has both direct alpha adrenergic agonist activity and an indirect sympathomimetic activity. Metaraminol can deplete norepinephrine stores on repeated administration to cause tachyphylaxis.

Metaraminol is administered intravenously, intramuscularly, or subcutaneously, the onset of action being 1 to 2 minutes, 10 minutes, and 15 to 20 minutes, respectively. The activity persists for 20 to 60 minutes. Larger doses are administered by intravenous infusion, and care must be taken to avoid leakage of the drug at the infusion site. Metaraminol produces a rise in diastolic and systolic blood pressure, but heart rate is usually decreased as a result of reflex bradycardia. The force of contraction of the heart is increased. Metaraminol is used clinically only to treat certain acute hypotensive states, as in spinal anesthesia.

Metaraminol does not have any pronounced central nervous system effects. Otherwise side effects, contraindications, and drug interactions are identical to those described for ephedrine.

Mephentermine (Wyamine)

Mephentermine is an indirect-acting sympathomimetic drug. The major effect of mephentermine is an increased blood pressure resulting from increased cardiac output and peripheral vasoconstriction. The effects of mephentermine persist for 30 to 60 minutes after subcutaneous administration and continue for up to 4 hours after intramuscular administration. Mephentermine can also be administered as a single intravenous dose. Mephentermine does not cause the tissue irritation characteristic of most vasopressor drugs.

Side effects of mephentermine are minimal and include drowsiness, weeping, incoherence, and, occasionally, convulsions. Contraindications and drug interactions are those described for other vasopressor drugs.

Vasodilator drugs

■ DRUG THERAPY FOR ANGINA

■ Nature of angina

Blood circulation to the heart. The heart has a very high requirement for oxygen and nutrients. These needs are met by the coronary circulation (Fig. 12-1) because the heart muscle cannot use the blood pumped through its chambers. The right and left coronary arteries originate at the aorta as it leaves the heart. The left coronary artery divides into the circumflex branch and the anterior descending branch. The three major vessels of the heart are thus the right coronary artery, circumflex coronary branch of the left coronary artery, and the anterior descending branch of the left coronary artery. These vessels divide and subdivide to the capillaries that finally service the individual cardiac cells. Ordinarily, the heart receives an adequate supply of blood through these coronary vessels.

FIG. 12-1

Coronary arteries. The three major coronary arteries are the right coronary artery and two branches of the left coronary artery: the circumflex coronary branch and the anterior descending branch. These arteries supply blood for heart muscle. Occlusion of one or more of these arteries can cause angina.

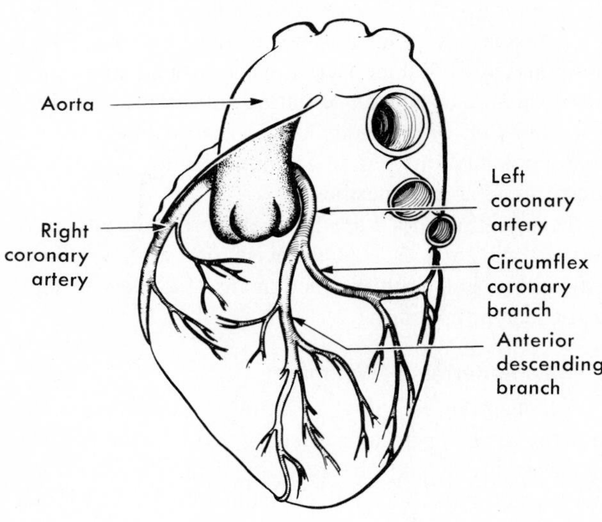

Coronary atherosclerosis. In about 1 of 50 American adults the coronary arteries become narrowed by fatty deposits that develop just underneath the inner lining of the vessel. This condition is called coronary atherosclerosis. The flow of blood in affected vessels is reduced, and the dependent heart muscle no longer receives an adequate blood supply. As the atherosclerosis worsens, the vascular system in the heart compensates by developing additional blood vessels (collateral circulation) to bypass the affected vessel. If a large enough area of the heart muscle does not receive sufficient oxygen, pain results. *Angina pectoris,* which literally means a choking of the chest, is the result of a temporary insufficiency of oxygen to the heart. In 98% of the cases, this insufficiency of oxygen is the result of coronary atherosclerosis in which the coronary vessels cannot supply sufficient blood to meet increased cardiac needs. Classic anginal pain is a sudden, severe, and pressing pain, which begins behind the breast bone and radiates up to the left shoulder and arm. This pain may often initially be a feeling of acute chest discomfort and appear in the neck, jaw, teeth, arms, or elbows, areas to which cardiac pain is physiologically referred. The pain gradually wears off when the person stops and rests.

■ Therapeutic options

The treatment of angina depends on the recognition that the supply of oxygen to the heart does not meet the demand. Chronically, the demand for oxygen can be decreased by altering secondary factors that are known to affect the heart adversely. These factors include smoking, excess weight, hypertension, arrhythmias, anxiety, anemia, and lack of regular exercise. The major risk factors for the progression of atherosclerosis are cigarette smoking, hypertension, and high serum cholesterol levels. There is evidence that alteration of these risk factors in patients with angina secondary to coronary atherosclerosis does prolong life. In the 1970's a surgical treatment of severe angina became popular: the aorta–coronary artery bypass procedure. One or more of the three main coronary vessels is bypassed with a graft from the aorta to the lower end of the vessel. One indication for the surgery is the demonstration that one or more of the vessels is severely narrowed by atherosclerosis. Replacement of such a major vessel with a graft greatly improves coronary blood flow and usually provides relief of angina. It is not known, however, whether this bypass surgery prolongs survival. The main value of the surgery may be to improve the quality of life.

The medical treatment of angina pectoris rests with two classes of drugs: the nitrates and nitrites for acute relief of angina and drugs that block beta adrenergic receptors for long-term relief of angina. The beta adrenergic antagonists propranolol, metoprolol, and naldolol are also widely used in the treatment of chronic hypertension and are discussed in detail in Chapter 13. The effectiveness of beta adrenergic receptor blockade in treating angina arises from the reduction in heart rate and contractility to produce a fall in cardiac output. This decreases the work of the heart and therefore reduces the need for oxygen, particularly during exercise. The beta adrenergic receptor antagonists are taken during the working hours and decrease dramatically the need for nitroglycerin.

Nitrates and nitrites (Table 12-2)

Mechanism of action. The nitrates and nitrites were originally believed to dilate the coronary blood vessels, thereby increasing blood flow in the heart. It is now appreciated that most patients with angina have atherosclerosis of the coronary vessels and that atherosclerotic vessels cannot dilate. Furthermore, insufficient oxygen (ischemia) is itself a potent vasodilator; thus the coronary vessels are already dilated during an anginal attack. The nitrates and nitrites do dilate arterioles and veins in the periphery thereby lowering blood pressure. The reduced blood pressure means that the work on the heart is greatly reduced. This reduced work load lowers the oxygen demand of the heart. The nitrates and nitrites, particularly nitroglycerin, are the mainstay of antianginal medication. The nitrates and nitrites are most effectively used as needed to relieve an acute anginal attack. Pa-

TABLE 12-2. Vasodilators prescribed for relief of angina pectoris

Generic name	Trade name	Dosage and administration	Comments
Amyl nitrite	Amyl Nitrite Vaporole	INHALATION: 0.18 to 0.3 ml Onset: immediate. Duration: 5 min.	Relief of acute angina attacks. Glass pearls are crushed and the volatile liquid inhaled. The odor is unpleasant. Headache, orthostatic hypotension, and reflex stimulation of the heart usually occur.
Erythrityl tetranitrate	Cardilate	SUBLINGUAL: 5 mg 3 times daily. ORAL, CHEWABLE: 10 mg 3 times daily. If required, the dose may be increased every 2 to 3 days up to 30 mg 3 times daily. Onset: 5 min for sublingual or chewable; 30 min for oral. Duration: 4 hr.	Prophylactic treatment to prevent anginal attacks. Hypotension, headaches, and tolerance to nitrates are possible side effects.
Isosorbide dinitrate	Angidil Iso-Bid Isordil Isotrate Sorbide Sorbitrate	SUBLINGUAL: 2.5 to 5 mg. CHEWABLE: 5 to 10 mg. Onset: 2 to 5 min. Duration: 1 to 2 hr.	Relief of acute angina attacks. "Possibly effective" prophylactically especially if taken in anticipation of a stressful situation. Hypotension is the side effect limiting the dose.
		ORAL: 5 to 30 mg 4 times daily. Timed-release forms, 40 mg 2 to 4 times daily. Onset: 15 to 30 min. Duration: 4 to 6 hr.	"Possibly effective" as prophylactic treatment to prevent anginal attacks. Headaches can be severe. Tolerance to nitrates may develop.
Mannitol hexanitrate	Nitranitol	ORAL: 30 to 60 mg every 4 to 6 hours.	Prophylactic treatment of angina pectoris.
Nitroglycerin	Nitroglycerin Nitrostat	SUBLINGUAL: tablets of 0.15 to 0.3 mg initially, up to 0.6 mg as required in individual patients. Individual dosages may be repeated at 5 min intervals, up to 3 tablets in 15 min. Peak action: 3 min. Duration: 10 min.	Direct-acting vasodilator. Drug of choice for angina pectoris. Take at the onset of acute anginal episodes or in anticipation of an episode, as before exercise or sex. Storage containers should be kept cool to prevent disintegration and airtight to prevent volatilization.
	Many trade names	ORAL, SUSTAINED-RELEASE: 2.5 to 6.5 mg every 8 to 12 hrs. Onset: slow variable. Duration: 8 to 12 hours.	A prophylactic administration of nitroglycerin. The effectiveness of this mode of therapy is not established. Tolerance to nitrates may develop.
Nitroglycerin ointment, 2%	Nitro-Bid Nitrol	TOPICAL: initially 1 inch is spread over an area of skin. This is increased by ½-inch increments as required. Absorption is improved by covering the area with plastic. Onset: 30 to 60 min. Duration: up to 3 hr.	A prophylactic administration of nitroglycerin. The effectiveness of this mode of therapy is not established. An excessive dose may cause a violent headache. The area of administration will be irritated and should be rotated. On terminating treatment, the area and frequency of administration should be reduced gradually over 4 to 6 weeks to prevent withdrawal reactions.

Continued.

TABLE 12-2. Vasodilators prescribed for relief of angina pectoris—cont'd

Generic name	Trade name	Dosage and administration	Comments
Pentaerythritol tetranitrate	Petn Plus Peritrate Many others	ORAL: Initially 10 to 20 mg 4 times daily. If required dosage may be adjusted up to 40 mg 4 times daily. Onset: 30 min. Duration: 4 to 5 hr.	"Possibly effective" as prophylactic treatment for angina pectoris. Hypotension, headaches, and tolerance to nitrates are possible side effects. Tablets are taken 30 min before meals or 1 hr after and at bedtime.
		SUSTAINED RELEASE: 30 to 80 mg twice a day. Onset: 30 to 60 min. Duration: 12 hr.	Taken on an empty stomach.
Trolnitrate phosphate	Metamine	ORAL: 10 mg 2 to 4 times daily.	Prophylactic treatment of angina pectoris.

tients who understand the factors that precipitate their own anginal attacks can take these medications prophylactically just before those activities.

Administration and fate. The organic nitrates will rapidly relieve anginal attacks when administered sublingually. These organic nitrates include nitroglycerin, isosorbide dinitrate, and erythrityl tetranitrate. All these drugs produce a general vasodilation by acting directly on blood vessels. The side effects of sublingual nitrates are also a result of the generalized vasodilation. These side effects include flushing, headache, and dizziness. The flushing is a result of the vasodilation in the "blush" area of the neck and face. The headache is a result of the pressure imposed by dilated blood vessels in the brain. The incidence of headaches decreases 2 to 3 weeks after initial therapy. The dizziness is the result of the generalized hypotension. The patient should sit or lie down to avoid fainting after taking one of these drugs. Indeed, if the hypotension is severe enough, a reflex increase in heart rate may occur. This will increase the cardiac work and make the pain worse.

The organic nitrates are frequently administered orally in large doses to provide prophylactic treatment for angina. Large doses are required because organic nitrates are rapidly degraded by the liver.

■ Specific drugs

Nitroglycerin

Nitroglycerin is considered the drug of choice for angina. When nitroglycerin is taken sublingually, its effect begins in 30 seconds, is maximal in 3 minutes, and lasts for about 10 minutes. A drawback to nitroglycerin is that it decomposes when exposed to light or heat. Nitroglycerin can also volatilize from the tablets and therefore must be kept in airtight containers. Nitroglycerin will cause a sting when placed under the tongue, and this sting can be used as an indication that the drug is still present.

Longer action from nitroglycerin has been achieved with oral doses up to 10 times those taken sublingually. Nitroglycerin is very lipid soluble and probably enters the body from the gastrointestinal tract through the lymphatics rather than the portal blood. Nitroglycerin is said to be effective for 8 to 12 hours when taken orally. Another route of administration for nitroglycerin is through the skin. A measured amount of nitroglycerin ointment is spread on a nonhairy part of the body and is held in place with plastic wrap taped over the area. This route of administration is said to produce relief for up to 3 hours.

Amyl nitrite

Amyl nitrite is the only nitrite used to treat angina. It is a volatile liquid packaged in an easily crushed vial with a woven cover and is self-administered by inhalation. Amyl nitrite is effective 30 seconds after inhalation and lasts for 3 to 5 minutes. Amyl nitrite has an unpleasant odor, is expensive, and is conspicuous to use. The side effects of headache, orthostatic hypotension, and reflex tachycardia can be pronounced. For these reasons amyl nitrite is seldom used. The "rush" felt when amyl nitrite is inhaled has caused this drug to be abused.

Erythrityl tetranitrate

Erythrityl tetranitrate is the longest-acting of the sublingual or chewable organic nitrates. It is effective in 5 minutes and lasts for 4 hours. This is a long onset compared to nitroglycerin or even isosorbide dinitrate, and therefore the use of erythrityl tetranitrate is more for prophylactic than for relief of acute attacks. Erythrityl tetranitrate is also available for oral administration.

THE NURSING PROCESS FOR ANTIANGINAL DRUGS

Assessment

Patients with angina pectoris have a primary single complaint: chest pain. In the majority of patients, pain is associated with exertion, exposure to cold, stress, eating a heavy meal, or other relevant activities; a few patients have no associated cause. The nurse should obtain a thorough patient assessment, focussing on the subjective and objective signs. The pulse, respiration, blood pressure, and level of consciousness should be determined. The history relevant to the onset and duration of the pain should be taken, asking about previous similar episodes and treatments. A detailed description of the nature and location of the pain should be obtained with an electrocardiogram and appropriate laboratory work, including serum enzyme concentrations. The degree of patient distress and previous history of cardiac problems will also determine the amount and focus of assessment. When in doubt as to the cause of chest pain, the usual practice is to treat the patient as if a myocardial infarction had occurred.

Management

Once the diagnosis of angina pectoris is made and a myocardial infarction is ruled out, the treatment is with one or more of the nitrates or nitrites or with a beta adrenergic antagonist, and the patient is observed and monitored for additional angina attacks. Instruction is begun about the prescribed drugs, and the patient and family are aided in identifying stresses that may precipitate attacks and in planning possible ways to decrease or alleviate these stresses. Additional measures that may be prescribed include losing weight, stopping smoking, controlling blood pressure, and a regular exercise program. Appropriate referrals may be to such members of the health care team as the dietician, the local heart association, or the visiting nurse association. For additional information about the treatment of patients with angina pectoris and other forms of heart disease, see appropriate textbooks of nursing.

Evaluation

The drugs used to treat angina are successful if the pain is relieved and the patient experiences no side effects resulting from drug therapy. The drugs do not halt the progression of disease. Before discharge the patient should be able to explain when and how to take the medications prescribed, to describe the side effects resulting from the drugs and how to treat them, and to explain what to do if drug therapy does not relieve the symptoms, how to correctly store the medication, and how to test for its continued effectiveness. In addition, the patient should be able to explain adequately why and how other therapies should be implemented, including weight loss, exercises, stopping smoking, and the treatment of hypertension or other medical problems. Finally, for some patients it may be appropriate to evaluate whether the family or close friends are able to explain how to administer a medication (e.g., sublingual nitroglycerin) if the patient were to be unable to do it. For additional specific guidelines, see the patient care implications section at the end of this chapter.

Isosorbide dinitrate

Isosorbide dinitrate is another organic nitrate that can be taken sublingually or chewed. It is effective in 2 to 5 minutes and can act for 1 to 2 hours.

Other agents

Additional organic nitrates marketed for prophylactic treatment of angina include mannitol hexanitrate, pentaerythritol tetranitrate, and trolnitrate phosphate. None of these drugs has been proven effective.

■ PERIPHERAL VASCULAR DISEASE AND VASODILATOR DRUGS

■ Vasospastic disorders

Blood flow to the arms and legs, particularly the hands and feet, can be limited by peripheral vascular disease. Basically, the blood vessels may be narrowed by arteriosclerosis or by spasm of the vessels (vasospasm). If the vessel narrowing is a result of arteriosclerosis, vasodilator drugs will be of little value. Vasodilator drugs may worsen the condition because vessels narrowed by arteriosclerosis will not dilate; adjacent vessels will dilate and shunt the blood away from the occluded area. The occluded vessel therefore has its blood flow reduced, not increased, by vasodilator drugs. On the other hand, if the narrowing of the vessel is a result of vasospasm, drugs will be of benefit.

Raynaud's disease is the classic vasospastic disease in which primarily the fingers and toes are affected. In Raynaud's disease, the blood vessels of the digits are readily thrown into spasm by cold or emotion and turn blue or white. Warming restores blood flow. Currently, the most successful drug treatment of Raynaud's disease is reported with two drugs that have been used to treat hypertension: reserpine or guanethidine. These drugs interfere with sympathetic innervation. Reserpine depresses sympathetic tone by depleting stored norepinephrine in the neurons. Guanethidine acts at the sympathetic neuron by blocking the release of norepinephrine as well as depleting norepinephrine stores. These drugs and their side effects are discussed fully in Chapter 13.

Unfortunately, a large number of ''vasodilator'' drugs are advertised for treating peripheral vascular spasm that are of doubtful clinical value. These drugs include cyclandelate, isoxsuprine, niacin, nylidrin, papaverine, and tolazoline.

■ Impaired cerebral blood flow

Vasodilator drugs are sometimes prescribed to improve blood flow in the brain, particularly in elderly patients with arteriosclerosis of cerebral vessels who have suffered strokes or show signs of mental impairment. The problem is cerebral ischemia: insufficient oxygen to areas of the brain. Controlled medical trials are showing that this drug therapy is of little value. There is some medical opinion that vasodilator drugs may make the situation worse by shunting blood away from the unreactive, damaged vessels to areas with adequate blood flow already, as described for peripheral vascular insufficiency resulting from arteriosclerosis. Cyclandelate, dihydrogenated ergot alkaloids, and papaverine are sometimes prescribed to improve cerebral blood flow. There is no evidence that these drugs alter the progression of cerebral arteriosclerosis. They may improve some symptoms on a short term basis.

■ Specific drugs (Table 12-3)

Cyclandelate

Cyclandelate acts directly on vascular smooth muscle to cause relaxation. In the laboratory, cyclandelate is a more effective vasodilator than papaverine, but the clinical effectiveness of cyclandelate is considered doubtful. Side effects include belching and heartburn, flushing, headache, weakness, and an increased heart rate.

Dihydrogenated ergot alkaloids

Dihydrogenated ergot alkaloids produce vasodilation in contrast to the ergot alkaloids, which produce vasoconstriction (Chapter 37). Dihydrogenated ergot alkaloids are of definite value in treating brain disease secondary to hypertension, but the benefit is related to the fall in blood pressure. These alkaloids act centrally to reduce vascular tone and slow heart rate. They act peripherally to block alpha adrenergic receptors. These alkaloids are available in a sublingual dosage form. Sublingual irritation, nausea, and gastrointestinal upset are side effects. The dihydrogenated ergot alkaloids can markedly reduce heart rate through their central effect of lowering sympathetic tone.

Isoxsuprine

Isoxsuprine was originally thought to stimulate beta receptors, but its vasodilating action is not blocked by drugs that are antagonists of the beta receptors. Clinical tests have not demonstrated any usefulness for isoxsuprine. Side effects include flushing, hypotension, dizziness, an increased heart rate, and, occasionally, a rash.

Niacin

Niacin (nicotinic acid) and nicotinyl alcohol have been used as vasodilators but without good evidence of clinical effectiveness. These drugs cause a pronounced flushing, postural (orthostatic) hypotension, and gastrointestinal upset. They can also cause a rash.

Nylidrin

Nylidrin is the classic example of a drug that stimulates blood flow in muscle. The rationale is to stimulate the beta receptors of the blood vessels to produce vasodilation. However, muscle blood vessels, not the blood vessels of the skin, have beta receptors, so the approach is of little value in vasospastic disorders of the digits. The beta-blocking drug propranolol does not entirely reverse this stimulation, so nylidrin is believed to also act directly on smooth muscle. Side effects attributed to nylidrin include trembling, nervousness, weakness, dizziness, palpitations, and nausea and vomiting.

TABLE 12-3. Drugs prescribed for vasodilation

Generic name	Trade name	Dosage and administration	Comments
Cyclandelate	Cyclospasmol Cyclanfor Cydel	ORAL: 300 to 400 mg 4 times daily. Can be decreased gradually to 100 to 200 mg 4 times daily.	A direct vasodilator for use in vasospastic disorders. May cause gastrointestinal disturbances.
Dihydrogenated ergot alkaloids	Hydergine	SUBLINGUAL: 1 mg 3 times daily.	Can cause marked bradycardia. Relieves symptoms in hypertensive brain disease by lowering blood pressure.
Isoxsuprine	Vasodilan Isolait Vasoprine	ORAL: 10 to 20 mg 3 to 4 times daily. INTRAMUSCULAR: 5 to 10 mg 2 to 3 times daily.	A direct acting vasodilator. No proven use.
Nicotinyl alcohol	Roniacol	TIMED-RELEASE: 300 to 400 mg every 12 hr.	A direct vasodilator that causes pronounced blushing. Gastrointestinal disturbances, tingling sensation, and rashes are side effects. Use has not been proven effective for any vasospastic disorders.
Nylidrin hydrochloride	Arlidin Circlidrin Rolidrin	ORAL: 3 to 12 mg 3 to 4 times daily.	Stimulates beta-adrenergic receptors and also directly dilates vessels. May cause dizziness, tachycardia, and hypotension.
Papaverine hydrochloride	Many trade names	ORAL: 100 to 300 mg, 3 to 5 times daily. TIMED-RELEASE: 150 mg every 12 hr. Can give up to 150 mg every 8 hr or 300 mg every 12 hr. INTRAVENOUS: 30 to 120 mg, over 1 to 2 min. INTRAMUSCULAR: 30 to 120 mg.	Depresses heart. Relaxes smooth muscle directly, particularly of the large blood vessels. Use is to relieve smooth muscle spasm in vascular disease or colic, but its effectiveness has not been proven.
Tolazoline hydrochloride	Priscoline Tolzol	ORAL: 25 mg 4 to 6 times daily, up to 50 mg, 6 times daily. TIMED-RELEASE: 80 mg every 12 hr. INTRAMUSCULAR, SUBCUTANEOUS, INTRAVENOUS: 10 to 50 mg 4 times daily.	A direct-acting vasodilator. May relieve vasospastic disorders.

Papaverine

Papaverine relaxes smooth muscle. In large doses, papaverine also depresses cardiac muscle, slowing conduction and prolonging the refractory period. Papaverine has long been used as a smooth muscle relaxant for ischemia of the brain, periphery, or heart. As with the other vasodilator drugs, there is little good evidence that papaverine improves peripheral vascular circulation. Side effects of papaverine can include flushing of the face, malaise, gastrointestinal upset, and headache. Other reported side effects include excess perspiration, loss of appetite, increased heart rate, and increased depth of respiration. Rarely, a hypersensitivity reaction involving the liver is seen. Symptoms of the liver damage include jaundice, eosinophilia, and altered results of liver function tests.

Tolazoline

Tolazoline is an alpha adrenergic antagonist that has an additional direct vasodilating effect. In theory a drug that blocks the action of norepinephrine at the alpha receptors of the blood vessels should be helpful, but in practice, alpha adrenergic antagonists are not very effective in relieving or preventing vasospasm. Tolazoline is not very effective by itself, but will potentiate the action of other drugs. Side effects are frequent with tolazoline therapy and include headache, nausea, chills, flushing, tingling of the skin, especially the scalp, and gastrointestinal disturbances. Occasionally irregular heart function is noticed; an arrhythmia or a pounding heart is the most common cardiac symptom.

■ THE NURSING PROCESS FOR VASODILATOR THERAPY IN PERIPHERAL VASCULAR DISEASE

■ Assessment

Patients with signs and symptoms of decreased peripheral blood flow come to the hospital with a variety of symptoms, some of which may be decreased or absent peripheral pulses, complaints of decreased or altered sensation in the extremities, ulcers on the extremities, poor healing of local injuries, absence of hair on the feet and toes, coolness to touch of the extremities, and change in color of the extremities. Patients with reduced cerebral blood flow may have a history of recent or old stroke, transient ischemic attacks, fluctuation in the level of consciousness, confusion, or other signs of decreased cerebral blood flow.
A complete patient assessment should be done, and a complete history about onset and course of vascular disease should be obtained. The nurse should assess the blood pressure and pulses, including peripheral pulses, and should make observations relative to the signs just described. Any deviation from normal should be recorded. A mental status examination should be obtained if decreased perfusion of the brain is suspected.

■ Management

Vasodilators are used to treat the symptoms and prevent recurrences resulting from altered or decreased perfusion. The nurse should monitor the presenting signs and symptoms, especially blood pressure and pulses, and look for drug side effects. If leg ulcers or other problems associated with vascular disease are present, treatment of these should be carried out. In addition to instruction on the medications, the nurse should begin teaching the patient about prevention of trauma to areas with decreased perfusion. Other therapies would include treatment of other medical problems, a prescribed exercise program, weight loss, and restriction of certain activities. An individualized plan of care should be devised by the health care team.

■ Evaluation

It is difficult to measure the effectiveness of these drugs. They do not alter the course of vascular disease, and it is often difficult to ascertain that they have played a role in alleviation of symptoms. Before discharge, the patient should be able to explain when and how to take the ordered medications, the possible side effects that might occur, and the situations that would require notification of the physician. If other therapies have been prescribed, the patient should be able to explain how to carry out the prescribed regimen. If the patient is going home and will continue to treat manifestations of peripheral vascular disease, the patient should be able to demonstrate how to carry out the prescribed therapies, such as warm soaks or heat that might be applied to ulcers on the legs. For more specific guidelines, see the patient care implications section at the end of this chapter.

■ PATIENT CARE IMPLICATIONS

Sympathomimetic drugs

1. Safe care of the patient receiving intravenous sympathomimetic drugs for the treatment of shock or hypotension includes the following:
   a. A microdrip intravenous administration set should be used to regulate the dose being administered more accurately.
   b. The patient's blood pressure and pulse should be monitored every 2 to 5 minutes until the blood pressure and rate of drug administration are stable, then every 15 minutes. The patient should not be left unattended.
   c. An electronic IV monitor or regulator should be used to accurately control the rate of IV fluid and drug administration.
   d. If possible, the central venous pressure should be monitored as frequently as the blood pressure is monitored.
   e. Monitor the fluid intake and output. Urinary output should be monitored and recorded every 30 to 60 minutes.

f. Read the labels of the drug ampules carefully, since not all forms of a drug may be administered intravenously. Some forms of epinephrine and ephedrine solutions are safe for IV administration, whereas others are not. Do not use any solution or medication if discolored or sediment is present.
g. Most adrenergic drugs are incompatible with many other drugs. For this reason, they are not added to IV solutions containing other medications, including sodium bicarbonate, and they are not added to blood. If in doubt, consult the pharmacist.
h. All patients should be observed for hypertensive crisis. If this does occur, the adrenergic drug should be slowed or discontinued, the physician notified, and the specific drug antidote administered as ordered. Phentolamine, an adrenergic blocking agent, may be ordered, if necessary.
i. If available, cardiac monitoring should be done while the patient is receiving intravenous adrenergic drugs.
j. Data such as the pulmonary capillary wedge pressure, cardiac output, and other hemodynamic parameters that can be measured via a balloon flotation catheter should be obtained, when possible, on a regular basis during administration of adrenergic drugs. These data will assist in evaluating the success of the drug therapy.

2. Extravasation of intravenous levarterenol, dopamine, or methoxamine may cause tissue necrosis and sloughing. For this reason, it is preferable to administer these drugs in a large central vein if possible. The intravenous insertion site should be inspected frequently. In the event of extravasation, the physician may order the site of injury infiltrated with a solution of 5 to 10 mg of phentolamine, an adrenergic blocker, diluted in 10 to 15 ml of normal saline solution.
3. Adrenergic drugs should be given cautiously to patients who have been receiving monoamine oxidase inhibitors or tricyclic antidepressants because a hypertensive crisis may be precipitated.
4. Propranolol, a beta adrenergic blocking agent, may interfere with the beta activity of levarterenol, epinephrine, dopamine, isoproterenol, and dobutamine.
5. Solutions of dopamine, dobutamine, or metaraminol should be discarded if over 24 hours old.
6. Patients who are markedly hypotensive or in shock may be anxious as a response to inadequate oxygenation of the brain and have a sense of "impending doom," symptoms that can accompany circulatory failure. As administration of adrenergic medications begins, the anxiety may continue as a response to the medication. In addition, palpitations and tachycardia may occur, which may also make the patient feel anxious. Provide calm reassurance to patients being treated with these drugs. In addition, encourage them to notify the health care personnel of new signs and symptoms that may appear.

Epinephrine and isoproterenol

1. The usual dose of epinephrine used for treating anaphylactic shock is 0.1 to 1 ml (0.1 to 1 mg) of 1:1000 solution given subcutaneously.
2. Epinephrine and isoproterenol are both strong cardiac stimulants and should not be administered simultaneously; they may be used alternately.
3. Epinephrine causes hyperglycemia, which may result in an increased insulin requirement in patients with diabetes mellitus.
4. Some forms of epinephrine solutions are safe for IV administration, whereas others are not. Do not use any solution or medication if discolored or sediment is present.

Antianginal drugs—general guidelines for patients receiving antianginal therapy

1. Proper use of antianginal agents is only a part of the usual recommended plan for satisfactory management of angina pectoris. Patients will often find additional relief by losing weight until the desired weight for their height is achieved, ceasing smoking, and becoming involved in a therapeutic exercise program if one is available and if the physician feels it is appropriate.
2. With help from the health care team, the patient can begin to identify situations or activities that precipitate anginal attacks. These activities often include eating a heavy meal, engaging in strenuous activity (work, play, or sports), lifting heavy objects, exposure to cold air or weather, certain stressful job situations, and sexual activity. If possible, the patient should try to learn to avoid the angina-producing situations or learn how to regulate the medications to prevent pain.
3. It is not clear what, if any, effect a low cholesterol diet has on angina pectoris, but it may be helpful for patients with high serum levels of cholesterol or triglycerides to modify their diets; consultation with a dietician will be helpful.
4. Encourage the patient to report to the physician any pain that differs from the patient's characteristic anginal attack. Differences might occur in duration, location, intensity, response to medication, or precipitating event.
5. Assessment of complaints of chest pain would include evaluation of blood pressure and pulse; aus-

cultation of lungs and heart; intensity, duration, location, and quality of pain; response to medication; presence of diaphoresis; electrocardiogram changes; precipitating factors; patient's objective degree of distress; patient history; and subjective patient complaints. Chest pain in the patient with a history of angina pectoris is not always due only to that cause.

6. Alcohol should be avoided because it potentiates the hypotensive effects of the antianginal agents.
7. Hypotension may be potentiated in patients receiving antianginal medications who are also receiving other drugs that can cause hypotension, such as diuretics, antihypertensives, central nervous system depressants, narcotics, and sedatives. Instruct the patient to keep all health care practitioners informed of all medications being taken.
8. Antianginal drugs used on a regular basis, that is, *not* on a prn basis, should be discontinued slowly to decrease the possibility of a withdrawal reaction in the form of more anginal attacks.
9. The presence of a severe headache in response to antianginal drugs may indicate too high a dosage; notify the physician.
10. Remind patients to keep these and all medications out of the reach of children.

Sublingual (rapidly acting) antianginal agents

1. The standard guideline for the use of sublingual antianginal agents is to have the patient use 1 tablet. If relief is not obtained, the dose may be repeated at 5-minute intervals until a total of 3 tablets has been taken. If the pain persists, the patient should call the physician or seek medical care. There are exceptions to this guide based on the individual patient's condition and the physician's preference. The practitioner should ascertain that the patient clearly understands how to use the medication.
2. There are very few medications taken via the sublingual route. Make certain that the patient knows to let the tablet completely dissolve under the tongue before swallowing.
3. The patient who experiences syncope (fainting) or hypotension characterized by dizziness, light-headedness, or weakness, should be instructed to lie down before taking one of these agents.
4. Because nitroglycerin decomposes rapidly, it is usually dispensed in small quantities (e.g., 100 tablets) and in light-resistant containers. Instruct the patient to obtain a new supply every 6 months or when the pills have lost their potency. Fresh (nondecomposed) nitroglycerin will cause a tingling sensation when used; old tablets will not. The patient should have a supply of pills available at all times but may not want to carry a full bottle. A fewer number can be carried in a light-resistant, airtight container; the pharmacist may be able to help in procuring a small bottle.
5. Family members should be instructed about the need for and use of sublingual agents. The patient's family should know to place a tablet in the patient's mouth if the patient is unable to do so.
6. When the patient with angina pectoris is in the hospital, it is often customary to keep a small supply (e.g., 10 tablets) of sublingual tablets at the bedside for the patient to use as necessary. The patient should be instructed to notify the staff as each tablet is used. In addition, the bedside supply should be counted and restocked every 8 hours. The frequency of tablet use, in addition to a brief patient assessment, should be recorded in the patient's record.

Oral antianginal agents

1. Taking oral antianginal preparations with meals may reduce gastric irritation.
2. Note that there are several dosage forms for the oral agents. There are tablets and capsules designed to be swallowed, and there are tablets that are designed to be chewed before swallowing; in addition, there are many dosage strengths. The physician's orders should be checked carefully to avoid error. The patient should be instructed clearly on how to take the prescribed medication. Make certain the patient knows the difference between the sublingual and oral preparations if both have been prescribed.

Amyl nitrite

1. Amyl nitrite is packaged in glass ampules wrapped in a protective covering. Instruct the patient to wrap the ampule in a cloth or handkerchief (to protect the fingers) and to crush the ampule to use. The medication is very strong smelling, but the patient should take a few deep inhalations.
2. Family members should be instructed how to break and use the ampules if the patient is unable to do so.

Antianginal ointment

1. These ointments are usually ordered in inches. Small sheets of paper with one-half inch markings supplied by the manufacturer are provided for measuring the correct dose.
2. Sites of application should be rotated. The rate of absorption does vary slightly depending on the site used, but there is no reason to limit application to one spot. Application to the chest wall provides no added benefit, except perhaps a psychological one to the patient. Markedly hairy areas should be avoided, if possible, because they interfere with absorption. On

the other hand, the area should not be shaved because it may increase the chance of skin irritation.

3. Although the ointment should cover a large surface area (several inches by several inches) the goal of application is not to rub in or to massage the ointment. Spreading the correct dose onto the plastic wrap before applying it to the skin will help prevent this.
4. The ointments do discolor clothing; choice of site should take this into account.
5. To protect the clothing and bed linens, plastic wrap is usually placed over the ointment and taped or wrapped in place.
6. To avoid absorption through the fingertips, the practitioner should apply the ointment with the measuring guide or the plastic wrap.
7. Skin irritation or contact dermatitis should be reported to the physician. If it is severe enough, it may be necessary to discontinue the medication.
8. This is an unusual route of administration; make certain that the patient can perform it correctly before discharge.

Beta adrenergic antagonists

Propranolol, metoprolol, and naldolol are discussed in Chapter 13.

Drugs prescribed for vasodilation

1. Vasodilators should be used with caution in patients with glaucoma.
2. Because vasodilators can cause hypotension, patients should be monitored carefully when first beginning a vasodilator or when dosages are changed. Symptoms of hypotension include vertigo, dizziness, light-headedness, syncope, increased heart rate, and decreased blood pressure. In some individuals, the hypotension is severe enough to warrant reduction of dose or discontinuation of the drug; other patients may have no problems with it. If postural hypotension occurs, instruct patients to move slowly from lying to sitting positions, and from sitting to standing. If a dose of medication is missed, patients should not ''double up'' on the next dose to catch up.
3. Alcohol should be avoided because it potentiates the hypotensive effects of vasodilators.
4. Hypotension may be potentiated in patients receiving vasodilators who are also receiving other drugs that can cause hypotension, such as diuretics, antihypertensives, central nervous system depressants, narcotics, and sedatives. Instruct the patient to keep all health care practitioners informed of all medications being taken.
5. The sublingual route of administration may be unfamiliar to patients taking dihydrogenated ergot alkaloids. Teach patients to let the tablet dissolve completely before swallowing.
6. Taking oral preparations with meals will reduce gastric irritation.
7. The safety of the vasodilators during pregnancy and lactation has not been established. Women of childbearing age may wish to use birth control measures during vasodilator therapy, or at least discuss with their physicians the benefits versus risks of taking these preparations.
8. Isoxsuprine has been used to relax the uterus in cases of premature labor. Because of the undesirable side effects (maternal hypotension, maternal and fetal tachycardia) patients should be monitored carefully with frequent determinations of blood pressure and pulse and supervised ambulation. Fetal heart tones should be measured frequently.
9. Most of the vasodilators can cause flushing; forewarn patients that this is an expected effect of therapy.
10. Parenteral administration of papaverine is as follows:
    a. Papaverine may be given intramuscularly or intravenously.
    b. For intravenous administration, it may be given undiluted or mixed with equal parts of sterile water for injection. Do not add to intravenous solutions. It is compatible with lactated Ringer's solution and protein hydrolysate. Before mixing with other medications, consult with the pharmacy.
    c. Administer slowly intravenously—1 ml (30 mg) over a period of 2 minutes.
    d. If possible, monitor the electrocardiogram during administration because the drug can produce ectopic ventricular rhythms (usually transient).
    e. Monitor the pulse, respirations, and blood pressure during administration and for an hour afterwards.
11. Parenteral administration of tolazoline hydrochloride is as follows:
    a. Tolazoline hydrochloride may be given intravenously, intramuscularly, subcutaneously, and, in rare instances, intraarterially (by a physician).
    b. In the event of overdose or severe hypotension, place the patient in the Trendelenburg position, administer fluids, and administer a vasopressor such as ephedrine; avoid epinephrine or norepinephrine.
    c. Marked hypertension has been reported in rare instances. Monitor the blood pressure for at least an hour after parenteral administration.
12. Niacin is discussed in Chapter 18.

■ SUMMARY

Sympathomimetic drugs are used in selected situations to improve blood flow in shock. Activation of alpha adrenergic receptors will cause vasoconstriction and increase blood pressure by increasing peripheral vascular resistance. Activation of the beta-1 adrenergic receptors of the heart will increase cardiac output.

Drugs administered primarily to activate alpha adrenergic receptors include the direct-acting sympathomimetics levarterenol (norepinephrine), methoxamine, and phenylephrine, and the indirect-acting sympathomimetics metaraminol and mephentermine.

Epinephrine is used to treat anaphylactic shock because epinephrine not only stimulates alpha receptors to restore blood pressure but also stimulates beta-2 receptors to dilate the bronchioles.

Dopamine is administered at low doses for its unique action to dilate renal arterioles and thereby prevent kidney failure secondary to shock. At intermediate doses, dopamine stimulates the cardiac beta-1 adrenergic receptors to increase cardiac output, and at high doses dopamine is also an indirect-acting sympathomimetic.

Dobutamine is relatively specific at low doses for stimulation of cardiac contractility without stimulation of heart rate, a selective action among cardiac beta-1 receptors. At high doses, dobutamine becomes a nonselective beta adrenergic receptor agonist, stimulating both beta-1 and beta-2 receptors.

Isoproterenol is a nonselective beta adrenergic receptor agonist. Its major use is as a bronchodilator, and its use as a cardiac stimulant is a minor one.

Angina is the pain that results when the oxygen demand of the heart is not met. Nitrates and nitrites, particularly nitroglycerin, offer acute and prophylactic relief. These vasodilators reduce the work load on the heart, which lowers the oxygen demand. In severe cases of angina, the beta adrenergic receptor antagonists propranolol, nadolol, or metoprolol may be effective. These drugs decrease the work of the heart by inhibiting sympathetic stimulation of the heart.

Several vasodilators are used to treat selected cases of impaired circulation of the digits or brain. The vasodilators used include cyclandelate, the dihydrogenated ergot alkaloids, isoxsuprine, niacin, nylidrin, papaverine, and tolazoline. The therapeutic effectiveness of these drugs is not clear.

■ STUDY QUESTIONS

1. List the direct-acting sympathomimetic drugs. What is their receptor selectivity and what physiological actions result?
2. List the indirect-acting sympathomimetic drugs. What is their receptor selectivity and what physiological actions result?
3. Which drug is used to treat anaphylactic shock?
4. Which drug is used as a renal vasodilator?
5. Which drug is used as a selective stimulant of cardiac contractility?
6. Why are sympathomimetic drugs sometimes administered during spinal anesthesia?
7. What is the origin of angina?
8. How do the nitrates and nitrites relieve angina?
9. What are two causes of insufficient blood flow to the digits? Which cause is amenable to drug therapy? What role do vasodilators play?
10. List the seven drugs used as vasodilators for improving peripheral circulation. What are some of their common side effects?

■ SUGGESTED READINGS

Andreoli, K.G., Fowkes, V.H., Zipes, D.P., and Wallace, G.G.: Comprehensive cardiac care, ed. 4, St. Louis, 1979, The C.V. Mosby Co.

Borow, K.M., Alpert, J.S., and Cohn, P.F.: The natural history and treatment of coronary artery disease: a perspective, Cardiovascular Medicine **3**(1):87, 1978.

Cain, R.S., Ferguson, R.M., and Tillisch, J.H.: Variant angina: a nursing approach, Heart & Lung **8:**1122, 1979.

Chandraratna, P.A.N.: Clinical pharmacology and mechanisms of action, Practical Cardiology **5**(5):161, 1979.

Combatting cardiovascular diseases skillfully. Nursing skillbook, Horsham, Pa., 1978, Intermed Communications.

Czerwinski, B.S.: Manual of patient education for cardiopulmonary dysfunction, St. Louis, 1980, The C.V. Mosby Co.

Fuller, E.O.: The effect of antianginal drugs on myocardial oxygen consumption, American Journal of Nursing **80:**250, 1980.

Giving cardiovascular drugs safely. Nursing skillbook, Horsham, Pa., 1978, Intermed Communications.

Gronim, S.S.: Helping the client with unstable angina, American Journal of Nursing **78:**1677, 1978.

Hansen, M.S., and Woods, S.L.: Nitroglycerin ointment—where and how to apply it, American Journal of Nursing **80:**1122, 1980.

Hoffman, G.S.: Raynaud's disease and phenomenon, American Family Physician **21**(1):91, 1980.

Koch-Weser, J., and Coffman, J.D.: Vasodilator drugs in peripheral vascular disease, New England Journal of Medicine **300:**713, 1979.

Latts, J.R., and Goldberg, L.I.: Dopamine in the management of shock, Drug Therapy **9**(1):25, 1979.

Naide, D.: Vasodilators for arterial insufficiency, American Family Physician **22**(1):128, 1980.

Richtsmeier, T.E., and Preston, T.A.: Drug management of stable angina pectoris, Postgraduate Medicine **62**(5):91, 1977.

Smith-Collins, A.: Dobutamine: a new inotropic agent, Nursing '80 **10:**62, March, 1980.

Sonnenblick, E.H., Frishman, W.H., and LeJemtel, T.H.: Dobutamine: a new synthetic cardioactive sympathetic amine, New England Journal of Medicine **300:**17, 1979.

Spitz, P.: Kids in crisis: common emergencies—correct actions to take, Nursing '78 **8:**26, April, 1978.

Stemerman, M.B.: Atherosclerosis: the etiologic role of blood elements and cellular changes, Cardiovascular Medicine **3:**17, 1978.

Walton, C.: Angina: teaching your patient how to prevent recurrent attacks, Nursing '78 **8:**32, Feb., 1978.

Zelis, R., Liedtke, J.A., Leaman, D.M., Babb, J.D., and Roberts, B.H.: Angina pectoris: diagnosis and treatment, Postgraduate Medicine **59**(5):179, 1976.

13 Antihypertensive drugs

■ OVERVIEW

■ Definition of hypertension

Hypertension is generally defined as a resting diastolic blood pressure greater than 90 mm Hg in an adult. In the United States it is estimated that this condition may apply to 15% of adults. High blood pressure reflects an increased tone of the arteries and arterioles. Renal, endocrine, or neurogenic diseases are found to be the cause of hypertension in 10% of patients with hypertension. The hypertension in these patients is treated by treating the cause of the hypertension. No primary cause of the hypertension can be found in the remaining 90% of patients with hypertension, and this hypertension of unknown origin is called *essential* hypertension. The patient with hypertension may have no symptoms of this disease but does have an increased risk of stroke, blindness, and heart and renal disease after 10 or more years of sustained high blood pressure that produces vascular and organ damage. The incidence of hypertension is higher in men than in women, higher in blacks than in whites, higher in older than in younger adults, and higher in those with diabetes mellitus, hyperlipidemia, or a family history of hypertension.

Patients with essential hypertension must take drugs for the rest of their lives to control the hypertension. It is rare that drug therapy can be discontinued after the blood pressure is brought into a normal range. Frequently the drug dosage can be reduced with time. This is important since antihypertensive drugs can produce uncomfortable side effects, whereas the hypertension itself may not produce uncomfortable symptoms, a situation that can make patient compliance with drug therapy difficult. Obesity and high salt diet are factors that aggravate hypertension. If a patient reduces weight and salt intake, drug requirements frequently may also be reduced.

■ Factors controlling blood pressure and pharmacological mechanisms for treating hypertension

The major factors regulating blood pressure are diagrammed in Fig. 13-1. These factors center around those influencing the circulating volume through adjustments of body salt and water (renal mechanisms) and those influencing the activity of the heart and blood vessels (cardiovascular mechanisms).

Renal mechanisms. The kidney plays an important role in maintaining blood pressure through control of the salt and water content of the body (Chapter 14). A decrease in blood pressure stimulates the release of renin from the kidney. Renin release may be partly controlled by beta adrenergic receptors. Renin is a proteolytic enzyme that acts on a protein in the blood to produce the peptide angiotensin I. Angiotensin I is converted to angiotensin II, a small peptide that is a potent vasoconstrictor and therefore increases blood pressure. Angiotensin II also acts on the adrenal cortex to stimulate the secretion of aldosterone. Aldosterone is the mineralocorticoid hormone that acts on the kidney to decrease the excretion of sodium and to increase potassium excretion. The resulting sodium retention expands the plasma and extracellular fluid volumes, which contribute to the elevation of blood pressure.

A diuretic, usually one of the thiazide or thiazide-like diuretics, is commonly the first drug prescribed to control hypertension. Diuretics inhibit renal tubular sodium reabsorption, causing diuresis leading to reduction of body salt and water (extracellular fluid). The loss of extracellular fluid is associated with reduction of arterial blood pressure, but the mechanism of this hypotensive action remains obscure. This hypotensive effect is not seen in normotensive patients. The volume depletion also produces a reduction in plasma volume, although it is not clear that this reduction in plasma volume persists after the first month of therapy. In addition, most of the antihypertensive drugs (other than diuretics) cause fluid retention, an action that limits their antihypertensive effect. Diuretics are therefore commonly given with the other antihypertensive drugs. Diuretics are discussed in detail in Chapter 14.

Cardiovascular mechanisms. Within the blood vessels, the blood pressure depends on the cardiac output and the resistance to blood flow in the blood vessels. Baroreceptors in the aorta and carotid sinus monitor the blood pressure and send the information to the brain. The brain integrates this information and adjusts the heart

FIG. 13-1

Numbers in diagram refer to mechanisms by which various antihypertensive drugs appear to act. *(1)* Drugs acting centrally to depress sympathetic tone: clonidine, alpha methyldopa, reserpine. *(2)* Drug blocking ganglionic receptor for acetylcholine: trimethaphan. *(3)* Drugs interfering with norepinephrine storage or release: guanethidine, reserpine. *(4)* Drugs blocking alpha adrenergic receptor: prazosin, phenyoxybenzamine, phentolamine. *(5)* Drugs directly dilating smooth muscle: hydralazine, minoxidil, sodium nitroprusside, diazoxide. *(6)* Drugs decreasing cardiac output by beta adrenergic receptor blockade: propranolol, metoprolol, nadolol. *(7)* Drugs blocking sodium reabsorption: diuretics.

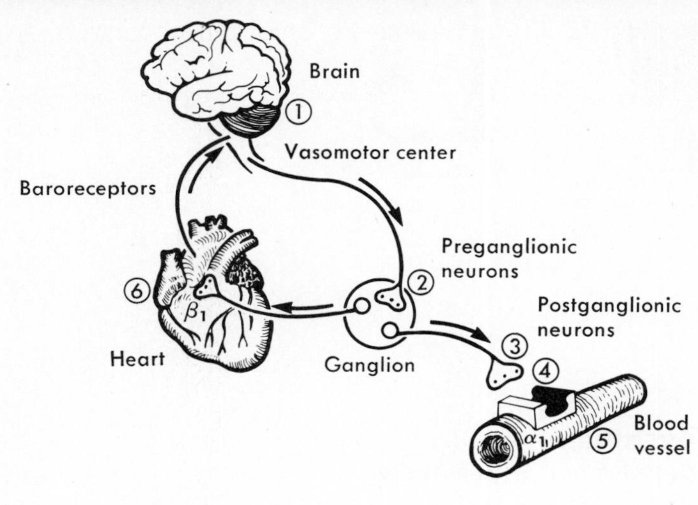

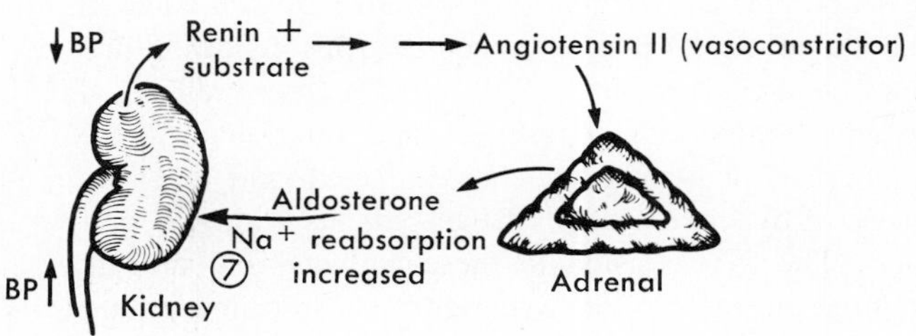

rate and resistance of the blood vessels, largely through the sympathetic nervous system, to fine-tune the blood pressure. The vasomotor center in the medulla is a major center in the brain controlling blood pressure. As the neurotransmitter of the sympathetic nervous system, norepinephrine raises blood pressure by stimulating the beta-1 receptors of the heart to increase cardiac output and by stimulating the alpha-1 receptors of the blood vessels, which causes constriction and increases the resistance to blood flow. In the central nervous system, norepinephrine is the neurotransmitter for nerve tracts that ultimately decrease blood pressure.

Antihypertensive drugs. Drug mechanisms that modify the activity of the sympathetic nervous system are reviewed in Chapter 8. Adrenergic drugs can lower blood pressure by decreasing the activity of the sympathetic nervous system peripherally or centrally.

Beta-1 adrenergic receptor antagonists are used as antihypertensive agents. Their antihypertensive action results from the reduction in cardiac output produced by the blockade of beta-1 receptors of the heart. These beta receptor antagonists also reduce renin release from the kidney. Beta-1 adrenergic receptor antagonists may additionally have an antihypertensive action in the central nervous system, but this action is not well understood.

Alpha-1 adrenergic receptor antagonists are used selectively as antihypertensive agents. The main pharmacological action is to prevent endogenous norepinephrine from constricting blood vessels to increase resistance to blood flow.

Drugs with *other mechanisms* that interfere with adrenergic innervation of blood vessels are also used as antihypertensive agents. Several drugs interfere with the storage and/or release of norepinephrine. A few antihypertensive drugs are believed to act in the vasomotor center of the medulla to inhibit peripheral sympathetic activity.

Several antihypertensive drugs are potent vasodilators that act by mechanisms not dependent on the alpha-1 receptor.

■ DRUGS ALTERING SYMPATHETIC ACTIVITY

■ Beta adrenergic receptor antagonists

(Table 13-1)

Propranolol (Inderal)

Mechanism of action. Propranolol blocks both beta-1 and beta-2 adrenergic receptors. The actions of propranolol are therefore to slow the heart rate and conduction velocity and to decrease the contractility of the heart and to block the beta-2 receptors of the bronchial smooth muscle and skeletal blood vessels.

Administration and fate. Propranolol can be administered orally or parenterally. It is readily metabolized by the liver and the metabolites are excreted in the urine. About 90% to 95% of the circulating drug is

TABLE 13-1. Drugs for treatment of chronic hypertension

Generic name	Trade name	Dosage and administration	Comments
BETA ADRENERGIC RECEPTOR ANTAGONISTS			
Propranolol hydrochloride	Inderal	For hypertension: ORAL: 20 mg 3 times daily with a diuretic. Dosage may be increased to 480 mg daily to control hypertension.	A beta receptor blocking drug that reduces cardiac output and aids in the control of essential hypertension. Used with a thiazide diuretic. Hydralazine may be added if low doses are not effective.
		For angina: ORAL: 10 mg 3 or 4 times daily, initially; increase to control symptoms. Usual range is 160 to 240 mg daily.	
		For pheochromocytoma: ORAL: 30 mg three times daily with an alpha-adrenergic blocking drug to control symptoms from pheochromocytoma. Dosage is increased to 60 mg 3 times daily for 3 days prior to surgery to remove pheochromocytoma.	Propranolol blocks the beta action on the heart from excess epinephrine produced by a tumor of the adrenal medulla called a pheochromocytoma. An alpha receptor blocking drug must also be used to control the hypertension.
		For arrhythmias: ORAL: 10 to 80 mg 3 to 4 times daily. INTRAVENOUS: 0.1 to 0.15 mg/kg body weight administered in increments of 0.5 to 0.75 mg every 1 to 2 min with ECG and blood pressure monitoring.	
Nadolol	Corgard	ORAL: *Adults*—40 mg once daily to start. Dosages are increased by 40 to 80 mg every 3 to 7 days until optimal blood pressure control is achieved. The dose range for maintenance is 80 to 120 mg daily.	A beta receptor blocking drug like propranolol. Used with a thiazide diuretic. Hydralazine may be added if low doses are not effective.
Metoprolol	Lopressor	ORAL: 50 mg 2 times daily. Dosage may be increased to 200 mg daily to control hypertension, maximum 450 mg.	A beta receptor blocking drug that specifically blocks beta-1 (cardiac) adrenergic receptors. Used with a thiazide diuretic for the control of essential hypertension.
ALPHA ADRENERGIC RECEPTOR ANTAGONISTS			
Phentolamine hydrochloride; phentolamine mesylate	Regitine Hydrochloride; Regitine Mesylate	ORAL: *Adults*—50 mg every 4 to 6 hr. *Children*—25 mg every 4 to 6 hr. INTRAMUSCULAR, INTRAVENOUS: *Adults*—5 mg. *Children*—1 mg.	Alpha adrenergic blocker. To diagnose hypertension from pheochromocytoma. To treat a hypertensive crisis secondary to pheochromocytoma, clonidine withdrawal, or tyramine ingestion during monoamine oxidase therapy. To reverse ischemia of levarterenol infiltration.
Phenoxybenzamine hydrochloride	Dibenzyline	ORAL: 10 mg daily. May be increased by 10 mg/day to a maximum dose of 60 mg daily.	Irreversible alpha adrenergic blocker. To treat hypertension secondary to pheochromocytoma. To improve peripheral circulation in Raynaud's disease, ulceration frostbite, and diabetic gangrene.

Continued.

TABLE 13-1. Drugs for treatment of chronic hypertension—cont'd

Generic name	Trade name	Dosage and administration	Comments
Prazosin hydrochloride	Minipress	ORAL: initial dosage 2 to 3 mg in divided doses. Dosage may be increased gradually to 20 to 30 mg/day.	A drug that blocks alpha adrenergic receptors and is usually added to a diuretic and a sympathetic depressant (particularly the beta adrenergic antagonists).
DRUGS INTERFERING WITH THE STORAGE AND/OR RELEASE OF NOREPINEPHRINE			
Reserpine	Lemiserp Rau-Sed Reserpoid Sandril Serpasil	ORAL: *Adults*—initial dosage 0.25 to 0.5 mg daily; maintenance dosage 0.1 to 0.25 mg daily. *Children*—0.25 to 0.5 mg daily.	A drug that depletes norepinephrine stores. Used with a diuretic for the control of essential hypertension. Reserpine is also used to treat the vasospasm of Raynaud's disease (Chapter 12).
Rauwolfia	Raudixin	ORAL: initial dosage 200 to 400 mg daily in 1 or 2 doses; maintenance dosage 50 to 300 mg daily in 1 or 2 doses.	Active ingredient is reserpine.
Alseroxylon	Rauwiloid	ORAL: initial dosage 2 to 4 mg daily; maintenance dosage 2 mg daily.	Active ingredient is reserpine.
Deserpidine	Harmonyl	ORAL: initial dosage 0.75 to 1 mg daily; maintenance dosage 0.25 mg daily.	A drug chemically related to reserpine.
Rescinnamine	Moderil	ORAL: initial dosage 0.5 mg 2 times daily; maintenance dosage 0.25 to 2 mg daily.	A drug chemically related to reserpine.
Guanethidine sulfate	Ismelin	ORAL: *Adults*—initial dosage 12.5 mg daily. Dosage may be increased every 7 days by increments of 12.5 mg to a maximum daily dosage of 100 mg. Further increments of 25 mg to the daily dosage may then be made every week to a maximum of 300 mg daily. *Children*—initial dosage 0.2 mg/kg of body weight daily. Increments of 0.2 mg/kg may then be made of the daily dosage every 7 to 10 days.	A drug that inhibits the release of norepinephrine and eventually depletes neuronal stores of norepinephrine. Used with a diuretic to control severe hypertension. Guanethidine does not enter the central nervous system to cause depression. Common side effects include orthostatic hypotension and diarrhea.
CENTRALLY ACTING ANTIHYPERTENSIVE DRUGS THAT INHIBIT THE ACTIVITY OF THE SYMPATHETIC NERVOUS SYSTEM			
Clonidine hydrochloride	Catapres	ORAL: 0.1 mg 2 or 3 times daily. Dosage may be increased daily in increments of 0.1 to 0.2 mg. Maintenance doses are commonly 0.2 to 0.8 mg daily and are seldom larger than 2.4 mg daily. Withdrawal symptoms will occur when doses are larger than 1.2 mg daily unless doses are reduced gradually.	A centrally acting drug reducing sympathetic output. Used with a diuretic for the control of essential hypertension.

TABLE 13-1. Drugs for treatment of chronic hypertension—cont'd

Generic name	Trade name	Dosage and administration	Comments
Methyldopa	Aldomet	ORAL: *Adults*—initial dose 250 mg in the morning. After 1 week, the dose may be doubled, giving the second 250 mg at bedtime. Dosage may then be increased to a maximum of 2 Gm daily. *Children*—initial dosage 10 mg/kg body weight divided into 2 to 4 doses. Dosage may be increased gradually after 2 days in increments to a maximum dosage of 65 mg/kg daily.	A drug that acts centrally to depress sympathetic tone. Used with a thiazide diuretic for the control of essential hypertension.
VASODILATORS			
Hydralazine hydrochloride	Apresoline	ORAL: *Adults*—initial dosage 10 to 25 mg 2 or 3 times daily. Dosage may be increased by 10 to 25 mg daily. Maximum dosage, 400 mg in 4 divided doses. *Children*—initial dosage 0.75 mg/kg body weight in 4 divided doses. Dosage may be increased over 3 to 4 weeks to a maximum dosage of 7.5 mg/kg daily.	A vasodilator drug usually added to a diuretic and a sympathetic depressant (particularly the beta adrenergic antagonists) for the control of essential hypertension.
Minoxidil	Loniten	ORAL: *Adults*—initial dosage 2.5 mg twice daily, increased to 5 mg twice daily after 1 week if needed. Up to 40 mg daily may be given. *Children*—initial dosage 0.1 to 0.2 mg/kg body weight daily in 2 doses. Increase gradually to 1.4 mg/kg of body weight daily if required.	A vasodilator drug like hydralazine. Usually added to therapy with a diuretic and a beta adrenergic antagonist.

bound to plasma protein, and plasma levels of propranolol cannot be readily correlated with therapeutic effectiveness. Dosages of propranolol must be individualized.

Uses. Propranolol was the only clinically used beta adrenergic receptor antagonist available in the United States until the late 1970's and became known as a wonder drug. Propranolol is a widely used antihypertensive drug because of its effectiveness in controlling mild to moderate hypertension. The effectiveness of propranolol is believed to be largely the result of the decrease in cardiac output that results in the generation of a lower systemic pressure. This direct blocking action on the heart also makes beta receptor antagonists particularly effective when combined with hydralazine. Hydralazine produces a transient hypotension that triggers a reflex stimulation of the heart (reflex tachycardia). This reflex stimulation is blocked by beta receptor antagonists, and therefore there is no increase in cardiac output to compensate for the fall in blood pressure.

Propranolol is a drug of choice for the prophylactic treatment of angina pectoris (Chapter 12). The decrease in the work of the heart decreases the demand of the heart for oxygen. Angina is the pain resulting when the heart is deficient in oxygen. Propranolol is a useful antiarrhythmic drug, effective for arrhythmias caused by catecholamines, such as during surgery (Chapter 15).

Propranolol is useful in treating the symptoms of hyperthyroidism resulting from catecholamine supersensitivity: nervousness, tremors, and a fast heart rate (Chapter 36). Propranolol, given with digitalis, slows the heart rate in atrial flutter or fibrillation.

A new use for propranolol is as a prophylaxis for migraine.

Side effects and contraindications. Side effects of propranolol are those predicted from its blockade of the beta adrenergic receptor. A slow heart rate (bradycardia) and hypotension are especially prominent when propranolol is given intravenously to treat arrhythmias. Propranolol is contraindicated for patients who already show signs of heart failure or atrioventricular conduction disturbances because of the further cardiac depression caused by propranolol. Propranolol can also precipitate an attack of asthma in patients with this disease. Propranolol favors the retention of sodium, and a diuretic is given concurrently to overcome this side effect. Hypoglycemia normally elicits the discharge of epinephrine. The effects of this released epinephrine will not be noticed easily in a patient taking propranolol. This is an important point for those patients with diabetes mellitus taking insulin or an oral hypoglycemic drug.

Nadolol (Corgard)

Nadolol is a new nonselective beta adrenergic receptor antagonist. Nadolol differs from propranolol primarily in that nadolol is not metabolized and is only slowly excreted in the urine. Since the plasma half-life of nadolol is 20 to 24 hours, oral administration once a day is sufficient. Nadolol is approved as an antihypertensive drug and as an antianginal drug.

Metoprolol (Lopressor)

Metoprolol is a new beta adrenergic receptor antagonist relatively selective for the beta-1 adrenergic receptor and approved as an antihypertensive drug. Metoprolol is effective when taken orally but is readily metabolized by the liver. The plasma half-life is only about 3 hours.

Metoprolol by itself can make respiratory symptoms worse in patients with asthma, but unlike propranolol, metoprolol does not interfere with the action of bronchodilator drugs.

■ Alpha adrenergic receptor antagonists

(Table 13-1)

Phentolamine (Regitine)

Phentolamine is a short-acting and reversible alpha adrenergic receptor antagonist. The major effects of phentolamine are vasodilation resulting from blockade of alpha-1 adrenergic receptors, and cardiac stimulation believed to be secondary to blockade of the presynaptic alpha-2 adrenergic receptors. (The presynaptic alpha-2 adrenergic receptors are associated with uptake of norepinephrine; see Chapter 8.)

Phentolamine is not well absorbed orally, and intravenous or intramuscular administration is more common.

Phentolamine has specific clinical uses as a vasodilator. One use is to lower blood pressure in patients with a tumor of the adrenal medulla, which secretes large amounts of epinephrine (the tumor is called a pheochromocytoma). Another use is to lower blood pressure in patients who are being treated with a monoamine oxidase (MAO) inhibitor and are suffering from the "cheese" reaction, a hypertensive crisis that can be reversed with phentolamine. (See Chapter 26 for a discussion of the "cheese" reaction.) A third use is to treat patients being withdrawn from the antihypertensive drug clonidine, who may suffer a temporary hypertensive crisis.

A major use of phentolamine is to infiltrate a site where levarterenol (norepinephrine) or metaraminol has leaked into the tissue surrounding the infusion site. Phentolamine reverses the profound vasoconstriction that can otherwise cause tissue death.

Side effects of the systemic use of phentolamine include hypotension, a fast heart rate (tachycardia) as a reflex response of the body to the hypotension, nasal congestion secondary to the vasodilation, and general gastrointestinal upset.

Phenoxybenzamine (Dibenzyline)

Phenoxybenzamine is an irreversible alpha receptor antagonist with a duration of action lasting several days. The prominent side effect of phenoxybenzamine is postural hypotension, which refers to a fall in blood pressure when rising from a recumbent to a standing position. In a normal person, postural hypotension is not seen because compensatory vasoconstriction redirects blood flow so that blood does not drain from the head to the legs on standing to cause fainting. In a person treated with phenoxybenzamine or other drugs that deplete peripheral norepinephrine, the compensatory vasoconstriction is lost. Reflex tachycardia, nasal congestion, and gastrointestinal upset are other common side effects of phenoxybenzamine resulting from its alpha adrenergic antagonist activity.

Phenoxybenzamine is used to control the high blood pressure caused by the elevated plasma levels of epinephrine in patients with the adrenal tumor pheochromocytoma when they are not yet ready for surgical removal of the tumor. Phenoxybenzamine is also used to dilate blood vessels in the skin, as in the treatment of Raynaud's phenomenon in which there is a prominent neurogenic vasoconstriction of the blood vessels of the skin, particularly in the hands and feet (Chapter 12).

A major source of drug interactions with phenoxybenzamine is overstimulation of beta adrenergic receptors by drugs like epinephrine that have both alpha and beta adrenergic receptor agonist activity. The blockade of alpha receptors allows beta receptor activation to go unopposed. Tachycardia (fast heart rate) is exaggerated. The vasodilator activity of drugs (such as, for example, of the opioids) is exaggerated in the presence of phenoxybenzamine.

Prazosin (Minipress)

Mechanism of action. Prazosin is a newly introduced vasodilator for the treatment of hypertension that acts primarily by blockade of alpha-1 adrenergic receptors. Prazosin does not cause the reflex stimulation of the heart seen with hydralazine. Prazosin can lower blood pressure in hypertension when administered alone, but prazosin does cause fluid retention and an increased plasma volume, which decrease the usefulness of the drug alone, so a diuretic is given concurrently.

Side effects. Side effects of prazosin common to the first dose include faintness, dizziness, palpitation, and occasional fainting. All the symptoms can be explained by a drop in blood pressure. Other side effects noted for prazosin include headache, drowsiness, dry mouth, fluid retention, depression, rashes, difficulty in urination, and pain in the joints (arthralgia).

Drug interactions. Because prazosin lowers blood pressure to a degree that can interfere with the perfusion of blood in the heart, prazosin can precipitate attacks of angina. On the other hand, because prazosin is a vasodilator, prazosin can interact with nitroglycerin taken to relieve an anginal attack to produce a profound hypotensive response from which the patient may pass out.

Prazosin is administered with a diuretic and a beta blocking drug for the control of moderate to severe hypertension.

■ Drugs interfering with the storage and/or release of norepinephrine (Table 13-1)

Reserpine (Serpasil)

Reserpine and related drugs are often called rauwolfia alkaloids because reserpine was originally isolated from the *Rauwolfia serpentina* bush of India. Reserpine was originally used as an antipsychotic drug but has been replaced in this use by the phenothiazine tranquilizers. Reserpine is effective in lowering blood pressure because it depletes stores of norepinephrine from neurons both in the central and in the peripheral nervous systems. The central action produces sedation and tranquilization. Occasionally, patients taking reserpine will become severely depressed to the point of attempting suicide. More commonly, patients complain of a lethargic feeling, an increased appetite, and increased dreaming. Nightmares are sometimes a complaint.

Other side effects of reserpine can be related to the decreased sympathetic tone: vasodilation, resulting in a flushed, warm feeling, and nasal congestion. Some side effects of reserpine can be related to the predominant parasympathetic tone when sympathetic tone is depressed: salivation, stomach cramps, and diarrhea. Since reserpine augments gastric acid secretion through the increased parasympathetic tone, reserpine should not be used in patients with a peptic ulcer.

Guanethidine (Ismelin)

Mechanism of action. Guanethidine is a very potent antihypertensive drug that is restricted for use in controlling severe hypertension. Guanethidine enters peripheral sympathetic neurons, being taken into the cell by the same mechanism as for the reuptake of norepinephrine. Inside the neuron, guanethidine blocks norepinephrine release. Guanethidine does not cross the blood-brain barrier and therefore produces no central effects. Because norepinephrine is not available for release from peripheral sympathetic neurons, both the peripheral vascular resistance and the cardiac output are decreased.

Administration and duration. The effects of guanethidine may take 1 to 2 weeks to reach the maximal therapeutic response to a given dosage regimen. Moreover, effects of guanethidine persist for 7 to 10 days after therapy is discontinued.

Side effects. A number of uncomfortable side effects arise from the depletion of peripheral norepinephrine stores. Orthostatic (postural) hypotension, as described for phenoxybenzamine, is a special problem with guanethidine therapy, too. The tone of blood vessels is abolished by guanethidine and, if the patient moves suddenly from a reclining to a standing position, the appropriate vascular changes cannot take place quickly enough for proper blood redistribution. The blood stays in the periphery and drains from the head on standing, resulting in fainting. Patients taking guanethidine must be instructed to change body positions slowly. Other side effects resulting from the depletion of norepinephrine include a slow heart rate (bradycardia) and diarrhea. This diarrhea can be severe and of an explosive nature after meals. In men, failure of erection or ejaculatory failure may arise secondary to the loss of vascular tone. Guanethidine also causes sodium retention, so a diuretic is administered concurrently.

Contraindications. Contraindications for guanethidine therapy include the presence of angina, cerebral insufficiency, or coronary artery disease, conditions that are further compromised by the loss of vascular tone.

Drug interactions. A number of drug interactions have been noted for guanethidine. Patients taking guanethidine are supersensitive to administered catecholamines. Patients become less responsive to guanethidine when an indirect-acting adrenergic drug such as amphetamine or ephedrine is taken or when a tricyclic antidepressant drug is taken. These indirect-acting adrenergic drugs release stored norepinephrine from neurons, an action that overcomes the effect of guanethidine to block release of norepinephrine. Tricyclic antidepressants block the uptake of guanethidine into the neuron so that guanethidine cannot reach its site of action.

■ Centrally acting antihypertensive drugs that inhibit the activity of the sympathetic nervous system (Table 13-1)

Methyldopa (Aldomet)

Methyldopa is taken into sympathetic neurons and metabolized to methylnorepinephrine. Methylnorepinephrine is stored in granules and released on stimulation of the neuron. Methylnorepinephrine is called a *false transmitter,* since it takes the place of norepinephrine. Until recently the antihypertensive effect of methylnorepinephrine was believed to result from the ineffectiveness of methylnorepinephrine as a vasoconstrictor. Recently it has been shown that methylnorepinephrine is a potent vasoconstrictor, so the action of methylnorepinephrine as a false transmitter for peripheral sympathetic neurons does not account for the antihypertensive effects of methyldopa. The effect of methyldopa in the central nervous system to decrease the activity of the sympathetic nervous system is now believed to account for the antihypertensive effect of the drug. Methyldopa decreases sympathetic tone and has a tranquilizing effect on behavior.

Side effects common to methyldopa are related largely to the decrease in central sympathetic activity. Drowsiness is common at the beginning of treatment. Unpleasant sedation, depressed mood, and nightmares are occasional complaints. Tiredness and fatigue may be noted. Peripheral effects include a slow heart rate (bradycardia), diarrhea, dry mouth, and occasional ejaculatory failure in men.

Occasionally, methyldopa causes a false positive Coombs' test. A positive Coombs' test indicates hemolytic anemia, but it is rare for the patient taking methyldopa to have hemolytic anemia in spite of the positive test. Methyldopa may also cause a mild alteration of liver function tests. Methyldopa is therefore not a drug to use for patients who already have impaired liver function, since the drug will interfere with evaluating the course of the disease. This alteration of liver tests ordinarily occurs during the first 6 weeks of therapy and is reversed by discontinuing methyldopa.

Clonidine (Catapres)

Clonidine has an antihypertensive effect as a result of its action in the central nervous system. Clonidine activates alpha receptors in the vasomotor center of the medulla, an action that inhibits activity of the sympathetic nervous system. Heart rate and cardiac output are decreased and account for the reduction in blood pressure.

Common side effects of clonidine therapy include drowsiness, dry mouth, and constipation. Sudden discontinuance of clonidine can be dangerous. After discontinuing therapeutic doses of clonidine for 12 to 48 hours, many patients experience symptoms of a sympathetic rebound: restlessness, insomnia, tremors, increased salivation, and increased heart rate (tachycardia). If clonidine is not reinstated, further symptoms follow: headaches, abdominal pain, and nausea. The most severe reaction is a hypertensive crisis that is best treated in the hospital with a combination of alpha-blocking and beta-blocking drugs: phentolamine and propranolol. To avoid these withdrawal problems, clonidine therapy is gradually reduced over a week or more.

■ Vasodilators used for treating chronic hypertension (Table 13-1)

Hydralazine (Apresoline)

Hydralazine acts directly on arteriolar smooth muscle to cause relaxation. The mechanism is not known. The drop in arterial blood pressure is great enough to activate the baroreceptors of the aorta. This activation causes a reflex stimulation of the heart, which increases cardiac output and partially compensates for the fall in blood pressure (reflex tachycardia). Hydralazine also causes sodium retention. Because hydralazine causes reflex stimulation of the heart and increases sodium retention, hydralazine is most effective in reducing hypertension when added to a regimen of a diuretic to counteract the sodium retention and a beta adrenergic receptor antagonist (propranolol, nadolol, or metoprolol) to block the reflex stimulation of the heart. Side effects common to hydralazine include headache, palpitation, loss of appetite, nausea, vomiting, and diarrhea. In the absence of a beta antagonist, hydralazine can cause angina in susceptible individuals as a result of the reflex stimulation of the heart. Hydralazine is not a good drug for a patient with angina, coronary artery disease, or congestive heart failure because of the indirect cardiac effects.

The main problem that has been documented in the past after long-term therapy at high doses of hydralazine is the appearance of a "lupus-like" syndrome. Lupus erythematosus is an autoimmune disease with symptoms of fever, joint pain, chest pain, edema, and circulating antibodies to DNA. The syndrome induced by hydralazine is similar but is reversed when the drug is discontinued. The appearance of "lupus-like" symptoms is infrequent when smaller doses of hydralazine are used in combination with the diuretic and sympathetic blocking drug. Patients on hydralazine therapy are monitored for the appearance of the anti-DNA antibodies and for lupus erythematosus (LE) cells.

Minoxidil (Loniten)

Minoxidil is a direct-acting vasodilator like hydralazine, but minoxidil is more potent. This new drug must be given with a diuretic to control fluid retention and a beta receptor blocker to prevent reflex tachycardia. A side effect of minoxidil is excessive hairiness that may develop after a few weeks of treatment. Some patients experience transient nausea, headaches, or fatigue when treatment is started.

TABLE 13-2. Drugs used in hypertensive emergencies

Generic name	Trade name	Dosage and administration	Comments
Diazoxide	Hyperstat	INTRAVENOUS: *Adults*—300 mg or 5 mg/kg body weight. *Children*—5 mg/kg body weight. The drug is injected within 30 sec. The injection may be repeated after 30 min.	A direct-acting vasodilator. Acts rapidly (2 to 5 min) and lasts 2 to 12 hr. Increases venous return and cardiac output. Blood pressure fall is rarely excessive, so blood pressure monitoring is not critical.
Sodium nitroprusside	Nipride	INTRAVENOUS: dissolve 50 mg in 500 to 1000 ml of 5% dextrose. Infuse 0.5 to 8 μg/kg/min. Solution must be protected from light and discarded after 4 hr.	A direct-acting vasodilator. Acts rapidly (1 to 2 min). Continuous infusion is necessary to maintain hypotensive effect. Decreased venous return with no change in heart rate. Blood pressure must be carefully monitored and infusion rate adjusted to maintain desired level.
Trimethaphan camsylate	Arfonad	INTRAVENOUS: administered as a 0.1% (1 mg/ml) infusion in 5% dextrose. The rate of infusion is begun at 0.5 to 1 mg/min and increased gradually until the blood pressure falls by 20 mm Hg. After several minutes, the rate is again increased until the blood pressure reaches the desired level.	A rapidly acting drug that blocks acetylcholine receptors in the ganglia. Inhibits both sympathetic and parasympathetic nervous systems. Decreases venous return and cardiac output. Blood pressure must be carefully monitored, since the hypotensive effect is variable and unpredictable.

■ DRUGS USED IN HYPERTENSIVE EMERGENCIES (Table 13-2)

■ Vasodilators

A hypertensive emergency cannot be simply defined. The blood pressure may be severely elevated or only moderately elevated. The important feature is that there is impending end-organ damage, usually of the brain, heart, or eyes. Unstable neurological symptoms suggesting damage to the brain include headache, restlessness, confusion, and even convulsions. Hemorrhaging may be apparent in the eye. Drugs that are currently used to treat hypertensive emergencies by rapidly lowering blood pressure are diazoxide (Hyperstat), sodium nitroprusside (Nipride), and trimethaphan (Arfonad).

Diazoxide (Hyperstat)

Diazoxide acts directly to relax arteriolar smooth muscle. This action lowers blood pressure but does not affect the venous side of circulation. Diazoxide is therefore not useful for those conditions requiring the decreased venous return produced by trimethaphan.

The advantage of diazoxide treatment is that a bolus of the drug can be given IV over 30 seconds and will usually be effective in 5 minutes and remain effective for 2 to 12 hours. Blood pressure does not have to be continuously monitored as with trimethaphan treatment. The patient rarely becomes excessively hypotensive. Diazoxide causes retention of sodium and water, which must be treated with a diuretic. Diazoxide also causes hyperglycemia.

Sodium nitroprusside (Nipride)

Sodium nitroprusside acts directly on the smooth muscle of both arterioles and venous vessels. The result is an immediate decrease in blood pressure with no increase in venous return. There are no real side effects with short-term use of nitroprusside. Blood pressure must be constantly monitored, and the drug is administered by intravenous drip. Nitroprusside is unstable to light, so it should not be used more than 4 hours after it is dissolved. Side effects arise from the use of nitroprusside for several days. Some of the nitroprusside is metabolized to thiocyanate, which can produce ringing in the ears (tinnitus), blurred vision, and hypothyroidism.

■ Ganglionic blocking drug (Table 13-2)

Trimethaphan (Arfonad)

Trimethaphan blocks the receptors for acetylcholine in the ganglia and is a ganglionic blocking drug. Ganglionic blocking drugs inhibit both sympathetic and parasympathetic activity and therefore have limited clinical uses. Trimethaphan is used in treating some hypertensive emergencies. Because trimethaphan has a short duration of action, it is administered by continuous intravenous drip during which blood pressure must be constantly monitored. Side effects result from the inhibition of both

■ THE NURSING PROCESS FOR ANTIHYPERTENSIVE DRUGS

■ Assessment

Patients with a persistent blood pressure exceeding 90 mm Hg of mercury diastolic pressure and/or an excessively high systolic pressure may be appropriate candidates for antihypertensive therapy. In some cases the cause of the hypertension may be clearly identified, as in renal disease, but most of the time it is not. Additional baseline data that should be obtained in these patients include weight, usual dietary practices related to salt intake, serum electrolyte concentration, blood urea nitrogen, and measures of renal and cardiovascular function.

■ Management

In cases of hypertensive crisis, patients may be admitted to the acute care setting for pharmacological manipulation of the blood pressure. The use of a cardiac monitor, standby availability of a vasopressor agent, and the use of sophisticated vascular monitoring may all be appropriate. In less acute situations, therapy may be started in the hospitalized or ambulatory patient. Parameters to monitor include the blood pressure and other vital signs, fluid intake and output, weight, serum electrolyte concentration, serum and urinary glucose levels, and other laboratory data specific to side effects of individual drugs, for instance, a blood count and liver function studies with methyldopa. Planning should be started for patient self-management at home, including determination by the health care team of other medications such as diuretics or potassium that may be needed, when sodium and/or caloric restrictions are required, and instruction about the potential dangers of hypertension.

■ Evaluation

Ideally, therapy with antihypertensive drugs will allow the patient's blood pressure to remain below 140/90 and the patient will be free of side effects such as orthostatic hypotension, drowsiness, and impotence (see text). In many, if not in most cases, it is not possible to achieve all these goals. The patient should be able to explain the hazards of untreated hypertension, why therapy is necessary, how to take the prescribed medications safely, why additional drugs such as diuretics or potassium may be needed, possible anticipated side effects and what to do about them, how to follow any dietary restrictions prescribed, and what situations warrant calling the physician. If the patient or family is to record weight or blood pressure on a regular basis, the ability to do this correctly should be demonstrated. The patient should be able to state the desired body weight. For more specific guidelines, see the patient care implications section at the end of this chapter.

---

sympathetic and parasympathetic tone. Severe hypotension can result from the inhibition of sympathetic tone. The intravenous drip is then discontinued until the blood pressure begins to rise again. Side effects from the loss of parasympathetic tone include pupillary dilation, loss of accommodation, drying of mucous surfaces, constipation, and urinary retention.

The disadvantages of trimethaphan therapy are that blood pressure must be carefully followed and that the loss of pupillary reflexes makes it difficult to monitor ongoing neurological damage to the brain, when neurological damage was the presenting set of symptoms. Also trimethaphan can be unpredictable in its effects: patients already on antihypertensive medication or with a reduced blood volume may be unusually sensitive to trimethaphan. Some patients do not respond readily to trimethaphan; other patients are initially responsive but become unresponsive.

Trimethaphan does decrease venous return of blood and lower cardiac output. These actions are helpful when the patient has a condition such as a dissecting aortic aneurysm, hypertensive encephalopathy, acute left ventricular failure, or cerebral hemorrhage, since the pressure is removed from the weakened tissue.

■ PATIENT CARE IMPLICATIONS

General guidelines for patients receiving antihypertensive drugs

1. Losing weight and adhering to a low sodium diet may decrease the need for antihypertensives.
2. The poor compliance frequently seen in drug therapy for hypertension results in part from the fact that patients do not feel any better while on antihypertensives and may in fact feel worse.
3. Hypotension is a common side effect of antihypertensive therapy, especially when the patient moves rapidly from a supine to a sitting or upright position (postural hypotension). Symptoms include dizziness, light-headedness, weakness, and syncope (fainting). If symptoms occur, instruct the patient to sit or lie down until symptoms pass, then to rise slowly. Postural hypotension is often worse in the mornings, and it may be aggravated by long periods of standing, hot weather, hot showers or baths, ingestion of alcohol, and exercise, especially if the exercise is followed by immobility. Hypotension is also worse when patients are begun on therapy and during periods of dosage adjustment.
4. When beginning a patient on antihypertensive therapy, during periods of dosage adjustment, or when other medications are being added to the regimen, the blood pressure should be monitored frequently, at least every 4 hours in the ambulatory hospitalized patient, and whenever a patient complains of the symptoms of hypotension. The blood pressure is often ordered to be measured with the patient in the lying, sitting, and standing positions. The outpatient may need to return frequently for blood pressure monitoring. In some instances the patient or family can be taught to measure the blood pressure at home.
5. Supervise the ambulation of hospitalized patients to guard against injury should the patient become dizzy or faint.
6. The elderly are more sensitive to the antihypertensives and find hypotension to be more of a problem.
7. When antihypertensives are given to patients taking other drugs that also cause hypotension, the incidence of hypotensive episodes may be increased. Such drugs might include other antihypertensives, diuretics, central nervous system depressants, and barbiturates. For the same reason, patients should be instructed not to take over-the-counter medications without clearance from their physicians.
8. When used alone, the antihypertensives often contribute to fluid retention and weight gain. Weigh patients daily under standard conditions (same time, same scales, same amount of clothing). Other signs of fluid retention are pitting edema (edema characterized by indentations that remain in the skin for seconds to minutes after pressure has been applied by the examiner's finger) and pulmonary rales. The patients at home should also monitor their weight if they have access to a scale and can read it accurately. A daily weight gain of 2 pounds or more should be reported to the physician.
9. Adherence to a low sodium diet will reduce the possibility of fluid retention. If indicated, refer the patient to a dietitian for instruction about sodium restriction. The degree of sodium restriction will depend on the patient's general medical condition and usual dietary habits. Instruction to the person who cooks the meals may be beneficial, in addition to instructing the patient, if the patient does not cook.
10. If a diuretic is added to the drug therapy regimen, liberalization of salt (sodium) intake is often necessary to reduce the possibility of electrolyte imbalance. Monitor serum electrolyte concentrations frequently. See Chapter 14 for a discussion of diuretics.
11. Measure the fluid intake and output of hospitalized patients.
12. It is sometimes necessary to help the patient find a creative way to remember to take the medications as ordered. One way might be to devise some sort of calendar on which the patient must indicate each dose that is taken.
13. If a dose of antihypertensive drug is missed, the patient should be instructed not to "double up" to make up for the missed dose but to resume the prescribed schedule the next time the medication is due.
14. There are preparations available containing a combination of an antihypertensive with a diuretic (one example is Aldoril, containing methyldopa and hydrochlorothiazide). Patients taking combination products are potentially at risk for side effects resulting from any of the component drugs and should be taught about them.
15. Many of the antihypertensives cause drowsiness or sedation, especially when first being used or when dosages are increased. Warn patients about this side effect, and caution them to avoid or to at least perform carefully any activity that requires mental alertness, such as driving, operating dangerous equipment, or engaging in any potentially dangerous activity. Concomitant use of other drugs that produce central nervous system depression may enhance the drowsiness (examples include alcohol, barbiturates, and sedatives).
16. The use of antihypertensives during pregnancy is

not recommended unless the mother's condition warrants it; women should discuss the benefits versus risks with their physicians. Women of childbearing age may wish to consider the use of birth control measures. The drugs are not recommended for use during lactation.

17. Intravenous administration
    a. Measure the blood pressure frequently (every 3 to 5 minutes) until stable, then every 15 to 30 minutes.
    b. An electronic infusion monitoring device should be used when constant infusion is required.
    c. A microdrip infusion set should be used for constant infusions.
    d. Monitor the pulse.
    e. Depending on the patient's general medical condition, it may be appropriate to attach the patient to a cardiac monitor.
    f. Patients should remain in bed for up to 3 hours after the drug has been administered.
18. Many antihypertensives cause tachycardia or bradycardia. Monitor the pulse when the blood pressure is monitored.
19. If possible, antihypertensives should be discontinued before the patient has surgery because control of blood pressure may be difficult for the patient receiving general anesthesia.
20. Careful and sympathetic questioning of patients taking antihypertensive medication, particularly those patients exhibiting poor compliance, may help health care personnel to develop a more individualized plan for reducing the patient's blood pressure. Side effects such as impotence may be difficult for the patient to accept and to acknowledge. If side effects that are bothersome to the patient are occurring, it may be possible to change the drug regimen.
21. Remind patients to keep these and all medications out of the reach of children.

Propranolol

1. During IV propranolol administration, the ECG and central venous pressure should be carefully monitored. Oral administration is preferred.
2. Patients with diabetes mellitus receiving propranolol should be instructed that this drug often causes hypoglycemia; a change in diet or insulin requirements may be needed.
3. Propranolol antagonizes the action of antihistamines, isoproterenol, and other beta adrenergic stimulating drugs. Its action is potentiated by general anesthesia and phenytoin sodium (Dilantin).
4. Propranolol should not be mixed in a syringe with any other medication. In addition, it should not be given simultaneously with other antihypertensives or with monoamine oxidase inhibitors.
5. Because propranolol decreases the heart rate, patients receiving this drug and a digitalis preparation should have their pulses monitored carefully.
6. Serious side effects may occur even with oral administration of propranolol, including hypotension, bradycardia, and bronchospasm. Antidotes would include epinephrine for hypotension, atropine for bradycardia, and a bronchodilator for bronchospasm.
7. Propranolol should not be suddenly discontinued. Patients should be instructed to consult with their physicians before changing the dose or discontinuing the drug.
8. The dose for propranolol should be checked carefully. Usual oral doses are in the range of 20 to 40 mg; IV doses in the range of 0.5 to 3 mg.

Metoprolol and nadolol

1. Metoprolol is similar in action and effect to propranolol, but it is thought to be less dangerous for patients with obstructive lung disease and may interfere less with glucose tolerance than does propranolol.
2. Common cardiovascular side effects include shortness of breath and bradycardia (which if severe can be treated with atropine). Other side effects include dizziness, tiredness, insomnia, gastrointestinal upset, ankle edema, and weight gain.
3. Absorption may be improved if metoprolol is taken with meals.
4. Nadolol is similar to propranolol; its major advantage may be that it needs to be taken only once a day by most patients.

Phentolamine

1. Every 2 to 5 minutes monitor the blood pressure, pulse, central venous pressure, and cardiac rhythm of the patient receiving intravenous phentolamine until the patient's condition stabilizes, then monitor every 15 minutes. The patient should not be left unattended.
2. The treatment of shock caused by hypotension after use of phentolamine is intravenous levarterenol.
3. An electronic IV monitor or regulator should be used to accurately control the rate of intravenous fluid and drug administration when IV phentolamine is being used.
4. Urinary output should be monitored and recorded every 30 to 60 minutes during IV administration of phentolamine.
5. Phentolamine can be mixed with most IV solutions but should probably not be mixed with other drugs. Solutions are stable for 48 hours but should then be discarded. If in doubt, consult the pharmacist.

Prazosin

1. Patients beginning therapy, adding a diuretic to the drug regimen, or increasing the dose of prazosin are susceptible to the "first dose" syndrome. Although characterized by hypotension, this syndrome can be severe enough to result in syncope and loss of consciousness. This hypotensive response usually occurs 30 to 90 minutes after taking the dose; it is more common with a first dose of 2 mg than 1 mg, so patients are usually started on the lower dose. Treatment is to lie the patient flat; the condition is self-limiting. In rare cases the episode is preceded by a tachycardia in which rates of heartbeat up to 180 beats per minute are reported.
2. Because "first dose" syndrome effects may occur for a couple of days after initiating or changing the dose of therapy, patients should be cautioned to avoid activities in which a syncopal episode might be dangerous.
3. To minimize the possibility of the first dose syndrome, patients may be instructed to take their first dose at bedtime and to remain lying down for at least 3 hours after the dose has been taken.
4. Families of patients receiving prazosin should also be instructed about the hypotensive effects, both to allay anxiety should it occur and also to ensure that the patient will receive correct treatment of the problem.

Reserpine and related drugs

1. Patients may find this group of drugs convenient to take because once a day therapy is usually sufficient.
2. Reserpine has a delayed onset of action and may require 4 to 6 weeks of therapy before its full effect can be seen. When discontinued, effects may persist for several weeks.
3. Serious mental depression is a side effect. Evaluate patients carefully for changes in mood or affect; it may be necessary to also question the patient's family. Signs of depression can include anorexia (loss of appetite), insomnia, impotence, self-deprecation, and mood swings. The use of barbiturates may enhance the central nervous system depression. Reserpine and related compounds should not be given to patients with a history of depression.
4. Taking reserpine with meals may reduce gastric irritation. Reserpine should not be used by patients with a history of ulcer disease or ulcerative colitis.
5. Reserpine changes the seizure threshold and should be used cautiously in patients with epilepsy.
6. Reserpine can cause bradycardia; this may be a problem in patients who also receive digitalis or other drugs causing bradycardia.
7. Cardiac arrhythmias have occurred in patients receiving the rauwolfia preparations; use cautiously in patients taking digitalis or quinidine.
8. Reserpine is available in a form suitable for intramuscular injection, but this is rarely used today because of the possibility of delayed hypotension and mental depression.
9. Parenteral reserpine, if given to treat eclampsia, crosses the placental barrier, causing drowsiness, nasal congestion, cyanosis, and anorexia in the newborn infant.
10. In an overdose serious enough to require vasopressor therapy, phenylephrine, levarterenol, or metaraminol should be used.

Guanethidine

1. Although orthostatic hypotension can affect patients taking any of the antihypertensives, it is a much more common problem with this drug.
2. Postural blood pressure determinations (blood pressure taken with the patient in lying, sitting, and standing positions) should be obtained with this drug, since the maintenance dose is partially determined by the standing blood pressure. The standing blood pressure should be determined after the patient has been standing for at least 10 minutes.
3. Guanethidine causes bradycardia; be especially careful when the patient is taking this drug along with digitalis.
4. Monoamine oxidase (MAO) inhibitors should be stopped for at least a week before initiating therapy with this drug.
5. If diarrhea is severe enough, it may be necessary to treat it. Also be alert to electrolyte imbalances in patients with severe chronic diarrhea.

Methyldopa

1. If sedation is a problem, instructing the patient to add any increases in dosage in the evening rather than the morning may help reduce sedation interfering with work.
2. Dry mouth and drowsiness will usually decrease over time.
3. Depression has been reported as a side effect; evaluate patients carefully for changes in mood or affect.
4. Urine may darken when left exposed to the air.
5. Although most patients who develop a positive Coombs' test while on methyldopa therapy are exhibiting a false positive result, it cannot be assumed that this is so. Evaluation for possible hemolytic anemia includes blood counts done before initiating therapy and at regular intervals during therapy. Liver function tests should also be performed at regular intervals.

6. Intravenous administration
   a. Intramuscular or subcutaneous administration is not recommended because of the erratic absorption that occurs.
   b. Methyldopa is not the drug of choice for intravenous antihypertensive control.
   c. Dilute the medication with enough 5% dextrose in water to make 100 ml.
   d. Administer the ordered dose over 30 to 60 minutes. See general guidelines.
   e. The patient should be switched to oral doses as soon as possible.

Clonidine

1. The side effects of therapy (dry mouth, drowsiness, and sedation) often diminish with continued therapy.
2. Impress on patients that stopping the drug suddenly can be dangerous. Patients should learn to have prescriptions refilled before their supply on hand runs out. Unreliable patients should not take this drug.
3. Patients taking clonidine should have regular eye examinations because in animal studies the drug has produced retinal degeneration.
4. Depression has been reported as a side effect; evaluate patients carefully for changes in mood or affect.

Hydralazine

1. Hydralazine seems to be better tolerated when used in combination with other drugs than when used alone.
2. This drug does not cause sedation or other central nervous system effects as commonly as do other antihypertensives.
3. Hydralazine can cause tachycardia.
4. There are parenteral forms available for intravenous and intramuscular use, but these are rarely used. Consult the pharmacy with questions.

Minoxidil

1. Minoxidil can cause tachycardia.
2. This drug can cause hypertrichosis (excessive hairiness) after several weeks of therapy. Instruct patients to report this side effect. For some patients, it may not be bothersome. The hair can be shaved, bleached, or removed, depending on the severity and locations. Some patients may prefer to change drugs. Caution patients not to discontinue the medications without contacting their physician.
3. Fluid retention can be a serious problem. Observe patients for edema.
4. Observe patients for pericardial effusion, a rare side effect. The patient may complain of chest pain or pain in the shoulder or arm. There may be dyspnea, tachycardia, distended jugular veins, and changes in heart sounds.

Diazoxide

1. Diazoxide is administered undiluted and fairly rapidly. The usual adult dose (300 mg in 20 ml) should be administered over 30 seconds.
2. Severe hypotension is uncommon, but can be treated with a sympathomimetic agent such as norepinephrine.
3. As always in hypertensive emergencies, appropriate drugs and equipment should be available for treating possible side effects.
4. Hyperglycemia is common. Monitor the blood and urine glucose levels. For the patient with diabetes mellitus, it may be necessary to increase the insulin dosage; in other patients it may not be necessary to treat hyperglycemia since diazoxide therapy is usually only continued for a couple of days.
5. The medication is highly alkaline and should not be given intramuscularly or subcutaneously. Extravasation should be avoided.
6. Monitor the vital signs, fluid intake and output, and weight.

Sodium nitroprusside

1. This drug should not be given undiluted. Dissolve 50 mg of drug in 2 to 3 ml of 5% dextrose in water. There are reports that sterile water may be safely used, but it *must not contain a preservative* (if in doubt, consult the pharmacy). The concentrated solution should then be further diluted in 500 or 1000 ml of 5% dextrose in water to make concentrations of 100 or 50 μg/ml. The solution may have a faint brownish tint; if highly colored, the solution should be discarded. The diluted solution should be covered with foil and the infusion tubing covered to protect from light. The solution should be used immediately; discard solution over 4 hours old. Do not mix with any other medications.
2. The rate of infusion should be prescribed by the physician and be based on the response of the blood pressure, but the usual rate is 0.5 to 8 μg/kg over a period of 1 minute.
3. Monitor the fluid intake and output.
3. This drug should only be administered in an acute care setting where appropriate equipment and drugs are available should an emergency arise.
5. To treat an overdose discontinue the infusion of nitroprusside. Administer amyl nitrite (Chapter 12) for 15 to 30 seconds each minute until a sodium nitrite solution for intravenous administration can be prepared. A 3% sodium nitrite solution should be administered intravenously at a rate of 2.5 to 5 ml per minute up to a total dose of 10 to 15 ml. After this, inject sodium thiosulfate intravenously, 12.5 Gm in 50 ml of 5% dextrose in water over a 10-minute

period. Monitor the patient carefully throughout. Signs of overdose can reappear for up to several hours, and sodium nitrite and sodium thiosulfate can be repeated at half the dose listed.

Trimethaphan camsylate

1. This drug *must* be diluted before administration. This is usually done by adding one ampule (500 mg or 10 ml) to 500 ml of 5% dextrose injection to make a concentration of 1 mg/ml. The use of other diluents is not recommended.
2. The drug is administered via constant infusion, and the dose is titrated in response to the blood pressure, which should be measured at 2- to 3-minute intervals. The physician should determine the goal of therapy, that is, the acceptable blood pressure.
3. This drug should be used in an acute care setting where equipment and drugs are available for treatment of any possible side effects.
4. If the blood pressure does not come down as anticipated with the patient in the supine position, the head of the bed can be raised. Do so carefully, however, as cerebral anoxia is to be avoided.
5. Note that the drug produces pupillary dilation so this parameter may not be helpful in evaluating the patient.
6. Monitor the pulse and respiration frequently.
7. In the event of overdose or severe hypotension requiring vasopressors, phenylephrine or mephentermine should be used, with norepinephrine reserved for refractory cases.
8. Monitor the fluid intake and output.
9. Trimethaphan camsylate should not be mixed with any other drugs.

■ SUMMARY

The control of hypertension by the selected use of drugs is an outstanding example of planned drug synergism. Mildly elevated blood pressure may be brought down to the normal range with the use of a diuretic alone. If further drug treatment is required, a drug that depresses the activity of the sympathetic nervous system is added (methyldopa, clonidine, propranolol, nadolol, metoprolol, or reserpine). The action of the diuretic to decrease vascular smooth muscle tone by volume depletion and sodium reduction is now supplemented by a drug action to reduce the sympathetic tone of blood vessels. If further drug treatment is required, a vasodilator (hydralazine) or an alpha adrenergic receptor antagonist (prazosin) is administered. The drug action added here is a direct one on the vascular smooth muscle to cause relaxation. In severe cases of hypertension, guanethidine is used to interfere with the release of norepinephrine from peripheral neurons or a potent vasodilator, minoxidil, is substituted for hydralazine.

Unfortunately, the drugs used to control hypertension can also cause annoying side effects. The knowledgeable health professional can offer sympathetic understanding to the patient adjusting to these medications. Gastrointestinal disturbances are common with all of the drugs. The drugs depressing sympathetic tone tend to produce weakness or lethargy and occasionally impotence in men. Impotence is most common with guanethidine treatment and rare with propranolol treatment. The vasodilators hydralazine and prazosin tend to cause headaches, dizziness, and palpitations.

Hypertensive emergencies are treated with rapidly acting drugs. Diazoxide and sodium nitroprusside, which are vasodilators, or trimethaphan, which is a ganglionic blocking drug, are the drugs most frequently used in treating hypertensive emergencies. The alpha adrenergic receptor antagonists phentolamine and phenoxybenzamine are used in selected cases of hypertensive emergency resulting from excessive endogenous norepinephrine.

■ STUDY QUESTIONS

1. Describe the renal mechanisms controlling blood pressure.
2. Describe the cardiovascular mechanisms controlling blood pressure.
3. Name the beta adrenergic receptor antagonists used as antihypertensive drugs. How does blockade of the beta receptors lower blood pressure? What are the side effects of these drugs?
4. For what situations is phentolamine used as an antihypertensive drug? What is the mechanism of action?
5. How does the action of phenoxybenzamine differ from that of phentolamine?
6. How does the use of prazosin differ from that of phentolamine?
7. List which antihypertensives act by interfering with storage and/or release of norepinephrine.
8. List which antihypertensives act centrally to inhibit sympathetic activity.
9. List which antihypertensives used in the chronic treatment of hypertension are direct-acting vasodilators.
10. List three drugs and their mechanisms of action that are used to control a hypertensive emergency.
11. What is a limiting side effect of reserpine?
12. What is orthostatic hypotension? Which antihypertensive drugs are commonly associated with orthostatic hypotension as a side effect?
13. Which antihypertensive is associated with the synthesis of a false transmitter?
14. What reaction may occur with the sudden discontinuance of clonidine?
15. Describe reflex tachycardia. Which antihypertensive drugs may cause reflex tachycardia?
16. Why is patient compliance with antihypertensive therapy frequently poor?

■ SUGGESTED READINGS

Essential hypertension

Andreoli, K.G., Fowkes, V.H., Zipes, D.P., and Wallace, A.G.: Comprehensive cardiac care, ed. 4, St. Louis, 1979, The C.V. Mosby Co.

Bharadwaja, K., and Promisloff, R.: Clinical pharmacology of propranolol, Drug Therapy **7**(3):22, 1977.

Bravo, E., Chrysant, S., Harris, T.R., Krakoff, L.R., Lothian, G., and Streeten, D.H.P.: Drug switching in hypertension regimens, Patient Care **11:**78, Oct. 15, 1977.

Caldwell, J.R.: Practical approach to hypertension. 1. Diagnostic evaluation, Postgraduate Medicine **65:**66, 1979.

Caldwell, J.R.: Practical approach to hypertension. 2. Treatment, Postgraduate Medicine **65**(5):81, 1979.

Combating cardiovascular diseases skillfully. Nursing skillbook, Horsham, Pa., 1978, Intermed Communications.

Czerwinski, B.S.: Manual of patient education for cardiopulmonary dysfunction, St. Louis, 1980, The C.V. Mosby Co.

Daniels, L.M.: What influences adherence to hypertension therapy, Nursing Forum **18:**231, 1979.

Engleman, K., Holland, B., Julius, S., and Moser, M.: Opt for propranolol in hypertension? Patient Care **11:**38, Oct. 15, 1977.

Frohlich, E.D.: Methyldopa: mechanisms and treatment 25 years later, Archives of Internal Medicine **140:**954, 1980.

Gifford, R.W.: Managing hypertension, Postgraduate Medicine **61**(3):153, 1977.

Giving cardiovascular drugs safely. Nursing skillbook, Horsham, Pa., 1978, Intermed Communications.

Graham, R.M., and Pettinger, W.A.: Drug therapy: prazosin, New England Journal of Medicine **300:**232, 1979.

Haslam, P.: Hypertension: anithypertensives and how they work, Canadian Nurse **75:**26, April, 1979.

Hill, M.: Helping the hypertensive patient control sodium intake, American Journal of Nursing **79:**906, 1979.

Jones, M.B.: Hypertensive disorders of pregnancy, JOGN Nursing **8:**92, 1979.

Karch, F.E.: Propranolol: something for everyone, Drug Therapy **8**(7):28, 1978.

Kolata, G.B.: Treatment reduces deaths from hypertension, Science **206:**1386, 1979.

Kopin, I.J.: CNS actions of antihypertensive drugs, Drug Therapy **9**(12):30, 1979.

Laragh, J.H.: Hypertension, Drug Therapy **10**(1):47, 1980.

Lowenstein, J., and Steele, J.M.: Prazosin: mechanism of action and role in antihypertensive therapy, Cardiovascular Medicine **4:**885, 1979.

Lowenstein, J.: Drugs five years later: clonidine, Annals of Internal Medicine **92:**74, 1980.

Lowenthal, D.T.: New beta-adrenergic blockers, American Family Physician **22**(2):142, 1980.

Maloney, R.: Helping your hypertensive patients live longer. Nursing '78 **8:**26, Oct., 1978.

Manzi, C.C.: Edema. How to tell if it's a danger signal, Nursing '77 **7:**66, April, 1977.

Marcinek, M.B.: Hypertension. What it does to the body, American Journal of Nursing **80:**928, 1980.

Marx, J.L.: Hypertension: a complex disease with complex causes, Science **194:**821, 1976.

Mehta, J.: Adrenergic blockade in hypertension, Journal of the American Medical Association **240:**1759, 1978.

Morgan, T., Myers, J., and Carney, S.: Salt restriction and hypertension, Practical Cardiology **6**(1):37, 1980.

Moser, M.: Hypertension. How therapy works, American Journal of Nursing **80:**928, 1980.

Pettinger, W.A.: Minoxidil and the treatment of severe hypertension, New England Journal of Medicine **303:**922, 1980.

Reeves, R.L.: Metoprolol—a new beta blocker for mild-to-moderate hypertension, Cardiovascular Medicine **4:**381, 1979.

Reid, J.L., Dean, C.R., and Jones, D.H.: Central actions of antihypertensive drugs, Cardiovascular Medicine **2:**1185, 1977.

Report of the task force on blood pressure control in children, Pediatrics **59**(suppl.):797, 1977.

Ross, A.M., Ryan, T.J., and Segal, M.S.: Beta-blockers: new uses, new benefits, Patient Care **13:**16, Dec. 15, 1979.

Schoof, C.S.: Hypertension. Common questions patients ask, American Journal of Nursing **80:**926, 1980.

Stokes, G.S., and Oates, H.F.: Prazosin: new alpha-adrenergic blocking agent in treatment of hypertension, Cardiovascular Medicine **3:**41, 1978.

Vidt, D.G.: Combination therapy in hypertension: a rational approach, Drug Therapy **8**(8):33, 1978.

Ward, G.W., Bandy, P., and Fink, J.W.: Treating and counseling the hypertensive patient, American Journal of Nursing **78:**824, 1978.

Weinshilboum, R.M.: Antihypertensive drugs that alter adrenergic function, Mayo Clinic Proceedings **55:**390, 1980.

Williams, S.R.: Essentials of nutrition and diet therapy, ed. 2, St. Louis, 1978, The C.V. Mosby Co.

Wollam, G.L., and Vidt, D.G.: The patient with resistant hypertension, Drug Therapy **8**(2):36, 1978.

Hypertensive emergencies

Brest, A.N.: Current concepts in the management of hypertensive emergencies, Practical Cardiology **6:**31, 1980.

Hartshorn, J.C.: What to do when the patient's in hypertensive crisis, Nursing '80 **10:**36, July, 1980.

Moore, M.A.: Hypertensive emergencies, American Family Physician **21**(3):141, 1980.

Segal, J.L.: Hypertensive emergencies: practical approach to treatment, Postgraduate Medicine **68**(2):107, 1980.

Shearer, J.K., and Caldwell, M.: Use of sodium nitroprusside and dopamine hydrochloride in the postoperative cardiac patient, Heart & Lung **8:**302, 1979.

Thomson, G.E.: The recognition and treatment of hypertensive emergencies, Drug Therapy **9**(4):24, 1979.

14 Diuretics

Diuretics are drugs that increase urine flow. There are several mechanisms by which drugs may produce this effect, but the clinically important drugs of this class act on the kidney. This chapter reviews pertinent renal physiology and discusses the mechanism of action and clinical properties of diuretic drugs.

■ THE FUNCTION OF THE NEPHRON IN SALT AND WATER BALANCE

The functional unit of the kidney is the nephron (Fig. 14-1). Glomerular filtration is the first step in the production of urine. Blood is brought into contact with a filtering surface in the glomerulus, where water and small molecules may pass into the tubule, leaving behind most proteins and protein-bound small molecules. The remainder of the nephron adjusts the salt and water content of the tubular fluid to achieve homeostasis, a balanced condition in which the body retains the salt and water required for proper body function and eliminates the excess. For the purpose of understanding diuretic drugs we can limit ourselves to a discussion of six ions or molecules: sodium (Na^+), chloride (Cl^-), potassium (K^+), water (H_2O), bicarbonate (HCO_3^-), and organic ions.

Sodium ion sites. Sodium ion freely enters the tubular fluid from the glomerulus so that the fluid entering the proximal convoluted tubule has the same sodium ion content as blood. The proximal convoluted tubule actively removes sodium ion from the tubule. No further sodium ion is removed in the descending limb of Henle's loop, but in the ascending limb, sodium ion passively follows chloride ion out of the tubule. In the distal convoluted tubule, sodium ion is removed by two processes, one an active pump like that in the proximal convoluted tubule. The second sodium ion pump in the distal convoluted tubule is a pump that exchanges sodium ion for potassium ion so that as sodium ion is reabsorbed, potassium ion is excreted.

Chloride ion sites. The major site for chloride ion removal from tubular fluid is in the ascending limb of Henle's loop. This active removal of chloride ion draws sodium ion along with it and effectively dilutes the tubular fluid.

Potassium ion sites. Potassium ion is not the primary ion involved in the action of any diuretic drug; those drugs are designed to alter sodium ion excretion patterns. Nevertheless, potassium excretion is altered by some of these agents, and the effects on some patients may be detrimental. Potassium ion may be reabsorbed in the ascending limb of Henle's loop. Secretion of potassium occurs in the distal convoluted tubule, where the ion is exchanged for sodium ion (Fig. 14-1).

Water sites. The kidney is the primary site for maintenance of water balance. Water may be recovered from the tubule by diffusion in the proximal convoluted tubule and in the descending limb of Henle's loop. The ascending limb of Henle's loop and the distal convoluted tubule are relatively impermeable to water. Final concentration of the urine is achieved in the collecting duct. Removal of water at this site is regulated by antidiuretic hormone (ADH), which increases permeability of the tissue to water and thereby increases water retention.

Bicarbonate sites. Bicarbonate, which is the main buffer for the blood, freely enters tubular fluid from the glomerulus and must be recovered for the body to maintain proper acid-base balance. Reabsorption of bicarbonate occurs in the proximal convoluted tubule. Reabsorption of bicarbonate is not direct but involves the action of the enzyme carbonic anhydrase. Carbonic anhydrase converts hydrogen ion and bicarbonate ion in the tubular fluid to carbon dioxide and water. Carbon dioxide may freely pass into the tubular epithelial cell and is reabsorbed, whereas bicarbonate ion stays in the tubule. The reabsorbed carbon dioxide is quickly reconverted to bicarbonate within the kidney cell and becomes available to the bloodstream.

Organic ion pumps. The kidney has the capacity to rapidly secrete complex ions such as amino acids and other natural compounds. This process occurs near the proximal convoluted tubule in the cortical portion of the descending limb of Henle's loop. Many drugs, including several diuretics, enter tubular fluid by this mechanism, which is referred to as an organic ion pump. Since some diuretics work only from within the tubule, the action of the drug depends at least in part on the proper function of this active secretion mechanism.

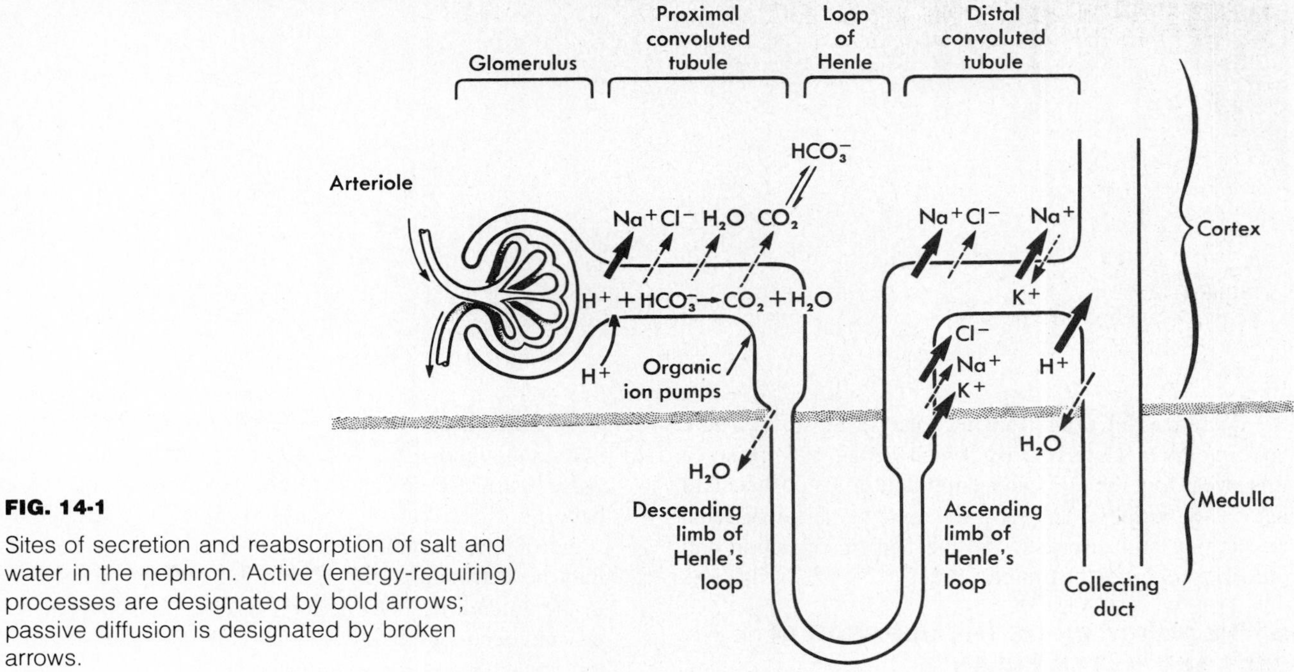

FIG. 14-1

Sites of secretion and reabsorption of salt and water in the nephron. Active (energy-requiring) processes are designated by bold arrows; passive diffusion is designated by broken arrows.

Mechanism of diuretic action. The diuretics considered in this chapter achieve their effects by increasing sodium ion excretion. Since water tends to follow sodium ion in the kidney, when sodium ion is excreted, so is water. Several distinct mechanisms for increasing sodium ion excretion exist and all may be understood in terms of the renal physiology just discussed. Specific mechanisms are discussed with the individual drugs and summarized in Table 14-1. Clinical properties of individual drugs are summarized in Tables 14-2 to 14-4.

■ PROPERTIES OF DIURETIC DRUGS

Ethacrynic acid (Table 14-2)

Mechanism of action. Ethacrynic acid inhibits the active reabsorption of chloride ion in the ascending limb of Henle's loop. Since chloride ion reabsorption is prevented, the passive reabsorption of sodium ion is also blocked. Therefore NaCl is retained in the tubule and excreted in the urine, carrying body water with it. Whereas ordinarily 99.4% of the sodium ion entering the tubule is reabsorbed, under the influence of ethacrynic acid only 70% to 80% is reabsorbed, along with an equivalent amount of chloride ion. Potassium ion is also excreted in higher than normal amounts in response to this drug (Table 14-1). Ethacrynic acid is one of the most potent diuretics known. Its rapid, powerful action must be carefully monitored to avoid profound dehydration and salt depletion in treated patients.

Since ethacrynic acid promotes the loss of excess salt and body water, it is a useful agent for controlling edematous states such as those occurring in congestive heart failure, renal disease, cirrhosis of the liver, lymphedema, nephrotic syndrome, and ascites associated with malignancies.

Absorption, distribution, and excretion. Ethacrynic acid is well absorbed from the gastrointestinal tract, producing a diuretic effect within an hour of administration. The drug is also appropriate for intravenous administration, producing diuresis within 2 to 10 minutes when given by that route. Ethacrynic acid should not be given by intramuscular or subcutaneous injection, since the drug can cause severe pain and irritation at the injection site.

Ethacrynic acid is bound to proteins in the bloodstream, and in the protein-bound form is not available for glomerular filtration. The drug is, however, secreted into the tubule by the organic anion pump in the descending limb of Henle's loop (cortical portion). The effectiveness of ethacrynic acid depends on being able to enter the tubule, since diuresis is produced from within the tubule. About two thirds of the normal dose of ethacrynic acid is excreted in the kidney, the remainder being eliminated by the liver. In the kidney, ethacrynic acid exists primarily as the free drug and as a complex with cysteine. The cysteine–ethacrynic acid complex formed in the body is many times more effective than the free drug.

Toxicity. The most likely toxic reaction to ethacrynic acid is actually an excess of the action for which the drug is prescribed. Ethacrynic acid is so potent that excessive salt and water loss may occur quickly in a patient. Dehydration with reduction in blood volume may precipitate circulatory collapse. Vascular thromboses and emboli may be generated, especially in elderly pa-

TABLE 14-1. Summary of diuretic effects on tubular transport

	Excretion increased					Excretion blocked		
Ethacrynic acid	Na^+	H_2O	K^+	Cl^-	—	Uric acid	Li^+	—
Furosemide	Na^+	H_2O	K^+	Cl^-	—	Uric acid	Li^+	—
Thiazides	Na^+	H_2O	K^+	Cl^-	HCO_3^-	Uric acid	Li^+	—
Acetazolamide	Na^+	H_2O	K^+	—	HCO_3^-	Uric acid	—	—
Organomercurials	Na^+	H_2O	—	Cl^-	—	Uric acid	—	—
Spironolactone	Na^+	H_2O	—	—	HCO_3^-	—	—	K^+,H^+
Triamterene	Na^+	H_2O	—	—	HCO_3^-	—	—	K^+,H^+
Osmotic diuretics	(Na^+)*	H_2O	(K^+)*	(Cl^-)*	—	—	—	—

*Large doses.
NOTE: The effects on ion transport shown are those commonly observed in humans during chronic therapy with normal clinical doses. With prolonged therapy, those ions whose excretion is increased may become depleted from the body, whereas those whose excretion is blocked may accumulate. Lithium ion accumulation is clinically important only for those patients receiving lithium carbonate therapy for mania. Uric acid accumulation is usually important only for those patients predisposed to gout.

TABLE 14-2. Summary of diuretic drugs: ethacrynic acid and furosemide

Generic name	Trade name	Dosage and administration	Diuretic effect: Onset	Peak	Duration
Ethacrynic acid	Edecrin	ORAL: *Adults*—50 to 100 mg initially; thereafter 50 to 200 mg daily. *Children*—25 mg initially, increasing by 25 mg to maintain.	30 min	1 to 2 hr	6 to 8 hr
		INTRAVENOUS: *Adults*—50 mg. Not recommended for children by this route.	5 to 10 min	15 to 20 min	1 to 3 hr
Furosemide	Lasix	ORAL: *Adults*—20 to 80 mg once or twice daily. *Children*—2 mg/kg initially, increasing by 1 or 2 mg/kg after 6 to 8 hr; maximum dose, 6 mg/kg.	60 min	1 to 2 hr	6 to 8 hr
		INTRAVENOUS: *Adults*—20 to 40 mg once or twice daily. *Children*—1 mg/kg initially, increasing by 1 mg/kg after 2 hr; maximum dose 6 mg/kg.	5 to 10 min	15 to 20 min	1 to 3 hr

tients. Electrolyte depletion may be a more gradual process marked by weakness or lethargy, dizziness, leg cramps, anorexia, vomiting, and possibly mental confusion.

Ethacrynic acid increases the loss of ions other than sodium and chloride, such as potassium and calcium. Excessive potassium loss impairs proper functioning of the heart, skeletal muscle, kidneys, and other tissues. Many physicians routinely prescribe some form of potassium replacement for their patients receiving ethacrynic acid for prolonged periods. Loss of calcium may rarely be sufficient to produce tetany. Most patients will not require calcium replacement, but serum calcium levels should be observed periodically.

Uric acid excretion is partially blocked by ethacrynic acid (Table 14-1). Therefore in certain susceptible patients gout may arise. For most patients the increase in serum uric acid produces no symptoms.

Ethacrynic acid has produced various gastrointestinal disturbances in a few patients, especially those receiving the drug continuously for several months. A sudden, severe, watery diarrhea indicates the drug should be withdrawn. The physician may discontinue the drug permanently if these symptoms arise.

Ethacrynic acid affects ion transport in several body tissues other than the kidney. Altered sodium and potassium transport may be associated with toxicity to certain cell types in the inner ear. Transient or permanent deafness has been observed in patients receiving ethacrynic acid, especially those receiving very high doses or those patients with reduced renal function who suffer drug accumulation.

Drug interactions. The potassium-depleting effect of ethacrynic acid makes this drug dangerous for patients receiving digitalis. Lowered potassium content in the tissue predisposes the heart to toxicity from the cardiac glycosides, which may include fatal arrhythmias. Note that corticosteroids are also potassium-depleting agents and may add to the danger of electrolyte imbalance when given with ethacrynic acid.

Ethacrynic acid lowers the renal clearance of lithium, a drug used for the control of manic cycles in manic-depressive psychosis (Table 14-1). Under these conditions lithium may accumulate, and severe toxicity may occur. These drugs are ordinarily not given together.

Ethacrynic acid has an antihypertensive action that may be additive with that of other antihypertensive agents. Care may be required to prevent excessive hypotension when these drugs are used together.

The ototoxic effect of ethacrynic acid may be potentiated by aminoglycoside antibiotics (Chapter 44), which are themselves ototoxic. Since permanent deafness may result from this combination, it is ordinarily avoided if at all possible.

Ethacrynic acid is strongly bound to serum proteins and may therefore displace other drugs from protein-binding sites. The result of this action is to increase the concentration of the free, active form of the displaced drug. The anticoagulant warfarin is known to be displaced in this manner by ethacrynic acid. Higher concentrations of unbound warfarin produce greater anticoagulant effects and may produce toxicity.

Furosemide (Table 14-2)

Mechanism of action. The clinically important action of furosemide is inhibition of the active reabsorption of Cl^- in the ascending limb of Henle's loop, a mechanism virtually identical to that of ethacrynic acid. Furosemide has the same potent effects on salt and water excretion previously described for ethacrynic acid. The only difference in action between the two drugs is that furosemide at high doses may occasionally increase bicarbonate excretion, whereas ethacrynic acid has no direct effect on bicarbonate excretion.

Furosemide is used like ethacrynic acid for the control of edematous states produced by various medical conditions. In addition, furosemide may be used for the control of hypertension either alone or in combination with other antihypertensive agents.

Absorption, distribution, and excretion. Furosemide is well absorbed from the gastrointestinal tract, producing diuresis within an hour of administration. Diuresis occurs within minutes of an intravenous dose of the drug. Furosemide may also be administered intramuscularly.

A significant proportion of furosemide in the bloodstream is bound to protein. Free drug is filtered in the glomerulus; furosemide also enters the tubular fluid by the organic anion pump. As with ethacrynic acid, it is only the drug within the tubule that is active in producing diuresis. About two thirds of an ingested dose of furosemide is ultimately found in the kidney, with most of the remainder being excreted in the feces. A small amount of administered furosemide is metabolized.

Toxicity. Furosemide is capable of producing the same acute dehydration, salt depletion, and potassium depletion as previously described for ethacrynic acid. Calcium loss and uric acid accumulation also occur with furosemide as for ethacrynic acid.

Various types of dermatitis and occasional blood dyscrasias have been reported for furosemide. The brisk diuresis produced by furosemide may be associated with urinary bladder spasm, thirst, perspiration, muscle cramps, weakness, and/or dizziness. Furosemide also impairs glucose tolerance in some patients, and rarely the drug has precipitated diabetes mellitus.

Gastrointestinal effects and ototoxicity are less common with furosemide than with ethacrynic acid.

Furosemide may produce an allergic interstitial nephritis that can produce reversible renal failure.

Drug interactions. Furosemide causes potassium depletion to the same extent as ethacrynic acid and for this reason should also be used with great care in patients receiving digitalis or potassium-depleting steroids. Furosemide, like ethacrynic acid, blocks lithium excretion and may lead to toxic lithium accumulation. The ototoxic potential of furosemide may be enhanced by aminoglycoside antibiotics or other ototoxic drugs.

Furosemide may increase the nephrotoxicity of antibiotics such as cephaloridine (Chapter 42). Furosemide also may increase the effect of tubocurarine, which can lead to muscle paralysis and paralysis of respiration. For this reason furosemide is usually discontinued a few days before surgery, if possible.

Furosemide and salicylates are both secreted by the organic anion pump. Since this pump system has limited capacity, furosemide may block the excretion of salicylates. Clinically, this process may be important for patients receiving high doses of salicylates for rheumatoid diseases. If these patients are also given furosemide, salicylates may accumulate and cause salicylate toxicity.

Thiazide diuretics (Table 14-3)

Mechanism of action. Thiazide diuretics have multiple effects on the nephron. These diuretics block sodium and chloride reabsorption in the distal convoluted tubule. This action leads to an increased excretion of NaCl and body water and establishes a new state of salt and water balance in which there is a lower level of body sodium maintained than before the drug was given. In

TABLE 14-3. Summary of diuretic drugs: thiazide diuretics

Generic name	Trade name	Dosage and administration	Diuretic effect		
			Onset	Peak	Duration
Chlorothiazide	Diuril Ro-chlorozide	ORAL, INTRAVENOUS: *Adults*—0.5 to 1 Gm once or twice daily. *Children*—10 mg/lb daily in 2 doses, oral route only. Intravenous not recommended.	2 hr	4 hr	6 to 12 hr
Hydrochloro-thiazide	Delco-Retic Diaqua Esidrix HydroDiuril Ro-Hydrazide	ORAL: *Adults*—25 to 200 mg once or twice daily. *Children*—1 mg/lb daily in 2 doses.	2 hr	4 hr	6 to 12 hr
Benzthiazide	Aquastat Aquatag Exna Hydrex Proaqua Rola-Benz Urazide	ORAL: *Adults*—50 to 200 mg; once daily for low doses, divide doses over 100 mg daily. *Children*—1 to 4 mg/kg daily in 3 doses initially; dose reduced for maintenance.	2 hr	4 to 6 hr	12 to 18 hr
Methyclothia-zide	Aquatensen Enduron	ORAL: *Adults*—2.5 to 10 mg once daily. *Children*—0.05 to 0.2 mg/kg daily.	2 hr	6 hr	24 hr
Trichlormethi-azide	Diurese Metahydrin Naqua Rochlo-methiazide	ORAL: *Adults*—1 to 4 mg once daily. *Children*—0.07 mg/kg daily in single or divided dose.	2 hr	6 hr	24 hr
Polythiazide	Renese	ORAL: *Adults*—1 to 4 mg once daily. *Children*—0.02 to 0.08 mg/kg daily.	2 hr	6 hr	36 hr
Quinethazone	Hydromox	ORAL: *Adults*—50 to 100 mg once daily.	2 hr	6 hr	18 to 24 hr
Hydroflu-methiazide	Diurcardin Saluron	ORAL: *Adults*—50 to 200 mg; once daily for low doses; divide doses over 100 mg daily. *Children*—1 mg/kg daily.	1 to 2 hr	3 to 4 hr	24 hr
Bendroflu-methiazide	Naturetin	ORAL: *Adults*—2.5 to 5 mg once daily. *Children*—0.4 mg/kg daily in 2 doses; reduce dose for maintenance.	1 to 2 hr	6 to 12 hr	18 to 24 hr
Metolazone	Zaroxolyn	ORAL: *Adults*—5 to 20 mg once daily.	1 hr	2 hr	12 to 24 hr
Chlorthali-done	Hygroton	ORAL: *Adults*—50 to 100 mg daily.	2 hr or less	2 hr	48 to 72 hr
Cyclothiazide	Anhydron	ORAL: *Adults*—1 to 2 mg once daily.	6 hr	7 to 12 hr	18 to 24 hr

addition to this action, thiazide diuretics also inhibit carbonic anhydrase in the proximal convoluted tubule, thereby elevating the excretion of bicarbonate and an additional increment of sodium. This minor component in the action of thiazide diuretics is lost after a few days. Potassium excretion is also enhanced by the thiazide diuretics, but this effect is not required for diuresis and is usually considered a toxic side effect.

Thiazide diuretics are less potent than ethacrynic acid and furosemide and are more suitable for use in outpatients. The drugs may be used to control edema associated with heart or kidney disease. Edema produced by corticosteroid or estrogen therapy may also be controlled with thiazide diuretics. The use of thiazide diuretics in controlling hypertension is discussed in Chapter 13.

Absorption, distribution, and excretion. Thiazide diuretics are well absorbed from the gastrointestinal tract and may begin to take action in the kidney within an hour of ingestion. Peak diuretic action may occur anytime from 2 to 6 hours or more after the oral dose, depending on which individual thiazide preparation is used. The various thiazide preparations differ in the timing and duration of diuretic effects (Table 14-3). In general, the longer-acting thiazide diuretics are highly bound to serum proteins. Their long duration of action is related to their slow elimination from these protein-binding sites.

Thiazide diuretics are primarily concentrated in the extracellular water in the body except for the drug concentrated in the kidney. Thiazides are secreted into the renal tubule by the organic anion pump. Most of the administered dose leaves the body by this route. Some drug, however, is eliminated by the liver, which secretes these drugs into the bile.

Chlorothiazide is available for intravenous dosage. The onset of action is somewhat more rapid by this route, but the duration of effect is not greatly altered from that observed with oral doses. This preparation must never be administered intramuscularly or subcutaneously. Great care should be taken to prevent leakage of the drug into the tissues when it is given intravenously.

Toxicity. Long-term administration of thiazide diuretics can lead to fluid and electrolyte imbalance, which may produce the classic signs: thirst, weakness, lethargy, restlessness, muscle cramps, and fatigue. The electrolyte imbalance most likely to be observed in patients receiving thiazide diuretics is excessive potassium and chloride ion loss. The loss of these ions leads to a metabolic alkalosis. Potassium supplements may be required to remedy this situation. Chloride loss alone is usually mild and is not treated.

Calcium excretion is blocked by thiazide diuretics, and increased serum calcium levels may result. The parathyroid glands may also be affected by long-term therapy with these diuretics. Uric acid excretion is also blocked by the thiazide diuretics, and the increased blood levels of this compound may precipitate an attack of gout in susceptible individuals.

Thiazide diuretics have a direct irritative effect on the gastrointestinal tract and may produce a variety of symptoms, ranging from simple nausea and vomiting to constipation, jaundice, and pancreatitis.

Thiazides have a direct effect on the central nervous system. Mild symptoms include dizziness, headache, and paresthesia. At very high concentrations such as those found in drug overdose, mental lethargy may progress to coma, although heart function and respiration are not markedly depressed.

Blood dyscrasia and various allergic reactions have been observed with thiazide diuretics. Although urticaria or other mild forms of allergy are more common, severe serum sickness and anaphylactic reactions have been noted.

Thiazides cause hypotension by a mechanism apparently unrelated to their action as diuretics. Some patients may suffer orthostatic hypotension when receiving these drugs. Thiazides occasionally lower glomerular filtration rates when given intravenously. This effect is of little consequence to most patients, although a patient with already reduced renal function may be adversely affected.

Drug interactions. Since thiazide diuretics have an intrinsic hypotensive activity, they may potentiate the action of other antihypertensive agents, especially those that act at ganglionic or peripheral adrenergic sites (Chapter 13).

Potassium loss is enhanced when thiazide diuretics are given with corticosteroids or adrenocorticotropic hormone (ACTH). Hypokalemia (low concentration of potassium in the blood) may render the patient more sensitive to digitalis toxicity.

Thiazides may increase the response to tubocurarine, a muscle relaxant commonly used in surgery. Patients receiving both of these drugs should be carefully observed for signs of excessive tubocurarine activity.

Thiazide diuretics frequently alter the requirement for insulin or other hypoglycemic agents. Any diabetic who must receive one of the thiazides should be carefully observed during the first few days of thiazide therapy to prevent loss of diabetic control.

Lithium excretion is blocked by thiazides and other diuretics. The increased danger of lithium toxicity prevents the safe use of both these drugs at once in a patient.

Carbonic anhydrase inhibitors (Table 14-4)

Mechanism of action. Diuretics that inhibit carbonic anhydrase in the kidney prevent the secretion of hydrogen ion into the renal tubule and the reabsorption of carbon dioxide from the renal tubule. As a result, the excretion of bicarbonate is rapidly increased and the urine becomes alkaline. The diuretic action of these carbonic anhydrase inhibitors arises from the fact that sodium ion accompanies the excreted bicarbonate. However, bicarbonate excretion is much greater than sodium ion excretion, and these drugs are classified as weak diuretics. Moderate amounts of potassium, phosphate, and chloride ion are also lost in the urine. When carbonic anhydrase inhibitors are given over a long period of time, metabolic acidosis may occur. Since metabolic acidosis prevents the action of these diuretics, these drugs are not suitable for long-term continuous administration as diuretics.

TABLE 14-4. Summary of diuretic drugs: carbonic anhydrate inhibitors, organomercurials, and potassium-sparing diuretics

Generic name	Trade name	Dosage and administration	Diuretic effect		
			Onset	Peak	Duration
CARBONIC ANHYDRASE INHIBITORS					
Acetazolamide	Diamox Rozolamine	ORAL, INTRAVENOUS: *Adults*—250 to 375 mg once daily; alternate-day therapy may be used.	About 1 hr	2 to 3 hr	About 12 hr
Ethoxzolamide	Cardrase Ethamide	ORAL: *Adults*—62.5 to 250 mg daily; alternate-day therapy may be used.	About 1 hr	2 to 3 hr	About 12 hr
ORGANOMERCURIALS					
Mersalyl with theophylline	Mercurasol Mercutheolin Mer-Im Mersalyn Salyrgan-Theophylline Theo-Syl R	INTRAMUSCULAR, INTRAVENOUS: *Adults*—initial dose 50 mg mersalyl and 25 mg theophylline; thereafter, 100 to 200 mg mersalyl and 50 to 100 mg theophylline (1 to 2 ml of drug as supplied) once or twice weekly. *Children*—doses are half those of adults.	30 to 40 min	2 to 4 hr	About 12 hr
Mercaptomerin sodium	Thiomerin Sodium	INTRAMUSCULAR, SUBCUTANEOUS: *Adults*—25 to 250 mg daily (0.2 to 2 ml of drug as supplied).	30 to 40 min	2 to 4 hr	12 hr
Merethoxylline procaine	Dicurin Procaine	INTRAMUSCULAR, SUBCUTANEOUS: *Adults*—50 to 200 mg mercurial, 25 to 100 mg theophylline (0.5 to 2 ml drug as supplied) daily or as needed.	30 to 40 min	2 to 4 hr	12 hr
POTASSIUM-SPARING DIURETICS					
Spironolactone	Aldactone	ORAL: *Adults*—25 to 200 mg daily in divided doses. *Children*—3.3 mg/kg daily in divided doses.	Effects build over a period of days		
Triamterene	Dyrenium	ORAL: *Adults*—100 mg twice daily after meals; do not exceed 300 mg daily. *Children*—2 to 4 mg/kg daily in divided doses.	2 to 4 hr (maximal effect not seen for several days)	6 hr	7 to 9 hr

Carbonic anhydrase inhibitors are primarily used in the treatment of glaucoma, congestive heart failure, and convulsive disorders.

Absorption, distribution, and excretion. The carbonic anhydrase inhibitors used for their diuretic action are chemically related to the sulfonamide antibiotics. These drugs tend to be well absorbed from the gastrointestinal tract. The most widely used drug of this class, acetazolamide, has a plasma half-life of 100 minutes and is rapidly concentrated in the kidney. Tissue levels in the kidney may be 2 to 3 times the plasma concentration within ½ to 2 hours of an oral dose of the drug. Acetazolamide enters the tubule by the organic anion pump. The drug also inhibits carbonic anhydrase in other tissues of the body.

Acetazolamide and other carbonic anhydrase inhibitors are sometimes given on alternate days rather than continuously (Table 14-4). The intent of this type of therapy is to prevent the kidney from becoming resistant to the action of the drug, that is, to prevent metabolic acidosis from occurring. During the day without the drug, the carbonic anhydrase inhibitors are cleared from the body and kidney function returns to its predrug condition. When the drug is readministered on the following day, it is as effective as when first given.

Toxicity. Reactions to these drugs are not very common, especially when they are used in intermittent or short-term therapy. These sulfonamide derivatives are capable of causing a variety of blood dyscrasias, fever, and rash. Drug precipitation in the urine has occurred, causing the formation of stones.

These drugs have direct actions on a number of tissues, including the central nervous system. Paresthesia, nervousness, sedation, lassitude, depression, headaches, vertigo, and other symptoms have been reported.

The conditions of patients already suffering from respiratory acidosis may worsen from these drugs, which tend to produce metabolic acidosis.

Drug interactions. Acetazolamide and other carbonic anhydrase inhibitors produce more marked potassium excretion than sodium excretion. Potassium depletion is therefore likely to occur. This possibility is made even more likely by corticosteroids or ACTH given concomitantly. Digitalis toxicity is increased in the presence of low serum potassium.

Organomercurial diuretics (Table 14-4)

Mechanism of action. The organomercurial compounds achieve diuretic action by inhibiting active chloride ion transport in the ascending limb of Henle's loop. Chloride excretion therefore increases and causes an increase in the excretion of sodium ion and water. Chronic administration of these compounds may ultimately deplete chloride and produce metabolic alkalosis. This condition renders the patient insensitive to the diuretic effect of the organomercurial compounds.

Potassium and ammonium ions may also be excreted in increased amounts, although organomercurial effects on potassium secretion depend on the original rate of secretion in the untreated patient. A patient with a high rate of potassium secretion before treatment may actually show a fall in potassium ion secretion with organomercurial diuretics. Excretion of calcium and magnesium ions is elevated by these drugs.

Organomercurial diuretics are seldom used in modern clinical practice, since newer and more convenient agents have become available.

Absorption, distribution, and excretion. Organomercurial compounds are irritative to the gastrointestinal tract and are unreliably absorbed by the oral route. For this reason, these drugs are usually best administered intramuscularly. Mersalyl may be administered intravenously, but care must be taken to administer the drug slowly, since too rapid an injection can cause transient high concentrations of drug, which may produce fatal arrhythmias. Subcutaneous use of mersalyl may produce severe local pain and irritation. Other organomercurials may be given subcutaneously (Table 14-4).

Organomercurial diuretics bind to sulfhydryl groups on albumin and are carried in the bloodstream primarily by that protein. Thirty to 40 minutes after an intravenous injection, sufficient drug will have reached the kidney so that sodium loss begins. Peak action of the drug is reached in 2 to 4 hours, but significant effects may be observed for several hours beyond that time.

Organomercurial diuretics act from within the renal tubule but do not enter the tubule by the organic ion pumps. Although the route of entry is not well established, more than two thirds of a parenterally administered dose of an organomercurial diuretic is eliminated by the kidney, with the remainder being excreted by the biliary route into the gut.

Toxicity. The potency of the organomercurial diuretics is great enough that electrolyte imbalance may be produced with improper or long-term use of these drugs. In addition to the irritative effects on skin and gastric mucosa, organomercurial diuretics may cause allergic responses with urticaria, pruritus, and occasionally anaphylactic shock. Bone marrow depression and kidney toxicity have also been observed.

Since these compounds contain mercury, a toxic metal, there is the potential for mercury poisoning under certain circumstances. This risk is increased in patients with impaired renal function who cannot eliminate the mercury rapidly from the body. For most people the mercury in these drugs exists in the body in complex with sulfur-containing compounds and is thus rendered harmless. However, great excesses of mercury may overwhelm the ability of the body to hold the metal in an inactive form.

One of the organomercurial diuretics, mersalyl with theophylline, may produce toxic reactions different from those seen with other diuretics of this class. Patients receiving mersalyl with theophylline should be observed for chills, fever, rashes, vomiting, or convulsions. This drug should be given in small test doses, which may be gradually increased until one of the symptoms just mentioned arises, in which case the drug should be discontinued. Theophylline, a xanthine-like drug chemically related to caffeine, has mild diuretic action of its own.

Potassium-sparing diuretics (Table 14-4)

Mechanism of action. Potassium-sparing diuretics inhibit the pump mechanism that normally exchanges potassium for sodium in the distal convoluted tubule (Fig. 14-1). This pump is under the control of mineralocorticoid hormones such as aldosterone, which increase sodium retention and promote potassium loss. Aldosterone is present in greater than normal amounts in edematous states resulting from congestive heart failure, nephrotic syndrome, and hepatic cirrhosis. Spironolactone, one of the potassium-sparing diuretics, competitively blocks the action of aldosterone on the sodium-potassium exchange pump, thereby causing sodium to remain in the tubule and be excreted. Potassium is not pumped into the tubule and so is spared from excretion. Another diuretic of this class, triamterene, produces the same effects as spironolactone but by a different mechanism that is not dependent on aldosterone. These properties explain the fact that spironolactone is most effective under circumstances in which aldosterone is elevated, whereas the more rapidly and directly acting triamterene is effective when aldosterone is low, high, or normal.

Since the sodium-potassium pump in the distal convoluted tubule is ordinarily responsible for reabsorbing only a small fraction of the sodium from the tubule, blockade of this pump increases sodium excretion only slightly. This fact limits the effectiveness of the potassium-sparing diuretics.

Spironolactone is used to control edema in congestive heart failure, cirrhosis of the liver, and nephrotic syndrome. Spironolactone may ameliorate the effects of excessive aldosterone levels in patients suffering from the endocrine disorder hyperaldosteronism. The drug may also be useful in treating hypertension and reversing potassium loss arising from various conditions. Triamterene is used in many of the same situations as spironolactone.

Absorption, distribution, and excretion. Spironolactone is a steroid derivative related in structure to natural mineralocorticoids (Chapter 35). As expected from the structure, spironolactone is not very water soluble. Early forms of the drug were not well absorbed from the gastrointestinal tract, but the pharmaceutical formulation has been improved by using very fine particles of the drug. In this form the drug is adequately absorbed from the gastrointestinal tract. Peak therapeutic effects with spironolactone are observed several days after dosage is begun (Table 14-4). This delay is related to the mechanism of action of the drug and is not a result of delay in absorption or other pharmacokinetic properties of the drug.

Spironolactone is extensively metabolized much the same as the natural steroids it chemically resembles. Metabolites of spironolactone appear in the urine and in lesser quantities in the bile.

Triamterene, although not a steroid like spironolactone, is also relatively insoluble in water. Intestinal absorption of this drug is somewhat variable but usually satisfactory. Most of the orally administered dose appears in the urine within 24 hours. The drug enters the renal tubule both by glomerular filtration and tubular secretion. Unlike spironolactone, the peak effect of this drug is observed within hours of an oral dose.

Toxicity. Spironolactone and triamterene may cause serum potassium levels to increase dangerously. Patients with impaired renal function or excessively high potassium intake are especially at risk. Fatal cardiac arrhythmias may result.

Spironolactone may cause various endocrine alterations, since the drug chemically resembles not only mineralocorticoids but also androgens and progestins. Females may observe menstrual irregularities, hirsutism, and deepening of the voice. Males may observe gynecomastia (breast development) and have difficulty in achieving or maintaining erection. Symptoms in both sexes are usually reversed when the drug is discontinued.

Spironolactone produces tumors in rats exposed to the drug for long periods. For this reason, use of the drug should be restricted to cases in which the benefit clearly outweighs this risk. Spironolactone should not be used in an attempt to control edema in pregnancy. If the drug is used in lactating women, breast-feeding should be discontinued, since metabolites of spironolactone appear in breast milk.

Triamterene may produce blood dyscrasias and a reversible azotemia revealed by an increased blood urea nitrogen (BUN). Gastrointestinal disturbances, skin rashes, and drug fever have been observed in patients receiving either spironolactone or triamterene.

Drug interactions. Two potassium-sparing diuretics should neither be concomitantly administered to the same patient nor should either drug be administered to a patient receiving potassium supplements or ingesting a diet rich in potassium.

Use of the potassium-sparing diuretics with antihypertensive agents may require reduction in doses of the latter drugs, since spironolactone and triamterene may have additive antihypertensive effects with these agents.

When spironolactone is combined with other diuretics, dosages may have to be reduced. Spironolactone can prevent the distal tubular reabsorption of sodium, making the diuretics that act early in the nephron even more effective.

Spironolactone reduces vascular responsiveness to norepinephrine. This effect may be important in patients receiving norepinephrine under local or general anesthesia.

Osmotic diuretics

Osmotic diuretics are nonelectrolytes of various types that are filtered by the glomerulus but not significantly reabsorbed or metabolized. Therefore osmotic diuretics enter the renal tubule and are highly concentrated in renal tubular fluid. The high osmolality in the tubule reduces the reabsorption of water with the result that urine production is increased. At high doses some increase in sodium excretion is produced, but this is not observed in most clinical circumstances. These drugs are therefore exceptions to the generalization that sodium excretion precedes water excretion during diuretic therapy.

Osmotic diuresis may be used clinically to prevent

■ THE NURSING PROCESS

■ Assessment

Patients with a variety of medical conditions may require diuretic therapy, including those patients with cardiac, renal, or hepatic insufficiency, hypertension, and other problems characterized by too much retained fluid or poor fluid mobilization. These patients may come to the hospital with such signs and symptoms as edema, congestive heart failure, pulmonary edema, elevated blood pressure, altered level of consciousness, and weight gain. In addition, patients with problems of fluid balance may display serum electrolyte abnormalities. The nurse should perform a total patient assessment, focusing on the presenting signs and symptoms and appropriate laboratory and other objective data that would help further define the nature of the patient's problems.

■ Management

Choice of diuretic depends on the patient's condition, the speed with which fluid needs to be eliminated, available routes of administration, and other drugs the patient may be receiving. The nurse should ascertain what actions are required to aid drug therapy. For example, dietary and fluid restrictions may be required to speed the process of fluid removal and to prevent reaccumulation. Monitoring of fluid intake and output, serum electrolyte levels, blood urea nitrogen, uric acid, body weight, blood pressure, and observing for the appearance of new signs or symptoms may be required with individual patients. The nurse should watch for side effects known to occur with a specific drug, such as ototoxicity with ethacrynic acid. For a patient who is not fully alert or who is immobilized, the insertion of a Foley catheter will decrease the discomfort of using the bedpan and facilitate accurate measurement of urine output. Use of cardiac monitoring may assist in the treatment of critically ill individuals.

■ Evaluation

Diuretic therapy is effective when excess fluid is lost and blood pressure is maintained, without producing abnormalities in electrolyte status or side effects resulting from the medication. For some patients, it is necessary to tolerate minor side effects to achieve required diuresis. The most common electrolyte imbalance, potassium depletion, may be overcome by administering a potassium supplement. As minimal preparation for discharge, the nurse should teach the patient why the medication is necessary, major possible side effects, and symptoms that should be reported to the physician. The nurse should also discuss why additional medications such as potassium supplements may need to be taken and how to monitor the general physical condition relative to diuretic therapy by performing activities such as recording the daily weight, fluid intake and output, and blood pressure. The patient should be able to repeat and to explain the appropriate information. If a restricted diet has been prescribed, the patient should demonstrate an ability to choose menus within the limits of the diet plan.

For specific clinical information about individual agents, the student should refer to the patient care implications section at the end of this chapter.

permanent damage during acute renal failure. The usefulness of osmotic diuresis in these cases frequently depends on maintaining adequate urine volume without altering electrolyte balance. Osmotic diuretics are also used to increase the osmolality of the plasma, which allows reduction of osmotic pressure inside the eye and in the cerebrospinal fluid.

The two agents currently used as osmotic diuretics, mannitol and urea, are usually administered intravenously. Mannitol is the preferred agent in most circumstances.

Toxicity produced by these agents depends on the amount of drug administered and how much the drug affects fluid balance in the body. These drugs are retained within the extracellular space and on intravenous administration can cause an acute expansion of extracellular fluid volume. This volume expansion may be hazardous to a patient with reduced cardiac reserve.

Fluid and electrolyte imbalances may be produced by osmotic diuretics, especially if a degree of renal impairment exists. Under these circumstances the diuretics tend to accumulate in the blood and may cause dangerous shifts in salt and water balance. Pulmonary congestion, acidosis, thirst, blurred vision, convulsion, nausea and vomiting, diarrhea, tachycardia, fever, and angina-like pain may be noted occasionally. Local irritation with thrombophlebitis can also occur with these drugs.

Urea should not be used in a patient with liver failure, since the high levels of urea may place additional demands on liver function.

■ PATIENT CARE IMPLICATIONS

General guidelines for diuretic therapy

1. Intake and output should be carefully measured and recorded for patients receiving diuretics. Any unexpected change should be reported to the physician. For example, oliguria (scanty urine output) or anuria (no urine output) would be unexpected after an increase in a diuretic dose. The patient at home is usually not required to measure intake and output except in the case of severe kidney or cardiovascular disease, but patients should be encouraged to report output that seems to be abnormal.
2. Weigh the patient daily or more often in the acute care setting to evaluate diuretic effectiveness. Weighing should be done under standard conditions: same time daily (usually early in the morning) and after urinating or emptying the urinary drainage bag but before eating. The same amount of clothing should be worn and the same scales used each day. The patient at home is often asked to keep a daily or weekly weight record so the patient should be instructed how to do this.
3. Monitor the blood pressure regularly. Although all patients receiving diuretic therapy would be expected to experience an initial drop in blood pressure, the elderly, those receiving intravenous diuretics, and those also taking antihypertensives may experience a precipitous fall in blood pressure, and in rare instances go into shock. Other drugs that can cause hypotension and thus can be potentiated by the addition of diuretics include central nervous system depressants, barbiturates, and narcotics. Some physicians prefer that the blood pressure be monitored with patients in both lying and sitting positions. Symptoms secondary to hypotension (low blood pressure) include dizziness, syncope (fainting), and light-headedness.
4. The use of alcohol enhances hypotension; the patient taking diuretics should be cautioned to avoid the use of alcohol.
5. Patients who experience postural hypotension (low blood pressure that occurs after moving suddenly from lying to sitting or standing) need to be instructed to do these activities slowly. If the problem persists, the physician may wish to change the dose of medication.
6. Monitoring of body fluid retention may include daily measurement of abdominal girth or circumference of one or both legs. To ensure accuracy of measurement, the patient's skin may be marked with ink to indicate the correct placement of the tape measure. For cosmetic reasons, the marks should be small and inconspicuous.
7. Check dependent areas daily for the presence of or change in the amount of pitting edema. (In pitting edema, an indentation or depressed area remains in the skin for seconds to minutes after pressure has been applied by the examiner's finger.) Dependent areas where this is more likely to occur include the sacral area and the feet and legs.
8. Dehydration can occur with any diuretic. Symptoms include thirst, decreased skin turgor, nausea, light-headedness, weakness, increased pulse, oliguria, decreased blood pressure, elevated hemoglobin level, hematocrit, and blood urea nitrogen (BUN).
9. Several electrolyte abnormalities can occur as a result of diuretic therapy. The practitioner needs to observe patients for these problems and teach the patient to report any of the symptoms that may indicate electrolyte abnormalities. (Serum electrolyte values are included as a guide, but interpretation of any patient's laboratory values should be done on an individualized basis.)
   a. Hypokalemia. Serum potassium level less than 3.5 mEq/L. Signs and symptoms include vomiting, leg cramps, muscle weakness, apathy, ab-

dominal distention, paralytic ileus, and electrocardiogram (ECG) changes such as sagging S-T segments, depressed T waves, and elevated U waves.

b. Hyperkalemia. Serum potassium level greater than 5.0 mEq/L. Signs and symptoms include weakness, spasticity, flaccid paralysis (late sign), nausea, colic, diarrhea, oliguria, and ECG changes such as tall, tent-shaped T waves, decreased amplitude of P waves, and, later, atrial asystole, widening of the QRS, and irregular ventricular rhythms.

c. Hyponatremia. Serum sodium level below 135 mEq/L. Signs and symptoms include muscle weakness, leg cramps, irritability or confusion, lethargy, headache, hypotension, nausea, vomiting, and abdominal discomfort.

d. Hypocalcemia. Serum calcium level below 4.3 mEq/L. Signs and symptoms include tingling of the fingers, toes, nose, and ears, muscle spasms (tetany), and convulsions.

e. Hypomagnesemia. Serum magnesium level below 1.5 mEq/L. Signs and symptoms include confusion, hallucinations, tremors, muscle spasms, paresthesia, convulsion, and hyperactive reflexes.

f. Metabolic alkalosis. Arterial pH above 7.45. Signs and symptoms include mental confusion, dizziness, tetany, and convulsions. When a result of diuretic therapy it is often related to potassium loss, and the symptoms are similar to hypokalemia.

g. Metabolic acidosis. Serum pH below 7.35. Signs and symptoms include headache, mental dullness, rapid and deep respirations, stupor, coma, and eventually death. Whereas diuretics may cause this, there are many other conditions that do also; it is not uncommon in an acute care setting.

h. Hypercalcemia. Serum calcium level above 5.5 mEq/L. Signs and symptoms include thirst, polyuria, anorexia, nausea, vomiting, constipation, and altered level of consciousness.

10. If a potassium supplement is prescribed, teach the patient the importance of taking it as ordered, and work with the patient to find a preparation the patient is willing to take. Many effervescent preparations are unpalatable. Enteric-coated tablets (sometimes found in combination with a thiazide diuretic) have been implicated in small bowel ulceration and should not be used. Oral solutions are the preferred form of therapy, but the solutions are often unpleasant tasting. These solutions should be diluted in juice or milk to reduce the risk of gastric irritation and to make the taste tolerable. Taking potassium with meals also helps to reduce gastric irritation.

11. Dietary sources of potassium include citrus fruits and juices; grape, cranberry, apple, pear, and apricot juices; bananas; meat, fish, and fowl; cereals; and tea and cola beverages. Some patients who have borderline low potassium levels can maintain their potassium levels by increasing their daily intake of potassium-rich foods. Note, however, that some potassium-rich foods are also high in sodium and may be contraindicated on that basis.

12. Other drugs that cause potassium loss are steroids and amphotericin B. Digitalis preparations are quickly and seriously toxic in the presence of hypokalemia. When any of these drugs are being used concurrently with a potassium-losing diuretic, the dangers of hypokalemia are increased.

13. In hypertension, cardiovascular disease, and renal disease, good dietary control by the patient is often as important as correct use of medications. The patient may need extensive teaching about the diet, including special requirements for calories, sodium, potassium, carbohydrates, cholesterol, and other components. Consultation with a dietitian is often necessary, and follow-up with a visiting nurse referral may be helpful to promote compliance.

14. Teach patients about their need for diuretic therapy, and prepare them for its effects. Poor compliance is sometimes a result of annoyance with frequent and excessive urination. If a diuretic is ordered once a day, it should be taken in the morning to prevent interruption of sleep for urinating. A twice daily dose could be taken at 8 AM and 2 PM for the same reason.

15. The safety of many diuretics during pregnancy is not known. Women of childbearing age should be encouraged to use birth control measures during diuretic therapy and to consult with their gynecologist before attempting pregnancy. Since some diuretics are excreted in breast milk, women on diuretic therapy should consult with their obstetricians before deciding to breast-feed their infants.

16. Dehydration and hypovolemia can contribute to thromboembolic disorders. Observe the patient for pain in the chest, calves, and pelvis that might indicate thromboembolism.

17. When the patient's condition will allow, the use of intermittent therapy (every other day) with diuretics decreases the occurrence of side effects.

18. Caution the patient to avoid over-the-counter preparations unless the physician has given clearance. The drugstore pharmacist can also be helpful to the patient in teaching about drugs that should not be

used concurrently. Patients should always be counselled to keep all their health care providers informed of all medications they are taking and any changes in dosages that have been made. Finally, teach the patient not to ''double up'' if a dose has been missed; if in need of guidance about missed doses of any medication, the patient should contact the physician.

19. Thirst is a frequent patient complaint after diuretic therapy has begun, especially if diuresis has been rapid and dramatic, as in the acute care setting. Before allowing the patient to drink fluids as desired, consult with the physician to obtain any specific guidelines necessary. Ingestion of too many fluids may compound the possible electrolyte imbalances and defeat the purpose of the diuresis. Assisting the patient with mouth care on a frequent basis will help a little; lemon and glycerin swabs, however, may increase the patient's thirst.

Furosemide

1. See the general guidelines just given.
2. Hypokalemia can be a problem; potassium supplements are often necessary. In addition to taking the potassium supplements, patients should be taught to report diarrhea, vomiting, and anorexia (loss of appetite) because these conditions increase potassium loss. Any form of gastric suctioning contributes to potassium loss.
3. This drug may cause hyperglycemia. Occasionally check the patient's urine for sugar; diabetics may require an increase in insulin dosage.
4. Use cautiously in patients taking lithium because furosemide decreases lithium excretion. (See Chapter 26 for signs of lithium toxicity.)
5. Side effects include agranulocytosis (depressed production of white blood cells). Instruct the patient to report any unexplained fever, chills, sore throat, or enlarged lymph nodes.
6. Signs and symptoms of ototoxicity include tinnitus (ringing in the ears), reduced hearing acuity, and vertigo.
7. Hypocalcemia occurs rarely.
8. Uric acid excretion is reduced. Monitor uric acid levels, observe for signs of gout, and instruct the patient to report any symptoms of gout.
9. Parenteral administration.
   a. Furosemide is incompatible with acidic solutions but will mix with isotonic saline solution, 5% dextrose in water, and lactated Ringer's solution. If in doubt, consult the pharmacy; flush the tubing before administering intravenously.
   b. Furosemide may be given intravenously undiluted. The rate should not exceed 20 mg over a period of 2 minutes.
   c. Do not mix with any other medication in a syringe.
   d. Use only fresh solutions and discard after 24 hours.
   e. Store at room temperature. Do not use if the solution has turned yellow.
   f. Intramuscular injection may produce transient pain at the injection site.

Ethacrynic acid

The same precautions observed with furosemide should be applied to ethacrynic acid with the following additions and exceptions:

1. Hyperglycemia occurs less often than with furosemide.
2. Hypokalemia, hyponatremia, hypocalcemia, and hypochloremic alkalosis all have been reported. See the general guidelines for signs and symptoms.
3. Safe doses in infants have not been determined; furosemide is preferred for this age-group.
4. Ethacrynic acid displaces warfarin from binding sites, causing overcoagulation and bleeding (Chapter 17). In patients receiving both drugs, the dose of warfarin may have to be reduced.
5. Oral administration: Giving the medicine with meals or immediately after eating may reduce gastric irritation.
6. Parenteral administration:
   a. Ethacrynic acid should not be given intramuscularly or subcutaneously.
   b. The usual dilution is 50 mg of ethacrynic acid in 50 ml of 5% dextrose in water or sodium chloride injection. Hazy or opalescent solutions should not be used.
   c. A single dose should not exceed 100 mg (100 ml).
   d. Ethacrynic acid may be administered by direct intravenous injection or by running infusion. Do not mix with other medications, do not add to intravenous solutions, and do not mix with blood or its derivatives. If in doubt, consult the pharmacy.
   e. The rate of administration should not exceed 10 mg (10 ml) per minute.
   f. Check the infusion site carefully; extravasation causes pain and tissue irritation.
   g. Discard solutions after 24 hours.

Thiazide diuretics

1. See the general statements about diuretic therapy and the text of this chapter.
2. The thiazides may cause hypokalemia, hypochloremic alkalosis, hyponatremia, and hypomagnesemia.

3. The thiazides promote potassium loss, but some patients stabilize their serum potassium level at 3 to 3.5 mEq/L without potassium supplementation as long as dietary sources of potassium are used regularly. The decision to use potassium supplements should be based on the serum potassium level, general physical conditions, usual dietary practices, and other medications that the patient may be taking.
4. Thiazides may elevate the blood glucose level. Monitor urine sugar levels regularly. Diabetics may need to increase their insulin dosage.
5. The uric acid level may be increased. Asymptomatic elevations need not be treated. Symptomatic elevations (gout) are treated with colchicine (Chapter 20).
6. The BUN may be transiently elevated.
7. The serum lipid level may be elevated in some patients; the significance of this is not known.
8. The routine use of thiazides for treatment of edema in pregnancy (before the development of preeclampsia) is under scrutiny. There have been some reports of electrolyte imbalance and thrombocytopenia in infants of mothers receiving thiazides during pregnancy.
9. Hypercalcemia has occurred after thiazide administration in hypoparathyroid patients receiving vitamin D and in patients with hyperparathyroidism. Thiazides should be discontinued before testing parathyroid functioning.
10. Licorice causes potassium excretion and should be avoided by patients receiving thiazides.
11. The thiazides can cause a paradoxical antidiuretic effect in patients who have diabetes insipidus (Chapter 34).
12. Exacerbation of systemic lupus erythematosus has been reported.
13. Oral administration: Administration with food or after meals will help reduce gastric irritation.
14. Parenteral administration:
    a. Chlorothiazide is not safe for intramuscular or subcutaneous administration.
    b. Dilute each vial (0.5 Gm) with at least 18 ml of sterile water. Further dilution may be done with 5% dextrose in water or sodium chloride injection.
    c. Unused solutions should be discarded after 24 hours.
    d. Administer slowly (0.5 Gm over a period of 5 minutes).
    e. This medication is incompatible with many other drugs and with blood or its derivatives. If in doubt, consult with the pharmacy.
    f. Check the intravenous insertion site carefully; avoid extravasation.

Carbonic anhydrase inhibitors

1. See the text and general guidelines.
2. Long-term therapy with the carbonic anhydrase inhibitors is usually limited to patients with primary open-angle glaucoma and other chronic glaucomas.
3. With chronic therapy, the diuretic effect of the carbonic anhydrase inhibitors subsides, probably because of the metabolic acidosis the drugs create. Signs and symptoms of this acidosis include headache, mental dullness, and increased respiratory rate with characteristic deep respirations; the arterial pH is below 7.35. In the most severe cases, disorientation, coma, and death will occur. Other side effects of these drugs, which may or may not be related to the acidosis, include anorexia, nausea, vomiting, diarrhea, weakness, decreased libido, impotence, and malaise. In infants, failure to thrive may result from acidosis. To reduce the problem with acidosis, intermittent therapy is often used. Because many of these side effects may be mild and develop insidiously, the practitioner needs to question patients carefully about their response to the drugs.
4. Rarely, carbonic anhydrase inhibitors can produce drug fever, thrombocytopenia (abnormally low number of platelets), agranulocytosis (depressed production of white blood cells), and aplastic anemia. The patient should be instructed to report any unexplained fever, rash, sore throat, bruising, or bleeding.
5. Patients with chronic obstructive lung disease, who are often already in a state of chronic acidosis, may be acutely worsened with these drugs.
6. Renal colic (severe flank pain), hematuria (blood in the urine), and oliguria are signs and symptoms of renal calculus formation.
7. Because they interfere with excretion of some other drugs, carbonic anhydrase inhibitors increase the risk of toxicity from quinidine, tricyclic antidepressants, amphetamines, erythromycin, procainamide, and salicylates. Carefully observe patients receiving these drugs for signs of toxicity.
8. The use of potassium supplements depends on the patient's response. In many patients, the serum potassium level drops initially but returns to normal within a couple of weeks unless another potassium-losing drug is also being given.
9. Elevation of serum uric acid levels has been reported, but exacerbation of gout is rare.
10. Hyperglycemia and glycosuria are rare but may require a change in insulin dose for diabetics.
11. Because carbonic anhydrase inhibitors alter electrolyte balance, clients receiving lithium should be watched carefully for alterations in serum lithium levels.

12. Oral administration: Note that there are two oral forms of acetazolamide, a regular tablet and a sustained-release capsule or sequel. The physician should specify which form should be used.
13. Parenteral administration:
    a. Dilute each 500 mg of acetazolamide with at least 5 ml of sterile water for injection.
    b. Administer slowly via intravenous injection (500 mg over a period of 5 minutes). It may be added to intravenous solutions and administered over 4 to 8 hours. Consult with the pharmacy before mixing with other medications. It is incompatible with protein hydrolysate.
    c. Because of an alkaline pH, intramuscular injection is very painful; the intravenous route is preferred.

Organomercurial diuretics

1. See the text and general guidelines.
2. Because of the possibility of an allergic reaction, patients should be skin tested before receiving a full dose or at least should be started on a low test dose. This allergic, sometimes fatal, reaction is characterized by a precipitous fall in blood pressure, dyspnea, gasping, cyanosis, and cardiac irregularities. If an allergic reaction occurs, discontinue the drug, notify the physician, and treat symptomatically.
3. Mercury poisoning can also occur after prolonged use. Symptoms include cardiac arrhythmias, an ashen gray appearance around the mouth and pharynx, a metallic taste, diarrhea, stomatitis, sore gums, foul breath, and excessive salivation. Treatment includes discontinuing the drug and administering dimercaprol (BAL).
4. The organomercurials can produce hypochloremic alkalosis, hyponatremia, hypokalemia, hypocalcemia, and hypomagnesemia.
5. Several organomercurials are produced in combination form with theophylline (Chapter 22).
6. Acute urinary retention has been reported (rarely). Patient complaints include pain in the bladder area, bladder distention, and inability to urinate. Notify the physician.
7. Oral administration: Oral preparations are no longer available.
8. Intravenous administration:
    a. The organomercurials are not recommended for intravenous administration because they may produce ventricular fibrillation. If necessary, however, mersalyl with theophylline may be given via this route.
    b. Dilute 0.5 ml of the medication with 5 to 10 ml of sterile water.
    c. Do not mix with any other medication in a syringe or add to an infusion.
    d. Administer each 0.5 ml of actual medication over a period of at least 2 minutes.
    e. Monitor the ECG while administering.
    f. Check the intravenous insertion site carefully because extravasation can cause tissue necrosis and sloughing.
    g. Mersalyl with theophylline should not be given subcutaneously.
9. Intramuscular administration: Injection sites should be rotated, but the gluteus maximus is the preferred site for injection.

Potassium-sparing diuretics

1. See the general guidelines and the text of this chapter.
2. The potassium-sparing diuretics may cause hyperkalemia or hyponatremia, although the latter may only result from excessive water ingestion.
3. Because of the likelihood of hyponatremia, a fairly liberal salt intake (sodium intake) may be permitted for these patients.
4. There are many combination products containing both a potassium-sparing diuretic and a potassium-losing diuretic. The goal of the combination products is to promote diuresis while maintaining normal serum potassium levels. Patients receiving a combination drug are potentially at risk for side effects resulting from any of the component drugs. Example combinations are Aldactazide, which combines spironolactone with hydrochlorothiazide, and Dyazide, which contains triamterene and hydrochlorothiazide.
5. It is theoretically possible that the potassium-sparing diuretics may alter the serum levels of lithium, so patients receiving both drugs should be monitored carefully.

Osmotic diuretics

1. See the general guidelines and the text of this chapter.
2. Mannitol is preferred over urea in most situations because it is easier to administer, has fewer side effects, and causes less rebound edema in cerebral edema when discontinued.
3. Mannitol can cause congestive heart failure and pulmonary edema resulting from the fluid shift from the intracellular to the extracellular space. In addition, angina-like chest pain has been reported. Assess patients frequently for signs of pulmonary or cardiac difficulty by monitoring such parameters as the pulse, blood pressure, respiratory rate, color, ECG, and subjective complaints.
4. Hyponatremia is possible with mannitol.
5. Diuresis occurs rapidly and copiously after adminis-

tration of mannitol or urea; it is usually necessary to insert a urinary catheter (Foley). If the urine output should fall below 30 to 50 ml per hour, notify the physician.
6. Deafness has been reported in patients receiving mannitol who are also receiving kanamycin. Signs of hearing difficulty include tinnitus, decreased hearing acuity, and vertigo.
7. Because both mannitol and urea affect electrolyte balance, serum lithium levels may be altered (Chapter 26).
8. Urea can cause both hyponatremia and hypokalemia.
9. Osmotic diuretics are often administered to patients who have a decreased level of consciousness. It is therefore up to the practitioner to assess the onset of side effects; thus patients should be monitored frequently and carefully.
10. Do not confuse the drug mannitol with mannitol hexanitrate, an antianginal drug (Chapter 12).
11. Administration of mannitol:
    a. Dilution of mannitol is not necessary. It should not be added to other intravenous solutions or medications or mixed with blood.
    b. The rate of administration is usually 1 to 2 Gm/kg over 30 to 90 minutes, but up to 3 Gm/kg has been given.
    c. Mannitol comes in several concentrations, ranging from 5% solutions to 25% solutions. If in doubt about the dosage, consult the physician and pharmacist.
    d. Before administering, check the bottle or ampule for crystallization, a frequent problem. If crystals are present, warm the container under running water until the crystals dissolve. Let cool to body temperature before administering. An in-line intravenous filter should be used.
12. Administration of urea:
    a. Urea must be diluted to make a 30% solution (30% solution equals 30 Gm of urea/100 ml or 300 mg/1 ml). Dilution may be done with 5% or 10% dextrose in water or with 10% invert sugar in water; some manufacturers supply the diluent. Patients with hereditary fructose intolerancy (aldolase deficiency) may have a severe reaction to the invert sugar solution if it is used as diluent. Symptoms include hypoglycemia, nausea, vomiting, tremors, coma, or convulsion.
    b. The rate of infusion should not exceed 4 ml per minute (1200 mg per minute).
    c. Only fresh solution should be used; discard any unused portion.
    d. Do not mix urea with blood or other drugs in the same syringe. If in doubt about the dilution or the compatibility, consult the pharmacy.
    e. Check the intravenous insertion site frequently and avoid extravasation. Venous irritation is more common with urea than mannitol. The use of hypothermia while urea is being administered increases the risk of venous thrombosis and hemoglobinuria (hemoglobin in the urine).

■ SUMMARY

Passive diffusion in the glomerulus allows water and small molecules to enter the renal tubule. In the proximal convoluted tubule, bicarbonate ion is reclaimed from the fluid by the action of carbonic anhydrase. Sodium is also actively reabsorbed, bringing along chloride ion and water. Water is removed in the descending limb of Henle's loop, whereas chloride and potassium are actively reabsorbed in the ascending limb of Henle's loop. Active sodium ion reabsorption occurs in the distal convoluted tubule, and potassium is secreted into the tubule. Final water removal from the tubular fluid occurs in the collecting duct. Diuretics increase urine flow by increasing the loss of sodium in the urine, which causes the concomitant loss of water.

Ethacrynic acid blocks chloride reabsorption in the ascending limb of Henle's loop, thereby passively blocking sodium reabsorption. This potent diuretic may be given orally or intravenously. Toxicity may involve dehydration, potassium loss, deafness, and gastrointestinal disturbances. Digitalis toxicity may be increased with ethacrynic acid.

Furosemide has the same mechanism of action as ethacrynic acid. Furosemide may be given orally, intravenously, or intramuscularly. Toxicity includes acute dehydration, dermatitis, and blood dyscrasias. Furosemide may increase the toxicity of digitalis and nephrotoxic antibiotics.

Thiazide diuretics block sodium and chloride reabsorption in the distal convoluted tubule, increasing salt and water excretion. These drugs also inhibit carbonic anhydrase, although this action contributes little to their long-term action. Thiazide diuretics are primarily oral agents, although chlorothiazide is available for intravenous use. These drugs should not be administered intramuscularly or subcutaneously. Thiazide diuretics may produce potassium loss and chloride loss, leading to metabolic alkalosis. Thiazides have central nervous system effects, allergic reactions, and hypotensive effects. Thiazide diuretics frequently alter the requirement for insulin or other hypoglycemic agents in diabetics.

Carbonic anhydrase inhibitors prevent the secretion of hydrogen ion into the renal tubule and the reabsorption of bicarbonate. Sodium ion is excreted along with the bicarbonate ion. These drugs ultimately produce metabolic acidosis, which in turn prevents their diuretic action. Carbonic anhydrase inhibitors are used in the treatment of glaucoma, congestive heart failure, and convulsive disorders. These drugs are administered orally and may affect the central nervous system. Potassium excretion is also increased.

Organomercurial diuretics inhibit chloride ion transport in the ascending limb of Henle's loop. The increased excretion of chloride and sodium produces diuresis but ultimately may lead to metabolic alkalosis, which terminates the diuretic action. Organomercurial diuretics are administered by intramuscular injection. These drugs are rarely used in modern therapy.

Potassium-sparing diuretics inhibit the sodium-potassium exchange mechanism in the distal convoluted tubule. Spironolactone blocks the action of aldosterone on this exchange mechanism, whereas triamterene acts independently of aldosterone. These weak diuretics have the advantage that, unlike most of the other diuretics, they do not cause excessive loss of potassium. One possible toxic reaction to these drugs is high concentrations of potassium in the blood. Spironolactone produces tumors in laboratory animals.

Osmotic diuretics cause increased osmotic concentrations within the renal tubule, thereby drawing water from the bloodstream into the tubule. These agents are given intravenously. Mannitol and urea have been used in this manner.

■ STUDY QUESTIONS

1. What is the nephron?
2. What is the function of the glomerulus?
3. What is the renal tubule?
4. Where is sodium reabsorbed from the renal tubule?
5. Where is chloride reabsorbed from the renal tubule?
6. Where is potassium reabsorbed, and where is it secreted in the renal tubule?
7. Which parts of the tubule are most permeable to water?
8. What is the mechanism by which bicarbonate ion is recovered from the tubular fluid? Where does this occur?
9. What is the general mechanism by which all diuretics act?
10. What is the specific mechanism of action of ethacrynic acid?
11. How may ethacrynic acid be administered?
12. What toxicity is characteristic of ethacrynic acid?
13. What drug interactions occur with ethacrynic acid?
14. What is the mechanism of action of furosemide?
15. How may furosemide be administered?
16. What toxicity is characteristic of furosemide?
17. What drug interactions occur with furosemide?
18. What is the specific mechanism of action of thiazide diuretics?
19. How may the thiazide diuretics be administered?
20. What toxicity is characteristic of thiazide diuretics?
21. What drug interactions can occur with thiazide diuretics?
22. How do carbonic anhydrase inhibitors produce diuresis?
23. How are carbonic anhydrase inhibitors administered?
24. What toxicity is characteristic of carbonic anhydrase inhibitors?
25. What drug interactions occur with carbonic anhydrase inhibitors?
26. What is the specific mechanism of action of organomercurial diuretics?
27. How may the organomercurial diuretics be administered?
28. What toxicity is associated with the organomercurial diuretics?
29. What is the specific mechanism of action of the potassium-sparing diuretics?
30. How may the potassium-sparing diuretics be administered?
31. What toxicity is associated with the potassium-sparing diuretics?
32. What drug interactions occur with the potassium-sparing diuretics?
33. How are the osmotic diuretics administered?
34. What reactions occur with the osmotic diuretics?

■ SUGGESTED READINGS

Aspinall, M.J.: A simplified guide to managing patients with hyponatremia, Nursing '78 **8**(12):32, 1978.

Brummett, R.E.: Drug-induced ototoxicity, Drugs **19:**412, 1980.

Elbaum, N.: Detecting and correcting magnesium imbalance, Nursing '77 **7**(8):34, 1977.

Giving cardiovascular drugs safely. Nursing skillbook, Horsham, Pa., 1978, Intermed Communications.

Harrington, J.T.: Diuretics, Drug Therapy Reviews **1:**100, 1977.

Hartshorn, J.C.: What to do when the patient's in hypertensive crisis, Nursing '80 **10**(7):36, 1980.

Haughey, E.J., and Sica, F.M.: Diuretics. How safe can you make them? Nursing '77 **7**(2):34, 1977.

Jellett, L.B.: Potassium therapy: when is it indicated? Drugs **16:**88, 1978.

Kemp, G., and Kemp, D.: Diuretics, American Journal of Nursing **78:**1006, 1978.

Lawson, D.H.: The clinical use of potassium supplements, Drug Therapy Reviews **1:**137, 1977.

Maloney, R.: Helping your hypertensive patients live longer, Nursing '78 **8**(10):26, 1978.

Manzi, C.C.: Edema. How to tell if it's a danger signal, Nursing '77 **7**(4):66, 1977.

Metheny, N.M., and Snively, W.D., Jr.: Nurse's handbook of fluid balance, ed. 3, Philadelphia, 1979, J.B. Lippincott Co.

Monitoring fluid and electrolytes precisely. Nursing skillbook, Horsham, Pa., 1978, Intermed Communications.

Quest, D.O.: Dehydrating agents commonly used in neurosurgery: advantages and disadvantages, Journal of Neurosurgical Nursing **11**(3):141, 1979.

Tucker, R.M., VanDenBerg, C.J., and Knox, F.G.: Diuretics: role of sodium balance, Mayo Clinic Proceedings **55:**261, 1980.

Williams, S.R.: Essentials of nutrition and diet therapy, ed. 2, St. Louis, 1978, The C.V. Mosby Co.

15 Cardiotonic drugs: the cardiac glycosides

■ FUNCTIONS OF THE HEART

■ Terms used to describe cardiac function

To understand the action of drugs on the heart, the student must understand the following terms relating to cardiac physiology.

Automaticity is the property of certain cells in the heart to depolarize spontaneously to initiate a beat (contraction of the whole heart). Normally a heartbeat is initiated in the sinoatrial node (SA node), but any of the conductive fibers of the heart are capable of spontaneously depolarizing and initiating beats and in fact do so in certain types of heart disease.

Depolarization is the process by which cells become less negatively charged than extracellular fluid. Depolarization occurs when sodium rushes into the cell as the first event in the generation of the action potential.

Excitability of a cell or fiber in the heart is defined as a measure of the ease with which that cell may be stimulated to depolarize. Certain drugs increase the excitability of cells, that is, they reduce the energy necessary to depolarize the cell, and some drugs can decrease the excitability of cells.

Action potential is a term describing a burst of electrical activity in a cell. Frequently described as cell "firing," the process is similar to that involved in the conduction of impulses along a nerve fiber. The cell undergoes rapid depolarization followed by a slower repolarization phase, and in the process stimulates adjacent cells to do likewise. In the heart, the generation of an action potential initiates ionic changes inside the cell that cause the myocardial fibers to contract.

Conduction velocity is defined as the rate at which an electrical impulse is passed through the atrioventricular (AV) node. There is a delay in transmission of the impulse to beat from the atrium to the ventricle produced by the AV node. This delay regulates the temporal separation in atrial and ventricular contractions.

Rate is defined as the number of beats or ventricular contractions per minute. In normal hearts this is the rate of SA node firing. Bradycardia means a slow heart rate. Tachycardia means a fast heart rate.

Contractility is measured as the strength of the muscular contraction of the heart. *Inotropic* is a commonly used term to refer to factors affecting the strength of cardiac contraction. A positive inotropic response is an increase in cardiac contractility. A negative inotropic response is a decrease in cardiac contractility.

■ The anatomy of the heart

Conductive tissues of the heart. The heart is formed of muscle similar in many respects to skeletal muscle but different in that many of the fibers are conductive as well as contractile. This property facilitates rapid conduction of action potentials. The action potentials do not pass directly between the atria and ventricles, however, because these two portions of the heart are insulated from each other by a ring of nonconductive tissue. The independence of the atria and ventricles as contractile units is important in regulating the heartbeat.

Within the heart the impulse to beat normally originates at the SA node, a specialized group of automatic cells in the right atrium (Fig. 15-1). Another group of specialized fibers, the AV node, transmits this impulse to the ventricles after an important delay.

The heart is innervated by both the sympathetic and parasympathetic branches of the autonomic nervous system (Fig. 15-2). The vagus nerve is part of the parasympathetic system; its action is localized in the nodes. Stimulation of the vagus nerve releases acetylcholine, which decreases the rate of depolarization and also makes the cells less excitable. In the SA node these actions decrease the rate of firing and hence reduce heart rate. Stimulation of the vagus nerve also tends to decrease conduction velocity through the AV node. This slowing of conduction velocity increases the temporal separation between contraction of atria and ventricles, and therefore also slows heart rate.

Sympathetic nerve fibers innervate both the atria and the ventricles. Stimulation of the sympathetic nerves releases norepinephrine, which activates the beta-1 adrenergic receptors of the heart. Activation of the beta-1 receptor in the conducting tissue of the heart speeds the repolarization of the cells. An increase in heart rate (positive chronotropic effect) and an increase in con-

FIG. 15-1

Transmission of action potentials through the heart. Initiation of a heart beat occurs at SA node and the action potential is transmitted throughout atrium before passing through AV node to ventricles. The numerals designate seconds it takes for impulse to travel from the SA node to the anatomical site designated by the numeral. Note that all parts of the atria have received the impulse within 0.09 seconds but that transmission to ventricles is delayed during its passage through the AV node so that ventricles do not begin to contract until 0.16 second after SA node firing. This delay allows the atria to contract and fill the ventricles before ventricles begin to contract to force blood from the heart.

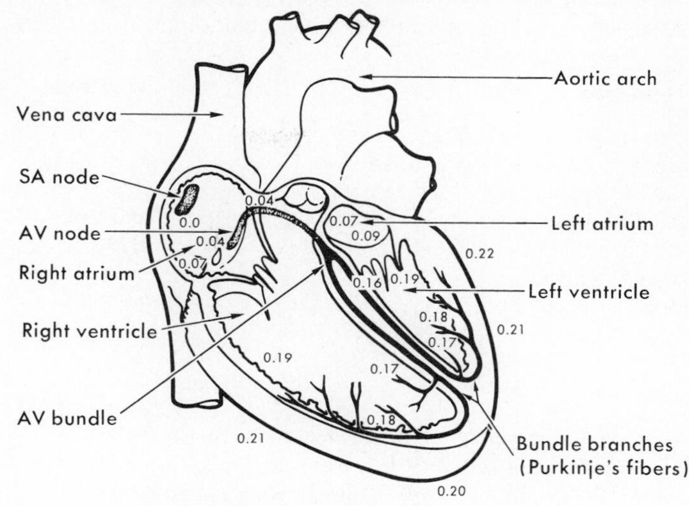

duction velocity (positive dromotropic effect) are the two consequences. Stimulation of the beta-1 adrenergic receptors in the ventricular muscle increases the force of contraction (positive inotropic response).

■ Regulation of myocardial output

Frank-Starling law. The volume of blood that the heart must deliver per second to the arteries varies with stress, exertion, and other factors. How the heart regulates its output to meet these variable demands is described by the *Frank-Starling law* of the heart. This principle of physiology states that the force of muscular contraction is directly related to the stretch of the muscle; the more a muscle is stretched, within mechanical limits, the stronger is its subsequent contraction. With respect to the heart, this principle means that when the ventricles are filled with larger than normal volumes of blood, they contract with greater than normal force to deliver their entire contents to the arteries. Normally blood does not accumulate in the veins, and all the blood coming to the heart is pumped into the arteries.

As the healthy heart responds to acute exercise, the Frank-Starling law applies. The heart increases its force of contraction and hence its output. In addition, sympathetic stimulation increases the rate of contraction; this is the second basic mechanism by which the healthy heart increases its output. The peak efficiency of the heart under these conditions is reached at about 150 to 175 beats per minute. Faster rates result in incomplete filling of the ventricles and reduce the overall efficiency of the pump.

Cardiac hypertrophy. If the heart is subjected to chronic demands for increased output, the heart may enlarge. This condition is called *hypertrophy of the myocardium* and may be a normal response to chronic stress. For example, athletes such as long-distance runners and tennis players may have enlarged hearts. In other cases the enlargement of the heart may signal a pathological process. For example, in chronic heart failure the myocardial output gradually falls below the required level resulting from the failure of the myocardium as a pump. As the output falls, the normal regulatory mechanisms come into effect. Hypertrophy of the heart may occur as the body seeks to increase the efficiency of the pump. Sympathetic stimulation may also be increased to increase the heart rate and hence the output. In many

FIG. 15-2

Autonomic innervation of the heart.

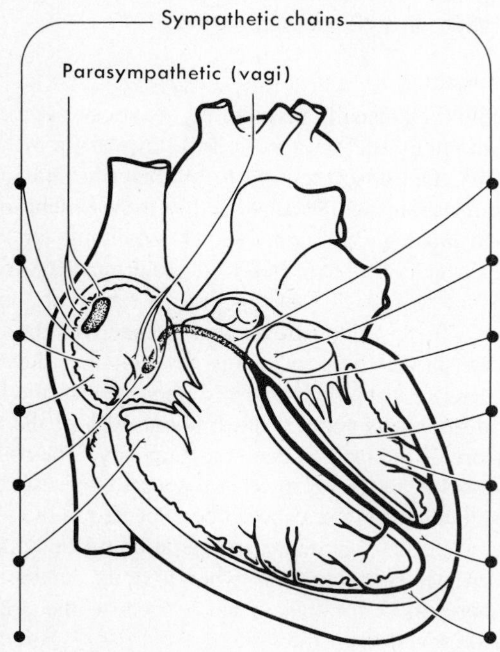

TABLE 15-1. Comparison of pharmacokinetics of cardiac glycosides

Properties	Digitoxin	Digoxin	Ouabain
Absorption after oral dose	90% to 100%	60% to 85%	Unreliable
Onset of action after oral dose	6 to 12 hr	About 1 hr	—
Intravenous loading dose	1.2 to 1.6 mg	0.75 to 1.5 mg	0.25 to 0.5 mg
Onset of action after intravenous dose	0.5 to 2 hr	15 to 30 min	5 to 10 min
Plasma protein binding	97%	30%	Less than 25%
Plasma half-life	5 to 7 days	36 hr	21 hr
Route of excretion	Hepatic	Renal	Renal

cases, in the absence of acute demands on the heart, these mechanisms will enable a weakened heart to maintain sufficient output. These patients may not complain of symptoms but on examination have enlarged hearts and high heart rates.

Congestive heart failure. If the mechanisms just described fail and cardiac output falls below venous return, the result is congestive heart failure. The symptoms arise directly as a result of the insufficient cardiac output. The blood pooled in the veins produces increased venous pressure. The kidneys do not receive sufficient blood flow to maintain salt and water balance. As a result of these conditions, edema of the lungs and periphery develops as fluid leaks into the tissues from the capillaries. The typical patient in congestive heart failure is therefore short of breath and has a rapid pulse resulting from sympathetic stimulation of the heart, obvious swelling of the hands and feet, and an enlarged heart. All of these symptoms may be erased by increasing the cardiac output. It is for this purpose that the drugs discussed in the next section are primarily used.

■ CARDIOTONIC DRUGS

■ Cardiac glycosides

The most commonly used drugs to increase cardiac output are the cardiac glycosides. These cardiac glycosides are named for the plant species from which they were extracted. Plants of the *Digitalis* species, which include the foxglove plant, produce the clinically useful glycosides digitoxin and digoxin. Plants of the *Strophanthus* species produce other glycosides, including ouabain from the seed of *S. gratus* and acetyl strophanthidin from the seed of *S. kombe*. Various other glycosides used in research but not in the clinic are derived from the bulb of the sea onion and from the skin of toads.

The three most clinically useful cardiac glycosides are digitoxin (Crystodigin), digoxin (Lanoxin), and ouabain (Table 15-1). The term *digitalis* may refer to a specific drug such as the elixir prepared from the leaf of *Digitalis purpurea;* more commonly today it is used as a generic term to refer to all cardiac glycosides derived from digitalis species. The digitalis preparations are primarily used in therapy of congestive heart failure; they are also widely used as antiarrhythmic drugs (Chapter 16). Ouabain is occasionally used intravenously in the hospital in emergency treatment of heart failure.

Actions of cardiac glycosides. The cardiac glycosides act directly on the heart cells to promote the accumulation of the calcium necessary for contraction. The action of cardiac glycosides is thus to increase contractility. As a result of increased contractility, cardiac output is increased, blood flow to the kidneys and periphery is improved, venous pressure falls, and excess fluid begins to be excreted as edema clears. This diuretic effect of digitalis is secondary to its action on the heart; diuretics alone may help to alleviate the edema associated with congestive heart failure but they do not directly improve the performance of the heart.

Administration of the cardiac glycosides. Digoxin and digitoxin are similar in intrinsic potencies but differ in their disposition in the body (Table 15-1). Because of these differences, these drugs offer a good example of the clinical application of the principles of pharmacokinetics discussed in Chapter 2. The differences in pharmacokinetics determine the dosage and frequency of administration of digitoxin and digoxin.

Digitoxin

Digitoxin is usually given orally in a dose to produce and to maintain the therapeutic level in plasma of 14 to 26 ng/ml. The dose required to produce the maximum therapeutic effect varies considerably from patient to patient and must be individualized. Digitalizing, or loading, doses would be expected to range around 0.8 to 1.2 mg per day. Since 97% of this drug is reversibly bound to protein in the bloodstream and is inactive, the dose given the patient must take into account that only 3% of the dose in the bloodstream is active. Since the half-life of digitoxin is about 6 days, about 10% of the total body store of the drug is excreted each day. The routine daily dose of the drug must compensate for this drug loss. Maintenance doses should be expected in the range of 0.05 to 0.2 mg per day. Consideration of the half-life of the drug is also important when toxicity occurs; toxicity may persist for long periods because the drug is slowly removed from the system.

■ THE NURSING PROCESS

■ Assessment

Patients who require cardiac glycosides have inadequate cardiac function. These patients include those with congestive heart failure, pulmonary edema, congenital cardiac defects, cardiac valve abnormalities, or postmyocardial infarction damage to the heart. The nurse should obtain baseline data, including the temperature, pulse, respiration and blood pressure, fluid intake and output, weight, serum electrolyte level, blood urea nitrogen, electrocardiogram, and other appropriate laboratory data. The nurse should auscultate the heart and lungs and observe the presence and location of edema, as well as the general condition of the patient. The nurse should obtain a subjective history of recent functioning, noting such things as dyspnea on exertion, shortness of breath, and the need to sleep with the head of the bed elevated.

■ Management

In some situations the patient will be critically ill when cardiac glycoside therapy is begun, but in other situations these drugs may be one in a list of several being gradually added to manage a chronic problem. Safe use of the drug involves monitoring the weight, fluid intake and output, electrocardiogram, serum electrolyte level (with specific focus on potassium), blood pressure, and other parameters of cardiovascular functioning. The nurse should auscultate the heart and lungs when a decrease in fluid in the lungs is anticipated. The nurse should also monitor the pulse when a decrease in the pulse is anticipated, but true bradycardia is often to be avoided. The parameters of the desired goal of therapy should be determined in consultation with the physician. Discharge planning should include determination of the names and dosages of all drugs to be taken, necessary dietary and activity restrictions, and referral to other appropriate departments or agencies such as the dietitian and the public health department for visiting nurse follow-up.

■ Evaluation

Successful use of cardiac glycosides should lead to weight loss through diuresis, increased cardiac output, decreased pulse, increased feeling of well-being, better tolerance of exertion, and less fluid in the lungs. For safe self-management the patient should be able to explain why and how to take all prescribed medications, any interrelations that may exist (e.g., the need to take potassium supplements if certain diuretics and cardiac glycosides are prescribed together), how to plan meals within prescribed dietary limitations, possible anticipated side effects of each drug, and situations requiring contact with a physician. If appropriate, the patient should know how often to record weight or pulse, be able to demonstrate how to accurately measure the pulse, and know what to do with the data obtained. For more specific guidelines, see the patient care implications section at the end of this chapter.

Digoxin

Digoxin is usually given orally in a dose to produce and to maintain the therapeutic plasma level of 0.8 to 1.6 ng/ml. Dosage regimens with this drug must also be individualized for the patient. Digitalizing doses should be expected to be in the range of 1 to 2.5 mg per day. This drug is less highly bound to plasma protein than digitoxin and has a much shorter half-life. The maintenance dose of digoxin must replace the 37% of the total body store of the drug that is lost every day. Maintenance doses should be expected to be in the range of 0.125 to 0.75 mg per day.

Because of the low therapeutic index and long half-life of digitalis preparations, patients are usually started at relatively high doses (loading or digitalizing doses) and then switched within a few days to a lower dose, called a *maintenance* dose, to replace the daily loss of the drug through excretion or biotransformation. This regimen is designed to achieve therapeutic serum levels rapidly and then maintain them for long periods of time while minimizing the danger of overdose. Patients taking digitalis frequently take maintenance doses of the drug for the rest of their lives.

Toxicity of the cardiac glycosides. There is such a small difference between the therapeutic dose and doses that cause side effects that at one time or another most patients taking digitalis will experience drug-related difficulties. The symptoms may be neurological, visual, cardiac, or even psychiatric, and often tend to be vague symptoms easily confused with the symptoms of congestive heart failure itself.

The neurological or central nervous system effects of digitalis are now recognized as significant sources of much of the toxicity observed with digitalis. The anorexia, nausea, and vomiting that the drug may produce result from stimulation of the chemoreceptor trigger zone in the central nervous system. Weakness, fatigue, fainting, and other neurological symptoms also point to an origin in the central nervous system. Visual disturbances such as dimness of vision, double vision, blind spots, flashing lights, or altered color vision also occur. Psychiatric disturbances range from mood alterations to psychoses or hallucinations.

The toxic action of digitalis on the heart may also partly result from central nervous system effects. Whatever the mechanism, the result is bradycardia (slow heart rate), various arrhythmias that may occasionally induce tachycardia, and ultimately ventricular fibrillation and death (Chapter 16). Patients receiving digitalis must be checked frequently for heart rate and for the appearance of extra beats or other arrhythmias. It is routine practice in many hospitals to omit the digitalis dose if the heart rate is less than 60 beats per minute.

The toxic reactions caused by digitalis are dose related and are therefore somewhat predictable (Chapter 2). For this reason, many hospitals have established an assay to measure digitalis in the blood of patients as an aid in establishing safe doses for individual patients and in diagnosing drug toxicity.

Digitalis toxicity may be increased by certain drugs a patients may be receiving. For example, potassium-depleting diuretics such as the thiazides, furosemide, and ethacrynic acid may predispose a patient to digitalis toxicity, since a low intracellular potassium level increases the likelihood of arrhythmias developing in the heart.

Accidental poisoning of children with digitalis preparations is not uncommon. Patients who are around small children should be warned of the potential danger their medicine poses to curious toddlers.

■ PATIENT CARE IMPLICATIONS

1. Patients receiving cardiac glycosides need careful observation to validate the effectiveness of the drug and dosage and to diagnose early toxicity. Desired effects of the cardiac glycosides might include a decrease in pulse and heart rate; slower, less labored respirations; diuresis with accompanying weight reduction; less coughing; less distended neck veins; and better tolerance of exertion.
2. Toxicity of the cardiac glycosides may produce any of the following signs or symptoms: anorexia, nausea, vomiting, diarrhea, visual changes (blurred or yellow vision, flickering lights, colored dots), abdominal discomfort, headache, fatigue, confusion, disorientation, restlessness, gynecomastia, decreased pulse rate, perceived changes in cardiac rhythm (premature ventricular contractions, bigeminy, occasionally tachycardia). Note that many signs of toxicity are exaggerations of desired effects (e.g., reduced pulse) or symptoms that are difficult to evaluate objectively (e.g., nausea, fatigue), so the patient needs careful, frequent, thoughtful evaluation.
3. Low serum potassium levels predispose to digitalis toxicity. The serum potassium level should be checked by the nurse whenever the measurement is obtained and prior to administration of the prescribed dose of medication. If the potassium level is excessively low, notify the physician. Signs of hypokalemia include weakness, thirst, depression, anorexia, nausea, vomiting, abdominal distention, postural hypotension, and hypoactive reflexes. Vomiting, chronic diarrhea, nasogastric suctioning, and any state of alkalosis can cause excessive potassium loss from the body. In addition, potassium loss can occur as a side effect associated with the administration of potassium-losing diuretics, chronic steroids, amphotericin B, and chronic glucose infusions.
4. Increased toxicity of cardiac glycosides is also seen when there is preexisting low serum magnesium levels, elevated serum calcium levels, or with hypothyroidism.
5. The concomitant use of a cardiac glycoside with some drugs has the following effects:
   a. With cholestyramine or barbiturates, diminished effectiveness of the glycoside may result.
   b. With antacids or Kaopectate, decreased absorption of the glycoside may result.
   c. With reserpine or sympathomimetics, increased frequent of arrhythmias may result.
   d. With propranolol, excessive bradycardia may result.
6. If digitalis toxicity occurs, the drug is withheld until the patient's condition is no longer toxic. Any arrhythmias that occur are treated with appropriate drugs (Chapter 16).

7. Take the apical pulse for 1 minute before administering a digitalis preparation. The usual rule states that if the apical pulse is less than 60 beats per minute in an adult or 90 to 110 beats per minute in a child, the dose should be omitted and the physician notified. Decisions about the lowest acceptable limit for the pulse need to be made based on individual assessment of each patient, however, and knowledge of the patient's usual pattern and the physician's goals of therapy for the patient need to be considered. Some physicians and institutions still prefer that an apical-radial deficit determination be obtained before administering a cardiac glycoside. This requires that two nurses be at the bedside. One nurse counts the apical pulse while the other nurse obtains the radial pulse during the same minute. The difference in the two rates is the apical-radial deficit.
8. If a serum digitalis level determination has been ordered, check the value before administering the drug.
9. If the patient is on a cardiac monitor or is having frequent electrocardiogram (ECG) tracings done, it is possible to monitor the effects of the cardiac glycoside on the heart by checking these tracings. Digitalis preparations can cause prolongation of the P-R interval, S-T segment sagging, any degree of atrioventricular block, atrial tachycardia with or without atrioventricular block, bigeminal pulse, ventricular tachycardia, and premature ventricular contractions.
10. Check carefully the name and dose of digitalis preparations because there are several different preparations that have similar spellings.
11. The patient's overall response to his heart disease should be monitored daily. Physical assessment should include daily weight, intake and output, breath sounds, checking for edema, especially in the sacral area and lower extremities, as well as other signs, symptoms, and measurements previously discussed.
12. Taking digitalis preparations with meals may reduce gastric irritation.
13. Before discharge, the patient needs thorough teaching about the cardiac glycoside as well as any other prescribed medications. In addition to knowledge about side effects, correct dosage, and frequency for each individual medication, the patient must understand the interaction of the medications. For example, if the patient is to be discharged on a digitalis preparation, a potassium-losing diuretic, and a potassium replacement, the patient should understand how the potassium replacement is essential to help reduce the possibility of digitalis toxicity and to prevent the electrolyte imbalance that the diuretic may create. If appropriate, the patient needs to be taught to measure and record the apical or radial pulse at regular intervals (e.g., daily, or once a week). A visiting nurse referral may be appropriate for follow-up.
14. Intravenous digitalis preparations need to be administered slowly (usually 1 ml per minute or more slowly). They should not be mixed with infusion fluids. Check with the pharmacy if in doubt.
15. Ouabain is the fastest acting cardiac glycoside. It is usually reserved for emergencies and may only be given intravenously. Administer slowly, 0.5 ml per minute, and do not mix with other infusion fluids.
16. Instruct patients that if a dose of medication is missed, they should not try to "double up" the next time a dose is taken to catch up. On the other hand, every effort should be made to help the patient find a way to remember to take the medication as ordered.
17. It may be appropriate to instruct patients to weigh themselves at home on a regular basis and record these weights. Weight gain in excess of 2 to 5 pounds per week, or as determined by the health care provider, should be reported by the patient. Consult the physician.
18. Instruct patients to keep all health care providers informed of all drugs being taken. Instruct patients to avoid the use of over-the-counter preparations unless the drug and dose are first cleared with the physician. Many over-the-counter preparations have cardiac effects, which may be undesirable for the patient or may alter the rate of absorption of the cardiotonic drug.
19. Remind patients to keep these and all medications out of the reach of children.

■ SUMMARY

The pumping action of the heart depends on the ability of the heart to contract at the proper time with sufficient strength to force blood from the chambers of the heart into the great arteries and then to the rest of the body. The signal for initiating contraction comes from the SA (sinoatrial) node and spreads to the ventricles through the AV (atrioventricular) node. The frequency of signals from the SA node is lowered by vagus nerve stimulation and increased by sympathetic nerve stimulation. The strength of contraction of the heart is regulated by sympathetic innervation of the ventricles and by the Frank-Starling law, which states that the more a muscle is stretched, the more forceful is its subsequent contraction.

Digitalis glycosides in use in the clinic include digoxin, digitoxin, and ouabain. All three drugs increase the strength of contraction of the failing heart by promoting the accumulation of calcium within the heart cells. Ouabain is an emergency medication suitable only for intravenous use. Both digitoxin and digoxin may be given intravenously or orally. Digitoxin is very highly bound to plasma protein and is eliminated by the liver. The half-time for elimination of digitoxin is 5 to 7 days. Digoxin is less tightly bound to plasma proteins, is excreted by the kidney, and has a half-time for elimination of about 36 hours. Both drugs are frequently given at high doses initially, then at lower doses intended to replace the amount of drug that is lost daily through normal elimination processes.

Cardiac glycosides have a very low therapeutic index, producing toxic reactions of increasing severity as concentrations of the drug rise in the bloodstream. As concentrations of digitalis in the bloodstream increase over therapeutic levels, nausea, visual disturbances, central nervous system effects, and cardiac arrhythmias may arise. Bradycardia (excessively slowed heart rate) is a common sign of digitalis toxicity. Pulse rates should be taken before each dose of digitalis is administered, and the dose may be omitted if heart rates drop below 60 beats per minute.

■ STUDY QUESTIONS

1. How does heart muscle differ from skeletal muscle?
2. What is the purpose of the ring of nonconductive tissue that separates the atria from the ventricles?
3. Where does the impulse to beat originate in the healthy heart?
4. What structure transmits the impulse to beat from the atria to the ventricles?
5. What is the effect of parasympathetic stimulation on the heart?
6. What is the effect of sympathetic stimulation on the heart?
7. What is the Frank-Starling law of the heart?
8. What symptoms are typical of congestive heart failure?
9. What is digitalis?
10. What is the physiological effect of digitalis on the heart?
11. What is the mechanism of action of digitalis?
12. What is the mechanism by which digitalis produces diuresis in a patient with congestive heart failure?
13. How do digitoxin and digoxin differ in plasma protein binding and route of excretion?
14. Which digitalis preparation has the longest elimination half-time?
15. What is the purpose of the loading dose at the beginning of digitalis therapy?
16. What is the purpose of the maintenance dose in digitalis therapy?
17. Does digitalis have a high or low therapeutic index?
18. What toxicity is common with digitalis therapy?
19. Why are pulse rates measured *before* administering each prescribed dose of digitalis?
20. What drugs increase the likelihood of digitalis toxicity?

■ SUGGESTED READINGS

Andreoli, K.G., Fowkes, V.H., Zipes, D.P., and Wallace, A.G.: Comprehensive cardiac care, ed. 4, St. Louis, 1979, The C.V. Mosby Co.

Arbeit, S.: Recognizing digitalis toxicity, American Journal of Nursing **77:**1935, 1977.

Brown, D.D., Spector, R., and Juhl, R.P.: Drug interactions with digoxin, Drugs **20:**198, 1980.

Cavanaugh, A.L., and Mancini, R.E.: Drug interactions and digitalis toxicity, American Journal of Nursing **80**(12):2170, 1980.

Czerwinske, B.S.: Manual of patient education for cardiopulmonary dysfunctions, St. Louis, 1980, The C.V. Mosby Co.

Drugs used in the care of the cardiac patient, Nursing Clinics of North America **13:**473, 1978.

Giving cardiovascular drugs safely. Nursing skillbook, Horsham, Pa., 1978, Intermed Communications.

Goldberg, P.B.: How do digitalis tolerance and toxicity change with age? Geriatric Nursing **1:**142, July-Aug., 1980.

Harvey, S.: Drugs in cardiovascular emergencies, Nurses' Drug Alert **2**(special issue):65, June, 1978.

Haslam, P.: Digitalis: antiarrhythmic and toxic effects, Canadian Nurse **74:**44, 1978.

Horvath, P.T., and Depew, C.C.: Toward preventing digitalis toxicity, Nurses' Drug Alert **4**(special report):25, March, 1980.

Huffman, D.H.: The clinical use of digitalis glycosides, Drug Therapy Reviews **1:**172, 1977.

Kumpuris, A.G., Raizner, A.E., and Luchi, R.J.: The role of serum digitalis levels in clinical practice, Heart & Lung **8**(4):711, 1979.

Lindemayer, G.E.: Cellular mechanism of action of digitalis, Drug Therapy **8**(6):91, 1978.

Meissner, J.E., and Gever, L.N.: Reducing the risks of digitalis toxicity, Nursing '80 **10**(9):32, 1980.

Spitz, P.: Kids in crisis. Common emergencies—the correct action to take, Nursing '78 **8**(4):26, 1978.

Taggart, A.J., and McDevitt, D.G.: Digitalis: its place in modern therapy, Drugs **20:**398, 1980.

16 Drugs used to control cardiac arrhythmias

■ ELECTROPHYSIOLOGY OF THE HEART

Cardiac arrhythmias are defined as any deviation from the normal rate or pattern of heartbeat. Heart rates that are too slow (bradycardia), too fast (tachycardia), or irregular are all included in this classification.

To understand the pharmacological control of arrhythmias, we must recall the physiological control mechanisms of the heart. The impulse to beat originates in the SA node, spreads through the atria, causing them to contract, passes through the AV node, and finally enters the ventricles and causes contraction of that tissue (Chapter 15).

Normal action potential. Typical action potentials for three types of cardiac tissue are illustrated in Fig. 16-1. Atrial and ventricular patterns are quite similar. Both begin with a rapid depolarization, marked by 0 on the curves, which is caused by a rapid rush of sodium ion (Na^+) into the cells. The inside of the cell therefore becomes more positive as the electrical potential shifts from about −90 mV to about +20 mV. Shortly thereafter, chloride ion (Cl^-) begins to enter the cardiac cell so the electrical potential becomes more negative. This phase is marked by 1 on the curve. During the relatively long plateau period, marked phase 2 on the curve, sodium ion and calcium ion (Ca^{++}) slowly enter the cell while potassium ion goes out. As time progresses, the sodium ion and calcium ion stop flowing in but potassium ion continues to flow out (phase 3). During this phase the electrical potential continues to become more negative. In the last phase of the action potential, sodium ion flows out of the cell in exchange for potassium ion, which enters the cell. At the end of this cycle, the cell has returned to the resting potential of about −90 mV and has regained the ability to generate another normal action potential. From the beginning of phase 0 until somewhere in the middle of phase 3, the cell is completely refractory and cannot be stimulated to beat again.

Automaticity of normal SA nodal cells. The action potential for the SA nodal tissue differs from that of the atrial and ventricular cells in several ways. Most important in terms of cardiac physiology is the gradual depolarization that occurs during phase 4 (Fig. 16-1). This ability to gradually shift from a potential of about −70 mV to −50 or −40 mV is what triggers the start of the action potential (phase 0) in these cells. Because of this trait these cells are termed *automatic:* they need no externally applied stimulus to initiate an action potential.

Electrocardiograph (ECG). Measurements of action potentials are performed in laboratories on experimental animals and are very helpful in revealing what happens when a heart beats. However, in the clinical setting, information about the function of a patient's heart is gained from electrocardiogram (ECG) tracings (Fig. 16-2). These ECG tracings may be related to action potentials in various parts of the heart. The change in potential marked in Fig. 16-2 as P (the P wave) is produced by the initial depolarization of atrial cells (phase 0 on the action potential). Very shortly after this wave of depolarization, the atrium contracts to complete filling of the ventricles. The waves marked Q, R, and S (the QRS complex) result from depolarization of the ventricles. Repolarization of the atria occurs at this time but is masked by the large changes produced by the ventricles. Ventricular contraction occurs between the QRS complex and the midpoint of the T wave. The T wave is generated by the repolarization (phases 1 through 3 of the action potential) of the ventricles.

■ Mechanisms producing arrhythmias

Arrhythmias occur because of disorders in the pacing of the heartbeat or disorders in conducting the impulse to beat through the heart tissues, or a combination of these causes.

Disorders in heart pacing are frequently related to changes in the automaticity of the heart. For example, the normal pacemaker of the heart, the SA node, may become overstimulated by the sympathetic nervous system. The catecholamine neurotransmitters for this branch of the nervous system increase the automaticity of the SA node. As a result, phase 4 on the action potential curve is steepened and shortened, phase 0 is triggered more frequently, and the heart beats more rapidly. In contrast, if the vagus nerve is predominant and sympathetic stimulation is removed, heart rates decrease. This action occurs because acetylcholine from the vagus nerve decreases the automaticity of the SA node.

FIG. 16-1

Typical action potential for three types of cardiac tissues. These action potentials are determined in the laboratory in tissues from experimental animals.

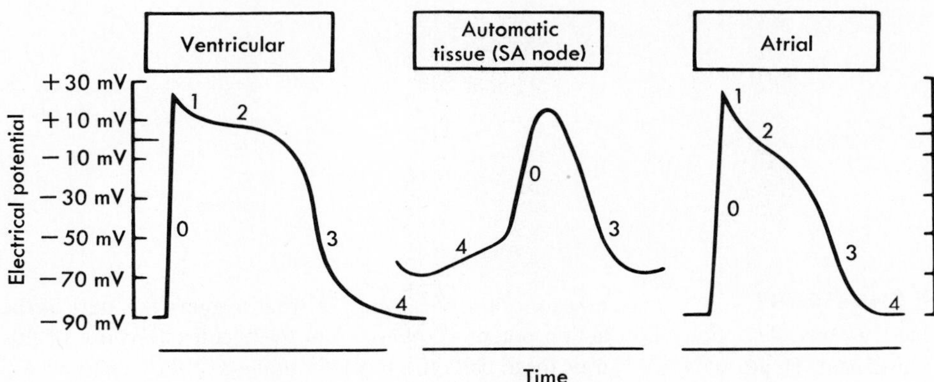

In addition to these disorders in automaticity at the SA node, the heart may suffer altered heart rates resulting from *ectopic foci* of automatic cells. These ectopic foci are groups of cells either in the atrium or ventricles that spontaneously begin to beat independently of the SA node. These groups of automatic cells may replace the SA node as the primary pacer for the heart, they may work in combination with the SA node so that the heart responds to both pacemakers, or they may interfere with SA nodal pacing with the result that neither pacing system is effective.

Conduction disorders are primarily of two types. One involves an alteration in the conduction time across the AV node. The function of the AV node is to prevent the ventricles from receiving the impulse to beat until the atria have contracted and filled the ventricles (Chapter 15). If the ventricles contract prematurely, ineffective pumping action occurs, since the chambers will be only partially filled. If the delay in transmission through the AV node becomes too long, skipped heartbeats may occur, since the AV node may still be in the refractory period from the last beat when the next impulse arrives from the SA node.

The second type of conduction disorder involves conduction through the contracting tissue. If an area of heart muscle becomes ischemic (oxygen starved) or damaged, it may not only fail to contract but it may also fail to properly conduct an action potential. Ordinarily the action potential spreads across the tissue in a pattern that allows all parts of the tissue to contract at the proper time so that the heart pumps efficiently. The presence of this damaged region alters the pattern of stimulation, and the subsequent contraction may not be rhythmic or effective. Occasionally the damaged area may alter conduction so that a phenomenon called *reentry* occurs. In this condition, the action potential from a single impulse to beat passes more than once through the same group of cells. In the extreme case, reentry may produce a continuous cycle or loop of electrical activity through part of the tissue that prevents the heart from contracting properly.

FIG. 16-2

Electrocardiogram (ECG) tracing showing the patterns typical of normal heart function.

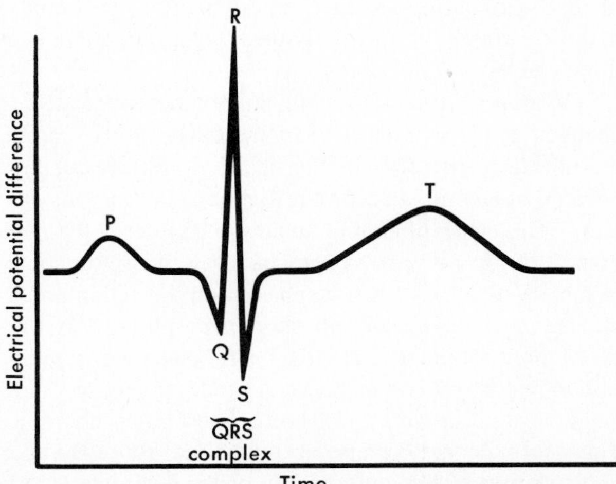

■ ANTIARRHYTHMIC DRUGS

Several classes of drugs possess properties that make them useful for controlling cardiac arrhythmias (Table 16-1). Some of the agents discussed in this section also have other clinically important uses that are discussed in the appropriate chapters.

Digitalis

Digitalis is primarily a cardiotonic agent (Chapter 15). However, in addition to its ability to strengthen

TABLE 16-1. Mechanism of action of antiarrhythmic drugs

Drug	Mechanism of antiarrhythmic action	Summary of cardiac actions: Conduction velocity	Auto-maticity	Con-tractility	Adverse reactions
CARDIAC STIMULANT					
Digitalis	Slows conduction through the AV node	Slowed	Increased at high doses	Increased	Bradycardia, premature ventricular beats, AV nodal tachycardia, anorexia, nausea, vomiting
CHOLINERGIC BLOCKER					
Atropine	Blocks the effects of vagus nerve stimulation	Hastened	Increased	No change	Effects due to muscarinic blockade throughout the body: dry mouth, cycloplegia, mydriasis, fever, urinary retention, central nervous system disturbances
DEPRESSANT ANTIARRHYTHMICS					
Propranolol	Beta adrenergic blockade and membrane-stabilizing effects that alter ion flow	Slowed	Decreased	Decreased	Bradycardia, lowered cardiac output; congestive heart failure; bronchospasm in persons with asthma
Quinidine	Suppresses automaticity, especially in ectopic foci, by membrane-stabilizing and anticholinergic effects	Slowed	Decreased	Decreased	Peripheral vasodilation, hypotension, paradoxical ventricular tachycardia, decreased cardiac output, cinchonism, allergy, fever, gastrointestinal distress
Procainamide	As for quinidine	Slowed	Decreased	Decreased	Hypotension, decreased cardiac output, ventricular tachycardia, lowered resistance to infection, allergy, gastrointestinal distress; chronic use causes collagen disorders resembling systemic lupus erythematosus
Disopyramide	As for quinidine	No change or slightly slowed	Decreased	Decreased	Anticholinergic effects: dry mouth, constipation, urinary hesitancy or retention, blurred vision; myocardial depression may be unexpectedly severe in critically ill patients
NONDEPRESSANT ANTIARRHYTHMICS					
Lidocaine	Increases the electrical threshold for ventricular stimulation	No change or slightly hastened	Decreased	No change	Central nervous system effects such as confusion, drowsiness, convulsions

Continued.

TABLE 16-1. Mechanism of action of antiarrhythmic drugs—cont'd

Drug	Mechanism of antiarrhythmic action	Summary of cardiac actions: Conduction velocity	Automaticity	Contractility	Adverse reactions
Phenytoin	Depresses spontaneous depolarization in ventricular and atrial but not nodal tissue	No change or slightly hastened	Decreased	No change	Rapid intravenous injection causes severe myocardial toxicity; chronic use produces cerebellar degeneration and gingival hyperplasia
Bretylium	Prolongs the effective refractory period	No change	No change	No change or slight increase	Bradycardia, hypotension, and precipitation of anginal attacks

TABLE 16-2. Pharmacological properties of drugs used to control cardiac arrhythmias

Generic name	Trade name	Dosage and administration	Comments
DIGITALIS			
Digitoxin	Crystodigin Purodigin	ORAL, INTRAVENOUS: *Adults*—load with 0.6 mg, followed by 0.4 mg, then 0.2 mg every 4 to 6 hr until total dose of 1.2 to 1.8 mg; maintain with 0.05 to 0.2 mg daily. *Children*—doses are lower than adults, individualized for age and body weight.	Effective serum levels 14 to 26 ng/ml; degraded by the liver; half-time for elimination about 7 days.
Digoxin	Lanoxin	ORAL: *Adults*—load with 0.5 to 0.75 mg, followed by 0.25 to 0.5 mg every 6 to 8 hr up to a total dose of 1 to 1.5 mg; maintain with 0.125 to 0.5 mg daily. *Children*—doses are lower than adults, individualized for age and body weight. INTRAVENOUS: *Adults*—load with total dose of 1 mg delivered in divided doses over 8 to 12 hr; maintain with 0.125 to 0.5 mg daily. *Children*—doses are lower than adults, individualized for age and body weight.	Effective serum level 1 to 2 ng/ml, toxic at 3 ng/ml; excreted by the kidney; elimination half-time about 36 hr.
Deslanoside	Cedilanid-D	INTRAMUSCULAR, INTRAVENOUS: *Adults*—1.6 mg total dose. (Intravenous dose should be in two sites.)	Onset of action within 30 min; maximal effect within 12 hr of dose.
Ouabain	G-Strophanthin	INTRAVENOUS: *Adults*—250 μg for loading, 100 μg hourly to maintain, with total dose no more than 1 mg daily.	Onset of action within 10 min; maximal effect within 2 hr of dose.
ANTICHOLINERGIC			
Atropine		INTRAVENOUS: *Adults*—0.4 to 1 mg every 1 to 2 hr as needed. *Children*—0.01 to 0.03 mg/kg of body weight.	Rapidly effective; excreted by the kidney within 12 hr of administration.
DEPRESSANT ANTIARRHYTHMICS			
Quinidine sulfate	Cin-Quin Quinora	ORAL: *Adults*—200 to 400 mg 4 times daily. *Children*—6 mg/kg every 4 to 6 hr.	Serum half-life about 6 hr.

TABLE 16-2. Pharmacological properties of drugs used to control cardiac arrhythmias—cont'd

Generic name	Trade name	Dosage and administration	Comments
Quinidine gluconate	Duraquin Quinaglute	ORAL: *Adults*—324 to 972 mg (1 to 3 tablets) 2 or 3 times daily. INTRAMUSCULAR: *Adults*—200 to 400 mg every 4 to 6 hr. INTRAVENOUS: *Adults*—10 mg each minute up to 400 mg with ECG and blood pressure monitoring.	More slowly absorbed than quinidine sulfate.
Quinidine polygalacturonate	Cardioquin	ORAL: *Adults*—as for quinidine sulfate (1 tablet of 275 mg is equivalent to 200 mg of quinidine sulfate).	Less irritating to gastrointestinal tract than other forms of quinidine.
Procainamide	Pronestyl	ORAL: *Adults*—250 to 500 mg every 3 to 6 hr. *Children*—50 mg/kg daily in 4 to 6 divided doses. INTRAMUSCULAR: *Adults*—250 to 1000 mg every 6 hr. INTRAVENOUS: *Adults*—100 mg over 5 min as needed.	Serum half-life about 3½ hr.
Disopyramide	Norpace	ORAL: *Adults*—100 to 150 mg every 6 hr, after 200 to 300 mg loading dose.	Effective serum level 2 to 4 μg/ml; serum half-life less than 4 hr; kidneys eliminate 80% of the active drug and metabolites.
Propranolol	Inderal	ORAL: *Adults*—10 to 80 mg 4 times daily. INTRAVENOUS: *Adults*—1 mg each minute up to 10 mg or 0.1 to 0.15 mg/kg administered in increments of 0.5 to 0.75 mg every 1 to 2 minutes with ECG and blood pressure monitoring.	Effective serum level 200 μg/ml; serum half-life 2½ to 4 hr; metabolized in the liver.
NONDEPRESSANT ANTIARRHYTHMICS			
Phenytoin	Dilantin	ORAL: *Adults*—1 Gm every 12 hr to load, then 100 mg every 6 hr. *Children*—initially 10 to 15 mg/kg daily in 2 or 3 doses; maintain with 5 to 10 mg/ kg daily in 2 or 3 doses. INTRAVENOUS: *Adults*—100 mg given over 10 min. Dose held under 1 Gm.	Effective serum level 10 to 18 μg/ml; serum half-life 2 days; phenobarbital increases liver metabolism of phenytoin; coumarin anticoagulants, isoniazid, and paraaminosalicylic acid (PAS) may increase serum levels of phenytoin
Lidocaine	Xylocaine without epinephrine	INTRAMUSCULAR: *Adults*—emergency use, 4 to 5 mg/kg, or 3 ml of 10% solution (300 mg). INTRAVENOUS: *Adults*—50 to 100 mg bolus, then drip at 1 to 5 mg per min. *Children*—5 mg/ml infused to give a dose of 0.03 mg/kg each min.	Effective serum level 1 to 5 μg/ml; serum half-life 15 to 20 min; metabolized in liver; toxicity increased by reduced liver blood flow or function.
Bretylium	Bretylol	INTRAMUSCULAR: *Adults*—5 to 10 mg/kg repeated in 1 to 2 hr, then every 6 to 8 hr. One site should receive no more than 5 ml of undiluted drug. INTRAVENOUS: *Adults*—5 to 10 mg/kg repeated every 15 to 30 min to a maximal dose of 30 mg/kg.	Bretylium is excreted unchanged by the kidneys.

contraction of the heart muscle, digitalis also increases vagal tone at the AV node. Through this action and direct effects on nodal tissue, digitalis slows conduction through the AV node. This action is the primary one sought when digitalis is used as an antiarrhythmic.

As with all the other antiarrhythmic drugs, at higher concentrations digitalis may also *cause* arrhythmias of various types. The most characteristic arrhythmias produced by digitalis are bradycardia and premature ventricular contractions. Bradycardia may be a sign of impending heart block (no impulse passes through the AV node to the ventricles). Premature ventricular contractions arise because digitalis increases the spontaneous rate of ventricular depolarization (phase 4 of the action potential). Automaticity of Purkinje's fibers in the ventricles is increased by digitalis.

Any digitalis preparation might potentially be used as an antiarrhythmic agent. However, in practice digoxin is commonly used intravenously in an emergency and then continued orally for maintenance or prophylaxis (Table 16-2). *Deslanoside* (Cedilanid-D) and *ouabain* (G-Strophanthin) are emergency medications that are sometimes used.

Atropine

Atropine, a drug previously discussed for its ability to block muscarinic cholinergic receptors, may also be used to treat certain arrhythmias. The action of atropine as an antiarrhythmic drug depends on the ability of atropine to reduce the effects of vagus nerve stimulation, primarily on the SA node. Atropine is therefore able to increase heart rate. Since atropine also speeds conduction through the AV node, it may lessen heart block in certain cases.

Depressant antiarrhythmics

The drugs propranolol, quinidine, procainamide, and disopyramide are usually considered together as depressant antiarrhythmics. The term *depressant antiarrhythmic* comes from the fact that these drugs all depress contractility of the heart as well as decrease conduction velocity and automaticity.

Quinidine and procainamide

Quinidine and procainamide have virtually identical mechanisms of action. Both drugs alter calcium distribution within the cardiac cell, thereby decreasing contractility of the heart muscle. Both quinidine and procainamide have atropine-like effects on the heart and block the effect of parasympathetic innervation on the heart. Finally, both drugs alter ion flow in and out of cardiac cells, resulting in a prolonged refractory period and prolonged spontaneous depolarization of automatic tissues. The ability of these drugs to prolong the refractory period of cardiac tissues may explain the ability of the drugs to suppress ectopic foci.

Absorption, distribution, excretion. Quinidine sulfate is relatively rapidly absorbed by oral routes. The half-life of quinidine in serum is about 6 hours; effective serum concentrations are 2 to 5 μg/ml. Quinidine gluconate is somewhat more slowly absorbed orally, and hence slightly longer acting. Quinidine polygalacturonate is reported to be less irritative to the gastrointestinal tract than other forms of quinidine. Quinidine is excreted unchanged in the urine, and the drug may accumulate in patients with renal failure.

Procainamide reaches effective concentrations in the serum (4 to 8 μg/ml) within 1 to 3 hours of an oral dose or within 30 minutes of an intramuscular dose. The half-life of the drug in serum is 3½ hours and about half the drug dose is eliminated unchanged in the kidney.

Side effects. The anticholinergic effects of quinidine and procainamide in some ways oppose the direct action of the drugs. The dual effects of quinidine have caused serious complications in the treatment of atrial fibrillation. Although the direct effects of quinidine might be expected to slow the atrial rate, the first observed effect may be an anticholinergic action producing increased conduction through the AV node, with the result that ventricular rates soar dangerously high before quinidine can slow atrial rates.

Toxic effects. The primary difference between quinidine and procainamide is in the toxic effects produced.

Quinidine is commonly associated with gastrointestinal reactions, but the most serious reactions include allergic responses and cardiovascular toxicity. When the drug is given intravenously, hypotension may result. Quinidine is an arteriolar and venous dilator. This action may account for the fact that quinidine significantly reduces cardiac output in some patients. At higher doses, usually resulting in blood levels above 6 μg/ml, quinidine may produce ventricular arrhythmias, including ectopic beats, tachycardia, and fibrillation.

Like quinidine, procainamide may cause gastrointestinal discomfort to patients receiving the medication orally. Procainamide is less completely bound to plasma proteins than is quinidine and therefore less subject to unexpected drug interactions resulting from displacement from plasma protein binding sites (Chapter 2). Allergic and immunological reactions are among the most striking adverse effects of procainamide. With long-term use the drug may produce a syndrome that resembles lupus erythematosus, including symptoms such as arthritis and arthralgias, myalgias, fever, and pericarditis. Direct toxic effects on the heart usually relate to changes in conduction within the heart, especially at the AV nodal tissue and the conducting fibers of the ventricles. These direct toxic effects on the heart are usually produced when blood levels exceed 12 μg/ml. Since normal therapeutic concentrations range from about 4 to 8 μg/ml, it is obvious that this drug, like the other arrhythmic drugs, has a very narrow safety margin.

Disopyramide phosphate

Disopyramide phosphate is a newer antiarrhythmic drug similar in action to procainamide and quinidine, although its mechanism has not been as thoroughly studied. Disopyramide, like procainamide, is excreted in about equal amounts by the kidney and liver. Like the other depressant antiarrhythmic drugs, disopyramide may dangerously suppress cardiac action in a patient already weakened by loss of cardiac function.

Propranolol

Propranolol is classified as a depressant antiarrhythmic drug since it decreases conduction, contractility, and automaticity in the heart. One mechanism by which propranolol produces these effects is a quinidine-like action affecting electrical activity of the heart cells. In addition, propranolol is an antagonist of beta adrenergic receptors of the sympathetic nervous system. Since sympathetic stimulation increases automaticity of the heart, propranolol may decrease automaticity in the heart by blocking these influences.

The most important dangers attendant on the use of propranolol as an antiarrhythmic agent result from the beta adrenergic blockade the drug produces. These effects are especially dangerous in patients with a significant degree of heart failure that has been compensated by increased sympathetic stimulation of the heart. Blockade of these sympathetic influences may produce bradycardia or heart arrest, especially if partial AV block is already present. In addition, propranolol may precipitate severe bronchospasm, since the beta receptors in the lung are also blocked by propranolol (Chapter 22). This latter reaction is more common in patients with a history of asthma or allergies.

■ Nondepressant antiarrhythmic drugs

Phenytoin and lidocaine are considered together as nondepressant antiarrhythmic agents. These drugs do not decrease cardiac contractility and have either no effect on conduction velocity or speed it slightly.

Phenytoin

Phenytoin, a drug also used as an anticonvulsant agent (Chapter 31), improves AV conduction. By changing membrane responsiveness, phenytoin may reduce the possibility for reentry, a process that contributes to severe arrhythmias. The major use of phenytoin is for digitalis-induced arrhythmias. Phenytoin is less effective than the other antiarrhythmic drugs for arrhythmias of other types.

Although phenytoin is a nondepressant antiarrhythmic agent, it is capable of producing dangerous myocardial depression if it is administered intravenously too rapidly. Bradycardia, hypotension, AV blockade, and cardiac arrest have been observed when the drug is injected into a vein more rapidly than 50 mg/min. The patient may be observed for nausea, dizziness, or drowsiness, which are signs of excessive blood levels of the drug. Chronic use of phenytoin for its antiarrhythmic action causes the same type of side effects produced when the drug is used as an anticonvulsant (Chapter 31).

Lidocaine

Lidocaine seems to exert its antiarrhythmic action more on ventricular than atrial or nodal tissues. The drug apparently does not alter AV conduction but may slow conduction along the Purkinje fibers within the ventricles, especially when the tissue is ischemic. Lidocaine is eliminated primarily by the liver, with over 90% of a dose being rapidly destroyed in that tissue. For this reason the drug is useful primarily when administered as a continuous infusion. Lidocaine causes a variety of central nervous system reactions ranging from muscle twitching and drowsiness to paresthesias, respiratory depression, convulsions, and coma. Toxic reactions to lidocaine are more common in patients with reduced hepatic function, since the drug may accumulate in these patients.

When administering lidocaine it is important to recall that the drug has two separate clinical uses and is packaged differently for those uses. When intended for use as a local anesthetic, lidocaine is frequently packaged in solution with epinephrine (Xylocaine with epinephrine; other trade names). When used as a local anesthetic, the epinephrine acts as a vasoconstrictor to reduce local blood flow and prolong the action of the anesthetic. If lidocaine with epineprhine were inadvertantly used for a cardiac arrhythmia, the epinephrine might well trigger severe arrhythmias by stimulating automaticity of the heart. Lidocaine intended for use in cardiac emergencies is labelled as "Lidocaine without preservatives" or as "Xylocaine for cardiac arrhythmias."

Bretylium

Bretylium has a different mechanism of action than other antiarrhythmic drugs. Bretylium increases the action potential duration and hence prolongs the refractory period. The drug does not directly suppress automaticity or conduction velocity. Bretylium accumulates in sympathetic neurons and causes an initial release of norepinephrine that may stimulate contractility, heart rate, and automaticity, but ultimately the drug produces an adrenergic blockade by preventing norepinephrine release. Bretylium is used intravenously or intramuscularly, primarily for ventricular tachycardia. The major reactions to this drug reported are precipitation of anginal attacks, bradycardia, and hypotension.

Pharmacological therapy of arrhythmias

Atrial flutter and fibrillation are usually serious arrhythmias that demand treatment. The drug of choice is digitalis. The rationale for this therapy is that by lowering the conduction of impulses through the AV node, digitalis protects the ventricles from overstimulation. The short-term therapeutic goal is not to slow the atrial rate but to produce a partial heart block that allows fewer of the impulses from the atria to stimulate the ventricles to beat. The patient may therefore be maintained with rapid atrial rates but with ventricular rates from 60 to 80 beats per minute. Many patients spontaneously convert to normal sinus rhythm after a few days of treatment.

If digitalis alone is not effective in slowing ventricular rates, propranolol may be added to the drug regimen. Propranolol aids in prolonging AV conduction times and since it blocks beta adrenergic receptors may also reduce catecholamine stimulation of the heart. Both effects tend to slow heart rate.

Occasionally quinidine may be selected to control atrial flutter or fibrillation. Since the anticholinergic action of quinidine may speed conduction through the AV node, the first result of this therapy may be a dramatic increase in the ventricular rate. Digitalis should always be used before quinidine in this case to prevent a dangerous overstimulation of the ventricles during the initial phases of treatment. Once atrial rates have been sufficiently reduced, this action of quinidine on the AV node poses no particular problem to the patient.

Sinus tachycardia, a rapid atrial rate, may not be harmful unless the ventricular rate is also abnormally increased. Many physicians do not administer antiarrhythmic drugs to patients with rapid atrial rates and no other symptoms. Sinus tachycardia may be produced in normal persons by anxiety, by ingestion of coffee, tea, or alcoholic beverages, or by smoking. Drugs such as nitrites, sympathomimetics, anticholinergics, or phenothiazines may also induce transient sinus tachycardia.

Sinus bradycardia is usually of minor importance and not treated. If bradycardia is associated with reduced cardiac output, atropine or isoproterenol may be prescribed. Atropine will increase the heart rate by blocking the effects of vagal nerve stimulation, whereas isoproterenol directly stimulates the heart through the beta adrenergic receptors.

Ventricular premature contractions occur when the ventricles beat in response both to the SA node and an abnormal pacemaker. The ECG pattern shows a normal QRS complex following a P wave (Fig. 16-2) and an abnormal QRS complex that is isolated from a P wave. These arrhythmias are found even among normal persons. If these premature contractions are rare, they are ordinarily not treated, unless the patient is recuperating from a myocardial infarction. If the patient complains of palpitations with the premature ventricular contractions, mild sedatives may be prescribed. Abstaining from coffee, tea, and cigarettes may also control the condition.

When ventricular premature contractions occur frequently or in rapid succession or when they occur in association with other signs of cardiac disease, treatment is usually instituted with lidocaine, quinidine, or procainamide. If these ventricular premature contractions are caused by a previous myocardial infarction, lidocaine is the drug of choice in the hospital.

Ventricular tachycardia is usually related to the presence of ectopic foci stimulating premature ventricular contractions. Lidocaine is again the drug of choice and may be used to control or to prevent this arrhythmia. Lidocaine is most useful for these ventricular arrhythmias, since the drug seems to be more specific for ventricular tissues than are the other antiarrhythmic agents.

Digitalis-induced arrhythmias constitute a significant fraction of arrhythmias seen in most clinics, usually arising in patients receiving digitalis as a cardiotonic agent. Digitalis may induce any type of arrhythmia but the most common seem to be bradycardia, ventricular premature contractions, and AV nodal tachycardia. The first step in therapy is to discontinue the digitalis. If the arrhythmia is not severe, no further therapy may be required. However, digitalis preparations routinely used as cardiotonics are relatively long-acting drugs, and it may be necessary to treat the arrhythmia while the digitalis is being eliminated from the system. Potassium levels should be assessed in these patients, since a low potassium level increases the sensitivity of the heart to digitalis and may predispose the tissue to develop arrhythmias. Potassium supplements may be given if required.

Phenytoin is the drug most often selected to treat digitalis-induced arrhythmias of all types. Empirically, phenytoin seems more effective in most patients than the other drugs, although a mechanistic explanation for this observation is lacking. If phenytoin does not control the arrhythmia satisfactorily, lidocaine or propranolol may be tried.

■ THE NURSING PROCESS

■ Assessment

Antiarrhythmic therapy is used in patients coming to the hospital with certain cardiac arrhythmias. Diagnosis of the rhythm is made by use of the electrocardiogram (ECG), although patients may seek medical evaluation with complaints such as "missed beats," "fluttering" in the chest, pounding in the chest, irregular heartbeat (rates), and other subjective complaints. The nurse should perform a thorough cardiovascular assessment to determine the patient baseline, identify possible causes, and determine if other cardiac problems exist.

■ Management

Treatment of the acute or most serious arrhythmias is usually done in the coronary care unit or other acute care setting, where bedside cardiac monitoring, emergency drugs, and equipment for resuscitation are readily available. For less serious arrhythmias, therapy is begun in the nonacute care setting, although the only accurate way to monitor the effect of the drugs on the rhythm is through cardiac monitoring. After the patient is stabilized and the dose adjusted, cardiac monitoring is needed only intermittently by periodic ECG tracings.

The nurse should ascertain the goal of therapy after consultation with the physician, but in general the goal would be to eliminate a potentially life-threatening arrhythmia and change the patient's arrhythmia to a less serious form or to restore normal sinus rhythm, if possible. The possible goal of therapy will be tempered by the specific arrhythmia displayed, its cause, the general condition of the heart, other physiological problems the patient has, other drugs being used, and the incidence of side effects of therapy. In preparing for discharge, the health care team should decide on the drugs and doses for chronic management, and other treatments that would be appropriate (e.g., dietary restrictions, activity restrictions). During dosage adjustment, the nurse should monitor the vital signs and blood pressure, weight, fluid intake and output, serum electrolyte levels, and laboratory work appropriate for the drug being used. The nurse should also observe the general physical condition of the patient and watch for the appearance of side effects.

■ Evaluation

Before discharge, it would be desirable to have the patient in a stable cardiac rhythm, either normal sinus rhythm or a nonthreatening arrhythmia. The nurse should evaluate the patient to see if this goal has been met and evaluate for the side effects of therapy. The patient should be able to explain or to demonstrate why and how to take the prescribed drugs, interactions between drugs, how to plan meals within prescribed dietary restrictions, how to manage persistent side effects (e.g., constipation with atropine, hyperglycemia with phenytoin), the signs and symptoms of toxicity, what situations warrant notifying the physician, and what side effects may occur. For more specific information, see the patient care implications section at the end of this chapter.

■ PATIENT CARE IMPLICATIONS

Digitalis preparations

Digitalis preparations are discussed at length in Chapter 15.

Atropine

1. Atropine is contraindicated in patients with glaucoma.
2. The side effects are often dose related: dry mouth, flushed skin, blurred vision, and tachycardia. Giving hard candy or gum to the patient, if appropriate, may help to relieve the dry mouth.
3. Assess pulse and blood pressure after administering.
4. With long-term administration, constipation may be a problem, but it can often be relieved with dietary manipulation such as increasing the fluid intake (may be contraindicated in cardiac patients), increasing the roughage intake, or drinking prune juice. Sometimes a stool softener needs to be prescribed.

5. Intravenous administration:
   a. Atropine may be given undiluted but can be diluted in at least 10 ml of sterile water. Do not add to intravenous infusions. It is incompatible with many medications, so do not mix with other medications in a syringe; consult the pharmacy.
   b. Administer at a rate that does not exceed 0.6 mg per minute.
   c. If possible, the patient should be attached to a cardiac monitor during intravenous administration.
6. Atropine is also discussed in Chapter 7.

Propranolol

Propranolol is discussed in Chapter 13.

Quinidine

1. It is recommended that a test dose of 1 tablet or 200 mg intramuscularly always precede full-dose administration to test for idiosyncrasy.
2. Side effects include nausea, vomiting, abdominal cramps, diarrhea, cold sweat, urge to defecate or urinate, and apprehensiveness. Many side effects will diminish with chronic administration.
3. When initiating therapy, it is preferable to have the patient on a cardiac monitor. The drug should be discontinued, at least temporarily, if any of the following occur: disappearance of P waves; widening of the QRS complex by more than 25%; resumption of sinus rhythm; or severe side effects.
4. Quinidine effectiveness is enhanced by normal potassium levels; the effectiveness is reduced in the presence of hypokalemia. Monitor the electrolyte levels.
5. Hypotension can be a problem; monitor the blood pressure at regular intervals until the patient's condition is stabilized.
6. Agranulocytosis has been reported. Teach the patient to report any unexplained fever, sore throat, fatigue, or infection.
7. Parenteral administration:
   a. The oral and intramuscular routes are preferred over the intravenous.
   b. Dilute 10 ml (800 mg) in 40 to 50 ml of 5% dextrose in water.
   c. Do not add to intravenous solutions or mix with other drugs in a syringe.
   d. Administer at a rate not to exceed 1 ml per minute.
   e. Taking oral quinidine with meals or food may help to decrease gastric irritation and side effects.

Procainamide

1. Minor side effects include anorexia, nausea, vomiting, skin rash, and fever. Major side effects include precipitous drop in blood pressure, prolongation of the P-R interval, widening of the QRS, prolongation of the Q-T interval, ventricular tachycardia or fibrillation, and agranulocytosis. Monitor the electrocardiogram when initiating therapy and at regular intervals while the patient is on long-term therapy. Teach the patient to report any unexplained fever, sore throat, rash, or fatigue.
2. A syndrome resembling lupus erythematosus is not uncommon as a side effect. Symptoms include polyarthralgia, pleuritic pain, and arthritis. Antinuclear antibody titers (ANA titers) should be measured before beginning therapy and at regular intervals.
3. Administration of oral doses with meals may reduce gastric irritation.
4. Parenteral administration:
   a. Dilute before intravenous administration. For direct infusion, dilute 100 mg with 10 ml of 5% dextrose in water or sterile water for injection. For constant infusion, add 1 Gm to 500 ml 5% dextrose in water.
   b. The rate of administration should not exceed 25 to 50 mg per minute.
   c. If being given via infusion, use a microdrip infusion administration set and an electronic infusion monitor.
   d. Monitor the blood pressure; if a drop of greater than 15 mm Hg occurs, stop the infusion and notify the physician.
   e. Keep the patient supine.
   f. Do not mix with other drugs or infusions.
   g. The antidote for hypotension is phenylephrine or levarterenol.

Disopyramide

1. This medication should be used cautiously in patients with glaucoma or possible problems with urinary retention (e.g., patients with benign prostatic hypertrophy). During early therapy, monitor intake and output to check for urinary retention.
2. This drug can cause hypotension. Monitor the blood pressure frequently until the dose is established.
3. Side effects include dry mouth and urinary hesitancy.
4. If widening of the QRS complex is greater than 25% of the original value or if prolongation of the Q-T interval or first-degree heart block develop, the drug should be discontinued and the patient reevaluated.
5. There is no specific antidote. An overdose or exaggerated response should be treated symptomatically.

Lidocaine

1. Do not use lidocaine with epinephrine as an antiarrhythmic.
2. Side effects include light-headedness, drowsiness, tinnitus, sensations of hot, cold, or numbness, and hypotension.
3. Depression of cardiac activity as manifested by pro-

longed P-R intervals and widened QRS complexes are indications for discontinuing therapy.

4. Intramuscular injection:
   a. The intravenous route is preferred over the intramuscular route.
   b. The deltoid is the preferred site of intramuscular injection.
   c. Intravascular injection must be avoided; aspirate before injecting any medication and pause during injection to aspirate again several times.
   d. The patient should be attached to a cardiac monitor.
   e. Monitor the pulse and blood pressure frequently.
   f. Emergency drugs and resuscitation equipment should be available.
   g. The intramuscular route can result in elevations of the serum creatinine phosphokinase (CPK), thus reducing the value of this diagnostic test in patients who may have myocardial damage.
5. Intravenous administration:
   a. A 100 mg bolus can be given at a rate of 25 to 50 mg per minute.
   b. For infusion, add 1 Gm of lidocaine to 1000 ml of 5% dextrose in water (results in a concentration of 1 mg/ml) or add 1 Gm to 500 ml of 5% dextrose in water, giving a concentration of 2 mg/ml.
   c. A microdrip infusion set and an electronic infusion monitor should be used for constant infusion.
   d. The patient should be attached to a cardiac monitor.
   e. The rate of infusion is determined by the cardiac response seen on the monitor.
   f. The blood pressure and pulse should be monitored.
   g. Emergency drugs and resuscitation equipment should be available.

Phenytoin

1. Phenytoin is also discussed in Chapter 31.
2. Early signs of toxicity include nystagmus, vertigo, ataxia, nausea, and vomiting. Overdose should be treated symptomatically.
3. Hyperglycemia has been reported. Monitor the blood glucose and urine glucose levels. Adjustment of insulin dosages in diabetics might be necessary.
4. Concomitant use of coumarin anticoagulants, disulfiram, phenylbutazone, or isoniazid may increase the risk of phenytoin toxicity.
5. The safety of this drug in pregnancy is not known. The pregnant woman should discuss the benefits versus risks of therapy with her physician.
6. Parenteral administration:
   a. The intramuscular route should be avoided because of erratic absorption with this route.
   b. Use only the diluent supplied by the manufacturer. Do not add to intravenous infusions or mix with other drugs.
   c. Do not exceed an intravenous administration rate of 50 mg per minute.
   d. The patient should be on a cardiac monitor; intravenous administration can cause cardiac arrest.

■ SUMMARY

Cardiac arrhythmias are any deviation from the normal rate or pattern of heart pacing: sympathetic overstimulation of the SA node produces tachycardia, whereas vagal nerve overstimulation produces bradycardia. Heart rates and ECG patterns may be altered when ectopic foci develop and begin to compete with the normal pacing of the heart by the SA node. Prolonged conduction times through the AV node can result in skipped beats and heart block.

Digitalis is widely used not only as a cardiotonic drug but also as an antiarrhythmic. As an antiarrhythmic, digitalis is used primarily to slow conduction through the AV node. Digitalis may induce arrhythmias, the most common of which is bradycardia.

Atropine is a drug capable of blocking muscarinic cholinergic receptors. As an antiarrhythmic agent, atropine is used to block the action of the vagus nerve on the SA node. Atropine increases heart rates.

The depressant antiarrhythmics all depress automaticity, conduction velocity, and contractility of the heart. Quinidine and procainamide have virtually identical mechanisms of action, altering calcium distribution, prolonging refractory periods of automatic tissues, as well as producing an atropine-like blockade of parasympathetic innervation on the heart. Quinidine may produce allergic reactions and cardiac toxicity. Procainamide can produce a syndrome resembling lupus erythematosus with prolonged use. Disopyramide is a newer depressant antiarrhythmic. The mechanism of action of disopyramide seems similar to that of quinidine and procainamide.

Propranolol is an antagonist of beta adrenergic receptors but is also classed as a depressant antiarrhythmic agent. Blocking beta adrenergic effects in the heart may lower automaticity, but it may be dangerous in heart failure when sympathetic stimulation may be critical in maintaining cardiac output.

Nondepressant antiarrhythmic drugs decrease automaticity but do not lower contractility and have either no effect on conduction velocity or speed it slightly. Phenytoin, a drug also used as an anticonvulsant, is especially useful in treating digitalis-induced arrhythmias. Lidocaine, a local anesthetic, is useful as an antiarrhythmic because of its direct effects on ventricular tissue. Lidocaine is very rapidly destroyed by the liver and so must be used by continuous intravenous infusion.

■ STUDY QUESTIONS

1. What is an action potential?
2. What tissues in the heart are normally automatic?
3. Describe how the waves on an ECG are related to electrical activity of different portions of the heart.
4. What is the normal pacemaker of the heart?
5. What is the effect of vagus nerve stimulation on the heart?
6. What is the effect of sympathetic stimulation on the heart?
7. What is the refractory period?
8. What is reentry?
9. What is the mechanism of action of digitalis as an antiarrhythmic agent?
10. What toxicity is associated with the use of digitalis as a antiarrhythmic agent?
11. What is the mechanism of action of atropine as a antiarrhythmic agent?
12. What characteristics do the depressant antiarrhythmic agents have in common?
13. What is the mechanism of action of quinidine and procainamide as antiarrhythmic agents?
14. What secondary action do both quinidine and procainamide share?
15. How do the toxic effects of quinidine and procainamide differ?
16. What is the mechanism of action of disopyramide?
17. What is the mechanism of action of propranolol as an antiarrhythmic agent?
18. What side effects does propranolol produce when the drug is used as an antiarrhythmic agent?
19. How does the mechanism of action of the nondepressant antiarrhythmics differ from that of depressant antiarrhythmic agents?
20. For what type of arrhythmia is phenytoin especially useful?
21. Lidocaine is most effective on which tissue in the heart?
22. What is the mechanism of action of bretylium used as an antiarrhythmic agent?

■ SUGGESTED READINGS

Andreoli, K.G., Fowkes, V.H., Zipes, D.P., and Wallace, A.G.: Comprehensive cardiac care, ed. 4, St. Louis, 1979, The C.V. Mosby Co.

Danahy, D.T., and Aronow, W.S.: Propranolol and lidocaine. Clinical uses as antiarrhythmic agents, Postgraduate Medicine **61**(1):113, 1977.

Federman, J., and Blietstra, R.E.: Antiarrhythmic drug therapy, Mayo Clinic Proceedings **54:**531, 1979.

Giving cardiovascular drugs safely. Nursing skillbook, Horsham, Pa., 1978, Intermed Communications.

Graboys, T.B.: Clinical pharmacology of antiarrhythmic agents, Heart & Lung **8**(4):706, 1979.

Greenblatt, D.J., and Miller, R.R.: The clinical use of procainamide, Drug Therapy Reviews **1:**6, 1977.

Greenblatt, D.J., and Smith, T.W.: Digitalis: clinical implications of new facts about an old drug, Postgraduate Medicine **59**(5):134, 1976.

Harvey, S.: Drugs in cardiovascular emergencies, Nurses' Drug Alert, **2**(special issue):65, June, 1978.

Lipman, B.S.: Aberrancy, ectopy, and reentry in the electrocardiogram, Practical Cardiology **4**(11):107, 1978.

Morgan, J., and Kupersmith, J.: Pharmacology and clinical use of newer antiarrhythmic agents, Practical Cardiology **5**(2):89, 1979.

Stanford, J.L., Felner, J.M., and Arensberg, D.: Antiarrhythmic drug therapy, American Journal of Nursing **80:**2188, 1980.

Vera, Z., Mason, D.J., Awan, N.A., and Amsterdam, E.A.: The newer antiarrhythmics: bretylium, Drug Therapy **10**(9):71, 1980.

Vera, Z., Mason, D.J., Awan, N.A., and Amsterdam, E.A.: The newer antiarrhythmics: disopyramide, Drug Therapy **10**(9):57, 1980.

Wenger, T.L., and Strauss, H.C.: When and how to treat arrhythmias, Drug Therapy **10**(9):40, 1980.

Winkle, R.A.: The clinical pharmacology and use of antiarrhythmic drugs, Practical Cardiology **4**(11):169, 1978.

17 Agents affecting blood coagulation

■ THE ROLE OF PLATELETS IN BLOOD COAGULATION

Platelets (thrombocytes) are the small cell fragments in blood that are derived from giant bone marrow cells called megakaryocytes. Ordinarily platelets do not stick to each other or to the endothelial lining of the blood vessels. When there is a break in the endothelial lining, however, platelets readily attach to the collagen in the exposed tissue. This attachment causes the platelets to aggregate, rapidly forming a plug that stops the bleeding and aids in the formation of a blood clot (thrombus). This aggregation of platelets in the presence of abnormal surfaces is the initial step in the normal repair system for the blood vessels. Drugs that interfere with this process have been termed "antiplatelet" or "antithrombic" drugs.

In the late 1970's, it was discovered that when the platelets adhere to a surface, they synthesize thromboxane A_2, a substance related to the prostaglandins. Thromboxane A_2 is a potent stimulus for the further aggregation of platelets and thereby accelerates the formation of the platelet plug. Therefore drugs blocking the synthesis of thromboxane A_2 inhibit the aggregation of platelets to form a plug. Aspirin and sulfinpyrazone (Anturane) are inhibitors of thromboxane A_2 synthesis. Dipyridamole (Persantine) and sulfinpyrazone prolong the survival of platelets in persons with thromboembolic diseases so that platelets do not initiate thrombus formation as readily.

■ CLINICAL USE OF ANTIPLATELET DRUGS

The role of platelet aggregation as the initial step leading to blood coagulation is well established. In particular, the blood clots forming in the arterial system, as opposed to the venous system, are highly linked to conditions promoting platelet aggregation. Patients readily identified as at risk for arterial clots are those who have already suffered a myocardial infarction or a stroke. Clinical trials are in progress to test whether aspirin, sulfinpyrazone, or dipyridamole will decrease the incidence of recurrent strokes or heart attacks when taken prophylactically by patients who have already experienced a heart attack or stroke. The clinical use of antiplatelet drugs at present is established only for heart valve disorders and shunts. Much exciting work remains to be done in this new area of therapy.

The dose of aspirin may be important to its effectiveness in preventing thrombus formation. A low dose of aspirin (80 to 180 mg per day) inhibits the synthesis of thromboxane A_2 by the platelets as just discussed. A higher dose of aspirin (1000 mg per day) also inhibits the synthesis of prostacyclin (prostaglandin I_2) by the epithelial lining of the blood vessel. Prostacyclin inhibits the aggregation of platelets, an action directly opposite that of thromboxane A_2. Prostacyclin therefore prevents the formation of a platelet plug. For this reason, a high dose of aspirin may be less effective than the low dose in preventing the formation of a thrombus.

■ BLOOD COAGULATION AND THE MECHANISMS OF ANTICOAGULANTS

The scheme for blood coagulation is diagrammed in Fig. 17-1. The initial step can be an event in the intrinsic pathway, the activation of the blood component factor XII (the Hageman factor) by contact with exposed collagen, or an event in the extrinsic pathway, that is, the release of tissue factor by damaged tissue. Either pathway results in the activation of factor X. Factor Xa (activated factor X) forms a complex with platelet phospholipids, calcium, and factor V. This complex, which is sometimes called thromboplastin, catalyzes the conversion of prothrombin (factor II) to thrombin. Thrombin then catalyzes the conversion of fibrinogen to fibrin. After crosslinking of fibrin by factor XIIIa, fibrin becomes insoluble, forming a mesh that is the blood clot.

Blood clots in the arterial system are initially composed largely of platelets with a fibrin mesh (white thrombus). Blood clots in the venous system have only a few platelet aggregates and are composed largely of fibrin with trapped red blood cells (red thrombus). A thrombus in either the arterial or venous system may dislodge, becoming an embolus. Venous emboli often lodge in the small arteries of the pulmonary circulation,

FIG. 17-1

The stages of blood coagulation are diagrammed. Actions of drug classes discussed in this chapter include four stages.

Stage I:

a. Antiplatelet drugs inhibit platelet aggregation in the intrinsic pathway.
b. Citrate and EDTA, which chelate calcium, prevent the formation of factor Xa.
c. Heparin, by activating antithrombin III, neutralizes factor Xa and stops coagulation at stage 1.
d. Oral anticoagulants prevent the synthesis of factors VII, IX, and X, which are necessary for stage 1.
e. Local hemostatic agents provide a contact to activate the intrinsic pathway.

Stage II: Oral anticoagulants prevent the synthesis of prothrombin.

Stage III: Heparin activates antithrombin III to prevent thrombin activity.

Stage IV:

a. Aminocaproic acid inhibits the activation or profibrinolysin and so inhibits clot degradation.
b. Streptokinase and urokinase activate profibrinolysin to aid clot digestion.

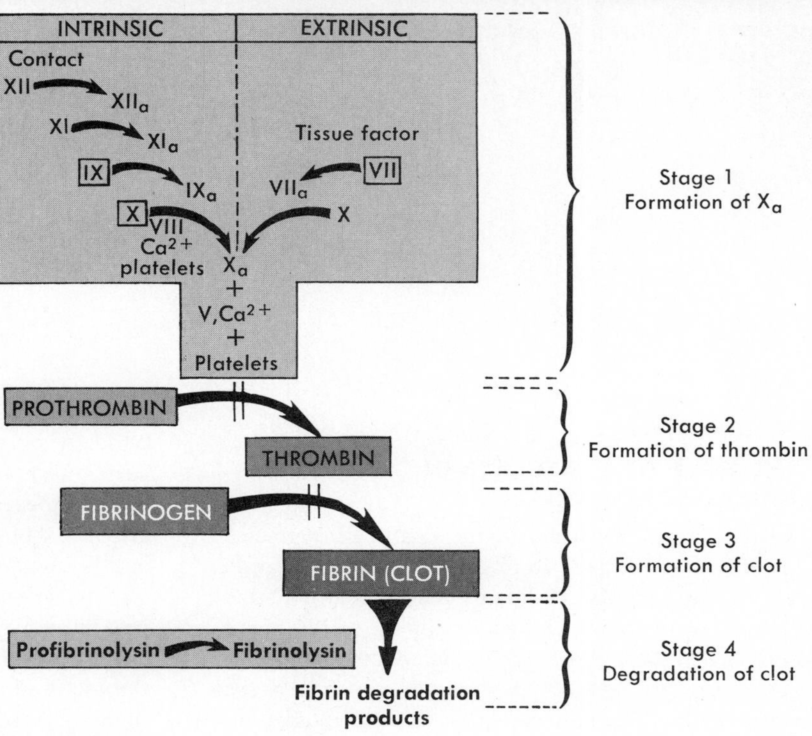

thereby markedly blocking the oxygenation capacity of the lungs and increasing the blood pressure in the pulmonary system, a life-threatening situation. Thrombi tend to form in veins when blood flow is low, favoring the accumulation of activated clotting factors. Patients at risk for venous thrombosis include anyone immobilized as a result of trauma or surgery or anyone with a history of thromboembolism.

Anticoagulant drugs are those drugs that interfere with any of the steps in Fig. 17-1, leading to the formation of fibrin. Blood coagulation is often referred to as a cascade phenomenon, since the process becomes magnified at every step. Each activated factor is a catalyst leading to the formation of many molecules of the next activated factor. The earlier in the process that a step can be blocked, the more efficient will be the inhibition of blood coagulation.

■ ANTICOAGULANTS

Anticoagulant drugs can be classified into three groups: (1) agents that remove calcium, (2) the drug heparin and (3) oral anticoagulants.

■ Agents that remove calcium

Calcium is a cofactor for each of the steps through the activation of prothrombin. The removal of calcium will prevent the coagulation of blood. *Citrate* and *ethylenediamine tetracetic acid (EDTA)* are compounds that will complex calcium, making calcium unavailable for blood coagulation. When blood is drawn for testing or storage, citrate or EDTA may be present to keep the blood from clotting in the container. Since calcium is essential for many biochemical events, anticoagulants that complex calcium can only be used in storage containers (in vitro), not in a patient (in vivo).

■ Heparin (Table 17-1)

Heparin is an anticoagulant that can either be administered to the patient or added to a storage container.

Mechanism of action. Heparin activates a plasma protein, antithrombin III. As the name indicates, antithrombin III will neutralize thrombin. However, antithrombin III also neutralizes factor Xa, the step before the activation of prothrombin to thrombin. This inhibition of factor Xa, rather than the inhibition of thrombin,

TABLE 17-1. Anticoagulant drugs

Generic name	Trade name	Dosage and administration	Comments
HEPARIN	Hepathrom Heprinar Lipo-Hepin Liquaemin Panheprin	SUBCUTANEOUS: 10,000 to 20,000 units, then 8000 to 10,000 units every 8 hr or 15,000 to 20,000 units every 12 hr. INTRAVENOUS: *Intermittent*—10,000 units, then 5000 to 10,000 units every 4 to 6 hr. *Continuous*—20,000 to 40,000 units daily in 1000 ml. SUBCUTANEOUS: 5000 units 2 hr before surgery, then every 8 to 12 hr until ambulatory.	High dose for therapeutic anticoagulation. Low dose for prophylaxis of postoperative thromboembolism.
ORAL ANTICOAGULANTS: COUMARINS			
Dicumarol (bishydroxycoumarin)		ORAL: 200 to 300 mg day 1; 25 to 200 mg daily for maintenance.	The prototype oral anticoagulant. Half-life is 1 to 2 days. Peak effect in 1 to 4 days. Anticoagulant effect persists 2 to 10 days after discontinuance. This coumarin is poorly and erratically absorbed.
Phenprocoumon	Liquamar	ORAL: 24 mg day 1; 0.75 to 6 mg daily for maintenance.	Half-life is 6½ days. Peak effect in 2 to 3 days. Anticoagulant effect persists 4 to 7 days after discontinuance.
Warfarin	Athrombin Coumadin Panwarfin	ORAL, INTRAMUSCULAR, INTRAVENOUS: 10 to 15 mg daily until prothrombin time is in therapeutic range. 2 to 10 mg daily for maintenance. A loading dose of 40 to 60 mg (20 to 30 mg in the elderly) may be given initially.	Half-life is 2 days. Peak effect in 1 to 3 days. Anticoagulant effect persists 4 to 5 days after discontinuance.
ORAL ANTICOAGULANTS: INDANDIONES			
Anisindione	Miradon	ORAL: 300 mg day 1, 200 mg day 2; 100 mg day 3, 25 to 250 mg daily for maintenance.	Half-life is 3 to 5 days. Peak effect in 2 to 3 days. Anticoagulant effect persists 1 to 3 days after discontinuance. Dermatitis is a side effect. Drug imparts an orange color to an alkaline urine.
Phenindione	Hedulin	ORAL: 300 mg day 1, 200 mg day 2, 100 mg daily for maintenance.	Half-life is 5 hr. Peak effect in 1 to 2 days. Anticoagulant effect persists 2 to 4 days after discontinuance. Blood cell values need to be monitored. Drug imparts an orange color to an alkaline urine.

appears to be primarily responsible for the effective anticoagulant action of heparin in low doses. Heparin may also serve as an antiplatelet drug. In vitro, heparin actually stimulates platelet aggregation. In vivo, however, heparin appears to coat the endothelial lining of the vessels. Since heparin is a very negatively charged polymer, heparin adds a negative charge to the endothelium that keeps platelets from attaching and forming a thrombus.

Clinical uses of heparin. There are three clinical uses of heparin that differ in the dose and route of administration: (1) to achieve anticoagulation (in high doses), (2) to prevent postoperative thromboembolism (in low doses), and (3) to prevent coagulation of laboratory samples and stored blood in vitro.

High-dose administration. Heparin is used in the hospital to prevent the further growth of venous thrombi. Large doses (35 to 100 units/kg) must be administered intravenously to achieve this anticoagulation. Heparin cannot be taken orally, since it is not absorbed and it will cause a painful hematoma if administered intramuscularly. Heparin may be given as an intravenous injection, achieving immediate anticoagulation, with the same or lesser dose repeated every 4 to 6 hours. Blood levels of heparin decrease by half every 1½ hours. Intermittent intravenous administration results in virtual incoagulability after administration and is associated with a higher risk of bleeding than continuous intravenous infusion. Thus an initial intravenous injection followed by continuous infusion at approximately 1000 units per hour is commonly given. An intravenous drip must be carefully monitored if used to deliver heparin, or overdosing may result, so an infusion monitor is usually used.

Low-dose administration. Heparin may also be given subcutaneously to achieve a slow, continual administration of heparin over an 8- to 12-hour period of time. Low-dose heparin is used for patients over 40 years of age undergoing thoracoabdominal surgery who are known to be at increased risk. It is not used in brain, spinal cord, or eye surgery, in which even minor hemorrhage could be catastrophic. It is not effective in hip replacement surgery. Heparin is administered subcutaneously (5000 units) 2 hours before surgery, and then another 5000 units is administered every 8 to 12 hours until the patient is walking. This regimen can reduce the incidence of deep leg vein thrombosis by 50% in these patients without markedly affecting their bleeding or clotting times. The effectiveness of this therapy appears to result from heparin activating antithrombin III, which in turn rapidly inactivates newly formed factor Xa. After antithrombin III has inactivated factor Xa, the heparin can dissociate from this inactive complex and act again to cause further inactivation.

In vitro use. Heparin will prevent the coagulation of blood after it leaves the body. Tubing used to shunt blood can be pretreated with heparin to prevent clotting. The negative charge of the heparin coated on the wall of the tubing preventing platelet adherence is probably the effective anticoagulant mechanism. Heparin is also preadded to containers used in the collection of blood. For transfusions, 4 to 6 units of heparin/ml of blood is used. For laboratory samples, 7 to 15 units of heparin/ml of blood is used.

Side effects. The major side effect of heparin is hemorrhage. Since the half-life of intravenously administered heparin is only 1½ hours, discontinuing heparin therapy is usually sufficient to reverse a hemorrhagic episode. If hemorrhaging must be stopped immediately, protamine sulfate may be given by slow intravenous infusion. Protamine is a highly positively charged molecule that complexes the negatively charged heparin. Protamine is itself an anticoagulant and has a longer half-life than does heparin. Protamine may persist and be the cause of bleeding after heparin is eliminated. One milligram of protamine sulfate neutralizes 100 units of heparin. No more than 50 mg of protamine sulfate should be administered in a 10-minute period.

Heparin is a natural compound, extracted from animal lungs or intestines for use in human beings. Some patients become allergic to heparin. The usual symptoms of heparin hypersensitivity are chills, fever, and urticaria, but other allergic reactions such as asthma, rhinitis, lacrimation, or even anaphylaxis have been reported. In some patients heparin has caused thrombocytopenia, so the platelet count should be measured daily after therapy.

■ Oral anticoagulants (Table 17-1)

Four clotting factors, II (prothrombin), VII, IX, and X, are synthesized in the liver, with vitamin K as a necessary cofactor. If vitamin K is deficient, these clotting factors will be synthesized in a functionally inactive manner, impairing blood coagulation.

Two classes of drugs, the *coumarins* and the *indandiones,* interfere with the regeneration of active vitamin K in the liver and thereby produce an effective vitamin K deficiency. Since it is the synthesis of functional clotting factors II, VII, IX, and X that is inhibited, the anticoagulant effect will not appear until preexisting factors II, VII, IX, and X are removed by normal degradation. This takes a day or longer. Factor II, prothrombin, is the longest lived of these clotting factors, and 24 hours is required to deplete half the existing prothrombin. A one-stage prothrombin test is frequently used to determine if the dose of oral anticoagulants is appropriate. Therapeutic doses of the oral anticoagulants increase the prothrombin time by 1½ to 2½ times the baseline values. Anticoagulant therapy must be individualized for each patient.

Anticoagulants that are vitamin K antagonists are ineffective in preventing coagulation of blood after it is drawn, since the clotting factors are already synthesized and present.

Coumarins

The coumarins are the major class of oral anticoagulants used in the United States. The most widely used coumarins are dicumarol, phenprocoumon, and warfarin. Only warfarin can be administered IM or IV in addition to orally.

Importance of protein binding to the pharmacokinetics of coumarins. The coumarins stay in the body a long time because they are bound tightly to plasma albumin. This tight binding to albumin has several consequences. First, only a small amount of the total drug in the body is free to diffuse to the site of action in the liver. Second, the liver also degrades the coumarin to inactive forms that are then excreted in the urine, so only a small amount of the total coumarin is available for

■ THE NURSING PROCESS FOR ANTICOAGULANT DRUGS

■ Assessment

Anticoagulants are used in patients with a recent thrombus, who are immobilized after certain types of surgeries, have certain cardiac valve diseases, or require hemodialysis. Anticoagulation is done to prevent clot formation and does not dissolve existing clots. Baseline data to obtain would be related to the general physical condition of the patient, the history of problems with clots, and blood coagulation studies that include prothrombin time (PT), partial thromboplastin time (PTT), platelet count, and clotting times. In addition, the presence of any bleeding should be documented.

■ Management

The blood coagulation studies should be monitored carefully, and the drug dosage titrated to maintain the desired range of anticoagulation. The patient should be monitored for bleeding from any site, and stools should be checked for occult blood. Any symptoms signaling possible embolus formation, such as chest pain or leg pain, or any symptom of internal bleeding, such as a headache, should be evaluated. An infusion monitoring device should be used for constant infusions of heparin, and dosages should be checked carefully. Discharge planning should be started by anticipating the level of anticoagulation desired, the drug to be used, and the length of time it will be taken. The antidotes for the drugs being used should be readily available during therapy.

■ Evaluation

The goals of anticoagulation therapy are to maintain the appropriate coagulation times within the desired range, to prevent thromboembolic problems, and to avoid side effects associated with bleeding. Before beginning self-management, the patient should be able to explain why the drug is needed, how to take the drug, the signs and symptoms of bleeding that should be reported, how to avoid injury and bruising, the side effects which may be related to the drug but that do not involve bleeding, and which additional side effects require notification of the physician. Finally, the patient should be able to state other drugs, such as aspirin, that should not be used while taking anticoagulants. For additional guidelines, see the patient care implications section at the end of this chapter.

---

degradation. Third, several other drugs can displace coumarins from albumin. This displacement dramatically increases the effective concentration of coumarin. This can be appreciated by considering that if only 1% of the total coumarin is not bound and displacement causes another 1% to be free, the concentration of free coumarin drug has doubled. Fourth, the albumin-bound coumarin acts as a reservoir for the drug. Even after administration is discontinued, several days will be required for the drug to dissociate from the albumin and to be degraded by the liver.

Drug interactions. Drugs interactions are especially numerous with the coumarins. Many drugs will alter the effectiveness of the coumarins. No drug should be added to or deleted from a therapeutic regimen that includes a coumarin without considering drug interactions and appropriately modifying dosages.

The anticoagulant action of heparin and coumarins is *enhanced* by drugs that decrease platelet adhesion, that is, aspirin, clofibrate, dextran, dipyridamole, hydroxychloroquine, ibuprofen, indomethacin, and phenylbutazone. The anticoagulant action of coumarins is *enhanced* by drugs that inhibit coumarin degradation, such as clofibrate, disulfiram, metronidazole, oxyphenbutazone, phenylbutazone, and trimethoprim; drugs that displace bound anticoagulant, such as chloral hydrate, oxyphenbutazone, and phenylbutazone; and drugs that interact by unknown mechanisms, for example, anabolic steroids, cimetidine, D-thyroxine, glucagon, quinidine, and sulfinpyrazone. The anticoagulant action of coumarins is *diminished* by drugs that accelerate coumarin degradation, such as barbiturates, ethchlorvynol, glutethimide, griseofulvin, and rifampin; drugs that decrease gastrointestinal absorption of coumarins, for example, cholestyramine; and drugs that interact by unknown mechanisms, such as 6-mercaptopurine. Dicumarol is known to *en-*

TABLE 17-2. Thrombolytic drugs

Generic name	Trade name	Dosage and administration	Comments
Streptokinase	Streptase	Loading dose of 250,000 IU in 30 min, then intravenous infusion of 100,000 IU hr. Dosage is continued for 24 to 72 hr for pulmonary embolism and for 72 hr for deep vein embolism.	Thrombin times are monitored every 12 hr. Allergic reactions are common (15% of patients), usually of the milder variety: itching, flushing, nausea, headache. Treat with antihistamines.
Urokinase	Abbokinase	Loading dose of 2000 IU/lb in 10 min by intravenous infusion, then 2000 IU/lb/hr for 12 hr.	Isolated from human urine. Not as allergenic as streptokinase, but very expensive.

hance the action of phenytoin. This summarizes the major drug interactions but is by no means exhaustive.

Side effects. The principal side effect of coumarins is hemorrhage. Signs of coumarin overdose can include blood in the urine or blood in the stools, causing them to turn red or black. The drug can be discontinued temporarily when minor hemorrhaging occurs. When hemorrhaging is severe, fresh or frozen plasma may be transfused to replace clotting factors immediately. Less severe hemorrhage may also be treated by administering 10 mg (up to 50 mg) of vitamin K_1, phytonadione. This adds excess vitamin K to overcome the block caused by the coumarins. Clotting factors are then again synthesized by the liver, returning the prothrombin time to normal about 24 hours later.

Side effects other than hemorrhaging are rare with the coumarins. For this reason, one of the coumarins is commonly used as an oral anticoagulant in spite of the numerous drug interactions.

Indandiones

The indandiones more frequently cause side effects, including rashes, depression of the bone marrow, hepatitis, and renal damage than do the coumarins and are not widely used in the United States. Drug interactions are not prominent with the indandiones.

■ THROMBOLYTIC DRUGS

■ Mechanisms and use

Thrombolytic drugs are those drugs that promote the digestion of fibrin, thereby dissolving the clot. As shown in Fig. 17-1, the plasma contains the enzyme fibrinolysin (also called plasmin), which degrades the fibrin into small, soluble pieces. Fibrinolysin normally exists in an inactive form, profibrinolysin (also called plasminogen). Profibrinolysin is activated to fibrinolysin by various factors in the plasma. Degradation products of fibrin act as anticoagulants, thereby limiting further clot formation.

Although the coagulation steps are very rapid, the dissolution step may take several days. Two drugs are available that speed the degradation of fibrin by activating profibrinolysin. These drugs are the enzymes *urokinase* and *streptokinase* (Table 17-2). Human fibrinolysin, which contains profibrinolysin activated with streptokinase, is also available, but the thrombolytic capacity seems to be related to the streptokinase content rather than to the fibrinolysin content, and fibrinolysin is seldom used. Thrombolytic therapy is reserved for use in acute pulmonary embolism, deep vein thrombosis, or peripheral arterial occlusion. Thrombolytic therapy may also be used locally to clear arteriovenous shunts in patients on long-term renal dialysis, but clots usually return. Following treatment with streptokinase or urokinase, the patient is then treated with heparin and then a coumarin to prevent the extension of existing clots and the formation of new clots.

■ HEMOSTATIC AGENTS

■ Systemic hemostatic drugs (Table 17-3)

Epsilon aminocaproic acid (Amicar)

Epsilon aminocaproic acid inhibits the activation of profibrinolysin (plasminogen) to the active enzyme fibrinolysin. The lack of fibrinolysin inhibits the dissolution of blood clots. Aminocaproic acid is used primarily in selected instances in which it is desirable to protect blood clots, such as surgery on the prostate, following a ruptured cerebral aneurysm, or for patients with hemophilia after a tooth extraction.

Aminocaproic acid can be given orally or intravenously. It is rapidly excreted in the urine. Most of the side effects are transient and minor: nausea, cramps, dizziness, headache, ringing in the ear, or stuffy nose. When intravenous therapy is used, aminocaproic acid can irritate the veins and give rise to thrombophlebitis. This may be minimized by diluting the drug before use and careful placement of the needle.

Vitamin K

Vitamin K is a fat-soluble vitamin required for the synthesis of clotting factors II, VII, IX, and X in the liver.

■ THE NURSING PROCESS FOR THROMBOLYTIC DRUGS

■ Assessment

The difference between anticoagulant therapy and thrombolytic therapy is that the goal of anticoagulant therapy is clot prevention and a clot already present will not be altered; in thrombolytic therapy, the clot is already present and the goal is clot dissolution. Both groups of drugs, however, alter the normal coagulation mechanism to cause anticoagulation. Baseline data needed for thrombolytic therapy are similar to those needed with heparin or coumarin therapy, with emphasis on assessment of the size and location of the clot and the signs and symptoms caused by the clot. A recent patient history of streptococcal infection would influence the choice of agents and should be documented.

■ Management

Thrombolytic drugs are used only in acute care settings and never on an outpatient basis. The use of an infusion monitoring device may be appropriate. Appropriate drugs to counteract bleeding, such as aminocaproic acid, should be available. The correct dose is calculated by patient size and should be done carefully in consultation with the pharmacy. The nurse should monitor the patient for signs of clot dissolution. As soon as possible, the patient will be switched to heparin therapy. In addition to monitoring the usual tests for blood coagulation, the hematocrit should be checked daily because it may drop even when bleeding is not present. The nurse should check the patient frequently for signs of bleeding from any body orifice; hemorrhage is the major complication of therapy.

■ Evaluation

If effective, a thrombolytic drug will dissolve the existing clot without causing any hemorrhaging in the patient. The patient will not be discharged while still on thrombolytic therapy. For additional specific guidelines, see the patient care implications section at the end of this chapter.

Vitamin K is contained in many foods. Humans cannot synthesize vitamin K, but bacteria in the gastrointestinal tract can synthesize vitamin K for absorption by the host. A variety of conditions that can produce vitamin K deficiency are given in the following list:

1. Long-term intravenous feeding
2. Debilitation resulting from poor diet
3. Prolonged oral antibiotic therapy
4. Malabsorption syndrome
5. Acute diarrhea in infants
6. Biliary disease

In addition, the oral anticoagulant drugs, the coumarins and the indandiones, produce a relative vitamin K deficiency by inhibiting the reactivation of vitamin K.

Administration and side effects. Vitamin K is available as vitamin K_1, phytonadione, and vitamin K_3, menadione, for replacement therapy, but only vitamin K_1 is effective as an antidote for severe bleeding episodes caused by an overdose of one of the oral anticoagulants. Vitamin K_1 or K_3 is safest when taken orally. Intravenous injection must be made slowly with a dilute solution and even then may cause a severe reaction. Reactions to intravenous injection include flushing, a heavy feeling on the chest, sweating, vascular collapse, and an anaphylactic reaction. Intramuscular and subcutaneous administration may cause pain and bleeding at the injection site.

In infants and anyone with a deficiency of the enzyme glucose-6-phosphate dehydrogenase, menadione (K_3) can produce hemolysis but phytonadione (K_1) does not. Vitamin K_1 or K_3 will not promote clotting in a patient with liver disease or a hereditary deficiency of one of the vitamin K–dependent clotting factors.

■ Local absorbable hemostatics (Table 17-3)

Local absorbable hemostatics provide a surface that promotes platelet adhesion and thereby promotes blood clotting where the agent is applied.

Absorbable gelatin sponge (Gelfoam)

Gelfoam is a sterile material that is moistened with sterile saline solution and applied to bleeding capillary beds that cannot be readily sutured. It is absorbed in 4 to 6 weeks.

TABLE 17-3. Hemostatic agents

Generic name	Trade name	Dosage and administration	Comments
SYSTEMIC HEMOSTATIC AGENTS			
Aminocaproic acid	Amicar	ORAL, INTRAVENOUS: *Adults*—5 to 6 Gm initially orally or by slow intravenous infusion, then 1 Gm hourly or 6 Gm every 6 hr. Maximum in 24 hr is 30 Gm. Reduced dosage is used with low renal output or renal disease. *Children*—100 mg/kg body weight every 6 hr for 6 days.	Prevents activation of plasminogen (fibrinolysis) so that blood clots are not broken down. Used in special surgical situations.
Phytonadione (vitamin K_1)	Aquamephyton Konakion Mephyton	ORAL, INTRAMUSCULAR, SUBCUTANEOUS: *Adults and children*—2.5 to 25 mg. INTRAMUSCULARLY, SUBCUTANEOUSLY, INTRAVENOUSLY: *Newborns*—0.5 to 1 mg immediately after birth. Alternatively the mother is given 1 to 5 mg 12 to 24 hr before delivery.	Intravenous route can be dangerous. Use only in emergencies for oral anticoagulant overdose, and dilute so that no more than 1 mg is given per minute. Subcutaneous and intramuscular injection may be painful.
Menadione (Vitamin K_3)		ORAL, INTRAMUSCULAR: *Adults and children*—2 to 10 mg daily.	Insoluble. Contraindicated in newborns, women in advanced pregnancy, and patients with glucose-6-phosphate dehydrogenase deficiency, as menadione may cause hemolysis.
Menadiol sodium diphosphate	Synkayvite	ORAL, INTRAMUSCULAR, SUBCUTANEOUS, INTRAVENOUS: *Adults*—5 to 15 mg once or twice daily. *Children*—5 to 10 mg once or twice daily.	To correct secondary hypoprothrombinemia.
Menadione sodium bisulfite	Hykinone	INTRAMUSCULAR, SUBCUTANEOUS, INTRAVENOUS: 2.5 to 10 mg daily.	To correct severe vitamin K deficiency.
LOCAL HEMOSTATIC AGENTS			
Absorbable gelatin sponge	Gelfoam	Blocks and cones of various sizes. Also a sterile (surgical) and nonsterile (dental) powder.	To control bleeding in a wound or at an operative site.
Absorbable gelatin film	Gelfilm	Thin film strips.	To repair membranes in neural, thoracic, and ocular surgery.
Oxidized cellulose	Oxycel	Gauze-type pads or strips. Also as sponges 2 × 1 × 1 inch.	To control hemorrhage and absorb blood. May be left in wound. Not for packing around bone fractures or to be left on skin.
Oxidized regenerated cellulose	Surgicel	Knitted fabric strips.	Like oxidized cellulose, but may be left on skin.
Microfibrillar collagen hemostat	Avitene	Sterile powder. 1 Gm should cover 50 × 50 cm (20 × 20 inches) to control light bleeding.	To control bleeding in a wound or at an operative site. May be used on skin. Discard unused material, since it cannot be resterilized.
Thrombin	Thrombin, Topical	Sterile powder. Packaged by units. May be dissolved in sterile saline solution and applied in absorbable gelatin sponge.	To control bleeding in a wound or at an operative site. Discard unused material, since it cannot be resterilized and the solution is unstable.

■ THE NURSING PROCESS FOR HEMOSTATIC AGENTS

■ Assessment

Patients requiring hemostatic therapy are those in whom the retention or formation of a blood clot is desirable or who have been overmedicated by a drug causing anticoagulation. Baseline data would include assessment of the type, location, and amount of bleeding; the symptoms related to the bleeding such as pain, swelling, and level of consciousness; appropriate blood coagulation tests such as partial thromboplastin time, prothrombin time, clotting time, and platelet count; the hematocrit; and general physical condition of the patient. In most cases, these patients, by the nature of their presenting problems, will be in acute care units, and extensive monitoring will be ongoing.

■ Management

The route of administration depends on the drug being used. The nurse should monitor the appropriate coagulation studies and hematocrit. The patient is observed for signs that bleeding is stopping and for side effects of the drugs. Overmedication with the systemic hemostatic agents is also possible, so care should be taken to assure that the patient receives the correct dose.

■ Evaluation

The goal of therapy with hemostatic agents is to stop bleeding without causing excessive coagulation or side effects resulting from the drug therapy. These patients will rarely be sent home on hemostatic therapy but should be able to explain what to do if bleeding should recur. For more specific guidelines, see the patient care implications section at the end of this chapter.

Absorbable gelatin film (Gelfilm)

Gelfilm is a thin sterile material used in neurological, thoracic, and ocular surgery to repair membrane surfaces. Reabsorption may take from 1 week to 6 months depending on the size and site of the film.

Oxidized cellulose (Oxygel) and oxidized regenerated cellulose (Surgicel)

Oxidized cellulose material is used much like the absorbable gelatin sponge. Both celluloses interfere with bone regeneration and therefore cannot be packed around fractures.

Oxygel retards formation of new skin and cannot be used as a surface dressing. Small implants are reabsorbed in a week, but large ones may require 6 weeks for reabsorption.

Microfibrillar collagen hemostat (Avitene)

Collagen hemostat is a water-insoluble powder that is applied to a bleeding surface to activate natural clotting. The collagen is absorbed in 7 weeks. Microfibrillar collagen is used in surgery to control bleeding in capillary beds, in the liver, and in skin graft sites. It does not interfere with the healing of skin or bone. Microfibrillar collagen must be kept dry and cannot be resterilized after the container is opened.

Thrombin

Thrombin is an activated clotting factor (Fig. 17-1). Thrombin is applied topically only as a sterile protein powder to bleeding surfaces. It must be kept cold and dry until use or it becomes inactive. Thrombin can be applied topically as a solution but it must not be injected.

■ PATIENT CARE IMPLICATIONS

General guidelines for patients receiving anticoagulants

1. Teach patients receiving anticoagulants (''blood thinners'') why they are taking the medication, the importance of taking the correct dose as directed, and precautions to observe to avoid bleeding.
2. Caution patients to avoid contact sports and activities associated with a high chance of injury such as construction work, carpentry, or foundry work. Obviously, patients are not usually able to change occupations, but they should be cautioned to avoid injury if at all possible.
3. Patients should use electric razors while taking anticoagulants because there is less risk of cutting themselves.
4. Teach patients to report any signs of bleeding from any site: nosebleeds, hematuria, bloody or tarry stools, bleeding gums, change in menstrual flow,

excessive bruising, or excessive bleeding from any cut or scratch.

5. Patients should not go barefoot.
6. Patients should brush their teeth gently, with a soft-bristle brush, and floss gently. Patients may find it necessary to forego flossing while on anticoagulant therapy, and some may even have to give up tooth-brushing because of excessive bleeding from gums. If patients cannot brush their teeth, assist them to find other acceptable ways to provide oral hygiene, such as swabbing the mouth or using mouthwashes. Note that excessive bleeding may indicate over-medication and should be reported.
7. Remind patients to keep all health care providers informed of any medications they are taking. Specifically point out that dentists need to know if patients are receiving anticoagulants.
8. Patients should obtain and wear a medical alert bracelet or tag stating their anticoagulant medication.
9. Women of childbearing age should be informed of the risks associated with the use of anticoagulants and should consider the use of birth control measures while on therapy. If in the first trimester when beginning therapy, some women may elect to terminate the pregnancy. Advise women to discuss the question of pregnancy with their physicians.
10. Health care providers should always keep in mind the possibility of drug interactions between the anticoagulants and many other drugs (Table 17-2). Patients should be cautioned not to take any medications without clearance from their physicians because of the many possible interactions. Point out to the patient that this includes even over-the-counter preparations such as aspirin, cold remedies, and cough remedies. Aspirin is of particular danger because of its potent antiplatelet effects.

Heparin therapy

1. Except in rare situations, heparin is used on an inpatient basis only.
2. Many hospitals require that heparin doses be checked by two professionals before administration.
3. Blood tests used to monitor heparin therapy include the Lee-White clotting time (desired goal of therapy is 20 minutes or the physician's preference) and the partial thromboplastin time (PTT) or activated PTT (aPTT), the desired goal of therapy being 1½ to 2 times normal.
4. Hospitals vary in their procedure, but it is often customary to obtain the necessary coagulation studies daily or more often when therapy is being initiated. The blood is drawn before a scheduled time of heparin administration, and based on the laboratory results, the heparin dose for that day is determined. Patients on continuous intravenous heparin therapy are usually monitored with at least daily laboratory work. The health care practitioner should check for new laboratory results and new heparin orders before *each* dose of heparin is administered. The physician should always be notified if the level of anticoagulation is not within the therapeutic range.
5. Patients on low-dose heparin therapy will have slight, if any, alteration in the clotting time or PTT. Platelet counts need to be monitored to detect thrombocytopenia secondary to heparin therapy. Thrombocytopenia increases the risk of hemorrhage.
6. When a patient is on heparin therapy while an oral anticoagulant is begun, it is necessary to monitor the anticoagulant activity resulting from both drugs. In addition to the clotting time and PTT, the prothrombin time (PT or pro time) will be added to the necessary lab work. The PT should be within the therapeutic range before heparin is discontinued. (See section on oral anticoagulants.)
7. Read the label on the heparin carefully because there are many strengths available.
8. The antidote for heparin overdose is protamine sulfate, which should be kept available. This drug can be difficult to administer (see text), so unless there is frank hemorrhage, most physicians will choose to discontinue the heparin and observe the patient carefully. If anticoagulation is still needed, heparin therapy can be resumed after 24 to 36 hours.
9. If possible, intravenous heparin therapy should be discontinued a couple of days before surgery.
10. If possible, the intramuscular route of administration for any medications should be avoided during heparin therapy because of the danger of intramuscular bleeding. If absolutely unavoidable, intramuscular injections should be scheduled for times when the coagulation time is the shortest, such as ½ to 1 hour before the next dose of heparin. This is of little concern for patients on low-dose heparin therapy.
11. Some hospitals or physicians prefer that routine analyses of stool and urine for occult blood be done on patients receiving heparin.
12. There are some infrequent and unusual side effects of heparin including anaphylaxis; hair loss (alopecia), which is temporary; burning sensation of the feet; myalgias; and bone pain.
13. In some patients, heparin therapy may cause thrombocytopenia. Monitor the platelet count, in addition to the usual blood studies for monitoring heparin activity. Symptoms of severe thrombocytopenia would be bleeding from the gums, urinary tract, or gastrointestinal tract and bruising; these are the same symptoms seen with heparin overdose.

14. Subcutaneous administration of heparin:
    a. Any commonly used subcutaneous site may be chosen, but the abdomen is preferred because there are few muscles there and bruising is not as much of a cosmetic problem. The arms are rarely chosen because of the possibility of unsightly bruises.
    b. Rotate sites, even if the abdomen is used most frequently.
    c. If using the abdomen, avoid the area 2 inches on any side of the umbilicus and avoid any abdominal scars.
    d. Efforts should be directed at avoiding bruising, but even with the best technique, occasional bruising will occur.
    e. Do not inject the skin with the same needle used to draw up the medication.
    f. Inject at a 45- to 90-degree angle with a ⅝- to ½-inch needle after careful assessment of the patient to avoid muscle and reach subcutaneous tissue.
    g. There is disagreement about pinching the skin, as would be done in administering insulin because pinching may cause more bruising.
    h. Do not aspirate before injecting the medication.
    i. Do not rub the site after administration. Apply firm pressure over the site for 2 minutes after administration.
15. Intravenous administration of heparin:
    a. Check the intravenous catheter frequently to ascertain that it is still in the vein.
    b. If the heparin is being given via constant infusion, an electronic infusion monitor should be used to regulate the flow. The infusion rate should be checked frequently (at ½- to 1-hour intervals) to ascertain that the patient is receiving the prescribed dose.
    c. Heparin is incompatible with many other medications. It should be administered via fresh tubing, or the tubing should be flushed before and after administration. Consult with the pharmacy if in doubt.
16. How to establish and use the heparin well (heparin lock):
    a. Intermittent intravenous heparin may be administered via heparin well. One method for this procedure is described. The heparin well should be inserted into the vein using the accepted sterile venipuncture technique, secured in place with tape, and "primed" with a small amount (1 to 2 ml) of heparin of the same dosage strength as will be used for anticoagulation. Each prescribed dose of heparin is injected via the heparin well. The injected dose displaces the heparin remaining in the well each time a dose is given, so flushing the well after the dose is administered is not necessary. Of course, individual hospital procedures should be followed if different from the above procedure.
    b. Heparin wells can be used for other medications administered via intermittent infusion. One method for doing this is described. The heparin well is inserted and secured as just described and then primed with 1 ml of a solution containing 100 units of heparin/ml. Solutions of 100 units/ml are available in prepackaged syringes, multiple dose vials, or can be prepared by the pharmacy or the nurse mixing the heparin with normal saline solution to achieve the desired concentration. Each time a drug is administered, the procedure would be to flush the well with 1 to 2 ml of normal saline solution (this may be omitted if the drug to be administered is compatible with heparin); to administer the prescribed medication via push or infusion; to flush the well with 1 to 2 ml of normal saline solution; and finally, to administer 1 ml of the solution containing 100 units of heparin/ml. The exact procedure of the individual hospital should be followed.
    c. When administering any drug via heparin well, it is important that the needle be in the vein so that infiltration does not occur. It may be difficult to ascertain the placement of the needle and procedures for checking this vary, but it should be possible to aspirate blood from the well if it is in the vein. In addition, drugs being injected should go in smoothly, with no patient discomfort and little resistance to the infusion. Finally, there should be no swelling, discoloration, redness, or tenderness around the insertion site. If there is doubt that the heparin well is in the correct place, it should be removed and a new one inserted.

Coumarins and indandiones

1. Oral anticoagulants are the choice for outpatient therapy.
2. The anticoagulant activity of the coumarins and indandiones is monitored by using the prothrombin time (PT or pro time), the desired goal being 1½ to 2½ times normal, or when expressed as a percent, 20% to 30% of the normal prothrombin activity.
3. Patients taking oral anticoagulants should avoid the use of alcohol because it alters the anticipated anticoagulant effect.
4. Oral anticoagulants cross the placenta and cause birth defects, so pregnant women needing anti-

coagulation should be treated with heparin. This may be stopped at about the thirty-seventh week of pregnancy to decrease the danger of hemorrhage during delivery.

5. Side effects of the coumarins are gastrointestinal discomfort, including diarrhea; dermatitis; hair loss (alopecia); and, rarely, agranulocytosis and elevated serum transaminase levels. Instruct the patient to report any of these side effects and any unusual fatigue, sore throat, chills, and fever (signs of infection resulting from agranulocytosis).
6. Infrequent side effects of the indandiones include agranulocytosis, jaundice, hepatitis, severe exfoliative dermatitis, and red cell aplasia. Caution patients to report unexplained fever, chills, sore throat, rash, fatigue, jaundice, abdominal pain, appearance of skin changes, or any other unusual symptoms that might indicate a drug side effect.
7. The indandiones may turn alkaline urine orange, and this may be mistaken for blood.
8. Overdose of the coumarins and indandiones is treated with vitamin K_1, phytonadione (Aquamephyton), if further therapy with the anticoagulant is necessary. If immediate and/or partial reversal of hemorrhage is necessary, fresh frozen plasma is transfused.
9. Patients taking oral anticoagulants should be instructed not to "double up" if a dose is missed. It may be necessary to help the patient devise a way to remember to take the daily dose of medication. An example of a helpful device might be a calendar that the patient marks each day the medication is taken.
10. The patient and family should be helped to understand the importance of returning for regular follow-up visits to monitor the anticoagulant activity. Blood work should be done routinely to evaluate the prothrombin time, liver function tests, hemoglobin, white cell count, and platelet count.
11. The patient on long-term anticoagulant therapy should wear a necklace or bracelet and have a card available indicating that anticoagulants are being used.
12. Parenteral administration of warfarin:
    a. Warfarin is available for intravenous or intramuscular use, although this use is much less common than oral administration.
    b. Diluent is supplied by the manufacturer and makes a solution of 25 mg/ml.
    c. For intravenous use, give via intravenous injection and do not mix with intravenous fluids. Flush tubing before and after administration.
    d. Warfarin is compatible with heparin in a syringe but incompatible with many other medications; consult the pharmacy.
    e. Rate of administration should not exceed 25 mg (1 ml) per minute.

Streptokinase and urokinase

1. The use of these two agents should be restricted to the acute care setting.
2. Bleeding is the most common and serious side effect, and is seen more frequently than with heparin therapy.
3. Contraindications to use include recent surgery (within 10 days), recent delivery, liver or kidney biopsy, spinal (lumbar) puncture, or when a dissecting aneurysm or active tuberculosis with cavitation is suspected.
4. Use during pregnancy is contraindicated unless absolutely necessary because it may cause premature separation of the placenta during the first couple of months.
5. If bleeding occurs, the drug should be stopped. Red blood cells and plasma volume expanders other than dextran may be given. Aminocaproic acid can be used.
6. A drop in hematocrit will be experienced by 20% to 30% of patients even if clinical bleeding has not occurred.
7. About 1/3 of the patients receiving streptokinase will develop a fever.
8. Streptokinase is derived from catabolic products of beta-hemolytic streptococci. Antibodies from a prior streptococcal infection may inactivate the streptokinase. Thus the efficacy of therapy should be checked by a prolonged thrombin time demonstrating fibrin breakdown products. Rarely, in persons having recently recovered from streptococcal infections, the drug may be completely inactivated and urokinase should be used.
9. Instructions are supplied by the manufacturer for the correct dose of medication based on the desired dose and the patient's weight. Collaborate with the pharmacy in the use of these drugs.
10. The same precautions that would be observed in administering heparin via constant infusion should be observed with either of these drugs.
11. After initial treatment with either of these drugs, the patient is then switched to heparin therapy.
12. Intramuscular injections of any medication are absolutely contraindicated because of the possibility of intramuscular bleeding. Venipunctures should be minimized, and pressure must be applied to the site for a minimum of 15 minutes.

Aminocaproic acid

1. Aminocaproic acid may be used as an antidote for streptokinase or urokinase overdose.
2. Parenteral administration of aminocaproic acid:
   a. The drug is supplied at a concentration of 1 Gm/4 ml, but should be diluted before administration with normal saline, sterile water, 5% dextrose in water or saline, or lactated Ringer's solution. Dilute until the ordered dose is in a volume of 50 to 100 ml.
   b. The dose is usually 5 to 6 Gm during the first hour and then 1 Gm per hour afterwards. The patient should be reevaluated after 8 hours of therapy if not before.
   c. Rapid infusion of the undiluted drug can cause hypotension, bradycardia, or arrhythmias. Monitor the pulse and pressure frequently during administration, and, if possible, have the patient attached to a cardiac monitor.
3. Safe use during pregnancy has not been established. Women of childbearing age or who are pregnant should discuss the benefits of therapy versus risks with their physician.

Vitamin K preparations

1. The daily requirement for vitamin K has not been established but has been estimated at 0.03 μg/kg for adults and 5 μg/kg for children. Although it is not stored in the body for long periods, vitamin K deficiency is rare in adults on the basis of dietary deficiency alone. Dietary sources include tomatoes, green leafy vegetables, meats, dairy products, cereals, and fruits.
2. Vitamin K, except the water-soluble salts menadiol diphosphate sodium and menadione bisulfate sodium, is absorbed from the gastrointestinal tract only in the presence of bile salts and pancreatic lipase. Therefore patients with bile deficiency who are receiving oral phytonadione or menadione need concomitant administration of bile salts for drug absorption.
3. Regular determinations of the plasma prothrombin time (PT or pro time) will be made to evaluate the effectiveness of therapy.
4. Menadione (K_3) and phytonadione (K_1) are preferred for treatment of hypoprothrombinemia secondary to oral anticoagulant overdose.
5. For treatment and prevention of hemorrhagic disease in the newborn, phytonadione is preferred.
6. Intramuscular injection of vitamin K_1 or K_3 can cause pain at the injection site, nodule formation, and bleeding from the injection site. In older children and adults, the gluteus maximus is the preferred intramuscular injection site. In infants and small children, the anterolateral aspect of the thigh is preferred.
7. Vitamins K_1 and K_3 are light sensitive and should be stored in a dark place. Doses should be administered as soon as prepared and unused portions discarded. If K_1 is being administered via the intravenous route, the tubing and container should be covered with foil or light-resistant paper.
8. The concomitant use of red blood cells and fresh frozen plasma may be necessary in cases of frank or severe hemorrhage resulting from excessively prolonged prothrombin times.
9. Intravenous administration of vitamin K_1, phytonadione:
   a. Read the labels carefully; vitamin K_3, menadione (Konakion), is for intramuscular use only.
   b. Vitamin K_1, phytonadione (Aquamephyton), should be diluted for intravenous administration with normal saline solution, 5% dextrose in water, or 5% dextrose in normal saline solution only; other diluents should not be used.
   c. The rate of administration should not exceed 1 mg per minute.
   d. The intravenous route should be used only in emergencies because severe reactions and fatalities have occurred with this route of administration. Reactions have included anaphylaxis, shock, cardiac arrest, respiratory arrest, and, less seriously, flushing, excessive sweating (hyperhidrosis), and a feeling of chest constriction. Patients should be monitored carefully during and after intravenous administration, including evaluation of vital signs, blood pressure, and electrocardiogram.
   e. The drug is incompatible with many drugs; check with the pharmacy if in doubt.
10. Both menadiol diphosphate sodium and menadione bisulfate sodium can be administered intravenously and produce a rapid response via this route, but phytonadione is usually the preparation of choice for intravenous administration. Menadiol phosphate sodium may be given undiluted or added to most intravenous infusions; the rate of administration should not exceed 75 mg per minute. Menadione bisulfate sodium may be given undiluted but should *not* be added to intravenous solutions; the rate of administration should not exceed 2 mg per minute. Both drugs are incompatible with several other drugs; consult the pharmacy if in doubt. Although severe side effects are less frequent with these preparations than with phytonadione, side effects are still possible, and patients should be monitored carefully (see discussion of phytonadione).

■ SUMMARY

Blood coagulation is a complex process and is outlined in Fig. 17-1.

Platelets are cell fragments capable of binding to an appropriate surface and aggregating to form a plug. This process appears to be a key step not only in the intrinsic pathway for blood coagulation, but also in initiating atherosclerotic plaques important in the etiology of strokes and myocardial infarctions. The recent elucidation of factors governing platelet aggregation has prompted clinical trials to determine whether drugs that inhibit platelet aggregation (antiplatelet or antithrombic drugs) will provide prophylaxis for patients with previous strokes or myocardial infarctions.

Anticoagulants in use include the following:

1. Drugs such as citrate and EDTA, which complex calcium and are used to prevent coagulation of stored blood
2. Heparin, which in low doses inhibits platelet adhesion in vivo and in high doses inhibits the activation of thrombin. Heparin is also an effective anticoagulant in vitro
3. Oral anticoagulants, the coumarins and indandiones, which inhibit the vitamin K–dependent synthesis of clotting factors by the liver

The prolonged onset of the oral anticoagulants (1 to 2 days) reflects the time for previously synthesized clotting factors to be destroyed. The coumarins are highly bound to plasma albumin and consequently have a long duration of action in the body. Coumarins interact with many other drugs because of protein binding, drug metabolism, and other factors, as described in the text.

Hemorrhaging is the most common toxicity of anticoagulants. Heparin has a short half-life (about 2 hours), and discontinuing administration is usually sufficient to control hemorrhaging. Protamine specifically complexes heparin and can be administered as an antidote. Vitamin K_1 is the specific antidote for an overdose with the oral anticoagulants, but in an acutely critical situation, transfusion of clotting factors is necessary.

Streptokinase and urokinase are enzymes used as thrombolytics to degrade blood clots in selected cases.

Hemostatic agents are systemic or local. Systemic hemostatics include aminocaproic acid, which inhibits the activation of profibrinolysin so that blood clots are not degraded, and vitamin K, the vitamin necessary for the synthesis of certain of the clotting factors by the liver. Local hemostatics include sponges and films of gelatin or cellulose, which can be sterilized and applied to areas to prompt blood clotting during surgical procedures. Thrombin and collagen can be applied as powders to promote blood clotting.

■ STUDY QUESTIONS

1. How do platelets initiate clot formation?
2. What drugs inhibit platelet aggregation?
3. What roles do thromboxane A_2 and prostacyclin play in platelet aggregation?
4. Describe the major steps in blood coagulation.
5. What are the three groups of anticoagulants and what is the mechanism of action of each group?
6. Describe the use of heparin in high-dose and low-dose therapy.
7. Which anticoagulants are effective when added to blood drawn for storage?
8. How do protamine and vitamin K each function as antidotes for hemorrhaging induced by drugs?
9. How does protein binding affect the pharmacodynamics of the coumarins?
10. What are the therapeutic limitations of the indandiones?
11. What is the action of thrombolytic drugs? Name the thrombolytic drugs.
12. What is the mechanism of action of aminocaproic acid? of vitamin K?
13. List the agents used as local hemostatics. What is their mechanism of action?

■ SUGGESTED READINGS

General references

Andreoli, K.G., Fowkes, V.H., Zipes, D.P., and Wallace, A.G.: Comprehensive cardiac care, ed. 4, St. Louis, 1979, The C.V. Mosby Co.

Giving cardiovascular drugs safely. Nursing skillbook, Horsham, Pa., 1978, Intermed Communications.

Jennings, B.M.: Improving your management of DIC, Nursing '79 **9**(5):60, 1979.

Moore, K., and Maschak, B.J.: How patient education can reduce the risks of anticoagulation, Nursing '77 **7**(9):24, 1977.

O'Brian, B.S., and Woods, S.: The paradox of DIC, American Journal of Nursing **78:**1878, 1978.

Zalumas, J.D., and Simon, C.: Anticoagulants: accepted treatment and current trends, Nurses' Drug Alert **3**(special report):105, Sept., 1979.

Antiplatelet drugs

Andes, A., and Weksler, B.: Can antiplatelet agents avert MI and stroke? Patient Care **13:**131, July 15, 1979.

Anturane Reinfarction Trial Research Group: Sulfinpyrazone in the prevention of cardiac death after myocardial infarction, New England Journal of Medicine **298:**289, 1978.

Anturane Reinfarction Trial Research Group: Sulfinpyrazone in the prevention of sudden death after myocardial infarction, New England Journal of Medicine **302:**250, 1980.

Canadian cooperative study group: A randomized trial of aspirin and sulfinpyrazone in threatened stroke, New England Journal of Medicine **299:**53, 1978.

Czervionke, R.L., Smith, J.B., Fry, G.L., Hoak, J.C., and Haycraft, D.L.: Inhibition of prostacyclin by treatment of endothelium with aspirin: correlation with platelet adherence, Journal of Clinical Investigation **63:**1089, 1979.

Hirsh, J.: Antiplatelet drugs in thromboembolism, Postgraduate Medicine **66**(3):119, 1979.

Koch-Weser, J., and Weiss, H.J.: Antiplatelet therapy (two parts), New England Journal of Medicine **298:**1344, and **298:**1403, 1978.

Marcus, A.J.: How useful is antiplatelet therapy? Drug Therapy **9**(10):53, 1979.

Marcus, A.J.: The role of prostaglandins in occlusive vascular disorders, Practical Cardiology **5**(12):66, 1979.

Marx, J.L.: Blood clotting: the role of the prostaglandins, Science **196:**1072, 1977.

McKee, P.A.: The prevention of thromboembolism, Drug Therapy **9**(9):25, 1979.

Mehta, J., and Mehta, P.: Status of antiplatelet drugs in coronary heart disease, Journal of the American Medical Association **241:**2649, 1979.

Needleman, P., and Kaley, G.: Cardiac and coronary prostaglandin synthesis and function, New England Journal of Medicine **298:**1122, 1978.

Heparin

Chamberlain, S.L.: Low-dose heparin therapy, American Journal of Nursing **80:**1115, 1980.

Jaques, L.B.: Heparin: an old drug with a new paradigm, Science **206:** 528, 1979.

Rosenberg, R.D., and Rosenberg, J.S.: The anticoagulant function of heparin, Drug Therapy **9**(9):87, 1979.

Sherry, S.: Preventing pulmonary embolism with heparin in low doses, Postgraduate Medicine **59**(5):80, 1976.

Simon, T.L.: The rationale for continuous heparin infusion, Drug Therapy **8**(11):17, 1978.

Oral anticoagulants

Ascione, F.J.: Oral anticoagulants with aspirin alternatives, Drug Therapy **8**(10):63, 1978.

Brignoli, E.T.B., editor: Using the antithrombotic agents, Patient Care **14:**62, July 15, 1980.

Furie, B.: Using oral anticoagulants effectively, Drug Therapy **9**(9): 108, 1979.

Honig, G.R.: Coagulation vitamin deficiencies, Drug Therapy **5**(3): 108, 1975.

Suttie, J.W.: How coumarin anticoagulants work, Drug Therapy **9**(9): 117, 1979.

Clot dissolution

Marder, V.J.: When to consider thrombolytic therapy, Patient Care **12:**190, July 15, 1978.

Marder, V.J.: The use of thrombolytic agents: choice of patient, drug administration, laboratory monitoring, Annals of Internal Medicine **90:**802, 1979.

Sasahara, A.A., Ho, D.D., and Sharma, G.V.R.K.: When and how to use fibrinolytic agents, Drug Therapy **9**(12):67, 1979.

Streptokinase and urokinase, The Medical Letter **20:**37, April 12, 1978.

18 Drugs to lower blood lipid levels

■ ORIGIN OF BLOOD LIPIDS AND THEIR ROLE IN ATHEROSCLEROSIS

There are two main types of lipids in the blood: triglyceride and cholesterol. These lipids are bound to special proteins to form soluble lipoproteins. There are four major classes of lipoproteins: chylomicrons, very low density lipoproteins (VLDL), low density lipoproteins (LDL), and high density lipoproteins (HDL). Chylomicrons and VLDL are composed largely of triglycerides and function to transport triglycerides to tissues for metabolic use or storage. LDL and HDL serve to transport cholesterol. The role and composition of the lipoproteins are summarized in Fig. 18-1.

■ Chylomicrons

Chylomicrons are very large lipoproteins that contain about 90% triglyceride by weight. After a meal the ingested fat is processed by the intestine into chylomicrons, which are transported through the lymphatic system to the plasma. Chylomicrons are normally found in the blood only during the 8 to 12 hours after a meal. Since chylomicrons represent dietary fat, patients being evaluated for triglyceride abnormalities should not eat for 12 to 16 hours before a blood sample is drawn.

■ Very low density lipoproteins (VLDL)

The VLDL are 60% triglyceride by weight. This triglyceride pool is synthesized by the liver from carbohydrate sources for export as fuel to other tissues. Triglycerides cannot be transported directly into cells for use. Tissues that use triglycerides, particularly muscle and fat tissues, secrete an enzyme called *lipoprotein lipase,* which breaks down the triglycerides to fatty acids and glycerol, compounds that can be taken into the cells.

■ Low density lipoproteins (LDL)

The LDL are only 5% triglyceride but are 50% cholesterol by weight. The LDL are the remains of the VLDL after removal of triglycerides and some protein. When cells need cholesterol, they synthesize receptors for LDL. The LDL bind to these receptors and are taken into the cell by pinocytosis and degraded. Most cells are also capable of synthesizing cholesterol, but this synthesis is turned off when the cholesterol from LDL is being utilized. When the cell has sufficient cholesterol, the cell stops making LDL receptors.

Role of LDL in atherosclerosis. Recent studies have examined the role of LDL in atherosclerosis because the concentration of LDL reflects the total cholesterol concentration. An increased total plasma cholesterol concentration is linked to an increased incidence of atherosclerosis. When there is an injury to the epithelial cells of arteries or when the amount of circulating LDL becomes very high, the receptor mechanism controlling LDL uptake no longer operates properly and the cell becomes overwhelmed with cholesterol. This is believed to be one beginning of atherosclerotic plaques. Platelets from the blood may also play a role in initiating atherosclerosis. Aggregated platelets release factors that stimulate smooth muscle growth. This stimulation of growth heals the minute breaks in the normal blood vessel. When the epithelial cells are overloaded with cholesterol and aggregated platelets stimulate an overgrowth of smooth muscle cells, an atherosclerotic plaque is formed. The eventual outcome of atherosclerosis is the narrowing of an artery so that the blood flow is reduced and may not be sufficient to maintain tissue function. Reduced blood flow also favors the formation of a clot that may completely obstruct flow. A stroke may result when the cerebral arteries are involved, or a myocardial infarction may result when the coronary arteries are involved. When the legs are involved, limbs may be lost from gangrene. Renovascular hypertension is associated with atherosclerosis.

■ High density lipoproteins (HDL)

The last major category of lipoproteins is the high density lipoproteins (HDL). The HDL are 50% protein, 20% cholesterol, and 5% triglyceride by weight. Only about 20% of the total plasma cholesterol is found in HDL. Until recently the HDL were not widely studied. It now appears that the HDL play a very important role in removing excess cholesterol from peripheral tissues. HDL can remove cholesterol from cells and can inhibit the uptake of LDL by cells. Recent studies indicate that persons with high concentrations of HDL have a lower incidence of atherosclerosis and the related problems of heart disease and strokes.

FIG. 18-1

Diagram of origin and fate of lipids. Sites of action of drugs that can lower excessive plasma concentrations of lipids: *(1)* Drugs that lower cholesterol by increasing the excretion of bile acids—cholestyramines and cholestipol. *(2)* Drugs that lower triglycerides by inhibiting hepatic triglyceride synthesis—clofibrate and niacin. *(3)* Drug that lowers cholesterol by stimulating LDL degradation—dextrothyroxine. *(4)* Drug that lowers cholesterol by inhibiting synthesis—probucol. *(5)* Drug that lowers cholesterol by inhibiting cholesterol absorption—beta sitosterol. Within the circles the clear areas denote the proportion of triglyceride; the stippled area denotes protein; the dark area denotes cholesterol; and the cross-hatched area denotes phospholipid.

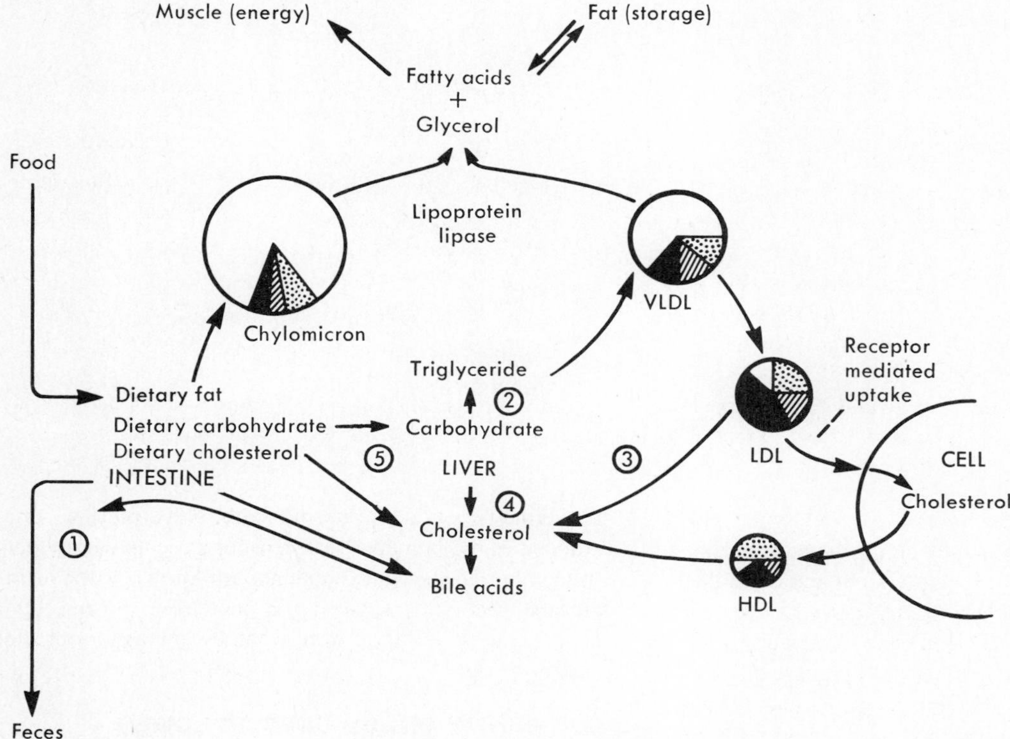

The liver can degrade cholesterol to bile acids, which are excreted into the small intestine. Bile acids emulsify lipids to aid in fat absorption. Some bile acids are absorbed into the portal vein for transport back to the liver. This circulation between the liver and small intestine is called *enterohepatic circulation*.

■ HYPERLIPIDEMIA

■ Origin and types of hyperlipidemia

Hyperlipidemia is associated with an abnormal concentration of one or more of the four lipoproteins. Five major types of hyperlipidemia have been described, depending on which lipoproteins are present in abnormally high concentrations. Since it is easier to measure cholesterol than to measure LDL and easier to measure triglyceride than to measure VLDL, hyperlipidemias are usually detected by measuring cholesterol and triglyceride. The characteristics of the five types of hyperlipidemia are given in Table 18-1. All hyperlipidemias can be genetically determined but may also be secondary to diabetes, obesity, alcoholism, hypothyroidism, and liver and kidney disease. Only two kinds of hyperlipidemias are commonly encountered: type II and type IV.

Type II hyperlipidemia is characterized by high concentrations of LDL but normal or modestly increased amounts of VLDL. Persons with elevated LDL are those most at risk for atherosclerosis. In genetically determined type II hyperlipidemia, patients who are homozygous for the type II trait have evidence of severe heart disease by age 20. In addition, type II hyperlipidemia can occur in individuals who are obese, are hypothyroid, or suffer from liver or kidney disease.

Type IV hyperlipidemia is characterized by high concentrations of VLDL with relatively normal levels of LDL. It is the most common lipid abnormality and also carries a high risk of coronary artery disease. Type IV hyperlipidemia is common among patients who have diabetes, are obese, or are alcoholics. Oral contraceptives or estrogen can elicit type IV hyperlipidemia in some women.

The two common types of hyperlipidemia are associated with a high production of triglycerides (type IV) or

TABLE 18-1. Types of hyperlipidemias

	Type I	Type II	Type III	Type IV	Type V
Lipoprotein content of fasting plasma					
1. Chylomicrons	Markedly increased	Absent	May be present	Absent	Increased
2. VLDL	Normal or decreased	Normal or increased	Increased	Increased	Increased
3. LDL	Normal or decreased	Increased	Increased	Normal	Normal or decreased
Lipids					
Cholesterol	Increased	Increased	Increased	Normal or increased	Increased
Triglyceride	Increased	Normal or increased	Increased	Increased	Increased
Incidence	Rare	Common	Relatively uncommon	Common	Relatively uncommon
Usual age at detection	Early childhood	Early adulthood (can be detected in infancy or childhood)	Early adulthood	Adulthood (middle age)	Early adulthood
Risk of atherosclerosis	Normal	Greatly increased	Greatly increased	Probably increased	Unknown

cholesterol (type II) by the liver. Type IV hyperlipidemia (high VLDL) is often well controlled by calorie restriction with emphasis on losing weight and on reducing carbohydrates from which the liver synthesizes triglycerides. A decrease in foods high in cholesterol such as egg yolk, liver, and shellfish and a decrease in saturated fats are recommended dietary modifications for patients with type II hyperlipidemia. When diet alone does not reduce blood lipid levels to acceptable ranges, a few drugs have been found effective for lowering the concentration of blood lipids. The type of hyperlipidemia determines which drug may be effective. These drugs have not been in use long enough to evaluate whether they have long-term side effects or indeed whether their use lowers mortality.

■ Role of drug therapy in treating hyperlipidemia

The Coronary Drug Project trial studied men with coronary atherosclerosis who were treated with clofibrate, dextrothyroxine, or niacin to lower blood lipid concentration. None of the drugs reduced mortality, and dextrothyroxine increased mortality. This study was limited, but it should be emphasized that at present there is no proof that lowering blood lipid concentrations in a patient with atherosclerosis will reverse or even halt atherosclerosis. Moreover, there are no prospective studies proving that intervention by diet or drugs to lower high blood lipid concentration in those persons at risk through family history, obesity, or diabetes will improve the person's long-term health. Nevertheless, some authorities recommend treatment for patients with hyperlipidemia because these patients are known to be at increased risk and because the increased plasma lipid levels can be reduced somewhat by therapy with diet and/or drugs.

■ SPECIFIC DRUGS USED TO LOWER BLOOD LIPID LEVELS (Table 18-2)

Cholestyramine resin

Cholestyramine (Questran) is a resin with a sandlike texture that stays in the intestine and binds bile acids. Bile acids are the degradation products of cholesterol produced in the liver and excreted into the intestine through the biliary tract. The binding of bile acids by cholestyramine decreases the reabsorption of bile acid through the enterohepatic circulation and therefore increases the amount of fecal bile acid. Thus the effect of cholestyramine is to increase the excretion of cholesterol, but the drug must be taken several times a day to achieve this goal. Cholestyramine is effective in treating type II hyperlipidemia (high LDL) only.

The patient may experience bloating, nausea, and constipation at the beginning of therapy with cholestyramine. During therapy cholestyramine may interfere with the absorption of fat-soluble vitamins (A, D, K), digitalis, thyroxine, and coumarin anticoagulants.

Colestipol hydrochloride

Colestipol (Colestid) is a new drug similar to cholestyramine.

TABLE 18-2. Drugs lowering blood lipid concentrations

Generic name	Trade name	Dosage and administration	Comments
Cholestyramine resin	Questran	ORAL: *Adults*—4 Gm 4 times daily (at meals and bedtime). May be increased to 6 Gm 4 times daily. Alternatively, the dosage may be divided into 2 or 3 doses. Material must be mixed with a liquid (1 oz for each gram). *Children*—over 6 yr, 8 Gm twice daily with meals. Total maximum dosage, 24 Gm daily.	Type II hyperlipidemia (high LDL). This resin stays in the intestine removing bile acids and thereby increasing cholesterol degradation by the liver.
Colestipol hydrochloride	Colestid	ORAL: *Adults*—15 to 30 Gm daily in 2 to 4 doses with meals. Mix 1 oz liquid with each 4 to 6 Gm. *Children*—not established.	Like cholestyramine.
Clofibrate	Atromid-S	ORAL: *Adults*—500 mg 3 to 4 times daily.	Types III, IV, and V hyperlipidemia. Type II hyperlipidemia if VLDL is elevated. Inhibits triglyceride synthesis in the liver and inhibits the breakdown of triglycerides in fat tissue.
Niacin (nicotinic acid)	Nicobid* Niac* Nicolar Wampocap	ORAL: *Adults*—initially 100 mg 3 times daily, increasing to a total of 2 to 6 Gm daily in divided doses with or after meals.	Types II, III, IV, and V hyperlipidemia. Inhibits the synthesis of VLDL by the liver.
Aluminum nicotinate	Nicolex	ORAL: *Adults*—2.5 to 7.5 Gm in 3 divided doses with or after meals.	Like niacin.
Dextrothyroxine	Choloxin	ORAL: *Adults*—with normal thyroid function, initially, 1 to 2 mg daily. May be increased monthly by 1 to 2 mg to a maximum of 8 mg daily (4 mg daily maximum in patients taking digitalis). *Children*—initially, 0.05 mg/kg body weight. May be increased monthly by 0.05 mg/kg to a maximum daily dose of 4 mg.	Type II hyperlipidemia. Lowers cholesterol by increasing LDL degradation.
Probucol	Lorelco	ORAL: *Adults*—500 mg twice daily (with breakfast and dinner). *Children*—not established.	Type II hyperlipidemia. Lowers cholesterol probably by inhibiting cholesterol biosynthesis in the liver.
Beta sitosterol	Cytellin	ORAL: *Adults*—12 to 24 mg daily. Divide to take just before meals and snacks.	Type II hyperlipidemia. Inhibits cholesterol uptake in the intestine. An aid when a low-cholesterol diet is indicated.

*Timed-release forms.

Clofibrate

Clofibrate (Atromid S) inhibits triglyceride synthesis by the liver and thereby reduces the formation of VLDL. Cholesterol synthesis may also be inhibited. Clofibrate is used to treat type IV hyperlipidemia, type II if there is elevated VLDL, and the rare types III and V.

Clofibrate produces few side effects. About 10% of patients initially experience some gastrointestinal upset. Long-term use of clofibrate has not been shown to reduce mortality and does increase the incidence of gallstones. Clofibrate may cause muscle cramps and impotence in men and should be used with caution in patients with liver or kidney disease. It is contraindicated during pregnancy or for nursing mothers. Clofibrate displaces several drugs from albumin, including coumarins, phenytoin, and tolbutamide. The higher concentration of displaced drug can cause toxic effects.

Niacin (nicotinic acid) and aluminum nicotinate

Niacin is a B vitamin for which the minimum daily requirement (MDR) is 20 mg. At doses 10 to 20 times higher than the MDR, niacin is a vasodilator (Chap-

■ THE NURSING PROCESS

■ Assessment

The need for drugs to lower blood lipid levels is often diagnosed as an incidental finding in patients when blood is drawn for another purpose and elevated cholesterol and/or triglyceride levels are found. Occasionally a suspected family history of hyperlipidemia leads to the diagnosis. Finally, some physicians may elect to use these drugs in patients with a history of atherosclerosis, regardless of triglyceride or cholesterol levels. Baseline assessment would include a general assessment of the patient, including the following: weight, serum cholesterol and triglyceride levels, blood pressure, and dietary history.

■ Management

These drugs have few associated side effects when used in usual doses. Any new sign or symptom the patient develops should be evaluated. Discharge planning should include instruction by the dietitian, particularly if the type of hyperlipidemia can be better treated by a dietary restriction and/or weight loss.

■ Evaluation

Ideally, effective use of these drugs would be validated by longer life span, but this cannot be easily proven. These drugs can be regarded as effective if the serum triglyceride or cholesterol levels approach normal. By the time of discharge, the patient should be able to explain why and how to take the prescribed drug, when it should be taken in relation to meals, anticipated side effects and what to do about them, which symptoms should be reported immediately to the physician, and how to plan meals within prescribed dietary restrictions. Finally, the patient should recognize that since the prescribed drug may interfere with other drugs, all health care providers should be kept informed about the drugs the patient is taking.

---

ter 13). At doses 100 to 200 times higher than the MDR, niacin depresses the synthesis of VLDL by the liver and thereby reduces LDL as well. Niacin is effective in treating types II, III, IV, and V hyperlipidemias. However, the high doses needed produce troublesome side effects in most patients, and only a few patients can tolerate continued use of niacin. Most patients experience marked flushing due to the vasodilator action of niacin. Itching and gastrointestinal upset are also frequent side effects. Tolerance may develop to all of these symptoms, so the dosage is usually started low and increased gradually to avoid severe reactions to the high doses. Aluminum nicotinate (Nicolex) is formulated to be hydrolyzed to niacin and aluminum hydroxide in the intestine to avoid gastric irritation. Aluminum hydroxide can interfere with the absorption of other drugs, however. Niacin can cause or aggravate peptic ulcer, glucose intolerance (diabetes), and high plasma uric acid (gout).

Dextrothyroxine

Dextrothyroxine (Choloxin) is the inactive stereoisomer of the hormone thyroxine. Dextrothyroxine enhances the degradation of LDL and thereby lowers plasma cholesterol levels. Since the action is to lower LDL, dextrothyroxine is only useful for type II hyperlipidemia. When plasma cholesterol levels are high, dextrothyroxine will produce a 20% to 30% decrease in 1 to 2 months. Side effects during this time include dizziness, diarrhea, and an altered sense of taste. Some patients show symptoms of hyperthyroidism: weight loss, nervousness, insomnia, sweating, and menstrual irregularities. Some patients may show hypersensitivity to iodine with itching or a rash. Angina may be aggravated.

Dextrothyroxine can decrease glucose tolerance in diabetic patients. The action of coumarin anticoagulants is enhanced by dextrothyroxine. Contraindications for dextrothyroxine include pregnancy and hypertension, as well as heart, renal, or liver disease. Since these latter conditions are common among patients with type II hyperlipidemia, the use of dextrothyroxine is limited.

Probucol

Probucol (Lorelco) is a new drug that inhibits cholesterol synthesis. Probucol decreases plasma LDL and cholesterol and therefore is potentially useful for type II hyperlipidemia. The main side effects of probucol are those of gastrointestinal upset: diarrhea, gas, abdominal pain, nausea, and vomiting. The long-term effects and effectiveness of probucol have not yet been established.

Beta sitosterol

Beta sitosterol (Cytellin) is a mixture of plant compounds resembling cholesterol. Sitosterols interfere with the absorption of cholesterol from the gastrointestinal tract. Patients with type II hyperlipidemia who must maintain low cholesterol intake may benefit from beta sitosterol. The main side effect is that bulky, loose stools are produced.

■ Other drugs used as lipid-lowering agents

Conjugated estrogens

Conjugated estrogens have been used as lipid-lowering agents because of the observation that premenopausal women have a low incidence of heart attacks. However, recent studies show that estrogen given to men not only feminizes them but also increases the incidence of heart attacks.

Progestins and androgens

Progestins may decrease hyperlipidemia in women with the rare type V hyperlipidemia. Progestins make other types of hyperlipidemia worse and cannot be used for men. Anabolic androgens may reduce elevated plasma triglyceride concentrations in men only. Androgens can cause water retention and therefore must be used with care in men with heart, kidney, or liver disease.

Neomycin

Neomycin is an antibiotic that is not well absorbed. Neomycin prevents cholesterol absorption in the intestine, thereby promoting bile acid secretion. These effects may lower elevated LDL levels in some patients with type II hyperlipidemia.

■ PATIENT CARE IMPLICATIONS

General guidelines for patients with hyperlipidemia

1. Patients requiring diet modification will probably benefit from referral to a dietitian. Diet requirements can become very complicated if patients need to limit calories, carbohydrates, saturated fats, cholesterol, sodium, potassium, and other component parts of their diet based on other medical needs. Patient education is important for patient compliance.
2. Even the most health-oriented patients will on occasion stop following their diets. Eating habits are usually developed over many years and for many reasons, and eating habits are also strongly influenced by family traditions and habits. Health care practitioners should not view noncompliance with dietary restrictions as an indication of personal or patient failure. Instead the health care team should maintain patience, try to put themselves into the patient's place (many severely restricted diets are boring, bland, and unpalatable), provide positive reinforcement when the patient persists with a diet, be nonjudgmental when a patient fails, and continue to individualize the health care teaching and patient approaches.
3. In hereditary hyperlipidemia, it will be necessary to screen children for the presence of the hyperlipidemia and to place them on special diets also.
4. Many of the drugs used to lower blood lipid levels need to be taken for 3 months or more before effects can be seen. Drugs should not be continued indefinitely if there is no positive response to them.
5. If a drug does produce a desired effect in lowering blood lipid levels, it is important that the patient understand that it may be necessary to continue treatment for years.
6. The safe use of these drugs during pregnancy has not been established. Women of childbearing age may wish to use birth control measures while receiving drug therapy with these drugs and to continue birth control for several months after drug therapy is discontinued to protect against possible birth defects. The use of these drugs during lactation is not recommended. Women should discuss the risks versus benefits with their physicians.
7. Remind patients to keep these and all medications out out of the reach of children.

Cholestyramine and colestipol

1. These two drugs should be taken before meals.
2. Oral administration of cholestyramine or colestipol:
   a. Neither drug should be taken in its dry form. Always mix with fluid or with food or fruit having a high fluid content.
   b. Fill a glass with 4 to 6 ounces of water, milk, or juice. Put the correct dose of medication on top of the fluid and let it stand, without stirring, for 1 to 2 minutes. This allows the medicine to absorb moisture and will help prevent lumps. Stir and drink the mixture while the drug is still suspended. Add a little more of the selected beverage to rinse the glass, and drink this also.
   c. Applesauce, crushed pineapple, and soups with high fluid content may also be used.
   d. Carbonated beverages may be used, but the addition of the medication will cause excessive foaming initially, so a large glass should be used.
3. Because these two drugs interfere with absorption of the fat-soluble vitamins, supplemental vitamins may be necessary. Vitamin K deficiency would be manifested by a tendency to bleed (Chapter 17).
4. Because cholestyramine or colestipol may adsorb other drugs given with them, other medications that

the patient receives should be given 1 hour before or 4 to 6 hours after but not at the same time as cholestyramine or cholestipol. If therapeutic dosage levels for a drug have been determined while a patient was receiving cholestyramine or colestipol and the antilipemic drug is then discontinued, the dose of the other medication may then be too high. This has occurred with digitalis preparations and oral anticoagulants.

5. If constipation is a chronic problem, dietary manipulation (daily prune juice, increasing fluid intake, increasing the intake of roughage) may help, or a stool softener can be prescribed. It may be necessary to reduce the dose of the antilipemic drug.
6. These two drugs may be prescribed to treat the pruritus of biliary stasis. When the drug is discontinued, the pruritus may reappear.

Clofibrate

1. The side effects most frequently seen are abdominal distress, flatulence, loose stools, muscle cramps, headache, fatigue, and urticaria. Less frequently reported side effects include hair loss (alopecia), increased or decreased incidence of angina, cardiac arrhythmias, impotence and decreased libido, and proteinuria. Reported alterations in blood values include elevations of serum transaminase levels. Long-term follow-up of the effects of clofibrate therefore includes careful questioning about side effects and blood analysis, urinalysis, and cardiac assessment.
2. The patient with chest pain may have elevated serum transaminase levels because of chronic clofibrate use, myocardial damage, or both.
3. Caution must be used in titrating the dose of other drugs, which may be displaced from albumin binding sites by clofibrate (see text). A specific example is coumarin. As little as one half the usual dose of a coumarin anticoagulant may produce adequate anticoagulation in a patient receiving clofibrate. Frequent prothrombin level determinations are needed until the correct coumarin dose is established. See Chapter 17 for a discussion of anticoagulation.
4. Displacement of tolbutamide may result in more frequent episodes of hypoglycemia (Chapter 39).

Niacin preparations

1. Review the discussion in the text.
2. Some patients will find that taking niacin preparations with meals or in a sustained-release form will decrease the severity of side effects.
3. Patients taking beta adrenergic antagonists such as propranolol (Inderal) for hypertension may have an increased incidence of hypotensive episodes when niacin is added to their medications.
4. Many patients with type III, IV, and V hyperlipidemias already suffer from gout or diabetes and will be unable to tolerate aggravation of these diseases by the niacin preparations.
5. Nicotinamide (niacinamide), the niacin component of many multivitamin preparations, does not produce the characteristic blushing (vasodilation) seen with other niacin formulations. Nicotinamide does not lower plasma cholesterol levels, so this preparation is useful only in vitamin replacement or in treatment of pellagra, a disease caused specifically by niacin deficiency. For additional information about the role of dietary niacin, refer to a text on nutrition.
6. Preparations are available for intramuscular and intravenous administration, although oral administration is the usual route. Intravenous nicotinic acid may be given undiluted or diluted in sodium chloride. The rate of administration should not exceed 2 mg per minute.

Dextrothyroxine

1. Refer to Chapter 36. Treatment with dextrothyroxine mimics treatment with any thyroid medication. Overdose would result in symptoms of hyperthyroidism. The necessary dose of anticoagulant is usually less in patients receiving this drug, and diabetics will often find it necessary to readjust their insulin dosage.
2. Note that patients taking digitalis preparations are particularly susceptible to cardiac side effects when both drugs are being taken concomitantly. The patient receiving digitalis should not exceed a total dose of 4 mg of dextrothyroxine. The effects of both drugs should be monitored carefully (Chapter 15).

Probucol

1. Absorption of probucol is increased if the drug is taken with meals.
2. So far there have been no reported drug interactions with anticoagulants or hypoglycemic agents in patients also receiving probucol.

Beta sitosterol

1. This drug may interfere with the absorption of other drugs. The practitioner should assess the effectiveness of other drugs the patient is receiving. Taking other drugs 1 hour before or 4 to 6 hours after taking beta sitosterol may help alleviate the problem.
2. Loose stools are a problem caused, at least in part, by the methylcellulose derivative that is used as a dispersing agent. Reducing the amount of roughage in the diet may help with this problem.

3. Oral administration of beta sitosterol:
   a. The drug is supplied as a suspension. Mixing it with coffee, tea, fruit juices, or milk may increase the palatability.
   b. Teach patients to spread out their total daily dose so that some is taken before each meal or large snack. A suggested way of dividing the dose would be 1 T (1 tablespoonful equals approximately 15 ml) before an average sized meal, 1½ to 2 T before a large meal, and ½ to 1 T before a snack.

■ SUMMARY

Hyperlipidemia refers to greater than normal concentrations of plasma cholesterol or plasma triglycerides. High concentrations of plasma cholesterol are associated with an increased incidence of atherosclerosis, whereas high concentrations of plasma triglycerides are associated with an increased incidence of coronary heart disease. Genetics, diet, and metabolic disease each can be linked to hyperlipidemia.

Diet modification is the major therapeutic approach for treating the common types of hyperlipidemia. Drugs may be added if diet alone is not effective. Drugs acting to lower plasma cholesterol levels include cholestyramine, colestipol, dextrothyroxine, probucol, and beta sitosterol. Drugs acting to lower plasma triglyceride concentrations include clofibrate and niacin.

■ STUDY QUESTIONS

1. List the four categories of lipoproteins and describe the role of each.
2. What is hyperlipidemia? What causes hyperlipidemia?
3. Name five drugs and their mechanism of action for lowering plasma cholesterol.
4. Name two drugs and their mechanism of action for lowering triglycerides.

■ SUGGESTED READINGS

Blackburn, H.: The public health view of diet and mass hyperlipidemia, Cardiovascular Review and Reports **1**:361, 1980.

Coronary Drug Project Research Group: Clofibrate and niacin in coronary heart disease, Journal of the American Medical Association **231**:360, 1975.

Czerwinski, B.S.: Manual of patient education for cardiopulmonary dysfunctions, St. Louis, 1980, The C.V. Mosby Co.

Eder, H.A.: What to do about the lipids to-do, Patient Care **14**:14, Oct. 30, 1980.

Giving cardiovascular drugs safely, Nursing Skillbook, Horsham, Pa., 1978, Intermed Communications, Inc.

Marx, J.L.: Atherosclerosis: the cholesterol connection, Science **194**: 711, 1976.

Williams, S.R.: Essentials of nutrition and diet therapy, ed. 2, St. Louis, 1978, The C.V. Mosby Co.

19 Drugs to treat nutritional anemias

■ IRON

■ Functions of iron

Iron is an essential component of several key proteins that function to carry oxygen or to utilize oxygen. Over 70% of body iron is part of hemoglobin, the protein of red blood cells that transfers oxygen to tissues and carbon dioxide away from tissues. The red color of blood is due to the iron-oxygen complex in the heme portion of hemoglobin. Iron is also part of myoglobin, the oxygen-carrying protein of muscle, and part of several of the electron transport enzymes of the mitochondria responsible for the oxidation-reduction reactions so essential to every functioning cell.

■ Absorption, storage, and excretion of iron

Given the importance of iron, it is not surprising that the body uses iron efficiently. The total iron content of a 70 kg man is about 4 Gm, yet iron is reused so efficiently that less than 1 mg of iron is lost daily. This small requirement is due to the extreme conservation of iron by the body. Not only is the iron of the red blood cell reused after degradation of the cell, but 10% to 35% of the body's iron is in a storage form for use when required. Iron is lost only as body cells are lost through shedding of cells from the gastrointestinal tract, skin, fingernails, and hair and as fluids such as bile, urine, and sweat are lost.

The absorption of iron from food is regulated. Iron is taken up by active transport into the mucosal cells of the duodenum and upper jejunum in the small intestine. These cells contain the protein ferritin, which binds the iron. When the ferritin is saturated with iron, further absorption of iron is limited. Iron remains in the mucosal cells unless transferred to the plasma protein transferrin. Iron not transferred within 5 days is lost in the feces as the mucosal cell is sloughed. Iron bound to transferrin is carried in the plasma and transferred to the proteins ferritin and hemosiderin, which act as storage forms of iron within the liver, spleen, and bone marrow.

■ Iron as a therapeutic agent

Iron deficiency anemia. When the intake of iron is inadequate to meet the demand, iron is first taken from the iron stores in hemosiderin and ferritin. Absorption of iron from the gastrointestinal tract can increase twofold when the ferritin within the mucosal cells is no longer saturated with iron. When iron stores are exhausted and the intake of iron is still inadequate, the newly made red blood cells are small (microcytic) and do not have much color (hypochromic) because there is not enough iron to make an adequate amount of hemoglobin to fill the cells. Iron deficiency anemia is therefore a microcytic, hypochromic anemia.

Requirements for iron. Iron deficiency anemia commonly results from one of two causes: blood loss or rapid growth. This is reflected in the varying requirements for dietary iron. The average American diet contains about 6 mg of iron/1000 calories, and only 10% of dietary iron is actually absorbed, although up to 20% may be absorbed in an individual who is deficient in iron. Adult men and postmenopausal women have the lowest daily requirement for dietary iron (5 to 10 mg). Menstruating women have a higher daily requirement, depending on the amount of blood loss they have during menstruation (7 to 20 mg). Pregnant women have the highest daily iron requirement because of the added demand of the placenta and developing fetus (20 to 58 mg). Children and adolescents have a higher requirement per unit weight than adults because of their rapid growth (4 to 20 mg total).

Administration of replacement iron. Iron for replacement therapy is most commonly given orally as a ferrous salt. Iron preparations are listed in Table 19-1. Ferrous sulfate is the standard for these preparations. The usual daily dose for iron replacement in iron deficiency anemia is 50 to 100 mg of iron. The amount of iron per tablet depends on the ferrous salt used. A 300 mg tablet of ferrous sulfate contains 60 mg of iron and 240 mg of sulfate; a 300 mg tablet of ferrous gluconate contains 37 mg of iron and 263 mg of gluconate; and a 300 mg tablet of ferrous fumarate contains 99 mg of iron and 201 mg of fumarate.

Iron is absorbed most readily in the ferrous form in the presence of acid. Therefore optimal absorption occurs when a tablet of ferrous sulfate or other soluble ferrous salt is taken before meals. However, iron is also

TABLE 19-1. Drugs to treat nutritional anemias

Generic name	Trade name	Dosage and administration	Comments
IRON SALTS FOR IRON DEFICIENCY ANEMIA			
Ferrous sulfate (20% elemental iron)	Feosol Fer-In-Sol Fero-Gradumet Mol-Iron	Replacement therapy requires 90 to 300 mg of elemental iron daily in divided doses before meals if tolerated or with meals.	Timed-release or enteric coated forms considered less effective because of poor iron absorption beyond the duodenum.
Ferrous gluconate (11.6% elemental iron)	Fergon Ferralet Plus Entron	See above.	See above.
Ferrocholinate (12% elemental iron)	Chel-Iron Ferrolip Plus Kelex	See above.	See above.
Ferrous fumarate (33% elemental iron)	Ferranol Fumerin Feostat Various others	See above.	See above.
Ferroglycine sulfate (16% elemental iron)	Ferronord	See above.	See above.
Iron-dextran injection	Imferon	INTRAVENOUS: *Adults and children*—no more than 100 mg daily, no faster than 50 mg (1 ml) per minute of the undiluted solution, or dilute in 500 to 1000 ml normal saline solution and administer by drip over 10 hr.	Reserved for use in severe iron deficiency anemia when oral iron is contraindicated (gastrointestinal disease) or unsuccessful. Serious toxic effects, including anaphylaxis, may accompany parenteral administration and are more common with intramuscular than with intravenous administration.
ANTIDOTE FOR IRON TOXICITY			
Deferoxamine mesylate	Desferal Mesylate	INTRAMUSCULAR: preferred route; 1 Gm followed by 0.5 Gm at 4 hr and 8 hr. INTRAVENOUS: in face of cardiovascular collapse; as for intramuscular but infused at 15 mg kg/hr. Not to exceed 6 Gm in 24 hr.	A specific chelator for iron. To manage acute iron intoxication. Will turn urine pink to red. Can be administered long term to manage secondary hemochromatosis.
VITAMIN B_{12} (CYANOCOBALAMIN) FOR PERNICIOUS ANEMIA			
Vitamin B_{12} (cyanocobalamin)	Betalin 12 Crystalline Redisol Rubramin PC Sytobex	INTRAMUSCULAR: 30 to 50 μg daily for 5 to 10 days, then 100 to 200 μg monthly.	For pernicious anemia, only intramuscular injection is effective. Oral forms may be taken for dietary deficiency.
Hydroxocobalamin	AlphaRedisol	As for cyanocobalamin.	Like cyanocobalamin. Somewhat longer acting.
FOLIC ACID FOR ANEMIA			
Folic acid	Folvite	ANY ROUTE: *Adults or children*—1 mg daily.	
Leucovorin calcium	Leucovorin Calcium	For megaloblastic anemia: 1 mg daily. To counter folic acid antagonists: give in amounts equal to the weight of antagonist.	The metabolically active form of folic acid. The expense does not justify its use for anemia, but protects normal tissue when given with methotrexate (antineoplastic drug) or pyramethamine (antimalarial drug)

highly irritating to the gastrointestinal tract, and many patients cannot tolerate iron tablets taken on an empty stomach and have to take iron with meals. Enteric forms of iron are not satisfactory, since they generally dissolve past the duodenum of the small intestine where there is little capacity for the absorption of iron. Infants and children given iron-supplemented formula or vitamins may develop an acute diarrhea from the gastrointestinal irritation.

Patients with iron deficiency anemia respond to iron therapy in the first 2 days with increased energy and appetite. Since this is too soon to correct the hemoglobin deficiency, the response may be due to restoration of the cellular enzymes containing iron. After 1 week there is an increase in the number of reticulocytes (immature red blood cells) and the rate of hemoglobin synthesis. Although the microcytic anemia of iron deficiency is eliminated after a few weeks of therapy, at least 6 months of therapy is necessary to restore iron storage sites.

Iron may also be given parenterally as iron dextran when oral administration is not possible. Slow intravenous injection is preferred. Deep intramuscular injection is painful and can discolor the injection site. An anaphylactic response is more common after intramuscular than after intravenous injection.

Food and drug interactions. Absorption of iron salts is increased with ingestion of large doses of ascorbic acid (vitamin C). Cereal and eggs decrease iron absorption as do antacids, particularly magnesium trisilicate, and tetracyclines because all of these bind iron and prevent its uptake by the mucosal cells in the small intestine.

■ Iron toxicity

Acute toxicity from excess iron. Acute toxicity from iron is uncommon in adults and is primarily seen in young children. The population most likely to be taking iron tablets are pregnant women who may also have small children. Many iron tablets are brightly colored and look like candy, leading young children to swallow many tablets at once. Most commonly the child experiences acute nausea and vomiting 30 to 60 minutes after ingestion of the tablets. The primary treatment is gastric lavage with sodium phosphate or sodium bicarbonate to remove undissolved tablets, to create an alkaline environment that retards absorption, and to complex the ferrous iron into insoluble salts.

Within a few hours of ingestion, metabolic acidosis is common and cardiovascular collapse can occur. If supportive treatment carries the child through these stages, the next stage originates from tissue injury. The high concentration of iron overloads the uptake capacity of the mucosal cells so that a high concentration of free ferrous iron enters the portal circulation. Signs of extensive damage to the liver and kidney are evident in children who die of iron toxicity after 24 hours.

To avoid damage from high plasma concentrations of iron, a specific antidote, *deferoxamine mesylate (Desferal),* is given as soon as possible and concurrently with lavage and supportive measures. Deferoxamine is given intramuscularly or intravenously, and in the plasma it combines with iron to form a water-soluble complex that is excreted in the urine (67%) and in the bile (33%). This complex gives a pink to red color to the urine and is evidence of elevated concentrations of iron in the plasma. The free deferoxamine gives no color to the urine.

Chronic toxicity from iron overload. Since the body has no mechanisms to get rid of excess iron, excess intake of iron can cause iron overload, called *hemosiderosis* after the storage protein for iron. Chronic iron overload can occur in patients treated with parenteral iron or in patients who receive frequent blood transfusions, since each milliliter of blood contains 0.5 mg of iron. Some patients have a genetic tendency to store excess iron; this genetic disorder is called *hemochromatosis*. Iron overload traditionally causes a bronze color of the skin of the face, neck, upper chest, genitalia, hands, and forearms. The pancreas is especially sensitive to damage, and diabetes mellitus can result. Liver damage is seen on biopsy but is generally not serious unless superimposed on liver disease. Patients with iron overload generally die of heart failure. Treatment of iron overload is weekly bleeding (phlebotomy).

■ MEGALOBLASTIC MACROCYTIC ANEMIAS

Both vitamin B_{12} and folic acid are required for a key reaction in the synthesis of thymidylate, a component of deoxyribonucleic acid (DNA). Whereas folic acid is the immediate cofactor in this synthesis, vitamin B_{12} is necessary to regenerate the active form of folic acid. A deficiency of either folic acid or vitamin B_{12} results in the release of too few red blood cells. Those red blood cells that are released are large and immature because of the deficiency of DNA synthesis required for cell division and maturation. This is a *megaloblastic* (immature) *macrocytic* (large cell) anemia. Other tissue cells that turn over rapidly and require an active DNA synthesis include some white cells and mucosal cells of the gastrointestinal tract. A deficiency in white cell counts may therefore appear, as can gastrointestinal upset in vitamin B_{12} or folic acid deficiency.

■ Vitamin B_{12} and pernicious anemia

Vitamin B_{12} is a unique vitamin because it requires a special binding protein for transport into the intestinal cells. This binding protein is called *intrinsic factor,* and it is produced and released by the parietal cells of the stomach. (Parietal cells also release hydrochloric acid.) Pernicious anemia is the relative or complete lack of intrinsic factor so that vitamin B_{12} is no longer absorbed. The body has a large store of vitamin B_{12}, 4 to 5 mg, and a deficiency will not occur for 2 to 5 years after intrinsic factor is no longer released. Stomach atrophy is a normal part of the aging process, and pernicious anemia appears more frequently in patients over 50 years old than in younger patients. Any condition that damages the stomach can also cause pernicious anemia.

Origin, absorption, and distribution of vitamin B_{12}. A diet including animal protein, eggs, and dairy products contains adequate vitamin B_{12}. The usual American diet contains 5 to 15 μg of vitamin B_{12}, although the minimum daily requirement is only 1 to 2 μg of vitamin B_{12}. Only strict vegetarians may develop dietary vitamin B_{12} deficiency over a period of several years. Vitamin B_{12} bound to intrinsic factor is absorbed in the distal ileum, the part of the small intestine just before the large intestine, and this absorption requires a slightly alkaline pH. Conditions in which the distal ileum is damaged or removed or in which the pancreas fails to secrete sufficient bicarbonate to keep the intestine at a slightly alkaline pH will slow absorption of vitamin B_{12}. After absorption, vitamin B_{12} is carried to storage sites. Some vitamin B_{12} is excreted in the bile but is then reabsorbed.

Neurological damage from vitamin B_{12} deficiency. A deficiency of vitamin B_{12} is especially serious because neurological damage may result. This damage arises because vitamin B_{12} is a cofactor for an enzymatic step necessary for producing the myelin sheath of nerves. A frequent initial neurological symptom of vitamin B_{12} deficiency is a tingling sensation of the extremities (paresthesia) from this neurological damage. Neurological damage becomes irreversible if vitamin B_{12} deficiency persists.

Administration of replacement vitamin B_{12} (Table 19-1). The intramuscular injection of vitamin B_{12} to bypass the intestine for systemic absorption is the treatment for pernicious anemia. Initial therapy is administered daily for about 1 week, then monthly throughout life. Oral vitamin B_{12} is indicated only for the rare dietary deficiency of vitamin B_{12} when there is an adequate amount of intrinsic factor released.

Vitamin B_{12} injections have been given indiscriminately to older patients as a general tonic, which it is not. Vitamin B_{12} injections are also not of therapeutic value for general neurological disorders, psychiatric disorders, general malnutrition, or loss of appetite. It is important also to realize that folic acid taken in large doses will overcome the block in DNA synthesis caused by the deficiency of vitamin B_{12}. Folic acid will thereby cure the anemia, but folic acid cannot affect the vitamin B_{12}–dependent reaction necessary for myelin synthesis. If folic acid is taken indiscriminately, the anemia of vitamin B_{12} deficiency will never appear but neurological damage may proceed until damage is irreversible.

Vitamin B_{12} injections are virtually free of side effects. Patients receiving vitamin B_{12} injections for pernicious anemia must understand that injections must be continued for the rest of their lives to avoid irreversible neurological damage.

■ Folic acid and anemia

Folic acid is found in most meats, fresh vegetables, and fresh fruits but is destroyed when these are cooked for longer than 15 minutes. Folic acid preparations are listed in Table 19-1. The minimum daily requirement is 50 μg, and the average American diet contains 200 μg to 300 μg. Unlike stores of vitamin B_{12}, stores of folic acid are not large and can be depleted in a few weeks when the diet is deficient in folic acid. Individuals with poor diets and chronic alcoholics can be deficient in folic acid. Pregnant women and nursing mothers have an increased requirement for folic acid, and folic acid is commonly given as a routine supplement to these women. Folic acid is readily absorbed in the intestine and is given orally.

Some drugs interfere with the utilization of folic acid: phenytoin, oral contraceptives, glucocorticoids, and aspirin. Methotrexate, antineoplastic drugs, and pyrimethamine, an antimalarial drug, are folic acid antagonists. When these drugs are used, *folinic acid (leucovorin),* the metabolically active form of folic acid, can be given to protect normal tissues from folic acid deficiency. Folic acid itself is nontoxic. The greatest danger of indiscriminate ingestion of folic acid is that it may correct the anemia of pernicious anemia but leave the neurological damage untreated.

■ THE NURSING PROCESS

■ Assessment

Patients requiring iron therapy frequently are those with poor nutritional intake, blood loss, or excessive growth; they may be vegetarians, and they are often female. They may appear with fatigue, pallor, and lethargy. Folic acid deficiency and vitamin B_{12} deficiency are usually diagnosed from blood studies but may be seen in patients with iron deficiency anemia. Baseline data would include vital signs; weight; diet history; blood studies including hemoglobin, peripheral blood smear, and reticulocyte count; and the presence of any neurological symptoms such as tingling in the fingers or toes.

■ Management

In the usual prescribed dosages there are few side effects with these drugs. In planning for discharge, dietary instruction should be given when the source of the anemia is dietary. Since cyanocobalamin has occasionally produced anaphylaxis, appropriate drugs and equipment for resuscitation should be available when this drug is administered.

■ Evaluation

The goal of therapy is the return to and the maintenance of a normal blood count and blood profile. Before discharge the patient should be able to explain the kind or kinds of anemia present, the reasons for drug therapy, how to correctly take the prescribed medications, the anticipated side effects and what to do about them, and which symptoms related to the anemia can be expected to improve and which will not. (The neurological damage in pernicious anemia is occasionally permanent.) In addition, the patient should be able to identify dietary sources of needed iron or folic acid. For additional information, see the patient care implications section at the end of this chapter.

■ PATIENT CARE IMPLICATIONS

General guidelines for patients receiving iron therapy

1. Ideally, iron preparations should be taken on an empty stomach, but many individuals cannot tolerate the gastrointestinal irritation that may result. If the drug cannot be taken on an empty stomach, then the patient may be advised to take the drug with meals. Absorption is significantly reduced in the presence of milk, antacids, tetracycline, many cereals, and eggs. Since the absorption is increased with the ingestion of ascorbic acid (vitamin C), some patients may wish to take the iron with orange or another citrus juice.
2. Inform the patient that the color and consistency of feces may change during iron therapy. Feces will be dark green or black in color and more tarry in consistency than usual. If there is doubt about whether the cause of a change in color or consistency in stools is due to blood or to ingestion of iron, the stool should be tested for blood.
3. Some patients will find that regular use of iron preparations will cause diarrhea, whereas others may complain that the iron causes constipation. If the latter occurs, instruct patients to increase their daily fluid intake to at least 3000 ml, to add fiber or roughage to the diet, and to add to the diet foods known by the patient to stimulate defecation, such as coffee, prune juice, or other foods.
4. Decreasing the dose of iron while increasing the frequency of taking the iron may decrease the incidence or severity of side effects.
5. Liquid iron preparations may stain the teeth so should be taken through a straw. Dilute the preparation well with water or fruit juice (see the individual manufacturer's suggestions), and rinse the mouth out well after taking the dose.
6. Intramuscular iron dextran: These preparations should only be administered in the large muscle mass of the buttocks to avoid possible staining of the skin in more frequently visible areas. The following method of administration is suggested to help reduce the possibility of staining. After drawing up the ordered dose, add 0.1 ml of air to the syringe. Discard the needle used to draw up the medication and obtain a new one. Use the Z-tract

method of intramuscular administration, and inject all of the medication and the 0.1 ml of air, the desired effect of the air being to flush any remaining medication out of the needle; then withdraw the needle. For an illustration of the Z-tract method, refer to a fundamentals of nursing textbook.

7. Side effects of parenteral iron may include allergic or anaphylactic responses. In addition, patients may experience febrile reactions, arthralgias, myalgia, headache, transitory paresthesia, nausea, shivering, and rash. Pain often occurs at the injection site. Intravenous administration may cause flushing, hypotension, and phlebitis. Monitor the vital signs. To decrease the possibility of severe anaphylactic reaction, it is suggested that a small test dose of 0.5 ml be given the first day, with the full strength doses begun on the next day. Appropriate drugs (epinephrine, antihistamines, steroids) and resuscitation equipment should be readily available in any setting where parenteral iron is being administered.
8. After an initial test dose, intravenous iron should be injected slowly via direct intravenous push at a rate not to exceed 1 ml (50 mg) per minute.
9. Parenteral iron preparations should not be used concurrently with oral preparations, as the incidence of toxic reactions to the parenteral forms is increased in this situation.
10. Review with the patient the dietary history and instruct as appropriate about modifications that could be made to increase the intake of iron-rich foods. Good sources of dietary iron include fish and meat, especially organ meats (liver, kidney, heart). Beans, prune juice, and iron-enriched cereals and breads are also good sources of iron. If appropriate, refer the patient to a dietitian in the hospital or health department for additional instruction.
11. Remind patients to keep iron preparations and all drugs out of the reach of children. Instruct patients about the signs and symptoms of acute iron overdose (see text), and emphasize the importance of seeking prompt medical attention if overdose is suspected. Because iron preparations are available so readily in over-the-counter preparations, adults may not realize the severity of overdose in children.

Deferoxamine mesylate (Desferal)

1. Patients receiving deferoxamine on a chronic basis should be checked periodically for cataracts.
2. Flushing of the skin, urticaria, and hypotension may occur after rapid intravenous administration. Other side effects of the drug include allergic reactions such as itching, rash and anaphylaxis, dysuria, abdominal discomfort, diarrhea, tachycardia, and fever.
3. The intramuscular route is preferred, although it may cause pain at the injection site. If administered intravenously, the rate of administration should not exceed 15 mg/kg/per hour. Monitor the vital signs.
4. Treatment of iron overdose should be done in the acute care setting where equipment and personnel are available for appropriate monitoring of cardiovascular functioning and treatment of possible circulatory collapse.

Vitamin B_{12}

1. Patients with pernicious anemia need to be taught about the disease. It is often hard for patients to understand why the vitamin B_{12} cannot be taken orally and why it must be continued for life.
2. Cyanocobalamin should never be given intravenously.
3. Side effects are rare but can occur and include diarrhea, itching, feeling of swelling of the entire body, pulmonary edema, congestive heart failure, and anaphylactic shock. Monitor the vital signs after parenteral administration. Observe the patient carefully following the first couple of doses, and instruct the patient to report any unusual signs or symptoms. It may be appropriate to administer a small test dose the day before the first full dose is administered to check for serious reactions to the drug.
4. Note that cyanocobalamin is a component of many multivitamin preparations, whether available by prescription or over the counter.
5. In those rare cases in which vitamin B_{12} is due to dietary causes, review the diet with the patient and instruct the patient about possible sources of the vitamin from the diet. Sources of vitamin B_{12} include animal protein, eggs, and dairy products. If appropriate, refer the patient to the hospital or health department dietitian for additional instruction.

Folic acid

1. Review with patients their usual dietary intake, and instruct as needed about sources of folic acid. Good sources of folic acid include meats, fresh vegetables, and fresh fruits.
2. Note that folic acid is a component of many multivitamin preparations.
3. Leucovorin should be reconstituted as directed on the vial. Use the reconstituted solution as soon as possible; precipitation may occur if it is left standing.

■ SUMMARY

The most common causes of nutritional anemias are deficiencies of iron, vitamin B_{12}, and folic acid.

Iron deficiency anemia is a microcytic, hypochromic anemia. Iron is a required part of hemoglobin, the red-colored protein that carries oxygen in the red blood cells. Normally the body stores 10% to 35% of its iron in reserve, but growth, pregnancy, and menstruation, in addition to a poor diet, can deplete these reserves.

The absorption of iron from the gastrointestinal tract is highly regulated. Because iron is so highly conserved, no route of excretion of any capacity exists for iron. Children ingesting an overdose of iron pills will suffer acute toxicity, which may cause death secondary to damage of the kidney and liver. Deferoxamine is a water-soluble iron chelator, which allows iron to be excreted into the urine and bile.

Pernicious anemia is a deficiency of vitamin B_{12} arising from a lack of intrinsic factor, a protein secreted by the parietal cells of the stomach and required to transport vitamin B_{12} into the body from the gastrointestinal tract. Pernicious anemia will give rise to a megaloblastic anemia because vitamin B_{12} is required to regenerate the folic acid needed for DNA synthesis. More serious is the damage to the myelin sheath of nerves, arising from the lack of vitamin B_{12}. This neurological damage can become irreversible if pernicious anemia is not treated. Replacement of vitamin B_{12} for pernicious anemia must be made by intramuscular injection.

A deficiency of folic acid gives rise to a megaloblastic anemia because folic acid is required for DNA synthesis and the maturation of red blood cells. Folic acid deficiency is most common during pregnancy and in alcoholics.

■ STUDY QUESTIONS

1. What is the role of iron?
2. Describe the factors governing the absorption of iron.
3. What are the symptoms of iron toxicity?
4. How does deferoxamine function as an antidote for iron toxicity?
5. What is pernicious anemia?
6. Why does vitamin B_{12} have to be injected intramuscularly to treat pernicious anemia?
7. What role do vitamin B_{12} and folic acid play in red blood cell maturation?
8. Why is folic acid contraindicated for treatment of pernicious anemia?

■ SUGGESTED READINGS

Fisher, D.S., Parkman, R., and Finch, S.C.: Acute iron poisoning in children, Journal of the American Medical Association **218:** 1179, 1971.

Flynn, K.T.: Iron deficiency among the elderly, Nurse Practitioner **3:**20 (Nov.-Dec.), 1978.

Green, J., III, and Trowbridge, A.: Hematologic and oncologic implications of alcoholism, Postgraduate Medicine, **71:**140, 1977.

Herbert, V.: The nutritional anemias, Hospital Practice, p. 65, March, 1980.

Katz, A.J.: Transfusion therapy: its role in the anemias, Hospital Practice, p. 77, June, 1980.

Peterson, C.: Problems of iron imbalance, Drug Therapy **9**(2):61, 1979.

Robinson, L.A., Brown, A.L., and Underwood, T.: Iron therapy: helps and hazards, Pediatric Nursing **4:**9 (Nov.-Dec.), 1978.

Rosner, F.: Shotgun hematinic therapy, Archives of Internal Medicine **138:**1129, 1978.

Steinberg, S.E., and Hillman, R.S.: Adverse hematologic effects of alcohol, Postgraduate Medicine **67:**139, 1980.

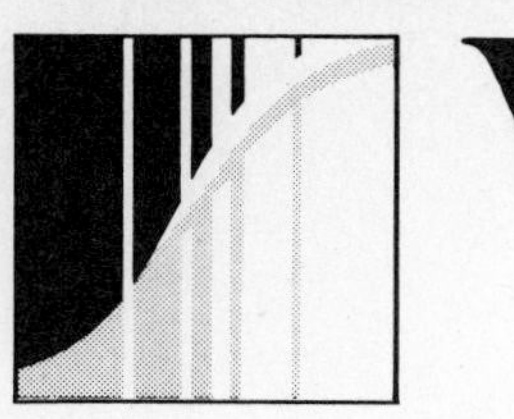
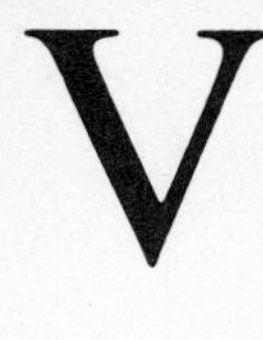

V DRUGS TO TREAT MILD PAIN AND FEVER, INFLAMMATION, ALLERGY, AND RESPIRATORY OBSTRUCTION

One area in classic pharmacology is that of the autacoids, those diverse "local mediators" whose functions are often poorly understood. This section covers the pharmacology of mild pain and fever, inflammation, allergy, and respiratory obstruction in which autacoids play a major role.

The subject matter of Chapter 20, **Analgesic-antipyretic, Nonsteroidal Antiinflammatory Drugs and Specific Agents to Treat Rheumatoid Arthritis and Gout,** may seem diverse but in fact relates the different uses of aspirin. Aspirin is now recognized as an inhibitor of the synthesis of one class of autacoids, the prostaglandins. Certain prostaglandins play a role in inflammation. Another autacoid is histamine; hence Chapter 21, **Antihistamines.** Chapter 22, **Bronchodilators and Other Drugs to Treat Asthma,** deals with the therapeutics of a disease, asthma, in which autacoids play a major role but for which the therapeutic pharmacology principally involves adrenergic mechanisms. Chapter 23, **Drugs to Control Bronchial Secretions,** includes classes of drugs for treating respiratory problems, including nasal congestion, cough, and thickened mucus, to complete the coverage of respiratory pharmacology.

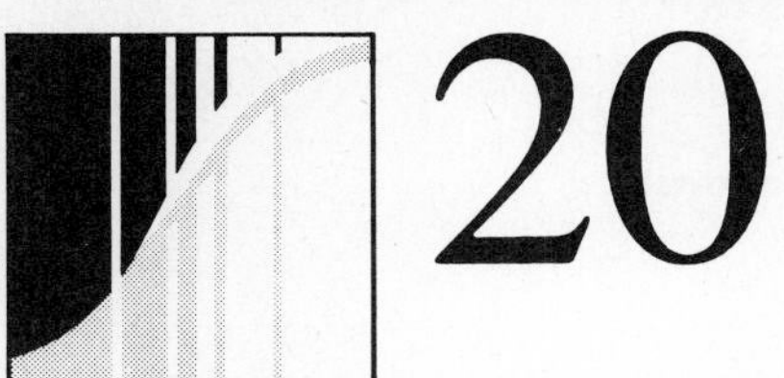

20 Analgesic-antipyretic, nonsteroidal antiinflammatory drugs and specific agents to treat rheumatoid arthritis and gout

This chapter is divided into four sections: analgesic-antipyretic drugs, nonsteroidal antiinflammatory drugs, drugs to treat rheumatoid arthritis, and drugs to treat gout. These are all classifications for the actions of aspirin, although aspirin is no longer used to treat gout. Aspirin is used for three basic pharmacological actions: antipyresis (reducing fever), analgesia for mild to moderate pain, and reducing inflammation. Although aspirin has been found to be an effective inhibitor of prostaglandin synthesis (Chapter 17), it is not clear that this explains more than the antiinflammatory action. In addition to aspirin each of the four sections considers other drugs that are used clinically.

■ ANALGESIC-ANTIPYRETIC DRUGS

■ Analgesia

The analgesics discussed in this chapter, also called the *nonnarcotic analgesics,* all act by a peripheral mechanism through which they interfere with local mediators released in damaged tissue to stimulate nerve endings. In the presence of the nonnarcotic analgesics, the nerves are not stimulated. Objective pain, the component of pain that arises from stimulation of peripheral nerve endings, is therefore not felt. This mechanism is in contrast to that of the narcotic analgesics, which interfere with subjective pain at the level of the central nervous system (Chapter 28).

■ Antipyresis

An antipyretic drug is one that reduces a fever. Normally the balance between heat production and heat dissipation is carefully balanced by the brain. An area of the preoptic anterior hypothalamus is considered the thermostat of the body. Fever results from an increase in the "set point" of this hypothalamic center for body temperature. An endogenous fever-producing agent (pyrogen) is released by white cells engulfing foreign matter (phagocytic leukocytes). This endogenous pyrogen is the major, if not the only, final product that acts on the hypothalamic center to produce fever in response to infections, hypersensitivity, or inflammation. Even though it is clear that fever is produced by a protein synthesized by the body as part of an immunological reaction, it is not clear how fever is a beneficial response, although phagocytosis is enhanced by a higher body temperature. The nonnarcotic analgesics act as antipyretics by reversing the effect of the endogenous pyrogen on the hypothalamus so that the "thermostat" is returned to normal.

■ Classes of analgesic-antipyretic drugs

Two drug classes, the paraaminophenols and the salicylates, are similar not only in producing both analgesia and antipyresis but also in being safe enough to be available without a prescription. The paraaminophenols, including acetaminophen (Datril, Tylenol, and others) and phenacetin, and several salicylates, including aspirin, are so widely used by the public that a patient may not think to mention them when asked, "What drugs have you taken recently?" Like all drugs, however, they do have side effects and can interact with other drugs. In addition to the paraaminophenols and the salicylates, the nonsteroidal antiinflammatory drugs discussed in the next section are also antipyretics and analgesics. However, they are prescription drugs and are used primarily to treat inflammation and its pain.

■ Paraaminophenol derivatives (Table 20-1)

Acetaminophen and phenacetin

Mechanism of action. Acetaminophen and phenacetin act at the hypothalamus to reduce fever and at peripheral pain receptors to block activation. Although the paraaminophenols are identical to aspirin in their antipyretic and analgesic properties, there is no evidence that these drugs effectively inhibit prostaglandin synthesis. These drugs are not effective in reducing the inflammation of rheumatoid arthritis.

Administration and use of acetaminophen (Datril, Tylenol, and others). Acetaminophen is used for the same spectrum of analgesic-antipyretic actions as is aspirin and can be combined with other analgesics, including codeine, or formulated as a liquid for infants and young children. Acetaminophen has become popular as an analgesic-antipyretic alternative to aspirin because acetaminophen does not produce gastric irritation or alter platelet function and bleeding times as does aspirin. Furthermore, acetaminophen does not interact with the oral anticoagulants or other drugs.

TABLE 20-1. Analgesic-antipyretic drugs

Generic name	Trade name	Dosage and administration	Comments
SALICYLATES			
Aspirin (acetyl-salicylic acid)	A.S.A. Aspergum Bayer Aspirin Children's Aspirin Dacaprin Ecotrin Measurin	FOR ANALGESIA OR ANTIPYRESIS: ORAL, RECTAL: *Adults*—650 mg every 4 hr, or 1.3 gm of timed-release every 8 hr. *Children*—65 mg/kg over 24 hr in divided doses, every 4 to 6 hours, OTC.*	Oral doses should be taken with a large glass of water or milk to decrease stomach irritation. Some patients may have to take aspirin after a meal to avoid gastrointestinal distress.
Aspirin, buffered	Aluprin Ascriptin Bufferin Alka-Seltzer Various others	Same as for aspirin. There are no smaller dose tablets for children. OTC.	Alka Seltzer contains 1.9 Gm sodium bicarbonate and 1 Gm citric acid per tablet. To avoid acid-base disturbances, limit ingestion to occasional use only. Remaining products contain magnesium and aluminum antacid salts. These salts are not absorbed systemically to any great extent.
Aspirin, aluminum		Same as for aspirin. These are chewable tablets (75 mg) for children. OTC.	Palatable, but poorly absorbed from gastrointestinal tract.
Calcium carbaspirin	Calurin	Same as for aspirin. OTC.	A complex of calcium, aspirin, and urea which is supposed to be less irritating than aspirin alone.
Sodium salicylate	Uracel Salbid	Same as for aspirin. OTC. An injectable form is available by prescription.	Less effective than an equal dose of aspirin. May be tolerated by patients with an allergic reaction to aspirin. Does not affect platelet function, but does retain vitamin K antagonist effect, which can increase prothrombin time.
Salicylamide	Salrin Salicylamide	ORAL: *adults and children over 12 yr*—650 mg every 6 hr. OTC.	Not as effective as aspirin.
OTHER ANALGESIC-ANTIPYRETICS			
Acetaminophen	Tylenol Datril Various others	ORAL: *Adults*—325 to 650 mg every 6 to 8 hr. No more than 2.6 Gm in 24 hr. *Children*—7 to 12 yr, ½ adult dose; 3 to 6 yr, 1/6 adult dose. OTC.	Analgesic and antipyretic only. Little antiinflammatory action. No inhibition of platelets. Contraindicated in patients with glucose-6-phosphate dehydrogenase deficienty. Not used for arthritis. A paraaminophenol.
Mefenamic acid	Ponstel	ORAL: *Adults and children over 14 yr*—500 mg initially, then 250 mg every 6 hr as needed. Prescription drug.	Should be taken with food. Should not be given for more than 1 wk.

*OTC, Over the counter; available without prescription.

Side effects of acetaminophen. Acetaminophen can be the cause of allergic reactions, usually involving skin rashes. People with a known glucose-6-phosphate dehydrogenase deficiency can develop hemolytic anemia if they take acetaminophen. When taken on a long-term basis, acetaminophen can cause methemoglobinemia, which impairs the oxygen-carrying capacity of the blood. This is only serious in infants.

Toxicity of acetaminophen. Overdose of acetaminophen produces liver damage in adults. Children rarely suffer permanent liver damage from acetaminophen, but adults who take more than 2.6 Gm in 24 hours may show mild symptoms of liver damage such as loss of appetite, nausea, vomiting, and slight jaundice. In deliberate overdoses of 10 Gm or more, adults are very susceptible to a dangerous degree of liver damage. Death has been reported following ingestion of 15 Gm. This toxicity arises because the liver normally conjugates toxic metabolites of acetaminophen with a sulfhydryl compound, glutathione, to produce an inactive, readily excreted compound. The amount of glutathione available for conjugation is exceeded when large amounts of acetaminophen are ingested. The unconjugated metabolites bind to and kill liver cells.

Recent success in preventing liver damage with acetylcysteine has been reported. Acetylcysteine is a drug used in respiratory therapy to degrade bronchial mucus (Chapter 23). Its use as an antidote for acetaminophen poisoning is at present experimental. Acetylcysteine provides the missing sulfhydryl groups to conjugate and inactivate the toxic metabolites of acetaminophen. Since acetylcysteine has the pervasive flavor of rotten eggs, it must be disguised in a flavored soft drink. Even then it may be vomited and have to be regiven. The traditional method of treating acetaminophen overdose is to remove undissolved tablets by gastric lavage followed by the administration of cathartics or activated charcoal.

Phenacetin. Phenacetin is a paraaminophenol used only in combination with aspirin and other analgesics and is therefore not included in Table 20-1. The most widely used over-the-counter preparation of phenacetin is A.P.C. tablets (aspirin, phenacetin, and caffeine). There is no advantage in combining aspirin and phenacetin for analgesia. The amount of caffeine per tablet is less than that in a half cup of coffee.

Phenacetin is converted to acetaminophen in the body, so the toxic effects of acetaminophen are produced by overdoses of phenacetin. Phenacetin causes renal damage when taken on a long-term basis.

■ Salicylates (Table 20-1)

Acetylsalicylic acid (aspirin)

Aspirin is effective in low doses (325 to 650 mg or 1 to 2 adult tablets) for reducing fever and relieving mild pain. Two aspirin tablets are considered the analgesic equivalent of 60 mg of codeine. Aspirin is an effective analgesic for most common mild to moderate headaches and for relieving generalized mild muscular aches. Aspirin or aspirin-codeine combinations are also useful for treating mild to moderate pain of tooth extractions, episiotomies, cancer, and bone fractures. A dose of 1.2 Gm per day of aspirin produces the maximum analgesic effect. At much higher doses (3 to 6 Gm per day) aspirin is the drug of choice in the treatment of the inflammation of rheumatoid arthritis. At this concentration, aspirin is the prototype for the nonsteroidal antiinflammatory drugs, which will be discussed in the next section.

Absorption and distribution. Aspirin is a weak acid and is rapidly absorbed from the stomach and upper small intestine. Buffering agents are present in several aspirin brands to hasten dissolution of the tablet and to reduce gastric irritation from the tablet. These advantages of buffering agents are minimal, and if several doses are to be taken, the buffering agents may cause loose stools. The Alka-Seltzer brand contains so much sodium and bicarbonate that it should be used only on a short-term basis.

Once aspirin is absorbed, 50% to 90% binds loosely to plasma albumin. Aspirin can displace oral anticoagulants, oral hypoglycemic drugs, phenytoin, and methotrexate. Since the unbound drug is the effective concentration, the free drug may reach toxic levels when displaced by aspirin.

Metabolism and excretion. Aspirin is rapidly hydrolyzed in the blood. The acetyl group of aspirin is readily transferred to the enzyme cyclooxygenase of the blood platelets. Cyclooxygenase is the key enzyme for the formation of prostaglandins. The acetylation of cyclooxygenase is irreversible and therefore persists for the 3- to 7-day lifetime of the platelet. Acetylated cyclooxygenase is inactive, and the synthesis of the prostaglandin thromboxane A_2 is therefore blocked. Thromboxane A_2, which is a potent agent promoting platelet aggregation, is normally synthesized by platelets when platelets begin to aggregate. Even one aspirin tablet inhibits blood clotting by inhibiting platelet aggregation. This observation has led to the examination of aspirin as a prophylactic agent to prevent heart attacks and strokes, processes associated with an increased tendency toward platelet aggregation (Chapter 17).

Salicylic acid is the other product of the hydrolysis of aspirin. Salicylate (the basic salt to which salicylic acid dissociates at the pH of blood) is an analgesic-antipyretic and a reversible inhibitor of prostaglandin synthesis. Salicylate does not affect platelet aggregation, and therefore a salicylate salt is sometimes used in place of aspirin.

In an acidic urine, salicylic acid is uncharged and therefore diffuses back into the blood. Vitamin C (ascorbic acid) maintains an acidic urine when taken in large doses and can therefore delay the excretion of salicylic acid. This can be a dangerous drug interaction if large doses of aspirin are being taken, as for arthritis. In an alkaline urine, salicylic acid dissociates to salicylate, which is charged, cannot diffuse back into the blood, and is therefore eliminated in the urine. Salicylate is metabolized to inactive salicyluric acid by the liver. However, a single 325 mg aspirin tablet will saturate this liver inactivation system. This means that the liver cannot readily metabolize large doses of aspirin.

Side effects. Approximately 2% to 10% of people taking an occasional aspirin tablet will experience gastrointestinal upset. This may be felt as heartburn or nausea. Aluminum and calcium-urea salts of aspirin have been formulated to be less irritating to the stomach than aspirin. When aspirin is taken regularly in large doses for arthritis, this incidence becomes 30% to 50% and may be the factor limiting the use of aspirin. Sometimes antacids are prescribed to minimize stomach irritation, but antacids also raise the pH of the urine and increase the rate of excretion of salicylic acid. Alternatively, therefore, enteric-coated or timed-release preparations may be tried to decrease gastric irritation.

Aspirin is directly irritating and damaging to gastric mucosal cells. Since alcohol also has these gastric effects, aspirin should not be taken when alcohol is in the stomach. The combination of alcohol and aspirin is greater than additive in producing gastric bleeding. Patients with active peptic ulcers should be advised not to use aspirin.

Long-term aspirin ingestion can cause the loss of 10 to 30 ml of blood a day from gastrointestinal irritation. This may lead to iron deficiency anemia in women with heavy menses. Rarely, massive gastrointestinal bleeding has been encountered in patients taking aspirin on a long-term basis.

Some people develop an allergy to aspirin. The most common form of aspirin intolerance is a rash. Patients with a skin rash caused by aspirin may tolerate other salicylates. A few people develop nasal polyps and sometime later develop an asthma that is triggered by aspirin.

Patients who are sensitive to aspirin may be sensitive to a variety of other compounds. Most commonly, individuals sensitive to aspirin may show *cross-sensitivity* to

1. Salicylin-containing foods, for example, apples, oranges, and bananas
2. Processed foods or drugs containing tartrazine dye or sodium benzoate
3. Iodide-containing substances
4. Other nonsteroidal antiinflammatory agents: indomethacin, mefenamic acid, ibuprofen, and phenylbutazone

As can be seen from this list, the origin of these cross-sensitivities is not always the classic cross-reactivity due to structural similarities of the agents.

Salicylism. Mild intoxication with aspirin is called *salicylism* and is commonly experienced when the daily dosage is more than 4 Gm. Tinnitus (ringing in the ears) is the most frequent effect and may be accompanied by some reversible hearing loss. Since salicylate stimulates the respiratory center, hyperventilation (rapid breathing) may be seen. Fever may even result because salicylate interferes with the metabolic pathways coupling oxygen consumption and heat production.

Toxicity. An acute overdose of aspirin causes serious disturbances in the acid-base balance of the blood. A child is more likely to die from a large overdose of aspirin than is an adult. Fatalities among children have been dramatically reduced since 1970 when the Poison Prevention Packaging Act required that orange-flavored "baby" aspirin (81 mg tablets) be limited to 36 tablets per bottle with safety caps. If it has been determined that a child has ingested more than 150 mg/kg (36 baby tablets [one bottle] or 9 adult tablets for a 45 lb child), vomiting may be induced or gastric lavage is carried out to get rid of undissolved tablets. Charcoal will absorb about half its weight in aspirin and is therefore given orally to reduce the absorption of aspirin.

Children, particularly those under 4 years of age, can rapidly develop metabolic acidosis. This is both because of the acidic nature of aspirin and its metabolites and because salicylate inhibits metabolism in a manner that favors the accumulation of organic acids, which would normally have been metabolized to carbon dioxide and water. The hyperthermia that is also produced with this metabolic block must be treated with sponge baths. The profuse sweating can produce dehydration. The supportive treatment of aspirin toxicity therefore consists of careful monitoring of the acid-base and electrolyte levels of the blood and appropriate fluid administration. Intravenous sodium bicarbonate can counter the tendency toward metabolic acidosis and produce an alkaline urine that hastens the excretion of salicylate. Osmotic diuretics or dialysis may be necessary in extreme cases to remove salicylate.

Salicylate is a weak vitamin K antagonist and in large doses will act like an oral anticoagulant. A day or two after massive aspirin ingestion, an increased bleeding tendency and signs of minor hemorrhaging may be noticed. See the box on page 232 for a summary of the treatment of aspirin poisoning.

Drug interactions. The drug interactions characteristic of aspirin are especially important because of the widespread and uncritical use of aspirin. The mechanisms of the drug interactions with aspirin have been described and are summarized here.

Drug interactions arise because aspirin

1. Enhances the potential for gastrointestinal bleeding and ulcers with glucocorticoids, alcohol, and phenylbutazone
2. Enhances anticoagulation with coumarins
3. Antagonizes the uricosuric effect of probenecid and sulfinpyrazone

■ THE NURSING PROCESS FOR ANALGESIC-ANTIPYRETIC DRUGS

The nursing process for the use of these drugs as analgesics only will be covered in the next section on nonsteroidal antiinflammatory drugs. This section will cover only the use of these drugs for reducing fever.

■ Assessment

The patient requiring a drug to reduce fever is one who has a temperature above 38.5° C (101° F) or above the locally accepted limit of normal. Fever is not a disease itself but is a symptom of an underlying process such as infection, some cancers, and drug reactions. Patient assessment relative to the fever includes determining the temperature and other vital signs; noting the presence of diaphoresis, chills, and/or seizures; and assessing the level of consciousness and the fluid intake and output. Since fever itself is a symptom, the nurse must evaluate the patient relative to the possible causes of fever. Thus the nurse should determine the respiratory status for possible pulmonary infections; wound status for possible wound infection; genitourinary system status for possible urinary tract infection; and so on.

■ Management

The treatment of fever is twofold. Attempts are made (1) to reduce the fever and (2) to determine the cause of the fever and to treat or eliminate the cause. To reduce the fever, antipyretics are given either when the temperature exceeds the ordered upper limit or every 4 hours around the clock. The temperature should be monitored every 4 hours, adequate fluid intake maintained, fluid intake and output measured, blood counts monitored, and other vital signs checked. Maintaining patient comfort is important. If antipyretics are not successful, additional measures may be employed, including cool water or alcohol baths and use of cooling mattresses. If aspirin is being used, the patient should be monitored for bruising or bleeding.

■ Evaluation

Success with antipyretic therapy is a return of the patient's temperature to normal range. Hospitalized patients are rarely discharged with a fever. Antipyretics are used often as self-medication by the public for ailments such as colds and flu. Patients should be able to state the correct dose and frequency of administration, when medical assistance should be sought for fever, the possible side effects of antipyretics, and the other drugs and substances that should be avoided during antipyretic therapy. For more specific guidelines see the patient care implications at the end of this chapter.

■ Other over-the-counter salicylates
(Table 20-1)

Salicylamide

Salicylamide (Salrin) is a chemically modified form of salicylate. Salicylamide is not hydrolyzed to salicylic acid. Salicylamide is a less effective analgesic than aspirin or salicylic acid.

Sodium salicylate

Sodium salicylate does not alter platelet function as does aspirin. Salicylates bind to plasma albumin and displace other drugs, particularly the oral anticoagulants.

Methyl salicylate (oil of wintergreen)

Methyl salicylate is used topically only and is not listed in the drug table. Methyl salicylate causes vasodilation in the applied areas and thereby creates a warmth that relieves muscle or joint stiffness.

■ Fenamates (Table 20-1)

Mefenamic acid

Mefenamic acid (Ponstel) is not chemically related to aspirin. It is a prescription drug, but it is no more effective than aspirin for relief of mild to moderate pain, and a number of side effects are associated with its use, including gastrointestinal upset, diarrhea, and rash. Mefenamic acid is contraindicated for patients with gastrointestinal, kidney, or liver disease. Therapy with mefenamic acid is limited to 1 week because of a high incidence of toxicity associated with the gastrointestinal, kidney, and blood-forming systems. Mefenamic acid can prolong prothrombin times, thereby potentiating the

TREATMENT OF ASPIRIN TOXICITY

Toxic salicylate plasma concentrations

Mild	45 to 65 mg/dl
Moderate	65 to 90 mg/dl
Severe	90+ mg/dl
Usually fatal	> 120 mg/dl

Treatment steps

1. Undissolved tablets are removed through induced vomiting or absorption with charcoal.
2. Plasma salicylate, acid-base, glucose, sodium, and potassium concentrations are determined every 4 to 5 hours.
3. Hyperthermia is treated with sponge baths, and dehydration is treated with fluid replacement.
4. Fluids are administered as required to treat electrolyte imbalances and acidosis.
5. If the salicylate concentration is dangerously high or does not fall with supportive treatment, dialysis or exchange transfusions may be used.

action of coumarins (oral anticoagulants), and increases the insulin requirements of diabetic patients.

■ NONSTEROIDAL ANTIINFLAMMATORY DRUGS

Aspirin is the prototype of the nonsteroidal antiinflammatory drugs. For many years aspirin has been the first drug used to control the pain and inflammation of rheumatoid arthritis. During the past few years several new drugs have been developed, which like aspirin are analgesic, antipyretic, and antiinflammatory. These new drugs are all prescription drugs. They are prescribed as analgesic antiinflammatory drugs for patients with rheumatoid arthritis who cannot tolerate aspirin. In addition they are prescribed for patients with painful joint disorders, with or without inflammation, such as osteoarthritis, ankylosing spondylitis, low back pain, and gout.

■ Mechanism of action

The primary mechanism of action of the nonsteroidal antiinflammatory drugs is believed to be the inhibition of the enzyme cyclooxygenase so that the prostaglandins are not formed. As discussed earlier, aspirin is an irreversible inhibitor of cyclooxygenase because cyclooxygenase is acetylated by aspirin. Other salicylates and nonsteroidal antiinflammatory drugs also inhibit cyclooxygenase but reversibly, for they do not acetylate cyclooxygenase.

How prostaglandins affect pain receptors is not known. The actions of one prostaglandin, prostaglandin E_2, include vasodilation and increased bone resorption. Large amounts of prostaglandin E_2 have been shown to be present in the synovial fluid of affected joints of patients with rheumatoid arthritis, synthesized by cells in the mesenchymal synovial lining. Presumably this production of prostaglandin E_2 contributes to the swelling and eventual bone erosion of rheumatoid arthritis. In addition, inflammation at other sites may involve the synthesis of prostaglandin E_2.

Prostaglandins act to protect gastric mucosa and inhibit gastric acid secretion. The gastrointestinal irritation common to aspirin and the other nonsteroidal antiinflammatory drugs may arise because this protection of gastric mucosa and inhibition of acid secretion is eliminated when these drugs, which are prostaglandin synthesis inhibitors, are present in the stomach. These gastric effects may be minimized by taking the drugs with meals.

Dysmenorrhea (menstrual cramps) appears to be due to the overproduction of prostaglandins by the uterus at the time of menstruation. The prostaglandins can cause the uterus to contract to the point of cramping, producing dysmenorrhea. Aspirin is not a very effective drug for treating dysmenorrhea, but the nonsteroidal antiinflammatory drugs are proving very effective in eliminating menstrual cramps, particularly if therapy is begun a few days before menses begins.

■ Specific drugs (Table 20-2)

Aspirin

Aspirin is the first drug tried to control the symptoms of arthritis. Doses of 2.6 to 7.8 Gm per day are required to produce the plasma concentrations of 20 to 30 mg/dl needed for an effective antiinflammatory response. As previously discussed, these doses are associated with a high incidence of gastric irritation with or without bleeding, salicylism, decreased platelet aggregation, and interactions with other drugs. Aspirin must be taken continuously for at least 2 weeks before an improvement may be noted. Timed-release or enteric-coated formulations may improve patient compliance by decreasing the number of times each day aspirin must be taken and by bypassing the stomach for dissolution and absorption, thereby reducing gastric irritation.

Because aspirin is highly irritating to the stomach, a number of salicylate salts have been introduced that substitute for aspirin and produce less gastrointestinal upset. These salicylates do not affect platelet aggregation but do displace oral anticoagulants from albumin.

Salicylate salts

Sodium salicylate, sodium thiosalicylate, magnesium salicylate, and *choline salicylate* are all salicylate salts that produce less gastrointestinal upset than aspirin.

TABLE 20-2. Nonsteroidal antiinflammatory drugs

Generic name	Trade name	Dosage and administration	Comments
ASPIRIN AND SALICYLATES			
Aspirin	Bayer Timed-Release Bufferin, Arthritis strength Decaprin Measurin Various others	ORAL: *Adults*—arthritis: 2.6 to 5.2 Gm daily in divided doses (every 8 hr for timed-release forms). For acute rheumatic fever, up to 7.8 Gm daily in divided doses. *Children*—65 mg/kg over 24 hr in divided doses every 6 hr. OTC.*	Dose needed to achieve blood levels for antiinflammatory activity (20% to 30 mg%) may vary from person to person. The doses given are average doses.
Choline salicylate	Arthropan	ORAL: *Adults and children over 12 yr*—870 mg (1 teaspoon) every 3 to 4 hr, up to 6 times daily. OTC*	A mint-flavored liquid formulated for patients with arthritis.
Magnesium salicylate	Lorisal Magan Mobidin	Same as aspirin. No pediatric forms. Prescription drug.	Contains no sodium; low incidence of gastrointestinal upset. Contraindicated in renal failure.
Salsalate	Disalcid	ORAL: *Adults only*—1 gm 3 times daily. Prescription drug.	A dimer of salicylate. Absorption is from the intestine only after hydrolysis to salicylic acid. Delayed onset compared to free salicylic acid.
Sodium salicylate	Salbid	Same as aspirin. OTC.* An injectable form is available by prescription.	Less effective than an equal dose of aspirin. May be tolerated by patients with an allergic reaction to aspirin. Does not affect platelet function, but does retain vitamin K antagonist effect, which can increase prothrombin time.
Sodium thiosalicylate	Arthrolate Nalate Thiodyne Thiolate Th-Sal	INTRAMUSCULAR: *Adults*—prescription drug. For arthritis, 100 mg daily. For musculoskeletal disorders, 50 to 100 mg daily or every other day. For rheumatic fever, 100 to 150 mg every 4 to 6 hr for 3 days, then 100 mg twice daily.	An injectable, longer acting form of salicylate that can be given in doses lower than for oral aspirin.
PHENYLBUTAZONE AND OXYPHENBUTAZONE			
Phenylbutazone	Azolid Butazolidin	ORAL: *Adults*—300 to 600 mg daily in divided doses every 6 to 8 hr. Not for children under 14 yr.	Administer immediately before or after meals or with a glass of milk to minimize stomach upset. Toxicity increases with age. Patients over 60 yr should not take this drug for more than 7 days, and those younger should not take this drug for more than 14 days.
Oxyphenbutazone	Oxalid Tandearil	ORAL: *Adults*—300 to 600 mg daily in divided doses every 6 to 8 hr. Not for children under 14 yr.	Same precautions as with phenylbutazone.

*OTC, over the counter; available without prescription.

Continued.

TABLE 20-2. Nonsteroidal antiinflammatory drugs—cont'd

Generic name	Trade name	Dosage and administration	Comments
INDOLE AND PYRROLE DERIVATIVES OF PARACHLOROBENZOIC ACID			
Indomethacin	Indocin	ORAL: *Adults*—25 mg 2 to 3 times daily. If necessary, the total daily dose can be increased 25 to 50 mg daily at weekly intervals, but the total daily dose should not exceed 150 to 200 mg. Not for children under 14 yr.	Administer with meals or with antacids to minimize gastric irritation.
Sulindac	Clinoril	ORAL: *Adults*—initially, 150 to 200 mg twice a day. Dose is adjusted for therapeutic response. Not for children under 14 yr.	Administer with food.
Tolmetin sodium	Tolectin	ORAL: *Adults*—initially, 400 mg 3 times daily, then adjust. Usual maintenance dose is 0.6 to 1.8 Gm daily. *Children over 12 yr*—initially, 20 mg/kg body weight daily in divided doses. Usual maintenance dose is 15 to 30 mg/kg daily.	Incidence of gastrointestinal upset is less with tolmetin than with aspirin or indomethacin, but it is advisable to administer tolmetin with milk or meals.
Zomepirac	Zomax	ORAL: *Adults*—100 mg every 4 to 6 hr.	New drug for relief of mild to moderate pain. Not recommended for chronic therapy or for use by children or lactating women because safety for these groups is not established.
PHENYLPROPIONIC ACID DERIVATIVES			
Fenoprofen	Nalfon	ORAL: *Adults*—600 mg 4 times daily.	Best administered 30 min before a meal or 2 hr after a meal because this drug is poorly absorbed in the presence of food. Milk or antacids may be used if there is gastrointestinal upset.
Ibuprofen	Motrin	ORAL: *Adults*—600 mg 4 times daily. Not for children under 14 yr.	Usually well tolerated. Gastrointestinal upset is the most frequent complaint.
Naproxen Naproxen sodium	Naprosyn Anaprox	ORAL: *Adults*—500 to 750 mg divided in 2 doses daily. Not for children under 14 yr.	Longer acting than many of the other drugs in this class.
FENAMATE			
Meclofenamate	Meclomen	ORAL: *Adults*—200 to 400 mg divided in 3 to 4 doses daily.	New drug for relieving symptoms of rheumatoid arthritis or osteoarthritis. Gastrointestinal upset is common, sometimes with severe diarrhea.

Salsalate

Salsalate (Disalcid) is a dimer of salicylic acid. It is slowly hydrolyzed to two molecules of salicylic acid in the small intestine and absorbed into the bloodstream.

Thiosalicylate

Thiosalicylate (Arthrolate and others) is a chemically modified form of salicylate for intramuscular injection.

Phenylbutazone and oxyphenbutazone

Phenylbutazone (Azolid, Butazolidin) and oxyphenbutazone (Oxalid, Tandearil) are potent antiinflammatory agents with a long (2 to 3 days) plasma half-life. They cause fluid retention and gastric irritation and prolong platelet function, thereby inhibiting blood clotting. Occasionally, they cause liver damage or bone marrow suppression. Phenylbutazone binds strongly to plasma

■ THE NURSING PROCESS FOR NONSTEROIDAL ANTIINFLAMMATORY DRUGS

■ Assessment

Patients requiring analgesic and/or antiinflammatory drugs will have a wide variety of complaints, including headache, menstrual cramps, arthritis, musculoskeletal injury, and postoperative pain. Many of these patients will seek medical assistance for relief of their problem, whereas others will self-medicate with such drugs as aspirin or acetaminophen. Assessment should include a thorough collection of data related to the specific patient complaint. These data would include such things as temperature, pulse, respiration, blood pressure, blood counts, a brief neurological examination, and other laboratory data relevant to the possible or probable diagnosis. Assessment of ability to perform activities of daily living may assist in planning for discharge.

■ Management

In general management is directed toward providing relief of the pain, improving the patient's condition, and determining a way to prevent and/or treat recurrences in the future. Individualized planning requires that the health care team and the patient work together to develop a plan to reach the goal or goals of drug therapy, and therapy in addition to drugs is often required. Examples of additional therapy include application of heat or cold, immobilization, special exercises, and restricted activity. A plan may be proposed for the patient to begin a course of prophylactic drug therapy at a specific time in the future with the hope of preventing the problem; this is done for certain types of headache disorders and with menstrual cramps. By the time the patient is ready to begin self-management, goals and plan of therapy should be understood by the patient and the health care team. During the management phase, the nurse should monitor the vital signs and subjective and objective data related to the specific problem and the laboratory data appropriate to the problem and the drug therapy. For example, in the patient experiencing menstrual cramps associated with heavy bleeding who is being treated with mefenamic acid (Ponstel), the hematocrit and hemoglobin level might be monitored because of the heavy bleeding, whereas the prothrombin time and the blood sugar concentration would be monitored because of the mefenamic acid.

■ Evaluation

The question to ask in evaluation of drug therapy with analgesics and antiinflammatory drugs is whether the short-term goal has been reached or will soon be reached while the patient remains free of side effects due to the medication. Before discharge the patient should be able to explain why and how to take the prescribed drugs and other therapies being used to treat the problem, which other drugs should be avoided while receiving therapy, whether alcohol should be avoided, what are reasonable expectations of the regimen (e.g., will joint pain disappear or only diminish), which are possible side effects and what to do if they occur, how to implement a plan for prophylactic treatment, and when to return for follow-up or assistance. For more specific guidelines see the patient care implications section at the end of this chapter.

---

albumin and can displace other bound drugs, particularly oral anticoagulant and oral hypoglycemic drugs. Because of these many problems, phenylbutazone or oxyphenbutazone are commonly prescribed for 1 to 2 weeks only to treat an acute inflammatory response.

Indomethacin

Indomethacin (Indocin) is prescribed for its analgesic and antiinflammatory actions. Gastrointestinal disturbances such as nausea, vomiting, loss of appetite, indigestion, or diarrhea are common among patients taking indomethacin, but the incidence can be reduced by taking the drug after meals. Occasionally, indomethacin can cause ulcerations in the gastrointestinal system, which can become serious if bleeding or perforation results. Headaches and dizziness are the most common side effects of indomethacin. These effects can often be minimized if the dose is lowered and then raised gradually. Other central nervous system disturbances that can limit the use of indomethacin include confusion, lightheadedness, fainting, drowsiness, coma, convulsions, and behavioral changes.

Sulindac, tolmetin, and zomepirac

Sulindac (Clinoril), tolmetin (Tolectin), and zomepirac (Zomax) are new antiinflammatory drugs chemically related to indomethacin.

Tolmetin was released in 1975. It has fewer side effects in the central nervous system than indomethacin. Tolmetin is absorbed rapidly and has a plasma half-life of only 1 hour. It does not interfere with the binding of oral anticoagulants but does prolong bleeding time by inhibiting platelet functions.

Sulindac was released in 1979. It has a plasma half-life of 8 hours and can therefore be taken less frequently. Sulindac does not affect platelet aggregation and therefore does not affect bleeding time.

Zomepirac was released in 1980. It is reported to be well tolerated and requires administration every 4 to 6 hours. Zomepirac prolongs bleeding time by inhibiting platelet function.

Ibuprofen, naproxen, and fenoprofen

Ibuprofen (Motrin), naproxen (Naprosyn), and fenoprofen (Nalfon) are arylalkanoic acids. Ibuprofen was released in 1974. Naproxen and fenoprofen were released in 1975. These drugs are approved for the treatment of rheumatoid arthritis. They provide good analgesic and antiinflammatory action. Their use for conditions such as dysmenorrhea, osteoarthritis, and gout is being evaluated.

Ibuprofen is rapidly absorbed and has a plasma half-life of 2 hours. It appears to be well tolerated. Fenoprofen and ketoprofen appear similar in half-life to ibuprofen. Naproxen has a half-life of 13 hours and needs to be taken only twice a day.

The most frequent side effects are those common to the other antiinflammatory drugs: gastrointestinal disturbances and dizziness or headaches. These drugs bind tightly to albumin and can displace other drugs. Like aspirin, these drugs inhibit platelet aggregation and increase bleeding time. These effects are reversible, however. Tinnitus (ringing in the ears) is also a frequent but reversible side effect.

Meclofenamate

Meclofenamate (Meclomen) was released in 1980. It is chemically similar to mefenamic acid, which was discussed in the section on the analgesic-antipyretic drugs. The half-life of meclofenamate is 2 to 3 hours. It is effective for relief of the symptoms of rheumatoid arthritis and osteoarthritis. It is reported to cause less fecal blood loss than aspirin, but it is associated with a high incidence of other gastrointestinal symptoms, including severe diarrhea.

■ DRUGS FOR RHEUMATOID ARTHRITIS

■ Rheumatoid arthritis

Rheumatoid arthritis is a highly variable disease process. It frequently goes into remission for months or years. In early rheumatoid arthritis the synovial membranes only are inflamed, causing a painful swelling. In this situation aspirin and the other nonsteroidal antiinflammatory drugs may be effective in reducing the inflammation. This effect added to the analgesic effect will ease the pain and help to increase the mobility of the affected joint. In mild cases of rheumatoid arthritis, the nonsteroidal antiinflammatory drugs may be sufficient to control symptoms. These drugs do not affect the progression of rheumatoid arthritis, however, which is marked by erosion of the bone at the joint and eventual bone deformation. Drugs that may be effective in altering the progression of joint erosion include gold therapy, hydroxychloroquine, penicillamine, and the immunosuppressive drugs, tried in that order. Glucocorticoids have a restricted role in treating rheumatoid arthritis. All these antirheumatic drugs have potentially serious side effects, which must be monitored carefully.

■ Specific drugs (Table 20-3)

Aurothioglucose and gold sodium thiomalate

Aurothioglucose (Solganal) and gold sodium thiomalate (Myochrysine) are injectable gold salts. It is not known how gold affects the synovial tissues to suppress rheumatoid arthritis. Therapy is started with weekly injections into the gluteal muscle until 1 Gm has been given. Further therapy depends on the patient's response. Gold requires a long time to come to plateau levels in the tissues, and it usually takes 2 to 6 months to see a response to gold therapy. Only 30% to 60% of patients treated with gold respond over a 2 to 3-year course of treatment. Patients in whom remission is induced usually continue receiving monthly injections.

The most common reason for discontinuing successful gold therapy is the appearance of serious side effects: skin reactions, mouth ulcers, fever, kidney damage, or abnormalities in the blood count. About 40% of patients develop an adverse reaction. The skin reactions and

TABLE 20-3. Drugs specific for rheumatoid arthritis

Generic name	Trade name	Dosage and administration	Comments
Aurothioglucose Gold sodium thiomalate	Solganal Myochrysine	INTRAMUSCULAR (GLUTEAL): *Adults*—Weekly injections of 10 mg week 1, 25 mg week 2, 25 to 50 mg week 3, 50 mg each week thereafter until a total of 800 mg to 1 Gm has been administered. If the patient has improved and there are no toxic signs, 50 mg injections are continued every 2 wk (4 doses) then every 3 wk (4 doses), then every 3 to 4 wk. *Children*—1 mg/kg (up to 25 mg) weekly for 20 wk, then every 2 to 4 wk if the therapy is beneficial.	About 40% of patients develop serious side effects, most commonly an allergy marked by skin reactions or mouth ulcers. Blood counts and urinalysis are done routinely to monitor for suppression of blood cells and kidney damage. Therapy is discontinued if no improvement is seen in 5 mo.
Hydroxychloroquine sulfate	Plaquenil Sulfate	ORAL: *Adults*—200 mg once or twice daily at meals, not more than 3.5 mg/lb.	Regular ocular examination for retinopathy is required.
Penicillamine	Cuprimine Depen	ORAL: *Adult*—initially 125 to 250 mg daily as a single dose. May be raised every 2 to 3 mo by 250 mg daily to 500 to 750 mg daily.	Patient must be carefully monitored for suppression of blood cells and autoimmune responses.

mouth ulcers are the most common side effects. If these are mild, the gold therapy may be halted temporarily and then tried again. Blood counts and a urinalysis for protein should be done before each dose early in gold therapy and continued periodically throughout therapy.

Hydroxychloroquine

Hydroxychloroquine (Plaquenil) is an antimalarial drug, which is also used as an alternative to gold therapy or when gold therapy has failed. A response may not be seen for 3 to 6 months after the start of therapy, and therapy is discontinued after 1 year if no response is seen. This drug is taken orally, and some drug remains in the body for months or years. Occasionally, patients develop retinopathy which can progress to blindness even when the drug is discontinued. Therefore, regular ophthalmic examination is necessary. Skin rashes, peripheral neuropathy, and a depressed white cell count are other side effects.

Penicillamine

Penicillamine (Cuprimine, Depen) is being evaluated for the treatment of rheumatoid arthritis. Side effects are frequent but are reversible when the dosage is reduced or discontinued. These side effects include the loss of taste, nausea, depression of platelets and white cells, and proteinuria. Side effects are minimized by starting with a low dose and increasing the dose every 4 to 6 weeks until a response is obtained or a total of 1 Gm per day is given.

Immunosuppressive agents

Rheumatoid arthritis is believed to be an autoimmune disease. When the drugs discussed (aspirin and other nonsteroidal antiinflammatory drugs, gold, hydroxychloroquine or penicillamine) have failed to alleviate symptoms and ease the patient into a remission, immunosuppressive agents may be used. In this country the drugs currently used are azathioprine and cyclophosphamide (Chapter 50). The use of these drugs for severe arthritis is experimental.

Glucocorticoids

Glucocorticoids will relieve inflammation and the accompanying pain of arthritis in a dramatic fashion. One action of glucocorticoids is to inhibit prostaglandin E_2 synthesis by an indirect action. However, glucocorticoids do not alter the course of rheumatoid arthritis. The long-term administration of glucocorticoids suppresses the pituitary-adrenal axis and leads to serious side effects (Chapter 35). Although the oral administration of glucocorticoids is rarely used to treat the symptoms of rheumatoid arthritis, the injection of a glucocorticoid into the articular space of the joint may relieve acute inflammatory episodes without systemic side effects. Glucocorticoids may be used to treat some of the nonarticular manifestations of rheumatoid arthritis, such as vasculitis and rheumatoid lung. Very small doses may sometimes be used to treat joint symptoms. *Hydrocortisone acetate, triamcinolone hexacetonide,* or depot *methylprednisone* are the glucocorticoids used because

■ THE NURSING PROCESS FOR DRUGS TO TREAT RHEUMATOID ARTHRITIS

■ Assessment

The patient with rheumatoid arthritis has a chronic illness. Assessment of an individual patient will vary in depth, depending on the frequency of patient contact with the health care team and whether the disease is in remission or exacerbation. A careful history of the presenting problem should be obtained in addition to vital signs, weight, and subjective and objective data related to the complaint and the overall condition of the patient. Laboratory work would include determining the hematocrit and hemoglobin level; blood counts; tests to confirm the diagnosis or to monitor the disease such as the rheumatoid factor, antinuclear antibody (ANA), complement, and erythrocyte sedimentation rate (ESR); and tests to monitor the activity or side effects of drugs the patient is taking. Finally regular assessment of joint function and ability to perform activities of daily living should be done.

■ Management

There are no drugs that can cure rheumatoid arthritis. Goals of drug therapy are to provide analgesia, to reduce inflammation, which will in turn help to decrease pain, and to maintain or increase joint function. Management involves combining drugs with rest, application of heat, special exercises, and other therapies to improve or at least to maintain the patient's condition. The specific drugs used for a patient will be determined by response to previous drugs or dosages and the severity of the disease. The nurse should monitor the patient's response to the therapeutic regimen including such factors as pain, joint function, subjective and objective data related to the patient's complaints, new signs and symptoms possibly due to the therapy, and laboratory work specific for the drugs being used or the patient's problems. It is important for the nurse to engage in goal planning with the patient so that patient management is directed to a mutually satisfactory outcome. Maintaining ideal weight is less stressful to joints in cases of arthritis; dietary restriction and instruction may be necessary. Referral to occupational therapy, physical therapy, and visiting nurses may be helpful.

■ Evaluation

Because of the nature of the disease, evaluation of drug effectiveness will vary with the patient. That is, a specific drug used with a patient early in the disease process may decrease pain and inflammation and help increase joint mobility. In another patient the same drug may decrease pain and inflammation, but the bony changes may be too severe to allow for much if any improvement in joint function. Finally most of these drugs have frequent and serious side effects. Before discharge and self-management, the patient should be able to explain the disease process and why specific drugs are being used, possible side effects of the drugs and what action to take if they should appear, how to take ordered drugs correctly, the need for frequent follow-up and data that will be obtained at these visits to monitor for effectiveness and side effects, and the need to avoid self-medication with over-the-counter drugs unless cleared by the physician. For additional specific information see the patient care implications section at the end of this chapter.

---

they have a longer duration of action than other injectable glucocorticoids. The use of injected glucocorticoid should be accompanied by the warning to avoid strenuous use of the affected joint. This is because the glucocorticoid masks the normal signals of stress at the joint, and therefore inadvertent damage can be done to the stressed joint.

■ DRUGS FOR GOUT

■ Gout

Gout is a metabolic disease in which total body pools of uric acid (a product of DNA and RNA degradation) are elevated. The uric acid crystallizes in joints or less commonly in tendons or bursae. The joint at the base of the big toe is most commonly affected. In an

TABLE 20-4. Drugs used to treat gout

Generic name	Trade name	Dosage and administration	Comments
Allopurinol	Zyloprim	ORAL: *Adults*—200 to 300 mg daily as a single dose; maximum, 800 mg daily. Dose is reduced if there is renal insufficiency.	Inhibits the formation of uric acid from hypoxanthine or xanthine; these are excreted instead.
Colchicine	—	ORAL: *Adults*—0.5 to 0.6 mg hourly or 1 to 1.2 mg initially and 0.5 to 0.6 mg every 2 hr. This is regimen for an acute gouty attack and is continued until the pain subsides or gastrointestinal symptoms appear. Maximum dose, 7 to 8 mg. For prophylaxis, 0.5 to 1 mg daily.	To terminate an acute gouty attack. Appearance of gastrointestinal distress usually limits the amount given.
		INTRAVENOUS: for an acute attack, 1 to 2 mg initially, then 0.5 mg every 3 to 6 hr or 1 dose of 3 mg; maximum dose, 4 mg.	Dilute the drug 10-fold with sterile saline solution before injecting to minimize tissue damage.
Probenecid	Benemid	ORAL: *Adults*—250 mg 2 or 3 times daily the first week, then 500 mg twice daily thereafter. May increase to 2.0 Gm daily if necessary.	Inhibits reabsorption of uric acid by the kidney. A prophylactic drug to reduce existing trophi and to prevent recurrence of a gouty attack.
Sulfinpyrazone	Anturane	ORAL: *Adults*—100 to 200 mg 2 times daily with meals or with milk at bedtime. The dosage is raised as needed to control blood urate levels (400 to 800 mg daily). The dose is then reduced to the minimum effective level, usually 300 to 400 mg daily.	Acts like probenecid. May also prevent the recurrence of a myocardial infarction.

attack of acute gouty arthritis there is a marked inflammation of the joint accompanied by much pain. This acute attack is treated with the drug colchicine, which acts in an unknown manner to relieve the pain of gouty arthritis, with one of the nonsteroidal antiinflammatory drugs already discussed, or in special circumstances with ACTH (Chapter 35). Some patients develop a tophus in a joint—crystals of uric acid with fibrous tissue grown over them. Patients with tophi or patients with recurrent attacks of gouty arthritis need to receive long-term treatment, often for the rest of their lives, with drugs that will reduce the uric acid levels in the body.

Aspirin was once used as a drug to treat gout based on the action of salicylates, in doses over 5 Gm, to increase excretion of uric acid. Lower doses have no effect, and doses of 1 to 2 Gm may decrease uric acid excretion. If trophi are present, they will often regress with long-term therapy, thereby restoring the joint to a normal range of function. About 25% of such patients will be found to overproduce uric acid. These patients are treated with the drug allopurinol, which prevents the formation of uric acid from xanthine and hypoxanthine, the purine metabolites of DNA and RNA metabolism. The remainder of the patients are treated with an uricosuric drug, probenecid or sulfinpyrazone. These drugs increase the renal excretion of uric acid by inhibiting its reabsorption from the proximal kidney tubule.

■ Specific drugs (Table 20-4)

Colchicine

Colchicine provides relief from the pain of an acute attack of gouty arthritis, usually within 24 hours. The earlier in an episode colchicine is taken, the more effective it will be. (Antiinflammatory drugs are similarly more effective if taken early in an acute episode of gouty arthritis.) Colchicine taken orally at the doses required to treat an acute gouty attack may produce nausea and vomiting followed by diarrhea. These effects limit the amount of colchicine that can be taken. Alternatively, colchicine may be given intravenously to minimize these side effects. Since colchicine produces severe tissue inflammation, colchicine is diluted before intravenous administration to minimize the effect of any drug leakage.

Colchicine may be continued at reduced dosages once the acute episode is over. Continuance of colchicine is most common if one of the drugs to reduce body uric acid is begun. A sudden change in body uric acid concentration will often precipitate a new acute attack of gouty arthritis. This can often be avoided with prophylactic colchicine.

■ THE NURSING PROCESS FOR DRUGS TO TREAT GOUT

■ Assessment

Patients with gout may appear with the classic symptoms of pain in one or both large toes or other joints or be identified as individuals with high serum uric acid levels, even if asymptomatic. Assessment should include vital signs, weight, history of previous attacks and/or family history of gout, and assessment of subjective complaints and objective data. Blood work would include the serum uric acid level. X-ray films and joint aspiration may be required.

■ Management

The goals of drug therapy will be one or more of the following: symptomatic treatment of an existing attack, reducing the pool of urates and uric acid, and preventing recurrences. Drugs will be used to help achieve the goals in addition to rest for the affected joints, dietary restrictions to reduce purine intake on a short- or long-term basis, and a weight reduction diet if appropriate. To prevent the formation of kidney stones, a high urinary output should be maintained (2000 to 3000 ml per day), which requires a high fluid intake. A determination of fluid intake and output should be monitored in the hospitalized individual until it is certain that the high fluid output is being maintained. The nurse should monitor vital signs, blood pressure, the condition of affected joints, subjective complaints, objective signs, and appropriate laboratory work. Finally drugs or dietary manipulation may be necessary to increase the alkalinity of the urine to help prevent urate crystal formation.

■ Evaluation

Therapy with these drugs is considered effective if the discomfort associated with an acute attack lessens, if recurrent attacks are prevented, if the serum uric acid level drops toward normal and remains down, and if no kidney stones form as a result of therapy. It may be necessary to use two or more drugs to achieve these goals. Before discharge the patient should be symptomatically better or, if being treated as an outpatient, should be more comfortable in 2 to 3 days. The patient should be able to describe the disease, which medications have been prescribed and their actions, how to take the drugs to achieve maximum benefit, and the possible side effects and which ones should be reported immediately. In addition, the patient should be able to demonstrate how to plan meals within any prescribed dietary restrictions and be able to explain how to maintain a fluid intake that will ensure an adequate urinary output. For specific guidelines see the patient care implications section.

Allopurinol

Allopurinol (Zyloprim) inhibits the formation of uric acid from xanthine or hypoxanthine so that xanthine or hypoxanthine are excreted instead. A patient who produces a morning urine with a ratio of uric acid to creatinine of greater than 0.75 or whose 24-hour urine collection contains more than 600 mg of uric acid is classified as an overproducer of uric acid. These uric acid overproducers and those patients with renal uric acid crystals or with impaired renal function are those patients for whom allopurinol will be most effective. Allopurinol is also effective for patients with gout resulting from drug therapy that increases uric acid production, particularly cancer therapy. Side effects of allopurinol are rare, but those seen appear to be allergic reactions.

Probenecid and sulfinpyrazone

Probenecid (Benemid) and sulfinpyrazone (Anturane) inhibit the reabsorption of uric acid by the kidney tubules and thereby promote the excretion of uric acid in the urine. It is important that the patient drink at least eight glasses of water daily to keep the excreted uric acid dilute so that it does not crystallize in kidney tubules or bladder. Since these drugs flood the kidney tubules with uric acid, they are contraindicated in patients with renal failure or with a history of renal stones.

Probenecid is generally well tolerated but occasionally causes gastrointestinal upset or an allergic reaction. Probenecid interferes with the renal excretion of a number of compounds.

Sulfinpyrazone is also well tolerated. The incidence

of gastrointestinal upset is higher with sulfinpyrazone than with probenecid. Recent studies show that sulfinpyrazone decreases the incidence of sudden death in the first 8 months after a heart attack. This effect is believed due to decreased platelet aggregation. Since many patients with gout also have conditions such as diabetes, hypertension, or coronary artery disease, which are high-risk factors for a heart attack, sulfinpyrazone may be more desirable than probenecid in spite of the higher incidence of gastrointestinal upset.

■ Drug interactions in the therapy of gout

Factors that *diminish* the effectiveness of the uricosuric drugs probenecid or sulfinpyrazone include the following:

1. A diet high in purines produces too much uric acid. The patient should avoid animal organs, yeast, shellfish, and anchovies.
2. Inhibition of uric acid secretion counteracts the block in reabsorption by the uricosuric drugs.
   a. Heavy alcohol consumption produces enough lactic acid to inhibit uric acid secretion.
   b. Aspirin and other salicylates at low doses (300 to 650 mg) inhibit uric acid secretion. Acetaminophen should be substituted for simple pain relief.
   c. Diuretics, particularly the thiazides, furosemide, ethacrynic acid, triampterene, and spironolactone inhibit uric acid secretion.

Drugs used to treat gout can *potentiate* other drugs.

1. Probenecid inhibits the renal secretion of these drugs, keeping their plasma levels high: penicillin, indomethacin, methotrexate, sulfonylureas (oral hypoglycemics), sulfinpyrazone, salicylates, and rifampin.
2. Sulfinpyrazone inhibits the degradation of these drugs: sulfonamides, particularly sulfadiazine and sulfisoxazole, sulfonylureas (oral hypoglycemics), and coumarins.
3. Allopurinol inhibits the degradation of these drugs: azathioprine, 6-mercaptopurine, antipyrine, coumarins, and cyclophosphamide.

■ PATIENT CARE IMPLICATIONS

Analgesic-antipyretic drugs

1. Remind patients to keep these and all medications out of the reach of children. Children should never be encouraged to take medications by being told it is candy.
2. Both aspirin and acetaminophen are frequently used as antipyretics in children. Review with parents the dosages appropriate for children of various sizes and ages. These drugs are available in a variety of forms: tablets for swallowing, tablets for chewing, liquids, and suppositories. Assist parents in finding a drug form that is easy to administer. Note that absorption from a rectal suppository is variable, and there may be rectal irritation; this route of administration may be the least desirable.
3. As indicated in Table 20-1, aspirin should always be administered with a full glass of milk or water to decrease gastric irritation. Some patients may find that eating a few crackers or taking the drug with meals will help.
4. Review with patients the side effects associated with long-term use and the symptoms of salicylism (see text). Although these effects are often dose related, some individuals will find that tinnitus may be a problem at relatively low doses.
5. Review with patients the drug interactions and cross-sensitivities with aspirin discussed in the text.
6. In patients taking aspirin on a long-term basis, routine testing of the stool for the presence of occult blood may be appropriate. Patients should be instructed to report immediately any rectal bleeding or change in color (to black) or in consistency (more tarry) of stools.
7. Patients requiring long-term treatment with aspirin may find the timed-release preparations helpful, particularly at night, so that blood levels of the drug will not be so low in the morning.
8. Instruct patients to read labels carefully to check dosages. The names of drugs can be misleading. For example, Arthritis Strength Bufferin contains 7½ grains of aspirin per tablet in combination with a buffering agent. Ascriptin A/D (*A*rthritis *D*oses) contains 5 grains of aspirin per tablet, with an increase in the amount of buffering agent over the regular Ascriptin formulation.
9. Patients having difficulty tolerating aspirin may find that switching to a different brand will be helpful.
10. Aspirin is a component of many over-the-counter products, including cold remedies and products for menstrual cramps. Patients who are allergic to aspirin, those already taking aspirin on a long-term basis, those taking oral anticoagulants, or anyone routinely using over-the-counter drugs should be cautioned to read labels carefully and to avoid inadvertent overdose with aspirin.
11. Because of its effect on the platelets, aspirin is routinely prescribed by some physicians for immobilized patients, especially those who have had orthopedic surgery or trauma, to decrease the incidence of thromboembolism.
12. There are some products available that contain both aspirin and acetaminophen.
13. Patients taking oral anticoagulants should be cautioned to avoid the use of aspirin. If an analgesic-antipyretic agent is needed, acetaminophen may

ordinarily be used. If in doubt, consult the physician.

14. The long-term or excessive use of any of these medications is unwise. Patients who self-medicate with high or frequent doses of these drugs should be advised to seek regular medical follow-up.
15. Monitor the urine and blood sugar concentrations in patients receiving mefenamic acid. Patients with diabetes mellitus may find it necessary to increase the dose of insulin or oral hypoglycemic agent while receiving therapy with this analgesic.
16. Regular use of aspirin may help in the prevention of recurrent transient ischemic attacks; however the ideal dosage is not yet known (Medical Letter, p. 71, Aug. 22, 1980).

Nonsteroidal antiinflammatory drugs

1. Complete aspects of the nursing care for patients with rheumatoid arthritis, rheumatic fever, or other conditions for which these drugs are prescribed are beyond the scope of this book. Refer to appropriate nursing journals and texts.
2. In the treatment of arthritis, better results will be obtained if drugs are taken routinely, as ordered, and not on an intermittent or ''prn'' basis. Physical activity will often be better tolerated if delayed until 30 minutes after medication is taken. Rest, application of moist heat, prescribed exercises, and other treatment modalities will also assist in the management of inflammatory diseases.
3. These drugs should be used with caution during pregnancy or lactation; consult the physician.
4. Discuss with patients the fact that these drugs may improve symptoms but will not alter the long-term course of the disease being treated.
5. Administer these medications with food or antacids (except for fenoprofen) (Table 21-2).
6. There may be a cross-sensitivity that occurs in patients allergic to aspirin or any of the other nonsteroidal antiinflammatory drugs. Any of these drugs should be administered cautiously to a patient with a known allergy to any other drug in this group.
7. Remind patients to keep these and all medications out of the reach of children. Remind patients to keep all health care providers informed of all medications being taken.
8. Review the patient care implications for analgesic-antipyretic drugs for information about aspirin.

Phenylbutazone and oxyphenbutazone

1. As indicated in the text, these drugs are used only on a short-term basis because of the serious side effects that can occur. Among the hematological problems that may occur are aplastic anemia, agranulocytosis, and pancytopenia. Instruct patients to report any unusual sign or symptom, including fever, rash, sore throat, stomatitis (inflammation of or sores in the mouth), and malaise.
2. These drugs may cause gastric irritation, including ulceration. Instruct patients to report persistent dyspepsia, bleeding with stools, or a change in the color or consistency of stools. Monitoring stools for the presence of occult blood may be appropriate.
3. These drugs can cause fluid retention. Patients in whom fluid retention might be dangerous (e.g., those with cardiovascular, hypertensive, or renal disease) should be instructed to weigh themselves daily and to report weight gain in excess of 2 to 5 pounds (as determined by the health care provider).
4. Monitor the blood pressure of the hospitalized patient at least twice a day and of the outpatient on each return visit.
5. Instruct patients to report any signs of bleeding from the gums, urinary tract, or rectum; excessive bruising; or the development of petechiae. Patients who are also receiving oral anticoagulants will probably need a dosage adjustment of the anticoagulant.

Indomethacin

1. As indicated in the text, gastrointestinal disturbances are a major problem with this drug. Instruct the patient to report any bleeding with stools or changes in the color or consistency of stools. Monitoring stools at regular intervals for the presence of occult blood may be appropriate.
2. Corneal deposits and retinal disturbances have occurred in patients receiving long-term therapy. Instruct the patient to report any changes in vision. Periodic ophthalmic examinations should be performed for patients receiving long-term therapy.
3. Indomethacin may cause drowsiness. Caution patients to avoid activities requiring mental alertness (e.g., driving, operating machinery) until the effects of the medication can be evaluated.
4. A variety of other side effects may occur, including headache, dizziness, vertigo, insomnia, edema, weight gain, and rashes. Instruct the patient to report the appearance of any new sign or symptom.

Tolmetin and sulindac

1. Although eye changes have not been reported with these two drugs, the frequent eye changes seen with other nonsteroidal antiinflammatory drugs have caused the manufacturers to recommend that periodic ophthalmic examination be performed on patients receiving either drug on a long-term basis. Instruct patients to report any visual changes.
2. Both drugs occasionally cause fluid retention and peripheral edema. Patients in whom fluid retention

might be dangerous (e.g., those with cardiovascular, hypertensive, or renal disease) should be instructed to weigh themselves daily and to report weight gain in excess of 2 to 5 pounds (as determined by the health care provider). Monitor the blood pressure of hospitalized patients at least twice a day and of outpatients on each return visit.
3. Both drugs may alter coagulation studies. Instruct patients to report any unusual bleeding, bruising, or the appearance of petechiae. There is no indication that it is necessary to change the dosage of oral anticoagulants, but patients should be observed carefully, and appropriate blood studies should be done at regular intervals.
4. The most frequently seen side effects are gastrointestinal in origin, including nausea, vomiting, and diarrhea; ulceration is rare. Instruct patients to report the appearance of any new sign or symptom or change in the color or consistency of stools.
5. Headache has been reported as a side effect of these drugs, and patients should be instructed to report this if it occurs.
6. Sulindac may cause transient abnormalities in liver function tests, especially in the alkaline phosphatase level. If abnormal values persist or continue to increase, the drug should be discontinued.

Ibuprofen, naproxen, and fenoprofen

1. Periodic ophthalmic examinations should be performed on patients receiving these drugs on a long-term basis. Instruct patients to report any visual changes.
2. These drugs can cause fluid retention and peripheral edema. Patients in whom fluid retention might be dangerous (e.g., those with cardiovascular, hypertensive or renal disease) should be instructed to weigh themselves daily and to report weight gain in excess of 2 to 5 pounds (as determined by the health care provider). Monitor the blood pressure of hospitalized patients at least twice a day and of outpatients on each return visit.
3. These drugs may alter coagulation studies. Instruct patients to report any unusual bleeding, bruising, or the appearance of petechiae. There is no indication that it is necessary to change the dosage of oral anticoagulants, but patients should be observed carefully and appropriate blood studies done at regular intervals.
4. Headache has been reported as a side effect of these drugs, and patients should be instructed to report this if it occurs.
5. Gastrointestinal side effects may occur, including nausea, vomiting, diarrhea, and ulceration. Instruct patients to report the appearance of any new sign or symptom or change in the color or consistency of stools.
6. These drugs may cause dizziness or drowsiness. Caution patients to avoid hazardous activities (e.g., driving, operating machinery) until the effects of the medication can be evaluated.
7. Tinnitus and decreased hearing ability have been reported. Instruct the patient to report any ear problems. If hearing loss is suspected, audiometric testing should be done at regular intervals.
8. These drugs are being used increasingly for treatment of menstrual cramps.
9. Fenoprofen may cause increases in the blood urea nitrogen (BUN), serum transaminase, lactic dehydrogenase (LDH), and alkaline phosphatase levels. It is recommended that periodic liver and renal function tests be performed on patients receiving this drug on a long-term basis.
10. Patients receiving phenobarbital for whom fenoprofen is prescribed may require a dosage adjustment of phenobarbital.
11. Fenoprofen should not be taken with meals (Table 20-2).

Drugs for rheumatoid arthritis

Gold

1. There are a variety of contraindications to gold therapy, some of which are renal disease, marked hypertension, cardiovascular disease, uncontrolled diabetes, preexisting hematological diseases, eczema, colitis, and pregnancy. Elderly persons may not tolerate therapy well.
2. Review with patients the side effects of gold therapy and instruct them to report skin changes, rash, dermatitis, stomatitis, sore throat, malaise, excessive bruising or bleeding, the development of petechiae, or any new sign or symptom.
3. Review with patients aspects of good oral hygiene, including regular dental checkups and brushing and flossing of teeth. If stomatitis should occur, assess the advisability of continuing the usual oral care routine. It may be necessary to discontinue flossing and/or brushing until the stomatitis clears. Oral cleansing can be done with mouthwashes or gargles and by gently swabbing the mouth. Lemon-glycerin preparations should be avoided as they are often irritating if open blisters are present. The development of a metallic taste in the mouth may be an early sign of impending stomatitis. If the patient has dentures, these should be removed from the mouth, except for mealtimes, until the stomatitis clears.
4. An allergic reaction, manifested by flushing, fainting, dizziness, sweating, malaise, weakness, or even anaphylaxis, may occur after administration of any

dose. Patients should be observed for 15 to 30 minutes after a dose before being sent home. Instruct patients to report the development of any of these signs or symptoms. Epinephrine, corticosteroids, antihistamines, and oxygen should be readily available in any setting where gold therapy is administered. In some cases the allergic type reaction may be due to the solvent used in the gold preparation and not to the gold itself; switching to another preparation may be sufficient to eliminate the problem.
5. Dermatitis may be aggravated by exposure to the sun. Instruct patients receiving gold therapy to avoid prolonged exposure to the sun or other sources of ultraviolet light.
6. Urinalysis should be performed before each dose. If proteinuria or hematuria is present, the dose should be withheld and the patient's condition evaluated. Complete blood counts should be performed every other week.
7. Inform patients that several weeks or months of therapy may be necessary before improvement is seen.
8. Solganal is an oil-based suspension, and Myochrysine is an aqueous suspension. Both should be administered via deep intramuscular injection into the gluteal muscle. For directions on preparing an oil-based injection, refer to the discussion of vasopressin tannate (Pitressin tannate) in Chapter 34.

Hydroxychloroquine

See Chapter 49 for further discussion of this medication, which is also an antimalarial drug.

Penicillamine

1. Penicillamine is a copper chelating agent and is used for this action in the treatment of Wilson's disease, a disorder of copper metabolism.
2. Drug fever may occur, usually commencing about 2 to 3 weeks after the initiation of therapy. It may or may not require discontinuation of the drug. Instruct the patient to report the development of fever.
3. Patients with Wilson's disease or with poor dietary intake may require pyridoxine replacement during therapy.
4. Skin reactions, rashes, and dermatitis are common, and the patient should be instructed to report them to the physician.
5. Hematological side effects include bone marrow suppression, agranulocytosis, and thrombocytopenia. Frequent evaluation of the blood counts should be done. Instruct the patient to report any bleeding, bruising, sore throat, malaise, fever, or any new sign or symptom.
6. Oral ulcers have been reported as a side effect of therapy. Review the aspects of oral hygiene discussed under gold therapy, item 3.
7. Other signs and symptoms that have been reported include tinnitus, excessive wrinkling of skin, anorexia, diarrhea, and decrease in taste perception. The patient should be carefully assessed on each visit to the health care center.
8. Cross-sensitivity between penicillin and penicillamine does not always occur, but patients should be questioned about possible allergy to penicillin before therapy with penicillamine is begun. Patients with a history of penicillin allergy should be observed carefully when therapy with penicillamine is begun.
9. Remind patients to keep these and all medications out of the reach of children.

Drugs for gout

1. For additional information about the treatment of gout, including appropriate dietary restrictions, consult nursing or medical texts.
2. The patient should be instructed to stay well hydrated so that an output of at least 2000 to 3000 ml per day is maintained.
3. Better relief is obtained if these drugs are used consistently, that is, as prescribed, rather than intermittently.
4. Remind patients to keep these and all medications out of the reach of children.

Colchicine

1. Inform patients that nausea, vomiting, and diarrhea may occur and that if they do occur, the physician should be notified. These symptoms serve as a warning that the dose being used is too high and that a lower dose is needed.
2. Long-term administration may be associated with a variety of hematological problems. Instruct patients to report any sore throat, fever, rash, malaise, excessive bruising or bleeding, or the development of petechiae.

Probenecid and sulfinpyrazone

1. Patients taking either of these drugs should be taught to maintain a fluid intake of 3000 to 4000 ml per day.
2. There are several preparations available that contain both probenecid and colchicine. Patients taking these combination products should be taught about each of the separate drugs.
3. Review with patients taking either of these drugs the interactions outlined in the text. Remind patients to keep all health care providers informed of all medications being taken.

4. Gastrointestinal side effects are the most common with these drugs and may be indicative of overdosage. Advise patients to report the appearance of any new sign or symptom. Taking the drug with meals or milk may help decrease the side effects.
5. Because probenecid may prolong the action of oral hypoglycemic agents, patients taking these two drugs should be alerted to the possibility that hypoglycemia may be a problem and that it should be reported if it occurs.
6. Alkalinization of the urine helps prevent crystallization of the uric acid. For this reason sodium bicarbonate, potassium citrate, or other alkalinizing agents may be prescribed concurrently with probenecid or sulfinpyrazone. Once serum urate levels return to normal, it may be possible to discontinue the alkalinizing agent.
7. Sulfinpyrazone may potentiate the action of oral hypoglycemic agents or insulin. Patients with diabetes mellitus should be alerted to the possibility of hypoglycemia and should report it if it occurs.
8. Anturane brand of sulfinpyrazone contains FD&C coloring number 5 (tartrazine), which may cause an allergic response in some individuals. Although rare, this response is more common in individuals with aspirin hypersensitivity.
9. Sulfinpyrazone may potentiate the action of oral anticoagulants. Patients receiving both drugs should be cautioned to report any excessive bleeding or bruising.
10. Low doses of aspirin and other salicylates inhibit uric acid secretion. Instruct patients to avoid the use of aspirin; acetaminophen may be used.

Allopurinol

1. Instruct the patient to notify the physician if a rash appears, as this is often the first sign of an allergic reaction and usually warrants discontinuing the drug.
2. Drowsiness may be a side effect of this drug. Caution patients to avoid activities requiring mental alertness (e.g., driving, operating machinery) until the effects of the medication can be evaluated.
3. Long-term administration of this drug may be associated with elevations of alkaline phosphatase and serum transaminase levels. If these blood studies are elevated, evaluation of the patient is appropriate.
4. Patients receiving mercaptopurine or azathioprine who are then started on allopurinol will require a reduction in dose of the mercatopurine or azathioprine to one fourth to one half the previous dose.
5. Salicylates may apparently be used with this drug with no adverse interactions.
6. Allopurinol prolongs the half-life of coumarin oral anticoagulants. Caution patients receiving both drugs to be alert to excessive bleeding or bruising and to report them if they occur. It may be necessary to reduce the dose of the anticoagulant.
7. Hematological problems have been reported occasionally. Instruct the patient to report any sore throat, fever, malaise, rash, bruising, or bleeding.
8. Patients should be reminded to maintain a high fluid intake, especially if they are also receiving a uricosuric drug.

■ SUMMARY

Aspirin is the prototype of the analgesic-antipyretic and nonsteroidal antiinflammatory drugs.

Aspirin and acetaminophen are over-the-counter drugs widely used by the public for analgesia and for treating a fever. Analgesia results from the inhibition of peripheral pain receptors. Antipyresis results from an action on the hypothalamus to overcome the action of pyrogen, a fever-producing protein released by phagocytes. Acetaminophen does not produce gastrointestinal irritation and does not alter platelet function or bleeding times as does aspirin. Acetaminophen is also formulated as a liquid for infants and children.

Aspirin is well absorbed and is rapidly hydrolyzed in the blood to salicylic acid. Aspirin irreversibly inactivates the enzyme cyclooxygenase of platelets, a characteristic only of aspirin and not of other salicylates. This irreversible inactivation accounts for the inhibition of blood clotting characteristic of even low doses of aspirin. Gastrointestinal irritation is the other major side affect of aspirin. Salicylism is mild intoxication with aspirin. Symptoms of salicylism include tinnitus, hyperventilation, and, occasionally, fever. Drug interactions and cross-sensitivities for aspirin allergies are listed in the text.

Other analgesic-antipyretic drugs include the over-the-counter drugs salicylamide and sodium salicylate and the prescription drug mefenamic acid.

The major mechanism of action of the nonsteroidal antiinflammatory drugs is the inhibition of prostaglandin synthesis. The nonsteroidal antiinflammatory drugs are effectve in treating the pain and inflammation of rheumatoid arthritis, osteoarthritis, other kinds of arthritis, muscle injury, gout, and dysmenorrhea. A common side effect is gastrointestinal upset. These drugs are variable in affecting platelet function and blood clotting.

Aspirin is an effective antiinflammatory drug but at much larger doses than are required for analgesia-antipyresis. Salicylates may be used if gastrointestinal upset becomes a problem. The other nonsteroidal antiinflammatory drugs are prescription drugs. Phenylbutazone and oxyphenbutazone are potent. Because they have potentially severe side effects and drug interactions, they are used for only 2 weeks or less. Indomethacin and the related new drugs sulindac, tolmetin, and zomepirac are another group of nonsteroidal antiinflammatory drugs. Limitations of indomethacin include gastrointestinal upset, headache, and dizziness. The arylalkanoic acids include ibuprofen, naproxen, and fenoprofen. These new drugs have less severe side effects than the other nonsteroidal antiinflammatory drugs and are proving a suitable alternative for patients with arthritis who cannot tolerate aspirin. Meclofenamate is a new drug released as an nonsteroidal antiinflammatory drug. Its major side effect is gastrointestinal upset with diarrhea.

One role of selected nonsteroidal antiinflammatory drugs is to reduce the pain and inflammation of rheumatoid arthritis until a remission occurs. If a remission does not occur and joint damage continues, a drug may be tried to induce a remission. Those drugs include gold salts, hydrochloroquine, and penicillamine. Since each drug can produce serious side effects, careful monitoring of the patient is required during therapy. The immunosuppressive drugs azathioprine and cyclophosphamide and the glucocorticoids have restricted roles in the treatment of rheumatoid arthritis.

Gout is a metabolic disease with elevated concentrations of uric acid. Gouty arthritis arises when uric acid crystallizes in one or more joints. Treatment of gout is of two types: treatment of a acute attack marked by severe inflammation of the joint and long-term treatment designed to prevent the recurrence of an acute attack. An acute attack may be treated with a nonsteroidal antiinflammatory drug, traditionally phenylbutazone, oxyphenbutazone, or indomethacin, or by the drug colchicine, whose mode of action is unknown. Long-term therapy is with allopurinol to inhibit the formation of uric acid and/or probenecid or sulfinpyrazone to promote the excretion of uric acid. These drugs for long-term treatment cause a number of drug interactions, which are listed in the text.

■ STUDY QUESTIONS

1. List the three pharmacological actions characteristic of aspirin.
2. How do the nonnarcotic analgesics produce analgesia?
3. What is the mechanism of antipyresis?
4. Which two paraaminophenols are found in over-the-counter analgesic-antipyretic drugs?
5. Why is acetaminophen considered safer than aspirin?
6. What are the side effects of acetaminophen?
7. What is the mechanism of acetaminophen toxicity?
8. What is the dosage difference for aspirin taken for analgesia-antipyresis versus an antiinflammatory response?
9. How does aspirin affect the stomach?
10. How does aspirin affect platelets?
11. What factors determine the metabolism and excretion of salicylate?
12. Describe salicylism.
13. Describe aspirin toxicity.
14. What pharmacological actions are characteristic of the nonsteroidal antiinflammatory drugs?
15. Why are phenylbutazone or oxyphenbutazone used for 2 weeks or less?
16. What are the major side effects of indomethacin?
17. Which new nonsteroidal antiinflammatory drugs are chemically related to indomethacin?
18. Describe the uses of ibuprofen, naproxen, and fenoprofen.
19. Which three drugs may be used to induce a remission in progressive rheumatoid arthritis?
20. Describe the role of colchicine in treating gout.
21. Describe the mechanisms of allopurinol, probenecid, and sulfinpyrazone for lowering the uric acid concentration of the body.

■ SUGGESTED READINGS

Analgesic-antipyretic drugs

Acetaminophen

Bailey, B.O.: Acetaminophen hepatotoxicity and overdose, American Family Physician **22**(1):83, 1980.

Cote, J., Moriarty, R.W., and Rumack, B.H.: Facing toxic overdose of acetaminophen, Patient Care **12:**16, Aug. 15, 1979.

Gever, L.N.: A new treatment for a new problem: acetaminophen overdose, Nursing '80 **10**(6):57, 1980.

Holtman, D.J.: Acetaminophen overdose, Journal of Emergency Nursing **4:**50, May-June, 1978.

Macy, A.M.: Preventing hepatotoxicity in acetaminophen overdose, American Journal of Nursing **79:**301, 1979.

Aspirin

Aspirin for transient ischemic attacks, The Medical Letter **22:**71, Aug. 22, 1980.

Beaver, W.T., Kantor, T.G., and Levy, G.: On guard for aspirin's harmful effects, Patient Care **13:**48, Sept. 30, 1979.

Beaver, W.T., Kantor, T.G., and Levy, G.: Putting aspirin to its many good uses, Patient Care **13:**70, Sept. 30, 1979.

Czervionke, R.L., Hoak, J.C., and Fry, G.L.: Effect of aspirin on thrombin-induced adherence of platelets to cultured cells from the blood vessel wall, Journal of Clinical Investigation **62:**847, 1978.

Edwards, J.L., and Taylor, R.B.: Salicylate intoxication in family practice, Postgraduate Medicine **67:**183, 1980.

Levy, G., and Giacomini, K.M.: Rational aspirin dosage regimens, Clinical Pharmacology and Therapeutics **23:**247, 1978.

McCaffery, M.: How to relieve your patient's pain fast and effectively . . . with oral analgesics, Nursing '80 **10**(11):68, 1980.

McCain, H.W., and Teague, R.S.: Metabolic complications of salicylate overload, Drug Therapy **9**(1):70, 1979.

Pierce, P.F.: About analgesics and kidney damage, Nurses' Drug Alert, Special Report **4**(9):89, 1980.

A randomized, controlled trial of aspirin in persons recovered from myocardial infarction, Journal of the American Medical Association **243:**661, 1980.

Rothschild, B.M.: Hematologic perturbations associated with salicylate, Clinical Pharmacology and Therapeutics **26:**145, 1979.

Samter, M.: Intolerance to aspirin, Hospital Practice **3**(12):85, 1973.

Prostaglandins and nonsteroidal antiinflammatory drugs

Brune, K., Graf, P., and Glatt, M.: Inhibition of prostaglandin synthesis in vivo by nonsteroid anti-inflammatory drugs: evidence for the importance of pharmacokinetics, Agents and Actions **6:**159, 1976.

Caldwell, B., Heymann, M.A., Ramwell, P., and Weksler, B.: Practical prostaglandins? Coming up, Patient Care **13:**20, June 15, 1979.

DiRosa, M., and Persico, P.: Mechanism of inhibition of prostaglandin biosynthesis by hydrocortisone in rat leucocytes, British Journal of Pharmacology **66:**161, 1979.

Lewis, J.R.: Evaluation of new analgesics, Journal of the American Medical Association **243:**1465, 1980.

Marx, J.L.: Dysmenorrhea: basic research leads to a rational therapy, Science **205:**175, 1979.

Moncada, S., and Vane, J.R.: Arachidonic acid metabolites and the interactions between platelets and blood-vessel walls, The New England Journal of Medicine **300:**1142, 1979.

Robinson, D.R.: Prostaglandins and their relationship to rheumatic diseases, Resident & Staff Physician **25**(2):92, 1979.

Smith, M.J.H., Walker, J.R., Ford-Hutchinson, A.W., and Penington, D.G.: Platelets, prostaglandins and inflammation, Agents and Actions **6:**701, 1976.

Willkens, R.F.: The use of nonsteroidal anti-inflammatory agents, Journal of the American Medical Association **240:**1632, 1978.

Drugs for rheumatoid arthritis

Brooks, P.M.: Drug treatment of rheumatoid arthritis, Australian New Zealand Journal of Medicine **8**(suppl. 1):101, 1978.

Brown-Skeers, V.: How the nurse practitioner manages the rheumatoid arthritis patient, Nursing '79 **9**(6):26, 1979.

Bunch, T.W., and O'Duffy, J.D.: Disease-modifying drugs for progressive rheumatoid arthritis, Mayo Clinic Proceedings **55:**161, 1980.

Calin, A.: Rheumatoid arthritis, American Family Physician **18**(1):89, 1978.

Healey, L.A.: The management of rheumatoid arthritis, Resident & Staff Physician **24:**50, 1978.

Hudak, C.M.: A pyramidal treatment plan for the patient with arthritis, Nurse Practitioner **2**(3):19, 1977.

Lightfoot, R.W., Jr.: Therapy of rheumatoid disease, American Family Physician **19**(3):186, 1979.

O'Duffy, J.D.: Gold compounds in rheumatoid arthritis, Drug Therapy **9**(3):54, 1979.

Ridolfo, A.S.: Nonsteroidal anti-inflammatory agents in arthritis, American Family Physician **17**(2):131, 1978.

Spruck, M.: Gold therapy for rheumatoid arthritis, American Journal of Nursing **79:**1246, 1979.

Turner, R.: Aspirin and newer anti-inflammatory agents in rheumatoid arthritis, American Family Physician **16**(1):111, 1977.

Drugs for gout

Gordon, G.V., and Schumacher, H.R.: Management of gout, American Family Physician **19**(1):91, 1979.

Kweskin, S.: New and old options in gout therapy, Patient Care **13:** 124, Jan. 30, 1979.

Simkin, P.A.: Management of gout, Annals of Internal Medicine **90:** 812, 1979.

Talbott, J.H.: Treating gout: successful methods of prevention and control, Postgraduate Medicine **63**(5):175, 1978.

21 Antihistamines

THE EFFECTS OF HISTAMINE

Naturally occurring histamine

Histamine is a naturally occurring amine that is formed from the amino acid histidine. Histamine is found in three major sites. One site is in mast cells, which are numerous in the lung and skin, and basophils, the counterparts of mast cells in the blood. The histamine released from the mast cells causes many of the symptoms associated with allergic reactions. The second site is in the gastrointestinal tract where histamine is a potent stimulant for the secretion of acid in the stomach. The third site is in certain parts of the brain where histamine is believed to be a neurotransmitter. The role of histamine in the brain at present is speculative but may involve regulating the level of arousal.

In this chapter the focus is on the role of histamine in allergic reactions and the drugs available to treat these reactions. The role of histamine in the stomach is discussed in Chapter 11.

Histamine release

Histamine in the mast cells and basophils is complexed with heparin and stored in granules. The typical allergic reaction such as hay fever or contact dermatitis involves the release of these granules in response to an antigen. Antibodies of the IgE class fix to the mast cells and basophils, and, when an antigen appears and binds to the fixed IgE, the cells degranulate, releasing histamine, heparin, and other compounds, which alter capillary permeability and attract phagocytes to degrade the bound antigen. This process is illustrated in Fig. 21-1.

In addition to the antigen-induced degranulation, many drugs and venoms cause degranulation. These include drugs and dyes that carry a positive charge, large molecules as in animal sera and dextran solutions, and venoms and enzymes that damage tissue.

Allergic responses explained by the action of histamine

Local allergic responses involving histamine are as follows:

- Angioedema: swelling caused by plasma leakage and blood vessel dilation in the skin or mucous membranes. ''Giant hives.''
- Anaphylaxis: Systemic. Onset is usually heralded by a generalized itching and tingling sensation and a feeling of apprehension. A profound hypotension leading to shock may follow, and the bronchioles are constricted, causing a choking sensation.
- Asthma: spasm of the bronchial smooth muscle.
- Eczema: inflamed areas of skin.
- Purpura: red spots on the skin caused by the leakage of blood from small vessels.
- Rhinitis: inflammation of the nasal mucous membranes that allows fluid to escape.
- Urticaria: hives, which are large wheals caused by leakage of plasma and are accompanied by severe itching.

Two actions of histamine are prominent in explaining allergic responses. First, histamine is a potent dilator of arterioles and makes the capillaries more permeable so that fluid and protein are lost into the extravascular space. This explains the bump that appears after an insect sting. Initially, there is a red spot reflecting the dilation of the small blood vessels, and as fluid leaks into the extravascular space, the bump, representing local edema, appears. Second, histamine stimulates the contraction of smooth muscle, particularly the bronchial smooth muscle. When mast cells are degranulated in the lung, as in asthma, the airway is narrowed and it becomes difficult to breathe.

Histamine released systemically causes anaphylaxis, which is characterized by a profound fall in blood pressure resulting from vasodilation and severe constriction of the bronchioles making breathing difficult. The loss of fluid from circulation resulting from the increased capillary permeability causes the shock that develops in an untreated anaphylactic response. Edema in the mucous tissue of the upper windpipe (laryngeal edema) can block the airway altogether. The treatment of choice

FIG. 21-1

The immunological mechanism underlying the release of histamine from mast cells is pictured. Antibodies of the IgE class are bound to the surface of mast cells. Binding of an antigen to IgE triggers degranulation of the mast cell, releasing histamine and slow reacting substance of anaphylaxis (SRS-A). Histamine is responsible for many of the symptoms of allergies and asthma.

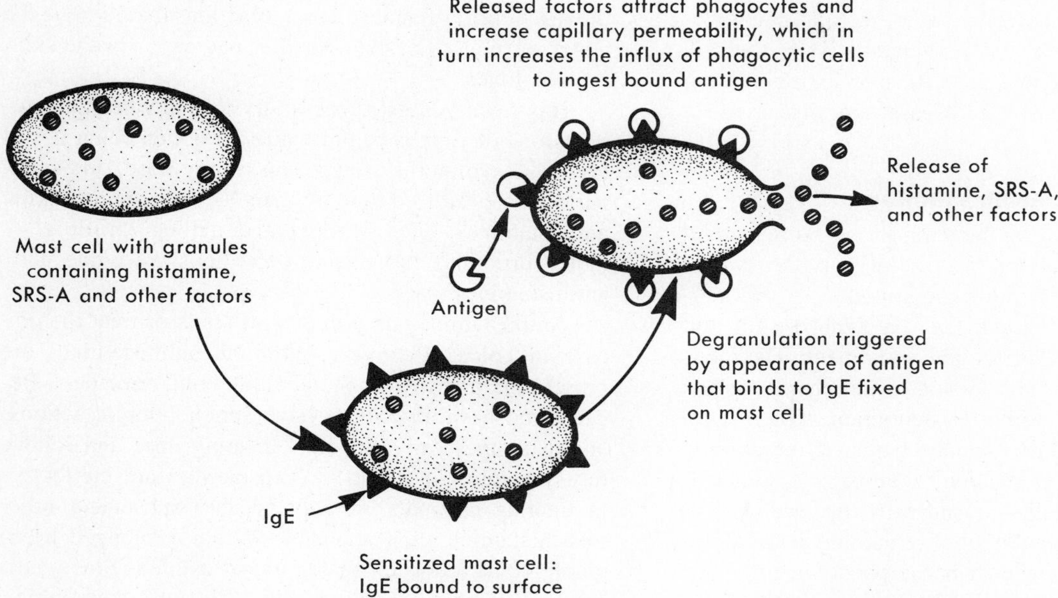

for anaphylactic shock is epinephrine. Epinephrine constricts blood vessels to raise the blood pressure and relieve laryngeal edema and dilates the bronchioles, actions that reverse those of histamine (Chapter 12).

■ Histamine metabolism

Once histamine is released, it is metabolized to inactive compounds in 5 to 15 minutes. One of the degradative pathways is inhibited by aspirin so that histamine may persist. This is the mechanism for one type of aspirin sensitivity.

■ ANTIHISTAMINES

Antihistamines have been available for about 40 years. Although these drugs are effective in blocking some actions of histamine, they are ineffective in blocking the histamine-mediated secretion of acid in the stomach. The explanation is that there are two types of histamine receptors: the H-1 receptors, acting principally on blood vessels and the bronchioles, and the H-2 receptors, acting principally on the gastrointestinal tract. The older antihistamines are specific antagonists for the H-1 receptors. One antagonist for the H-2 receptor is currently available clinically to reduce stomach acid: cimetidine (Tagamet), which is discussed in Chapter 11. In the present chapter, the term *antihistamine* will refer to drugs that specifically block the H-1 receptors.

■ Absorption and fate of antihistamines

Antihistamines are given orally and are well absorbed. Their action is seen in 10 to 30 minutes and lasts for 4 to 6 hours. Timed-release forms are active 8 to 12 hours. Antihistamines are metabolized to inactive compounds by the liver and kidneys.

■ Other pharmacological actions of antihistamines

Although the antihistamines are so named because they specifically compete with histamine for the H-1 receptors, the antihistamines have other pharmacological properties. The main secondary action is an anticholinergic or atropine-like action. This is the origin of side effects such as inhibition of secretions, blurred vision, urinary retention, fast heart rate (tachycardia), and constipation. In the central nervous system, the anticholinergic effect can cause insomnia, tremors, nervousness, and irritability. These effects are particularly predominant in children. Sedation and drowsiness, the central antihistaminic effects, are more commonly seen in adults. The spectrum of antihistaminic and anticholinergic properties depends on the drug, the dose, and the individual.

Most antihistamines have a local anesthetic effect, which might relieve the itching of skin rashes. Antihistamines are rarely used for this purpose because they tend to be good antigens, thereby causing skin rashes themselves. There are other clinically important pharmacological actions limited to a few of the antihistamines. Some antihistamines are effective in preventing nausea and vomiting, particularly from motion sickness. A few antihistamines prevent vertigo (the feeling of movement, particularly rotational movement, when there is none). Antihistamines that are effective in suppressing the tremors of Parkinson's disease are discussed in Chapter 32.

■ Toxic effects of antihistamines

An overdose of an antihistamine can cause central nervous system depression or central nervous system stimulation, the latter being more common in children. The atropine-like symptoms (i.e., a flushed skin and fixed, dilated pupils) also become prominent. The treatment is to maintain an airway and to treat hypotension. In children a high temperature is common, which is reversed with ice packs and sponge baths. If the antihistamine is not a phenothiazine, vomiting is induced, gastric lavage is carried out, and cathartics are used to empty the gastrointestinal tract of remaining drug. Vomiting should not be induced when a phenothiazine antihistamine is involved because phenothiazines can cause uncoordinated movements of the head and neck, which would cause aspiration of vomitus. The antihistamines that are phenothiazine derivatives are identified in the drug tables.

■ Drug interactions and contraindications for antihistamines

The main drug interaction associated with the antihistamines is the additive depression of the central nervous system when taken with alcohol, hypnotics, sedatives, antipsychotics, antianxiety drugs, or narcotic analgesics. Because of their atropine-like effects, the antihistamines should be used with caution in patients with glaucoma, hyperthyroidism, cardiovascular disease, or hypertension.

Antihistamines are contraindicated for nursing mothers because the drug is secreted in the milk. Antihistamines taken by young children can cause paradoxical excitement, whereas the elderly are sensitive to the sedative actions.

■ CLINICAL USES OF ANTIHISTAMINES

■ Antihistamines for allergic reactions

(Table 21-1)

Antihistamines are effective primarily in decreasing the discomfort of acute allergic reactions that involve the upper respiratory system, such as hay fever, or the skin, such as hives.

Hay fever is most successfully treated when the antihistamine therapy is begun while the pollen count is still low. The symptoms of sneezing, runny nose, and swollen eyes are reduced in more than 70% of patients taking antihistamines. The swelling and itching (pruritus) of hives (urticaria) and related conditions are reduced by antihistamines.

Antihistamines do not prevent colds or treat the disease of colds effectively, although antihistamines are present in many over-the-counter cold remedies. Because most antihistamines have anticholinergic actions, antihistamines can "dry up" a runny nose and relieve the symptoms of a cold. Antihistamines are ineffective in treating asthma, probably because substances other than histamine are responsible for the prolonged bronchiole constriction characteristic of asthma. Since antihistamines have a drying effect because they inhibit bronchial secretions, antihistamines can make asthma worse.

Antihistamines exert no effect of their own on histamine receptors. Because of this, some allergic responses are not effectively treated with antihistamines. Anaphylaxis, the response to the systemic release of histamine, represents a true emergency for which an antihistamine is inadequate because it neither acts fast enough nor can it reverse the histamine reactions. Epinephrine acts rapidly, and its pharmacological actions reverse those of histamine.

TABLE 21-1. Antihistamines used to control allergic reactions

Generic name	Trade name	Dosage and administration	Comments
Azatadine maleate	Optimine	ORAL: *Adults*—1 to 2 mg twice daily. *Children*—not established.	Drowsiness is the most common side effect.
Bromodiphenhydramine hydrochloride	Ambodryl	ORAL: *Adults*—25 to 50 mg 3 times daily.	
Brompheniramine maleate	Bromatane Dimetane Rolabromophen	ORAL: *Adults*—4 to 8 mg 3 to 4 times daily or 8 to 12 mg of sustained-release form 2 to 3 times daily. *Children*—over 6 yr, ½ adult dose; under 6 yr, 0.5 mg/kg daily divided into 3 to 4 doses.	Drowsiness is the most common side effect.
Carbinoxamine maleate	Clistin	ORAL: *Adults*—4 to 8 mg 3 to 4 times daily or 8 to 12 mg of sustained-release form 2 to 3 times daily. *Children*—over 6 yr, 4 mg 3 to 4 times daily; 3 to 6 yr, 2 to 4 mg 3 to 4 times daily; 1 to 3 yr, 2 mg 3 to 4 times daily.	Low incidence of drowsiness. Anticholinergic effect is weak.
Chlorpheniramine maleate	Chlormene Chlortab Chlor-Trimeton* Ciramine Pyranistan Trymegen	ORAL: *Adults*—4 mg 3 to 4 times daily or 8 to 12 mg of sustained-release form 2 to 3 times daily. *Children*—6 to 12 yr, 2 mg 3 to 4 times daily or 8 mg of sustained-release form once daily; 2 to 6 yr, 1 mg 3 to 4 times daily.	Low incidence of drowsiness. A common ingredient in cold remedies.
Clemastine	Tavist	ORAL: *Adults*—2.68 mg 3 times daily. Not intended for children.	Low incidence of drowsiness. Very weak anticholinergic effects.
Cyproheptadine hydrochloride	Periactin	ORAL: *Adults*—4 to 20 mg daily, not more than 0.5 mg/kg. Dose is started at 4 mg 3 times daily. *Children*—7 to 14 yr, 4 mg 2 to 3 times daily to a maximum of 16 mg daily; 2 to 6 yr, 2 mg 2 to 3 times daily to a maximum of 12 mg daily.	Used to relieve itching. Drowsiness is the most common side effect.
Dexchlorpheniramine maleate	Polaramine	ORAL: *Adults*—1 to 2 mg 3 or 4 times daily or 4 to 6 mg 2 times daily or 6 mg of timed-release form 3 times daily. *Children*—under 12 yr, 0.15 mg/kg daily divided into 4 doses.	Drowsiness is the most common side effect.
Dimethindene maleate	Forhistal Maleate Triten	ORAL: *Adults and children over 6 yr*—1 to 2 mg 1 to 3 times daily or 2.5 mg of sustained-release form 1 to 2 times daily.	High incidence of drowsiness.
Diphenhydramine hydrochloride	Benadryl Hydrochloride Bendylate Fenylhist Rohydra Valdrene	ORAL: *Adults*—25 to 50 mg 3 to 4 times daily. *Children*—over 20 lb, 2.5 to 25 mg 3 to 4 times daily; under 12 yr, 5 mg/kg in 4 divided doses each day.	High incidence of drowsiness with little paradoxical stimulation in children. Also used to treat motion sickness and mild Parkinsonism. Also used as an antitussive. May be used with epinephrine in treating an anaphylactic reaction.

*Available without a prescription.

Continued.

TABLE 21-1. Antihistamines used to control allergic reactions—cont'd

Generic name	Trade name	Dosage and administration	Comments
Diphenylpyraline hydrochloride	Diafen Hispril	ORAL: *Adults*—2 mg every 4 hr or 5 mg of sustained-release form every 12 hr. *Children*—over 6 yr, 2 mg every 6 hr or 5 mg of sustained-release form once daily; 2 to 6 yr, 1 to 2 mg every 8 hr.	
Doxylamine succinate	Decapryn*	ORAL: *Adults*—12.5 to 25 mg every 4 to 6 hr. *Children*—6 to 12 yr, 75 mg divided into 4 to 6 doses daily; under 6 yr, 2 mg/kg body weight divided into 4 to 6 doses daily.	High incidence of drowsiness. Often included in nonprescription sleep aids.
Methdilazine hydrochloride	Tacaryl	ORAL: *Adults*—8 mg 2 to 4 times daily. *Children*—over 3 yr, 4 mg 2 to 4 times daily.	A phenothiazine derivative used primarily to relieve itching. Incidence of drowsiness is less than with other phenothiazines.
Promethazine hydrochloride	Phenergan Quadnite Remsed Zipan	ORAL: *Adults*—12.5 mg 4 times daily or 25 mg at bedtime. *Children*—½ adult dose.	A phenothiazine derivative with marked sedative action. Also used to treat motion sickness and to control nausea and vomiting.
Pyrilamine maleate	Allertoc* Zem-Histine*	ORAL: *Adults*—25 to 50 mg 4 times daily. *Children*—6 to 12 yr, ½ adult dose.	Low incidence of drowsiness.
Trimeprazine tartrate	Temaril	ORAL: *Adults*—2.5 mg 4 times daily or 5 mg of sustained-release form every 12 hr. *Children*—over 3 yr, 2.5 mg at bedtime or up to 3 times daily (over 6 yr can take 5 mg of sustained-release form once a day); 6 mo to 3 yr, 1.25 mg at bedtime or up to 3 times daily.	A phenothiazine derivative. Drowsiness is the most common reaction. Used primarily to relieve the itching of neurodermatitis, contact dermatitis, and chickenpox.
Tripelennamine citrate or hydrochloride	PBZ-SR Pyribenzamine Hydrochloride Ro-Hist	ORAL: *Adults*—25 to 50 mg every 4 to 6 hr or 100 mg of sustained-release form every 12 hr. *Children*—over 5 yr, 50 mg of sustained-release form every 12 hr; children and infants, 5 mg/kg daily divided into 4 to 6 doses.	Dizziness is a common side effect.
Triprolidine hydrochloride	Actidil	ORAL: *Adults*—2.5 mg 3 to 4 times daily. *Children*—over 6 yr, ½ adult dose; under 6 yr, 0.3 to 0.6 mg 3 to 4 times daily	Low incidence of side effects, with drowsiness being the most common side effect.

*Available without a prescription.

■ THE NURSING PROCESS FOR ANTIHISTAMINES USED IN TREATMENT OF ALLERGIC REACTIONS

■ Assessment

The patient requiring antihistamines for allergic reactions may be displaying nonacute symptoms such as red, watery eyes; nasal congestion; hives; or rash. Nausea, vomiting, and diarrhea may represent allergy to food or medications. An acute allergic response (anaphylaxis) manifests with rapidly developing edema of the face and hands, wheezing, bronchoconstriction, cyanosis, dyspnea, tachycardia, and hypotension, which can lead to death. Anaphylaxis is an emergency; the more delayed and chronic response may represent a source of annoyance to the patient but may never progress to an acute phase.

Vital signs, respiratory and cardiovascular status, relevant history of previous allergy and exposure to possible allergens, subjective symptoms, and objective data such as the extent and type of rash should be assessed.

■ Management

The acute allergic reaction anaphylaxis requires immediate diagnosis and treatment, usually with 1:1000 epinephrine injected subcutaneously or intramuscularly, followed by parenteral antihistamines. Supportive care is symptomatic and based on rapid assessment of the cardiovascular and respiratory response of the patient. Management of the less acute allergic response is not an emergency. The nurse should monitor the vital signs, respiratory status, cardiovascular status, platelet count, and white blood cell count. The patient is observed for side effects of drug therapy, especially drowsiness; the fluid intake and output are monitored to determine urinary retention; and frequency of bowel movements is monitored to determine constipation. At the same time, the patient may be undergoing tests to identify the specific allergens responsible.

■ Evaluation

Before discharge, the patient should be able to explain why and how to take the prescribed medication, the side effects that may appear and which of these should be reported immediately, and what to do for specific side effects such as dry mouth, constipation, hypotension, and drowsiness. If specific allergens have been identified, the patient should be able to name them. The patient should be able to state the importance of wearing a medical identification tag or bracelet identifying specific allergens. The goal of therapy is primarily to reduce the histamine response and improve patient comfort. Treatment with antihistamines does not eliminate any allergies. Ideally, the patient would be symptomatically improved and free of drug side effects. In fact, most patients have some side effects resulting from antihistamine therapy. For additional information, see the patient care implications section at the end of this chapter.

TABLE 21-2. Antihistamines used to control nausea and vomiting

Generic name	**Trade name**	**Dosage and administration**	**Comments**
Buclizine hydrochloride	Bucladin-S	ORAL: *Adults*—50 mg 30 min before travel, 50 mg 4 to 6 hr later for extended travel. 50 mg 2 to 3 times daily to control nausea. Not for children.	Most effective for preventing motion sickness. May alleviate nausea of disorders causing dizziness. Contraindicated in pregnancy. Drowsiness and anticholinergic effects are the most frequent side effects.
Cyclizine hydrochloride, cyclizine lactate	Marezine Hydrochloride and Lactate	ORAL: *Adults*—50 mg 30 min before travel, 50 mg 4 to 6 hr later for extended travel, maximum dosage 200 mg daily. *Children*—6 to 10 yr, ½ adult dose. INTRAMUSCULAR: *Adults*—50 mg every 4 to 6 hr as needed.	Most effective for preventing motion sickness. Used for treating postoperative nausea and vomiting. Drowsiness and anticholinergic effects are the most frequent side effects.
Dimenhydrinate	Dramamine* Dimenest Dramocen Dymenate Trav-Arex* Various others Vertiban*	ORAL: *Adults*—50 mg every 4 hr. *Children*—8 to 12 yr, 25 to 50 mg 3 times daily. INTRAMUSCULAR, INTRAVENOUS, RECTAL: same as oral, if required. Intravenous dose should take at least 2 min.	Most effective for preventing motion sickness. Drowsiness is the most frequent side effect.
Diphenhydramine hydrochloride	Benadryl Hydrochloride Fenylhist Rohydra Valdrene	ORAL: *Adults*—50 mg 30 min before travel, 50 mg every 6 to 8 hr during travel. *Children*—over 20 lb, ¼ to ½ adult dose (5 mg/kg every 12 hr). INTRAMUSCULAR: *Adults*—10 to 50 mg every 2 to 3 hr up to 400 mg/day. *Children*—5 mg/kg in 4 doses up to 300 mg/day.	Most effective for preventing motion sickness. Drowsiness is a frequent side effect.
Hydroxyzine hydrochloride, hydroxyzine pamoate	Atarax Vistaril	ORAL: *Adults*—25 to 100 mg 3 to 4 times daily. *Children*—over 6 yr, 50 to 100 mg daily in divided doses; under 6 yr, 50 mg daily in divided doses. INTRAMUSCULAR: *Adults*—25 to 50 mg. *Children*—0.5 mg/lb.	A sedative that controls nausea and vomiting.
Meclizine hydrochloride	Antivert Bonine* Eldezine* Roclizine* Vertrol* Weyvert*	ORAL: *Adults*—25 to 50 mg 1 hr before travel, repeated every 24 hr during the journey. Not recommended for children.	Most effective for preventing motion sickness and vertigo. Contraindicated in pregnancy. Drowsiness and anticholinergic effects are the most common side effects.
Promethazine hydrochloride	Fellozine Phenergan Promine Prorex Provigan Quadnite Remsed V-Gan Zipan-50	ORAL, RECTAL: *Adults*—25 mg 30 to 60 min before travel, repeat in 8 to 12 hr. During journey, 25 mg on arising and at dinner. *Children*—½ adult dose. *Postoperatively:* 25 mg every 4 to 6 hr; children's dose ½ adult dose. INTRAMUSCULAR: ½ oral dose.	A phenothiazine derivative. Used to treat motion sickness and postoperative nausea and vomiting.

*Available without a prescription.

■ THE NURSING PROCESS FOR PATIENTS TAKING ANTIHISTAMINES AS ANTIEMETICS

■ Assessment

There are a variety of conditions and situations that may produce nausea and vomiting in susceptible individuals, including the flu, motion sickness, general anesthesia, certain medications, pain, or odors. The nurse should assess the patient's overall condition, checking skin turgor, fluid intake and output, weight and weight changes, and vital signs. The history obtained should include the causes, amount, frequency, and characteristics of vomitus and subjective complaints.

■ Management

Nausea and vomiting from many causes are self-limiting. Antiemetic therapy is symptomatic until time cures the problem or a specific cause can be found. The nurse should monitor the vital signs, the fluid intake and output, the skin turgor, and the level of consciousness and should check for constipation.

The patient should be provided with a clear liquid diet. Comfort measures may be helpful, including decreasing or eliminating environmental odors, keeping food out of the patient's sight, applying a cool washcloth to the head, and providing regular mouth care. These measures should be individualized, based on the patient's response. Appropriate laboratory tests include the white blood cell count, the platelet count, and the serum electrolyte levels.

■ Evaluation

Ideally, antiemetics will decrease nausea and vomiting, permit the patient to eat without difficulty and to be more comfortable, without causing side effects. In fact, many patients have side effects with antihistamine therapy, although some patients may welcome drowsiness that permits sleeping if the nausea and vomiting have been severe. In most cases, antiemetics are needed on a short-term basis, usually only 1 week to 10 days, but this time period varies with the cause of the nausea. Before beginning self-medication, the patient should be able to explain what the prescribed dose is, and how to take the prescribed medication, what the side effects are and how to treat them, which side effects require immediate contact with a physician, what to do if the nausea and vomiting do not improve within a specified period of time, and what to do to prevent dehydration and fluid and electrolyte imbalance with continued vomiting.

■ Antihistamines to control vomiting (antiemesis) (Table 21-2)

Antihistamines are principally effective in preventing the nausea of motion sickness, but the drug must be taken before the motion starts. *Cyclizine (Marzine), meclizine (Antivert, Bonine),* and *dimenhydrinate (Dramamine)* are the antihistamines most effective in preventing motion sickness. Dimenhydrinate causes considerable sedation.

Nausea and vomiting caused by factors acting on the chemoreceptor trigger zone are best treated with the antipsychotic drugs, the phenothiazines. These drugs are chemically related to the antihistamines but also block the dopamine receptor in the chemoreceptor trigger zone. *Promethazine (Phenergan, Remsed)* is the antihistamine considered most effective as an antiemetic. It is chemically related to the phenothiazines.

■ Antihistamines as sedatives (Tables 21-1 and 21-2)

Sedation is a common side effect of antihistamines, and some are used principally for this purpose. Many over-the-counter sleeping aids use an antihistamine as the active agent.

Hydroxyzine (Vistaril, Atarax)

Hydroxyzine is a prescription drug sometimes used as an antianxiety agent when it is desirable to have the antiemetic and antihistaminic properties, such as in treating motion sickness, in an allergic skin reaction, or in a preanesthetic medication. See Table 24-2 for dosage and administration. For the nursing process for drugs used for sedation, see Chapter 24.

■ PATIENT CARE IMPLICATIONS

1. The side effects usually seen with the antihistamines are discussed in the text; these should be reviewed with the patient.
2. Caution patients taking antihistamines to avoid driving, operating machinery, or engaging in other activities in which sedation could be dangerous.
3. If constipation occurs, encourage the patient to increase the fluid intake to at least 3000 ml per day, to add roughage and fiber to the diet, and to add prune juice or other foods known to the patient to serve as stimulants to defecation. Constipation is also more common in the immobilized patient; encourage the patient to increase the amount of daily exercise. In rare instances, it may be necessary to add a laxative or stool softener to the drug regimen.
4. Urinary retention is more common in the elderly, the immobilized, or men with prostatic enlargement. Signs and symptoms include decreased output, palpable urinary bladder, and inability to empty the bladder during urination. Monitor the fluid intake and output. Instruct the outpatient to notify the physician if the patient suspects urinary retention.
5. Caution the patient that if blurred vision occurs, the patient should notify the physician and discontinue taking the antihistamine.
6. If dry mouth is a problem, the patient may find it helpful to chew gum or suck on sugarless candies or mints. A dry mouth can often lead to a bad taste in the mouth, which may be partly relieved by frequent oral hygiene, including brushing the teeth and/or rinsing with a mouthwash or gargle. Increasing the fluid intake may also help to decrease the dry feeling. Some patients may find the use of a commercially available saliva substitute to be helpful.
7. For patients in pain, antiemetics are often ordered with a narcotic analgesic. The two drugs together potentiate the central nervous system depressant effects of the narcotic and help to reduce nausea, a side effect that often accompanies narcotic use. When used together, the dose of the narcotic should be lower than the dose if the drug were used alone; ½ the usual dose is usually adequate.
8. Patients taking antihistamines should avoid the use of alcohol and other central nervous system depressants (see text) unless specifically prescribed by the physician.
9. Remind the patient to keep all health care providers informed of all drugs they are taking, including over-the-counter preparations.
10. In some individuals, hypotension may occur as a side effect of antihistamine therapy. Symptoms might include dizziness, visual changes, syncope, and light-headedness. If these symptoms occur, instruct the patient to notify the physician and to discontinue the antihistamine pending the advice of the physician. Monitor the blood pressure.
11. In the hospital, patients who have received antihistamines should have the side rails up. If the patient is unsteady or hypotensive, instruct the patient to call for assistance before ambulating.
12. Gastrointestinal side effects may be relieved by taking the antihistamine with a small snack or meals.
13. When used for motion sickness, antihistamines should be taken 30 minutes to 1 hour before the start of travel. If motion sickness occurs in automobiles, the affected individual may find riding in the front seat to be helpful in reducing the motion sickness.
14. Rarely, agranulocytosis and thrombocytopenia have been reported with some of the antihistamines. Instruct patients to report sore throat, fever, general malaise, bruising, or unexplained bleeding.
15. The antihistamines can themselves cause allergic responses. Instruct patients to report to the physician any unusual signs or symptoms that develop with antihistamine use.
16. Patients with allergies should be encouraged to carry medical information with them or to wear medical identification bracelets or tags indicating the nature of their allergies and who to contact for additional medical information.
17. Patients using over-the-counter preparations for colds, hay fever, sleep, and other uses should be cautioned to read the labels carefully, because many of these preparations contain two or more drugs. The patient may be inadvertently taking some unnecessary drugs found in combination with the desired drug. The pharmacist can be of assistance to the patient in helping to explain differences in drugs and dosages.
18. Dimenhydrinate (Dramamine) should be used with caution in patients receiving ototoxic drugs, since this anithistamine may mask the ototoxic symptoms of the other drug.
19. Remind patients to keep these and all medications out of the reach of children.
20. The use of antihistamines during pregnancy or lactation is not recommended unless the benefit clearly outweighs the possible risk. Instruct women to discuss the use of antihistamines with their physicians.

■ SUMMARY

Histamine is a naturally occurring amine in the body and plays a role in allergic reactions, in stomach acid secretion, and probably as a neurotransmitter in the central nervous system.

Two classes of receptors, the H-1 and H-2 receptors, have been identified for histamine. In humans, activation of the H-1 receptors by histamine results in vasodilation (blood vessels) and in constriction of bronchial smooth muscle, whereas activation of H-2 receptors (stomach) results in gastric acid secretion.

The term antihistamine refers to drugs that block the H-1 receptor. Antihistamines are effective for treatment of hay fever and hives. Selected antihistamines also produce anticholinergic, antiemetic, and sedative effects.

■ STUDY QUESTIONS

1. Describe the origin, location, and role of histamine.
2. What factors mediate histamine release?
3. What are five pharmacological actions of antihistamines?
4. What are the drug interactions and contraindications for the antihistamines?
5. Describe three clinical uses of the H-1 receptor antihistamines.
6. How does cimetidine differ from the H-1 receptor antihistamines?

■ SUGGESTED READINGS

Church, J.A., et al.: Pharmacology of respiratory allergy, Drug Therapy **7**(7):33, 1977.

Harvey, S.: Drugs in pulmonary and neurologic emergencies, Nurses' Drug Alert **2**(special issue):105, Sept., 1978.

Krausen, A.S.: Antihistamines: guidelines and implications, Annual Reviews of Otology, Rhinology and Laryngology **85:**686, 1976.

Pearlman, D.S.: Antihistamines: pharmacology and clinical use, Drugs **12:**258, 1976.

White, S.J.: Respiratory drugs: when to give them . . . what to watch for, RN **41**(6):46, 1978.

22 Bronchodilators and other drugs to treat asthma

In this chapter drugs that dilate the bronchioles (bronchodilators) and other drugs that are used to treat asthma are discussed.

ASTHMA

Asthma is a disease of reversible obstruction of the bronchioles. An attack of asthma involves not only constriction of the bronchioles but also edema of the bronchial mucosa and excess secretion of mucus, all of which combine to restrict the caliber of the airway as diagrammed in Fig. 22-1. Asthma is classified as *extrinsic* if an allergic response is the primary stimulus for bronchial constriction. When no such response can be identified, asthma is classified as *intrinsic*.

Mechanisms in extrinsic asthma

Extrinsic asthma involves an immunological mechanism. In patients with extrinsic asthma, the mast cells play a major role in precipitating the attack. In the lung, mast cells are primarily located in the epithelial layer and exposed to the surface. IgE antibodies bind to mast cells, and when an antigen appears it becomes bound to the IgE. The formation of the antigen-antibody complex causes the mast cells to degranulate, releasing several substances, including histamine and the slow-reacting substance of anaphylaxis (SRS-A), both potent bronchoconstrictors. Histamine also produces vasodilation and increases capillary permeability, which results in the mucosal edema characteristic of asthma. Drug therapy for extrinsic asthma includes one or more bronchodilator drugs in addition to cromolyn sodium, a drug that prevents the mast cells from degranulating so that an asthma attack does not start. In severe cases of asthma, glucocorticoids may be used to reverse the severe inflammation of the bronchioles. As discussed in Chapter 21, antihistamines play no role in the treatment of asthma, and because antihistamines have a drying effect that makes mucosal plugging worse, antihistamines are contraindicated for patients with severe asthma.

Adrenergic mechanisms in asthma

In the last 10 years, much has been learned about the molecular pharmacology of the bronchial smooth muscle and the mast cell. This knowledge has led to an understanding of some mechanisms involved in reversible airway obstruction. As diagrammed in Fig. 22-2, the beta adrenergic system plays a major role in determining the relaxation of bronchial smooth muscle and in inhibiting degranulation of the mast cells. Activation of the beta-2 receptor stimulates an enzyme, adenylate cyclase, to synthesize more cyclic adenosine 3′,5′-monophosphate (cyclic AMP), which is a second messenger for the beta-2 receptor (Chapter 8). Cyclic AMP activates intracellular pathways that result in (1) the relaxation of smooth muscle, (2) the inhibition of mast cell degranulation, and (3) the stimulation of the ciliary apparatus to remove secretions more effectively. This means that drugs which increase cyclic AMP are bronchodilators as well as inhibitors of mast cell degranulation and promoters of secretion flow in the bronchioles. Drugs that increase cyclic AMP include the beta adrenergic agonists, which stimulate the beta-2 receptor, and the phosphodiesterase inhibitors, which inhibit the breakdown of cyclic AMP. The xanthine compounds are used clinically as bronchodilators because of their inhibition of phosphodiesterase. Prostaglandins E_1 and E_2 also stimulate adenylate cyclase, but at present there are no drugs available clinically that mimic these prostaglandins.

Cholinergic mechanisms controlling bronchioles

In human beings the bronchioles have little if any direct innervation by the sympathetic nervous system. However, there is indirect involvement, since sympathetic nerve terminals in pulmonary blood vessels release norepinephrine, which can act on the beta-2 receptors in the bronchioles. Norepinephrine is not a potent stimulant of beta-2 receptors, however. The beta-2 receptors are activated by epinephrine released from the adrenal medulla in response to stress. Acetylcholine, the neurotransmitter of the parasympathetic nervous system, acts on the muscarinic receptors to cause bronchoconstriction through the intracellular second messenger, cyclic 3′,5′-guanyl monophosphate (cyclic GMP). Mast

FIG. 22-1

Factors restricting the airway. Major factors include hypersecretion of mucus, mucosal edema, and bronchoconstriction. Mucous plugs may form in the alveoli.

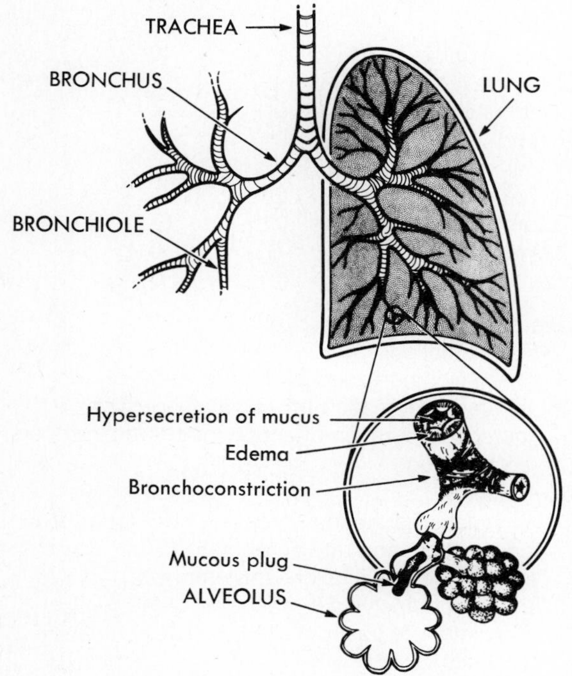

cell degranulation is also promoted by agents that stimulate the formation of cyclic GMP. Intrinsic asthma is believed to arise from a direct stimulation of the enzyme, guanyl cyclase, which synthesizes cyclic GMP. Irritants such as noxious gases can stimulate guanyl cyclase. Asthmatic individuals respond to low doses of inhaled methacholine, a cholinomimetic drug, with bronchospasm, whereas high doses are needed to induce bronchospasm in the nonasthmatic individual. Intrinsic asthma may therefore primarily involve a parasympathetic response, mediated by cyclic GMP, to inhaled bronchial irritants. Blocking the muscarinic receptor with atropine or scopolamine causes bronchodilation, but muscarinic antagonists do not at present play a major role in the treatment of asthma.

Prostaglandin F_{2a} is another potent bronchoconstrictor that acts by stimulating the synthesis of cyclic GMP. However, the factors causing the release of prostaglandin F_{2a} are not well understood at present, and it is not clear whether prostaglandin F_{2a} plays a major role in asthma.

FIG. 22-2

Histamine and slow-reacting substance of anaphylaxis (SRS-A) released from mast cells stimulate smooth muscle contraction to produce bronchoconstriction. Mast cell degranulation and smooth muscle contraction are both stimulated by acetylcholine and prostaglandin F. Smooth muscle relaxation and inhibition of mast cell degranulation are both promoted by beta-2 receptor agonists, phosphodiesterase inhibitors, and prostaglandin E.

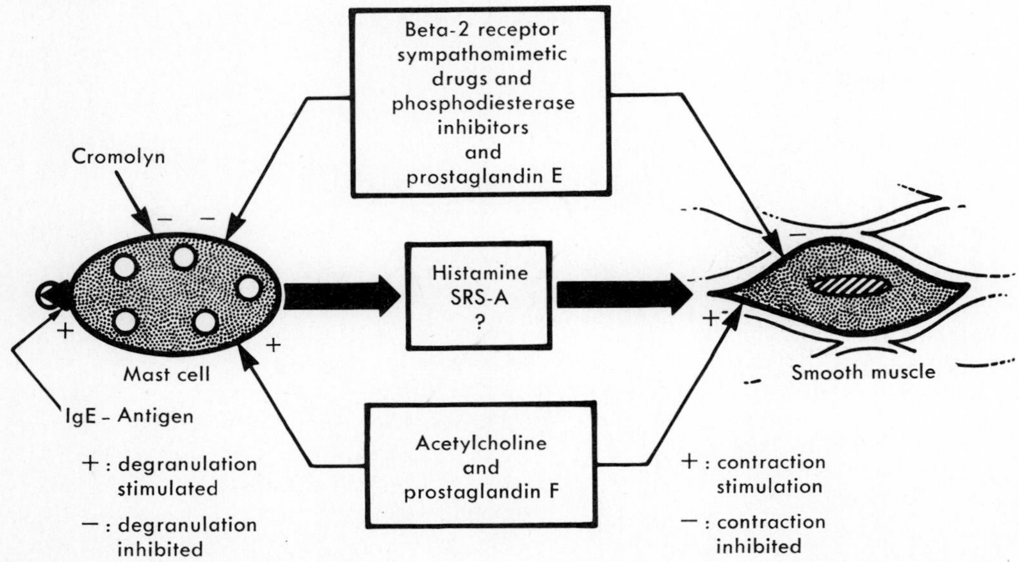

■ Other pulmonary diseases with airflow obstruction

Obstruction of airflow is a component of many pulmonary diseases. In long-standing pulmonary disease, irreversible changes take place so that the elastic smooth muscle tissue is replaced with inelastic scar tissue. This can take place in the bronchioles in chronic bronchitis or in the alveoli in emphysema. These irreversible changes cannot be modified with drugs. However, since the early stages of chronic bronchitis and emphysema often involve reversible bronchospasm, bronchodilators can provide some relief.

TABLE 22-1. Sympathomimetic bronchodilators' adrenergic receptor specificity*

Drug	Alpha effects	Beta-1 effects	Beta-2 effects
Albuterol/salbutamol	0	0	+
Carbuterol	0	0	+
Cyclopentamine	+	0	0
Ephedrine	+	+	+
Epinephrine	+	+	+
Fenoterol	0	0	+
Isoetharine	0	0	+
Isoproterenol	0	+	+
Metaproterenol	0	(±)	+
Phenylephrine	+	0	0
Terbutaline	0	0	+

Alpha effects
- Vasoconstriction—
  1. Systemic: increased blood pressure.
  2. Inhaled: Decreased bronchial congestion, increased duration of action for co-administered beta-2 drug.

Beta-1 effects
1. Stimulation of heart, increasing rate, force of contraction, and rate of repolarization. Overstimulation causes palpitations, arrhythmias.
2. Increased lipolysis (breakdown of fat).
3. Relaxation of gastrointestinal tract.

Beta-2 effects
1. Bronchiole dilation.
2. Stimulation of skeletal muscle to cause a tremulous or shaky feeling.
3. Vasodilation (mainly in blood vessels supplying muscle).
4. Glycogenolysis (breakdown of stored glucose).

Central nervous system effects
- Stimulation, causing nervousness, anxiety, insomnia, irritability, dizziness, sweating.

*0, No stimulation; +, stimulation; (±), modest stimulation.

TABLE 22-2. Adrenergic bronchodilators: onset and duration of action

Generic name	Trade name	Administration	Onset (min)	Duration (hr)
Ephedrine		Oral	15	2 to 4
Epinephrine hydrochloride		Subcutaneous Inhalation	5 2	1 to 3 2 to 3
Epinephrine suspension	Sus-Phrine	Subcutaneous	15	Up to 8
Isoetharine	Bronkometer Bronkosol Dilabron	Inhalation	2	1
Isoetharine and phenylephrine	Bronkosol-2	Inhalation	2	2
Isoproterenol	Isuprel Vapo-Iso	Inhalation	2	½ to 2
Isoproterenol and cyclopentamine	Aerolone Compound Aludrine	Inhalation	2	3½
Isoproterenol and phenylephrine	Nebu-Prel	Inhalation	2	3½
Metaproterenol	Alupent Metaprel	Inhalation Oral	2 15	2 to 4 3 to 4
Terbutaline	Bricanyl Sulfate	Oral Subcutaneous	10 15	4 to 7 2 to 4

■ BRONCHODILATORS

Beta adrenergic agonists

Mechanism of action. The mechanism by which the beta adrenergic agonists increase cyclic AMP to cause dilation of the bronchioles has been discussed. The beta receptors of the bronchial smooth muscle are beta-2 receptors, whereas cardiac beta receptors are beta-1 receptors. The goal has been to develop drugs that stimulate only beta-2 receptors because stimulation of the heart is not desirable and can limit the use of the drug. Stimulation of the alpha receptors in theory causes vasoconstriction of the blood vessels around the bronchioles, limiting the edema, a desirable action. However, systemic constriction of alpha receptors can cause an increase in blood pressure that is undesirable. Also there is some evidence that alpha receptors constrict bronchiolar smooth muscle, at least in disease states. Table 22-1 summarizes the alpha, beta-1, and beta-2 activities of the adrenergic drugs used as bronchodilators: ephedrine, epinephrine, isoetharine, isoproterenol, metaproterenol, and terbutaline and those under development: albuterol/salbutamol, carbuterol, and fenoterol.

Administration and fate. Also important to the selection of a bronchodilator is the route of administration and the onset and duration of action. Table 22-2 summarizes these points. Inhalation is a particularly effective route of administration for the bronchodilators. Not only are epinephrine, isoproterenol, and isoetharine degraded if swallowed, but inhalation places the drug near the site of action. When inhalation is the route of administration, alpha agonist activity is desirable both because it reduces congestion and because it limits systemic absorption of the drug. In fact, cyclopentamine or phenylephrine, which stimulate alpha but not beta receptors, are included in some inhalation preparations of isoproterenol to relieve congestion and to slow systemic absorption, thereby limiting cardiac effects while increasing the duration of action of the beta agonist.

Epinephrine, isoproterenol, isoetharine, and metaproterenol can be administered by inhalation. This requires that the drug be in a solution that is contained in a nebulizer or pressurized cartridge (aerosol), which will disperse the drug solution in tiny drops to be taken into the lungs by a deep inhalation. The metered aerosols are particularly easy to use and deliver a measured dose with each push of the cartridge. The disadvantage is that the inert carrier substances may irritate the bronchioles and cause bronchospasm. Also the patient must be well-instructed in the use of inhalation therapy so that the patient inhales the drug rather than gagging and swallowing the drug.

In a severe attack of asthma, the patient may not be able to inhale a drug. A subcutaneous injection of epinephrine or terbutaline would then be appropriate. An orally or subcutaneously administered bronchodilator would also be preferred if there is a great deal of mucosal edema and bronchoconstriction, which would limit the access of the inhaled drug.

■ Specific beta adrenergic bronchodilators

(Table 22-3)

Epinephrine (Asmolin, Medihaler-Epi, Adrenalin and others)

Epinephrine can be administered subcutaneously for the relief of an acute asthmatic attack. Epinephrine will not only cause bronchodilation but will also cause vasoconstriction, which relieves bronchial edema. Given subcutaneously, an aqueous suspension of epinephrine (Sus-Phrine) lasts 8 hours, whereas the hydrochloride salt lasts only 3 hours. Epinephrine is also available in metered-dose inhalers as an aerosol or in solution for use in a nebulizer.

The most common side effects of epinephrine are an increased heart rate, muscle tremors, and stimulation of the central nervous system to produce anxiety, nervousness, or excitability. Large doses can produce an acute hypertensive episode and cardiac arrhythmias.

Ephedrine

Ephedrine has a similar spectrum of action as epinephrine but is effective orally. Ephedrine is a weaker bronchodilator than epinephrine and of no use for an acute asthma attack. The major use of ephedrine is a prophylactic one for patients with mild to moderate asthma. Several formulations combine ephedrine with theophylline and a sedative in a single pill.

The major action of ephedrine is the release of stored norepinephrine from sympathetic neurons, an indirect sympathomimetic effect that explains the weak broncho-

TABLE 22-3. Bronchodilators and other drugs to treat asthma

Generic name	Trade name	Dosage and administration	Comments
BETA RECEPTOR AGONISTS			
Ephedrine sulfate	Ectasule Minus Slo-Fedrin	ORAL: *Adults*—25 to 50 mg every 3 to 4 hr as needed. *Children*—6 to 12 yr, 6.25 to 12.5 mg every 4 to 6 hr; 2 to 6 yr, 0.3 to 0.5 mg/kg every 4 to 6 hr.	Oral or parenteral administration only. Central nervous system stimulation is a common side effect. Not selective for beta-2 receptors.
Epinephrine (base)	Sus-Phrine (1:200)	INTRAMUSCULAR, SUBCUTANEOUS: *Adults*—0.1 to 0.3 ml not more often than every 4 hr, maximum test dose, 0.1 ml. *Children*—0.005 ml/kg body weight not more often than every 4 hr, maximum test dose, 0.15 ml.	Long-acting suspension. Effect may persist for 8 to 10 hr.
	Asmolin (1:400)	Double above volumes.	
Epinephrine bitartrate	Asthma Meter* Medihaler-Epi* Primatene Mist*	INHALATION: Aerosol nebulizers metered to deliver 0.2 mg epinephrine (0.1 mg for Medihaler-Epi) with each inhalation. Allow 1 to 2 min between inhalations.	Overuse can cause serious adverse effects, including death. Reduce dose if bronchial irritation or central nervous system stimulation arises. For symptomatic relief only.
Epinephrine (racemic)	microNEFRIN (2.25%)	As for epinephrine bitartrate.	
Epinephrine hydrochloride	Adrenalin Chloride (1:1000)	SUBCUTANEOUS: *Adults*—0.2 to 0.5 mg every 2 hr as needed for an acute asthma attack. *Children*—0.01 mg/kg body weight, maximum, 0.5 mg, every 4 hr as needed for an acute asthma attack. For severe acute attacks, may repeat initial dose every 20 min for 3 doses.	Short-acting injection. Do not expose drug to light. Do not use if brown or contains a precipitate. Reacts with many compounds.

*Available without a prescription.

TABLE 22-3. Bronchodilators and other drugs to treat asthma—cont'd

Generic name	Trade name	Dosage and administration	Comments
Epinephrine hydrochloride—cont'd	Adrenalin Chloride (1:100)* Vaponephrin (2.25%)*	INHALATION: Solutions for nebulization. Allow 1 to 2 min between inhalations.	Excessive use causes bronchial inflammation and stimulation of the heart and central nervous system.
Isoetharine hydrochloride Isoetharine mesylate	Bronkosol Bronkometer	INHALATION: nebulized solution; 3 to 7 inhalations. INHALATION: aerosol; 1 to 4 inhalations every 3 to 6 hr, maximum 12 inhalations daily.	A beta-2 selective drug. Phenylephrine is included to relieve congestion and prolong the duration of action.
Isoproterenol hydrochloride	Iprenol Isuprel Hydrochloride	SUBLINGUAL: *Adults*—10 mg initially. No more than 15 mg 4 times daily or 20 mg 3 times daily. *Children*—5 to 10 mg, not exceeding 30 mg daily.	Sublingual absorption is unreliable. Patients should not swallow saliva until tablet has completely disintegrated.
		INTRAVENOUS: *Children only*—initial infusion rate is 0.1 μg/kg/min. Increase by 0.1 μg/kg/min every 15 min until heart rate exceeds 180 or clinical improvement is seen or infusion rate is 0.8 μg/kg/min.	This route of administration is used only in pediatric intensive care units for children in respiratory failure.
   Isoproterenol sulfate	Isuprel Mistometer Norisodrine Aerotrol Medihaler-Iso Norisodrine Sulfate	INHALATION: (solution for nebulization, 0.5% to 1%): *Adults*—1 or 2 deep inhalations, repeated no more than every 4 hr. INHALATION (aerosol metered dose): *Adults*—1 or 2 deep inhalations repeated once or twice at 5 to 10 min intervals if necessary. Repeat after 4 hr. *Children*—5 to 15 deep inhalations of 1:200 aerosol repeated in 10 to 30 min if necessary.	Excessive use has caused refractory bronchial obstruction and tolerance to the drug. In some individuals inhalation precipitates a severe, prolonged attack of asthma.
Metaproterenol sulfate	Alupent Metaprel	ORAL: *Adults*—10 mg 3 or 4 times daily initially, increased to 20 mg 3 or 4 times daily over 2 to 4 wk. *Children*—6 to 9 yr, 10 mg 3 or 4 times daily; over 9 yr or over 60 lb, 20 mg 3 or 4 times daily.	Relatively selective for beta-2 (bronchial) receptors. More effective orally than ephedrine. Shakiness (a stimulation of skeletal muscle) is the most frequent side effect.
		INHALATION (metered aerosol): *Adults and children over 12 yr only:* 2 to 3 inhalations every 3 to 4 hr not to exceed 12 inhalations daily.	Longer-acting than isoproterenol. Patients are less likely to develop tolerance to metaproterenol than to isoproterenol.
Terbutaline sulfate	Brethine Bricanyl	SUBCUTANEOUS: *Adults*—0.25 mg repeated in 15 to 30 min if necessary, with no more than 0.5 mg administered in any 4 hr period. *Children*—0.01 mg/kg body weight to a maximum of 0.25 mg.	Subcutaneous route used for relief of an acute asthma attack.
		ORAL: *Adults*—initially 2.5 mg every 8 hr, increased to 5 mg every 8 hr 3 times daily over 2 to 4 wk. Dose may be lowered to 2.5 mg if side effects are too disturbing. *Children 12 yr and younger*—1.25 to 2.5 mg 3 times daily during waking hours.	Shakiness (a stimulation of skeletal muscle) is the most frequent side effect.

Continued.

TABLE 22-3. Bronchodilators and other drugs to treat asthma—cont'd

Generic name	Trade name	Dosage and administration	Comments
XANTHINES			
Aminophylline (theophylline ethylenediamine)	Sold mainly under generic name	For acute asthma attack: INTRAVENOUS: Solutions should be diluted to 25 mg/ml and injected no more rapidly than 25 mg/min to avoid circulatory collapse. Loading dose, 5.6 mg/kg over 30 min. Maintenance dose, no more than 0.9 mg/kg/hr by continuous infusion. Dose is determined by age, cardiac and liver status, and smoking history. RECTAL: *Adults*—250 to 500 mg 1 to 3 times daily. *Children*—5 mg/kg not more often than every 6 hr. ORAL: *Adults*—500 mg for an acute attack. Maintenance dose, 200 to 250 mg every 6 to 8 hr. *Children*—7.5 mg/kg for an acute attack. Maintenance dose, 5 mg/kg every 6 hr.	85% theophylline, so 116 mg of aminophylline is equivalent to 100 mg theophylline. Watch for nausea, wakefulness, restlessness, and irritability as early symptoms of toxicity. Serious toxic effects of intravenous administration include delirium, convulsions, hyperthermia, and circulatory collapse.
Dyphylline	Airet Circair Dilin Dilor Dyflex Emfabid Lufyllin Neothylline	ORAL: *Adults*—200 to 800 mg every 6 hr. *Children*—2 to 3 mg/lb/24 hr given in divided doses every 6 hr. Maximum dose, 15 mg/kg every 6 hr. INTRAMUSCULAR: *Adults*—250 to 500 mg.	Not a theophylline salt. Has a short half-life (2½ hr) and is not excreted in the urine without being metabolized.
Oxytriphylline (choline theophyllinate)	Choledyl	ORAL: *Adults*—200 mg every 6 hr. *Children 2 to 12 yr*—100 mg/60 lb every 6 hr.	64% theophylline, so 156 mg is equivalent to 100 mg theophylline.
Theophylline	Many names, elixirs, syrups, tablets, capsules, timed-release preparation, suppositories	ORAL: *Adults, children*—Initial dose, 3 to 5 mg/kg every 6 hr. For maintenance: *Adults*—100 to 200 mg every 6 hr. *Children*—50 to 100 mg every 6 hr. RECTAL: *Adults*—250 to 500 mg every 8 to 12 hr. *Children*—10 to 12 mg/kg/24 hr. Administered no more frequently than every 6 hr.	Headache, dizziness, nervousness, nausea, vomiting, and epigastric pain are the most common side effects of oral administration. Therapeutic levels are 10 to 20 mg/ml serum.
Theophylline monoethanolamine	Fleet Brand Theophylline	RECTAL: *Adults*—250 to 500 mg. Do not repeat in less than 8 hr. Do not administer more than 2 times in 24 hr.	75% theophylline, so 133 mg is equivalent to 100 mg theophylline.
Theophylline sodium glycinate	Glynazan Panophylline Forte Synophylate Theofort	ORAL: *Adults*—330 to 660 mg every 6 to 8 hr after meals. *Children*—over 12 yr, 220 to 300 mg; 6 to 12 yr, 165 to 220 mg; 3 to 6 yr, 110 to 165 mg; 1 to 3 yr, 55 to 110 mg every 6 to 8 hr after meals.	49% theophylline, so 200 mg is equivalent to 100 mg theophylline.

dilator effect. The major metabolite is phenylpropanolamine, an active alpha adrenergic drug by itself that is frequently used as a decongestant.

The most common side effect of ephedrine is stimulation of the central nervous system manifested as nervousness, excitability, and insomnia. The development of orally active, beta-2 selective bronchodilators is making the use of ephedrine obsolete.

Isoetharine

Isoetharine (Bronkosol, Bronkometer) is a beta adrenergic drug that has relative selectivity for beta-2 receptors. Isoetharine is only available for inhalation and is effective for 2 to 3 hours. Isoetharine is safer for patients with cardiovascular disease, hypertension, or diabetes mellitus than bronchodilators without relative beta-2 selectivity.

Side effects of isoetharine are those seen with other bronchodilators: increased heart rate, palpitations, headache, tremor, and anxiety.

Isoproterenol (Isuprel Hydrochloride, Vapo-Iso, Medihaler-Iso, Norisodrine Sulfate)

Isoproterenol was the first widely used adrenergic drug with selectivity for the beta receptors. It is not selective for beta-2 receptors and therefore stimulates the heart as well. Isoproterenol is primarily given by inhalation and is effective for up to 2 hours in relieving bronchoconstriction. If swallowed, it is degraded in the gut wall. Isoproterenol is available as a sublingual tablet, but the absorption is so erratic that this route is not often used.

Some side effects are related to stimulation of the heart: palpitation, fast heart rate, and arrhythmias. Isoproterenol can also cause tremors, headache, nervousness, and hypotension. Excessive inhalation can cause bronchial constriction for which the drug no longer has a bronchodilator effect. Drug effectiveness returns when isoproterenol is discontinued for a few days.

Metaproterenol (Alupent, Metaprel)

Metaproterenol is relatively specific for beta-2 receptors, can be given orally or by inhalation, and is effective for up to 5 hours. These properties make metaproterenol useful for the prophylactic treatment of asthma, and metaproterenol is replacing ephedrine as the oral adrenergic bronchodilator for prophylactic use. The most common side effect is a muscle tremor, which is attributed to a beta-2 effect on skeletal muscle. Also blood pressure can fall because of vasodilation in the blood vessels of skeletal muscle, and an increase in heart rate secondary to the decreased blood pressure is experienced.

Terbutaline (Brethine, Bricanyl)

Terbutaline is relatively specific for beta-2 receptors. At present it is available for subcutaneous or oral administration only. The subcutaneous route is used to treat a severe asthma attack. Taken orally, terbutaline is effective for up to 8 hours and can be used in the prophylactic treatment of asthma. Unfortunately, side effects can be prolonged when they occur.

New beta agonist bronchodilators

Three sympathomimetic bronchodilators that are widely used in Europe are being tested in the United States. These are *albuterol/salbutamol (Proventil), fenoterol (Berotec),* and *carbuterol.* These are highly selective for stimulation of the beta-2 receptor, can be taken orally or inhaled, and are effective for 4 to 6 hours.

■ Xanthines

Theophylline

Mechanisms of action. Theophylline is the prototype of the xanthines used to treat asthma. Like the beta adrenergic agonists, theophylline is thought to act by increasing cellular cyclic AMP concentrations, an action that relaxes bronchial smooth muscle and inhibits mast cell degranulation. Theophylline and the other xanthines accomplish this by inhibiting the degradation of cyclic AMP by the enzyme phosphodiesterase. This action complements that of the beta agonists, and the two kinds of agents may both be included in therapy when the effect of either drug alone is insufficient to control bronchospasm.

Administration and fate. Theophylline is an effective bronchodilator that can be given intravenously (as aminophylline) for the control of acute bronchospasm in status asthmaticus or can be given orally to control the bronchospasm of mild, moderate, or severe asthma. Theophylline is not very water soluble, and there are many formulations of theophylline to improve the solubility. Actually, recent studies show that theophylline tablets are well absorbed, with more than 96% of the drug appearing in the plasma within 2 hours. Aminophylline is the most common soluble form of theophylline and is the only form of theophylline that can be administered intravenously.

Several soluble salts of theophylline are available, and dosage is determined by the theophylline content. In addition, theophylline is available in slow-release preparations, a fast-release preparation, alcoholic or aqueous solutions, and suppositories. Only the suppository preparation is so erratically absorbed as to be unreliable, however; rectal solutions are well absorbed. Theophylline is combined with ephedrine and a sedative in several combination products for treating asthma. Most clini-

TABLE 22-4. Other drugs to treat asthma

Generic name	Trade name	Dosage and administration	Comments
Beclomethasone dipropionate	Vanceril	INHALATION (metered dose inhaler): each dose is 50 μg. *Adults*—2 inhalations 3 to 4 times daily. *Children 6 to 12 yr*—1 to 2 inhalations 3 to 4 times daily.	An inhaled glucocorticoid. Patients transferfering from oral glucocorticoids to beclomethasone must be carefully monitored because adrenal function is impaired and may require months to begin functioning adequately.
Cromolyn sodium	Aarane Intal	INHALATION: *Adults and children over 5 yr*—20 mg capsule inhaled 4 times daily.	Prophylactic drug to inhibit mast cell degranulation. Cough or bronchospasm is occasionally experienced after inhaling the dry powder.

cians prefer to individualize doses of each ingredient to minimize side effects while maximizing therapeutic effects and therefore do not favor combination drugs. Theophylline is not effective when administered by inhalation. Intramuscular injections of theophylline are not used because they are painful.

Variability of plasma levels. Theophylline is metabolized by the liver into inactive compounds that are excreted in the urine. There is a wide variability among individuals as to the plasma half-life of theophylline. In normal, nonsmoking adults, the plasma half-life is about 6 hours, but this can vary from 3 to 12 hours. In smokers and children, the plasma half-life is shorter, whereas in the elderly, premature infants, and patients with liver disease or congestive heart failure with pulmonary edema, the plasma half-life is prolonged.

Side and toxic effects. The most common side effects of theophylline after oral administration are nausea and epigastric pain. Headache, dizziness, and nervousness are also common. The effectiveness of theophylline is determined by its plasma concentrations, with the therapeutic range being 10 to 20 μg/ml. Agitation, exaggerated reflexes, and mild muscle tremors (fasciculations) are often seen when plasma levels are 20 to 30 μg/ml. Seizures and cardiac arrhythmias may be seen when plasma levels exceed 30 μg/ml but have been occasionally reported with plasma concentrations between 20 and 30 μg/ml.

Other actions of theophylline seen in the therapeutic dose range are dilation of blood vessels and a mild diuresis from the increased renal blood flow and glomerular filtration. Stomach acid secretion is increased, and this may be a problem for a patient with an ulcer. Another effect is stimulation of the medullary centers of respiration, which is beneficial if the asthmatic patient is hypoxic. Theophylline is useful for treating Cheyne-Stokes respiration, a condition in which the medullary sensitivity to hypoxia is decreased. Theophylline is administered to stimulate respiration in newborns who are not breathing well.

Dyphylline

Dyphylline (Airet, Dilor, Lufyllin, Neothylline) is related to theophylline but is less potent and shorter acting than theophylline. Dyphylline has a half-life of 2½ hours and is eliminated largely unchanged in the urine.

■ Other drugs

Cromolyn sodium (Table 22-4)

Cromolyn sodium (Intal, Aarane) is a prophylactic drug that acts by inhibiting mast cell degranulation and the release of bronchospastic agents caused by immunological (antigen IgE) or nonimmunological (exercise, hyperventilation) stimulation. Cromolyn is of no value in treating an ongoing asthma attack or in preventing asthma attacks brought on by vagal reflexes rather than by mast cell degranulation. By itself, cromolyn has no bronchodilator or antiinflammatory activity.

Cromolyn can be administered only by inhalation using a "Spinhaler," a hand-held and hand-operated device that when activated punctures a capsule, releasing a dry powder. This powder is dispersed by the air current from a small rotor blade and enters the lungs during deep inhalation. Given orally or parenterally, cromolyn is so rapidly excreted in the urine that effective drug levels cannot be maintained. Because of this rapid clearance, cromolyn is practically nontoxic. The major side effect that can limit use is bronchospasm caused by the dry powder in sensitive individuals. Some individuals become allergic to cromolyn.

Cromolyn is usually added to bronchodilator therapy to avoid the use of glucocorticoids or to allow the gradual reduction in dose of glucocorticoids. No tolerance develops to cromolyn. Cromolyn is reported to be more effective in treating children than in treating adults for asthma.

■ THE NURSING PROCESS FOR BRONCHODILATORS

■ Assessment

Patients requiring bronchodilator therapy are those with asthma or other respiratory diseases that have bronchospasm as a component, such as some cases of bronchitis and emphysema. Although a general assessment of the patient should be done, the focus is often on the respiratory system. The nurse should check the vital signs, the amount and characteristics of secretions, and the level of fatigue; auscultate breathing sounds; determine the arterial blood gas levels, the vital capacity, subjective complaints, and the ability to perform activities of daily living and tolerance for activity; and obtain relevant history such as smoking, exposure to irritants, infection, and stress. In addition, the nurse should monitor the level of consciousness and send the sputum for culture and drug sensitivity if ordered.

■ Management

The initial use of these drugs is to provide symptomatic relief of dyspnea, (shortness of breath) and inadequate oxygenation. Coupled with drug therapy are efforts to stabilize the patient for discharge. The vital signs are monitored, and an acute care unit may be appropriate for the patient in acute respiratory distress. The nurse should monitor the fluid intake and output, the level of consciousness, the blood gas levels, vital capacity, and the treatment of any infectious process. An infusion control device should be used for intravenous drugs. Serum xanthine levels are monitored and the blood glucose concentration is measured when patients receive xanthine therapy. In addition to drug therapy, the plan of care should be individualized to include instruction of any additional aspects of maintenance such as breathing exercises, irritants and inhalants to be avoided, and how to use supplies at home, including oxygen, nebulizers, and intermittent positive pressure breathing machines. The patient may be referred to appropriate agencies for respiratory therapy, social services, or the local visiting nurse association. Finally, the nurse should work with the physician and the patient to determine the best combination of drugs for management of the respiratory problem in the home setting.

■ Evaluation

These drugs are successful if the patient is both subjectively and objectively improved. The vital capacity should be increased, arterial blood gas levels should be closer to normal values, the respiratory rate should be decreased, and the patient should appear to be in less respiratory distress. Subjectively, the patient should be able to report easier breathing, less feeling of shortness of breath, less fatigue, and better tolerance for activities of daily living. Before discharge for home management, the patient should be able to explain which drugs are to be taken and how to take them correctly, to explain what situations would require notification of the physician either because of exacerbation of the disease process or because of effects resulting from drug therapy, and to demonstrate how to perform any other measures such as exercises for respiratory management and the correct use of oxygen. The patient should be able to demonstrate correct use of any equipment such as intermittent positive pressure breathing machines or drug administration devices such as an inhaler or nebulizer. The patient should be able to explain which specific respiratory irritants should be avoided.

Glucocorticoids (corticosteroids)

Glucocorticoids are used to treat the asthmatic patient who has severe symptoms that are not controlled by bronchodilator therapy. Initially, very high doses (up to 1 Gm of methylprednisolone) of a glucocorticoid may be administered for as long as 5 days to bring a severe asthma attack under control when intravenous aminophylline and sympathomimetics have proved inadequate. As discussed in Chapter 35, high doses of glucocorticoids can be tolerated for a short period of time, but on a long-term basis, glucocorticoids cause many severe side effects. Few patients with asthma will require glucocorticoids even after an acute attack. The mechanisms by which glucocorticoids specifically act to alleviate asthma are not known, but they do potentiate the action of the bronchodilators. To minimize the long-term toxic effects of glucocorticoids, they are administered in small doses (20 mg) every other day. This schedule minimizes suppression of adrenal function and also avoids giving enough glucocorticoid to cause the Cushing syndrome, which is characteristic of excessive glucocorticoid administration (Chapter 35).

Beclomethasone

Beclomethasone (Vanceril, Viarex) is an aerosol glucocorticoid that can be inhaled daily without producing adrenal suppression or the Cushing syndrome. As with other aerosol medications, the patient must be carefully instructed in the administration of the drug. The aerosol cannot be used during an episode of acute bronchospasm because the powder will only cause further irritation and the bronchospasm will prevent adequate inhalation. An oral glucocorticoid is indicated instead. Patients using the beclomethasone aerosol should gargle after use to prevent the drug trapped in the throat from being swallowed and absorbed systemically and to avoid a candidal infection (a type of fungal infection) in the mouth or throat.

Anticholinergic drugs

At present, no anticholinergic drug has been approved for the treatment of asthma. One such drug being tested is ipratropium bromide aerosol *(Atrovent)*. This drug may prove effective in the treatment of intrinsic asthma in which the vagal reflex bronchoconstriction seems dominant.

■ PATIENT CARE IMPLICATIONS

Bronchodilators: Beta receptor agonists

1. Review the side effects discussed in the text and the information in Tables 22-1 to 22-3.
2. Monitor the patient's pulse, blood pressure, and respiratory rate. The frequency with which these parameters should be measured will vary with the patient's condition, the dose of medication, and route of administration. During intravenous administration, monitor these parameters every 5 to 15 minutes; following subcutaneous administration, monitor every 30 minutes; following inhalation, monitor every 15 to 60 minutes.
3. Beta receptor agonists should be used with caution in the elderly and in those individuals with cardiovascular disease, hypertension, diabetes mellitus, or hyperthyroidism.
4. In acutely ill individuals or those with known cardiovascular disease, it may be appropriate to move the patients to intensive care units for treatment and to have the patients attached to cardiac monitors. Appropriate emergency drugs and equipment should be available to treat arrhythmias, exaggerated responses to the drug, and acute hypertension.
5. Anxiety, insomnia, fear, and other emotional responses may aggravate bronchospasm and air hunger in the patient. Maintain a calm but efficient attitude in caring for patients with bronchoconstriction. Do not leave the patient unattended for long periods.
6. For subcutaneous or intramuscular injection, aspirate carefully before administering the dose to avoid inadvertent intravenous administration.
7. For intravenous administration, the use of an infusion control device is recommended. Monitor the fluid intake and output. Monitor the vital signs frequently. The patient should be attached to a cardiac monitor in an acute care unit with emergency drugs and equipment nearby.
8. Sus-Phrine is a suspension. Shake the vial or ampule thoroughly before preparing the ordered dose and administer immediately so the drug does not settle out of the suspension.
9. The patient using an inhaler for the first time may need assistance. Instruct the patient to exhale deeply, then to put the mouthpiece into the mouth with the opening directed to the back of the throat. Grasp the mouthpiece with the teeth and lips. The patient should then inhale deeply while depressing the aerosol container or activating the spray mechanism. The patient should then try to hold the breath for as long as possible before exhaling. The patient should wait 2 to 3 minutes before repeating the

dose, depending on the physician's instructions. It may be necessary to hold the nose shut on children. Consult the manufacturer's literature for additional information.

10. If sublingual tablets are being used, instruct the patient to let the tablet dissolve under the tongue and not to swallow the saliva until the tablet is completely dissolved.
11. Before discharging a patient on a beta receptor agonist, ascertain that the patient understands how to take the prescribed medication. This includes correct use of the route of administration, the frequency with which the medication is to be used in a 24-hour period, and what to do if the patient does not obtain relief from the medication.
12. Caution patients not to increase the frequency of taking prescribed medications without the advice of the physician because the drugs lose their effectiveness with frequent repeated use. Also advise the patient not to switch to other drugs or inhalers because individual preparations vary in their strength and recommended frequency of use, and in some instances, mixing various drugs can be dangerous.
13. The use of these drugs during pregnancy is not recommended without the advice of a physician.
14. Drugs with beta-2 activity stimulate glycogenolysis and thus may cause patients with diabetes mellitus to have difficulty in maintaining control of their disease. Instruct patients with diabetes mellitus who are also taking beta receptor agonists to monitor their urine glucose levels closely.
15. Remind patients to keep these and all medications out of the reach of children.

Xanthines

1. The xanthines should be used with caution in patients with cardiac or hepatic disease, hypertension, or hyperthyroidism. Peptic ulcer disease may be aggravated.
2. To decrease gastric irritation with oral preparations, the patient may be able to take the preparation with or just after meals; check with the physician, because this will alter the rate of absorption.
3. These preparations may cause dizziness, lightheadedness, or vertigo. Supervise ambulation until it is clear that the patient is steady while up. Keep the siderails up on hospitalized patients.
4. Monitor the vital signs, specifically the pulse and blood pressure. In some patients, hypotension may be pronounced. If hypotension occurs, keep the patient in bed until the effects of the drug wear off.
5. Patients should be cautioned not to smoke because smoking alters the drug half-life of the xanthines and related drugs.
6. These drugs may produce hyperglycemia. Instruct patients with diabetes mellitus to monitor their urine glucose levels carefully. Persistent glycosuria may require a change in diet or insulin levels.
7. Instruct patients to avoid over-the-counter preparations unless cleared with the physician.
8. The use of xanthines during pregnancy should be restricted to those individuals in whom the benefit clearly outweighs the risk. Consult the physician.
9. Intravenous aminophylline: Too rapid infusion may cause arrhythmias, profound hypotension, and cardiac arrest. Monitor the vital signs every 5 to 15 minutes until stable. Use an infusion control device or volume control device; a microdrip infusion set is recommended. Monitor the fluid intake and output. In the acutely ill patient or one with known heart disease, it may be advisable to have the patient attached to a cardiac monitor. This drug should not be mixed with any other in a syringe, and it is compatible with only a few other drugs for infusion; consult the pharmacy. If in doubt, do not allow infusion fluids to mix at all.
10. Rectal aminophylline is poorly absorbed at best, but absorption is decreased if the rectum contains feces. Notify the physician if the suppository causes any anal or rectal irritation.
11. The serum theophylline concentration may be measured at regular intervals to check on the rate of theophylline clearance. Several drugs have been reported to interact with theophylline, for example, erythromycin and troleandomycin may inhibit theophylline clearance. Signs of high plasma levels in the patient may be agitation, exaggerated reflexes, and mild muscle tremors, progressing to seizures and cardiac arrythmias (see text). In monitoring for sources of theophylline, remember to consider oral preparations such as cough medicines that the patient might be taking. The agitation associated with high levels of the drug should be treated by reducing theophylline doses and not by sedating the patient.
12. Keep these and all medications out of the reach of children.

Cromolyn

1. Instructions for use of the Spinhaler are provided by the manufacturer and should be reviewed with the patient before using the device.
2. Side effects are infrequent, but should any of the following occur, the patient should contact the physician: bronchospasm, cough, nasal congestion, wheezing, dizziness, joint swelling and pain, nausea, headache, urticaria, or any other unexpected sign or symptom.

3. If the patient complains of irritation of the mouth or throat or dry mouth after use of cromolyn, instruct the patient to suck on a lozenge or drink a glass of water after each dose. If heartburn or esophageal irritation occurs, the patient may find that drinking a glass of milk or taking a dose of antacid before each dose of cromolyn may help. Before using antacids on a regular basis, the patient should consult with a physician.

Beclomethasone

1. Instructions for use of the beclomethasone inhaler are provided by the manufacturer and should be reviewed with the patient before use.
2. Side effects and problems associated with the long-term use of steroids are discussed more fully in Chapter 35. It is important to help patients understand that even though the beclomethasone is being taken via inhalation it is as important as other orally administered drugs, and since it is a glucocorticoid, should not be discontinued suddenly. Advise patients to take their medications only as directed by the physician, to return to the physician for problems or questions, and to report any unexpected signs or symptoms.
3. As indicated in the text, patients should gargle and rinse their mouths after each use of the inhaler to help prevent fungal infections.

■ SUMMARY

Asthma is a disease in which there is reversible obstruction of the bronchioles involving constriction of the bronchial smooth muscle, edema of the bronchial mucosa, and excessive secretion of mucus (Fig. 22-1). Extrinsic asthma is the best characterized form of asthma and involves an immunological mechanism that releases histamine and other active compounds from mast cells. Drugs acting to increase intracellular cyclic AMP have proven especially efficacious in treating extrinsic asthma. These drugs include the beta adrenergic receptor agonists and the xanthines. Beneficial actions mediated through cyclic AMP include (1) bronchial dilation, (2) inhibition of mast cell degranulation, and (3) stimulation of the ciliary apparatus to remove secretions.

Cholinergic mechanisms may be important in the etiology of intrinsic asthma and may involve the intracellular second messenger cyclic GMP. The pharmacology affecting cyclic GMP is not well developed at present.

Bronchodilators include beta adrenergic receptor agonists and the xanthines. Beta adrenergic receptor agonists vary in their effective route of administration and include inhalation, oral, sublingual, and subcutaneous routes. Uses vary from prophylaxis to treatment of an acute attack. The most common side effects include cardiovascular, muscular, and central nervous system stimulation. The beta receptor agonists are relatively specific for the beta-2 adrenergic receptors and have a lesser incidence of cardiac stimulation. Xanthines, chiefly forms of theophylline, are used both prophylactically and to control an acute attack.

Other drugs used in the therapy for asthma include cromolyn and beclomethasone. Cromolyn prevents mast cell degranulation and is a prophylactic drug only for asthma. Beclomethasone is a glucocorticoid administered by inhalation and reserved for use only by patients with severe extrinsic asthma not controlled by other drugs alone.

■ STUDY QUESTIONS

1. What are the three components that restrict the airway in extrinsic asthma?
2. Contrast the mechanisms responsible for extrinsic and intrinsic asthma.
3. What is the mechanism of action of the bronchodilators (beta adrenergic receptor agonists and theophylline)? List three beneficial responses attributed to this mechanism.
4. Which of the beta adrenergic agonists used as bronchodilators are relatively specific for the beta-2 receptor?
5. What are the side effects associated with the bronchodilators?
6. What role does cromolyn play in the treatment of extrinsic asthma? What is the mechanism of action?
7. What role does beclomethasone play in the treatment of extrinsic asthma? What is the mechanism of action?

■ SUGGESTED READINGS

Ahmad, M., and Lindquist, C.: Bronchial asthma: some aspects of pathogenesis and therapy, Postgraduate Medicine **62**(1):111, 1977.

Antacids reverse cromolyn-induced esophagitis, Nurses' Drug Alert **4**(3):21, 1980.

Bergner, R.K., and Bergner, A.: Outpatient management of asthma, American Family Physician **15**(5):141, 1977.

Bernstein, I.L., Johnson, C.L., and Ted Tse, C.S.: Therapy with cromolyn sodium, Annals of Internal Medicine **89:**228, 1978.

Billingsley, J.G., Kimbel, P., Morris, J.F., Renzetti, A.D., and Winterbauer, R.H.: Getting the most from bronchodilators, Patient Care **13:**63, May 30, 1979.

Bulger, J.J., Chai, H., Falliers, C.J., Kaiser, H.B., Neff, T.A., and Nordlund, H.M.: Asthma: individualizing drug therapy, Patient Care **11:**92, Aug. 15, 1977.

Chodosh, S.: Rational management of bronchial asthma, Archives of Internal Medicine **138:**1394, 1978.

Chrow, L.A.: On the use of selected bronchodilators in the asthmatic and non-asthmatic patient, AANA Journal **46:**389, 1978.

Fink, J.N.: The asthmatic, American Family Physician **18**(6):124, 1978.

Hanna, C.J., and Eyre, P.: On the action of combination bronchodilators, Agents and Actions **9:**301, 1979.

Harvey, S.: Drugs in pulmonary and neurologic emergencies, Nurses' Drug Alert **2**(special issue):105, 1978.

Imbeau, S.A., and Geller, M.: Aerosol beclomethasone treatment of chronic severe asthma, Journal of the American Medical Association **240:**1260, 1978.

Mancini, R.E.: Aminophylline: modern approaches to therapy, American Family Practice **21**(1):154, 1980.

Middleton, E.: A rational approach to asthma therapy, Postgraduate Medicine **67**(3):107, 1980.

Oslick, T.: Aerosol sympathomimetic amines, American Family Physician **15**(6):146, 1977.

Paterson, J.W., Woolcock, A.J., and Shenfield, G.M.: Bronchodilator drugs, American Review of Respiratory Disease **120:**1149, 1979.

Platshon, L.F., and Kaliner, M.: The effects of the immunologic release of histamine upon human lung cyclic nucleotide levels and prostaglandin generation, Journal of Clinical Investigation **62:**1113, 1978.

Plummer, A.L.: Choosing a drug regimen for obstructive pulmonary disease. 1. Agents to achieve bronchodilatation, Postgraduate Medicine **63**(4):36, 1978.

Richards, W., Church, J.A., and Lawrence, R.: Uses and limitations of corticosteroids in asthma, Drug Therapy **9**(5):52, 1979.

Rodman, J.J.: The drug interactions we all overlook, RN **43**(11):40, 1980.

Settipane, G.A., Klein, D.E., Boyd, G.K., Sturam, J.H., Freye, H.B., and Weltman, J.K.: Adverse reactions to cromolyn, Journal of the American Medical Association **241:**811, 1979.

Sexton, D.L.: The place of cromolyn sodium in the management of asthmas, Nurses Drug Alert **3**(special report):117, 1979.

Van Dellen, R.G.: Series on pharmacology in practice. 4. Theophylline: practical application of new knowledge, Mayo Clinic Proceedings **54:**733, 1979.

Webber-Jones, J.E., and Bryant, M.K.: Over-the-counter bronchodilators, Nursing '80 **10**(1):34, 1980.

Weinberger, M., and Hendeles, L.: Management of asthma. 1. Approach, Postgraduate Medicine **61**(5):85, 1977.

White, S.J.: Respiratory drugs: when to give them . . . what to watch for, RN **41**(6):46, 1978.

Wieczorek, R.R., and Horner-Rosner, B.: The asthmatic child: preventing and controlling attacks, American Journal of Nursing **79:**258, 1979.

Wolfe, J.D., Tashkin, D.P., Calvarese, B., and Simmons, M.: Bronchodilator effects of terbutaline and aminophylline alone and in combination in asthmatic patients, New England Journal of Medicine **298:**363, 1978.

Wyatt, R., Waschek, J., Weinberger, M., and Sherman, B.: Effects of inhaled beclomethasone dipropionate and alternate-day prednisone on pituitary-adrenal function in children with chronic asthma, New England Journal of Medicine **299:**1387, 1978.

23 Drugs to control bronchial secretions

Drugs to treat nasal congestion

■ ALPHA ADRENERGIC AGONISTS AS NASAL DECONGESTANTS

Mechanism of action. Nasal congestion results when the blood vessels in the nasal passage become dilated as a result of infection, inflammation, allergy, or emotional upset. This dilation increases capillary permeability and allows fluid to escape into the nasal passage. Drugs that stimulate alpha receptors cause blood vessels to constrict, thereby relieving the congestion. These drugs are alpha adrenergic agonists because they mimic the action of the neurotransmitter norepinephrine (Chapter 8).

■ Topical nasal decongestants

Several alpha adrenergic agonists are applied topically as drops or sprays. Because these nasal decongestants have an immediate and direct contact with the nasal mucosa, they have a rapid action and provide temporary symptomatic relief by opening up the nasal passages. However, when the effect of the drug wears off, the congestion reappears (rebound congestion). If the nasal decongestant is used with increasing frequency, it has less and less effect. The drug ultimately irritates the nasal passages and causes the congestion to become worse rather than better. For this reason, decongestants are most effective when used only occasionally and for no longer than 3 to 5 days. Nasal decongestants are available without a prescription.

Administration of nose drops. When a nasal decongestant is applied as drops into the nostril, the patient should be lying on a bed with the head hanging over the edge and turned to one side. The drops are then instilled into the upper nostril. After a few seconds the head is turned to allow administration to the other nostril. Use of this lateral, head-low position allows the drops to coat the nasal mucosa without being immediately swallowed. The drops may cause a stinging or burning sensation or induce sneezing.

With repeated use of a nasal congestant, more of the drug is absorbed and systemic effects become possible. The symptoms of an overdose are those expected from a sympathomimetic drug (Chapter 8): nervousness, dizziness, palpitation, and transient high blood pressure readings. Children are especially vulnerable to overdoses of nasal decongestants and may have reactions such as sweating, drowsiness, shock, or coma.

■ Orally active decongestants

Those alpha adrenergic agonists most commonly found in cold remedies include *phenylpropanolamine, phenylephrine,* and *pseudoephedrine*. Cold remedies are syrups, tablets, or capsules that may also include an antihistamine, an analgesic, or other miscellaneous ingredients. Cold remedies are discussed in Chapter 5.

Drug interactions with nasal decongestants. Patients with hyperthyroidism, diabetes mellitus, hypertension, or heart disease are vulnerable to the sympathomimetic side effects of nasal decongestants and should avoid these drugs. A hypertensive reaction to a nasal decongestant may occur in a patient taking a monoamine oxidase inhibitor. Patients receiving tricyclic antidepressants are vulnerable to the cardiac effects of sympathomimetic agents.

■ Specific sympathomimetic drugs used as nasal decongestants (Table 23-1)

Phenylephrine

Phenylephrine (Coricidin, Neo-Synephrine, and others) is a potent alpha adrenergic agonist that is administered orally or topically. It is available by itself but is also included in many combination cold preparations.

Phenylpropanolamine

Phenylpropanolamine (Propadrine) is used mainly in oral combination cold remedies. It is an alpha adrenergic agonist and also acts indirectly, releasing norepinephrine from nerve terminals.

Pseudoephedrine

Pseudoephedrine (Novafed, Sudafed, and others) is included in many oral combination cold remedies. It is a beta agonist as well as an alpha agonist.

TABLE 23-1. Nasal decongestants (nonprescription drugs)

Generic name	Trade name	Dosage and administration	Comments
Ephedrine sulfate	I-Sedrin	ORAL: *Adults*—25 to 50 mg every 3 to 4 hr. *Children*—3 mg/kg body weight daily in 4 to 6 divided doses. TOPICAL: *Adults* and *children*—3 to 4 drops of a 1% or 3% solution in each nostril every 3 to 4 hr, no more than 4 times daily. Also may apply as a pack or tampon.	Can cause central nervous system stimulation, transient hypertension, and palpitations, so contraindicated for patients with heart disease, diabetes, hypertension, and hyperthyroidism. Rebound congestion is common.
Epinephrine hydrochloride	Adrenalin Chloride	TOPICAL: 0.1% aqueous solution as a spray or 1 to 2 drops every 4 to 6 hr. Not recommended for children under 6 yr.	Short-acting. Frequently causes rebound congestion. Can cause central nervous system stimulation, headaches, and palpitations.
Naphazoline hydrochloride	Privine Hydrochloride	TOPICAL: 0.05% and 0.1% solutions. Two drops in each nostril no more than every 3 hr or 2 sprays every 4 to 6 hr.	An imidazoline. Can cause rebound congestion. Systemic effects from overuse include arrhythmias, transient hypertension, slowing of the heart rate, and drowsiness. Do not use in an atomizer with aluminum parts.
Oxymetazoline hydrochloride	Afrin	TOPICAL: *Adults*—2 to 4 drops or 2 to 3 sprays of 0.05% solution in each nostril at morning and at bedtime. *Children*—over 6 yr, as for adults; 2 to 5 yr, 0.025% solution is used as above.	An imidazoline. Long-acting. Side effects are mild, generally safe.
Phenylephrine hydrochloride	Coricidin Decongestant Nasal Mist Neo-Synephrine Hydrochloride Super Anahist Nasal Spray	TOPICAL: *Adults*—drops of 0.25% to 1% solution in each nostril (head in lateral, head-low position) every 3 to 4 hr. Nasal spray or nasal jelly may be used. *Children over 6 yr*—as for adults. *Infants and young children:* 0.125% solution is used as above.	Less potent and longer acting than epinephrine. No central nervous system stimulation, but can cause transient hypertension, headaches, and palpitations.
Phenylpropanolamine hydrochloride	Propadrine Hydrochloride	ORAL: *Adults*—25 mg every 3 to 4 hr or 50 mg every 6 to 8 hr. *Children 8 to 12 yr*—20 to 25 mg 3 times daily. Not recommended for children under 8 yr.	Similar to ephedrine but with less central nervous system stimulation.
Propylhexidrine	Benzedrex	TOPICAL (inhalation): 2 inhalations in each nostril as needed.	A volatile drug safe for adult use; children should be supervised. Inhaler should be warmed by the hands if cold.
Pseudoephedrine hydrochloride	Novafed Sudafed	ORAL: *Adults*—60 mg every 6 to 8 hr. *Children*—4 mg/kg body weight in 4 divided doses.	The stereosomer of ephedrine with a lesser incidence of central nervous system stimulation and hypertension than ephedrine. Useful for relief of a runny nose or congestion leading to an earache.
Pseudoephedrine sulfate	Afrinol Repetabs	As for pseudoephedrine hydrochloride.	

Continued.

TABLE 23-1. Nasal decongestants (nonprescription drugs)—cont'd

Generic name	Trade name	Dosage and administration	Comments
Tetrahydrolozine hydrochloride	Tyzine	TOPICAL: *Adults*—2 to 4 drops of a 0.1% solution in each nostril. Do not repeat more frequently than every 3 hr. *Children*—6 yr and over, as for adults; 2 to 6 yr, 2 to 3 drops of a 0.05% solution in each nostril every 4 to 6 hr.	An imidazoline. Adverse reactions can be severe: hypertension, drowsiness, sweating, rebound hypotension, bradycardia, and cardiac arrhythmias. May cause a high fever and coma in young children. Rebound congestion may persist a week after discontinuing.
Tuaminoheptane sulfate	Tuamine Sulfate	TOPICAL: *Adults*—4 to 5 drops of the 1% solution per nostril, 4 to 5 times daily for no more than 4 days. *Children*—6 yr and over, as for adults; 1 to 6 yr, as above but decrease to 2 to 3 drops per nostril. *Infants*—1 to 2 drops per nostril.	Relatively safe for young children if not abused. Patients with cardiovascular disease should use caution.
Xylometazoline hydrochloride	Neo-Synephrine II, Long-acting Otrivin Spray Sinutab Long-lasting Sinus Spray	TOPICAL: *Adults*—2 to 3 drops of 0.1% solution or 1 to 2 inhalations of 0.1% spray in each nostril every 8 to 10 hr. *Children*—6 mo to 12 yr, 2 to 3 drops of 0.05% solution in each nostril every 4 to 6 hr. *Infants*—1 drop of 0.05% solution in each nostril every 6 hr.	An imidazoline. A relatively safe, long-acting decongestant but should not be used excessively or for more than a few days. Do not use in atomizers with aluminum parts.

Propylhexedrine

Propylhexedrine (Benzedrex) is a volatile drug that stimulates alpha receptors. It causes little stimulation of the central nervous system and is therefore generally safer than some of the other nasal decongestants.

Tuaminoheptane

Tuaminoheptane (Tuamine sulfate) is applied as nasal drops and has a long duration of action. It is considered relatively safe for young children.

■ Imidazolines (Table 23-1)

There is a subgroup of four nasal decongestants that are chemically related, the imidazolines. These all stimulate the alpha adrenergic receptors to produce vasoconstriction. They are potent, and only xylometazoline is considered safe for young children. All are used topically. Naphazoline and xylometazoline will react with aluminum and should not be used in atomizers with aluminum parts.

Naphazoline

Naphazoline (Privine) is a very effective nasal decongestant but can also produce a severe rebound congestion resulting from irritation and swelling of the nasal mucosa. Overdosage of naphazoline has been reported to produce coma in children and to produce such systemic effects as hypertension, sweating, cardiac arrhythmias, and drowsiness in adults.

Oxymetazoline

Oxymetazoline (Afrin) is a relatively long-lasting nasal decongestant that has not been implicated in as many severe systemic effects as naphazoline. However, rebound congestion does occur with repeated use.

Tetrahydrozoline

Tetrahydrozoline (Tyzine) is an effective nasal decongestant similar to naphazoline in its adverse effects.

Xylometazoline

Xylometazoline (Neo-Synephrine II, Sinutab Long-Lasting Spray, and others) is similar to oxymetazoline in its effects.

■ Other drugs used to relieve nasal congestion

Nasal congestion is common with an allergy like hay fever. As discussed in Chapter 21, antihistamines are useful in treating hay fever because they block the receptors for histamine on the blood vessels and thereby prevent the dilation causing nasal congestion. Antihistamines are also frequently included in cold remedy preparations. The anticholinergic action characteristic of antihistamines aids in reversing the vasodilation of the nasal blood vessels. The same anticholinergic action inhibits bronchial secretions to inhibit a productive cough, so these drugs may not be helpful for alleviating the symptoms of a cold.

FIG. 23-1

Mucous layer at top is the lumen of the airway. Relative position of goblet cells and bronchial glands, secretions of which make up the mucus, are shown. Mucous layer is normally swept up toward the throat by the cilia to cleanse the airway.

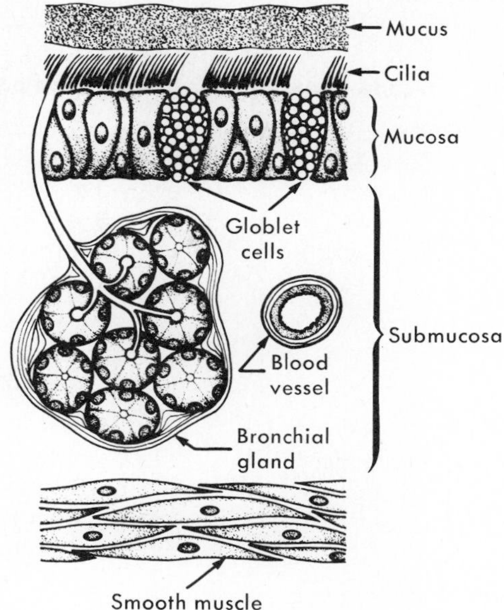

Drugs to treat a cough

■ EXPECTORANTS, ANTITUSSIVES, AND MUCOLYTIC DRUGS

■ Origin of secretions

Respiratory secretions in the trachea, bronchi, and bronchioles originate from the goblet cells and from the bronchial glands (Fig. 23-1). The goblet cells lie on the surface, making up part of the epithelial layer. The tracheal epithelium consists of about 20% goblet cells, whereas the bronchiolar epithelium consists of only 2% goblet cells. The goblet cells produce a gelatinous mucus that they periodically secrete. What factors normally control the goblet cells is not known, but chronic exposure to irritants increases the size, number, and activity of the goblet cells. An example is the phlegm coughed up by smokers. The bronchial glands lie several layers beneath the epithelium. The grapelike (acinar) cells are controlled by the cholinergic nervous system, and when stimulated these cells secrete a plentiful watery fluid into a duct that empties onto the surface.

The secretions of the goblet cells and bronchial glands combine to form a mucus called the *respiratory tract fluid*. Much of the water in the respiratory secretions evaporates to humidify the air taken into the lungs. If too much water is lost to humidification, the mucus forms thick plugs that cannot be readily eliminated. Normally the respiratory tract fluid forms a lining that is swept upward by the action of the ciliary hairs into the throat (pharynx) where it is swallowed. This activity, the *mucociliary escalator,* provides a cleansing mechanism for the lungs, since any foreign particles or bacteria are trapped in this viscous layer and eliminated. If the ciliary hairs are paralyzed by tobacco smoke or by alcohol, the secretions cannot be cleared naturally and give rise to the "smoker's cough."

■ Cough

A cough is a protective reflex initiated by irritation in the airway. As long as material is being brought up by the cough, it is beneficial. Several common situations cause an unproductive cough. The air of heated rooms can dry the airway enough to cause irritation. A sore throat can produce an unproductive cough and can be self-perpetuating when the cough itself further irritates the throat. A cough can result from irritants responsible for asthma or pulmonary edema, which also stimulate the cough receptors. Congestion of the nasal mucosa results in a postnasal drip, which irritates the throat and produces the cough associated with a cold or the flu.

When a cough is unproductive and disrupts sleep and rest, relief is sought. Therapy for a cough depends on the cause. If the air is dry, a vaporizer or steamer may be sufficient to liquify the secretions so that they do not become irritating. A dehydrated state limits respiratory secretions, so having the patient drink plenty of fluids prevents or overcomes the dehydration that accompanies common illnesses. Patients with sore throats can suck hard candies to increase the flow of saliva to coat the throat. If these simple measures do not eliminate the cough, expectorants may be used. An *expectorant* is a drug that increases the output of respiratory tract fluid to coat the trachea and bronchi. In addition, a cough suppressant or *antitussive* drug may be taken. Expectorants and antitussive drugs are widely available as over-the-counter drugs.

TABLE 23-2. Expectorants*

Generic name	Trade name	Dosage and administration	Comments
Guaifenesin (glycerol guaiacolate)	Anti-tuss Glycotuss Nortussin Robitussin Various others	ORAL: *Adults*—100 to 200 mg every 3 to 4 hr. *Children*—6 to 12 yr, 100 mg every 3 to 4 hr; 2 to 6 yr, 50 mg every 3 to 4 hr.	Use for symptomatic relief of a dry, unproductive cough. Occasionally causes nausea or drowsiness. Available without prescription.
Hydroiodic acid		ORAL: *Adult*—¼ to 1 tsp (17 to 70 mg) 2 or 3 times daily after meals. *Children over 1 yr*—1 to 10 drops (0.7 to 7 mg) diluted in water 1 to 3 times daily.	See potassium iodide.
Iodinated glycerol	Organidin	ORAL: *Adults*—20 drops of solution (50 mg) or a 60 mg tablet or 5 ml elixir (60 mg) 4 times daily. *Children*—no more than ½ adult dose daily.	See potassium iodide.
Potassium iodide	Potassium Iodide SSKI Pima Iodo-Niacin	ORAL: *Adults*—300 mg every 4 to 6 hr. *Children*—60 to 500 mg daily, divided in 2 to 4 doses.	Contraindicated for patients with hyperkalemia, hyperthyroidism, or hypersensitivity to iodide. Symptoms of hypersensitivity include a skin rash. Iodism (overdose of iodide) causes a metallic taste, fever, skin eruptions, nausea, vomiting, mucous membrane ulcerations, and salivary gland swelling.

*Only those expectorants available by themselves have been listed. Other drugs included in cough or cold mixtures as an expectorant include potassium guaiacolsulfonate, ammonium chloride, terpin hydrate, ipecac, calcium iodide, and citric acid.

■ Expectorants (Table 23-2)

Although many drugs are used as expectorants, no expectorant has been proven effective. Iodide, usually given as potassium iodide, is one widely used expectorant. After entering the bloodstream, potassium iodide is believed to stimulate the bronchial glands to secrete more fluid. Use of iodides is associated with a high incidence of adverse effects. Some people develop a skin rash. A few patients become hypothyroid. One symptom of iodide excess is a mumpslike swelling of the parotid glands, presumably a result of stimulation of the glands. Iodides are seldom used today.

Another mechanism that stimulates the secretion of respiratory tract fluid is the reflex activity carried by the vagal nerve characteristic of nausea. Some drugs used as expectorants are believed to initiate this reflex by irritating the stomach when swallowed. One such drug is *guaifenesin (glycerol guaiacolate),* a widely used expectorant for which there is some evidence of efficacy. Other drugs acting by this mechanism include *syrup of ipecac* and *ammonium chloride*. Potassium iodide is believed to act in part by this latter mechanism as well as by the secretory mechanism just described. Syrup of ipecac is more commonly used to induce vomiting (emesis) than as an expectorant.

Other agents added as expectorants to cough suppressant mixtures include *terpin hydrate, citric acid, sodium citrate, iodinated glycerol,* and *calcium iodide*.

■ Antitussives (Table 23-3)

Tussis is the Latin word meaning cough, and cough suppressants are called antitussives. *Codeine* and *hydrocodone* are good antitussives, but they are opiates and therefore capable of producing drug dependence. Hydrocodone has a greater potential for producing drug dependence than codeine. Most preparations containing codeine or hydrocodone are prescription drugs. Some preparations are available as Schedule V drugs and may be obtained by signing for them with a registered pharmacist. The opiates suppress a cough by directly inhibiting the medullary center for the cough reflex. The doses required to suppress a cough are less than those to produce analgesia or respiratory depression. Side effects at antitussive doses are uncommon, but include nausea, dizziness, and constipation.

TABLE 23-3. Antitussives

Generic name	Trade name	Dosage and administration	Comments
Codeine, codeine phosphate, codeine sulfate		ORAL: *Adults*—10 to 20 mg every 4 to 6 hr, no more than 120 mg in 24 hr. *Children*—6 to 12 yr, 5 to 10 mg every 4 to 6 hr, no more than 60 mg in 24 hr; 2 to 6 yr, 2.5 to 5 mg every 4 to 6 hr, no more than 30 mg in 24 hr.	A Schedule II drug. Codeine is included in some Schedule III and Schedule V combination formulations, usually including a decongestant, an antihistamine, and an expectorant. For adverse effects, see Chapter 28.
Hydrocodone bitartrate	Codone Dicodid	ORAL: *Adults*—5 to 10 mg every 6 to 8 hr. *Children*—0.6 mg/kg daily in divided doses.	A Schedule II drug. Hydrocodone is included in some Schedule III and Schedule V combination formulations, usually including a decongestant, an antihistamine, and an expectorant. For adverse effects, see Chapter 28.
Dextromethorphan hydrobromide	Coughettes Sucrets Cough Control Lozenge Romilar CF Various others	ORAL: *Adults*—10 to 20 mg every 4 hr or 30 mg every 6 to 8 hr. *Children*—6 to 12 yr, ½ adult dose; 2 to 6 yr, ¼ adult dose.	Nonnarcotic, available without prescription. No tolerance develops. Has no analgesic or hypnotic effect, does not depress respiration. Does not cause constipation as readily as codeine.
Diphenhydramine hydrochloride	Benylin Cough Syrup	ORAL: *Adults*—25 mg every 4 hr, no more than 100 mg in 24 hr. *Children*—6 to 12 yr, ½ adult dose. 2 to 5 yr, ¼ adult dose.	An antihistamine. Side effects include drowsiness and a drying effect.
Benzonatate	Tessalon	ORAL: *Adults*—100 mg 3 to 6 times daily. *Children*—over 10 yr, same as adults; under 10 yr, 8 mg/kg body weight in 3 to 6 divided doses.	Unlike other antitussives, works peripherally, anesthetizing stretch receptors in the respiratory mucosa.

Nonopiate antitussives include *dextromethorphan, diphenhydramine,* and *benzonatate.*

Dextromethorphan hydrobromide

Dextromethorphan hydrobromide is the most widely used antitussive in over-the-counter cough mixtures. It is related to the opiates but has no analgesic effect and causes no drug dependence. Dextromethorphan is an effective cough suppressant that inhibits the medullary center for the cough reflex. It is very well tolerated and only occasionally causes drowsiness or dizziness.

Diphenhydramine

Diphenhydramine *(Benylin)* is an antihistamine with antitussive action. Adverse effects include the drowsiness common to the antihistamines and the anticholinergic drying effect that hinders a productive cough.

Benzonatate

Benzonatate *(Tessalon)* is chemically related to the local anesthetics and is believed to act by depressing the peripheral receptors in the throat that are responsible for initiating a cough. This peripheral action of benzonatate is unique among the antitussives. Side effects include a "chilly" sensation, dizziness, and drowsiness.

■ Mucolytic drugs

The value of water, both drunk as liquid and inhaled as vapor, has already been mentioned as a useful method for keeping the mucus from becoming too viscous. The use of expectorants to stimulate the watery secretion of the bronchial glands has also been covered.

Mucolytics are agents that break up a viscous mucus so that it can be coughed up or otherwise drained. A viscous mucus is most likely to occur in the patient with a pulmonary infection or with chronic obstructive lung disease where the normal mechanisms for clearing the lungs are compromised.

Table 23-4 lists the dosages and administration of the mucolytic drugs.

Acetylcysteine

Acetylcysteine (Mucomyst) is a sulfhydryl compound that can break disulfide bonds. A viscous mucus

TABLE 23-4. Mucolytic drugs

Generic name	Trade name	Dosage and administration	Comments
Acetylcysteine	Mucomyst	NEBULIZATION USING A FACE MASK, MOUTHPIECE, OR TRACHEOSTOMY: 1 to 10 mg of a 20% solution or 2 to 20 ml of a 10% solution every 2 to 6 hr. DIRECT INSTILLATION: 1 to 2 ml of a 10% or 20% solution as often as every hour.	Has the odor of rotten eggs, which may cause gastrointestinal upset. Solutions can be diluted with sterile water for nebulization. Reacts with iron, copper, and rubber, so nebulization equipment should not have these materials.
Tyloxapol	Alevaire	Aerosol nebulization should be used. For administration into a tent, one 500 ml bottle (0.125% tyloxapol) is nebulized every 12 to 24 hr. For administration into a face mask, 10 to 20 ml is nebulized.	Solutions should not be diluted.

■ THE NURSING PROCESS FOR DRUGS MODIFYING RESPIRATORY SECRETIONS

■ Assessment

Patients that require drugs to modify bronchial secretions are those who are self-medicating for symptomatic treatment of colds and upper respiratory infections, those with serious upper respiratory problems, and those few patients with chronic pulmonary diseases characterized by problems with coughing or secretions. The nurse should assess the total patient in addition to focusing on the patient's subjective complaints. An appropriate history would include questions related to the onset of symptoms, possible irritants for the symptoms that are present, the times of the day when symptoms are worse (such as coughing, which is more troublesome at night), therapies used by the patient that have successfully relieved the symptoms, and the history of irritants or environmental conditions that may be aggravating the symptoms. Objective data might include the respiratory rate, the vital signs, the character and quantity of any secretions, an examination of the nose, throat, and ears, and an assessment of the lungs.

■ Management

Since the patient is usually being treated for relief of symptoms, the nurse needs to monitor these symptoms during the course of therapy. The nurse should monitor the vital signs, and in some patients it may be necessary to monitor the fluid intake and output. The nurse should work with the patient to identify nonmedical solutions for troublesome symptoms. For patients receiving mucolytic agents, a suction machine should be at the bedside if there is doubt that the patient can adequately handle secretions.

■ Evaluation

These drugs are successful if the patient's symptoms are relieved or if the underlying condition requiring the drugs has improved because of therapy. Before discharge for self-management, the patient should be able to explain how to take the drugs correctly, to demonstrate how to administer the drugs correctly, to explain what side effects might occur that would require notification of the physician, to explain the need to discontinue the drugs after symptoms have improved, and to explain what actions to take if the symptoms return or do not improve.

has long molecules linked by disulfide bonds; when these disulfide bonds are broken, the molecules separate, reducing the viscosity.

Acetylcysteine is administered by nebulization through a face mask, mouthpiece, or tracheostomy. Acetylcysteine has a rotten egg odor and may irritate the nasal passages.

Tyloxapol

Tyloxapol (Alevaire) is a detergent administered by an aerosol nebulizer as a fine mist. As a detergent, tyloxapol lowers the surface tension and viscosity of the secretions in the pulmonary tract. This loosens the secretions so that they may be cleared by the cilia or by coughing.

■ PATIENT CARE IMPLICATIONS

Nasal decongestants

1. Review the side effects discussed in the text.
2. Most patients buy cold remedies, antitussives, nasal decongestants, and expectorants as over-the-counter drugs. Instruct patients to read the ingredients in these preparations and to buy only formulations containing the desired drug(s), without unnecessary other drugs. The pharmacist can assist an individual in choosing an appropriate remedy for a specific problem.
3. Caution patients that rebound congestion can be a problem when discontinuing nasal decongestants. For this reason, decongestants should be used only as directed and for as few days as necessary.
4. Caution patients that rebound congestion can be a problem when discontinuing nasal decongestants. For this reason, decongestants should be used only as directed and for as few days as necessary.
5. Patients receiving monoamine oxidase inhibitors or tricyclic antidepressants should avoid using nasal decongestants (see text).
6. Patients with hyperthyroidism, diabetes mellitus, hypertension, or heart disease should use these drugs only with the approval of their physicians.
7. Caution patients to keep these and all medications out of the reach of children. Only preparations designed for pediatric doses should be used with children.
8. For best results with topical application, instruct the patient to blow the nose before using the medication. After instillation of the drops or spray, the patient may blot a runny nose, but should avoid blowing the nose for several minutes to allow the maximum amount of medication to be absorbed.
9. To prevent contamination, each patient or individual family member should have a different dropper or spray applicator. Applicators should be washed or rinsed with hot water after each use.

Expectorants and antitussives

1. Instruct patients about the difference between an expectorant and an antitussive and in what situations it might be desirable to use one rather than the other. Caution the patient to read labels carefully on over-the-counter preparations to avoid taking unnecessary medications.
2. Caution patients to keep these and all medications out of the reach of children. When using a formula for children, only the prescribed dose should be administered.
3. Review the side effects discussed in the text and in Tables 23-2 and 23-3.
4. If an antitussive causes a patient to be drowsy, caution the patient to avoid activities requiring mental alertness, such as driving or operating machinery. If the patient must continue these activities, it may be possible for the patient to reserve the medication for use at bedtime or during leisure hours and to control the cough during work time by sucking on hard candies, avoiding smoking and talking, and staying well hydrated (2500 to 3000 ml of fluid intake per day).

Mucolytic agents

1. Patients receiving mucolytic agents should be supervised carefully during and after treatment to see that the airway is still patent in the presence of increased pulmonary secretions. For patients who are elderly, immobilized, or not alert and those who are intubated, have a tracheostomy tube in place, or who are otherwise unable to cough or handle secretions, a suction machine should be at the bedside.
2. Before using a mucolytic agent the first time with a patient, the patient should be informed about the purpose of the agent and instructed to cough up and expectorate loosened secretions as needed.
3. Patients with asthma should be supervised carefully if acetylcysteine is being used, because it may cause varying degrees of bronchospasm. If bronchospasm occurs, discontinue the nebulization. In some cases, a bronchodilator administered via nebulization may be needed.
4. Other side effects associated with acetylcysteine include stomatitis, rhinorrhea, and nausea.

■ SUMMARY

A runny nose and cough are two of the most common cold symptoms for which people seek relief.

Nasal congestion and a runny nose result from dilation of the blood vessels in the nasal mucosa and leakage of fluid from these vessels. Drugs that stimulate alpha adrenergic receptors cause vasoconstriction and thereby relieve nasal congestion. Commonly these drugs are applied as drops or sprays. Abuse of these drugs results in the blood vessels becoming unresponsive, and rebound congestion occurs. A few sympathomimetic drugs are effective orally. The imidazolines are selective alpha receptor agonists for topical use.

Secretions arise from goblet cells and bronchial glands in the respiratory tract to form mucus. This mucus normally traps particulate matter in the lungs and is swept up to the throat by ciliary hairs. Expectorants are drugs such as iodides, guaifenesin, ipecac, and ammonium chloride that stimulate the production of these secretions.

Irritation of the throat causes a cough, which is a protective reflex mediated through the medullary cough center. Suppression of a cough may be desired to provide rest or when the cough is unproductive. Codeine, hydrocordone, dextromethorphan, and diphenhydramine all act at the medullary cough center to suppress a cough. Benzonatate acts as a local anesthetic to depress the receptors initiating a cough.

Mucolytic drugs are those drugs that break up a viscous mucus that cannot be coughed up or drained. Acetylcysteine breaks the disulfide bonds holding together the long molecules that compose mucus. Toloxapol is a detergent that lowers the surface tension and viscosity of mucus.

■ STUDY QUESTIONS

1. Explain how alpha adrenergic agonists act to relieve nasal congestion.
2. Describe the technique for administering topical nasal decongestants.
3. What are the side effects, drug interactions, and contraindications for the use of nasal decongestants?
4. What is rebound congestion?
5. Categorize the drugs used as nasal decongestants as topical sympathomimetics, oral sympathomimetics, and imidazolines.
6. Describe the origin and function of mucus.
7. List the expectorants and their mechanisms of action.
8. List the mucolytic drugs and their mechanisms of action.
9. List the antitussives and their mechanisms of action.
10. What are the nonmedicinal approaches for treating a cough?

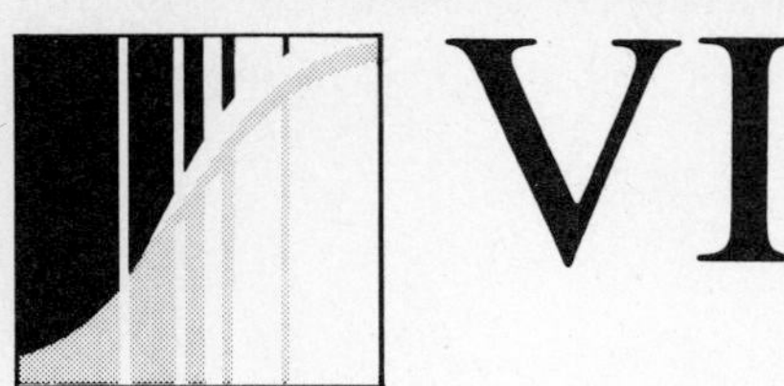

VI DRUGS USED FOR TREATING MENTAL AND EMOTIONAL DISORDERS

In this section drug classes used to affect behavior are presented. Chapter 24 includes the drugs used to treat insomnia and anxiety. Although the barbiturates are declining in use in favor of the benzodiazepines, the barbiturates remain an important example of factors determining drug disposition as well as drug tolerance. The benzodiazepines are discussed with respect to their highly favorable therapeutic index and low abuse potential. Other sedative-hypnotic, antianxiety drugs are not presented in great detail. A major emphasis of the chapter is the dependency potential of the drugs and their cross-tolerance. Because alcohol is a major drug with respect to these two points, alcohol is also presented in detail in this chapter. The importance of alcohol as a source of drug interactions as well as alcohol as a source of drug abuse are major points.

Chapter 25 presents the antipsychotic drugs, with emphasis on the importance of the antagonism of the central neurotransmitters dopamine, norepinephrine, and acetylcholine, in explaining the various effects of these drugs. Chapter 26 presents the major classes of antidepressant drugs: the tricyclic antidepressants, the monoamine oxidase inhibitors, and lithium. The role of these drugs in improving the neurotransmitter functions of norepinephrine and serotonin in the central nervous system is emphasized. Chapter 27 concentrates principally on the therapeutic roles of central nervous system stimulants in treating narcolepsy, hyperactivity, and obesity and in improving deficient respiratory drive. The abuse of amphetamine, cocaine, and caffeine is also presented.

24 Sedative-hypnotic agents, antianxiety agents, and alcohol

Sedative-hypnotic drugs and antianxiety drugs are considered together because they are not really different so much in their action as in their historic origin. The term *sedative-hypnotic* is used for the older drug classes, primarily the barbiturates. The barbiturates are a class of chemically related drugs developed in the early 1900's, effective both as sedatives and as hypnotics. A small dose to calm an anxious patients is called a *sedative*. A larger dose sufficient to induce sleep is a *hypnotic*.

After the 1950's, drugs were developed to be used specifically as sleep-inducing agents (hypnotics). Other drugs were developed for use as sedatives to treat anxiety. The benzodiazepines are the drug class most used today to treat anxiety. However, the term *minor tranquilizer,* used to describe these new sedative drugs, gives the impression that these sedative drugs have much in common with the major tranquilizers or antipsychotic drugs. Actually, the clinical use of the major and minor tranquilizers does not overlap, and these two drug classes have no common pharmacological mechanisms. To avoid confusion, minor tranquilizers are now called *antianxiety* drugs.

An additional drug appropriate to this chapter is alcohol because it has the pharmacological actions characteristic of a sedative-hypnotic or antianxiety drug. Indeed, the social use of alcohol is mainly as an antianxiety agent, self-prescribed. Furthermore, drug abuse and drug dependency are discussed in this chapter. Alcohol, when recognized as a drug, is seen to be a major source of drug abuse and dependency.

Psychopharmacology of general central nervous system (CNS) depressants

■ Behavioral changes with general CNS depressants

Role of the reticular activating system. The effects of a single dose of a sedative-hypnotic drug, an antianxiety drug, or alcohol are very much alike. All of these drugs act pharmacologically as *general depressants* of the CNS, since they depress the reticular activating system of the brain stem. The reticular activating system refers to those neural pathways in which incoming signals from the senses (sight, sound, smell, touch, taste, and balance) and viscera are collected, processed, and passed on to the higher brain centers (Fig. 24-1). Higher brain centers also have neural pathways to the reticular activating system to modulate activity. The reticular activating system determines the level of our awareness of our environment and therefore governs our reactions to our environment.

Stages of CNS depression. Depression of the reticular activating system by a general CNS depressant accounts for the behavioral changes seen in someone who has taken one of these drugs. The degree of depression depends on the amount of drug taken. At a low dose *sedation* is produced, which is characterized by decreased physical and mental responses to stimuli. With an increasing dose, *disinhibition* is the next level of depression reached. Disinhibition falsely appears as a stimulated state of awareness. This is because neurons inhibiting arousal become depressed. The result of disinhibition may be a feeling of euphoria, excitement, drunkenness, loss of self-control, and impaired judgment. The relief of anxiety produced by a general CNS depressant results from sedation and/or disinhibition. A loss of motor coordination (ataxia) and involuntary eye movements (nystagmus) may frequently be seen at this level of depression and are clues to look for if drug use is suspected. Pain can intensify disinhibition and result in paradoxical excitement in postoperative patients who

FIG. 24-1

Awareness is a function of the reticular activating system. Diagram illustrates the role of reticular activating system as an integration network. General central nervous system depressants act on the reticular activating system at some level although the mechanisms are not understood.

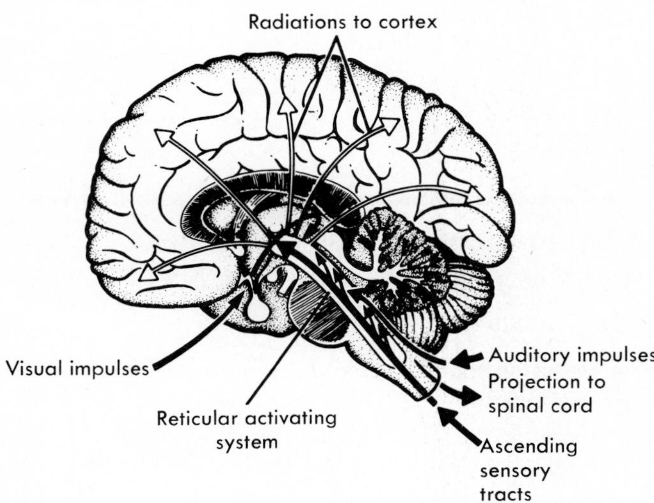

are given a sedative-hypnotic or an antianxiety drug. Increasing the drug dose further will produce *sleep* (hypnosis). *Anesthesia,* the loss of feeling or sensation, is achieved at very high doses of a general CNS depressant drug.

The effect seen from a single dose of a sedative-hypnotic drug, an antianxiety drug, or alcohol is therefore dependent on the dose taken. In practice, not much distinction can be made in the sedative versus hypnotic dose for drugs used primarily as hypnotics. Similarly, those drugs most popular as sedative or antianxiety drugs are those that produce minimal sleepiness at an effective dose.

■ Drug dependency with general CNS depressant drugs

Origin of drug dependence. Continued administration of a general CNS depressant drug can cause drug dependence. Drug dependence means that the body has adjusted to the continual depression of the CNS so that the body now requires the presence of the drug to function. If administration is discontinued abruptly, the body experiences withdrawal symptoms. The symptoms of withdrawal from a general CNS depressant drug reflect hyperactivity of the CNS. Mild withdrawal symptoms include agitation, tremulousness, and insomnia, whereas the major withdrawal symptom is convulsions, a life-threatening emergency. The symptoms disappear when the drug is retaken.

Dose to produce drug dependence. It is not possible to state simply what dose produces drug dependence because there is so much variation among individuals. Very broadly, the general CNS depressant drugs can produce drug dependence when taken at twice their prescribed doses for 2 to 8 weeks. The dependency potential does vary among the drug classes somewhat, as will be discussed more fully for each individual class. A thought-provoking observation is that each new sedative-hypnotic and antianxiety drug has been introduced with the conviction that it was not addicting, whereas in fact no drug of the general depressant type has turned out to be nonaddicting. The benzodiazepines, a class of drugs that account for at least 15% of all prescriptions written in the United States, have only recently been widely recognized as capable of producing drug dependence.

Development of drug abuse. The time required for drug dependency to develop depends on the drug dose. Chronic use of low doses does not have to lead to drug dependence. Many people take a low dose of a barbiturate to control epilepsy and do not experience withdrawal symptoms if their medication is changed. Moderate alcohol consumption, even on a daily basis, does not necessarily lead to alcohol dependence. However, tolerance does develop to the sedative and euphoric effects of the general CNS depressants. A person abuses the drug when the reaction to this tolerance is to increase the amount of drug taken. As the dose of drug increases, a point is reached at which failure to take the drug produces withdrawal symptoms. At this point, drug use may be continued as much to avoid withdrawal symptoms as to produce drug effects. It is this stage that we refer to as *drug dependency* or *drug addiction*. The individual's life may become centered around the drug, while personal, family, and social interactions assume a lesser importance.

Drug addiction cannot be simply explained by drug tolerance and physical dependency. In general, physical dependency can be overcome by decreasing the drug intake by 10% of the initial dose daily for 10 days. This gradual reduction prevents withdrawal symptoms from becoming severe. However, many patients revert back to drug abuse after they have been withdrawn from drug dependence. Drug addiction therefore involves social and psychological factors that underlie drug abuse.

Cross tolerance among CNS depressants. Tolerance to any one of the sedative-hypnotic drugs, antianxiety drugs, or alcohol results in tolerance to any other of these general CNS depressants. This property is called *cross tolerance* and is a major factor in drug abuse. The most common pattern of drug abuse is alcohol in combination with one or more sedative-hypnotic drugs or antianxiety drugs. This combination works in an additive fashion. This means that one way an individual can avoid taking more of the same drug to overcome tolerance is by adding a second drug, usually alcohol. This can be a lethal combination, for although it is relatively uncommon for someone to drink enough to die from alcohol alone, this becomes quite feasible when another drug such as a sedative-hypnotic drug or an antianxiety drug is added. Moreover, because of cross tolerance, a dose that would not lead to drug dependency by itself will contribute to drug dependency when added to a second drug of the general depressant type.

Mechanisms of general CNS depressants for insomnia and anxiety

■ Sleep and hypnotic drugs

Stages of sleep. What determines sleep is not well understood. Current sleep research makes use of the brain wave patterns and eye movements recorded during sleep, as shown in Fig. 24-2. Four stages of sleep are defined by these brain wave patterns. Stage 1 represents the lightest level of sleep and is accompanied by some muscle relaxation and slowing of the heart rate. Stage 4 represents the deepest level of sleep and is accompanied by marked muscle relaxation and slowing of the heart rate. During most of the sleep cycle the eye movements are not noticed under the closed lids. However, during about 20% of the average adult sleep time the eyeballs move rapidly back and forth under the closed eyelids. This is called *REM sleep* (*r*apid *e*ye *m*ovement), and it is superimposed on stage 1 or stage 2 sleep. The body is physiologically active during REM sleep so that the heart rate increases, breathing is irregular, stomach acid is secreted, and the clitoris or penis becomes erect. Muscles lose their tone during REM sleep, however, so that it is only the mind and autonomic nervous system that are active during this stage. Since dreaming occurs exclusively during REM sleep, this time is also called *dreaming* sleep. Many authorities believe that REM sleep is a period during which we integrate emotionally meaningful experiences.

FIG. 24-2

Normal sleep pattern. Sleep is cyclical. Deep sleep is more frequent during early cycles than later cycles. Dreaming occurs during rapid eye movement (REM) sleep and is associated with stage 1 and stage 2 sleep. Pattern shown is characteristic for adults. Children and elderly persons will often awaken more frequently. Most hypnotics will depress REM sleep.

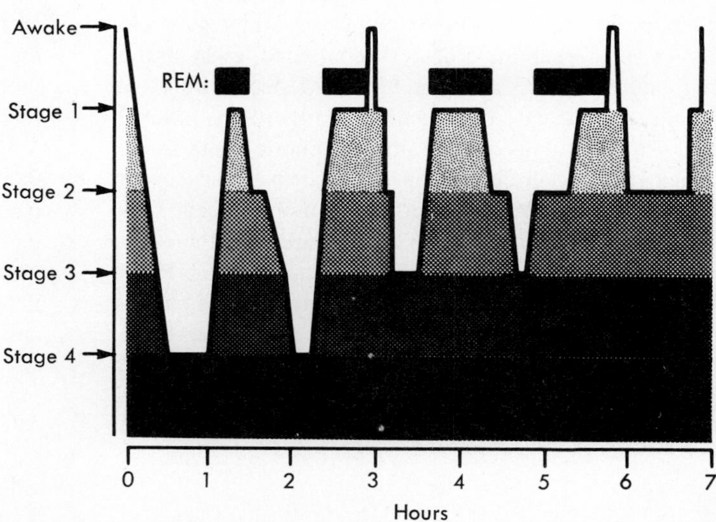

TABLE 24-1. Conditions in which insomnia is prominent

Condition	**Characteristic type of insomnia**
Depression	Early morning insomnia is common.
Chronic alcoholism	REM sleep and deep sleep are reduced.
Hyperthyroidism	Deep sleep is reduced.
Heart failure	Insomnia is an early complaint.
Pregnancy	Insomnia is common during the last trimester.
Renal insufficiency	
Many neurological disorders	

TABLE 24-2. Symptoms of anxiety

Appearance	**Complaints**
Excessively alert	Cardiorespiratory: heart palpitations, fast heart rate, breathlessness
Easily startled	Gastrointestinal: abdominal cramps, nausea, vomiting, diarrhea
Constantly in motion or inhibited in motion	Musculoskeletal: tension headaches, chest pain or tightness, backache
Excessive and disjointed speech	General: fatigue, weakness, insomnia
Eyes constantly scanning	
"Fussy" dress	
Tremors, restlessness	
Dilated pupils	

Sleep cycles. As indicated in Fig. 24-2, an individual normally cycles from stage 1 through stage 4 back to stage 1 every 90 minutes or so. Deep sleep (stages 3 and 4) occupies more of the early sleep cycles, whereas dreaming (REM sleep) occupies more of the late sleep cycles. Children spend more total time in deep sleep than do adults, whereas the elderly may spend little time in deep sleep. With increasing age it becomes more common to awake at the end of a sleep cycle, particularly the early morning cycles.

Insomnia. Insomnia, the inability to sleep, is the most common sleep complaint and can be characterized as either difficulty in getting to sleep or waking up and being unable to go back to sleep. Insomnia is not a disease but a symptom of physical or mental distress. Several conditions in which insomnia is prominent are listed in Table 24-1.

Action of hypnotic drugs. Hypnotic drugs are taken to fall asleep faster or to sleep longer. Studies in sleep laboratories show that most hypnotic drugs suppress REM sleep. When the drug is discontinued, even after a single dose, there is a rebound in REM sleep with vivid dreams and increased awakening. Furthermore, after 3 weeks of continuous therapy, most hypnotic drugs are no longer effective in decreasing the time to fall asleep or the duration of sleep. Nevertheless, if the patient now discontinues the drug, a worse insomnia and the associated anxiety will be experienced because of the REM rebound. This reaction may lead the uninstructed patient to continue the drug, perhaps at an increased dose, to regain the hypnotic effect. This is the beginning of drug abuse with hypnotic drugs. The fact that hypnotic drugs can make insomnia worse rather than better means that the cause of insomnia rather than the insomnia itself should be discovered and treated. Alcohol and antianxiety drugs can interfere with sleep patterns in a similar fashion if taken in large enough doses.

■ Anxiety and drug therapy

Anxiety means different things to different people. There is a constellation of symptoms associated with anxiety, listed in Table 24-2. An anxious individual will have some, though not all, of these physical symptoms. Anxiety may be generalized, in which the individual is unaware of a specific cause of anxiety and may even deny anxiety, or anxiety may be anticipatory, in which the individual is all too well aware of the origin of the anxiety.

Action of antianxiety drugs. As already discussed, the pharmacological action of drugs used as sedatives or antianxiety agents may be to decrease the general level of arousal by inhibiting the reticular activating system of the brain stem. This is not a "cure" for anxiety, although response is blunted. Rather there is general agreement that drug therapy for anxiety should be limited to a few weeks while psychotherapy or behavior modification therapy is begun to deal directly with the origin of the patient's anxiety. In part this recommendation rests on the fact that tolerance develops to these drugs after a few weeks so that effective therapy requires larger doses, the first step in drug abuse. Patients being given sedative or antianxiety drugs should be told that drug therapy will only offer limited relief.

Drugs prescribed for insomnia and anxiety

The drugs prescribed for insomnia and anxiety will be presented in three sections. The first section will present the barbiturates, a class of drugs used to cause a spectrum of CNS depression from sedation to anesthesia. The second section will present the benzodiazepines, the most popular drug class today for treating insomnia and anxiety. The third section will present miscellaneous drugs occasionally prescribed for insomnia or anxiety.

■ BARBITURATES

Over 50 derivatives of barbituric acid have been marketed for clinical use since the first part of this century, and 9 are still widely used. The barbiturates are classified according to their duration of action and have been traditionally divided into four classes: ultra short-acting, short-acting, intermediate-acting, and long-acting. Although traditional, this classification was derived from animal data and is somewhat arbitrary for the clinical setting where the variables of dose and patient expectations can modify the degree and duration of effectiveness. In particular, the contrast between short-acting and intermediate-acting sedative-hypnotics is not as striking in clinical practice as in drug tables.

■ Factors determining onset and duration of action

The ultra short-acting barbiturates are administered intravenously, but the other barbiturates are usually given orally and are well absorbed. The differences in the onset and duration of action among the barbiturates depend on their lipid solubility and protein binding. These properties are determined by the chemical structure. The ultra short-acting barbiturates are very lipid soluble, and on intravenous administration the concentration reaching the brain, which has a high blood flow, is large because the barbiturates readily cross the blood-brain barrier and depress the reticular activating system. Their action is quickly terminated, however, because they redistribute into organs with a lesser blood flow so that the concentration reaching the brain quickly drops. In fact, the ultra short-acting barbiturates may persist in body fat because of their high lipid solubility and in muscle, reflecting their high degree of protein binding.

Metabolism. Barbiturates are slowly released from muscle and fat back into the blood for eventual metabolism by the liver and excretion by the kidney. It is believed that the persistence of low concentrations of barbiturates in the body may account for the "hangovers" after the therapeutic effect has worn off. The short- and intermediate-acting barbiturates redistribute less rapidly into body fat and muscle, so they act for longer times. The long-acting barbiturate phenobarbital binds still less to protein and is very much less lipid soluble than the ultra short-acting barbiturates. Although the ultrashort-, short-, and intermediate-acting barbiturates must be metabolized by the liver to water-soluble metabolites for excretion by the kidney, 30% to 50% of a dose of phenobarbital will be excreted unchanged in the urine.

■ Side effects and toxicity

Mild withdrawal symptoms. As discussed for hypnotics in general, barbiturates are not effective as hypnotics after 3 weeks' use. Furthermore, even a single dose suppresses REM sleep and leads to rebound REM sleep when the barbiturate is discontinued. Mild withdrawal symptoms from short-term use of barbiturates include nightmares, daytime agitation, and a "shaky" feeling.

An *acute overdose* of barbiturates causes depression of the medullary centers controlling respiration and the cardiovascular system. The symptoms are a fast heart rate (tachycardia) and a fall in blood pressure (hypotension) that leads to shock. Reflexes disappear, and respiration is markedly depressed. The patient becomes comatose, and death may result from respiratory and cardiovascular collapse. There is no specific antagonist for barbiturates, thus treatment of barbiturate poisoning is to support respiration and to maintain blood oxygen levels.

■ Factors determining tolerance and drug dependency

Metabolic tolerance. Administration of barbiturates for a few days activates the liver to synthesize more of the drug-metabolizing enzymes. This activation is called *enzyme induction*. Since these enzymes are located in the microsomal fraction of broken cell preparations, these drug-metabolizing enzymes are usually referred to as the liver *microsomal enzyme* system. After induction of the microsomal enzymes, the barbiturates are themselves more rapidly metabolized, resulting in a decrease in average blood levels after a given dose. This is a classic example of *metabolic tolerance*. Since many other drugs are also metabolized by the same microsomal enzymes, barbiturates can induce tolerance of other drugs as well. Notable examples are the coumarins (anticoagulants) and the anticonvulsant phenytoin (Dilantin).

Pharmacodynamic tolerance. In addition to drug-induced tolerance, *pharmacodynamic tolerance* also develops with repeated administration of the barbiturates. This is the tolerance described earlier for all general CNS depressants in which the nervous system becomes adapted to the presence of the depressant. However, the medullary centers controlling respiration and the cardiovascular system do not become adapted to general CNS depressants, since they are not affected at the usual doses taken. The lethal dose for barbiturates therefore does not increase with drug dependence. This fact accounts for the accidental death of individuals dependent on high doses of barbiturates, since these doses can be lethal. The lethal dose for barbiturates in a nontolerant individual is about 15 times the hypnotic dose.

Abuse of barbiturates. Barbiturates are a class of widely abused drugs. As with other abused classes of drugs, those individual drugs with the most rapid onset are the most abused. This is because the euphoric feeling or "rush" depends on a rapid rate of altering perception. Among the barbiturates, secobarbital, pentobarbital, and amobarbital are on Schedule II (drugs having a high potential for abuse) of the Controlled Drugs list. Butabarbital is a Schedule III drug (lesser abuse potential), whereas phenobarbital and mephobarbital are Schedule IV (low abuse potential) drugs. (The Controlled Drugs list is discussed in Chapter 4.) With the Schedule II barbiturates, a daily consumption of 400 mg leads to severe drug dependency in about 6 weeks. With larger doses, the time decreases.

Severe withdrawal symptoms begin within 24 hours after the drug is discontinued in an individual with severe drug dependency. Grand mal convulsions and delirium are common symptoms; an elevated temperature, coma, and death are less common. Because of the danger associated with barbiturate withdrawal, gradual withdrawal is used to detoxify a dependent person. Withdrawal is achieved by reducing the dose of the barbiturate to zero over 10 to 20 days. Sometimes the long-acting barbiturate phenobarbital is substituted for a short-acting barbiturate for once-a-day administration. Phenobarbital (30 mg) is substituted for 100 mg of secobarbital, pentobarbital, or amobarbital.

■ Drug interactions

The depressant effect of barbiturates is not only additive with the other general CNS depressants, which include alcohol, sedative-hypnotic drugs, antianxiety drugs, and general anesthetics, but also is potentiated by the antipsychotics and the narcotic analgesics. These interactions are important to remember for the patient who is scheduled to undergo surgery. If secobarbital or pentobarbital is prescribed as the night-before sleeping pill, it should be given at least 8 hours before any of the major tranquilizers, narcotic analgesics, or general anesthetics are administered to avoid undue depression of the medullary control of respiration and the cardiovascular systems.

■ Individual barbiturates (Table 24-3)

Thiamylal, thiopental, and methohexital

Thiamylal (Surital), thiopental (Pentothal), and methohexital (Brevital) are ultra short-acting barbiturates administered intravenously for the induction and/or maintenance of anesthesia. These barbiturates will be discussed with the general anesthetics in Chapter 29.

Amobarbital, pentobarbital, and secobarbital

Amobarbital (Amytal), pentobarbital (Nembutal), and secobarbital (Seconal) are most frequently used as hypnotic drugs. The combination of secobarbital and amobarbital is sold under the name Tuinal as an hypnotic. Although these barbiturates are effective hypnotics for a few days, they lose their effectiveness by the second week of use. Since barbiturates depress REM sleep, there is a rebound in REM sleep when they are discontinued. As previously discussed, this REM rebound can itself lead to insomnia. Furthermore, drug dependency can develop with the usual hypnotic doses within 2 months, although this does not lead to severe withdrawal symptoms unless the dose has been raised above 400 mg daily.

Butabarbital

Butabarbital (Butisol) is an intermediate-acting barbiturate prescribed for daytime sedation and less commonly at night for inducing sleep. It is frequently combined in sedative doses with other drugs used to treat conditions with psychogenic overtones: allergies, ulcers, and inflammatory bowel disease.

Phenobarbital

Phenobarbital (Luminal) is the longest acting and most widely used of the barbiturates. Phenobarbital and *mephobarbital (Mebaral)* control some kinds of epilepsy (Chapter 31). Phenobarbital is infrequently abused because it is slower in onset of action and it does not give a "rush." Peak blood levels occur 6 to 18 hours after an oral dose, and the half-life of phenobarbital is 3 to 4 days. Phenobarbital is the barbiturate that most readily induces the liver microsomal enzyme system, thereby enhancing its own metabolism as well as that of many other drugs. Phenobarbital treatment enhances the degradation of bilirubin and is used in infants and children to lower elevated plasma bilirubin levels.

Phenobarbital may be substituted for other barbiturates or nonbenzodiazepine hypnotics when decreasing drug levels for withdrawal. The longer action of phenobarbital allows once-a-day therapy.

TABLE 24-3. Sedative-hypnotic and antianxiety drugs: barbiturates

Generic name	Trade name	Dosage and administration	Comments
Amobarbital*	Amytal	ORAL: *Adult*—as sedative, 50 to 300 mg daily in divided doses; as hypnotic, 65 to 200 mg at bedtime. *Children*—as sedative, 6 mg/kg body weight in 3 divided doses. INTRAVENOUS: *Adults and children over 6 yr*—as hypnotic, 65 to 500 mg, no more than 1 ml of a 10% solution per minute.	An intermediate-acting barbiturate that acts like a short-acting barbiturate in humans. Used for daytime sedation, preanesthetic sedation, and hypnosis. Precautions are like those for secobarbital. Schedule II substance.
Butabarbital	Butal Butazem Buticaps Butisol Sodium Sarisol	ORAL: *Adult*—as sedative, 50 to 120 mg/day in 3 or 4 divided doses; as hypnotic, 50 to 100 mg at bedtime. *Children*—as sedative, 6 mg/kg body weight in 3 divided doses daily.	An intermediate-acting barbiturate used for sedation or for insomnia when the need is to prolong sleep rather than to induce sleep. Schedule III substance.
Pentobarbital*	Nembutal	ORAL: *Adults*—as sedative, 30 mg 3 or 4 times daily or 100 mg in timed-release form in the morning; as hypnotic, 100 mg at bedtime. *Children*—as sedative, 6 mg/kg of body weight in 3 divided doses daily. RECTAL: *Adults*—120 to 200 mg as required for sedation or hypnosis. *Children*—as sedative, 6 mg/kg body weight in 3 divided doses. INTRAMUSCULAR: *Adults*—as hypnotic, 150 to 200 mg. INTRAVENOUS: *Adults*—as hypnotic, 100 mg. After 1 min, can administer small increments, but no more than 500 mg total. *Children*—as hypnotic, 50 mg initially.	A short-acting barbiturate used principally for insomnia and preanesthetic sedation, and occasionally for daytime sedation. Precautions are like those for secobarbital. Schedule II substance.
Phenobarbital*	Luminal Pheno-Square Solfoton Sedadrops	ORAL: *Adults*—as sedative, 30 to 120 mg daily in 2 or 3 divided doses; as hypnotic, 100 to 320 mg at bedtime. *Children*—as sedative, 6 mg/kg daily in 4 divided doses. INTRAMUSCULAR, INTRAVENOUS: *Adults*—as sedative, 30 to 120 mg; as hypnotic, 100 to 320 mg, with no more than 100 mg (2 ml of 5% solution) per minute IV. Full effect lasts 15 min. RECTAL: *Children*—as sedative, 6 mg/kg body weight divided in 3 doses.	A long-acting barbiturate used principally as a sedative. (For use as an anticonvulsant see Chapter 31.) Not readily addictive. Schedule IV substance.
Secobarbital*	Seconal	ORAL: *Adults*—as sedative, 30 to 50 mg; as hypnotic, 100 to 200 mg at bedtime; for preoperative sedation, 200 to 300 mg 1 to 2 hr before surgery. *Children*—as sedative, 6 mg/kg body weight in 3 divided doses; for preoperative sedation, 50 to 100 mg. RECTAL: *Adults*—120 to 200 mg as required for sedation or hypnosis. *Children*—6 mg/kg body weight in 3 divided doses. INTRAMUSCULAR: *Adults*—as hypnotic, 100 to 200 mg. *Children*—as hypnotic, 3 to 5 mg/kg body weight, up to 100 mg. INTRAVENOUS: *Adults*—as hypnotic, 50 to 250 mg, inject only 50 mg in 15 sec.	A short-acting barbiturate used principally for insomnia and as a preanesthetic sedative. Not indicated for repeated use because tolerance develops, rebound insomnia becomes marked, and the addiction potential is high. Schedule II substance.

*Also available as the sodium salt. Only the sodium salt is suitable for administration as a solution by the rectal, intramuscular, or intravenous route.

■ BENZODIAZEPINES

Safety. Benzodiazepines were introduced clinically in the 1960's as antianxiety drugs. By the early 1970's diazepam (Valium) was the most widely prescribed drug in the United States. The popularity of the benzodiazepines rests in part on the very high therapeutic index. Overdoses of 1000 times the therapeutic dose have been reported not to result in death. At therapeutic doses, side effects beyond drowsiness and motor incoordination (ataxia) are uncommon. No drug interactions are prominent beyond the additive effect with other CNS depressant drugs.

As listed in Table 24-4, seven benzodiazepines are available in the United States. Flurazepam (Dalmane) is marketed only as an hypnotic. The remaining benzodiazepines are marketed primarily as antianxiety drugs.

Metabolism. The benzodiazepines are metabolized by the liver. The metabolites of lorazepam (Ativin) and oxazepam (Serax) are inactive glucuronides that are excreted in the urine. These two benzodiazepines are therefore found in active form in the blood for only a few hours. The remaining benzodiazepines are metabolized to active metabolites that may persist for 1½ to 10 days, depending on the individual. This means that the person taking daily or nightly doses will have active forms of the drug accumulating in the body and may experience side effects after a few days of therapy rather than initially.

Side effects. Side effects common with the benzodiazepines include daytime sedation, motor incoordination (ataxia), dizziness, and headaches. Tolerance commonly develops quickly to these side effects. The elderly are more likely to experience these side effects to a degree that is disabling. Moreover, the elderly do not readily metabolize benzodiazepines, so that the drug persists 2 to 3 times longer. For these reasons the drug dose is reduced for elderly patients and for patients who have impaired liver function. Less common side effects of benzodiazepines include blurred or double vision, hypotension, tremor, amnesia, slurred speech, urinary incontinence, and constipation.

Acute toxicity. An acute overdose of benzodiazepines alone is seldom fatal. There are no specific antagonists for benzodiazepines, but patients frequently regain consciousness and normal vital signs with a large concentration of drug still in their body.

Abuse potential and withdrawal symptoms. Benzodiazepines are Schedule IV drugs, since their abuse potential is considered low. Daily use of 30 mg of diazepam in the absence of alcohol or other depressant drugs for 3 months seldom produces dependence. Whereas tolerance to sedation and ataxia develops rapidly, tolerance for the antianxiety effect develops slowly. If dependence is developed, the appearance of withdrawal symptoms after discontinuance will take several days for those benzodiazepines with active metabolites. An acute phase of chronic withdrawal symptoms, consisting of depression, insomnia, nightmares, agitation, and psychological distress, can persist for 6 weeks. Withdrawal begins during the first week following discontinuance of the drug, with symptoms of agitation, nausea and vomiting, nervousness, sweating, and muscular cramps. Seizures are seldom seen unless high doses have been abused, but if seizures do occur, they occur at the end of the first week.

Drug interactions and contraindications. Like the barbiturates, the sedative effect of the benzodiazepines is increased by other drug classes: alcohol and other general CNS depressants, tricyclic antidepressants, opiate analgesics, antipsychotics, and antihistamines. Unlike the barbiturates, benzodiazepines have only slight effects on the liver microsomal enzymes. Patients over 50 years old with a history of psychosis are the most likely to develop paradoxical excitement or aggression. Benzodiazepines may make glaucoma worse. Benzodiazepines are contraindicated for women in labor and nursing mothers because of adverse depression of the infant. An increased incidence of cleft lip has been reported among infants whose mothers took diazepam (Valium) during early pregnancy.

■ Individual benzodiazepines (Table 24-4)

Diazepam

Diazepam (Valium) is the most widely prescribed antianxiety drug in the United States. It is also used in the hospital as a preanesthetic medication for sedation. Alcohol withdrawal symptoms are sometimes relieved with diazepam. Diazepam has two unique uses among the benzodiazepines: (1) it is prescribed to relieve muscle spasticity in patients with cerebral palsy or other conditions, and (2) diazepam is the drug of choice for terminating continued convulsions (status epilepticus).

Diazepam is well absorbed orally and is effective within an hour. Absorption from intramuscular injection is erratic, and the injection site is painful, so the intramuscular route is seldom used. An intravenous injection of diazepam must be given slowly and carefully into a large vein to minimize irritation and swelling at the injection site, with possible phlebitis or thrombosis.

Flurazepam

Flurazepam (Dalmane) is prescribed as an hypnotic only and accounts for almost 60% of the hypnotic prescriptions. Flurazepam does suppress stage IV sleep but does not markedly depress REM sleep. Flurazepam is the only hypnotic in current use that has been demonstrated effective for more than 2 weeks. Furthermore, flurazepam does not produce rebound insomnia when it

TABLE 24-4. Sedative-hypnotic and antianxiety drugs: benzodiazepines

Generic name	Trade name	Dosage and administration	Comments
Chlorazepate	Tranxene Azene	ORAL: *Adults*—13 to 60 mg divided into 2 to 4 doses or at bedtime. *Elderly*—6.5 to 15 mg daily.	Used to treat anxiety. Half-life is 30 to 200 hr. Metabolites are active. Schedule IV substance.
Chlordiazepoxide	Libritabs Librium	ORAL: *Adults*—for anxiety, 15 to 100 mg divided in 3 to 4 doses or in 1 dose at bedtime. *Elderly*—5 mg 2 to 4 times daily. *Children*—0.5 mg/kg body weight daily in 3 to 4 doses. May be given IM. INTRAVENOUS: *Adults*—for alcohol withdrawal, 50 to 100 mg slowly over at least 1 min, then 25 to 50 mg every 6 to 8 hr, with the total dose not more than 300 mg.	Used to treat anxiety and alcohol withdrawal. Half-life is 24 to 48 hr. Metabolites are active. The hydrochloride salt is used for injection. Schedule IV substance.
Diazepam	Valium	ORAL: *Adults*—4 to 40 mg divided into 2 to 4 doses or a single dose of 2.5 to 10 mg at bedtime. *Elderly*—2 to 2.5 mg once or twice daily. *Children*—0.12 to 0.8 mg/kg body weight daily in 3 to 4 doses. INTRAVENOUS: administer no more than 5 mg/min. For severe anxiety, severe muscle spasm, status epilepticus, or recurrent seizures: *Adults*—5 to 10 mg initially, repeated in 3 to 4 hr if needed. *Children*—0.04 to 0.2 mg/kg body weight initially, repeat in 3 to 4 hr if necessary. For basal sedation for cardioversion or endoscopic procedures: *Adults*—10 to 20 mg as required. For acute alcohol withdrawal symptoms: *Adults*—5 to 20 mg, then 5 to 10 mg in 3 to 4 hr if necessary.	Used to treat anxiety, severe muscle spasm, status epilepticus, and acute alcohol withdrawal symptoms and to provide sedation. Half-life is 48 to 200 hr. Metabolites are active. Schedule IV substance.
Flurazepam	Dalmane	ORAL: *Adults*—as hypnotic, 15 to 30 mg at bedtime. *Elderly*—15 mg. Onset: 20 to 45 min. Duration: 7 to 8 hr.	Used as a hypnotic only. Active metabolite is formed with a half-life of 47 to 100 hr, so repeated use leads to cumulation of this metabolite and may impair daytime activity. Schedule IV substance.
Lorazepam	Ativan	ORAL: *Adults*—for anxiety, 1 to 2 mg 2 to 3 times daily, may increase dose to 10 mg maximum daily; as hypnotic, 2 to 4 mg at bedtime. *Elderly*—½ adult dose.	Used to treat anxiety and insomnia. Repeated use for insomnia can cause rebound insomnia. Half-life is 15 hr so there is little cumulation. Metabolites are inactive. Schedule IV substance.
Oxazepam	Serax	ORAL: *Adults*—for anxiety, 30 to 120 mg daily in 3 to 4 doses. *Elderly*—30 mg in 3 divided doses, increased if necessary to 45 to 60 mg.	Used to treat anxiety. Half-life is 3 to 21 hr, so there is little cumulation. Metabolites are inactive. Schedule IV substance.
Prazepam	Verstran Centrax	ORAL: *Adults*—20 mg in a single dose, increased to 40 to 60 mg daily in divided doses or once at bedtime. *Elderly*—10 to 15 mg.	Used to treat anxiety. Half-life is 30 to 200 hr. Metabolites are active. Schedule IV substance.

is discontinued, probably because of the long half-life of its active metabolites. The persistence of active metabolites accounts for the decreased mental alertness during the day, particularly after repeated use of flurazepam by the elderly and by patients with decreased liver function.

Chlordiazepoxide

Chlordiazepoxide (Libritabs) or chlordiazepoxide hydrochloride (Librium) is prescribed as an antianxiety drug, as a preanesthetic medication for sedation, and to treat the symptoms of alcohol withdrawal. Like diazepam, chlordiazepoxide is absorbed orally better than intramuscularly, and care must be used with intravenous injections. Chlordiazepoxide is metabolized by the liver into an active metabolite to give a persistent effect.

Chlorazepate

Chlorazepate (Tranxene, Azene) is not absorbed orally until it is converted by stomach acid to an active metabolite. Any condition or medication (such as antacids) that reduces stomach acidity will markedly interfere with the absorption of chlorazepate. The metabolite of chlorazepate persists in the body. Chlorazepate is prescribed to treat anxiety or alcohol withdrawal symptoms.

Prazepam

Prazepam (Centrax, Verstran) is prescribed to relieve anxiety. Prazepam is given orally and after absorption is metabolized by the liver to an active metabolite that persists for several days.

Oxazepam and lorazepam

Oxazepam (Serax) and lorazepam (Ativan) are given orally, but unlike the other benzodiazepines they are converted by the kidneys to inactive metabolites, which are then excreted. This makes these benzodiazepines suitable for the patient with liver disease. The effects of oxazepam or lorazepam do not persist for more than 24 hours. These benzodiazepines are presently used as antianxiety drugs and occasionally to treat insomnia. Lorazepam is also used as a preanesthetic medication, whereas oxazepam is also used to treat alcohol withdrawal symptoms.

Clonazepam

Clonazepam (Clonopin) is used only as an anticonvulsant (Chapter 31).

■ OTHER HYPNOTIC AND ANTIANXIETY DRUGS

■ General comparisons with the barbiturates

The miscellaneous hypnotic and antianxiety drugs listed in Table 24-5 are more like the barbiturates than the benzodiazepines in that they are generally shorter acting, which makes them more readily abused. Discontinuance will produce withdrawal symptoms resembling those described for the barbiturates. In fact, the degree of dependence is sometimes determined by giving 200 mg of pentobarbital every 2 hours until signs of intoxication appear. The patient is then detoxified with divided doses (4 to 6 per day) of pentobarbital, and the total daily dose is decreased by 100 mg per day. This approach is possible because pentobarbital is cross tolerant with these other drugs. Alternatively, the abused drug is decreased daily over a 10- to 20-day period or phenobarbital is administered in decreasing daily doses.

In addition to these drugs, several of the antihistamines have a pronounced sedative effect for which they are sometimes used (Chapter 21).

■ Specific drugs (Table 24-5)

Chloral hydrate

Chloral hydrate (Noctec) is the oldest of the currently used hypnotic drugs, having been introduced in the nineteenth century. While chloral hydrate is not effective for more than 2 weeks, it does not suppress REM sleep and therefore does not cause rebound insomnia. Chloral hydrate and its active metabolite trichloroethanol have a half-life of only 8 hours, so there is no persistent effect as with flurazepam.

Chloral hydrate has an unpleasant taste and odor, which are masked by capsules or by taking the drug as a chilled elixir or syrup or as a suppository. Chloral hydrate produces fewer side effects, particularly paradoxical excitement, among children or the elderly than other hypnotics, but it will cause gastric irritation in some patients and will displace the coumarin anticoagulants from plasma protein. Drug dependence is produced by long-term use of chloral hydrate. An acute overdose can produce a coma with pinpoint pupils. In folklore, chloral hydrate added to an alcoholic beverage produces a ''knock-out'' drink, the Mickey Finn, resulting from the additive effect of the two general CNS depressants.

Chloral betaine (Beta-Chlor) and Triclofos sodium (Triclos) are forms of chloral hydrate that do not have the disagreeable taste or odor. They behave otherwise like chloral hydrate, and all these drugs are Schedule IV (low abuse potential) substances.

TABLE 24-5. Sedative-hypnotic and antianxiety drugs: miscellaneous

Generic name	Trade name	Dosage and administration	Comments
Chloral hydrate	Noctec	ORAL, RECTAL: *Adults*—as sedative, 250 mg 3 times daily after meals; as hypnotic, 500 mg to 1 gm 15 to 30 min before bedtime. *Children*—as sedative, 25 mg/kg body weight in 3 to 4 doses daily; as hypnotic, 50 mg/kg as a bedtime dose, not to exceed 500 mg.	A generally safe hypnotic. The unpleasant taste and odor can be masked by chilling the drug or using the capsule form. Schedule IV substance.
Chloral betaine	Beta-Chlor	ORAL: *Adults and children over 12 yr*—for preoperative sedation or as hypnotic, 870 mg to 1.7 gm 15 to 30 min before bedtime or 60 to 90 min before surgery.	A chemical adduct of chloral hydrate that eliminates the unpleasant taste and odor of chloral hydrate. Schedule IV substance.
Triclofos sodium	Triclos	ORAL: *Adults*—as hypnotic, 1.5 Gm 15 to 30 min before bedtime. *Children*—over 12 yr, as hypnotic, as for adults; under 12 yr, for sleep induction, 20 mg/kg body weight.	A modified chloral hydrate that eliminates the unpleasant taste and odor of chloral hydrate.
Methaqualone	Quaalude Sopor Parest	ORAL: *Adults only*—for sedation, 70 mg 3 or 4 times daily; for hypnosis, 150 to 400 mg at bedtime.	
Methyprylon	Noludar	ORAL: *Adults*—for hypnosis, 200 to 400 mg at bedtime. *Children over 3 mo*—50 mg to 200 mg at bedtime.	
Ethchlorvynol	Placidyl	ORAL: *Adults only*—as hypnotic, 500 mg to 1 gm at bedtime.	
Ethinamate	Valmid	ORAL: *Adults only*—as hypnotic, 500 mg to 1 gm at bedtime.	
Glutethimide	Doriden	ORAL: *Adults only*—as hypnotic, 250 to 500 mg at bedtime.	
Hydroxyzine hydrochloride, hydroxyzine pamoate	Atarax Vistaril	ORAL: *Adults*—for anxiety, 75 to 400 mg daily divided into 4 doses. For allergic skin reactions: ORAL: *Adults*—25 mg 3 or 4 times daily. *Children under 6 yr*—50 mg daily in 3 to 4 divided doses. INTRAMUSCULAR: *Adults*—for anxiety, 50 to 100 mg every 4-6 hr.	An antihistamine that has antiemetic and antianxiety properties. It is used in treating allergic skin rashes, motion sickness, and as a preanesthetic medication. The usual doses of barbiturates or narcotics must be cut 50% if given concurrently.
Meprobamate	Equanil Meprospan Miltown	ORAL: *Adults*—for anxiety, 1.2 to 1.6 gm daily divided into 3 or 4 doses. *Children over 6 yr*—for anxiety, 25 mg/kg body weight daily divided into 2 or 3 doses.	

Methaqualone

Methaqualone (Quaalude, Sopor) is one of the many hypnotic drugs introduced in the 1950's. A distinguishing side effect is the occasional complaint of a tingling sensation (paresthesia). There is some evidence that the chronic use of methaqualone may occasionally produce a permanent nerve damage (peripheral neuropathy). Methaqualone is widely abused in part because it is believed to be an aphrodisiac (love potion) by the drug culture and in part because it is not detected in the usual urine tests performed on addicts in drug clinics. Methaqualone has a high potential for drug dependency and is a Schedule II substance.

An acute overdose of methaqualone characteristically produces increased muscle tone with exaggerated reflexes and repeated muscle contractions in addition to the expected effects of a CNS depressant.

■ THE NURSING PROCESS FOR SEDATIVE-HYPNOTIC AND ANTIANXIETY DRUGS

■ Assessment

Patients requiring sedative-hypnotics or antianxiety agents appear with a wide variety of complaints, diseases, and symptom complexes. Examples include patients with diagnosed anxiety, insomnia, other medical conditions that are treated in part with the use of mild sedatives (such as some forms of heart disease), and patients requiring preanesthetic medications. A systematic patient assessment should be done with attention to the vital signs, the level of consciousness, and the patient's affect. The nurse should investigate fully any subjective complaints and other medical diseases the patient has.

■ Management

The common denominator of all the drugs discussed in this chapter is that they produce CNS depression. The amount of depression depends on the patient's response to the drug and on the drug and dose used. The nurse should assess the level of consciousness, the affect, the vital signs, and the blood pressure. The underlying condition for which the medication has been prescribed should also be assessed. The use of other drugs that also cause CNS depression should be avoided if possible. The nurse should work with the patient to identify nonmedicinal treatments that may be helpful in controlling the underlying problem. For example, patients being treated with sedative-hypnotics to produce sleep may be aided by such traditional remedies as warm milk at bedtime, relaxing in a warm bath before bed, or reading briefly before going to sleep. The nurse should monitor the ability of hospitalized patients to ambulate safely, keeping siderails up if there is a chance the patient may become disoriented at night. The nurse should watch for side effects that may indicate that the prescribed dose is too high or too low; consult the physician when necessary. If these drugs are being used intravenously, appropriate equipment for resuscitation and a suction machine should be available.

■ Evaluation

The success of these drugs depends on the original purpose for which they were being used. The patient being treated for insomnia would regard as successful any medication that produces 6 to 8 hours of sleep at night without causing hangover effects in the morning. The patient being treated for anxiety would regard as successful a drug that produces a subjective feeling of calmness without producing sedation or a depressed level of consciousness. Before discharge for self-management, the patient should be able to explain how to take the prescribed medication correctly, what symptoms may occur indicating too high a dose of medication, what to do if the medication is no longer effective, and when to return to the physician for follow-up. The patient should be able to list other drugs or substances such as alcohol that should be avoided when sedative-hypnotics or antianxiety agents are being used. Patients should not be denied the use of these drugs if they are necessary for treating the patient's condition; at the same time, however, it is important to remember that many of the most frequently abused drugs in the United States fall into this category. The nurse should use judgment in pointing out to patients that continued prolonged use of these drugs, or use of these drugs in increasing amounts, can lead to drug dependence and/or addiction.

Methyprylon

Methypyrlon (Noludar) was introduced as a hypnotic in the 1950's. It is a Schedule II drug used like the short-acting barbiturates.

Ethchlorvynol

Ethchlorvynol (Placidyl) was introduced in the 1950's as a hypnotic. The most frequent patient complaint is an aftertaste. Occasionally patients show an exaggerated depression with deep sleep and muscular weakness. Some individuals have an idiosyncratic response of CNS stimulation that may be mild or hysteric. Ethchlorvynol is a Schedule IV drug with a duration of action similar to the short-acting barbiturates.

Ethinamate

Ethinamate (Valmid) was introduced in the 1950's as a hypnotic. It has a shorter duration of action than the short-acting barbiturates and is a Schedule IV drug.

Glutethimide

Glutethimide (Doriden) was also introduced in the 1950's and briefly became a popular hypnotic. Glutethimide is longer acting than many of the other sedative-hypnotic drugs introduced in the 1950's. Like phenobarbital, glutethimide induces the liver microsomal enzyme system. Chronic use of glutethimide is associated with atropine-like effects of dilated pupils (mydriasis) and a dry mouth. Glutethimide is widely abused, and an overdose after acute or chronic intoxication is less successfully treated than an overdose of barbiturates because of the higher incidence of cardiovascular collapse and because it is difficult to remove this highly fat-soluble drug by dialysis. Glutethimide is a Schedule III drug.

Hydroxyzine

Hydroxyzine (Atarax, Vistaril) is an antihistamine with sedative properties. Hydroxyzine is discussed in Chapter 21.

Meprobamate

Meprobamate (Equanil, Miltown) was introduced in the 1950's as the first widely prescribed antianxiety drug. Although physical dependency readily develops with abuse, meprobamate is a Schedule IV drug. Withdrawal symptoms range from insomnia and anxiety to hallucinations and grand mal seizures. Meprobamate is sometimes used as a centrally acting skeletal muscle relaxant although its effectiveness in this role is questionable.

Alcohol and its effects

■ Pharmacological actions and drug interactions

Alcohol is a drug that is widely used and abused in our society. In this section the important actions of alcohol and its interactions with other drugs are reviewed.

Alcohol as general CNS depressant. As a general CNS depressant, alcohol will cause all of the behavioral changes described in the introduction: sedation, disinhibition, sleep, and anesthesia. As summarized in Table 24-6, the amount of alcohol in the blood can be predicted from the amount consumed and produces characteristic behavioral effects. Alcohol also enhances the sedative and hypnotic effects of other drug classes, including all of the general CNS depressants discussed in this chapter and other drug classes with sedative side effects: the antihistamines, the phenothiazines, the narcotic analgesics, the tricyclic antidepressants, and the monoamine oxidase inhibitors. This enhancement of CNS depression means that irreversible coma or death can occur when alcohol is taken concurrently with other drugs, a fact not widely enough appreciated in our society.

Alcohol as a vasodilator. Acute ingestion of alcohol has effects in addition to those attributed to its general CNS depression. Rising levels of alcohol may activate the vomiting center. Alcohol acts centrally to produce vasodilation and a feeling of warmth. This vasodilation can produce a marked hypotensive response in persons taking guanethidine or nitroglycerin.

Factors affecting absorption. Alcohol is absorbed more readily from the small intestine than from the stomach. Absorption of alcohol is therefore decreased by food, which dilutes the alcohol and keeps it in the stomach longer. Alcohol in concentrations of 10% or less will stimulate gastric secretions, thereby aiding digestion, but larger concentrations of alcohol inhibit gastric secretions and damage the cells lining the stomach. This irritation may make some people nauseated the day after heavy drinking and accounts for the inflammation of the stomach (gastritis) and ulcers frequently seen in alcoholics. Aspirin is another drug that readily damages the stomach lining. The combination of aspirin and alcohol can produce bleeding in the stomach.

Metabolism. Over 90% of ingested alcohol is oxidized by the liver, with the remainder being excreted in the breath and urine. The oxidation of alcohol to carbon dioxide and water means that alcohol is a source of calories. Alcoholics may get most of their calories from alcohol but be malnourished because alcoholic beverages lack vitamins, minerals, and protein.

TABLE 24-6. Alcohol intake and its behavioral effects

Alcohol content (oz)	Beverage intake in 1 hr*	Blood alcohol level (mg/100 ml) in a 150-lb man	Behavioral effects
½	1 oz 100-proof spirits 1 glass wine 1 can beer	0.025	No noticeable effect
1	2 oz 100-proof spirits 2 glasses wine 2 cans beer	0.050	Lower alertness, impaired judgment, good feeling, less inhibited
2	4 oz 100-proof spirits 4 glasses wine 4 cans beer	0.100	Slow reaction time, impaired motor function, less cautious; should not drive; may activate vomiting reflex
3	6 oz 100-proof spirits 6 glasses wine 6 cans beer	0.150	Large increase in reaction times
4	8 oz 100-proof spirits 8 glasses wine 8 cans beer	0.200	Marked depression of sensory and motor abilities
5	10 oz 100-proof spirits 10 glasses wine 10 cans beer	0.25	Severe depression of sensory and motor abilities
6	12 oz 100-proof spirits 12 glasses wine 12 cans beer	0.30	Stuporous, unconscious of surroundings
7	14 oz 100-proof spirits 14 glasses wine 14 cans beer	0.35	Unconscious
8	16 oz 100-proof spirits 16 glasses wine 16 cans beer	0.40	Lethal dose in 50% of the population
12	24 oz 100-proof spirits 24 glasses wine 24 cans beer	0.60	Lethal dose in 95% of the population

*Since only ¼ to ⅓ oz of alcohol is metabolized each hour, alcohol will rapidly accumulate.

There are two enzyme systems in the liver that transform alcohol. The major enzyme for alcohol metabolism is alcohol dehydrogenase. This is also the enzyme that limits the rate of alcohol metabolism. In the average adult, the liver alcohol dehydrogenase can only metabolize about 10 ml of alcohol in an hour. This means that no matter how much someone has drunk, only 10 ml of alcohol can be metabolized in an hour, and alcohol readily accumulates in the body when this amount is exceeded. Neither coffee, fresh air, nor exercise will speed up alcohol metabolism to help someone "sober up."

The product of alcohol metabolism by alcohol dehydrogenase is acetaldehyde, a highly toxic compound. Ordinarily acetaldehyde does not accumulate because it is further metabolized by aldehyde dehydrogenase. Disulfiram (Antabuse) and other drugs can inhibit this enzyme so that acetaldehyde accumulates and produces unpleasant symptoms, which include headache, nausea, and vomiting.

The liver microsomal enzyme system described for the barbiturates can also degrade alcohol but ordinarily with a very limited capacity. Like phenobarbital, alcohol can induce this enzyme system so that the liver can metabolize not only more alcohol but more of other drugs as well, and this is one source of drug interactions. Alcoholics are able to metabolize twice as much alcohol as those who do not drink chronically.

TABLE 24-7. Sources of drug interactions with alcohol

Effect	Interacting drugs	Comments
Increased CNS depression	Barbiturates Meprobamate Hypnotics Antihistamines Narcotic analgesics Monoamine oxidase inhibitors Tricyclic antidepressants Benzodiazepines Chlorpromazine and other sedating phenothiazines	Any drug causing sedation or drowsiness will be potentiated by alcohol. Most of these drugs carry warnings not to drive or operate dangerous equipment and stating that the situation is made worse if alcohol is ingested. Alcohol can cause coma or death by respiratory depression when combined with CNS depressants even when the dose of either drug is not lethal by itself.
Increased liver metabolism	Barbiturates Phenytoin Tolbutamide Warfarin	When taken over a long period alcohol will induce the liver microsomal enzyme system for drug degradation. This speeds up the metabolism of drugs metabolized by these enzymes so that the effective therapeutic dose must be increased. Alternatively, if an alcoholic receiving one of these drugs becomes detoxified, the drug dose may have to be lowered.
Gastric and mucosal irritation	Aspirin Nicotine	Aspirin and alcohol act synergistically to irritate the stomach and cause bleeding. Alcoholic smokers have up to a 15-fold greater incidence of oral cancer.
Hypoglycemia	Insulin	Alcohol acts to lower blood glucose levels independently of insulin and may cause marked hypoglycemia when taken with insulin.
Disulfiram reaction	Disulfiram Sulfonylureas (oral hypoglycemic agents) Nitroglycerin	Disulfiram inhibits the degradation of acetaldehyde, which then accumulates and causes hypotension, gastrointestinal distress, and headache.
Vasodilation	Guanethidine Nitroglycerin	Alcohol acts centrally to produce vasodilation, which can potentiate the action of these drugs.

Drug interactions. Alcohol is a major source of drug interactions because it is so widely consumed. Alcohol in particular influences other CNS depressants, drug metabolism, gastric mucosal integrity, blood glucose levels, and vasodilation. These drug interactions are listed in Table 24-7. The importance of alcohol as a source of drug interactions can be appreciated by considering the estimate that 5% of adults in the United States are alcoholics and that 30% to 60% of hospitalized individuals are alcoholics.

Effects of an acute overdose. Unless a large amount of concentrated alcohol has been rapidly swallowed on an empty stomach or ingested with another CNS depressant drug, an acute overdose of alcohol commonly causes an individual to pass out before lethal doses can be drunk. However, note that a pint of 100-proof liquor is an $L.D._{50}$ dose for a small man (Table 24-6). With rapid drinking of straight liquor, someone can drink enough to die. The greatest danger of acute alcohol intoxication to nonalcoholic individuals is that they may involve themselves or others in traffic accidents (30,000 alcohol-related traffic deaths per year) or that they may fall and injure themselves.

A hangover is common on recovery from acute alcohol intoxication and includes such symptoms as an upset stomach, thirst, fatigue, headache, depression, anxiety, and generally feeling out of sorts. Many of these symptoms are caused by congeners, the natural products that are by-products of fermentation and aging. Vodka, which is a mixture of pure alcohol and water and contains few congeners, also produces few hangover symptoms relative to wines and aged spirits with higher congener contents.

TABLE 24-8. Degenerative changes common with chronic alcohol consumption

System	Comments
Brain	Lack of vitamin B_1 (thiamine) common to alcoholics produces *Wernicke's disease:* brain lesions manifested as an inability to learn or recall. *Korsakoff's psychosis* describes alcoholics who are confused and disoriented as to time or place. Wernicke's disease and Korsakoff's psychosis are considered variations of the same brain disease. Replacement of vitamin B_1 helps reverse symptoms in the early stages but will not restore lost function later.
Liver	Chronic drinking produces a fatty liver because in the presence of alcohol, fatty acids are stored in the liver rather than being metabolized. About 75% of alcoholics show some cirrhosis after 10 years. In cirrhosis, fibrous tissue replaces liver cells. Severe cases result in liver failure and death. Hepatitis (inflammation of the liver) is also common among alcoholics.
Stomach and gastrointestinal tract	Alcohol causes gastritis, which leads to ulcers and blood loss. Nonspecific diarrhea is common. Inflammation of the pancreas (pancreatitis) is common.
Heart	Some alcoholics develop an enlarged heart that functions poorly (cardiomyopathy).
Blood	Because of blood loss and lack of folic acid, alcoholics can have both iron-deficiency (microcytic) anemia and folate-deficiency (macrocytic) anemia. Liver disease may result in clotting factor deficiency. White cells and platelets are decreased.
Metabolic	Alcoholics are often hypoglycemic because alcohol inhibits glucose production by the liver. Since alcohol is converted to a substrate for carbohydrate and fat metabolism, high levels of lipids, lactic acid, uric acid, and ketone bodies may appear in the blood. Plasma magnesium, plasma phosphate, and plasma albumin concentrations are low in alcoholics.
Skin	The vasodilation produced by alcohol eventually produces a permanent rosy nose and cheeks. Skin ulcers are common.

■ Physiological changes associated with chronic drinking

Chronic drinking can produce characteristic degenerative changes in the body, as listed in Table 24-8. These changes are seen after about 10 years of drinking 150 ml of alcohol daily. In addition to these degenerative changes, some alcoholics may have blackout spells, periods in which they are awake and functioning but of which they have no memory. Heavy drinking during pregnancy is associated with a 63% incidence of neurological abnormalities in the offspring. A fetal alcohol syndrome is now recognized in the offspring of alcoholic mothers, a syndrome characterized by a face that is flat with widely spaced, small eyes and by mental retardation.

Withdrawal symptoms after chronic drinking. Chronic drinking also leads to the appearance of withdrawal symptoms when the person stops drinking. The severity of the withdrawal symptoms depends on the individual's drinking history, but are most common when a chronic drinker stays intoxicated for 2 or more weeks and then stops drinking. The first symptoms, which appear within a few hours, are tremors and anxiety. As the first stage progresses, the heart rate becomes rapid, the blood pressure increases, and there is heavy sweating, a loss of appetite, nausea and vomiting, and insomnia. The second stage of withdrawal is characterized by hallucinations, usually visual, but sometimes involving hearing or feeling things. The patient is still oriented and only mildly confused despite these hallucinations.

Untreated withdrawal. About 10% of untreated patients will go on to have seizures within the first 48 hours of withdrawal. Delirium tremens is a stage of withdrawal that occurs in about 10% of untreated alcoholics 2 to 7 days after the start of withdrawal. Delirium tremens lasts about 2 days, during which time the person is completely disoriented, extremely agitated, sweats, and has a fever and a changing pulse and blood pressure. The person usually has no memory of delirium tremens.

Treatment of withdrawal. A patient undergoing alcohol withdrawal is usually treated with one of the benzodiazepines: diazepam, chlordiazepoxide, chlorazepate, or oxazepam. This treatment is effective because alcohol is cross tolerant with the benzodiazepines.

Additional therapy during withdrawal is designed to restore normal metabolic parameters and overcome the vitamin B_1 (thiamin), B_{12}, and folic acid deficiencies. This supportive therapy will provide relief from neurological symptoms secondary to hypoglycemia, ketosis, and vitamin deficiency.

TABLE 24-9. Drug interactions with disulfiram

Drug	Action
Phenytoin (Dilantin), coumarins (oral anticoagulants)	Potentiated by disulfiram, which inhibits their degradation by the liver microsomal enzymes
Benzodiazepines	Potentiated by disulfiram, which inhibits their plasma clearance
Benzodiazepines and ascorbic acid (vitamin C)	Decreased alcohol-disulfiram reaction by protecting the acetaldehyde-oxidizing enzymes
Tricyclic antidepressants	Increased alcohol-disulfiram reaction by inhibiting the acetaldehyde-oxidizing enzymes
Isoniazid, metronidazole	Can cause neuropsychiatric symptoms by an unknown mechanism in the presence of disulfiram

Aversion therapy with disulfiram. One drug, disulfiram (Antabuse), is prescribed for the patient who has been detoxified and wishes to avoid drinking again. As previously described, disulfiram blocks the oxidation of acetaldehyde. The accumulation of acetaldehyde causes unpleasant reactions, which include flushing, throbbing in the head and neck, a throbbing headache, respiratory difficulty, nausea, copious vomiting, sweating, thirst, chest pain, rapid breathing, fast heart rate, fainting, weakness, vertigo, blurred vision, and confusion. These effects can be elicited by alcohol for 1 to 2 weeks after disulfiram is discontinued. The reaction lasts from 30 minutes to several hours. Severe reactions can cause death from cardiovascular collapse or respiratory failure. Because of the severity of the reactions, only well-informed, motivated patients are considered for disulfiram therapy, which is at best a supportive treatment when supplemented by psychiatric therapy. Patients whose drinking problem is lack of moderation after the first drink is taken are considered the best candidates for disulfiram therapy. By itself, disulfiram produces transient effects that usually disappear within 2 weeks: drowsiness, tiredness, impotence, headache, acne, and a metallic or garliclike aftertaste. A number of drug interactions with disulfiram have been described and are listed in Table 24-9.

■ PATIENT CARE IMPLICATIONS

General guidelines for the use of the antianxiety agents and sedative-hypnotics

1. Patients should be instructed to take their medications only as directed and not to increase the dose without prior physician approval.
2. Caution patients to keep all health care providers informed of all medications they are taking, so that inadvertent drug interactions can be avoided. Patients do not always view all their medications as being equally "important" and may consider the regular use of a hypnotic as being unimportant.
3. Caution patients using any of the drugs discussed to avoid the use of alcohol.
4. The barbiturates and miscellaneous hypnotics should be used with caution, if at all, in patients with chronic respiratory diseases such as chronic obstructive pulmonary disease, emphysema, and chronic bronchitis.
5. Urge patients to seek appropriate therapy for anxiety or insomnia and not to rely on the drugs alone, because the drugs provide only temporary, symptomatic relief.
6. Any of the CNS depressants can produce drowsiness, so these drugs should not be taken prior to driving, operating machinery, or engaging in other activities requiring mental alertness unless it is known that the patient can tolerate the particular dose of medication. For example, a patient who has been taking a chronic low dose of diazepam may safely drive; a patient who has received a single dose of a barbiturate for an outpatient surgical procedure could not safely drive home. Individual patient assessment should be done, though all patients should be cautioned of the hazards of drowsiness and reduced mental alertness. The elderly may not subjectively recognize sedation or decreased mental performance; careful objective evaluation is important.
7. Health care providers in the outpatient setting should be alert to patients who return for prescription refills on an increasingly frequent basis, because this may indicate improper use or abuse of the particular requested drug. In addition, depressed patients should be evaluated carefully for possible suicidal tendencies.
8. The usual dose of the medications discussed in this chapter should be reduced in the elderly, the debilitated, or those with known liver or renal disease.
9. Paradoxical restlessness, agitation, or even rage can occasionally occur with some of the drugs in

this chapter. If an unanticipated reaction occurs, the patient and family should be instructed to seek medical assistance.

10. As with all medications, patients should be reminded not to "share" drugs with friends or family.
11. Patients should be reminded to keep these and all medications out of the reach of children. Childproof caps on medications should be used.
12. Instruct patients not to keep these drugs on the nightstand or any other place where the patient could accidentally repeat a dose of medication if awakened during the night.
13. Hospitalized patients receiving any sleeping medication should have the siderails up during the night, and the patients should be instructed to call for assistance before getting up during the night. Keeping a night-light on in the room may be helpful to some patients. Report any symptoms of confusion or disorientation in the patient that occur during the night; these symptoms may indicate a need to change drugs or dosages.
14. Being hospitalized is stressful to most individuals, and for this reason, many physicians prescribe some form of sleeping medication that the patient may take on a p.r.n. basis (as needed), once or twice per night. The patient should not be denied needed medication, but on the other hand, patients should not automatically be given the sleeping medication without individual assessment. A back rub, a small snack, a glass of warm milk, or other aids to sleep may be more effective in promoting sleep in some individuals than the automatic consumption of medications.
15. With chronic use, some of the medications discussed in this chapter may produce changes in libido or sexual activity. Careful questioning of the patient may reveal this problem; it may justify changing the patient to a different medication.
16. The medications discussed in this chapter are generally not recommended for use during pregnancy or during lactation. Some women may wish to consider using birth control measures while taking these medications. If a woman suspects she may be pregnant, she should consult her physician immediately.

Barbiturates

1. Review the general guidelines just given.
2. The general actions of the CNS depressants are discussed in the text of the chapter. In addition to these effects, the barbiturates can occasionally cause allergic reactions. Instruct patients to report any rash, skin changes, photosensitivity, or any other unexpected sign or symptom.
3. Individuals taking phenobarbital for its anticonvulsant activity may find the drowsiness produced to be troublesome. Reassure these patients that with continued use, tolerance to the drowsiness will usually develop.
4. The barbiturates have no analgesic properties and should not be substituted for analgesics in the patient with pain. In fact, in the presence of pain the barbiturates may produce paradoxical restlessness and excitement. If used concomitantly with narcotic analgesics, the dose of barbiturate may need to be reduced because both groups of drugs cause CNS depression.
5. Explain to patients that the hangover effect seen with many barbiturates is a side effect of the medication and not an indication for increasing the dose the next night to "sleep better."
6. The barbiturates increase the metabolism of the tricyclic antidepressants, corticosteroids, digitoxin, phenothiazines, quinidine, doxycycline, oral anticoagulants, and phenytoin, so the dose of any of these medications may need to be increased while the patient is taking barbiturates.
7. Barbiturates are one of the most commonly used group of drugs for attempted suicide by drug overdose. For this reason, patients should be carefully assessed before barbiturates are prescribed. In addition, large quantities of the prescribed drug should not be dispensed to avoid potentially fatal overdose.
8. Intravenous barbiturates: The intravenous route is used infrequently, except in surgery. Administer the prescribed drug slowly, observing the patient carefully for respiratory depression, which might result in apnea, or vasodilation, which might produce shock. Monitor the pulse and blood pressure carefully. Use only in a setting where supportive emergency care is available. A suction machine should be at the bedside, as well as appropriate personnel and equipment for intubation. For instructions regarding dilution and rate of administration, see the manufacturer's literature.
9. Agranulocytosis and thrombocytopenia can occur rarely. Instruct patients to report a fever, sore throat, malaise, easy bruising, or unexplained bleeding.
10. Symptoms of barbiturate overdose include ataxia, decreased level of consciousness or mental dullness, nystagmus, and respiratory depression. Eventually coma will develop. Treatment should be supportive and should involve respiratory assistance as needed, intravenous fluids, appropriate drugs to correct cardiovascular difficulties, and oxygen. Dialysis may be used if necessary.

Benzodiazepines

1. Review the general guidelines just given.
2. The side effects associated with benzodiazepine therapy are discussed in the text and should be reviewed with the patient before the start of therapy. In addition, jaundice has occasionally been reported. Instruct patients to report the appearance of any side effect.
3. Benzodiazepines should be used with caution in patients with renal impairment. In addition, urinary retention may occur; monitor the fluid intake and output.
4. Blood dyscrasias have been reported with some of the benzodiazepines in long-term therapy. Instruct the patient to report any sore throat, fever, malaise, jaundice, bruising, or bleeding tendencies.
5. Gastrointestinal symptoms, should they occur, may be reduced by taking the medication with meals, immediately after eating, or with a small snack.
6. Cimetidine (Tagemet) potentiates the sedative effects of diazepam; the dose of the latter may have to be reduced.
7. After long-term therapy, even at relatively low doses, the benzodiazepines should be discontinued slowly. Review with patients the possible withdrawal symptoms (see text), and instruct the patient to report signs of withdrawal to the physician. It may be necessary to slow the rate at which the drug is being discontinued. Instruct patients on long-term therapy not to discontinue the drug without physician approval.
8. Although overdose with a single preparation of the benzodiazepines may not be fatal, patients who choose to attempt suicide by drug overdose often consume many different drugs and/or alcohol in their attempt. The combined effect of many CNS depressants may quickly be fatal.
9. Symptoms of benzodiazepine overdose are somnolence, confusion, coma, and diminished reflexes. In all cases of drug overdose, the vital signs should be carefully monitored and supportive care provided, usually in an acute care setting. Dialysis is of limited value with this group of drugs.
10. Intravenous diazepam: Intravenous diazepam should be given slowly, at a rate not exceeding 5 mg per minute. The drug should not be mixed with other drugs or intravenous solutions; administer as close to the venous insertion site as possible. Monitor respirations, blood pressure, and level of consciousness. Suction equipment should be at the bedside. Resuscitation equipment and intubation equipment should be readily available.
11. Intramuscular chlordiazepoxide: Prepare intramuscular chlordiazepoxide as directed by the manufacturer by using the diluent provided and administer immediately after it is reconstituted. When prepared with the supplied diluent, it should not be given intravenously. Any unused solution should be discarded.
12. Intravenous chlordiazepoxide: Dilute the sterile powder with 5 ml of sterile water for injection or normal saline solution added to 100 mg of powder. Agitate the ampule gently to reconstitute, and administer immediately over at least a minute. Any unused portion should be discarded. When reconstituted with sterile water or normal saline solution, the drug should not be administered intramuscularly.

Miscellaneous agents

1. Review the general guidelines just given.
2. Of the miscellaneous agents mentioned in the text, there are few side effects when the drugs are used as directed for short periods of time. In general, the most frequent side effects result from the CNS depression and include such things as ataxia, sedation, and, with some drugs, visual changes and hangover effects.
3. Glutethimide and chloral hydrate should be used with caution in patients taking oral anticoagulants because the dose of the latter may have to be altered to provide adequate anticoagulation.
4. Blood dyscrasias have been reported with some of the agents. Caution patients to report sore throat, fever, malaise, bruising, unexplained bleeding, or jaundice.
5. Taking the prescribed medication with a small snack may help to reduce gastric irritation.
6. Allergic reactions are rare but may occur. Instruct the patient to report any rash, skin changes, dermatitis, or any other unusual finding.
7. When giving medications at night to induce sleep, preparations for bed should be completed before taking the medication. Once a drug has been taken, its effects may begin within 15 to 30 minutes.
8. Abrupt withdrawal of any of the hypnotic drugs discussed, especially if the patient was receiving large doses or had been on long-term therapy, may result in withdrawal symptoms. Instruct patients to discontinue the medications only on the advice of their physicians.
9. Hydroxyzine is discussed in Chapter 21.

Disulfiram (Antabuse)

1. Patients who receive or have recently received metronidazole, paraldehyde, alcohol, or alcohol-containing preparations (e.g., cough syrups, over-the-counter tonics) should not be given disulfiram.
2. Disulfiram is contraindicated in severe myocardial disease and psychosis and is used with caution if patients have diabetes mellitus, epilepsy, nephritis, cirrhosis, hypothyroidism, or cerebral damage.
3. Patients should be taught about the effects of taking disulfiram and what will happen if alcohol is consumed while on the drug. Possible sources of alcohol ingestion should be reviewed: liquor, beer, wine, sauces used in cooking and desserts, vinegars, and some liquid medications. The effects of a single dose of disulfiram may last as long as 14 days.
4. In addition to ingested alcohol, the patient should be instructed to avoid topical applications of alcohol, such as after-shave lotions, back rubs, and some colognes.
5. Treatment with disulfiram is not a cure for alcoholism and should only be used with other forms of supportive therapy. Patients should be assessed carefully before this drug is prescribed. Only highly motivated, reliable patients may have success with disulfiram when used with other forms of therapy.
6. The usual side effects seen with disulfiram are discussed in the text. Usually patients are instructed to take their daily dose of disulfiram in the morning, but if the sedation produced by the drug is troublesome, some patients may find that taking the dose in the evening is better.
7. Review the drug interactions listed in Table 24-9.
8. Patients being treated with disulfiram should carry an identification card indicating that they are on disulfiram therapy and who should be notified in the event of an emergency. These cards can be obtained from the drug manufacturer.
9. Treatment of a severe disulfiram reaction may require hospitalization because the patient may go into shock. The patient's family should be instructed in detail about the effects of alcohol consumption while the patient is receiving disulfiram.

■ SUMMARY

Selected general CNS depressants are used as drugs to sedate or to induce sleep (hypnosis). The sedative-hypnotic drugs are used at a lower dose to sedate and at a higher dose to induce sleep. Newer drugs have been developed to be used as hypnotics only or as antianxiety agents (minor tranquilizers) only.

The mechanisms of action of these general CNS depressants are not well characterized. They do depress the reticular activating system, which controls the level of awareness. Tolerance develops to general CNS depressants and continued administration leads to drug dependence. With drug dependence, the body experiences withdrawal symptoms if the drug is abruptly discontinued. Drug dependence is reversed by gradually decreasing the dose of the drug. Drug abuse and drug addiction represent the continuance of drug use for nonmedical purposes. There is cross tolerance among the general CNS depressants, so that ingestion of alcohol or any one of the sedative-hypnotic or antianxiety drugs can prevent withdrawal symptoms from any other of these drugs.

The medical uses of the sedative-hypnotic and antianxiety drugs are to treat insomnia and anxiety. Although hypnotic drugs are widely used to induce sleep, they all alter normal sleeping patterns to some degree. The nature of sleep appears to be such that the body reacts to this alteration with disturbed sleeping patterns after the drug is discontinued. Furthermore, most hypnotic drugs are effective for only 3 weeks, after which tolerance has developed to the hypnotic effect. Similarly, chronic drug therapy for anxiety is effective for only a limited time. Medicinal therapy for insomnia or anxiety is thus limited and must be supplemented by other therapeutic treatments.

Barbiturates encompass a spectrum of onset and duration times determined by lipid solubility. The action of the highly lipid-soluble ultra short-acting barbiturates is terminated by redistribution because they rapidly cross membranes to distribute throughout the body. These barbiturates must be metabolized to be made water soluble and eliminated.

Overdose of a barbiturate produces depression of respiration and the cardiovascular system. Treatment is supportive. A severe drug dependence to barbiturates can develop over 6 weeks of daily use. Both metabolic and pharmacodynamic tolerance develop. Metabolic tolerance refers to the induction of the liver metabolizing enzymes that degrade many drugs. Since barbiturates are degraded by these enzymes, larger doses of barbiturates can be tolerated because the liver has a greater capacity for degradation. Pharmacodynamic tolerance refers to the adaptation of much of the CNS to the depressant action of the barbiturates. However, the medulla does not develop tolerance; thus as the "effective" dose increases, it approaches the lethal dose, which does not change, and increases the potential for lethal overdosing.

Withdrawal symptoms after discontinuance of the barbiturates can include seizures, so detoxification is achieved by gradual reduction of the dose.

Barbiturates have several uses depending on the onset and duration of action of the individual barbiturate. Ultra short-acting barbiturates are administered intravenously to provide induction for surgical anesthesia. Secobarbital, pentobarbital, and amobarbital are used as hypnotics. Butabarbital is used as a sedative. Phenobarbital is a long-acting barbiturate used as a sedative, as an anticonvulsant, and to manage drug withdrawal from barbiturates or other sedative-hypnotic drugs.

Benzodiazepines are widely used in the United States as antianxiety agents because their abuse potential is much lower than with the barbiturates and because by themselves, benzodiazepines do not cause death in overdose. However, benzodiazepines are cross tolerant with other CNS depressants and can decrease the lethal dose of alcohol or other depressant drugs when taken in combination with another CNS depressant.

Of the benzodiazepines, flurazepam is used as a hypnotic only. It appears to be effective for several weeks and does not appear to greatly alter REM sleep. Diazepam is the most widely prescribed drug in the United States. Diazepam is used primarily as an antianxiety drug, but is also used to treat spasticity. Administered intravenously, diazepam is the drug of choice for terminating status epilepticus.

Most benzodiazepines are metabolized into compounds that are also pharmacologically active and slowly excreted. Only oxazepam and lorazepam are metabolized into inactive compounds excreted in less than 24 hours.

Hypnotics introduced in the 1950's that are still used include methaqualone, methyprylon, ethchlorvynol, ethinamate, and glutethimide. Chloral hydrate has been used as a hypnotic for more than a hundred years. It is well tolerated by children and the elderly and does not markedly alter REM sleep. Meprobamate was the first antianxiety drug introduced in the 1950's but has a narrow margin of safety by today's standards.

Alcohol is a general CNS depressant. Alcohol is widely consumed and is therefore a major source of drug interactions (Table 24-7). The capacity of the liver to metabolize alcohol is limited, so continuous drinking over a few hours leads to the rapid accumulation of alcohol. Chronic drinking over a period of years produces physiological changes (Table 24-8) and the appearance of severe withdrawal symptoms when consumption is temporarily discontinued.

Disulfiram is a drug used in aversion therapy for alcoholism. Alcohol is normally metabolized to acetaldehyde, which is then rapidly degraded further. Disulfiram inhibits the degradation of acetaldehyde, and the rising plasma concentrations of acetaldehyde produce highly unpleasant symptoms, including a throbbing headache and extreme nausea.

■ STUDY QUESTIONS

1. Define sedative, hypnotic, and antianxiety drugs.
2. What is the reticular activating system and how is it affected by general CNS depressants?
3. Describe the stages of CNS depression.
4. What is drug dependence?
5. What are withdrawal symptoms?
6. What is cross tolerance?
7. Name the stages of sleep and describe which ones are affected by hypnotics.
8. What is anxiety?
9. Describe the four categories of barbiturates and list which drugs belong in each category.
10. What is redistribution?
11. Describe withdrawal symptoms from barbiturates.
12. Define metabolic tolerance.
13. Define pharmacodynamic tolerance.
14. What are the different uses of barbiturates?
15. What advantage do the benzodiazepines have over the barbiturates?
16. What drug interactions are seen with benzodiazepines?
17. Describe the uses of flurazepam and diazepam.
18. How does the metabolism of oxazepam and lorazepam differ from that of the other benzodiazepines?
19. What are the features of chloral hydrate as an hypnotic?
20. List the hypnotics introduced since the 1950's. Are they more like barbiturates or benzodiazepines?
21. What are the special features of the toxicity of methaqualone? of glutethimide?
22. What drug interactions are seen with alcohol?
23. What factors affect alcohol absorption?
24. Describe alcohol metabolism. How does disulfiram interfere with alcohol metabolism?
25. What are the side effects of alcohol ingestion with disulfiram?
26. What are the physiological changes associated with chronic drinking?
27. How is alcohol withdrawal treated?

■ SUGGESTED READINGS

Sleep and hypnotics

Brandner, J.A.: Help for the patient who can't sleep, Patient Care **10:**98, Feb. 1, 1976.

Jenkins, B.L.: A care against "sleeper," Journal of Gerontological Nursing **2**(2):10, 1976.

Kales, A., and Kales, J.D.: Recent findings in the diagnosis and treatment of disturbed sleep, New England Journal of Medicine **290:** 487, 1974.

Kales, J.D., Kales, A., Bixler, E.O., and Soldatos, C.R.: Sleep disorders: what the primary care physician needs to know, Postgraduate Medicine **67**(3):213, 1980.

Kales, A., Schart, M.B., Kales, J.D., and Soldatos, C.R.: Rebound insomnia: a potential hazard following withdrawal of certain benzodiazepines, Journal of the American Medical Association **241:** 1692, 1979.

Kramer, M., Kupfer, D.J., and Pollak, C.P.: Insomnia: when the patterns of sleep go askew, Patient Care **14:**122, Aug. 15, 1980.

Pagel, J.F.: Sleep disorders and insomnia, American Family Physician **17**(2):165, 1978.

Smith, R.J.: Study finds sleeping pills overprescribed, Science **204:** 287, 1979.

Solomon, F., White, C.C., Parron, D.L., and Mendelson, W.B.: Sleeping pills, insomnia and medical practice, New England Journal of Medicine **300:**803, 1979.

Anxiety and drug dependence

Anderson, G.D.: Benzodiazepines, Nurse Practitioner **5**(1):47, 1980.

Cline, F.W.: Psychotropic medication, Nurse Practitioner **3**(2):35, 1978.

Drugs for psychiatric disorders, Medical Letter **22:**77, 1980.

Eiland, D.C.: The chronically anxious patient, American Family Physician **9**(2):157, 1974.

Fink, R.D., Knott, D.H., and Beard, J.D.: Sedative-hypnotic dependance, American Family Physician **10**(3):116, 1974.

Franks, R.D.: The overtranquilized patient, American Family Physician **20**(4):105, 1979.

Fuller, E.: Clues to the diagnosis of anxiety, Patient Care **12:**158, July 15, 1978.

Hall, R.C.W., and Kirkpatrick, B.: The benzodiazepines, American Family Physician **17**(5):131, 1978.

Imboden, J.B., and Chapman, J.: Practical psychiatry in medicine. Part 10. Drug abuse and the addictions, Journal of Family Practice **6:**911, 1978.

Karstadt, E.: Valium use with abuse, Nurses' Drug Alert **3**(special report):113, Sept., 1979.

Kissin, B., Lowinson, J.H., and Millman, R.B.: Recent developments in chemotherapy of narcotic addiction, Annals of the New York Academy of Sciences **311:**59, 1978.

Koch-Weser, J., Greenblatt, D.J., and Shader, R.I.: Prazepam and lorazepam, two new benzodiazepines, New England Journal of Medicine **299:**1342, 1978.

Murphree, H.B.: The continuing problem of barbiturate poisoning, American Family Physician **8**(2):108, 1973.

Newton, M., Godbey, K.L., Newton, D., and Godbey, A.L.: Psychotropic drug therapy, Nursing '78 **8**(7):46, 1978.

Ramon de la Fuente, J., Rosenbaum, A.H., Martin, H.R., and Niven, R.G.: Lorazepam-related withdrawal seizures, Mayo Clinic Proceedings **55:**190, 1980.

Tallman, J.F., Paul, S.M., Skolnick, P., and Gallager, D.W.: Receptors for the age of anxiety: pharmacology of the benzodiazepines, Science **209:**274, 1980.

Vesell, E.S.: Elucidation of the pharmacokinetic interaction between acutely administered ethanol and benzodiazepines, Journal of Laboratory and Clinical Medicine **95:**305, 1980.

Williams, J.G.: Systematic management of the anxious patient, American Family Physician **15**(2):124, 1977.

Alcohol and alcoholism

Chafetz, M.E.: Alcohol and alcoholism, American Scientist **167:**293, 1979.

Feinberg, J.F.: The Wernicke-Korsakoff syndrome, American Family Physician **22**(5):129, 1980.

Knott, D.H., Fink, R.D., and Morgan, J.C.: The subacute phase of alcoholism, American Family Physician **15**(5):108, 1977.

Ray, O.: Drugs, society and human behavior, ed. 2, St. Louis, 1978, The C.V. Mosby Co.

Reilly, D.: Drug interactions with disulfiram, Drug Therapy **10**(4): 91, 1980.

Toutant, C., and Lippmann, S.: Fetal alcohol syndrome, American Family Physician **22**(1):113, 1980.

25 Antipsychotic drugs

One of the truly remarkable advances in pharmacology in the last 25 years has been the discovery and application of drugs effective in treating the major mental illnesses schizophrenia and depression. In this chapter the *antipsychotic* or *antischizophrenic* drugs are discussed. These drugs are also called *neuroleptic* drugs. The term *neuroleptic* refers to the ability of these drugs to cause a general quiescence and state of psychic indifference to the surroundings. Another term for these drugs is the *major tranquilizers*. However, many professionals feel that the term *tranquilizer* is misleading, since the major action of antipsychotic drugs is their unique reversal of the symptoms of psychosis.

■ MECHANISMS OF ANTIPSYCHOTIC DRUGS

■ Chemical classes of antipsychotic drugs

There are five chemical classes of antipsychotic drugs: the phenothiazines, the thioxanthines, the butyrophenones, the dibenzoxazepines, and the dihydroindolones. The latter three classes contribute only one drug each to clinical use at present. Twelve phenothiazine and two thioxanthene compounds are currently in clinical use as antipsychotic drugs.

Phenothiazines. The largest antipsychotic drug class is the phenothiazines. Chlorpromazine was the first phenothiazine introduced in the United States and is still the most widely used drug in this class. Chlorpromazine was originally licensed as an antiemetic drug, later as a drug to potentiate anesthesia, and finally as an antipsychotic drug. The thioxanthenes have a three-ringed main structure that differs by only one atom from that of the phenothiazines. The remaining three drug classes, the butyrophenones, the dibenzoxazepines, and the dihydroindolones are chemically quite different from the phenothiazines and from each other. However, the three classes behave the same pharmacologically with respect to potency and side effects as outlined in Table 25-1.

Subgroups of phenothiazines. The phenothiazines are subdivided into three subgroups based on the chemical differences in side groups on the three-ringed main structure. These subgroups are the *aliphatic,* the *piperidine,* and the *piperazine* phenothiazines. The three subgroups differ in potency and in the incidence of key side effects as summarized in Table 25-1.

■ Antipsychotic drugs as dopamine receptor antagonists

Four effects of antipsychotic drugs have been linked to the blockade of dopamine receptors in various parts of the brain. The *antipsychotic* effect arises from receptor blockade in the limbic system and the *antiemetic* effect from receptor blockade in the chemoreceptor trigger zone. Therapeutic use is made of these effects. *Extrapyramidal* effects arise from blockade in the corpus striatum of neurons from the basal ganglia and *endocrine* effects from blockade in the pituitary gland. These two effects are undesired actions of antipsychotic drugs.

The dopamine theory of psychosis. Current ideas on the neurochemical origin of psychotic behavior come from the understanding of the action of the antipsychotic drugs. These drugs block receptors in the central nervous system for the neurotransmitter dopamine. The hypothesis is that too much of this neurotransmitter in the limbic system produces psychotic symptoms. The limbic system is that area of the brain which regulates emotional behavior. Blocking the receptors for dopamine in the limbic system reverses psychotic symptoms.

Extrapyramidal reactions and dopamine deficiency. The antipsychotic drugs also cause the extrapyramidal reactions described in Table 25-2. These extrapyramidal reactions arise from the blockade of dopamine receptors in certain nuclei of the basal ganglia of the brain. This area of the brain is responsible for the coordination of movement. A common extrapyramidal reaction is drug-induced parkinsonism. In Parkinson's disease there is degeneration of dopamine neurons going to the basal ganglia, resulting in a local deficiency of dopamine (Chapter 32). The blockade of dopamine receptors in this area of the brain produces the same symptoms as a deficiency of dopamine.

TABLE 25-1. Antipsychotic drugs listed according to drug class, potency, and major side effects

Drug	Relative potency	Relative incidence of side effects: Sedative effect	Orthostatic hypotension	Anticholinergic effects	Extrapyramidal symptoms
PHENOTHIAZINES					
Aliphatic					
Chlorpromazine	100	High	Moderate	High	Moderate
Triflupromazine	25	High	Moderate	High	Moderate
Piperidine					
Mesoridazine	50	High	Moderate	Moderate	Low
Piperacetazine	10	Moderate	Low	Moderate	Moderate
Thioridazine	100	High	Moderate	Moderate	Low
Piperazine					
Acetophenazine	20	Moderate	Low	Low	High
Butaperazine	10	Moderate	Low	Low	High
Carphenazine	25	Moderate	Low	Low	High
Fluphenazine	2	Low	Low	Low	High
Perphenazine	8	Low	Low	Low	High
Prochlorperazine	10	Moderate	Low	Low	High
Trifluoperazine	4	Moderate	Low	Low	High
THIOXANTHENES					
Chlorprothixene	100	High	High	Moderate	Low
Thiothixene	4	Low	Low	Low	High
BUTYROPHENONE					
Haloperidol	2	Low	Low	Low	High
DIBENZOXAZEPINE					
Loxapine	20	Moderate	Low	Low	High
DIHYDROINDOLONE					
Molindone	20	Moderate	Moderate	Moderate	Moderate

Emesis and dopamine. Dopamine is the neurotransmitter involved in vomiting (emesis) in the medullary chemoreceptor trigger zone. Antipsychotic drugs are effective in preventing vomiting by blocking these dopamine receptors. As described in Chapter 11, several of the antipsychotic drugs are commonly used as antiemetic drugs.

Endocrine actions of dopamine. Dopamine inhibits the release of the hormone prolactin by the pituitary gland. Blockade of dopamine leads to the hypersecretion of prolactin and secondarily to endocrine disturbances of the reproductive system by mechanisms not yet understood.

■ Antipsychotic drugs as antagonists of adrenergic and cholinergic receptors

The phenothiazines and thioxanthenes block receptors for norepinephrine as well as receptors for dopamine. At one time the antipsychotic action was believed to be the blockade of central nervous system norepinephrine receptors. However, the finding that the butyrophenone haloperidol blocked only dopamine and not norepinephrine receptors solidified the data implicating the major role of dopamine rather than norepinephrine in psychotic disorders.

Central nervous system effects and adrenergic receptor blockade. Norepinephrine is a neurotransmitter associated with specific neurons in the central nervous system just as it is associated with the postganglionic neurons of the sympathetic nervous system. Neurons containing norepinephrine in the reticular activating system of the brain are associated with alertness. The sedative effect of the phenothiazines and the thioxanthenes may result from their blockade of these receptors for norepinephrine. The blockade of receptors for norepinephrine in the vasomotor center inhibits peripheral

TABLE 25-2. Side effects of antipsychotic drugs

Type of effect	Signs and symptoms	Comments
Adrenergic blockade (CNS)	Sedation	Usually transient
	Postural (orthostatic) hypotension	
Cholinergic blockade	Atropine-like effects: dry mouth, blurred vision, constipation, delayed micturition	Usually transient
Endocrine—dopamine blockade	Men: erection problems	Usually transient
	Women: menstrual irregularities, unexpected lactation	
Extrapyramidal—dopamine blockade	Acute dystonia: neck twisting, facial grimacing, abnormal eye movements, involuntary muscle movements	Most common during the first few days of therapy; usually disappears after brief treatment with antiparkinsonian drugs
	Akathisia: restlessness, difficulty in sitting still, strong urge to move about	Most common during the first few days of therapy; control with antiparkinsonian drugs or diazepam
	Parkinsonism: motor retardation, masklike face, tremor, rigidity, salivation, shuffling gait	Most common after the first week of therapy; control with antiparkinsonian drugs
	Tardive dyskinesia: protrusion of tongue, puffing of cheeks, chewing movements, involuntary movements of extremities, involuntary movements of trunk	Most common when dosage is lowered after prolonged therapy; elderly women at greatest risk; may not be reversible
Allergic reactions	Photosensitivity	Common
	Cholestatic hepatitis	
	Agranulocytosis	Rare

sympathetic tone and causes orthostatic hypotension. The sedative and hypotensive side effects of the phenothiazines and thioxanthenes appear early in therapy. If tolerance does not develop, the dosage can be lowered or another drug can be tried.

Anticholinergic actions of antipsychotic drugs. All of the antipsychotic drugs have some degree of anticholinergic action. The atropine-like effects of dry mouth, blurred vision, delayed micturition, and constipation are common side effects of the antipsychotic drugs. A central anticholinergic action is beneficial in controlling some extrapyramidal reactions, however. Extrapyramidal reactions such as the parkinsonian symptoms are believed to reflect a relative lack of dopamine and a relative abundance of acetylcholine in neuronal areas controlling movement coordination (Chapter 32). Since antipsychotic drugs produce extrapyramidal reactions by blocking the action of dopamine, those drugs that also have substantial ability to block the action of acetylcholine have less tendency to cause extrapyramidal reactions.

■ PHARMACOLOGY OF ANTIPSYCHOTIC DRUGS

■ Absorption and fate

The antipsychotic drugs are administered orally in tablet or syrup form. The syrup form is preferred for patients who hide or do not swallow pills. Many of the antipsychotic drugs come in an injectable form as well. Only fluphenazine is available in two different depot forms for intramuscular injection, which require administration only every 3 to 6 weeks. Normally antipsychotic drugs are given in divided daily doses initially and in daily doses when the patient has stabilized. Peak plasma levels of the drug are reached 2 to 3 hours after oral administration. Up to 90% of the drug may be bound to plasma proteins. The drugs are metabolized in the liver and excreted in the urine and feces. However, the excretion is very slow, and metabolites may be found in the urine as long as 6 months after the drug is discontinued. Apparently some of the metabolites are active. Improvement can last as long as 3 months after medication is halted, but it is not clear whether this reflects remission or the presence of persistent active metabolites.

Antipsychotic effects may not be seen for 7 to 10 days after the start of therapy, and 4 to 6 weeks are needed to see the full effect of a given dosage regimen. Dosages must be adjusted for individual patients.

The dosage requirement for use as an antiemetic is much smaller than for the antipsychotic effect, and the antiemetic effect is seen within 1 hour of administration.

■ Extrapyramidal reactions (Table 25-2)

The most important side effects of the antipsychotic drugs are the extrapyramidal reactions. The extrapyramidal reactions are most frequent with the piperazine phenothiazines and least frequent with the aliphatic phenothiazines. The origin of the extrapyramidal reactions is the dopamine blockade in areas of the brain governing motor coordination and movement. There are four extrapyramidal syndromes associated with antipsychotic drugs: acute dystonia, akathisia, pseudoparkinsonism, and tardive dyskinesia. *It is important to recognize these bizarre reactions as side effects of the drug therapy that require palliative medication or reduction or discontinuance of therapy rather than to see these bizarre reactions as manifestations of the psychotic disease being treated and raise the drug dosage.*

Acute dystonia. Acute dystonia is a spasm of muscles of the tongue, face, neck, or back and may mimic seizures. Dystonia is usually seen in the first 5 days of antipsychotic therapy. It may be treated with an antihistaminic or anticholinergic antiparkinsonian drug (Chapter 32). Injection of one of these drugs usually dramatically relieves the dystonia. Dystonia reactions are most common in patients under 25 years of age and rarely persist after treatment of the acute reaction. Some of the classic reactions seen in dystonia include torticollis (neck twisting), an oculogyric crisis (upward gaze paralysis), stereotyped motions of the jaw, and opisthotonus (a spasm in which the head and feet go back to make a U shape of the body).

Akathisia. Akathisia is motor restlessness and may be mistaken for psychotic restlessness or agitation. Akathisia commonly appears after the first few days of therapy, and if not recognized, the antipsychotic drug dosage may again be mistakenly increased to relieve the agitation. Patients experiencing akathisia will have difficulty in sitting still and may pace about, fidget, or constantly move their legs. Anticholinergic drugs or a muscle relaxant such as diazepam may be effective in treating these symptoms. If these treatments are not effective, a different antipsychotic drug may have to be tried. Tolerance does not quickly develop to akathisia, but akathisia disappears when the drug is discontinued.

Pseudoparkinsonism. Pseudoparkinsonism is marked by motor retardation and rigidity. The patient finds it difficult to initiate movements or to carry out movements. The face even appears like a mask because emotions do not register on the face. The patient will have a shuffling gait and will hypersalivate. A tremor is seen in the hands and legs. These parkinsonian symptoms commonly appear after a week of therapy and are treated with antiparkinsonian drugs. Tolerance does not develop to the parkinsonian symptoms. If they cannot be controlled with drug therapy, the antipsychotic drug has to be changed.

Tardive dyskinesia. Tardive dyskinesia is classically associated with long-term, high dose antipsychotic therapy. It is most common in elderly women and in stroke patients. Tardive dyskinesia is the worst of the extrapyramidal reactions because it cannot be readily treated, it is persistent, and it may not altogether disappear when drug therapy is discontinued. In fact tardive dyskinesia usually appears some months after therapy has been started when the drug dosage is reduced or discontinued. Tardive dyskinesia is believed to represent the development of receptors that are supersensitive to dopamine after prolonged blockade by the antipsychotic drugs. Thus removing the antipsychotic drug makes the condition worse, since dopamine then has ready access to these supersensitive receptors. Antiparkinsonian drugs also make tardive dyskinesia worse, since they either increase dopamine or block the acetylcholine opposing the effects of dopamine. Some of the common symptoms of tardive dyskinesia are protrusion of the tongue (flycatcher sign), puffing of the cheeks or the tongue in a cheek (bonbon sign), chewing movements, and involuntary movements of the extremities and trunk (choreoid or athetoid movements). The recent recognition that tardive dyskinesia is a common reaction (up to 50%) in patients treated for a long time with high doses of antipsychotic drugs has prompted reevaluation of long-term therapy with these drugs. The current choice is to use as low a dose as possible and to put the patient on a "drug holiday" during periods of remission.

■ Other side effects (Table 25-2)

A number of side effects are associated with the antipsychotic drugs.

Sedation and postural hypotension. Sedation and postural hypotension are most commonly seen early in treatment with the aliphatic phenothiazines, the class of phenothiazines with the most prominent adrenergic blocking activity. These side effects are most likely to be prominent in elderly or debilitated patients. If sedation and hypotension are not severe, the dosage can be reduced and then gradually increased to produce tolerance to these effects.

The antipsychotic drugs are not addicting.

ECG changes. The aliphatic phenothiazines are also the most likely to produce nonspecific changes in the T wave of the ECG. This change has no particular meaning but is undesirable for a patient with concurrent heart disease who is being monitored for ECG changes.

Seizure potential. The antipsychotic drugs must be used with caution in patients with epilepsy as convulsions can be precipitated by these drugs. This lowering of the convulsive threshold makes antipsychotic drugs unsuitable for the treatment of drug withdrawal likely to produce seizures, such as withdrawal from alcohol, barbiturates, and other sedative-hypnotic drugs.

Endocrine disturbances. The endocrine impairment that results in sexual dysfunction in men and women was discussed relative to the dopaminergic blocking action of the antipsychotic drugs. Women may experience delayed ovulation and menstruation, lack of menstruation (amenorrhea), milk production (galactorrhea), or weight gain. Men may experience impotence, decreased libido, retrograde ejaculation, or moderate breast growth (gynecomastia).

Allergic reactions. Photosensitivity and cholestatic hepatitis are allergic reactions that occasionally develop during therapy with antipsychotic drugs.

Photosensitivity. Photosensitivity is fairly common and represents an allergic reaction to a metabolite produced not by the body but by reaction with sunlight. The long half-life of the antipsychotic drugs and their metabolites have been discussed. These metabolites accumulate in the skin where exposure to sun causes chemical changes that can cause skin allergies. Patients taking antipsychotic drugs should not sunbathe for they run the risk of a painful skin rash. Some patients taking antipsychotic drugs develop slate-blue patches in their skin. This is an accumulation of drug metabolites that is not an allergy and is not dangerous.

Cholestatic hepatitis. Cholestatic hepatitis can develop with antipsychotic therapy. Jaundice develops when the bile duct becomes blocked by an allergic inflammation caused by metabolites excreted in the bile. Cholestatic hepatitis is commonly seen in the first month of therapy with one of the aliphatic phenothiazines. It is normally mild and self-limiting, but if jaundice is detected, the drug should be stopped and an antipsychotic drug from a different chemical class should be used.

Blood dyscrasias. A blood dyscrasia is the depression of the synthesis of one of the blood elements and occasionally occurs with antipsychotic therapy. Depression of leukocytes is common with antipsychotic therapy but is usually transient and not serious. Agranulocytosis, however, in which leukocytes are no longer produced, is serious and often fatal. Agranulocytosis is most common within 3 months of the start of therapy. Therefore blood counts should be done early in therapy, and any sign of fever or sore throat indicates the possible onset of agranulocytosis and should be immediately checked out.

■ CLINICAL USES OF ANTIPSYCHOTIC DRUGS

There are three major uses of antipsychotic drugs: to treat psychoses, to prevent vomiting, and to potentiate the action of other central nervous system drugs. The individual antipsychotic drugs are described in detail in Table 25-3.

■ Treatment of psychoses

The antipsychotic drugs are unique in allowing symptomatic treatment of psychoses. A psychosis is a major emotional disorder with an impairment of mental function great enough to prevent the individual from participating in the everyday matters of life. The hallmark of a psychosis is the loss of contact with reality. There is no one symptom of a psychosis. The symptoms may include agitation, hostility, combativeness, hyperactivity, as well as delusions, hallucinations, disordered thought and perception, emotional and social withdrawal, paranoid symptoms, and personal neglect. The antipsychotic drugs specifically decrease at least some of these symptoms so that the patient becomes able to think and function more coherently.

Psychoses account for most of the patients hospitalized for mental illness, disabling as many Americans as heart disease and cancer combined.

Functional psychoses. A functional psychosis may be an isolated "breakdown" due to a major traumatic event. This psychosis is usually very amenable to treatment with an antipsychotic drug. The acute manic phase of manic-depressive illness is treated with an antipsychotic drug and/or lithium (Chapter 26).

Schizophrenia. Schizophrenia is a chronic mental illness with psychotic episodes. Before the advent of the antipsychotic drugs in the 1950's, schizophrenia accounted for most of the large patient population in mental hospitals. Today with continued antipsychotic drug therapy, patients with schizophrenia do not usually require the degree of supervision found in mental hospitals. The current trend in treating schizophrenia is acute initial care in the psychiatric intensive care unit followed by minimum care in community facilities. Antipsychotic drugs do not cure schizophrenia. Treatment is lifelong, although patients may be taken off medication for several weeks or months during a disease remission.

Organic psychoses. Organic psychoses result from damage to the brain by such things as infectious diseases, deficiency diseases, lead poisoning, tumors, and injury through trauma or interrupted blood supply as in strokes.

Text continued on p. 314.

TABLE 25-3. Antipsychotic drugs

Generic name	Trade name	Dosage and administration	Comments
PHENOTHIAZINES			
Aliphatic			
Chlorpromazine hydrochloride	Thorazine Chlor-PZ Promapar Ormazine	Psychiatric outpatients: ORAL: *Adults*—12 to 40 yr, average dose 400 to 800 mg daily; over 40, a limit of 300 mg daily is suggested. Acutely psychotic, hospitalized patients: INTRAMUSCULAR: *Adults*—25 to 100 mg every 1 to 4 hr until symptoms are controlled. *Elderly or debilitated patients*—10 mg every 6 to 8 hr to control acute symptoms. *Children*—0.5 mg/kg every 6 to 8 hr, gradually increasing dose to a maximum of 40 mg for children under 5 years and 75 mg for those under 12 years. INTRAVENOUS: Not recommended because it is highly irritating. Drug must be diluted to at least 1 mg/ml and no more than 1 mg/min given. ORAL: *Adults*—200 to 600 mg daily in divided doses, increased every 2 to 3 days by 100 mg, up to 2 Gm if needed. *Elderly or debilitated patients*—⅓ to ½ of adult dose with 20 to 25 mg increments. *Children*—0.5 mg/kg every 4 to 6 hr.	Control of initial acute psychotic episodes is achieved with high doses, which are then tapered down to the lowest maintenance dose when the patient's condition stabilizes. Best tolerated by patients under 40 years old and those hospitalized less than 10 yr. Sedation is very pronounced at the start of therapy, which may be desired for highly agitated patients. Incidence of hypotension, ophthalmic changes, and dyskinesias is high in older patients. Anti-adrenergic and anticholinergic side effects usually diminish after the first week. Not for seizure-prone patients.
		To control nausea and vomiting: ORAL: 10 to 25 mg every 4 to 6 hr. INTRAMUSCULAR: 25 mg initially, then 25 to 50 mg every 3 to 4 hr to stop vomiting.	Severe nausea and vomiting can be controlled by low doses.
		Other uses: ORAL: *Adults*—25 to 50 mg 3 or 4 times daily INTRAMUSCULAR: 25 mg every 3 or 4 hr.	Other uses include intractable hiccups, tetanus, acute intermittent porphyria.
Triflupromazine hydrochloride	Vesprin	Psychotic disorders: ORAL: *Adults*—50 to 150 mg daily. *Elderly patients*—20 to 30 mg orally daily. *Children over 2½ yr*—0.5 mg/kg, up to 150 mg maximum. INTRAMUSCULAR: *Adults*—50 to 150 mg daily. *Elderly patients*—10 to 75 mg daily. *Children over 2½ yr*—0.2 to 0.25 mg/kg up to 10 mg maximum. All daily doses for children should be divided.	Management of psychotic disorders. Control of nausea and vomiting.
		Nausea and vomiting: INTRAVENOUS: *Adults*—1 mg up to 3 mg. INTRAMUSCULAR: *Adults*—5 to 15 mg every 4 hr up to 60 mg daily. ORAL: *Adults*—20 to 30 mg total daily. ORAL, INTRAMUSCULAR: *Children over 2½ yr*—0.2 mg/kg, up to 10 mg in 3 doses daily.	

TABLE 25-3. Antipsychotic drugs—cont'd

Generic name	Trade name	Dosage and administration	Comments
Piperidine			
Thioridazine	Mellaril Hydrochloride	Psychotic disorders: ORAL: *Adults*—50 to 100 mg 3 times daily, increasing up to 800 mg. *Elderly patients*—⅓ to ½ adult dose. *Children over 2 yr*—1 mg/kg in divided doses.	Management of psychotic disorders. Little antiemetic activity. Safe for patients with epilepsy.
		Depressive neurosis, alcohol withdrawal syndrome, intractable pain, senility: 10 to 50 mg 2 to 4 times daily.	"Possibly effective" in alcohol withdrawal syndrome, intractable pain, senility. Pronounced sedative and hypotensive side effects initially. One of the least likely of the antipsychotic drugs to cause extrapyramidal reactions because of the pronounced anticholinergic action. Photosensitivity has not been reported. Doses over 800 mg daily have produced serious pigmentary retinopathy.
Mesoridazine besylate	Serentil	ORAL: *Adults*—150 mg daily initially. Increased by 50 mg increments until symptoms controlled. *Elderly patients*—⅓ to ½ adult dose. INTRAMUSCULAR: *Adults and children over 12 yr*—25 to 175 mg daily in divided doses (irritating).	Management of psychotic disorders. This is a metabolite of thioridazine with antiemetic activity, and no reported retinopathy.
Piperacetazine	Quide	ORAL: *Adults and children over 12 yr*—20 to 40 mg daily, increased by increments of 10 mg up to 160 mg to control symptoms. *Elderly patients*—⅓ to ½ adult dose. INTRAMUSCULAR: *Adults and children over 12 yr*—2 to 10 mg repeated in 1 hr, then every 3 to 4 hr initially to control symptoms. *Elderly patients*—⅓ to ½ adult dose.	Management of psychotic disorders. Compared to the other piperidines, piperactazine causes fewer autonomic sedative effects but a greater incidence of extrapyramidal reactions.
Piperazine*			
Acetophenazine maleate	Tindal Maleate	ORAL: *Adults*—60 mg daily in divided doses that can be increased in 20 mg increments. Optimal level is usually 80 to 120 mg. Occasionally, severe symptoms require 400 to 600 mg. *Elderly patients*—⅓ to ½ adult dose. *Children*—0.8 to 1.6 mg/kg in divided doses. Maximum, 80 mg daily.	Management of psychotic disorders.
Butaperazine	Repoise	ORAL: *Adults*—15 to 30 mg daily in 3 doses, increased by 5 to 10 mg to a maximum daily dose of 100 mg. *Elderly patients*—⅓ to ½ adult dose.	Management of psychotic disorders.
Carphenazine maleate	Proketazine Maleate	ORAL: *Adults*—75 to 150 mg daily in 3 divided doses, increased weekly by 25 to 50 mg. Increments to 400 mg maximum. *Elderly patients*—⅓ to ½ adult dose.	Management of psychotic disorders.

*The piperazine phenothiazines are less sedative in effect and have fewer autonomic side effects than other phenothiazine classes. Extrapyramidal reactions are more common, particularly in large doses in patients over 40. Piperazine phenothiazines are less likely to produce allergic reactions and do not change ECG tracings.

Continued.

TABLE 25-3. Antipsychotic drugs—cont'd

Generic name	Trade name	Dosage and administration	Comments
PHENOTHIAZINES—cont'd			
Piperazine—cont'd			
Fluphenazine hydrochloride	Prolixin Permitil	ORAL: *Adults*—2.5 to 10 mg initially, reduced to 1 to 5 mg daily for maintenance. *Elderly patients*—⅓ to ½ adult dose. INTRAMUSCULAR: *Adults*—1.25 mg increased gradually to 2.5 to 10 mg daily in 3 or 4 doses. *Elderly patients*—⅓ to ½ adult dose.	Most potent of the phenothiazines used for the management of psychotic disorders.
Fluphenazine decanoate Fluphenazine enanthate	Prolixin Decanoate Prolixin Enanthate	INTRAMUSCULAR, SUBCUTANEOUS: *Adults under 50 yr*—12.5 mg initially, then 25 mg every 2 wk. Increase by 12.5 mg amounts if needed. Rarely require more than 100 mg every 2 to 6 wk.	Long-acting depot forms lasting at least 2 wk. Dosage should be stabilized in the hospital, since severe episodes of parkinsonism can appear. Not recommended for elderly patients or patients who have had difficulty with extrapyramidal reactions.
Perphenazine	Trilafon	ORAL: *Adults*—16 to 64 mg daily in divided doses. *Elderly patients*—⅓ to ½ adult dose. *Children over 12 yr*—6 to 12 mg daily INTRAMUSCULAR: *Adults*—5 to 10 mg initially, then 5 mg every 6 hr with 15 mg maximum daily in ambulatory and 30 mg daily in hospitalized patients. *Elderly patients*—⅓ to ½ adult dose. *Children over 12 yr*—Lowest adult dose.	For acute psychotic disorders. Lower doses needed when used as an antiemetic.
Prochlorperazine Prochlorperazine edisylate Prochlorperazine maleate	Compazine Compazine Edisylate Compazine Maleate	Psychiatric disorders: ORAL: *Adults*—5 to 10 mg 3 to 4 times daily. Raise dosage every 2 to 3 days as required. From 50 to 75 mg daily is common range for mild cases and 100 to 150 mg for severe cases. *Elderly patients*—⅓ to ½ adult dosage. *Children over 2 yr*—2.5 mg 2 to 3 times daily up to a total dose of 20 to 25 mg. Same dosage used rectally. INTRAMUSCULAR: *Adults*—10 to 20 mg in buttock; repeat every 2 to 4 hr up to 80 mg total. *Elderly patients*—⅓ to ½ adult dose. *Children over 2 yr*—0.06 mg/lb initial dose only, then switch to oral. Nausea and vomiting: ORAL: *Adults*—5 to 10 mg 3 or 4 times daily. *Children*—20 to 29 lb, 2.5 mg 1 to 2 times daily; 30 to 39 lb, 2.5 mg 2 to 3 times daily; 40 to 85 lb, 2.5 mg 3 times daily or 5 mg 2 times daily. INTRAMUSCULAR: *Adults*—5 to 10 mg every 3 to 4 hr. *Children*—0.06 mg/lb. RECTAL: *Adults*—25 mg twice daily. *Children*—same as oral dosage.	More widely used to control severe nausea and vomiting than for psychiatric treatment. Hypotension is seen when given i.v. for surgery.

TABLE 25-3. Antipsychotic drugs—cont'd

Generic name	Trade name	Dosage and administration	Comments
Trifluoperazine	Stelazine	ORAL: *Adults*—2 to 4 mg daily in divided doses (outpatient), 4 to 10 mg daily (hospitalized). *Elderly or debilitated patients*—⅓ to ½ adult dosage. *Children over 6 yr*—1 mg 1 to 2 times daily, gradually raised to maximum of 15 mg. INTRAMUSCULAR: *Adults*—1 to 2 mg every 4 to 6 hr, maximum 10 mg daily. *Elderly or debilitated patients*—⅓ to ½ adult dose. *Children over 6 yr*—same as oral dosage.	Management of psychotic disorders.
THIOXANTHENES†			
Chlorprothixene	Taractan	ORAL: *Adults and children over 12 yr*—75 to 200 mg daily in divided doses. Gradually increase if necessary, with total optimal dose usually being less than 600 mg daily. *Elderly patients*—½ adult dose. INTRAMUSCULAR: *Adults and children over 12 yr*—75 to 200 mg daily in divided doses. *Elderly patients*—½ adult dose.	Management of psychotic disorders. Incidence of side effects like aliphatic phenothiazines: high sedation, autonomic effects, low extrapyramidal effects.
Thiothixene hydrochloride	Navane Hydrochloride	ORAL: *Adults and children over 12 yr*—6 to 10 mg daily in divided doses. Gradually increase, with the usual optimal dose being 20 to 30 mg daily, rarely as high as 60 mg daily. *Elderly patients*—⅓ to ½ adult dose. INTRAMUSCULAR: *Adults and children over 12 yr*—4 mg 2 to 4 times daily; gradually increase if necessary to a maximum of 30 mg. *Elderly patients*—⅓ to ½ adult dose.	Management of psychotic disorders. Incidence of side effects is like the piperazine phenothiazines: low incidence of sedation and autonomic effects, high incidence of extrapyramidal effects.
BUTYROPHENONE			
Haloperidol	Haldol	Acute psychotic management: ORAL: *Adults and children over 12 yr*—1 to 15 mg in divided doses initially, which can be increased gradually up to 100 mg to bring symptoms under control. Dosage is then gradually reduced. Maintenance dose, usually 2 to 8 mg daily. *Elderly patients and children under 12 yr*—0.5 to 1.5 mg daily initially. Dosage increased by 0.5 mg increments if necessary. Usual maintenance dose, 2 to 4 mg daily. INTRAMUSCULAR: *Adults and children over 12 yr*—2 to 5 mg every 4 to 8 hr or every hour if acute state requires. Acute symptoms are usually under control in 72 hr, and 15 mg daily is usually sufficient. Chronic schizophrenia: ORAL: *Adults and children over 12 yr*—6 to 16 mg in divided doses gradually increased to achieve control. Doses as high as 100 mg may be necessary to achieve control. Doses are then gradually reduced to achieve maintenance of control, usually 15 to 20 mg daily. *Elderly patients*—0.5 to 1.5 mg initially, increased very gradually. Maintenance dosage, usually 2 to 8 mg daily.	Management of psychotic disorders. Very likely to produce extrapyramidal reactions in patients prone to neurological reactions. In severe cases of hyperkinetic, retarded patients, large doses may bring improvement in social behavior and concentration. Drug of choice for the treatment of Gilles de la Tourette's syndrome. Spectrum of side effects is like that of the piperazine phenothiazines: low incidence of sedation and autonomic effects, but high incidence of extrapyramidal reactions.

†The thioxanthenes are chemically related to the phenothiazines.

Continued.

TABLE 25-3. Antipsychotic drugs—cont'd

Generic name	Trade name	Dosage and administration	Comments
BUTYROPHENONE—cont'd			
Haloperidol—cont'd		Mental retardation with hyperkinesia: ORAL (given after intramuscular treatment as for acute psychoses): *Adults and children over 12 yr*—80 to 120 mg daily, gradually reduced to a maintenance dose of about 60 mg daily. *Elderly patients and children under 12 yr*—1.5 to 6 mg daily in divided doses; gradually increase dosage up to 15 mg daily for control, then reduce dosage for maintenance. Gilles de la Tourette's syndrome: Initial dosages to achieve control are like those for chronic schizophrenia. Maintenance dosages: adults and children over 12 yr—9 mg daily; children under 12 yr—1.5 mg daily.	
DIBENZOXAZEPINE			
Loxapine succinate	Loxitane Daxolin	ORAL: *Patients over 16 yr*—10 to 25 mg twice daily initially, with dosage increased rapidly over 7 to 10 days to achieve control. Dosage reduced for maintenance to 60 to 100 mg daily; maximum, 250 mg daily. *Elderly patients*—⅓ to ½ dose just listed.	A new drug presently reserved for patients refractory to established antipsychotic drugs.
DIHYDROINDOLONE			
Molindone hydrochloride	Moban Lidone	ORAL: *Adults*—15 to 40 mg daily initially, with increased dosage to control symptoms, up to 225 mg daily. Dosage should then be reduced for maintenance. *Elderly patients*—⅓ to ½ adult dose.	A new drug presently reserved for patients refractory to established antipsychotic drugs.

Organic psychoses are not as successfully treated with antipsychotic drugs as are functional psychoses.

Toxic psychoses. Toxic psychoses can arise during withdrawal from alcohol or other drugs. Some toxic psychoses are treated with diazepam, one of the antianxiety drugs, rather than with the antipsychotic drugs. Amphetamine can cause a toxic psychosis because it releases dopamine in the central nervous system, and therefore the blockade of dopamine receptors by antipsychotic drugs provides specific therapy for an amphetamine-induced psychosis.

■ Antiemetic use of antipsychotic drugs

Several of the antipsychotic drugs are prescribed to control vomiting. Chlorpromazine, triflupromazine, perphenazine, and prochlorperazine in particular are widely used as antiemetics. Chlorpromazine is also prescribed for intractable hiccups. Because of the numerous side effects of the antipsychotic drugs, their use as antiemetics is restricted to the management of postoperative nausea and vomiting, radiation and chemotherapy sickness, nausea and vomiting caused by toxins, and intractable vomiting.

■ Antipsychotic drugs and drug potentiation

Antipsychotic drugs potentiate the action of central nervous system depressant drugs including sedative-hypnotic drugs, narcotic analgesics, and anesthetic agents. The potentiation of sedative-hypnotic drugs (including alcohol) is an important drug interaction. The effects of an alcoholic drink or a sleeping pill will be greatly exaggerated in a patient who is taking an antipsychotic drug. A toxic overdose of the alcohol or sedative-hypnotic drug therefore becomes possible at a lower dose.

Clinical use is made of the potentiation of narcotic analgesic drugs by antipsychotic drugs. Terminal cancer patients in chronic pain can be relieved by lower doses of a narcotic analgesic drug when an antipsychotic drug is also given. This greatly slows the development of tolerance to the narcotics. The antipsychotic drug has the further advantage of controlling the vomiting produced by radiation therapy or chemotherapy.

Finally, droperidol, a drug related to the antipsychotic drug haloperidol, is widely used with a narcotic to produce a state of quiescence and indifference to stimuli, which allows such procedures as bronchoscopy, x-ray

THE NURSING PROCESS

Assessment

Patients requiring antipsychotic drugs are those who display some form of behavior that is characterized as abnormal or ill relative to accepted appropriate forms of behavior. The exact symptoms vary greatly. Assessment should include a total physiological assessment with a focus on the behavioral component of the patient. The nurse should assess the affect, the ability to interact with others, and the ability to initiate appropriate conversation; should assess abnormal thought processes such as hallucinations or delusions; and should observe any unusual mannerisms, or conversely, the lack of any outward activity. The nurse should evaluate such things as judgment, decision making, and overall thought processes. The depth and focus of the mental health examination will vary with the patient and the ability of the patient to assist in identifying some, if any, of the specific problems.

Management

Patients requiring antipsychotic drug therapy will also require psychiatric care, at least during the initial time of drug therapy. Initially the goals will be to stabilize the patient receiving medication sufficiently to allow the patient to begin appropriate interactions with the physician or nurse for the purpose of modifying behavior. The nurse should observe the patient closely for changes in the overall affect and behavior. The nurse should also monitor vital signs, level of consciousness, blood pressure, and signs of drug toxicity. Serious side effects would include the development of extrapyramidal reactions or acute dystonia. The appearance of these and other side effects may warrant decreasing the drug dose or switching to another drug. If side effects are not severe and if the patient's mental illness is being adequately controlled, the physician may elect to continue the drug and either treat the side effects or assist the patient in adapting to these side effects. A variety of forms of psychiatric therapy may be used in conjunction with medications; for additional information about the treatment of psychoses and schizophrenia consult appropriate textbooks of nursing.

Evaluation

Most patients will require continued use of these medications, with brief drug-free periods, for the rest of their lives. Ideally the patient's symptoms will be decreased, and the patient will be able to participate fully in the activities of daily living, interacting appropriately with the world around. This goal is achieved by some patients and not by others. Before discharge for self-management, if that is appropriate, the patient and/or family should be able to explain how to take the medication correctly, what symptoms or side effects should be reported immediately to the physician, what situations indicating either overdosage or underdosage should be reported to the physician, and what symptoms of disease exacerbation should be reported to the physician. If other medications are being used, either to treat the underlying condition or to treat side effects of the antipsychotic drugs, the patient and/or family should also be able to explain the necessary information about these drugs. For further specific guidelines, see the patient care implications section.

---

studies, burn dressing, and cystoscopy to be performed. Nitrous oxide can be added to this neuroleptic-narcotic combination to produce general anesthesia for surgery, neuroleptanesthesia. The anesthesia results from the synergistic effect of the drugs with nitrous oxide, for nitrous oxide alone is not potent enough to produce surgical anesthesia (Chapter 30).

PATIENT CARE IMPLICATIONS

1. Health care professionals should be knowledgeable about the side effects most frequently seen with each of the antipsychotic drugs (Tables 25-1 and 25-2).
2. In some instances sedation of the patient may be desirable, whereas in others it is not. Caution patients to avoid activities that require mental alertness (such

as driving or operating machinery) until it is clear the patient is not so sedated as to be dangerous. Keep the siderails up on the beds of hospitalized patients. Supervise ambulation and use discretion in supervising other possibly dangerous activities such as smoking.

3. Instruct the patient and family that the patient should not take other drugs while receiving antipsychotic drugs unless the drugs and dosages have been approved by the physician. Of particular concern are other drugs causing sedation or hypotension. Remind the patient that over-the-counter medications should be approved by the physician also; many combination products in this latter group contain drugs that may aggravate side effects of the antipsychotic drugs.
4. Patients taking antipsychotic drugs should avoid the use of alcohol.
5. If the patient is hospitalized, monitor the blood pressure every 4 hours until stable. This may require several days to 2 weeks as most of the antipsychotic drugs are cumulative and marked side effects may not appear in the first day or two of therapy. Some physicians may request that blood pressure be checked with the patient in lying, sitting, and standing positions.
6. Instruct the patients to move slowly from lying to sitting or standing positions. If orthostatic hypotension should occur, instruct the patient to lie or sit down. Symptoms include dizziness, lightheadedness, visual changes, and occasionally syncope. Hypotension may be accentuated with hot baths or showers, and these should be avoided. Having the patient wear elastic stockings may help; consult the physician.
7. Side effects may make the patient unsteady when ambulating. Supervise and assist with ambulation until the patient is stable and steady. Instruct the patient to call for assistance before getting up, whether at home or in the hospital, if the patient feels dizzy or unsteady.
8. The anticholinergic effect of dry mouth may be annoying to the patient. Offer fluid frequently. Chewing sugarless mints or gum or sucking on hard candies may help. Encourage frequent oral hygiene including brushing the teeth and rinsing with a pleasant tasting oral rinse or mouthwash. Keep the lips moist with application of a lip balm or ointment. The use of a commercially prepared saliva substitute may be helpful.
9. To monitor for delayed micturition monitor the fluid intake and output. This problem will be more common in immobilized patients, elderly persons, or men who already have an enlarged prostate gland.
10. To counteract constipation keep a record of the frequency of bowel movements and have the patient or the family do the same at home. Maintain an adequate fluid intake (2500 to 3000 ml per day), and encourage the patient to eat a diet that contains a variety of fruits, fiber, and vegetables. Adding prune juice or other foods known to stimulate defecation to the diet may be helpful for an individual patient. Constipation is more common in less active or immobilized patients, so frequent ambulation or exercise may help. If, despite trying the aforementioned measures, constipation is a frequent or constant problem, the addition or a daily stool softener, bulk-former, or other aid to defecation may be appropriate; check with the physician.
11. Instruct the patient to report blurred vision or other visual changes. If blurred vision occurs, it may necessitate reducing the drug dosage or changing drugs. The patient should avoid driving or other potentially dangerous activities until the vision improves. Because long-term therapy has been associated with ocular changes, patients receiving antipsychotic drugs on a long-term basis should be encouraged to have regular eye examinations.
12. The possible endocrine impairments and side effects (see text) should be explained to the patient and appropriate family members. Both the patient and spouse may need emotional support if impotence should occur. The patient should be asked to report the onset of amenorrhea, galactorrhea, gynecomastia, or menstrual irregularities. The institutionalized patient should be monitored for endocrine changes on a regular basis. For some patients the endocrine abnormalities are so disturbing as to cause the patient to want to discontinue therapy with the particular drug.
13. Weigh the patient regularly. This may mean weekly for the outpatient (the patient could do this at home and keep a record) or monthly for patients in the long-term care facility. Antipsychotics may contribute to fluid retention and/or increased appetite.
14. The various extrapyramidal symptoms are described in the text. Explain to the patient and family that these symptoms may occur and instruct the patient to report them if they do. For some patients the extrapyramidal symptoms may be the most bothersome side effects; emotional support of the entire family may be necessary. If other drugs are prescribed to alleviate some of the extrapyramidal symptoms, the use and side effects of these drugs should also be explained to the patient.
15. Evaluate the appearance of new behaviors and of new signs and symptoms in the patient carefully. What may appear to be increased agitation may be

akathisia or what may resemble anxiety may be early parkinsonian-type side effects. The decision to increase the dose of antipsychotic drug or add additional drugs to the patient's regimen should be made carefully and after thoughtful patient evaluation.

16. It is important to monitor the patient frequently for symptoms of tardive dyskinesia. Since there is no effective treatment for this unpleasant side effect, its early detection is imperative. Fine vermicular (wormlike) movements of the tongue have been cited as a possible early sign of tardive dyskinesia. Other classic signs of this side effect are described in the text.
17. As indicated in the text, photosensitivity may be a side effect. Caution patients to avoid exposure to the sun or ultraviolet light. The appearance of any skin changes or discoloration should be reported. Hyperpyrexia has been reported in some patients receiving phenothiazines; caution patients to avoid excessive heat.
18. Cholestatic hepatitis can occur. Instruct the patient to report any skin color changes (jaundice), right upper quadrant abdominal pain, fever, or change in the color or consistency of stools.
19. Instruct the patient to report any fever, sore throat, general malaise; these are symptoms of agranulocytosis.
20. Contact dermatitis with the phenothiazines has been reported. Personnel preparing and administering these drugs should be careful to avoid letting the drugs make contact with their skin, and they should wash the area carefully if contact should occur. It may be appropriate to have personnel wear gloves if they must work frequently with these drugs.
21. Women of childbearing age may wish to consider the use of birth control measures when taking antipsychotic drugs. Women should consult their physicians for appropriate advice about possible pregnancy.
22. Antipsychotic drugs have been associated with hyperglycemia and hypoglycemia. Patients with diabetes mellitus may require readjustment of diet and of drug therapy (insulin or oral hypoglycemics). Caution these patients to monitor their urine glucose concentration carefully and to report frequent episodes of hypoglycemia or excessive spilling of sugar in their urine.
23. Supervise the psychiatric patient carefully to ascertain that any dose of medication is actually swallowed and not hidden in the mouth to be discarded later or stored by the patient. Some of the antipsychotic drugs are available in syrup, injection, or depot injection forms to help ensure that the patient receives the prescribed dose. On an outpatient basis it may be necessary for a responsible family member to supervise the taking of medications.
24. As with all medications, the antipsychotics drugs should be kept out of the reach of children.
25. It has been suggested that taking the antipsychotic drugs with tea or coffee may greatly reduce the absorption of the drug (Hirsch, 1979; Kulhanek et al., 1979; Nurses Drug Alert, 1980). If a patient's response seems variable, it may be due to inactivation of the drug by food items, specifically coffee or tea. Consider giving the drug at a time other than with meals or give it only with water.
26. Antipsychotic drugs should be used with extreme caution in children or adolescents who display signs or symptoms suggestive of Reye's disease.
27. Many antipsychotic drugs have been implicated in suppression of the cough reflex. For this reason they should be used cautiously in patients with chronic obstructive lung disease, emphysema, or asthma; elderly persons; postoperative patients, individuals confined to bed, or anyone with a decreased level of consciousness.
28. The effect of antipsychotic drugs on the seizure threshold is variable. Monitor patients with a history of seizures carefully when administering an antipsychotic drug.
29. Antipsychotic drugs may produce false results (positives) in pregnancy tests. If there is a possibility of pregnancy, women should consult their physicians.
30. Although hypotension is the much more frequent side effect, chlorpromazine may counteract the antihypertensive effects of guanethidine. Monitor the blood pressure frequently.
31. There are concentrated oral forms of most of the antipsychotic drugs available for institutional use. The dose should be diluted to at least 60 ml in one of the diluents suggested by the manufacturer. Note that coffee and tea are listed by some manufacturers as acceptable diluents, although these may cause the drugs to precipitate (see item 25).
32. There are a variety of reasons for apparent drug treatment failures. The patient may take the drug erratically, there may be insufficient emotional care and support for the underlying condition, or the patient and/or family may not understand the disease or reasonable expectations of the medications. Apparent treatment failures require thoughtful investigation.
33. Antipsychotic drugs should not be discontinued suddenly. Encourage patients receiving long-term therapy to continue the ordered drugs, to report complaints about the drugs to the physician, and to report the appearance of new side effects.
34. The care of mentally ill individuals is complex and

involves the use of many treatment modalities. The reader is referred to appropriate texts and articles about psychiatric care.

35. Intramuscular injection of non–depot forms of phenothiazines may cause marked hypotension. The patient should be kept lying down for ½ to 1 hour, the blood pressure monitored, and the patient allowed to get up slowly. For rare severe reactions, levarterenol (Levophed) and phenylephrine (Neo-Synephrine) are the vasoconstrictors of choice; epinephrine and other agents should not be used.
36. With the exception of mild sedation, mild hypotension, and occasionally dry mouth, side effects are rare when the antipsychotic drugs are used for their antiemetic effects. On the other hand, any of the side effects mentioned in the patient care implications can occur in that rare individual who is extremely sensitive to the drug, so health care personnel should be alert to possible side effects. Remember that when the antipsychotic drugs are given with narcotic analgesics, they may potentiate the effects of the analgesics, including sedation and hypotension.
37. Mesoridazine (Serentil) contains a specific coloring, FD&C yellow number 5 (tartrazine) and may cause allergic-type reactions in some individuals. This allergic-type reaction is seen more often in individuals with aspirin hypersensitivity.

■ SUMMARY

Current antipsychotic drugs come from five chemical classes with the phenothiazines being the oldest and most numerous. The antipsychotic action is attributed to the blockade of dopaminergic receptors in the limbic system. Blockade of dopaminergic receptors in other areas of the brain accounts for the antiemetic action, extrapyramidal reactions, and endocrine disturbances characteristic of these drugs. Sedation and orthostatic hypotension are characteristic side effects of those antipsychotic drugs that also block adrenergic receptors. Some antipsychotic drugs also have anticholinergic activity, which gives rise to atropine-like effects but also decreases the incidence of extrapyramidal side effects.

Antipsychotic drugs are principally administered orally. Although the sedation characteristic of some antipsychotic drugs is seen within an hour, antipsychotic effects take a week to develop and require a month or more of continuous therapy for the full effect to be apparent. Extrapyramidal reactions are the main limitation of the antipsychotic drugs. These disorders in movement coordination, acute dystonia, akathisia, pseudoparkinsonism, and tardive dyskinesia, are described fully in the text and in Table 25-2. Other side effects associated with antipsychotic drugs include sedation and postural hypotension, ECG changes, a lowering of the seizure potential, endocrine disturbances, allergic reactions, and, rarely, blood dyscrasias.

The clinical uses of antipsychotic drugs are to treat psychoses and emesis and to potentiate other central nervous system depressants for surgery or analgesia. The psychoses responsive to antipsychotic drugs include functional psychoses, schizophrenia, and amphetamine-induced psychosis. Organic psychoses and withdrawal psychoses do not readily respond to antipsychotic drugs.

■ STUDY QUESTIONS

1. What is the major chemical class of antipsychotic drugs? List the three subclasses.
2. What are the four actions of antipsychotic drugs attributable to blockade of dopaminergic receptors?
3. What are two actions of antipsychotic drugs attributable to blockade of receptors for norepinephrine?
4. What are two actions of antipsychotic drugs attributable to blockade of cholinergic receptors?
5. List the four types of extrapyramidal reactions, the key features of each type, and when each type is likely to occur during antipsychotic drug therapy.
6. Describe the allergic reactions attributed to antipsychotic drugs.
7. For which types of psychoses are antipsychotic drugs generally effective therapy?
8. Name the two clinical uses of antipsychotic drugs other than for the treatment of psychoses.

■ SUGGESTED READINGS

Baldessarini, R.J.: The ''neuroleptic'' antipsychotic drugs. 1. Mechanisms of action. 2. Neurologic side effects, Postgraduate Medicine **65**(4):108, 1979.

Bernstein, J.G.: Prescribing antipsychotics, Drug Therapy **9**(11):85, 1979.

Bozzuto, J.C.: Use of antipsychotic agents for schizophrenia, Drug Therapy **7**(3):39, 1977.

Cline, F.W.: Psychotropic medication, Nurse Practitioner **3**(2):35, 1978.

Cohen, S.: 20 years with the major tranquilizers, Resident & Staff Physician **24**(2):67, 1978.

Crow, T.J.: Molecular pathology of schizophrenia: more than one disease process? British Medical Journal **280:**66, 1980.

Doller, J.C.: Tardive dyskinesia and changing concepts of antipsychotic drug use: a nursing perspective, Journal of Psychiatric Nursing and Mental Health Concepts **15**(11):23, 1977.

Drug interactions with beverages: coffee and tea reduce potency of antipsychotic drugs, Nurses Drug Alert **4:**20, March, 1980.

Drugs for psychiatric disorders, The Medical Letter **22:**77, 1980.

Ehrensing, R.H.: Tardive dyskinesia, Archives of Internal Medicine **138:**1261, 1978.

Gelenberg, A.J., and Klerman, G.L.: Outpatient treatment of schizophrenia, Drug Therapy **8**(9):71, 1978.

Goldfrank, L., and Bresnitz, E.: Phenothiazines, Hospital Physician **15**(6):42, 1979.

Granacher, R.P.: Tardive dyskinesia, American Family Physician **17**(4):163, 1978.

Hasan, M.K., and Mooney, R.P.: Reversible toxic psychosis, American Family Physician **20**(6):89, 1979.

Hirsch, S.R.: Precipitation of antipsychotic drugs in interactions with coffee or tea, Lancet **2**(8152):1130, 1979.

Hitchens, E.A.: Helping psychiatric outpatients accept drug therapy, American Journal of Nursing **77:**464, March, 1977.

Kline, N.S.: The perils of prescribing psychotropic drugs, Resident & Staff Physician **24**(8):57, 1978.

Kulhanek, F., Linde, O.K., and Meisenberg, G.: Precipitation of antipsychotic drugs in interaction with coffee or tea, Lancet **2**(8152):1130, 1979.

McAfee, H.A.: Tardive dyskinesia, American Journal of Nursing **78:**395, 1978.

Mills, J.: Dystonic reactions to phenothiazines, Journal of Emergency Nursing **4**(6):43, 1978.

Newton, M., Godbey, K.L., Newton, D.W., and Godbey, A.L.: Psychotropic drug therapy, Nursing '78 **8**(7):46, 1978.

Prevention and treatment of tardive dyskinesia, The Medical Letter **21:**34, 1979.

Snyder, S.H.: Antischizophrenic drugs and the dopamine receptor, Drug Therapy **8**(5):29, 1978.

Steinhart, M.J.: Psychotropic drugs, American Family Physician **12**(2):93, 1975.

Waring, E.M.: Psychiatric illness in the elderly, American Family Physician **21**(1):109, 1980.

White, J.H.: Handling psychiatric emergencies, Drug Therapy **7**(11):37, 1977.

26 Antidepressant drugs

Nature of depressive disorders

■ DEPRESSION

Depression is a disorder of mood (affect) that is estimated to occur in 15% to 30% of all adults at some time during their lives. Depression is not a single entity; rather it is a syndrome that can include various symptoms, as outlined in Table 26-1. Depression becomes a medical problem when normal functioning is significantly hampered. Three major categories of depression are recognized: reactive depression, endogenous depression, and manic-depressive disorder.

■ Reactive depression, endogenous depression, and manic-depressive disorder

Reactive depression is experienced after some significant loss in one's life. This depression is usually acute for a couple of weeks and resolves within 3 months. Therapy for reactive depression is to provide emotional support. One of the benzodiazepines, the antianxiety drugs, may be prescribed to relieve anxiety or insomnia if required. An antidepressant drug is not commonly needed.

Endogenous depression is depression with no apparent cause. Current views are that endogenous depression is a neurochemical disorder that can be treated with appropriate drug therapy. This concept arose from the observation in the 1950's that reserpine caused depression in patients treated for hypertension. Reserpine was found to deplete the neurotransmitter norepinephrine. About the same time, iproniazid, a drug then used to treat tuberculosis, was found to relieve depression in patients. Iproniazid was found to inhibit the degradation of norepinephrine by inhibiting the enzyme monoamine oxidase. These two observations suggested that a deficiency in the brain neurotransmitter norepinephrine is associated with depression. Current evidence favors a *biogenic amine* theory of depression in which a deficiency either in brain norepinephrine or in another amine neurotransmitter, serotonin, is associated with depression. The two drug classes currently used to treat depression, the tricyclic antidepressants and the monoamine oxidase inhibitors, have pharmacological mechanisms that restore norepinephrine and serotonin in the brain.

TABLE 26-1. Symptoms characteristic of depression

Parameter	Change
General mood	Low for a week or more
Behavior	Appetite or weight change
	Sleep change; early morning awakening is the most common insomnia; some patients may sleep more than usual, though level of activity is either exaggerated or depressed
	Loss of energy
	Loss of interest in activities and/or sex
	Feelings of guilt or self-reproach
	Inability to concentrate
	Thoughts of suicide

Manic-depressive is the third type of depressive disorder. The classic manic-depressive patient has a manic period characterized by excessive euphoria, overactivity, a flow of ideas, extreme self-confidence, and little need for sleep, alternating with a period of depression. Lithium is the specific drug treatment for mania.

■ Depression as a drug side effect

In addition to these three classes, depression can also be the side effect of some drugs, especially the antihypertensive drugs reserpine, methyldopa, guanethidine, and propranolol. Alcohol and antianxiety drugs often unmask depression by alleviating the anxiety that frequently accompanies depression. Steroids, particularly glucocorticoids and oral contraceptives, can cause depression. Drug-induced depression mimics endogenous depression but is treated by removing the drug or lowering the dose.

Drugs used in treating depressive disorders (Table 26-2)

■ Tricyclic antidepressants

Mechanism of action. The tricyclic antidepressants block the reuptake of norepinephrine and/or serotonin into their presynaptic neurons as depicted in Fig. 26-1. This action causes an increase in the synaptic concentration of these neurotransmitters, which is an early effect of the drug. However, clinically no antidepressant response is seen for 2 weeks. Recent research suggests that the tricyclic antidepressants also alter the sensitivity of brain tissue to the action of norepinephrine and serotonin. Since this effect takes 2 weeks to become established, this action more closely correlates with the onset of the clinical antidepressant action.

Administration and fate. The tricyclic antidepressants are commonly administered orally, although amitriptyline and imipramine are available in injectable forms. Metabolites of the tricyclic antidepressants are active, so that an active form of the drug persists in spite of the fact that the drug is well absorbed and readily metabolized by the intestine and liver. The rate of tricyclic metabolism decreases with age, and the dosage for people over 55 is generally started at half the regular adult dose.

TABLE 26-2. Antidepressant drugs

Generic name	Trade name	Dosage and administration	Comments
TRICYCLIC ANTIDEPRESSANTS			
Amitriptyline hydrochloride	Amitril Elavil Endep Rolavil	ORAL: *Adults*—begin with 50 mg at bedtime, increase dosage by 25 to 50 mg if necessary to 150 mg. Alternatively, start with 25 mg 3 times daily, increase to 50 mg 3 times daily. Total dosage should not exceed 300 mg daily. Maintenance doses are usually 50 to 100 mg at bedtime. These are outpatient dosages; inpatient dosages may be twice as much. *Adolescents and elderly*—10 mg 3 times daily plus 20 mg at bedtime (50 mg total) is usually sufficient. INTRAMUSCULAR: 20 to 30 mg 4 times daily.	Bedtime administration is preferred to lessen the discomfort of the sedation and anticholinergic effects prominent with this drug.
Desipramine hydrochloride	Norpramin Pertofrane	ORAL: *Adults*—begin with 25 mg 3 times daily, increase gradually to a total of 200 mg daily and not more than 300 mg daily; maintenance dosages usually 50 to 200 mg taken at bedtime. *Adolescents and elderly:* 25 to 50 mg daily; increased to 100 mg in divided doses if necessary.	Sedation and anticholinergic effects are not prominent. A metabolite of imipramine.
Doxepin hydrochloride	Adapin Sinequan	ORAL: *Adults*—75 mg, increased to 150 mg in divided doses or at bedtime; maintenance dose usually 25 to 150 mg daily and should not exceed 300 mg daily.	Bedtime administration is preferred to lessen the discomfort of the sedation and anticholinergic effects prominent with this drug. Doxepin is reported to have much less effect on the heart when compared to the other tricyclic antidepressants.

Continued.

TABLE 26-2. Antidepressant drugs—cont'd

Generic name	Trade name	Dosage and administration	Comments
TRICYCLIC ANTIDEPRESSANTS—cont'd			
Imipramine hydrochloride Imipramine pamoate	Imavate SK-Pramine Tofranil Tofranil-PM	ORAL: *Adults*—75 mg daily in divided doses or at bedtime. Dose may be increased up to 200 mg daily if required. These are outpatient doses; inpatient doses are ⅓ higher. *Adolescents and elderly*—30 to 40 mg daily, increased to a maximum of 100 mg/day. *Children*—over 6, for bed-wetting, 25 mg, 1 hr before bedtime; if no response in 1 week, increase to 50 mg; over 12, may receive up to 75 mg.	Imipramine is the prototype tricyclic antidepressant. Sedative and anticholinergic effects are moderate. Can be taken at bedtime.
Nortriptyline hydrochloride	Aventyl Pamelor	ORAL: *Adults*—initially, 40 mg in divided doses or at bedtime; maximum dose 100 to 150 mg daily. *Adolescents and children*—30 to 50 mg daily in divided doses.	A metabolite of amitriptyline. Sedative effect is moderate; anticholinergic effect mild. Can be taken at bedtime.
Protriptyline hydrochloride	Vivactil	ORAL: *Adults*—15 to 40 mg daily divided in 3 to 4 doses; maximum dose 60 mg daily. Increments are added to the morning dose. *Adolescents and elderly*—15 mg daily in 3 doses. No more than 20 mg total.	This is the only tricyclic antidepressant that has little sedative action and can cause insomnia if given at bedtime. Preferred for the patient who has been immobile and sleepy.
Trimipramine maleate	Surmontil	ORAL: *Adults*—75 mg daily increased to 150 mg in divided doses or at bedtime. These are outpatient dosages; inpatient dosages 100 mg daily increased to 200 mg daily with a maximum of 300 mg daily. *Adolescents and elderly*—50 mg daily increased to no more than 100 mg daily as required.	Newest tricyclic antidepressant released. Sedation is high, but the anticholinergic effect is moderate.
MONOAMINE OXIDASE (MAO) INHIBITORS			
Isocarboxazid	Marplan	ORAL: *Adults*—20 to 30 mg daily in divided doses; maintenance dose usually 10 to 20 mg daily.	Patient should be instructed in food and drug interactions with the MAO inhibitors.
Phenelzine sulfate	Nardil	ORAL: *Adults*—45 to 75 mg daily in 3 doses or 1 mg/kg body weight in divided doses. Daily dosage should not exceed 90 mg.	Patient should be instructed in food and drug interactions with the MAO inhibitors.
Tranylcypromine sulfate	Parnate	ORAL: *Adults*—20 to 40 mg daily in 2 doses for 2 weeks. Dosage is reduced after a response is obtained. Usually the maintenance dose is below 30 mg. Higher doses are not advised for out-patients.	Patient should be instructed in food and drug interactions with the MAO inhibitors. Has some psychomotor stimulant activity characteristic of amphetamine.
LITHIUM			
Lithium carbonate	Eskalith Lithane Lithonate Lithotabs	ORAL: *Adults*—initially 0.6 to 2.1 Gm daily divided into 3 doses. Increase or decrease dose by 0.3 Gm/day to obtain a blood level of 0.8 to 1.5 mEq/L.	Blood should not be drawn for determination of lithium levels earlier than 8 hr after the last dose. Levels above 2.0 mEq/L are toxic. Patients should be instructed not to "make up" a missed dose of lithium.
Lithium citrate	Lithonate-S	Maintenance dose usually 0.9 to 1.2 Gm daily in divided doses.	

FIG. 26-1

Depression is seen as resulting from too low a concentration of amine to act at the receptor; mania is seen as an overabundance of amine acting at the receptor. In the diagram the biogenic amine theory of depression is applied to the actions of the antidepressant drugs, the tricylic antidepressants and the monoamine oxidase inhibitors, and to the action of lithium, used to treat mania (the opposite of depression). *1,* Lithium inhibits the release of norepinephrine and serotonin. *2,* Tricylic antidepressants and monoamine oxidase inhibitors increase the receptor sensitivity to norepinephrine and serotonin. *3,* Tricyclic antidepressants block the reuptake of norepinephrine and serotonin. Lithium enhances the reuptake of norepinephrine and serotonin. *4,* Monoamine oxidase inhibitors prevent the degradation of norepinephrine and serotonin.

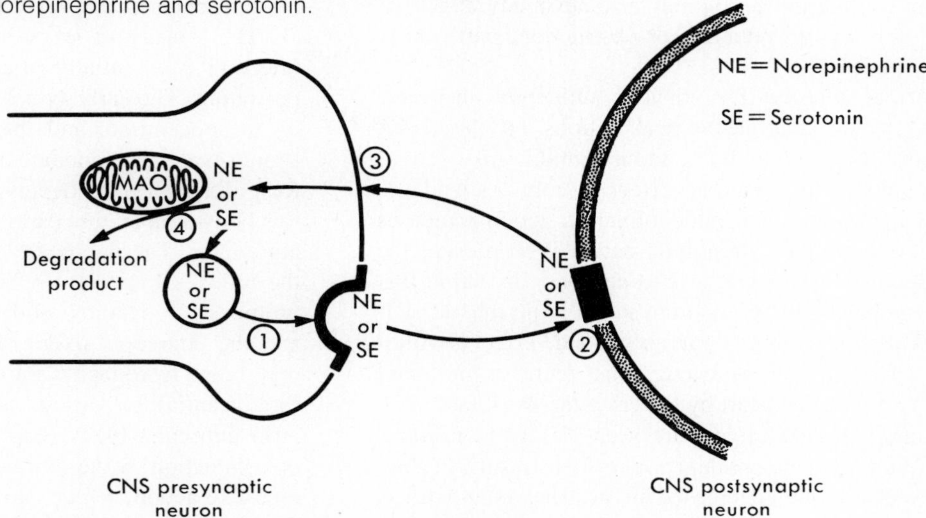

The major side effects of the tricyclic antidepressants are an atropine-like (anticholinergic) effect and sedation. The relative incidence of these side effects among the tricyclics is listed in Table 26-3. Because of these side effects the drug is usually given before bedtime so that the patient is asleep when the side effects are maximal. The more sedating tricyclics, amitriptyline and doxepin, are particularly effective in relieving the insomnia of depression when given as a bedtime dose. These drugs do not interfere with the normal sleep pattern described in Chapter 24.

The anticholinergic and sedative side effects are apparent with the first dose of a tricyclic antidepressant, although little lifting of the depression is seen before 2 weeks of therapy. For this reason, the dose is started at about one third the expected therapeutic dose to allow the patient to develop tolerance to the side effects. The dose is increased to the expected therapeutic dose over the first week. After 2 weeks of drug therapy, the dosage is reviewed in light of side effects and therapeutic response. The final dosage is individualized for the patient. Therapy is discontinued if there is no response after 1 month. If the patient's depression is relieved, the duration of therapy depends on the severity of the depression being treated. A mild depression might be treated for 2 to 3 months, whereas a severe depression might be treated for 1 to 2 years. The drug therapy is then gradually withdrawn. Reappearance of depression is a sign for reinstituting drug therapy. The spectrum of therapy for depression ranges from a few weeks to a lifetime, depending on the severity and recurrence of depression.

TABLE 26-3. Relative incidence of side effects of the tricyclic antidepressants*

Drug	Sedative activity	Anticholinergic activity
Amitriptyline	+++	+++
Desipramine	+	+
Doxepin	+++	+++
Imipramine	++	++
Nortriptyline	++	+
Protriptyline	+/0	++
Trimipramine	+++	++

*Number of + indicates relative activity; +/0 indicates no activity.

Anticholinergic side effects. The anticholinergic side effects include dry mouth, blurred vision, and constipation. Some patients may experience temporary confusion or speech blockage. Patients with glaucoma or disposed toward glaucoma must have this condition checked when taking tricyclic antidepressants because the anticholinergic effect may worsen this condition. The anticholinergic action may also adversely affect patients with urinary retention or obstruction, particularly elderly patients.

Cardiac effects. The tricyclic antidepressants have three separate pharmacological actions on the heart: anticholinergic, adrenolytic, and a quinidine-like action. Therefore the final cardiac effect is complex and depends on dosage. The anticholinergic action increases the heart rate. The adrenolytic action is to prevent the reuptake of norepinephrine into neurons, an action that tends to deplete norepinephrine stores in peripheral neurons. The most common adrenolytic side effect is orthostatic (postural) hypotension. This decrease in blood pressure affects the heart by lowering the work load. The quinidine-like side effects are seen at high concentrations of the tricyclic antidepressants. This results in a decreased heart rate, decreased myocardial contractility, and decreased coronary blood flow. For these reasons, tricyclic antidepressants are contraindicated for patients with a recent myocardial infarction and present special concern for the patient with cardiac disease. Hyperthyroid patients, who are at risk for developing cardiac arrhythmias, have this risk potentiated by the tricyclic antidepressants. Doxepin is a tricyclic antidepressant that has minimal cardiac effects.

Acute toxicity. The tricyclic antidepressants are not addicting, and their abuse potential appears very limited. A major problem is their acute toxicity when depressed patients overdose on the tricyclic antidepressant drug in a suicide attempt. Doses of 1 Gm of the sedating tricyclics are toxic, and doses of 2 Gm are often fatal. Those doses represent only a 5- and 10-fold margin, respectively, over the therapeutic dose.

The toxicity of an overdose of the tricyclic antidepressants is essentially an anticholinergic (atropine-like) poisoning. The early symptoms are confusion, an inability to concentrate, and, perhaps, visual hallucinations. More severe signs include delirium, seizures, and coma. Respiration may be depressed. The patient may have a low body temperature early but an elevated body temperature later. The pupils are dilated, the eyeballs restless, the reflexes hyperactive, and motor coordination compromised. Depending on the cardiac status of the patient and the degree of overdose, the overall cardiac effect may range from tachycardia to slowing of the heart rate (bradycardia) to various arrhythmias secondary to an atrioventricular block. Especially serious is the slowing of conduction in the atrioventricular node by the quinidine-like action, which can result in a heart block. Sudden death from cardiac arrhythmias may even occur several days after an overdose. Physostigmine (Antilirium), a peripherally and centrally active anticholinesterase agent, reverses the anticholinergic toxic symptoms of tricyclic overdose. Physostigmine, 2 mg, is given every 1 to 2 hours, as necessary. It must be given frequently because it is short acting, whereas the tricyclics are long acting.

The tricyclic antidepressants do not decrease the suicide potential among depressed patients during the early weeks of therapy. Depressed patients with suicidal thoughts are best hospitalized to begin drug therapy rather than being given quantities of drugs that may be used in a suicide attempt. Patients who have attempted or threatened suicide are frequently treated initially with electroconvulsive shock therapy. Since tricyclic antidepressants can increase the seizure potential, they are not administered concurrently with electroconvulsive shock therapy.

Drug interactions. Table 26-4 lists a number of drug interactions with the tricyclic antidepressants. The tricyclic antidepressants can potentiate central nervous system depression, anticholinergic effects, and sympathomimetic effects. The interaction of guanethidine and a tricyclic antidepressant is classic: the tricyclic antidepressant inhibits the uptake of guanethidine by the neurons so that guanethidine cannot get to its site of action and is therefore ineffective in lowering blood pressure. Clonidine is also blocked from its reuptake site in the central nervous system by the tricyclic antidepressants.

TABLE 26-4. Drug interactions with antidepressant drugs

Drug class	Effect on therapy with a tricyclic antidepressant
MAO inhibitors	Hypertensive crisis and/or high fever.
Guanethidine	Antihypertensive effect is blocked.
Clonidine	Antihypertensive effect is blocked.
Anticholinergics	Potentiation of anticholinergic effects.
Sympathomimetics	Potentiation of sympathomimetic effects.
Alcohol	Potentiation of CNS depression.
Barbiturates	Potentiation of CNS depression, increased metabolism of tricyclic antidepressants.
Benzodiazepines	Potentiation of CNS depression.
Methylphenidate	Decreased metabolism of tricyclic antidepressants.

Drug class	Effect on therapy with a monoamine oxidase inhibitor
Sympathomimetics* (amphetamine, alpha methyldopa, levodopa, dopamine, tryptophan, epinephrine, norepinephrine)	Hypertensive crisis
Tricyclic antidepressants	Hypertensive crisis
Alcohol	Central nervous system depression
Meperidine	Central nervous system depression
Sleeping pills	Central nervous system depression
Antihistamines*	Central nervous system depression
Antihypertensive drugs	Orthostatic hypotension
Diuretics (particularly thiazides)	Orthostatic hypotension
Insulin	Hypoglycemia
Oral hypoglycemic drugs	Hypoglycemia

*Preparations frequently containing sympathomimetic and/or antihistaminic drugs include asthma preparations, cold tablets or capsules, cough medications, nose drops or sprays, sinus preparations, and weight-reducing pills.

■ Specific tricyclic antidepressants

Amitriptyline

Amitriptyline (Elavil and others) is associated with a high incidence of sedation and anticholinergic effects. These properties are more pronounced than with other tricyclic antidepressants and can cause confusion in the older patient. Weight gain is sometimes seen with amitriptyline. Amitriptyline has a plasma half-life of about 1 to 2 days and is metabolized to nortriptyline, an active tricyclic antidepressant.

Desipramine

Desipramine (Norpramin, Pertofrane) has a low incidence of sedation and anticholinergic effects. It is a metabolite of imipramine and has a plasma half-life of ½ to 3 days.

Doxepin

Doxepin (Adapin, Sinequan) has a high incidence of sedative and anticholinergic side effects. Doxepin does not have the quinidine-like cardiac effect to the degree characteristic of the other tricyclic drugs and is therefore indicated when cardiac function must be considered.

Imipramine

Imipramine (Trofranil and others) has a moderate degree of sedative and anticholinergic side effects. It is metabolized to desipramine, which is also an active tricyclic antidepressant. Imipramine has a plasma half-life of ½ to 1 day. Imipramine is occasionally used to treat enuresis (bed-wetting) in older children or adults.

Nortriptyline

Nortriptyline (Aventyl, Pamelor) is moderately sedating and has minimal anticholinergic side effects. It is a metabolite of amitriptyline.

Protriptyline

Protriptyline (Vivactil) is the one tricyclic antidepressant with minimal sedating effect and is therefore most useful in depressed patients who seem physically immobilized by their depression or who sleep excessively. The plasma half-life of protriptyline is very long (4 to 9 days).

Trimipramine

Trimipramine (Surmontil) is a new tricyclic antidepressant with a high incidence of sedation and a moderate incidence of anticholinergic side effects.

Monoamine oxidase inhibitors

Mechanism of action. The monoamine oxidase (MAO) inhibitors were in use before the tricyclic antidepressants were discovered. The MAO inhibitors irreversibly inhibit the enzyme monoamine oxidase. According to the biogenic amine hypothesis of depression, the MAO inhibitors are effective because they prevent the degradation of norepinephrine and serotonin, so that the concentration of these central nervous system neurotransmitters is increased as diagrammed in Fig. 26-1. The MAO inhibitors are not as effective as the tricyclic antidepressants in treating common endogenous depression, but the MAO inhibitors are more effective in treating depressions exhibited as phobias.

Administration and fate. The MAO inhibitors are well absorbed orally. They are metabolized in the liver to inactive forms and excreted in the urine. In spite of this, the onset of action requires 2 to 3 weeks. The MAO inhibitors act by irreversible inhibition, and removal of enough enzyme to produce clinical effectiveness takes time. Similarly, the effect is persistent for 2 to 3 weeks after discontinuing the MAO inhibitors, reflecting the time to synthesize adequate monoamine oxidase.

Sedation and anticholinergic effects are common side effects associated with the MAO inhibitors, but these drugs are commonly administered in divided doses during the day because of their tendency to cause insomnia if given in the evening. Orthostatic hypotension is sometimes a side effect. At one time, MAO inhibitors were used as antihypertensive drugs.

Like the tricyclic antidepressants, the MAO inhibitors are not addicting.

Interactions leading to a hypertensive crisis. There are a number of clinically significant problems arising from the interaction of the MAO inhibitors with certain foods and other drugs (Tables 26-4 and 26-5). A hypertensive crisis may be precipitated when a food containing tyramine or a sympathomimetic drug is ingested. Sympathomimetic drugs and tyramine are normally degraded rapidly by the MAO of the liver. When MAO is inhibited, tyramine remains undegraded and triggers the release of accumulated norepinephrine, which in turn causes a hypertensive episode. The earliest symptom of such a hypertensive response may be a severe headache. A list of foods and drugs producing a hypertensive response is given in Tables 26-4 and 26-5. The necessity of avoiding these substances to avoid a life-threatening hypertensive crisis is the major limitation of the MAO inhibitors. Phentolamine, the alpha receptor antagonist, may be given to lower the blood pressure during a hypertensive crisis.

TABLE 26-5. Foods containing tyramine to be avoided by patients being treated with MAO inhibitors

Avocados	Papaya products, including meat tenderizers
Bananas	Pâté
Beer	Pickled and kippered herring
Bologna	Pepperoni
Canned figs	Pods of broad beans (fava beans)
Chocolate	Raisins
Cheese (except cottage cheese)	Raw yeast or yeast extracts
Cheese-containing food such as pizza or macaroni and cheese	Salami
Liver	Sausage
Meat extracts like Marmite, Bovril	Sour cream
Offal	Soy sauce
	Wine, Chianti
	Yogurt

Acute toxicity. After ingestion of an overdose of a MAO inhibitor, symptoms appear within 12 hours and reflect increased adrenergic activity: restlessness, anxiety, and insomnia, progressing to include a rapid heart rate and sometimes to convulsions. Dizziness and hypotension may be found, whereas some patients have severe headaches and develop a high blood pressure. Some patients develop a high fever that should be brought down with a sponge bath and external cooling. Treatment is supportive to maintain respiration and circulation. Because the effect of the MAO inhibitor is persistent, patients must be followed for at least a week.

Specific MAO inhibitors

Isocarboxazid

Isocarboxazid (Marplan) is not considered as effective as the other MAO inhibitors but is occasionally prescribed for depressed patients who are unresponsive to the tricyclic antidepressants and to electroconvulsive shock therapy.

Phenelzine

Phenelzine (Nardil) is regarded as the safest of the MAO inhibitors. Patients with a high level of anxiety who do not respond to a tricyclic antidepressant may respond to phenelzine. The dose must be individualized because there is a wide individual variability in the metabolism of phenelzine.

Tranylcypromine

Tranylcypromine (Parnate) can have a stimulatory action similar to amphetamine, and the antidepressant activity is seen more rapidly than with the other MAO inhibitors.

■ Lithium for manic-depressive disorder

Mechanism of action. Lithium acts to lower concentrations of norepinephrine and serotonin by inhibiting their release from and enhancing their reuptake by neurons (Fig. 26-1). These effects, along with the side effects and toxic effect of lithium, are believed to be related to the partial replacement of sodium by lithium in membrane reactions. Lithium is the drug of choice for treating the manic phase of a manic-depressive disorder.

If the patient is severely manic, an antipsychotic drug or electroconvulsive shock therapy may be used initially to subdue behavior. Lithium therapy alone will usually reverse mild to moderate manic symptoms in 1 to 3 weeks. The duration of lithium therapy depends on the individual. Patients with occasional manic periods may be treated only during those periods. Continuous lithium therapy is indicated for those individuals in whom lithium reduces the frequency and intensity of their manic-depressive disorder. There is evidence that lithium may be effective in treating the depression of the manic-depressive disorder and even endogenous depression per se. At this time, however, lithium is approved only for treating acute mania and as prophylaxis for recurrent mania. In research studies lithium is being tested for its effectiveness in treating a variety of psychiatric and neurological brain disorders.

Administration and fate. Lithium is administered orally as the carbonate or citrate salt. Since lithium is an element, related in the atomic table to sodium and potassium, lithium is not metabolized but is excreted by mechanisms similar to those for sodium and potassium. Of the lithium filtered in the kidney, 80% is reabsorbed in the proximal tubule and 20% is excreted in the urine. The half-life of lithium in the plasma is 24 hours and is increased to about 36 hours in the elderly so that the relative dose of lithium must be decreased to avoid the cumulation to toxic doses. Other factors that decrease lithium excretion include sodium deficiency, extreme exercise, diarrhea, and post partum status. Factors that increase lithium excretion include high sodium intake and pregnancy.

Toxicity. The therapeutic index for lithium is relatively small, and at the start of treatment patients taking lithium are tested at least weekly to assure that their plasma level of lithium is in the therapeutic range. The therapeutic range is 0.6 to 1.2 mEq/L but as low as 0.2 mEq/L in the elderly. Side effects common early in therapy include mild nausea, dry mouth, increased thirst, increased urination (polyuria), and a fine tremor of the hands. Toxic symptoms begin to appear at 1.5 to 2.0 mEq/L and by 4.0 mEq/L may be fatal. The toxic symptoms are listed in Table 26-6.

Acute lithium toxicity is treated by hastening lithium excretion while maintaining fluid and electrolyte balance. Lithium excretion is increased by administration of an osmotic diuretic such as urea or mannitol. The drugs aminophylline and acetazolamide increase lithium excretion, and one may be given concurrently with the osmotic diuresis. Peritoneal dialysis or, better, hemodialysis may be used for severe toxicity or when there is renal failure.

TABLE 26-6. Toxic symptoms of lithium

Blood level (mEq/L)	Symptoms
Below 1.5	Fine tremor of hands Dry mouth Increased thirst Increased urination Nausea
1.5 to 2.0	Vomiting Diarrhea Muscle weakness Incoordination (ataxia) Dizziness Confusion Slurred speech
2.0 to 2.5	Persistent nausea and vomiting Blurred vision Muscle twitching (fasciculations) Hyperactive deep tendon reflexes
2.5 to 3.0	Myoclonic twitches or movements of an entire limb Choreoathetoid movements Urinary and fecal incontinence
Above 3.0	Seizures Cardiac arrhythmias Hypotension Peripheral vascular collapse Death

Contraindications. Lithium therapy is contraindicated in early pregnancy because an increased incidence of congenital malformations in infants of treated mothers has been noted. The secretion of the thyroid hormone thyroxine is inhibited by lithium, and a few patients develop an enlarged thyroid gland and may become hypothyroid. A few patients on lithium therapy develop nephrogenic diabetes insipidus (Chapter 34), which is reversed when the lithium dose is lowered or discontinued. Paradoxically, administration of a thiazide diuretic may reverse this polyuria. More seriously, permanent renal damage (initially without symptoms) may develop with long-term lithium therapy. The incidence of this damage remains to be evaluated.

Drug interactions. There are several documented drug interactions with lithium. Lithium potentiates haloperidol, tricyclic antidepressants, the phenothiazines, the benzodiazepines, and the neuromuscular blocking drugs. Lithium is itself potentiated by methyldopa, sodium-depleting diuretics, and the phenothiazines.

■ THE NURSING PROCESS

■ Assessment

Antidepressants are used for patients with pronounced, prolonged depression or those with a diagnosis of manic-depressive disease. In addition to a thorough physiological assessment, the nurse should assess the patient's mental status, focusing on objective signs of depression that the patient may be displaying. The nurse should also monitor the vital signs, weight, and the blood pressure.

■ Management

During the management phase, the health care team will be observing the patient to determine the appropriate discharge drug level. The nurse should monitor the fluid intake and output, the weight, and the blood pressure. If serum blood levels of the drug have been obtained, these should be reviewed. The patient's level of consciousness should be observed with attention to excessive patient sedation. All patients with severe depression should be observed for possible suicidal tendencies. The nurse should look for side effects of the drugs, for example, the dry mouth and constipation that may occur with tricyclic antidepressants. Additional psychiatric therapies may be used in treating these patients; for additional information about psychiatric care, see an appropriate textbook of nursing.

■ Evaluation

Antidepressant drugs are considered successful if the patient's depression lessens and the patient is suffering few if any side effects resulting from drug therapy. Before discharging a patient for self-management, ascertain that the patient and/or the family can explain what drug is being taken, how to take it correctly, the side effects that may occur and those which should be reported immediately to the physician, any dietary restrictions associated with the medication being used, and the ways in which the success of the drug will be monitored. The patient or family should be able to explain why a follow-up is necessary and when to return for the follow-up visits. For more specific information, see the patient care implications section.

■ PATIENT CARE IMPLICATIONS

General guidelines for the use of antidepressants

1. Reassure patients and families that many of the side effects resulting from the antidepressants may diminish or disappear with continued use of the drug. On the other hand, some side effects may persist. Encourage the patient to keep the physician informed of the appearance or persistence of side effects, because it may be possible to adjust dosages or change medications to allow for fewer side effects.
2. Reassure patients and families that several weeks of drug therapy are needed in many cases to produce a significant change in the patient's condition.
3. Warn patients and families that as the patient begins to improve the medications still need to be taken as ordered, because it is the persistent blood levels of the drug causing the improvement. Permitting the patient to take the prescribed antidepressant only when the patient ''feels like it'' will not result in good control of the depression.
4. Patients should be warned to take the medication in the dose prescribed and not to change doses without the physician's approval. If a dose is missed, the patient should not try to ''catch up'' by doubling the dose at a later time.
5. The risk of suicide is present in seriously depressed patients and may persist for several weeks after the patient starts antidepressant therapy. For this reason, many antidepressants are dispensed or prescribed in small amounts to reduce the risk of a fatality should the patient attempt to commit suicide by overdose with the antidepressants. In some situations it may be appropriate for a responsible family member to supervise medication administration for some patients.
6. Patients should be cautioned to keep all their health care providers informed of all medications they are receiving. This is particularly important with anti-

depressants because of the many drug interactions seen with these drugs and others that may be prescribed (Table 26-4).

7. Caution the patient to avoid over-the-counter preparations unless they are first cleared with the physician.
8. As the patient's mood improves, there may be a significant improvement in appetite and some patients will find weight gain to be a problem. Have the patient keep a record of weekly weight. If weight gain is significant, a change in drug or dosage may be indicated, or the patient may need to be instructed in a calorie-restricted diet.
9. Treatment of depression is usually long-term and often requires more than just drug therapy. Encourage the patient and family to return to the physician for follow-up visits and not to hesitate in seeking assistance from appropriate health care personnel (psychiatrists, psychologists, psychiatric nurse clinicians, and others) in handling the depression and its effects.
10. Development of heart conditions in the patient may alter the patient's ability to tolerate antidepressants because of the effects of the drugs on the myocardium. If it is necessary to discontinue antidepressants because of heart disease or other conditions, both the patient and family may need emotional support in learning to cope with the patient's depression should it recur.
11. The most frequently seen side effects that occur with the antidepressants are discussed in this chapter. The patient and family should be instructed, however, to report any unusual sign, symptom, or change in patient behavior.
12. Antidepressants should be used with caution in women of childbearing age, and some women may choose to use a form of birth control while on antidepressants. Instruct women to discuss this with their physicians. If a woman suspects she is pregnant while on therapy, she should consult her physician.
13. Patients should be instructed to keep antidepressants and all medications out of the reach of children.
14. Caution patients not to discontinue antidepressant therapy suddenly but to do so only on the advice of their physician.

Tricyclic antidepressants

1. Because of marked sedation that may occur, caution the patient to avoid activities requiring mental alertness (driving or operating machinery) until the patient's response can be evaluated. Administration of some of the drugs at bedtime may alleviate daytime sedation. In some instances, sedation is a desired effect of a drug.
2. If dry mouth is a problem, chewing gum or taking sugarless mints or candies may make it more tolerable. Frequent oral hygiene such as toothbrushing or rinsing with a mouthwash or gargle may help to eliminate a bad taste in the mouth. Some patients may find the use of a commercially prepared saliva substitute to be helpful.
3. If blurred vision occurs, the patient should be instructed to report it immediately. In addition, that patient should not engage in activities requiring visual acuity, such as driving or operating machinery, until the visual disturbances clear.
4. Encourage the patient to have regular (annual or every 6 months) checks for glaucoma. Institutionalized patients should have regular eye examinations also.
5. Constipation may be a troubling side effect. Have the patient keep a record of bowel movements. If the frequency drops below one every 2 or 3 days, instruct the patient to increase fluid intake to 2500 to 3000 ml per day and pay special attention to choosing a diet with plenty of roughage. The addition of prune juice to the diet or other items known by the patient to stimulate defecation may help. In some instances it may be necessary to add a stool softener, bulk former, or other aid to defecation to the drug regimen; check with the physician.
6. Urinary retention is sometimes seen, although it is most common in the elderly, the immobilized, or men with prostatic enlargement. In the hospital, monitor intake and output until it can be seen that retention is not a problem. Symptoms of retention that the patient would experience include pain in the bladder area, an enlarged bladder on palpation, inability to initiate urination, or a feeling that the bladder does not empty at the time of urination. If this side effect should occur at home, the patient should notify the physician.
7. Hypotension may be a problem. Instruct patients to move gradually from lying to sitting or standing positions. Symptoms of orthostatic hypotension include dizziness, light-headedness, visual changes, and syncope. If the patient begins to feel hypotensive, the patient should lie or sit down. Prolonged periods of standing may contribute to hypotension. Hot showers and baths should be avoided because they may cause vasodilation and aggravate the problem.
8. Hospitalized patients should have their blood pressure and pulse monitored twice a day until stable.
9. Rarely agranulocytosis has been reported as a side effect. Instruct the patient to report any fever, chills, malaise, or sore throat.

10. Rarely thrombocytopenia may occur. Symptoms include unexplained bleeding or bruising, and the physician should be notified.
11. Both increases and decreases in the blood glucose level have been reported by patients taking tricyclic antidepressants. Monitor patients with diabetes mellitus carefully; it may be necessary to change the diet, dose of insulin, or oral hypoglycemic agent while on therapy.
12. Photosensitivity is a problem in some patients. Caution patients to avoid prolonged exposure to the sun or other sources of ultraviolet light, or to use a sunscreen ointment when outside.
13. The symptoms of tricyclic antidepressant overdose are described in the text of the chapter. Instruct the family to seek medical help for the patient if any of these symptoms occur.
14. Patients receiving tricyclic antidepressants should not receive ethclorvynol (Placidyl) because delirium may be precipitated.
15. Concentrated solutions are available for some of the tricyclic antidepressants; see the manufacturer's literature for appropriate diluents.
16. Tofranil and Norpramin both contain FD&C number 5 coloring (tartrazine), which in a few susceptible individuals can cause an allergic response, including an asthmalike reaction. This response is rare, but is seen most often in patients who also have a hypersensitivity to aspirin.
17. Imipramine is used for treatment of enuresis. In children treated for this problem, the most frequent side effects of the drug therapy are nervousness, sleep disorders, and gastrointestinal upset, although any of the side effects seen in antidepression therapy are possible. Treatment is continued for as short a period as possible to obtain relief, then the dose is tapered. Some patients do not respond to imipramine therapy for this condition. The drug should be taken about 1 hour before bedtime, although early-night bed-wetters may get a better response if part of the dose is given in the afternoon and part at bedtime; check with the physician. The treatment of enuresis can be complex, and the patient and family should receive emotional support from the health care team as attempts are made to resolve the problem. For additional information, see textbooks of pediatrics or pediatric nursing.

Monoamine oxidase inhibitors

1. Patient care implications related to anticholinergic effects, sedation, and hypotension are discussed under tricyclic antidepressants.
2. It is very important to review the necessary dietary restriction with the patient and family (Table 26-5). Excessive amounts of caffeine should be avoided, although caffeine in small amounts is acceptable.
3. Symptoms of hypertensive crisis that might occur after ingestion of tyramine-rich foods include headache, palpitations, visual changes, neck stiffness or soreness, nausea, vomiting, sweating, photophobia, pupillary changes, and bradycardia or tachycardia. Hypertensive crisis is an emergency, and the patient should seek medical assistance if these symptoms occur.
4. Phentolamine, the alpha-receptor antagonist, is used to reduce the blood pressure in hypertensive crisis.
5. When possible, monoamine oxidase (MAO) inhibitors should be discontinued 10 days to 2 weeks before elective surgery because of possible interactions with anesthetic agents or postoperative narcotics.
6. Because the effect on the convulsive threshold may vary from patient to patient, the MAO inhibitors should be used with caution in patients with a history of seizures. It may be appropriate to hospitalize these patients to initiate therapy.
7. The MAO inhibitors should be used with caution in patients with diabetes mellitus because these drugs may precipitate hypoglycemia. Monitor diabetics carefully; a change in the dose of insulin or oral hypoglycemic agent may be necessary.
8. Review the possible drug interactions outlined on Table 26-4, and instruct the patient about these.
9. Instruct the patient to report any jaundice, change in skin color, right upper quadrant abdominal pain, or change in the color of stools because these symptoms may indicate liver dysfunction.

Lithium

1. Review the general guidelines for the use of antidepressants just given.
2. Some patients will find the fine hand tremor that lithium produces to be embarrassing. Family and the hospital staff should provide appropriate reassurance and support.
3. It is very important for patients to return for follow-up visits to have their serum lithium levels monitored until the dose is stabilized. Emphasize this point to patients and families.
4. After several weeks of lithium therapy, the patient and family may find the change in affect a pleasant change from the previous manic-depressive state. If it is necessary at a later time to discontinue the medication, both the patient and family may need support and reassurance from the health care team.
5. Patients on a sodium- or fluid-restricted diet (e.g., patients with renal, cardiovascular, or hypertensive disease) will be unable to take lithium.
6. Polyuria may be a nuisance to the patient but may decrease with continued therapy. If polyuria persists, the patient should be evaluated for diabetes insipidus, the symptoms of which are polyuria of copious amounts of dilute urine, with a very low specific gravity, 1.000 to 1.005.
7. If the patient develops diarrhea from any cause, the physician should be notified; the ensuing electrolyte depletion may promote lithium toxicity.
8. Symptoms of lithium toxicity are varied, but should they appear, the patient should notify the physician (Table 26-6). They include fasciculations, ataxia, changes in level of consciousness (confusion, stupor), dizziness, anorexia, nausea, vomiting, glycosuria, sedation, and blurred vision.
9. Excessive weight gain or edematous swelling of wrists and ankles can occur. Have the patient keep a weekly weight record. Inspect patients for the appearance of edema; if necessary, measure the wrists and ankles. Monitor the blood pressure.
10. Some patients complain of a metallic taste in the mouth. This will remain throughout the course of therapy but is not serious, and the patient should be reassured not to worry about it.
11. Taking lithium with meals may decrease nausea associated with the drug. Ideally, patients should take their dose of lithium at the same time each day.
12. Nontoxic goiter has been reported. Outpatients should have their thyroid glands palpated regularly. Instruct patients to report any perceived change in size of the thyroid gland.

■ SUMMARY

According to the biogenic amine theory, depression represents too little norepinephrine or serotonin acting on certain receptors in the brain. Drugs acting as antidepressants restore active norepinephrine and serotonin; on the other hand, lithium, which is used to treat mania, the syndrome opposite to depression, lowers active norepinephrine and serotonin. The tricyclic antidepressants increase the sensitivity of the receptors to these neurotransmitters and block the reuptake of these neurotransmitters. The monoamine oxidase inhibitors prevent the degradation of norepinephrine and serotonin and also enhance receptor sensitivity to these neurotransmitters. Lithium, a chemical element related to sodium and potassium, inhibits the release of norepinephrine and serotonin and enhances their reuptake.

Both tricyclic antidepressants and monoamine oxidase inhibitors take 10 days or more to produce improvement. Sedation and atropine-like side effects are common with each drug class. Certain of the tricyclic antidepressants have distinct depressant effects on the heart. Acute toxicity of tricyclic antidepressants is related to atropine-like poisoning and to the complex cardiac effects. Monoamine oxidase inhibitors have a more complex toxicity. First, a number of foods and drugs that contain sympathomimetic amines, normally degraded by monoamine oxidase, can cause a hypertensive crisis when ingested. Second, an acute overdose disturbs cardiovascular regulation, frequently reflecting an increase in adrenergic activity, but because norepinephrine stores can be depleted secondarily to inhibition of monoamine oxidase, hypotensive episodes, reflecting a lack of norepinephrine, may also be present.

Lithium is a relatively toxic drug so that side effects are often found in the therapeutic range, and the toxic doses are only 2- to 3-fold higher than the therapeutic doses. Lithium is handled like sodium, and treatment of lithium toxicity is directed at increasing lithium excretion by the kidney.

■ STUDY QUESTIONS

1. What is the biogenic amine theory of depression?
2. How are the actions of the tricyclic antidepressants, monoamine oxidase inhibitors, and lithium consistent with the biogenic amine theory of depression?
3. How can some drugs cause depression?
4. What are the major side effects of the tricyclic antidepressants?
5. What is the acute toxicity of the tricyclic antidepressants?
6. What are the major drug interactions of the tricyclic antidepressants?
7. How can a hypertensive crisis be precipitated in a patient taking a monoamine oxidase inhibitor?
8. What are the common side effects of monoamine oxidase inhibitors?
9. What are the symptoms of lithium toxicity?

■ SUGGESTED READINGS

Ack, M., Bulger, J.J., Creson, D.L., Kimball, C.P., Lipinski, J., Talley, J.H., and Weiss, B.L.: Using the tricyclic antidepressants, Patient Care **12:**28, May 15, 1978.

Akiskal, H.S., and McKinney, W.T., Jr.: Depressive disorders: toward a unified hypothesis, Science **182:**20, 1973.

Annitto, W.J.: Recognizing lithium-associated neurotoxicity, Drug Therapy **9**(3):45, 1979.

Burgess, H.A.: When a patient on lithium is pregnant, American Journal of Nursing **79:**1989, 1979.

Claghorn, J.L., Greenberg, B.L., Eng, L., and Larson, J.W.: MAO inhibitors and tyramine don't mix, Patient Care **11:**87, April 1, 1975.

Cline, F.W.: Psychotropic medication, Nurse Practitioner **3**(2):35, 1978.

Cutler, N.R., and Heiser, J.F.: The tricyclic antidepressants, Journal of the American Medical Association **240:**2264, 1978.

De Montigny, C., and Aghajanian, G.K.: Tricyclic antidepressants: long-term treatment increases responsivity of rat forebrain neurons to serotonin, Science **202:**1303, 1978.

Drugs for psychiatric disorders, Medical Letter **22:**77, 1980.

Hall, R.C.W., Perl, M., and Pfefferbaum, B.: Lithium therapy and toxicity, American Family Physician **19**(4):133, 1979.

Koch-Weser, J., and Hollister, L.E.: Drug therapy: tricyclic antidepressants. Part 1, New England Journal of Medicine **299:**1106, 1978.

Koch-Weser, J., and Hollister, L.E.: Drug therapy: tricyclic antidepressants. Part 2, New England Journal of Medicine **299:**1168, 1978.

Kontos, P.G., and Steinhilber, R.M.: Using antidepressants effectively, Postgraduate Medicine **64**(2):55, 1978.

Lipscomb, P.A.: Cardiovascular side effects of phenothiazines and tricyclic antidepressants, Postgraduate Medicine **67**(3):189, 1980.

Maas, J.W.: Clinical and biochemical heterogeneity of depressive disorders, Annals of Internal Medicine **88:**556, 1978.

Newton, M., Godbey, K.L., Newton, D., and Godbey, A.L.: Psychotropic drug therapy, Nursing '78. **8**(7):46, 1978.

Pariser, S.F., Young, E.A., Jones, B.A., Pinta, E.R., and Paul, L.G.: Depression: a new approach to an old syndrome, American Family Physician **18**(4):127, 1978.

Ravaris, C.L., Robinson, D.S., Nies, A., Ives, J.O., and Bartlett, D.: Use of MAOI antidepressants, American Family Physician **18**(1):105, 1978.

Rosenbaum, A.H., Maruta, T., and Richelson, E.: Series on pharmacology in practice. 1. Drugs that alter mood. I. tricyclic agents and monoamine oxidase inhibitors, Mayo Clinic Proceedings **54:** 335, 1979.

Rosenbaum, A.H., Maruta, T., and Richelson, E.: Series on pharmacology in practice. 1. Drugs that alter mood. II. lithium, Mayo Clinic Proceedings **54:**401, 1979.

Sourkes, T.L.: Biochemistry of mental depression, Canadian Psychiatric Association Journal **22:**467, 1977.

Talley, J.H.: Treat depression as the curable disease it is! Patient Care **15:**20, March 1, 1977.

Thornton, W.E.: Tricyclic antidepressant and cardiovascular drug interactions, American Family Physician **20**(1):97, 1979.

Zisook, S., Hall, R.C.W., and Gammon, E.: Drug treatment of depression, Postgraduate Medicine **67**(5):153, 1980.

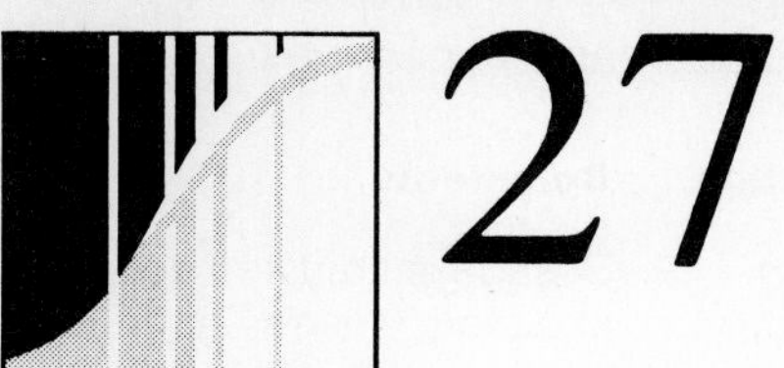

27 Central nervous system stimulants

The central nervous system regulates its level of activity by maintaining excitatory and inhibitory systems. Therefore excessive stimulation of the central nervous system may be produced either by excessive activity of excitatory neurons or by blockade of inhibitory neurons. Many types of chemicals at some dose produce a degree of central nervous system stimulation by one of these mechanisms. Few of these compounds have legitimate pharmacological uses. Central nervous system stimulants are currently medically accepted only for the treatment of narcolepsy, hyperkinetic behavior in children, and obesity. The drugs are also occasionally used to treat depression in geriatric patients and as agents to reverse respiratory depression produced by central nervous system depressants, although they are not generally recommended for these purposes.

In this chapter the mechanism of action of central nervous system stimulants used in clinical conditions and the properties of the central nervous system stimulants that make them prominent drugs of abuse are examined.

■ CENTRAL NERVOUS SYSTEM STIMULANTS USED IN NARCOLEPSY AND HYPERKINESIS

■ Narcolepsy: rationale for therapy

Narcolepsy is a condition in which patients unexpectedly fall asleep in the middle of normal activity, such as while typing, driving a car, or talking to someone. During an attack of narcolepsy, patients experience paralysis of the voluntary muscles similar to that experienced during the dreaming state. The onset of sleep is sudden in these attacks. Therefore, the patient may abruptly collapse and fall. Patients with this sleep disorder obviously should be advised to avoid operating cars or dangerous machinery.

The treatment of narcolepsy usually includes the use of central nervous system stimulants during active daytime periods. These agents have alerting effects and reduce the number of sleeping episodes. One class of central nervous system stimulants used for this purpose is amphetamines. The three most commonly used amphetamines are dextroamphetamine, amphetamine sulfate, and methamphetamine (Table 27-1).

The most commonly used central nervous stimulant in narcoleptic patients is methylphenidate (Table 27-1). This drug is frequently used in combination with imipramine (Chapter 26). The effect of imipramine on narcolepsy is not produced by the antidepressant effects of the drug. The reversal of narcolepsy is rapid, whereas the antidepressant effects of imipramine develop over a prolonged period.

Although drug therapy may be beneficial for many narcoleptic patients, most also require other therapy such as scheduled daytime naps. Psychological counseling may be helpful in assisting patients to reconcile their living patterns with the constraints imposed by the disease.

TABLE 27-1. Summary of central nervous system stimulants used for narcolepsy and hyperkinesis

Generic name	Trade name	Medical use	Dosage and administration	Comments
Amphetamine sulfate (also called racemic or *dl*-amphetamine sulfate)	Benzedrine	Narcolepsy	ORAL: *Adults and children over 6*—5 to 60 mg daily in divided doses. Sustained action formulations may be given once daily.	Dosage is adjusted according to patient's needs and tolerance. Sympathomimetic effects on the cardiovascular system as well as central nervous system toxicity may be noted with long-term use.
		Hyperkinesis	ORAL: *Children*—3 to 5 yr, 2.5 mg daily and increase by 2.5 mg increments weekly to achieve desired effect; 6 yr and older, initially 5 mg daily and increase by 5 mg increments weekly up to a maximum daily dose of 40 mg.	Dosage should be the minimal required for control of symptoms. Long-term continuous use should be avoided to prevent growth inhibition. Drugs may be withdrawn during less stressful periods, such as summer holidays. Schedule II substance.
Dextroamphetamine	Dexampex Dexedrine Diphylets Ferndex	Narcolepsy Hyperkinesis	Same as for amphetamine sulfate. Same as for amphetamine sulfate.	Same as for amphetamine sulfate, except less tendency to produce cardiovascular toxicity. Schedule II substance.
Methamphetamine	Desoxyn	Hyperkinesis	ORAL: *Children 6 yr and older*—2.5 to 5 mg once or twice daily; increase by 5 mg increments at weekly intervals to optimal dosage, usually 20 to 25 mg.	Has central nervous system and cardiovascular toxicity. Schedule II substance.
Methylphenidate	Ritalin Hydrochloride	Hyperkinesis	ORAL: *Children 6 yr and older*—5 mg before breakfast and lunch; increase by 5 to 10 mg at weekly intervals up to 0.3 to 0.5 mg/kg. Special cases may rarely require doses up to 2 mg/kg.	Drug of choice for most hyperkinetic children. Schedule II substance.
		Narcolepsy	ORAL: *Adults*—10 to 60 mg daily. Common dose is 10 mg twice or 3 times daily.	Frequently used along with imipramine to treat narcolepsy. Schedule II substance.
Pemoline	Cylert	Hyperkinesis	ORAL: *Children 6 and older*—37.5 mg daily in a single dose; increase weekly by 18.75 mg increments until response is obtained. Effective dosage range usually 56 to 75 mg daily. Do not exceed 112.5 mg daily.	Clinical effects develop over 3 to 4 wk period. Schedule IV substance.

■ Hyperkinesis: rationale for therapy

Hyperkinetic children display a variety of symptoms, which impair their ability to learn or to maintain appropriate social interactions. These children are excessively active, impulsive, and irritable. Their attention span is very short, and their activity is purposeless. Learning disabilities of various types are frequently encountered in these children. Many hyperkinetic children display abnormal EEG patterns and poorer coordination than normal children of the same age. Intelligence is not impaired. Because of the wide range of symptoms produced, this syndrome has been called by many names, including *minimal brain dysfunction, minimal brain damage, hyperkinesis, attention-deficit disorder with hyperkinesis,* and *hyperkinetic syndrome with learning disorder*.

Hyperkinetic children must receive psychotherapy and counseling, as well as remedial education adjusted to their own needs and abilities. Drug therapy to reduce the hyperactive behavior and lengthen the attention span may also be required. The drugs most effective in controlling this disorder are, paradoxically, central nervous system stimulants. These agents, which increase agitation and activity in adults, have a calming effect on hyperkinetic children. Amphetamines such as dextroamphetamine and methamphetamine have been used to control this disorder (Table 27-1). An equally effective drug with fewer peripheral side effects is methylphenidate. Pemoline is sometimes used but in general is less effective than either the amphetamines or methylphenidate (Table 27-1).

Controversy surrounds the diagnosis and treatment of children with hyperkinesis. Many authorities believe the syndrome is diagnosed more frequently than it exists and suggest that thousands of children may be receiving central nervous system stimulants unnecessarily. This problem remains to be resolved.

■ Pharmacological properties of individual agents

Amphetamines

Mechanism of action. Amphetamines increase the release and effectiveness of catecholamine neurotransmitters in the brain and in peripheral nerves by several mechanisms. These drugs seem to increase the release of neurotransmitters during normal nerve activity. In addition, amphetamines block the specific reuptake of catecholamine neurotransmitters into the presynaptic neuron. Since this reuptake system is normally a major mechanism for terminating the action of the neurotransmitter, blockade of the reuptake system produces prolonged and enhanced stimulation of the postsynaptic nerves. Norepinephrine and dopamine are thought to be the catecholamines whose actions are most enhanced by amphetamines.

Amphetamines may affect many sites within the brain. However, many of the clinically observed actions of amphetamines are probably related to activity in two particular regions of the brain. One of these regions is the reticular activating system. This complex of neurons regulates sensory input to the brain and thus controls the level of arousal. Amphetamines stimulate the reticular activating system, creating increased alertness and sensitivity to stimuli.

The second area of the brain that seems to be especially responsive to amphetamines is the reward center, or the medial forebrain bundle. The reward, or pleasure, center can be activated by amphetamines. The result to the user is a perception of pleasure unrelated to external stimuli. This stimulation of the pleasure center is thought to be the source of the addictive potential of amphetamines.

Absorption and fate. Amphetamines for medical uses are given orally. These drugs are well absorbed from the gastrointestinal tract and produce peak serum concentrations within 2 to 3 hours after ingestion. The half-lives of the various amphetamines in the bloodstream range from 7 to 14 hours. These simple uncharged compounds easily penetrate the blood-brain barrier to produce their central nervous system effects.

Amphetamines are excreted primarily by the kidneys. The rate of excretion is highly dependent on urinary pH. Excretion of these drugs can be greatly enhanced by acidifying the urine.

Toxicity. Amphetamines cause toxic reactions in a number of organ systems. Unpredictable effects can occur in the gastrointestinal tract, but vomiting, diarrhea, abdominal cramps, and dry mouth often occur. Anorexia may be produced, but this reaction is caused by the central nervous system effects of amphetamines.

Most of the central nervous system toxicity of amphetamines can be seen as an extension of the effects observed at therapeutic doses. At high doses amphetamines cause restless behavior, tremor, irritability, talkativeness, insomnia, and mood changes. Excessive aggressiveness, confusion, panic, and increased libido also may occur. More rarely, patients will suffer a syndrome resembling schizophrenia, with delirium or hallucinations. Long-term intoxication with amphetamines frequently causes this schizophrenia-like reaction, sometimes referred to as *toxic psychosis*.

Because of their sympathomimetic effects amphetamines can cause various reactions in the cardiovascular system. Patients report headache, chilliness, and palpitations. Either pallor or facial flushing may be present. Angina can be precipitated as well as various cardiac arrhythmias. Hypertension or hypotension may be observed at various stages during intoxication. The severely intoxicated patient may die in circulatory collapse.

Amphetamine toxicity differs somewhat, depending on which specific drug is used. The drug sold under the trade name of Benzedrine is a mixture of two forms of amphetamine called *d (dextro)* and *l (levo)*. The *d* form of amphetamine stimulates the central nervous system much more effectively than does the *l* form. Conversely, the *l* form stimulates the cardiovascular system slightly more effectively than does the *d* form. Benzedrine, being a mixture of *d* and *l* forms, causes both central nervous system and cardiovascular toxicity.

The drug sold under the trade name of Dexedrine is dextroamphetamine, the *d* form of amphetamine. This preparation is much more selective for the central nervous system and does not produce the same degree of cardiovascular toxicity observed with Benzedrine. Methamphetamine is the *d* form of a derivative of amphetamine. Methamphetamine is equivalent in its properties to dextroamphetamine.

Children receiving amphetamines may suffer growth retardation. This effect can be minimized by giving drug holidays during which drug therapy is suspended.

Drug interactions. Amphetamines interact with a number of other drugs. Amphetamines block the hypotensive effect of methyldopa and guanethidine. The metabolism of tricyclic antidepressants is blocked by amphetamines, causing these drugs to accumulate unless dosage is reduced. Sympathomimetic drugs can increase the effects of amphetamines. Monoamine oxidase inhibitors also increase catecholamine levels and potentiate the effects of amphetamines.

Methylphenidate

Mechanism of action. Methylphenidate is a mild central nervous system stimulant. The drug is sometimes called a *cortical stimulant,* since it tends to have greater effects on mental than motor activities.

The exact biochemical mechanism of methylphenidate action is unknown, but the drug appears similar in its effects to the amphetamines.

Absorption and fate. Methylphenidate is well absorbed orally and is usually prescribed to be given to adults 30 to 45 minutes before meals. Orally administered methylphenidate is extensively metabolized during the first pass through the liver. The metabolites of methylphenidate that are formed are not capable of stimulation of the central nervous system or sympathetic peripheral neurons. Most of the methylphenidate taken orally is excreted in the urine as inactive metabolites of the drug.

Toxicity. Methylphenidate commonly causes nervousness and insomnia. Insomnia may be minimized by not administering the drug in the evening. Nervousness is frequently controlled by reducing overall drug dosage. Anorexia, nausea, and abdominal pain may occur with methylphenidate as with the amphetamines. Cardiovascular effects similar to those produced by amphetamines are also seen.

Methylphenidate rarely produces toxic psychosis but may produce psychological drug dependence. Both effects are observed following long-term use of doses far in excess of those used therapeutically.

Methylphenidate can cause allergic reactions in sensitive patients. These reactions may range from mild skin rashes to exfoliative dermatitis and thrombocytopenic purpura.

Methylphenidate causes a temporary slowing of growth in prepubertal children. Most children seem to overcome the deficit and ultimately gain normal stature. Growth slowing can be minimized by giving the child a drug-free period during therapy.

Drug interactions. Methylphenidate, like the amphetamines, can interact with many other medications. Since methylphenidate causes its effects by release of catecholamines such as norepinephrine, the effects of methylphenidate may be greatly increased by monoamine oxidase inhibitors, sympathomimetic agents, or vasopressors. Methylphenidate also inhibits the metabolism of a variety of drugs including phenytoin, phenobarbital, primidone, phenylbutazone, imipramine, desipramine, and coumarin anticoagulants. Therefore these drugs must be given at reduced dosages to avoid drug accumulation and excessive toxicity when methylphenidate is also being administered. The antihypertensive medication guanethidine is made less effective by methylphenidate, apparently because guanethidine uptake into the nerve terminal is blocked.

Pemoline

Mechanism of action. Pemoline stimulates the central nervous system in a manner similar to amphetamines and methylphenidate but lacks the strong sympathomimetic effects of many of those stimulants. The exact biochemical mechanism for the action of pemoline is unknown.

■ THE NURSING PROCESS FOR CENTRAL NERVOUS SYSTEM STIMULANTS USED IN NARCOLEPSY AND HYPERKINESIS

■ Assessment

A small percentage of individuals in the United States are diagnosed as having narcolepsy or hyperkinesis, and these patients may be treated with central nervous system stimulants. In addition to obtaining a thorough history of the patient's presenting problem, the nurse should assess vital signs, weight, and height in children. A thorough mental status examination should be done.

■ Management

The nurse should spend time with the patient or family in identifying reasonable goals of therapy. The nurse should monitor the height, weight, and vital signs as well as obtain an indication of mental status at periodic intervals. The nurse may question the patient about subjective symptoms or problems not evident through observation, such as insomnia, agitation, dizziness, headache, and irritability. When children are being treated for hyperkinesis, the parents may be additional sources of information about the response of the patient to the drugs. If it is decided that the medication is beneficial and will be used in an outpatient setting, preparation of the patient and family for long-term therapy with the medication should be started.

■ Evaluation

In hyperkinesis these drugs are considered successful if the child becomes less hyperactive and approaches a more normal attention span. In narcolepsy the goal is to have an individual who is able to remain awake and alert, although not excessively active, during specified appropriate time periods. It may require some time to adjust the dosage to the right level for the patient. Before discharge, the patient or family should be able to state why the medication is being used, side effects that may occur, side effects that should cause notification of the physician, any allowable adjustments in dosage that can be made based on side effects (such as giving a nighttime dose at a different time for a child with hyperkinesis), and any activities or measures that should be employed to monitor the effectiveness of the drug in the home setting. Examples are keeping a weekly weight record and for the child a height record at regular intervals.

Absorption and fate. Pemoline is well absorbed orally, producing peak serum levels 2 to 4 hours after dosage. The serum half-life for the drug is about 12 hours. Therefore the drug may be given once daily. The kidney excretes most of the administered pemoline, both as unchanged drug and as metabolites.

Although the blood levels reach a plateau within a few days after therapy is begun, the therapeutic effects of pemoline are not immediately evident in hyperkinetic children. Dosage is gradually increased over a 2 to 4 week period when therapy is started. Significant clinical response may not be seen until the third or fourth week.

Toxicity. Pemoline, when used in properly selected children at recommended doses, seldom causes serious toxic reactions. Insomnia is frequently reported but is a transient reaction in most patients. Pemoline causes anorexia, stomach ache, and nausea, which may slow normal weight gain. Children do not seem to suffer permanent growth retardation with this drug, but careful records of the child's growth should be maintained to allow assessment during therapy.

Pemoline may produce skin rashes and altered liver function tests. These reversible reactions may be due to allergy.

Central nervous system signs such as irritability, mild depression, dizziness, headache, and hallucinations may be provoked by pemoline. Tachycardia and agitation usually result with overdosages.

Pemoline has not been as widely used as some of the other central nervous system stimulants. Toxic reactions to the drug may therefore not be fully defined. Since the drug is thought to alter dopamine systems within the central nervous system, signs of dyskinesia should be carefully watched for (Chapter 25).

TABLE 27-2. Drugs used to suppress appetite

Generic name	Trade name	Dosage and administration	Comments
Amphetamine sulfate	Benzedrine	ORAL: *Adults*—15 to 30 mg daily given as 5 to 10 mg doses 30 to 60 min before meals. Sustained-action formulations may be taken once daily in the morning.	Should be used on a short-term basis only. Tolerance develops within 4 weeks. Schedule II substance.
Benzphetamine	Didrex	ORAL: *Adults*—25 to 50 mg once daily; may be increased as needed up to 3 doses daily.	Similar to amphetamine. Schedule III substance.
Chlortermine hydrochloride	Voranil	ORAL: *Adults*—50 mg daily at mid-morning.	May be used in patients with mild cardiovascular disease. Central nervous system stimulation and insomnia are common reactions. Schedule III substance.
Dextroamphetamine	Dexedrine Diphylets Obotan	ORAL: as for amphetamine sulfate.	As for amphetamine sulfate. Schedule II substance.
Diethylpropion	o.b.c.t. Ro-Diet Tenuate Tepanil	ORAL: *Adults*—25 mg 1 hr before morning, noon, and evening meals and at mid-evening if needed. Timed-release formulations (75 mg) are taken once daily.	Safest anorexiant for use in patients with mild cardiovascular disease. Dry mouth and constipation are common reactions. Schedule IV substance.
Fenfluramine hydrochloride	Pondimin	ORAL: *Adults*—20 mg 3 times daily before meals. Dosage may be doubled if required.	Only anorexiant that depresses central nervous system activity. Sedation and depression may occur. Schedule IV substance.
Mazindol	Sanorex	ORAL: *Adults*—doses range from 1 mg daily at breakfast to 1 mg 3 times daily with meals. Minimum dose should be used.	Used in the same type of patients as diethylpropion. Insomnia, dizziness, and agitation occur. Schedule III substance.
Methamphetamine hydrochloride	Desoxyn Methampex Obedrin	ORAL: *Adults*—2.5 to 5 mg 30 min before each meal. Sustained-action formulations taken once daily in the morning.	As for amphetamine sulfate. Schedule II substance.
Phendimetrazine	Anorex Bacarate Ex-Obese Limit Melfiat Plegine Ropledge Statobex Various others	ORAL: *Adults*—35 mg 2 or 3 times daily taken before meals.	Stimulates the central nervous system in the same manner as the amphetamines. Gastrointestinal distress may occur. Schedule III substance.
Phenmetrazine	Preludin	ORAL: *Adults*—25 mg 2 or 3 times daily before meals. Sustained-action formulation (75 mg) is taken once daily at midmorning.	Similar in properties to amphetamine sulfate. Schedule II substance.

TABLE 27-2. Drugs used to suppress appetite—cont'd

Generic name	Trade name	Dosage and administration	Comments
Phentermine	Adipex Fastin Rolaphent Tora	ORAL: *Adults*—8 mg 3 times daily be-form meals or single dose of 15 to 37.5 mg may be taken 2 hr after breakfast.	Commonly causes insomnia. Schedule IV substance.
Phenylpropanolamine hydrochloride	Coffee Break Control Dex-A-Diet II Diadax Liquid-Trim Pro-Dax 21 P.V.M.	ORAL: *Adults*—25 mg 3 times daily before meals or 50 to 75 mg of sustained-action formulation once daily at midmorning.	Widely used as a nasal decongestant. Blood pressure increases occur. These diet preparations should never be used with cold or allergy medications. Nonprescription.

■ CENTRAL NERVOUS SYSTEM STIMULANTS USED IN OBESITY

■ Rationale for therapy

Many central nervous system stimulants suppress appetite even while stimulating other central nervous system functions. Because of this effect on appetite many of these drugs have been used to help control obesity.

■ Pharmacology of individual agents

Amphetamines were the original central nervous system stimulants used for controlling obesity. Long-term use of amphetamines produces many undesirable side effects, up to and including addiction, as will be discussed later in this chapter. Therefore if amphetamines are used for obese patients, they must be used for short periods and at appropriate doses (Table 27-2). At the low dosage ranges used in this type of patient, tolerance develops to the appetite suppressant properties of amphetamines within 4 to 6 weeks.

Efforts have been made to discover drugs that suppress the appetite but that do not produce general central nervous system stimulation, cardiovascular stimulation, or the danger of addiction. These attempts have met with some success. The systemic effects of appetite suppressants are summarized in Table 27-3. These agents can be divided into three classes. The first class includes those agents that resemble the amphetamines in activity and types of reactions but that produce these reactions less frequently and less severely. Drugs in this class include *benzphetamine, phenmetrazine,* and *mazindol.* The second class includes those agents that produce no significant cardiovascular stimulation and thus may be used in patients with various types of cardiovascular disease. Drugs in this class include *diethylpropion, chlortermine,* and *phendimetrazine.* The third class of anorexiant drugs is represented by *fenfluramine.* This agent is unlike the other anorexiant drugs in that it depresses the central nervous system while suppressing the appetite. *Phentermine* usually has no effect on mood but like the amphetamines does produce cardiovascular stimulation. Also included in Table 27-3 is phenylpropanolamine, a drug frequently used in nonprescription nasal decongestant preparations. *Phenylpropanolamine* mildly suppresses appetite and is included in a very wide array of nonprescription appetite suppressants. Phenylpropanolamine is used alone or in combination with a variety of other agents in these preparations.

Toxicity and side effects. The use of appetite suppressants in treating obesity is a controversial medical practice. All the available effective agents carry substantial risks for the patients taking the drugs. Many of the agents have a very high abuse potential. A high percentage of patients experience some level of dependence on these medications and may seek them from several physicians rather than following the advice of a single physician who may limit the use of the drugs to 2 or 3 months. Many of the appetite suppressants also carry the risk of producing psychotic reactions either as a result of overdosage or prolonged use. Amphetamines are obvious examples of agents that carry this danger, but other appetite suppressants also carry similar risks. Chlortermine and phenmetrazine are both known to produce psychotic reactions in some patients, for example. Fenfluramine may also produce dangerous mental imbalances, although with this drug the danger is depression rather than stimulation of the central nervous system. Fenfluramine should never be given to a patient with a previous history of depression or suicidal tendencies.

TABLE 27-3. Systemic effects of drugs used to suppress appetite

Generic name	Effects on				
	Mood	**Motor activity**	**Heart rate**	**Blood pressure**	**Abuse potential**
Amphetamine sulfate	Highly elevated	Increased	Increased	Increased	Very high
Benzphetamine	Elevated	May increase	May increase	May increase	High
Chlortermine	May be elevated	May increase	Unchanged	Unchanged	High
Dextroamphetamine	Highly elevated	Increased	May increase	May increase	Very high
Diethylpropion	May be elevated	May increase	Unchanged	Unchanged	Relatively low
Fenfluramine	Depressed	Depressed	Usually no change	May increase	Relatively low
Mazindol	May be elevated	May increase	Increased	Usually no change	High
Methamphetamine	Highly elevated	Increased	May increase	May increase	Very high
Phendimetrazine	Highly elevated	Increased	Usually no change	Usually no change	High
Phenmetrazine	Highly elevated	Increased	Increased	Increased	Very high
Phentermine	Usually no change	May increase	Increased	Increased	Relatively low
Phenylpropanolamine	Usually no change	Usually no change	May increase	May increase	None

■ THE NURSING PROCESS FOR CENTRAL NERVOUS SYSTEM STIMULANTS USED IN OBESITY

■ Assessment

Obesity is a major health problem in the United States. In addition to obtaining a thorough patient assessment, the nurse should focus on the vital signs, obtain the patient's weight, discuss usual eating habits, and evaluate any other existing medical conditions. The nurse should establish with the patient reasonable goals of therapy in terms of desired weight. Assessment also includes evaluating the mental status of the patient. The health care team may recommend that the patient seek counseling for behavior associated with obesity, as well as begin appropriate use of other treatments to assist in weight reduction such as use of a calorie restricted diet and a prescribed exercise program. The use of drug therapy alone in the treatment of obesity is rarely successful.

■ Management

The goal of therapy with central nervous system stimulants for the purposes of treating obesity is to promote weight reduction without producing any cardiovascular or mental status effects. The nurse should monitor the patient for these side effects and offer emotional support and information related to control of obesity.

■ Evaluation

When the patient is discharged to home therapy, the patient should be able to explain why the medication is being used and how to take it correctly, the hazards of overmedication, side effects that may occur, symptoms that should be reported to the physician, and how abuse of many of these drugs can cause addiction. In addition, the patient should be able to explain how to carry out other prescribed measures such as caloric dietary restriction and exercise. The nurse may be the member of the health care team who performs follow-up of these patients, monitoring weight and other signs and symptoms. The central nervous system stimulants are not used for long-term control of obesity.

Tolerance. Tolerance develops to all the appetite-suppressing drugs in clinical use. Effective weight reduction cannot be maintained by relying on drugs alone to control eating patterns. Persons seeking to lose weight must develop appropriate eating habits and develop an exercise plan adjusted to their own age and physical limitations. Drugs to suppress appetite may help a patient during the initial stages of a weight reduction program, but these agents are not the key to a successful long-term program. None of these drugs are intended for use in children.

Drug interactions. All the appetite-suppressing agents are capable of interacting with many other medications. For example, any sympathomimetic drug may have a much greater effect in patients receiving appetite suppressants, since the appetite-suppressing drugs tend to increase the effectiveness of catecholamines. This precaution should be mentioned to patients, and they should be warned to avoid cold remedies, allergy medications, and nasal decongestants that include sympathomimetic agents.

Blood pressure can be affected by appetite suppressants. Many of these agents may directly elevate blood pressure. Phenylpropanolamine is occasionally used clinically for its vasopressor effect. Patients receiving medications to treat high blood pressure should avoid appetite-suppressing drugs.

■ CENTRAL NERVOUS SYSTEM STIMULANTS USED TO STIMULATE RESPIRATION (Table 27-4)

■ Rationale for therapy

Certain central nervous system stimulants have generalized effects on the brain stem and spinal cord as well as on higher centers in the brain. These drugs may increase responsiveness to external stimuli and stimulate respiration. As a group these drugs are referred to as *analeptics*.

Analeptics have been used primarily to stimulate respiration when it has been artificially suppressed by drugs, asphyxiation, or electric shock. The use of these drugs has become less common, since modern techniques of respiratory therapy allow a patient to be adequately ventilated even when the natural reflex is temporarily absent. Respiratory paralysis caused by overdoses of narcotic agents is appropriately treated with specific narcotic antagonists and not with these generalized analeptic agents.

Two properties of the analeptic drugs make them especially hard to control. First, the drugs are nonspecific stimulants of the central nervous system and may produce unwanted effects in addition to respiratory stimulation. Second, all these drugs at a high enough dose or in a predisposed patient may produce convulsions.

■ Pharmacological properties of individual agents

Methylxanthines: caffeine and theophylline

Mechanism of action. Methylxanthines block the destruction of cyclic AMP, the compound that mediates the effects of beta adrenergic stimulation (Chapter 8). As a result of this action, these compounds affect many body systems, including the central nervous system. Caffeine and theophylline are the methylxanthines most often used clinically.

Caffeine may stimulate any level of the central nervous system, depending on the dose of the drug. Mild cortical stimulation is produced by low oral doses such as those available in coffee, tea, and cola or in the nonprescription alerting medications. At higher doses caffeine stimulates the medullary centers controlling respiration, vasomotor tone, and vagal tone. Very high doses of caffeine may stimulate the spinal cord and lead to generalized convulsions.

Theophylline also acts as a central nervous system stimulant but produces more action on the heart than does caffeine. Theophylline is most often used clinically as a means of relaxing bronchial smooth muscle. This action is useful in treating chronic obstructive pulmonary disease and asthma (Chapter 22). Theophylline has also been used as a respiratory stimulant, especially in newborn infants.

TABLE 27-4. Summary of central nervous system stimulants used for respiratory stimulation

Generic name	Trade name	Dosage and administration	Comments
Caffeine (citrated caffeine)		ORAL, NASOGASTRIC TUBE: 10 mg/kg initially, then 2.5 mg/kg daily.	Used especially in newborn infants.
Caffeine sodium benzoate injection		INTRAMUSCULAR, INTRAVENOUS: 500 mg as necessary.	Care must be taken to avoid overdosage.
Doxapram	Dopram	INTRAVENOUS: *Adults*—0.5 to 2 mg/kg intermittently as needed. For chronic obstructive pulmonary disease, 1 to 2 mg/min infusion for 2 hr.	Rapidly acting drug whose action is over within 10 min.
Nikethamide	Coramine	ORAL, INTRAVENOUS: *Adults* or *Children*—drug available as 25% solution. From 1.5 to 15 ml administered as necessary in emergency therapy.	Very narrow safety margin and may induce convulsions.
Theophylline		ORAL, NASOGASTRIC TUBE: 6 mg/kg initial dose, then 2 mg/kg every 12 hr. INTRAVENOUS: aminophylline is the only form for parenteral use. Doses are 5.5 mg/kg body weight initially, then infusion of 1.1 mg/kg until proper plasma level is reached.	Most commonly used to treat asthma but is also used to treat apnea in newborn infants.

Absorption and fate. Methylxanthines are absorbed from the gastrointestinal tract. Salt forms of these agents are better absorbed, since the salts are much more soluble in water than are the free alkaloids. The parenteral form of caffeine includes sodium benzoate to maintain solubility of the caffeine.

Caffeine has a half-life in the plasma of about 4 hours. The drug may be partially metabolized in the liver. A portion of a dose of caffeine appears in the urine as the unchanged compound or as metabolites of caffeine. Theophylline has a half-life in the plasma of 8 to 9 hours in adults.

The metabolism and clearance of methylxanthines may be much lower in neonates than in normal adults. When these drugs are used in newborn infants, it may be necessary to adjust the dose to allow for the longer persistence of the drugs in the body. Since neonates vary greatly in their ability to metabolize methylxanthines, it may be necessary to measure blood levels of these drugs. Clearance of methylxanthines is also lower in patients with liver disease or congestive heart failure. These patients may also require adjusted doses of methylxanthines.

Toxicity. Methylxanthines frequently irritate the gastrointestinal mucosa, producing bleeding. Bleeding may occur without other signs or may be accompanied by nausea and vomiting. High concentrations of methylxanthines in the blood can lead to excessive central nervous system stimulation and convulsions. At ordinary therapeutic concentrations, however, the most common reaction to caffeine is nervousness or jitteriness. Theophylline most commonly increases heart rate (tachycardia).

Doxapram

Mechanism of action. Doxapram stimulates respiration by two mechanisms. At low doses the drug seems to stimulate the peripheral carotid chemoreceptors. This action increases the sensitivity to carbon dioxide and thereby increases the impulse to breathe. At slightly higher doses doxapram stimulates the medullary centers controlling respiration.

Absorption and fate. Doxapram is administered intravenously. The drug is very rapid acting with effects being observed within the first minute after injection. The duration of respiratory stimulation is usually 5 to 12 minutes. Doxapram may be given repeatedly to sustain a patient throughout a period of respiratory depression.

■ THE NURSING PROCESS FOR CENTRAL NERVOUS SYSTEM STIMULANTS USED TO STIMULATE RESPIRATION

■ Assessment

Patients requiring drug therapy to stimulate respiration are primarily patients with burns and spinal cord injuries; these drugs are not used much in current practice. The nurse should complete a thorough patient assessment with a focus on the respiratory system. The nurse should auscultate the lungs, check the respiratory rate and depth of respirations, and evaluate the vital capacity. Arterial blood gas levels may be measured.

■ Management

These drugs will be used on a short-term basis until the patient develops adequate voluntary respiration. If the drugs are being administered via constant infusion, an infusion control device or volume control device may be helpful. The nurse should monitor the vital signs with an emphasis on the respiratory system. A suction machine should be at the bedside. The nurse should monitor any serum drug levels if they are being obtained. The mental status of the patient should be evaluated on a regular basis.

■ Evaluation

The goal of these drugs is to stimulate the respiratory system so that the patient breathes at a rate and depth approaching normal. These medications are for short-term use in the hospital.

Toxicity. Doxapram has a wider margin of safety than other analeptics. Nevertheless, doxapram can produce a variety of reactions. Dizziness, apprehension, and disorientation may be reported. Restless, involuntary muscle activity, and increased reflexes are frequently observed. Patients may report a feeling of warmth with flushing, sweating, and increased body temperature. Blood pressure is elevated. Chest pains and cardiac arrhythmias may occur. Extreme agitation, hallucinations, or convulsions usually occur only with overdose, but certain patients may be more susceptible to these reactions. The maximum cumulative dose for doxapram is 3 Gm.

Since doxapram increases blood pressure, this drug should not be used in combination with other drugs tending to elevate blood pressure (e.g., sympathomimetics). Adverse interactions can also occur between doxapram and the inhalation anesthetics that sensitize the heart to catecholamines (halothane, cyclopropane, enflurane). A delay of 10 minutes or more between the cessation of anesthesia with these drugs and the administration of doxapram is suggested to lessen the possibility of excessive cardiac toxicity.

Nikethamide

Mechanism of action. Nikethamide is a potent stimulator of the central nervous system at all levels. At low doses there may be a slight selectivity for stimulation of the medullary centers controlling respiration. This respiratory stimulation is the effect sought when nikethamide is used clinically. Unfortunately, there is a narrow margin of safety with this drug. Doses slightly in excess of those required for respiratory stimulation can cause convulsions.

Absorption and fate. Nikethamide may be administered by any route. It is most effective by the intravenous route. The duration of action of this drug is only 5 to 10 minutes. This short duration of action may necessitate repeated administration of the drug to sustain a patient throughout a period of respiratory depression.

Toxicity. Nikethamide produces a variety of predictable toxic reactions as a result of its ability to cause generalized central nervous system stimulation. Hypertension, tachycardia, and various arrhythmias may be produced. Tremors, sweating, flushing, and increased body temperature (hyperpyrexia) also occur. Itching, coughing, and sneezing may also signal excessive central nervous system stimulation.

Nikethamide causes convulsions at doses very near those used to stimulate respiration. Central nervous system depression follows these convulsions and may further complicate recovery of the patient.

■ CENTRAL NERVOUS SYSTEM STIMULANTS AS DRUGS OF ABUSE

Central nervous system stimulants most commonly come to the attention to the medical professional as drugs of abuse. The medical uses of these agents are limited. This section discusses the more commonly abused drugs of this class, dealing primarily with the symptoms and sequelae of abuse. The list of drugs covered is necessarily limited. References listed in Suggested Readings at the end of the chapter give more comprehensive coverage of unofficial or "street" drugs.

■ Amphetamines as drugs of abuse

Although the medical uses of the amphetamines are rather limited, amphetamines are produced in massive amounts by industry. The inevitable conclusion is that much of the drug produced ends up being used illegitimately. In 1970, the year before amphetamines were put on Schedule II, the Department of Justice reported that 38% of the manufactured amphetamines could not be traced and presumably went to illegal markets. Strong restrictions on the manufacture and sale of amphetamines followed, but amphetamine availability seemed to be virtually unimpaired. A Drug Enforcement Administration report in 1976 suggested that amphetamine abuse was increasing and that the source of the drug was largely physicians' prescriptions. Estimates of the extent of amphetamine abuse are obviously filled with uncertainties. However, most experts in the area agree that the most common amphetamine abuser is middle class, gets amphetamines from one or more medical sources, and takes the drugs orally. A minority of amphetamine abusers are the so-called "speed freaks," that is, members of the drug subculture who take high doses of amphetamines by injection.

Long-term use of low doses of amphetamines can produce psychological dependence. The drug user may have originally taken the drug intermittently to overcome fatigue or depression. Doses of 5 to 20 mg will be effective in the naive user. Persons who take these doses three or four times daily will begin to feel as if they cannot get along without the drug. If the person stops taking the drug, depression ensues. Whether amphetamines produce actual physical withdrawal symptoms is debatable, but this withdrawal depression is sufficiently unpleasant to induce many users to return to amphetamines.

Heavy use of amphetamines either orally or by injection can lead to severe reactions. Persons taking large doses of amphetamines may begin to show stereotyped behavior consisting of compulsive or repetitive actions. These actions frequently have no useful goal. For example, the user may repeatedly wax one fender of a car or count the pages of a book. This type of activity is usually harmless. Other behavior patterns induced by amphetamines are less benign. For example, chronic abusers often have the conviction that bugs are crawling under their skin and may mutilate themselves in an attempt to remove these imaginary bugs. Some amphetamine users develop feelings of paranoia and suspicion, feelings that frequently erupt into violent behavior. Many chronic abusers of amphetamines develop what is called *toxic psychosis,* or *paranoid psychosis*. This severe reaction involves visual and auditory hallucinations, and is frequently mistaken for schizophrenia. The toxic psychosis of amphetamines is specifically treated with an antipsychotic drug (Chapter 25).

■ Cocaine as a drug of abuse

Cocaine was introduced into medicine as a local anesthetic and is very effective for that purpose. Unfortunately, cocaine is also a central nervous system stimulant very similar to amphetamines in its mechanism of action and effects on the central nervous system.

Pure cocaine is very expensive, relative to the amphetamines, and is therefore favored by a more affluent group of drug abusers than are the amphetamines. Widely touted as a glamorous drug, cocaine use is very high among certain popular musicians and professional athletes. For the ordinary street user, the white powder bought as cocaine is usually an adulterated blend of active and inert ingredients. Amphetamines, phencyclidine, or LSD may be added to or substituted for cocaine in the material sold on the street.

An additional attraction of cocaine for middle class drug users is that the drug need not be injected. Most cocaine users sniff cocaine into the nose to coat the nasal mucosa. The drug is then absorbed through that membrane. Cocaine is a potent local vasoconstrictor and, when used on a long-term basis, irritates the nasal mucosa.

At moderate doses cocaine can increase heart rate and blood pressure, as well as produce general central nervous system stimulation. Like amphetamines, cocaine can produce convulsions if high enough doses are taken. Death by cocaine overdose is relatively rare, but when a fatal overdose is taken, convulsions, cardiovascular collapse, and death may occur within 2 or 3 minutes of the dose.

Chronic abuse of cocaine produces physical symptoms much like those produced by amphetamine abuse. Toxic psychosis, stereotyped behavior, and paranoia are also observed.

■ Caffeine as a drug of abuse

Caffeine may be the most widely abused drug in the United States, although the effects of this abuse are much less obvious and usually less devastating than those produced by other abused drugs. Caffeine abuse often takes place unwittingly. Consider the following example:

> John has a cup of coffee while dressing in the morning and a second cup at breakfast. At work John consumes another cup of coffee at the 10:30 AM coffee break. At lunch John drinks two glasses of iced tea. On afternoon coffee break John has a chocolate bar and a cola. Before he leaves work John takes two Excedrin for a headache. At dinner John drinks two cups of tea. Before bed John takes two more Excedrin.

Why is John unable to sleep? John cannot sleep because he ingested about 1 Gm of caffeine during this typical day.

Most people are aware of the caffeine content of coffee, which ranges from 80 to 150 mg per cup. Less well known is the fact that tea, colas, chocolate, and many nonprescription medications such as Excedrin also contain caffeine. In the example given, John took over half a gram of caffeine in these forms.

Ingestion of over 500 mg (half a gram) of caffeine daily produces a variety of central nervous system effects as well as cardiovascular reactions. Irritability or nervousness is a very common complaint, along with disturbances of sleep. Patients may report heart palpitations or that their heart is racing. These descriptions may suggest premature ventricular contractions and tachycardia, both common symptoms of chronic caffeine toxicity. Diarrhea and gastrointestinal irritation commonly accompany chronic overdosage with caffeine. Patients complaining of symptoms such as those just listed should be questioned about caffeine intake. The person taking the history should ask specifically about individual beverages, foods, and medications that contain caffeine to get an accurate estimate of intake. The caffeine content of common items is given in Table 27-5.

Psychological dependence on caffeine may occur. People have great difficulty in omitting the drug from their diets. Nevertheless, patients with peptic ulcer disease should avoid caffeine. Pregnant women may wish to avoid indulging in caffeine, since the drug freely passes to the fetus. Any person who takes more than 200 mg of caffeine daily should be encouraged to reduce intake to avoid the subtle onset of signs of chronic toxicity.

TABLE 27-5. Caffeine content of commonly ingested substances

Substance	Caffeine content
FOODS AND BEVERAGES	
Coffee	
Brewed	80 to 150 mg/5 oz cup
Instant	85 to 100 mg/5 oz cup
Decaffeinated	2 to 4 mg/5 oz cup
Tea, brewed	30 to 75 mg/5 oz cup
Cocoa	5 to 40 mg/5 oz cup
Cola soft drinks*	35 to 60 mg/12 oz bottle or can
NONPRESCRIPTION MEDICATIONS	
Analgesics (Anacin, Bromo-Seltzer, Cope, Midol, Vanquish)	32 mg/tablet
Excedrin	60 mg/tablet
APPETITE SUPPRESSANTS	
Hungrex plus	66 mg/tablet
Anorexin, Super Odrinex	100 mg/tablet
Bio-Slim-T, Permathene-12, Prolamine	140 mg/tablet
Dexatrim, Dietac, Slim One	200 mg/tablet
COLD MEDICATIONS	
Dristan, Dristan AF	16 mg/tablet
Triaminicin	30 mg/tablet
STIMULANTS	
Nodoz	100 mg/tablet
Vivarin	200 mg/tablet

*Many soft drinks other than colas contain caffeine as an additive. The label will reveal the presence of caffeine but not the amount.

■ PATIENT CARE IMPLICATIONS

General guidelines for patients receiving drugs to treat narcolepsy or hyperkinesis or for appetite suppression

1. Review with patients, parents of children, or other appropriate family members, the possible side effects of drug therapy. Significant alterations in mood, irritability, agitation, hallucinations, or any other behavioral change may represent poor patient tolerance to the prescribed drug(s) or inappropriate dosage, and the physician should be notified.
2. Because of the potential for abuse, many of these drugs are dispensed in small quantities, requiring the patient to return to the physician for refills.

3. These drugs should be taken only as directed. Patients should not try to "catch up" if a dose is missed.
4. Keep these and all medications out of the reach of children. Parents should supervise medication administration in children with hyperkinesis.
5. Remind patients to keep all health care professionals informed of all medications being taken, including over-the-counter preparations. Instruct patients to avoid taking any medications unless the drug and dose have been cleared by the physician.
6. After prolonged administration these drugs should be discontinued slowly and with the advice of a physician.
7. None of these drugs is appropriate for treatment of general fatigue.
8. Insomnia may decrease with continued use of a specific drug but may be better treated by eliminating the last dose of medication during the day; check with the physician.
9. Sucking on hard candy or chewing sugarless gum may help relieve dry mouth if it is a problem. Some patients may find the use of a commercially prepared saliva substitute to be helpful.
10. The hospitalized patient should have the blood pressure and pulse checked every 4 hours until the effects of the drug can be ascertained.
11. In addition to reviewing the most frequently seen side effects (see text), instruct patients to report any rash, skin changes, unusual bruising, diarrhea, constipation, impotence, visual disturbances, or any unusual sign or symptom.
12. Caution diabetic patients to monitor their urine sugar concentration carefully as it may be necessary to change insulin and/or diet requirements while receiving amphetamines or appetite suppressants.
13. Warn patients that there may be impairment of ability to engage in hazardous activities such as driving or operating machinery.
14. Except for treatment of hyperkinesis, the use of any of these drugs in children is not recommended.
15. The use of these drugs during pregnancy is not recommended. Some women may wish to consider the use of birth control measures while receiving any of these drugs. Consult with the physician.

Drugs for narcolepsy and hyperkinesis

1. When therapy is being initiated with these drugs, the patient should be weighed two to three times per week until the effects of the drug can be evaluated. Although not being given for the purpose of weight reduction, most of these drugs will suppress the appetite.
2. Careful weight and height records should be kept on a weekly or monthly basis for children being treated for hyperkinesis. Parents can be instructed to do this at home.
3. Caution parents that several weeks of therapy may be necessary in some cases before the results can be seen.
4. Drug therapy for hyperkinesis or narcolepsy should be accompanied by appropriate family and patient teaching, counseling, and support.
5. Review the text for possible drug interactions.
6. Methylphenidate may lower the seizure threshold in individuals with a history of seizures. Observe these patients carefully when therapy is initiated.
7. Ritalin contains FD&C yellow number 5 coloring (tartrazine), which may cause allergic-type responses in some individuals. Although the overall incidence is rare, persons with aspirin hypersensitivity seem to be more susceptible.
8. Signs of dyskinesia, a possible side effect of pemoline, include uncontrolled movements of the tongue, lips, face, and extremities.

Drugs for appetite suppression

1. As indicated in the text, although weight reduction will usually occur while patients are taking appetite suppressants, long-term weight reduction requires the concomitant use of patient counseling and patient alteration of dietary habits.
2. Inform patients that the rate of weight reduction will be greater during the first couple of weeks of therapy but will slow after that.
3. Didrex and Preludin Endurets, 75 mg, contain FD&C yellow number 5 coloring (tartrazine), which may cause allergic-type responses in some individuals. Although overall incidence is rare, persons with aspirin hypersensitivity seem to be more susceptible.
4. A few of these drugs have been reported to alter the seizure threshold. Observe patients with a history of seizures when initiating therapy.
5. If tolerance to the loss of appetite effects occurs after several weeks, the patient should be instructed to notify the physician. The treatment is to discontinue therapy rather than to increase the dose of the drug.
6. Fenfluramine should not be given to patients with a history of depression or suicidal tendencies or to patients with a history of alcohol abuse.
7. Phenylpropanolamine and its related side effects are discussed in greater detail in Chapter 23.

Central nervous system stimulants used to stimulate respiration

1. It should be anticipated that seizures may occur as a result of using these drugs. Have a suction machine at the bedside. Keep siderails up, use padded siderails, or by other means make certain that the patient cannot fall. The patient should not be left unattended.
2. Oxygen and resuscitation equipment should be readily available.
3. Monitor pulse, blood pressure, and respiration frequently. This may mean every 3 to 5 minutes with intravenous administration of a drug to every 15 to 30 minutes with nasogastric administration.
4. The patient should be attached to a cardiac monitor.
5. Monitor the patient's temperature when using doxapram or nikethamide.
6. Short-acting barbiturates (e.g., pentobarbital sodium) should be available to counteract the central nervous system stimulant effects of these drugs.
7. See the manufacturer's literature for specific guidelines about drug dilution, dose, and rate of administration for doxapram and nikethamide.
8. Theophylline is discussed in greater detail in Chapter 22.

■ SUMMARY

Narcolepsy, a condition in which a patient spontaneously falls asleep during active periods, may be treated with central nervous stimulants. Hyperkinesis, a condition characterized by overactivity in children, is also treated, paradoxically, with central nervous system stimulants.

Amphetamines increase the release and effectiveness of catecholamine neurotransmitters in the brain and in peripheral nerves. Amphetamines stimulate the reticular activating system of the brain, creating increased alertness, and stimulate the reward center, creating a perception of pleasure. Amphetamines for medical uses are administered orally. Excretion through the kidneys may be increased by acidifying the urine. Most of the toxicity of the amphetamines is in the central nervous system (restlessness, tremor, irritability, insomnia, confusion) or the cardiovascular system (headache, chilliness, palpitation, angina, cardiac arrhythmias). The *d* (dextro) form of amphetamine is more potent in the central nervous system than the *l* (levo) form, but the reverse is true in the cardiovascular system.

Methylphenidate stimulates the cortical levels of the brain more than the motor levels. The drug is well absorbed orally but is rapidly metabolized in the liver during the first pass. Many of the reactions to methylphenidate are similar to those seen with amphetamines.

Pemoline is a central nervous system stimulant with less sympathomimetic effects than other drugs of this type. The drug has a longer duration of action than methylphenidate. The effects of pemoline in reversing hyperkinesis take several weeks to be established. Pemoline seems to cause less central nervous system effects at normal doses than amphetamines, and cardiovascular toxicity is rare.

Many central nervous system depressants also suppress the appetite center in the brain. Amphetamines were the first drugs of this type used to treat obesity. Patients receiving amphetamines for obesity run the risk of central nervous system toxicity, cardiovascular effects, and drug dependency. Benzphetamine and phenmetrazine are nonamphetamine appetite suppressants that cause many of the same reactions as amphetamines. Diethylpropion and chlortermine cause less cardiovascular toxicity than other appetite suppressants. Fenfluramine is unique in this group of drugs in producing central nervous system depression rather than stimulation. Phenylpropanolamine is a mild appetite suppressant frequently found in over-the-counter preparations. Tolerance develops to all the appetite suppressing drugs in clinical use.

Some central nervous system stimulants are occasionally used to stimulate respiration by medullary stimulation. Methylxanthines such as caffeine and theophylline have been used in this way. Doxapram stimulates respiration also by increasing sensitivity to carbon dioxide. Nikethamide stimulates other areas of the brain in addition to the medulla. At higher doses all these drugs can produce excess central nervous system stimulation and convulsions.

Long-term use of amphetamines can produce psychological dependence. High doses cause stereotyped behavior, paranoia, and violent behavior. Chronic abusers may develop toxic psychosis. Cocaine produces similar symptoms when abused.

Excessive use of caffeine can produce an anxiety syndrome with signs of gastrointestinal irritation.

■ STUDY QUESTIONS

1. What is narcolepsy?
2. What is the treatment of narcolepsy?
3. What is hyperkinesis?
4. What is the treatment of hyperkinesis?
5. What is the mechanism of action of amphetamines in the central nervous system?
6. What two brain areas are especially affected by amphetamines?
7. What is the route of administration of amphetamines used in clinical medicine?
8. What toxic reactions are common with amphetamines?
9. How do the *d* (dextro) and *l* (levo) forms of amphetamines differ in toxicity?
10. What other drugs interact with amphetamines?
11. What is the mechanism of action of methylphenidate in the central nervous system?
12. What is the route of elimination of methylphenidate?
13. What toxicity is associated with the use of methylphenidate?
14. What is the mechanism of action of pemoline?
15. How does the duration of action of this drug differ from methylphenidate?
16. How long does it take for full therapeutic effects of pemoline to develop?
17. What toxic reactions are associated with pemoline?
18. Why are central nervous system stimulants used to treat obesity?
19. How do the nonamphetamine appetite suppressants differ from amphetamines?
20. Which nonamphetamine appetite suppressants produce reactions similar to those of amphetamines?
21. Which nonamphetamine appetite suppressants produce little cardiovascular stimulation?
22. Which nonamphetamine appetite suppressant produces central nervous system depression?
23. Which nonamphetamine appetite suppressant is most often found in over-the-counter obesity medications?
24. What toxic reactions may develop during therapy with the nonamphetamine appetite suppressants?
25. Why are central nervous system stimulants used to stimulate respiration?
26. What two methylxanthines are sometimes used to stimulate respiration?
27. What reactions are observed to the methylxanthines used to stimulate respiration?
28. What is the mechanism of action of doxapram?
29. How is doxapram administered?
30. What is the duration of action of doxapram?
31. What toxicity is observed with doxapram?
32. What is the mechanism of action of nikethamide?
33. How may nikethamide be administered?
34. What toxicity is associated with nikethamide?
35. What is the source of most amphetamine used in an abusive manner?
36. What is the effect of toxic doses of amphetamines in an amphetamine abuser?
37. How does cocaine differ from amphetamine?
38. Why may caffeine be considered a drug of abuse?
39. What are the effects of chronic overdosage with caffeine?

■ SUGGESTED READINGS

Beede, M.S.: Phencyclidine intoxication, Postgraduate Medicine **68**(5):201, 1980.

Byck, R., Weiss, B.L., and Wesson, D.R.: Cocaine: chic, costly, and what else? Patient Care **14**(15):136, 1980.

Carluccio, C.: Anxiety syndrome or caffeinism? Diagnosis **2**(9):74, 1980.

Cline, F.W.: Stimulants and their use with hyperactive children, Nurse Practitioner **2**(6):33, 1976.

Coke: nothing to sniff at, Emergency Medicine **7**(9):17, 1975.

Dawber, T.R., Kannell, W.B., and Gordon, T.: Coffee and cardiovascular disease. Observations from the Framingham Study, New England Journal of Medicine **291**:871, 1974.

DuPont, R.I., Goldstein, A., and O'Donnell, J., editors: Handbook on drug abuse. National Institute on Drug Abuse, Washington, D.C., 1979, U.S. Government Printing Office.

Ellinwood, E.H., Jr., and Kilbey, M.M., editors: Cocaine and other stimulants, New York, 1977, Plenum Press.

Gilbert, R.N.: Caffeine as a drug of abuse. In Gibbins, R.J., Israel, Y., Kalant, H., Popham, R.E., Schmidt, W., and Smart, K.G., editors: Research advances in alcohol and drug problems, vol. 3, New York, 1976, John Wiley & Sons, Inc.

Goldstein, A., Kaizer, S., and Warren, R.: Psychotropic effects of caffeine in man. II. Alertness, psychomotor coordination, and mood, Journal of Pharmacology and Experimental Therapeutics **150**:146, 1965.

Graham, D.M.: Caffeine—its identity, dietary sources, intake and biological effects, Nutrition Review **36**:97, 1978.

Hennekens, C.H., Drolette, M.E., Jesse, M.J., Davies, J.E., and Hutchison, G.B.: Coffee drinking and death due to coronary heart disease, New England Journal of Medicine **294**:633, 1976.

Mark, L.C.: Analeptics: changing concepts, declining status, American Journal of Medical Science **254**:296, 1967.

Martin, W.R., editor: Drug addiction. II. Amphetamine, psychotogen, and marihuana dependence, Handbuch der Experimentellen Pharmakologie vol. 45, Berlin, 1977, Springer-Verlag.

Petersen, R.C., and Stillman, R.C., editors: Cocaine: 1977, National Institute on Drug Abuse, Department of Health, Education, and Welfare Publ. No. (ADM) 77-471, Washington D.C., 1977, U.S. Government Printing Office.

Petersen, R.C., and Stillman, R.C., editors: PCP phencyclidine abuse: an appraisal. National Institute on Drug Abuse, Department of Health, Education, and Welfare Publ. No. (ADM) 78-728, Washington D.C., 1978, U.S. Government Printing Office.

Picchioni, A.L.: Clinical status and toxicology of analeptic drugs, American Journal of Hospital Pharmacy **28**:201, 1971.

Reichard, C.C., and Elder, S.T.: The effects of caffeine on reaction time in hyperkinetic and normal children, American Journal of Psychiatry **134**:144, 1977.

Safer, D., Allen, R., and Barr, E.: Depression of growth in hyperactive children on stimulant drugs, New England Journal of Medicine **287**:217, 1972.

Schnoll, S.H.: Guidelines for the care of the drug abusing patient, Hospital Medicine **12**(10):85, 1976.

Sroufe, L.A., and Stewart, M.A.: Treating problem children with stimulant drugs, New England Journal of Medicine **289**:407, 1973.

Turner, C.E.: Marijuana research and problems: an overview, Pharmacy International **1**(5):93, 1980.

Tyrala, E.E., and Dodson, W.E.: Caffeine secretion into breast milk, Archives of Disease in Childhood **54**:787, 1979.

Wang, S.C., and Ward, J.W.: Analeptics, Pharmacological Therapeutics [B]**3**:123, 1977.

Weathersbee, P.S., and Lodge, J.R.: Alcohol, caffeine, and nicotine as factors in pregnancy, Postgraduate Medicine **66**(3):165, 1979.

Weiss, G., and Hechtman, L.: The hyperactive child syndrome, Science **205**:1348, 1979.

Zarcone, V.: Narcolepsy, New England Journal of Medicine **288**:1156, 1973.

VII DRUGS TO CONTROL SEVERE PAIN

Section VII discusses those drugs that have made modern surgery possible. Chapter 28, **Narcotic Analgesics (Opioids),** focuses on the analgesic uses of opioids for surgery and other conditions in which pain is prominent. The remarkable insight recently gained on the endogenous morphine-like compounds, the endorphins, are reviewed. Since the opioids are also a major drug class for illicit use, attention is given to the features of opiate dependence, the role of the specific opiate antagonist naloxone in treating acute opiate overdose, and the role of the long-acting opioid methadone in treating opiate withdrawal. Chapter 29, **General Anesthetics,** presents the theories of anesthesia, the inhalation and intravenous anesthetics, and the combinations of drugs now widely used for ''balanced'' anesthesia and for neuroleptanesthesia. The limitations as well as desirable characteristics of each anesthetic are described. Chapter 30, **Local Anesthetics,** reviews both the surface use of local anesthetics as well as their use by injection for major surgery.

28 Narcotic analgesics (opioids)

■ HISTORICAL REVIEW OF THE NARCOTIC ANALGESICS

■ The nature of pain

Analgesics are drugs that relieve pain. Because there are two major components of pain, analgesics fall into two major classifications. One component of pain is *objective* and represents the stimulation of peripheral nerve endings when tissue is damaged. Nonnarcotic analgesics such as aspirin and acetaminophen (Datril, Tylenol) are believed to act by interfering with the local mediators that are released in damaged tissue to stimulate the nerve endings. In the presence of nonnarcotic analgesics, pain is not felt because the nerves are not stimulated and the pain message is therefore never delivered to the central nervous system. The nonnarcotic analgesics are discussed in Chapter 20. The second component of pain is *subjective* and represents how one reacts to pain, usually with fear, anxiety, and withdrawal. The subjective level of pain involves the spinal cord and brain, which collect and process the painful stimuli. The narcotic analgesics act to blunt this subjective component of pain. The individual treated with a narcotic analgesic may become unaware of pain and indifferent to all unpleasant stimuli.

■ The history of morphine

Opium has been used to produce analgesia and euphoria throughout the history of mankind. The word *opium* comes from the Greek word "opion," meaning poppy juice, and the source of morphine today is still the sticky brown gum (opium) collected from the seed pod of *Papaver somniferum,* a variety of poppy. About 10% of the content of opium is morphine. Codeine can also be extracted from opium, although in such small amounts that most of the medicinal codeine is derived from the methylation of morphine. Morphine was isolated in 1803 by a German pharmacist and named after Morpheus, the Greek god of sleep. Morphine was the first pure chemical substance that mimicked the pharmacological effects of the natural product after extraction from the natural product.

Even today morphine remains the prototype of the narcotic analgesics, a class of drugs more properly called the *opioids*. Some of the narcotic analgesics are chemical modifications of morphine. The term *opiate* as a drug class refers to codeine and to morphine and its semisynthetic derivatives. The purely synthetic narcotic analgesics with morphine-like activities were originally termed *opioids,* but today the term *opioids* is used by most pharmacologists as a general term for *narcotic analgesics*. In this chapter, the term *opioid* will be used in place of the term *narcotic analgesic,* although this more familiar phrase is used elsewhere in this book. The chief characteristic of the opioids is their ability to render the individual unreactive to pain even though the individual is conscious and the source of pain has not been removed. The term *narcotic* is derived from the Greek word meaning stupor or insensibility.

All opioids have abuse potential to a greater or lesser degree. In general, opioids come under the Controlled Substance Act as described in Chapter 4. The schedule under which each opioid falls is listed in the drug tables.

Drug dependency as a property of morphine was not appreciated in the United States until the Civil War, when morphine was widely used in treating wounded soldiers whose addiction subsequently became a significant social problem. Opium and morphine were readily available and were often ingredients of patent medicines. By the late 1800's, there were attempts to modify the structure of morphine to keep the analgesic property but eliminate the addictive potential. The first semisynthetic drug was heroin, but heroin soon proved to produce drug dependency more readily than morphine. Today heroin is not a legal drug in the United States although it is in other countries.

The first purely synthetic morphine-like compound was meperidine (Demerol), which came into clinical use in the 1940's. Because meperidine was not a chemical modification of morphine, there was widespread belief that meperidine did not cause drug dependency. Today meperidine is considered a drug with high abuse potential (Schedule II) like morphine. The most recent examples of opioids whose abuse potential was not originally recognized are pentazocine (Talwin) and propoxyphene (Darvon), which are now classified as drugs of low abuse potential (Schedule IV). The characteristics of opiate dependency and its treatment will be discussed later in this chapter.

■ Endorphins: the body's own morphine

The most recent development in the search for a better analgesic has been the discovery of how morphine acts in the body. It had long been suspected that morphine acted at very specific receptor sites. In the early 1970's scientists were able to demonstrate that specific receptors for morphine-like drugs did indeed exist in the brain, spinal cord, and gut. These receptors recognized only opioids and none of the known neurotransmitters. This suggested that there was a previously unknown, naturally occurring substance in the brain, spinal cord, and gut that is mimicked by morphine. Such substances have been identified and are termed *endorphins,* for *endo*genous mo*rphin*e-like substances. All endorphins are polypeptides and are found in those specific locations that have been long associated with the actions of morphine and in which opiate receptors can be identified. The smallest endorphins are the pentapeptides (five amino acids) called the *enkephalins,* a term meaning "from the head," referring to the first tissue from which they were isolated. The enkephalins seem to be neurotransmitters associated with (1) the mediation of pain and analgesia, (2) the release of growth hormone, prolactin, and vasopressin from the pituitary, (3) the modulation of locomotor activity, (4) the regulation of mood, and (5) the regulation of gut motility. It can be anticipated that these recent discoveries will clarify the nature of analgesia and the development of the opiate type drug dependency as well as provide the basis for understanding the role of endorphins in mental disorders, seizure activity, and behavior patterns involving the reward system, eating, and drinking.

The goal in developing analgesics has been to provide an effective analgesic that will not produce tolerance or drug dependence. This goal has not yet been fully realized. With the characterization of opiate receptors, it has become clear that the opioids such as pentazocine and nalbuphine, which have the least dependency potential, have not only agonistic properties (mimicking endorphin effects) but antagonistic properties as well (blocking endorphin effects). The search for a nonaddicting opioid may depend on finding the drug that has the right combination of agonist-antagonist properties without unpleasant side effects.

■ THE PHARMACOLOGY OF MORPHINE

The pharmacology of morphine provides the standard for comparing the actions of opioids.

■ Actions in the central nervous system

Many effects of morphine are in the central nervous system.

Analgesia. The analgesia produced by morphine has three characteristics. First, morphine raises the threshold for pain perception, making the individual less aware of pain. Second, morphine reduces anxiety and fear, which are the emotional reactions to pain. Third, morphine induces sleep even in the presence of severe pain.

The biochemical mechanism of pain relief by the opioids is their ability to mimic endogenous compounds, the endorphins, which act at many sites in the brain to modify the perception of and reaction to pain. Support for this concept has come from studies using naloxone (Narcan), which is a specific opioid antagonist. Naloxone blocks the placebo response and reduces the effectiveness of acupuncture anesthesia, two processes believed to reflect the activity of endorphins. The interpretation of these effects of naloxone is that naloxone blocks the effect of endorphins, which are released in response to pain to minimize the perception of pain. These studies also provide a biochemical explanation for the effectiveness of the acupuncture technique to reduce pain.

Medullary actions. Morphine affects several medullary centers. The most important is the respiratory center, which becomes less sensitive to carbon dioxide in the presence of morphine. Tolerance does develop to this effect so that an individual who abuses one of the opioids can tolerate doses of opioids that would cause fatal respiratory depression in the nondependent individual. Death from an overdose of an opioid is frequently from respiratory arrest; the victim simply stops breathing. Similarly, the most important drug interactions with morphine are those arising from a synergistic depression of the respiratory center, as with any of the sedative-hypnotic drugs, minor tranquilizers, alcohol, general anesthetics, or phenothiazines. Tolerance does not develop to the respiratory depression produced by these latter drug classes. An individual abusing an opioid and a drug of another class, such as alcohol or one of the other sedative-hypnotic drugs, can readily succumb to drug-induced respiratory depression.

A second medullary center depressed by morphine is the cough center. Morphine itself would seldom be prescribed as a cough suppressant but a related drug such as codeine would. Cough suppressants (antitussive drugs) are described in Chapter 11.

The third major medullary center affected by morphine is the chemoreceptor trigger zone. Morphine stimulates this center to produce nausea and vomiting. This is a transient effect, so repeated doses of morphine do not usually cause nausea and vomiting. Individuals vary in their sensitivity to this emetic action of morphine.

Behavior. The effect of morphine on behavior depends on the mental state of the individual. Euphoria may be experienced if the individual has been in pain or has been fearful and anxious. Therapeutic doses of morphine produce minimal sedation, but larger doses cause drowsiness, sleep, or, in very large doses, coma. A few individuals become excited rather than depressed by morphine.

■ Actions in the periphery

Gastrointestinal tract. Morphine has a profound depressant effect on the gastrointestinal tract so that constipation is a common side effect of morphine administration. Although morphine itself is not used to treat nonspecific diarrhea, related drugs such as codeine or diphenoxylate are so used. The common medicinal use of opium in ancient medicine was as a drug to stop diarrhea.

Secretions. Gastric, biliary, and pancreatic secretions are inhibited by morphine. Morphine is used to treat the pain associated with biliary colic, but morphine may exacerbate rather than relieve the pain in some patients. This is because the biliary tract may go into painful spasms in the presence of morphine.

Urinary retention. Urinary retention is another side effect of morphine. Morphine stimulates the release of vasopressin (antidiuretic hormone), so that more water is absorbed in the kidney tubules, decreasing urine volume. Morphine also reduces the perception for voiding.

Cardiovascular effects. Morphine commonly causes hypotension. In part, this may be a result of depression of the vasomotor center in the medulla. In addition, morphine causes histamine release, and histamine is a potent vasodilator. The concurrent administration of a phenothiazine or atropine can intensify the hypotension. In large doses, morphine slows the heart rate.

Ocular effect. A classic effect of morphine is to reduce the pupillary size. A pinpoint pupil is one characteristic of a narcotic overdose. However, if the victim is near death, hypoxia causes the release of epinephrine, which dilates the pupil.

■ Adverse reactions and contraindications to opioids

The common adverse reactions of the opioids are those predicted by their pharmacological actions: nausea and vomiting, constipation, urinary retention, itching, and hypotension resulting from histamine release.

Some of the actions characteristic of morphine are undesirable in certain patients. The respiratory depression caused by the opioids is one such action. Patients with impaired respiratory function may be severely compromised by an opioid because their respiratory drive is already impaired. Although in general the opioids relax bronchial smooth muscle, a few patients with asthma will experience severe bronchoconstriction and die. These drugs will also pass into the milk of a nursing mother and affect the infant.

Patients suffering from a head injury should not be given an opioid because the decreased respiration will increase carbon dioxide retention and carbon dioxide will dilate the intracranial blood vessels, further worsening the situation. Also the sedative and behavioral effects will obscure evaluation of the central nervous system.

Since the opioids can cause hypotension, they must be used cautiously in patients suffering from shock or blood loss, conditions worsened by a hypotensive action.

■ Tolerance and dependence with opioids

Drug tolerance. Drug tolerance refers to the situation in which repeated use of a drug results in a lesser response unless the dose is raised. Tolerance develops rapidly to the euphoric effect of the opioids. Individuals abusing the narcotic analgesics will keep raising the dose to maintain the "good" feeling associated with the drug. Patients receiving an opioid for severe pain over a limited period of time may also develop tolerance. The patient is unlikely to become drug dependent because as the pain subsides, so will the need for the opioid. However, the individual abusing an opioid will become drug dependent rather rapidly. Daily use of one of the opioids can produce drug dependence in 3 weeks.

Little or no tolerance develops to the pupillary constriction or to the constipating effect of the opioids. Pinpoint pupils are one characteristic of dependence on opioids.

Drug dependency. There are complex psychological and social components of drug dependency, but here we will only consider the pharmacological component. A drug-dependent person will experience distinct physical reactions if the drug is suddenly discontinued; these reactions make up the *abstinence syndrome*. Basically, the abstinence syndrome represents the readjustment of the body to function in the absence of the drug. The more quickly the drug is eliminated, the more pronounced will be the abstinence syndrome. The severity of the symptoms will be greater the longer the drug has been used and the higher the dose used.

Symptoms of the abstinence syndrome. The opiate abstinence syndrome following the sudden cessation of morphine or heroin use is predictable. The individual has a runny nose (rhinorrhea), goose flesh, tearing (lacrimation), sweating, and yawning 16 hours after the last dose. The pupils do not react readily to light. Over the next 20 hours the individual becomes restless, cannot sleep, and experiences muscle twitching. Hot and cold flashes and abdominal cramping occur. By 36 hours, the individual feels nauseous, vomits, and has diarrhea. The abstinence symptoms are generally the reverse of the drug effects described for the opioids. The body overcompensates when the drug is removed.

The opiate abstinence syndrome is unpleasant although not life threatening like the sedative-hypnotic abstinence syndrome. A major part of drug abuse behavior may be the search for more drug to stop the abstinence syndrome.

Methadone for maintenance and detoxification. The major approach in the United States for treating individuals dependent on heroin or another opioid is to substitute methadone, which can be given orally in a daily dose. Since tolerance has already developed to the ''kick'' from heroin in these individuals, the methadone maintains this tolerance while protecting against withdrawal symptoms. The goal of maintenance is to discourage the individual from continuing to seek drugs and to participate instead in rehabilitation programs. If detoxification (elimination of drug) is the goal, methadone will be administered first when withdrawal symptoms appear and then the dose of methadone will be gradually reduced to zero over a period of 1 to 3 weeks. Because methadone has a long half-life in the body, the abstinence symptoms are not as severe as with morphine or heroin.

■ Acute toxicity of the opioids and the use of opiate receptor antagonists (narcotic antagonists) (Table 28-1)

Respiratory depression is the usual cause of death from an acute overdose of an opioids. An overdose is most likely to occur in an individual who buys drugs for abuse on the street. Street drugs represent unknowns as to purity and concentration of the drug, so occasionally the drug content will be higher than anticipated.

The overdosed individual will be stuporous or in a deep sleep and will initially be warm with a flushed wet skin. The next stage will be a coma in which respiration is depressed and as the individual becomes hypoxic (starved for oxygen), the skin will become cold, clammy, and mottled, and the pupils will dilate. Death is then imminent.

Naloxone

When a patient is brought to the emergency room comatose from a drug overdose, the first goal is to support respiration and the second is to determine which drug was used. If an opioid is suspected, there is a specific test. Naloxone (Narcan) is administered intravenously, and if the overdose is a result of an opioid, the patient will respond in 2 to 3 minutes with improved respiration and return to consciousness. This response reflects that naloxone is a pure antagonist for the opiate receptor. Naloxone displaces the opioid from the receptor but produces no effect of its own. The result is a dramatic reversal of the drug overdose. The patient must still be carefully monitored, however, because naloxone has a short duration of action and its effect may wear off before the overdosed drug has been sufficiently eliminated. If the patient returns to a coma, naloxone must be given again.

Multiple drug abuse is common, and naloxone will only reverse the depression resulting from the narcotic analgesic. Naloxone will have no effect when the overdose is of a drug that is not a narcotic analgesic.

TABLE 28-1. Narcotic antagonists

Generic name	Trade name	Dosage and administration	Comments
Levallorphan tartrate	Lorfan	INTRAVENOUS: *Adults*—1 mg followed by 1 or 2 doses of 0.5 mg spaced every 10 to 15 min. *Neonates*—0.05 to 0.1 mg into umbilical vein on delivery.	Has agonist properties but acts as an antagonist in the presence of narcotic analgesics. Used to reverse respiratory depression in adults and in neonates of addicted mothers.
Nalorphine hydrochloride	Nalline Hydrochloride	INTRAVENOUS: *Adults*—5 to 10 mg to reverse respiratory depression, repeated if necessary every 10 to 15 min; maximum, 3 doses. *Neonates*—0.2 mg repeated if necessary to a total dose of 0.5 mg. SUBCUTANEOUS: *Adults*—1 to 3 mg to diagnose narcotic addiction. If no symptoms, repeat with 5 mg at 30 min, and if still no symptoms, repeat with 8 mg after 30 min.	Properties and uses are like those of levallorphan. Used to diagnose narcotic addiction because withdrawal symptoms will appear after injection. The more severe the addiction, the smaller the dose required to elect withdrawal symptoms.
Naloxone hydrochloride	Narcan	INTRAVENOUS, INTRAMUSCULAR, SUBCUTANEOUS: *Adults*—0.4 mg for respiratory depression caused by narcotic overdose. Repeated in a few minutes if necessary up to 3 doses. For narcotic depression of respiration after surgery: 0.1 to 0.2 mg every few minutes as necessary. INTRAVENOUS: *Neonates*—0.01 mg/kg body weight.	A pure narcotic antagonist used to reverse respiratory depression from narcotic overdose. Unlike nalorphine and levallorphan, naloxone produces no respiratory depression of its own.

Nalorphine and levallorphan

Nalorphine (Nalline) and levallorphan (Lorfan) are two other drugs used as opiate receptor antagonists. Both of these drugs are also narcotic agonists and are effective analgesics. However, they produce dysphoria (unpleasant feeling) rather than euphoria to a degree that makes them unacceptable analgesics. Both nalorphine and levallorphan, like naloxone, will reverse respiratory depression resulting from an overdose of an opioid. However, nalorphine and levallorphan do themselves produce respiratory depression, although to a much lesser degree than the other opioids. If the cause of drug overdose is not known, as is common in the emergency room, there is the risk that levallorphan or nalorphine will make the respiratory depression worse if any drug other than an opioid is involved. Naloxone has therefore become the drug of choice for reversing respiratory depression, since naloxone will not cause additional respiratory depression.

■ SPECIFIC OPIOIDS

There are 14 narcotic analgesics presently in use. They are compared as to efficacy, dose, onset, and duration of action in Table 28-2. In addition to those drugs listed in Table 28-2, there is fentanyl (Sublimaze), a short-acting narcotic analgesic used primarily in anesthesia; oxycodone, a Schedule II compound found only combined with a nonnarcotic analgesic; and hydrocodone, a Schedule II drug prescribed only as an antitussive agent.

The major use of the opioids is for the relief of moderate to severe pain. These drugs are most effective in relieving the constant dull pain associated with trauma, surgery, heart attack, biliary or ureteral colic, inflammation, or cancer. Isolated, sharp pain is not as effectively relieved by the opioids.

TABLE 28-2. Comparison of the narcotic analgesics

Level of pain	Drug	Equivalent analgesic dose (mg) given IM or SC	Time for peak effect (min)	Duration (hr)	Schedule
Severe	Morphine	10	30 to 90	Up to 7	II
	Hydromorphone hydrochloride (Dilaudid)	1.5	30 to 90	4 to 5	II
	Oxymorphone (Numorphan)	1 to 1.5	30 to 90	36	II
	Levorphanol tartrate (Levo-Dromoran)	2 to 3	60 to 90	58	II
	Methadone (Dolophine)	7.5 to 10	60 to 120	3 to 6	II
Moderate to severe	Alphaprodine (Nisentil)	40 to 60	30	1 to 2	II
	Anileridine (Leritine)	25 to 30	30 to 60	2 to 3	II
	Butorphanol (Stadol)	1.5 to 3.5	30	3 to 4	N.S.*
	Meperidine (Demerol)	75 to 100	30 to 60	2 to 4	II
	Nalbuphine (Nubain)	10	30	3 to 6	N.S.*
	Pentazocine (Talwin)	40 to 60	30 to 60	2 to 3	IV
Mild to moderate	Codeine phosphate	120	60 to 90	4 to 6	II
	Propoxyphene (Darvon)	180 to 240	60	4 to 6	IV

*N.S., Not yet scheduled as a controlled substance.

■ Opioids effective for relieving severe pain

(Table 28-3)

Morphine

Morphine has already been described as the prototype for the opioids. Chemically morphine is a base that is positively charged at the pH's in the gastrointestinal tract and therefore is not readily absorbed when taken orally. Furthermore, morphine is readily metabolized within the gut and by the liver. For these reasons, morphine is given intramuscularly or subcutaneously. Elderly patients usually require a smaller dose because they do not metabolize morphine as readily as do younger patients.

Morphine or meperidine is used to treat the pain of an acute myocardial infarction (heart attack). At analgesic doses morphine not only relieves the pain but also reduces the anxiety without altering the cardiovascular system. If undue reduction in respiration, heart rate, or blood pressure does occur secondary to morphine administration, these can be reversed by administering naloxone, the narcotic antagonist.

Morphine is the drug of choice to treat pulmonary edema. The beneficial actions of morphine include relief of anxiety and vasodilation, which reduces the work load of the heart so that the heart pumps more efficiently. This increased cardiac efficiency relieves the pulmonary edema that arises when the left side of the heart cannot adequately pump out the blood being supplied by the pulmonary veins. This inefficiency gives rise to hypertension and edema in the pulmonary system.

Hydromorphone

Hydromorphone (Dilaudid) is a semisynthetic derivative of morphine. It is more potent but shorter acting than morphine. Oral doses require more time to become effective but are longer acting than parenteral doses. The actions of hydromorphone are identical to those of morphine.

Oxymorphone

Oxymorphone (Numorphan) is a semisynthetic derivative of morphine that has all the actions of morphine except the antitussive (cough suppressant) action. Oxymorphone is more potent than morphine but must also be given by injection.

TABLE 28-3. Narcotic analgesics

Generic name	Trade name	Dosage and administration	Comments
Alphaprodine hydrochloride	Nisentil	SUBCUTANEOUS: *Adults and children over 12 yr*—0.4 to 1.2 mg/kg body weight not to exceed 240 mg in 24 hr. INTRAVENOUS: *Adults and children over 12 yr*—0.4 to 0.6 mg/kg body weight not to exceed 240 mg in 24 hr. Not for children under 12 yr.	Not for oral or intramuscular administration. When intravenous route is used, a narcotic antagonist and resuscitation equipment should be available, since respiration may be severely depressed. Schedule II substance.
Anileridine hydrochloride or phosphate	Leritine	ORAL: *Adults*—25 to 50 mg every 4 to 6 hr. INTRAMUSCULAR, SUBCUTANEOUS: *Adults*—25 to 50 mg up to 75 to 100 mg every 4 to 6 hr but no more than 200 mg in 24 hr. INTRAVENOUS, for use during anesthesia: 50 to 100 mg in 500 ml 5% dextrose solution, no faster than 0.6 mg/min (3 to 6 ml/min).	Schedule II substance.
Butorphanol tartrate	Stadol	INTRAMUSCULAR: *Adults*—1 to 4 mg every 3 to 4 hr. INTRAVENOUS: *Adults*—0.5 to 2 mg every 3 to 4 hr.	A new drug, not currently classified as a controlled substance.
Codeine sulfate, codeine phosphate		ORAL, INTRAMUSCULAR, SUBCUTANEOUS: *Adults*—30 to 60 mg every 4 to 6 hr. *Children*—0.5 mg/kg body weight every 4 to 6 hr.	Not for severe pain. Schedule II substance.
Hydromorphone hydrochloride	Dilaudid	ORAL: *Adult*—2 mg every 4 to 6 hr. INTRAMUSCULAR, SUBCUTANEOUS: *Adult*—1 to 1.5 mg every 4 to 6 hr. May be given by slow intravenous injection or as a suppository.	Schedule II substance.
Levorphanol tartrate	Levo-Dromoran	ORAL, SUBCUTANEOUS: *Adults*—2 mg.	Schedule II substance.
Meperidine hydrochloride	Demerol	ORAL, INTRAMUSCULAR, SUBCUTANEOUS, SLOW INTRAVENOUS: *Adults*—50 to 150 mg every 3 to 4 hr. *Children*—1 to 1.5 mg/kg body weight, maximum 100 mg, every 3 to 4 hr.	Schedule II substance.
Methadone hydrochloride	Dolophine Westadone	ORAL, INTRAMUSCULAR, SUBCUTANEOUS: *Adults*—2.5 to 10 mg. For pain relief, repeat every 6 hr.	Used as a replacement drug for opiate dependence or to facilitate withdrawal. Schedule II substance.
Morphine sulfate		ORAL: *Adults*—5 to 15 mg every 4 hr. INTRAMUSCULAR, SUBCUTANEOUS: *Adults*—5 to 20 mg every 4 hr. *Children* (subcutaneous only)—0.1 to 0.2 mg/kg body weight, maximum 15 mg. INTRAVENOUS: *Adults*—2.5 to 15 mg in 5 ml water, injected over 4 to 5 min. *Children*—0.1 to 0.2 mg/kg body weight.	Not well absorbed orally. Schedule II substance.

Continued.

TABLE 28-3. Narcotic analgesics—cont'd

Generic name	Trade name	Dosage and administration	Comments
Nalbuphine hydrochloride	Nubain	INTRAMUSCULAR, SUBCUTANEOUS, INTRAVENOUS: *Adults*—10 mg every 3 to 6 hr, maximum single dose 20 mg and maximum daily dose 160 mg.	Possesses both agonist and antagonist properties. A new drug, not classified as a controlled substance.
Oxymorphone hydrochloride	Numorphan	INTRAMUSCULAR, SUBCUTANEOUS: *Adults*—1 to 1.5 mg every 6 hr. INTRAVENOUS: *Adults*—0.5 mg. RECTAL: *Adults*—5 mg every 4 to 6 hr.	Schedule II substance.
Pentazocine hydrochloride	Talwin 50	ORAL: *Adults*—50 mg every 3 to 4 hr, maximum daily dose 600 mg.	Possesses both agonist and antagonist properties. Schedule IV substance.
Pentazocine lactate	Talwin Lactate	INTRAMUSCULAR, SUBCUTANEOUS, INTRAVENOUS: *Adults*—30 mg every 3 to 4 hr. Subcutaneous route is not recommended, may cause tissue damage.	
Propoxyphene hydrochloride	Darvon Dolene SK-65	ORAL: *Adults*—65 mg every 6 to 8 hr.	Schedule IV substance.
Propoxyphene napsylate	Darvon-N	ORAL: *Adults*—100 mg every 6 to 8 hr.	Schedule IV substance.

Levorphanol

Levorphanol (Levo-Dromoran) is an opioid that has actions identical to those of morphine. The effective dose of levorphanol is about one-fourth that of morphine.

Methadone

Methadone (Dolophine) is an opioid with actions similar to those of morphine. Methadone can be taken orally. Although the onset of action for a single analgesic dose of methadone is similar to that for morphine, methadone is highly protein bound and not readily metabolized. Methadone has a half-life of 25 hours.

Methadone, 40 to 120 mg daily, substitutes for other opioids in drug-dependent individuals and prevents withdrawal symptoms as discussed earlier. Methadone is currently used in the treatment of opioid dependency because it is effective orally and because only one dose per day is necessary. Also the long plasma half-life of methadone more easily allows the gradual reduction in dose without the appearance of side effects.

■ Opioids effective in relieving moderate to severe pain (Table 28-3)

Meperidine

Meperidine (Demerol) was the first of the synthetic narcotic analgesics. It is shorter acting than morphine and does not have an antitussive effect. Meperidine is widely used for obstetrical analgesia. To minimize respiratory depression in the infant, meperidine should be administered intramuscularly late in labor, within 1 hour of birth. Meperidine differs from morphine because high doses are excitatory and can cause convulsions.

Alphaprodine

Alphaprodine (Nisentil) is an opioid chemically related to meperidine but with a more rapid onset and shorter duration of action. Its use is primarily in situations in which the brief duration is desirable.

Anileridine

Anileridine (Leritine) is an opioid chemically related to meperidine. Anileridine is effective orally or parenterally and has a slightly shorter duration of action than meperidine.

Butorphanol

Butorphanol (Stadol) is a new opioid related to levorphanol. Since butorphanol has both agonist and antagonist properties, it may be less likely to produce tolerance and drug dependence than the older drugs. In general the actions of butorphanol resemble those of morphine except that butorphanol increases pulmonary arterial pressure and the cardiac work load, making this drug undesirable for treating the pain of a myocardial infarction or pulmonary edema.

Nalbuphine

Nalbuphine (Nubain) is a semisynthetic derivative of morphine that has both agonist and antagonist properties. The uses and limitations of nalbuphine are primarily those of meperidine or morphine. Nalbuphine may be preferable for treating the pain of a myocardial infarction, since nalbuphine appears to reduce the oxygen needs of the heart without reducing blood pressure. Nalbuphine is a stronger antagonist than pentazocine, suggesting that the degree of tolerance and drug dependence for nalbuphine should be low. However, withdrawal symptoms are seen when nalbuphine is abruptly discontinued, and nalbuphine causes withdrawal symptoms when administered to an individual already dependent on one of the more common narcotic analgesics.

Pentazocine

Pentazocine (Talwin) is an opioid with weak antagonist properties. For several years after pentazocine was introduced it was not believed to produce drug dependency. Pentazocine is now a Schedule IV drug, reflecting a low potential for producing drug dependency. Pentazocine does cause respiratory depression in the fetus when used in obstetrics. Unlike morphine, pentazocine increases blood pressure and cardiac work, properties that make pentazocine less desirable than morphine for treating the pain of myocardial infarction or pulmonary hypertension. Pentazocine causes a dysphoria rather than a euphoria. This dysphoria can include nightmares, feelings of depersonalization, and visual hallucinations. Large doses induce seizures. Although there are reports of individuals with a drug dependency for pentazocine, administration of pentazocine to an individual dependent on the usual narcotic analgesics will result in withdrawal symptoms because of the antagonistic properties of pentazocine.

Propiram

Propiram (Dirame) is a new opioid under investigational use. It is chemically unrelated to other opioids. It has only slight antagonistic activity, and its agonist activities are similar to those of morphine. Propiram is effective orally or parenterally and should be handled with the same precautions as the opiate analgesics.

■ Opioids effective in relieving mild pain

(Table 28-3)

Codeine

Codeine is not administered in doses large enough to be as effective as morphine because the high dose required to produce an equal degree of analgesia results in a high incidence of side effects. An oral dose of 32 or 65 mg of codeine is equivalent to 2 aspirin tablets (650 mg). At these low doses codeine seldom produces side effects. At high doses the side effects of codeine are similar to those of morphine.

Codeine causes significant histamine release if given intravenously, so codeine is given only intramuscularly or orally. A portion of a codeine dose is metabolized to morphine in the liver. Codeine is a Schedule II drug in analgesic doses. Codeine is also formulated with the nonnarcotic analgesics for pain relief, and these are usually Schedule III drugs. Codeine is an effective cough suppressant at low doses and is available for this purpose in dilute solutions as a Schedule V drug.

Propoxyphene

Propoxyphene (Darvon) is an opioid related to methadone. Propoxyphene is not a very potent analgesic. Propoxyphene at a dose of 65 mg is the analgesic equivalent of 2 tablets (650 mg) of aspirin or acetaminophen. Propoxyphene is commonly prescribed in combination with one of the nonnarcotic analgesics. Propoxyphene, alone or in combination, is a Schedule IV drug. Side effects are not common at analgesic doses. Propoxyphene has a low abuse potential but has been implicated as a cause of death when abused in combination with alcohol and other central nervous system depressant drugs.

■ Treatment of chronic pain

The use of opioids in treating chronic pain is only indicated for terminal cancer, since tolerance to the opioids will limit the effectiveness of these drugs in nontoxic doses. Even in treating the pain associated with terminal cancer, a case in which drug dependency is irrelevant, special care must be used to keep the dose as low as possible to prolong the effectiveness of the drug and to keep the patient alert. The opioids with low dependency liability are used first, and the total comfort of the patient is considered. A combination of drugs may be used to lessen the dose of a strong narcotic analgesic needed and thereby prolong the duration of effectiveness. One combination of drugs for oral administration that receive publicity is "Brompton's cocktail," consisting of heroin (morphine in the United States), cocaine, a phenothiazine, and ethyl alcohol. However, recent studies indicate that this combination may be no more effective than oral morphine alone.

■ THE NURSING PROCESS FOR THE USE OF OPIOIDS

■ Assessment

Narcotic analgesics are used primarily in the patient complaining of pain from any cause. The data base from which the nurse should begin the development of the plan for patient care should include information from a detailed discussion with the patient of the history, nature, and location of the pain. Objective data about the patient's position, facial expression, medical history, vital signs, and age are helpful. A brief neurological examination should be done. It is not possible to determine the patient's severity of pain by knowing only isolated facts such as what an injury looks like or the "usual" response of patients to a specific painful procedure or surgery; the subjective component of the pain is very important.

■ Management

Regular use of opioids at identified intervals around the clock usually provides better relief of pain than use on a p.r.n. (as needed) basis. Clarifying reasonable, possible goals of analgesic therapy with the patient will help to bring pain under control. No patient who needs medication for pain should be denied pharmacological assistance, but the professional nurse also employs other nursing care measures to promote comfort, including positioning, distracting, and touching the patient as well as introducing relaxation techniques. The patient care plan should include careful descriptions of what does or does not work in any specific patient. The possibility of addiction to these drugs should not be forgotten but should be kept in perspective. During administration of opioids, the nurse should monitor the vital signs, the level of consciousness, and the frequency of bowel movements and should check for nausea and vomiting and for urinary retention. Some side effects will necessitate discontinuing therapy, decreasing the dose, or using additional kinds of treatments. Narcotic antagonists should be available. If antiemetics or other drugs are ordered, monitor for the side effects of these drugs; also check compatibilities before administering two or more drugs in the same syringe. When using the opioids via the intravenous route, resuscitation equipment should be readily available, and a microdrip administration set and an infusion monitoring device should be used for constant intravenous infusion.

■ Evaluation

Ideally treatment with opioids results in relief of pain with no side effects, but this is not often possible. Usually the treatment is considered effective if the pain or its perception is lessened. The side effects that occur are treated if they interfere with the level of functioning appropriate for the patient. When the therapeutic goals specific for the patient are considered, the evaluation of the effectiveness will be easier. For example, to achieve pain relief one patient with cancer might not consider drug-induced drowsiness unpleasant whereas a second patient might. Before discharge, the patient should be able to explain the name and dose of drugs to be taken, the possible side effects that might occur and how to treat them, the signs indicating too large a dose, what to do if the pain worsens, and what drugs to avoid. The patient should be able to state that alcohol should be avoided while these drugs are being taken. For additional specific guidelines, see the patient care implications section.

■ Role of opioids in anesthesia

Additional uses of opioids include preanesthetic medication and surgical anesthesia. As a preanesthetic medication, the opioids relieve anxiety and provide sedation so that the patient is not in a fearful state before surgery. The more potent analgesics, morphine, meperidine, fentanyl, and hydromorphone, are widely used as components of surgical anesthesia with nitrous oxide. Nitrous oxide by itself is not potent enough for surgical anesthesia but is potentiated by a narcotic analgesic. A muscle relaxant such as tubocurarine is also used. This combination of an opioid, nitrous oxide, and a muscle relaxant is called "balanced anesthesia" (Chapter 29). The duration of anesthesia is controlled by the duration of action of the opioid used.

■ PATIENT CARE IMPLICATIONS

Narcotic analgesics

1. Although narcotic analgesics represent one of the most useful classes of medications available, they are also drugs with the potential for serious undesirable side effects and abuse. Because most narcotic analgesics are ordered on an "as needed" (p.r.n.) basis, it is important that health care personnel learn to assess each patient with sensitivity and objectivity. In addition, knowledge of the effects of each individual medication the patient is receiving should assist health care personnel in making the decision whether to administer a medication.
2. The meaning of pain to an individual is a complex process, influenced by heredity, culture, environment, expectations, diagnosis, location, previous experiences with pain, and other factors. This text can only address a few aspects of pain relief. The reader is referred to other sources listed in the suggested readings.
3. Administration of a narcotic analgesic is only one way to decrease a patient's discomfort. Remember that providing comfort can be aided by such activities as repositioning patients, straightening the sheets, touching, listening, providing food, drink, or reassurance, or even simply stopping by a patient's room frequently so the patient does not feel alone. Too often, the administration of a narcotic is substituted for other comfort measures.
4. Pain in the nonalert patient may be manifested by restlessness, increase in blood pressure or pulse, sweating, and facial grimaces. Patients who are unable to speak may have to depend on an alert health care provider to assess the need for pain medication.
5. Explain to the patient what results can reasonably be expected from the medications being taken and enlist the patient's aid in determining the best combination of drugs to be used in any anticipated situation. For example, some patients have a variety of p.r.n. medications available, including a narcotic analgesic, a less potent oral or nonnarcotic analgesic, an antiemetic, a mild tranquilizer, and a sedative-hypnotic. Each of these has advantages and disadvantages, but when given at the same time or too close together, might have serious side effects (e.g., hypotension, sedation, respiratory depression). Patients should not be denied appropriate pharmacological help, but neither should health care personnel overmedicate a patient through poor planning or lack of knowledge.
6. Although the theoretical possibility of narcotic addiction exists for all patients who receive narcotic analgesics, in fact only a very small percentage of patients do become dependent. Patients who persist in requesting frequent or large doses of pain medication beyond the "average time" postoperatively should not be automatically characterized as becoming addicted. Pain is a warning signal, and its unexpected persistence should be investigated. If it is suspected that the patient is becoming addicted, the health care team should plan as a group an individualized approach to the problem.
7. Some postoperative patients fear requesting any medication for pain because they fear addiction. Reassure patients that use of narcotics in decreasing amounts over 3 or 4 days will not cause addiction and that recovery will be easier if severe pain can be lessened.
8. Not all cancer patients have severe pain, and early in the course of the disease, many patients have no pain. If and when a patient with cancer begins to have pain, the choice of analgesic should be based on individual patient assessment and should begin with nonnarcotic analgesics, if possible. For many patients, high doses of aspirin may be adequate initially, and as this becomes ineffective, combination products with aspirin or acetaminophen and a mild narcotic (e.g., propoxyphene combinations, oxycodone combinations) can be tried. Finally, potent narcotic analgesics, either alone or in combination with antiemetics or tranquilizers, may be used.
9. The constraints influencing the use of analgesics with cancer patients are different than with other pain problems. The possibility of patient addiction is irrelevant with terminal cancer patients. Rather the goal should be pain relief, or at least lessening of the pain, but without serious side effects or marked sedation. Thus narcotic analgesics may relieve the pain, but their early use in the course of cancer treatment can cause an otherwise functional and active patient to become markedly sedated, to require higher and higher doses of narcotics, and to become less independent and functional. Recently time and effort have been directed at developing oral liquid combinations of a narcotic with one or more other medications in a fruit-flavored base. The original mixture, Brompton's cocktail, has been modified into many other combinations. The advantages of these oral preparations are that they can produce analgesia, often without marked sedation; can be modified to include other medications a patient might need (e.g., an antiemetic); are more easily taken than pills or injections, especially on an out-

patient basis; and the dose of narcotic needed by the patient can be adjusted easily.

10. Health care personnel should be knowledgeable about the component parts of all analgesic preparations they administer, and there are many combination products in use. For example, Tylox and Percocet both contain acetaminophen and oxycodone; Empirin compound with codeine previously contained aspirin, phenacetin, caffeine, and codeine, but now contains only aspirin and codeine; Mepergan Fortis contains meperidine and promethazine.
11. Narcotic overdose may be manifested by respiratory depression with a decreased rate of breathing, Cheyne-Stokes respirations, or cyanosis; cold, clammy skin; sleepiness progressing to stupor or coma; hypotension; and skeletal muscle flaccidity.
12. Other side effects of narcotic use may include flushing, palpitations, syncope, pruritus, rashes, urticaria, dry mouth, anorexia, and a variety of central nervous system effects, including euphoria, dysphoria, headache, insomnia, agitation, disorientation, and visual disturbances. Many narcotics will cause pain at intramuscular injection sites.
13. Narcotic antagonists, oxygen, and resuscitation equipment should be available whenever narcotic analgesics are regularly used.
14. Narcotic analgesics provide better pain relief if taken before pain becomes severe. For this reason, a pain medication is more effective if taken 30 to 60 minutes before a dressing change, ambulation, wound debridement, or other painful activity.
15. Because pain interferes with sleep and rest, can increase anxiety, and can decrease a patient's willingness to perform needed postoperative activities (turning, coughing, deep breathing), narcotics should be given every 4 hours (or as ordered) around the clock during the first 24 hours after major surgery. This decision, of course, should still be based on the individual patient's response.
16. Because of cough suppression and respiratory depression caused by anesthesia and narcotic analgesics, postoperative patients should be turned and made to cough and breathe deeply every 2 hours to prevent pulmonary complications.
17. If nausea and vomiting occur, it may be possible to administer an antiemetic with the analgesic. Although this reduces nausea, it may also potentiate hypotension and sedation.
18. Constipation can be a severe problem for patients taking narcotic analgesics. When possible, patients should be ambulated as soon as possible and frequently. Fluid intake should be increased to 2500 to 3000 ml per day. The diet should include a variety of vegetables, fruits, and fiber, if possible. It may be necessary to use cathartics and/or stool softeners in patients receiving narcotics on a long-term basis.
19. The elderly or patients receiving narcotic analgesics in moderate to large doses should be assisted to ambulate, and the blood pressure should be monitored every 4 hours. Keep the siderails up while the patient is in bed.
20. Narcotics should be used cautiously, if at all, in patients with chronic obstructive lung disease or asthma because of the possible respiratory depression that can occur. Monitor the respiratory rate, auscultate breath sounds, and if necessary, measure the tidal volume if concerned about an individual patient's response.
21. Patients receiving narcotic analgesics may have a decreased urge to void. Monitor the intake and output. Remind patients to void every 4 hours if they have not. Notify the physician if a patient with an adequate intake is unable to void in 8 hours.
22. Potent narcotic analgesics are not used in head injury or suspected head injury patients because of sedation and the possibility of an altered level of consciousness, respiratory depression, alteration in pupillary response, and the increased intracranial pressure that can result from the narcotics. Explain this to patients and family who may not understand why stronger medications are not being used to lessen the pain when there is an injured head.
23. For the hospitalized patient in severe pain, narcotics are sometimes ordered IV. In some situations, it is desirable to administer the dose via direct intravenous injection (IV push), such as for morphine in a patient experiencing an acute myocardial infarction. Often it may be desirable to infuse the medication slowly over 30 or more minutes. For slow infusion, dilute the medication as directed by the pharmacy, use a microdrip infusion set and/or a volume control device, and if appropriate, consider the use of an electronic infusion monitoring device. Calculation of the infusion rate is important. Too rapid infusion of a narcotic, whether by direct infusion or diluted, may produce marked sedation, hypotension, respiratory depression, circulatory collapse, and death. Monitor the vital signs, and slow or stop the infusion if undesirable side effects begin to occur. If an ordered dose for intravenous infusion seems excessively high, do not hesitate to question the physician.
24. Discharge teaching for any patient being sent home while taking analgesics needs to be individualized. The patient should be taught the name of the drug, the frequency with which it may be taken, what side effects may occur and what to do about them, and what to do if the pain worsens.

25. Although all medications should be kept out of the reach of children, it is especially important that adults keep narcotic analgesics out of the way to avoid overdose and death in children.
26. Patients taking narcotic analgesics on an outpatient basis should be warned that the drug may cause drowsiness and should be used with caution when it is necessary to be alert, such as for driving or operating machinery.
27. Patients should avoid the use of the central nervous system depressants (including tranquilizers, sedative-hypnotics, narcotic analgesics, and alcohol) while taking narcotic analgesics unless specific drugs and doses have been cleared by the physician.
28. The use of narcotic analgesics during pregnancy should be avoided unless the benefits outweigh the risks. Instruct the patient to discuss this with her physician.
29. Administer pentazocine with caution to patients dependent on narcotics, because the narcotic-antagonist properties of the pentazocine may precipitate narcotic withdrawal symptoms.
30. Meperidine should not be used in patients taking monoamine oxidase inhibitors or patients who have taken them within the previous 2 weeks. Meperidine may precipitate an unpredictable and occasionally fatal reaction.
31. Meperidine syrup should be taken in a glass of water, because when diluted, the syrup may cause temporary mucous membrane anesthesia.

Narcotic antagonists

1. In patients with suspected narcotic overdose, oxygen and resuscitation equipment should be available.
2. Monitor the vital signs frequently (every 5 to 15 minutes) until the patient's condition stabilizes after administration of a narcotic antagonist. The patient should not be left unattended. The effects of the narcotic antagonist may wear off before the effects of the narcotic does, and it may be necessary to repeat the dose.
3. No drug overdose should be treated lightly. If possible, the patient's condition should be checked by a cardiac monitor. The vital signs should be carefully monitored, as well as intake and output. Intubation equipment should be nearby, as well as suctioning equipment.

■ SUMMARY

Opioids, familiarly called narcotic analgesics, blunt the subjective reaction to pain by raising the threshold for pain perception, reducing anxiety and fear, and inducing sleep. Morphine is the prototypical opioid. Opioids mimic endorphins, naturally occurring polypeptides that serve as neurotransmitters for a number of functions including analgesia. Other characteristic actions of morphine include respiratory depression, cough suppression, nausea and vomiting, depression of gut motility, depression of gastric, biliary, and pancreatic secretions, urinary retention, hypotension, and constricted pupils.

Drug tolerance readily develops to the opioids, and in particular, the lethal dose for respiratory depression increases with tolerance. However, opioids enhance the respiratory depression of other drug classes. Drug dependency is characterized by a distinct abstinence syndrome when the drug is discontinued. The opioid abstinence syndrome is treated in the United States with methadone, an orally active, long-acting opioid. Methadone can be used for maintenance or for detoxification.

Overdose of an opioid is best treated with naloxone, a specific opiate receptor antagonist, which reverses the opioid-induced respiratory depression.

Over a dozen opioids are in use as analgesics. These are used to treat pain associated with surgery, broken bones, dental procedures, and obstetrics. Selected cardiovascular actions make morphine and butorphanol useful in treating pulmonary edema and morphine and nalbuphine useful in treating the pain of a heart attack. Opioids are also used as preanesthetic medication and as one component of "balanced anesthesia." Opioids are not used for chronic pain except in treating the pain of terminal cancer.

■ STUDY QUESTIONS

1. What are the two components of pain? Which is affected by opioids?
2. What are endorphins? What are enkephalins and what actions do they mediate?
3. What are the three characteristics of the analgesia produced by morphine?
4. What are the three major actions of morphine in the medulla?
5. What actions does morphine have on tissues outside the central nervous system?
6. What are five common adverse reactions to morphine?
7. Describe the abstinence syndrome for opioids.
8. What properties of methadone make it useful for maintaining or withdrawing from opioid dependence?
9. Why is naloxone a better drug for treating acute opioid toxicity than nalorphine or levallorphan?
10. What are the five opioids used to relieve severe pain?
11. What are the seven opioids used to relieve moderate pain?
12. What are the two opioids used to relieve mild pain?
13. Which opioids have antagonist as well as agonist activity?
14. Which opioids play a special role in treating pulmonary edema? pain of a heart attack?
15. When are opioids used to treat chronic pain?
16. What role do opioids have in anesthesia?

■ SUGGESTING READINGS

Aronoff, G.M., Wilson, R.R., and Sample, S.S.: Treating chronic pain: the team approach, Journal of Nursing Care **11:**12, 1978.

Bonica, J.J.: Cancer pain: a major national health problem, Cancer Nursing **1**(8):313, 1978.

DiBlasi, M., and Washburn, C.J.: Using analgesics effectively, Amercan Journal of Nursing **79**(1):74, 1979.

Dole, V.P.: Addictive behavior, Scientific American **243:**138, 1980.

Donovan, C.T.: Chronic pain management: transition from hospital to home, Nurses Drug Alert **3**(special report):145, Dec, 1979.

Eddy, N.B., and May, E.L.: The search for a better analgesic, Science **181:**407, 1973.

Fagerbaugh, S.Y., and Strauss, A.: Politics of pain management. Menlo Park, Calif., Addison-Wesley Publishing Co., 1977.

Fordyce, W.E.: Evaluating and managing chronic pain, Geriatrics **33**(1):59, 1978.

Gever, L.N.: Brompton's mixture: how it relieves the pain of terminal cancer, Nursing '80 **10**(5):57, 1980.

Goldfrank, M.D., and Bresnitz, E.: Opioids, Hospital Physician **14**(10):26, 1978.

Goldstein, A.: Opioid peptides (endrophins) in pituitary and brain, Science **193:**1081, 1976.

Grad, R.K., and Woodside, J.: Obstetrical analgesics and anesthesia: methods of relief for the patient in labor, American Journal of Nursing **77:**242, 1977.

Houde, R.W.: The rational use of narcotic analgesics for controlling cancer pain, Drug Therapy **10**(7):41, 1980.

Jacox, A.K., editor: Pain: a sourcebook for nurses and other health professionals, Boston, 1977, Little, Brown and Co.

Jacox, A.K.: Assessing pain, American Journal of Nursing **79:**895, 1979.

Kissin, B., Lowinson, J.H., and Millman, R.B.: Recent developments in chemotherapy of narcotic addiction, Annals of the New York Academy of Science **31k:**59, 1978.

Lipman, A.G.: Drug therapy in cancer pain, Cancer Nursing **3**(2): 39, 1980.

Lipton. S., editor: Persistent pain: modern methods of treatment, New York, 1977, Grune & Stratton, Inc.

Luce, J.M., Thompson, T.L., Getto, C.J., and Byyny, R.L.: New concepts of chronic pain and their implications, Hospital Practice **14:**113, 1979.

Marx, J.L.: Opiate receptors: implications and applications, Science **189:**708, 1975.

Narx, J.L.: Neurobiology: researchers high on endogenous opiates, Science **193:**1227, 1976.

Marx, J.L.: Analgesia: how the body inhibits pain perception, Science **195:**471, 1977.

Maxwell, M.B.: How to use methadone for the cancer patient's pain, American Journal of Nursing **80**(9):1606, 1980.

McCaffery, M.: Pain relief for the child, Pediatric Nursing **3**(4):11, 1977.

McCaffery, M.: Nursing management of the patient with pain, ed. 2, Philadelphia, 1979, J.B. Lippincott Co.

McCaffery, M.: Understanding your patient's pain, Nursing '80 **10**(5):57, 1980.

McCaffery, M.: Patients shouldn't have to suffer: how to relieve pain with injectable narcotics, Nursing '80 **10**(10):34, 1980.

McCaffery, M.: How to relieve your patients' pain fast and effectively . . . with oral analgesics, Nursing '80 **10**(11):58, 1980.

McMahon, M.A., and Miller, P.: Pain response: the influence of psycho-social-cultural factors, Nursing Forum **7**(1):58, 1978.

Neaderthal, R.L., and Calabro, J.J.: Treating heroin overdose, American Family Physician **11**(2):141, 1975.

Neal, H.: The politics of pain, New York, 1978, McGraw-Hill Book Co.

O'Neal, J.T.: Managing chronic pain, American Family Physician **10**(6):75, 1974.

Pace, J.B.: Helping patients overcome the disabling effects of chronic pain, Nursing '77 **7**(7):38, 1977.

Practical psychiatry in medicine. Part 10. Drug abuse and the addictions, Journal of Family Practice **6:**911, 1978.

Rogers, A.G.: Pharmacology of analgesics, Journal of Neurosurgical Nursing **10**(12):180, 1978.

Roland, E.J.: Nursing care for patients with pain, AORN Journal **27:**1180, 1978.

Sandoval, R.G., and Wang, R.I.H.: Narcotics and narcotic antagonists in clinical practice, Drug Therapy **1**(11):41, 1971.

Silman, J.: The management of pain. Reference guide to analgesics, American Journal of Nursing **79:**74, 1979.

Smith, R.J.: Federal government faces painful decision on Darvon, Science **203:**857, 1979.

Snyder, S.H.: Opiate receptors and internal opiates, Scientific American **236:**44, 1977.

Storlie, F.: Pointers for assessing pain, Nursing '78 **8**(5):37, 1978.

Valentine, A.S., Steckel, S., and Weintraub, M.: Pain relief for cancer patients, American Journal of Nursing **78:**2054, 1978.

Vandam, L.D.: Analgesic drugs—the potent analgesics, New England Journal of Medicine **286:**249, 1972.

29 General anesthetics

Modern surgery did not really begin until the introduction of nitrous oxide, ether, and chloroform as general anesthetics in the middle 1800's. The agents used today as general anesthetics include gases (nitrous oxide and cyclopropane), volatile liquids (diethyl ether, halothane, methoxyflurane, enflurane, and isoflurane), and intravenous agents (ketamine and narcotic analgesics). The ultrashort-acting barbiturates and benzodiazepines are used intravenously for induction of anesthesia.

■ MECHANISM OF ACTION

■ Lack of receptor mechanism

General anesthetics act on the central nervous system to abolish the patient's perception of pain and reaction to painful stimuli. The general anesthetics are unusual in their mechanism of action because they do not appear to act by a receptor mechanism. Instead general anesthetics are believed to alter the lipid structure of cell membranes so that physiological functions are impaired. The network of neurons making up the central nervous system is especially vulnerable because alteration of membrane structure interrupts the complex intercommunication necessary for function. The most sensitive system to such alterations is the ascending reticular activating system, the neuronal formation monitoring incoming stimuli from the body and determining what information is to be passed up to the brain for processing and response. Consciousness is lost when the ascending reticular activating system ceases to transmit information effectively.

■ Stages of anesthesia

For many years the general anesthetics have been classified purely as general central nervous system depressants, as discussed with the sedative-hypnotic drugs in Chapter 24. This scheme is diagrammed in Fig. 29-1. According to this scheme, the stages of anesthesia represent the increasing depression of the central nervous system and are labelled as follows:

Stage I: analgesia
Stage II: excitement (or delirium)
Stage III: surgical anesthesia
Stage IV: medullary paralysis

These stages represent what is observed in patients anesthetized with diethyl ether in the absence of other medication, a practice quite obsolete. Nevertheless, it is useful to review this classification.

Stage I (analgesia) begins with a conscious patient and ends when the patient is unconscious. This is the lightest stage of anesthesia, but the degree of analgesia is sufficient for some dental procedures and for the second stage of labor.

Stage II (excitement or delirium) represents a removal of the inhibition of the lower brain centers by the higher centers and is manifested by activity such as involuntary movement of the limbs, an irregular pattern of breathing, and pupillary dilatation. This stage is undesirable because reflex responses such as laryngospasm may begin, which are injurious or dangerous to the patient. The brief second stage of anesthesia during induction of anesthesia with inhalation anesthetics is the least stable and most dangerous period of anesthesia. This stage is less prominent with modern anesthetics such as halothane and enflurane, which induce anesthesia more rapidly than does ether, which has a very long induction time. In modern anesthetic practice, an induction agent such as an ultrashort-acting barbiturate is used for induction of anesthesia to bypass stage II altogether.

Stage III (surgical anesthesia) represents the gradual loss of muscle tone and reflexes as the central nervous system is further depressed. Not all anesthetics produce good muscle relaxation, so a muscle relaxant is commonly used. This stage ends as the muscles controlling

FIG. 29-1

This diagram of central nervous system excitation and depression demonstrates how drugs have been described as either causing stimulation or causing depression. The classic description of anesthesia is as a pure depressant action on the central nervous system. The four stages of anesthesia included in this diagram are those originally described for diethyl ether. (From Winter, W.: Effects of drugs on the electrical activity of the brain: anesthetics. Reproduced, with permission, from the Annual Review of Pharmacology and Toxicology **16:**413, 1976. © 1976 by Annual Reviews Inc.)

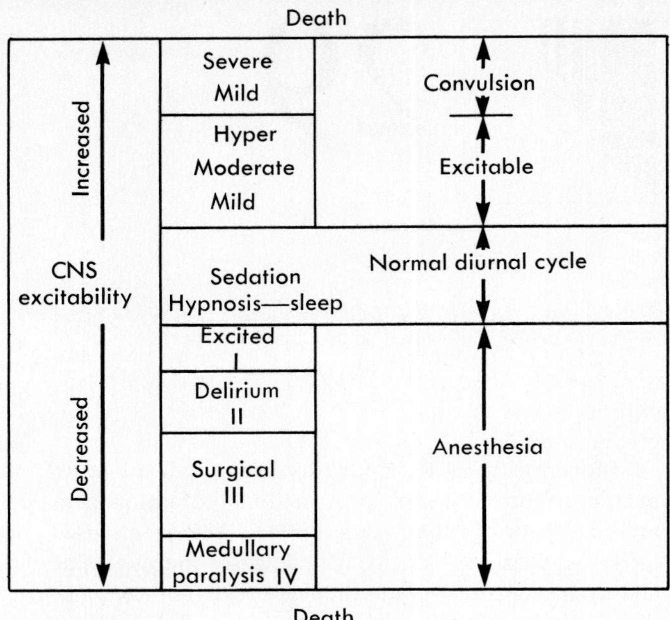

FIG 29-2

Winters has determined brain wave patterns of cats under anesthesia. Anesthesia is pictured as arising from central nervous system stimulation (ketamine) or depression (barbiturates). Each anesthetic produces its own characteristic pattern of central nervous system stimulation and depression. For instance, diethyl ether produces the pattern I ↔ II ↔ III ↔ IV, which includes both stimulant and depressant stages. (From Winter, W.: Effects of drugs on the electrical activity of the brain: anesthetics. Reproduced, with permission, from the Annual Review of Pharmacology and Toxicology **16:**413, 1976. © 1976 by Annual Reviews Inc.)

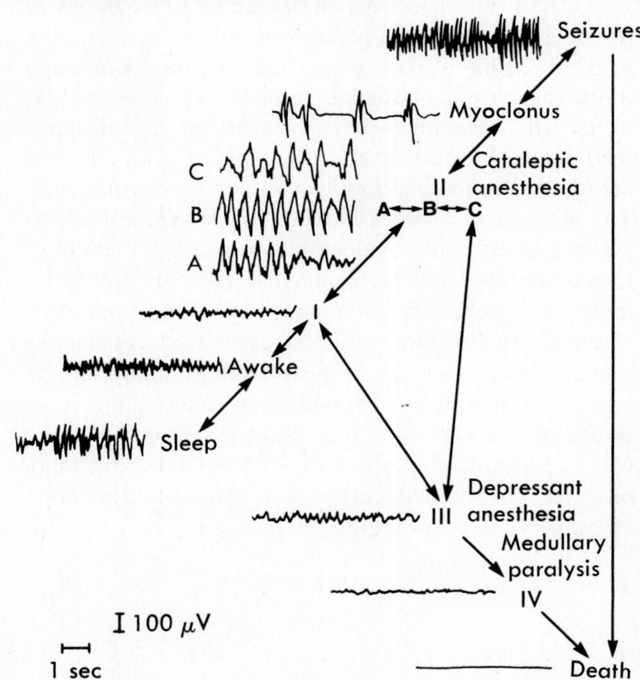

breathing are paralyzed, the intercostal muscles controlling the rib cage being paralyzed first followed by the diaphragm.

Stage IV (medullary paralysis) is the toxic state of anesthesia, characterized by the loss of spontaneous breathing and collapse of the cardiovascular system.

■ Stages of anesthesia based on brain wave patterns

Recently, Winter has proposed a new scheme for describing general anesthetics. This scheme is diagrammed in Fig. 29-2 and is based on brain wave patterns (electroencephalogram or EEG) observed during anesthesia. The concept of a correlation between surface electrode EEG changes and the depth of anesthesia is extremely complex, controversial, and not clinically useful. However, Winter's scheme does offer another approach toward the understanding of how anesthetics alter pain perception by including stimulant as well as depressant anesthetics. Each anesthetic drug can follow a different mechanistic route to abolish pain perception.

Stage I now represents a mild stimulation of the reticular activating system, producing motor excitement and then unconsciousness.

Stage II represents further stimulation as the reticular activating system becomes unable to screen incoming stimuli. The subclasses of stage II include the following: *subclass A,* hallucinations with recall; *subclass B,* hallucinations with no recall; and *subclass C,* catalepsy with no recall. Catalepsy is the state in which the patient neither moves nor reacts to stimuli. The stimulant anesthetics ketamine, enflurane, and nitrous oxide produce a cataleptic anesthesia. Ether, the prototype for the old scheme, produces initial excitement at stage IIC, then depression at Stage III.

Stage III is the same as in the old scheme, representing the level of surgical anesthesia produced by depression of the central nervous system. The anesthetics halothane and isoflurane and the barbiturates are purely depressant anesthetics, taking the patient from stage I to stage III.

Stage IV remains medullary paralysis.

■ Properties of the ideal anesthetic

The ideal anesthetic would produce (1) analgesia, (2) unconsciousness, (3) muscle relaxation, and (4) reduction of reflex activity. This anesthetic would be prompt to act and rapidly eliminated, remaining unmetabolized and producing no unwanted effects in body tissues. Since no anesthetic has all these desirable properties, several drugs are used in combination to achieve these goals.

■ CHARACTERISTICS OF INHALATION ANESTHETICS

■ Partial pressure as a measure of anesthetic concentration

The inhalation anesthetics are gases or volatile liquids administered as gases. The effective concentration of an inhalation anesthetic in the brain does not depend on the solubility of the anesthetic in blood or tissue. Rather the effective concentration depends on the partial pressure of the anesthetic, the partial pressure being the effective pressure of the gas in the atmosphere. If a constant partial pressure of anesthetic is inhaled, the partial pressure in the alveoli will rise toward the inhaled level. If the gas is not very soluble in blood, little of the gas will be removed by the blood circulating around the alveoli and the partial pressure of the gas in the blood will quickly reach the inhaled partial pressure. This anesthetic will have a rapid onset of action. However, if the gas is soluble in blood, the partial pressure of the gas in the alveoli will quickly drop because the gas is being removed more rapidly by the blood than can be replenished by breathing. A long time will be required to equilibrate the blood with the gas to the point where the partial pressure matches that coming into the alveoli. To shorten the time to reach this steady state, anesthesia is induced using a high partial pressure of the gas and then lowering the partial pressure to maintain anesthesia.

■ Minimum alveolar concentration (MAC)

The potency of an inhalation anesthetic is determined by the *m*inimum *a*lveolar *c*oncentration (MAC) that will produce anesthesia (insensitivity to a skin incision) in 50% of the patients. For instance, MAC of 10% is equivalent to a partial pressure of 0.1 atmosphere or 76 mm of mercury at standard conditions (sea level). A MAC of 10% means than when air in the alveoli has equilibrated with the body and incoming air, all of which are 10% anesthetic gas, the patient has a 50:50 chance of being unreactive to a skin incision. Surgery is conducted at about 1.4 times the MAC value of the anesthetic chosen.

■ Distribution and excretion of inhalation anesthetics

The distribution of the anesthetic is determined by the blood flow, so the brain, liver, and kidneys reach equilibrium first. Excretion of the inhalation anesthetics is largely through the lungs. The amount of anesthetic that is in solution is metabolized by the liver to a variable degree. Certain of the halogenated hydrocarbons (enflurane, halothane, methoxyflurane) are metabolized to products that may damage the liver and kidney.

Emergence is the time during which the patient regains consciousness after the anesthetic has been discontinued. The duration of emergence from the inhaled anesthetics depends on the same factors as induction. The patient's vital signs are carefully monitored in a recovery room and symptoms of pain or nausea and vomiting must be watched for and treated appropriately.

■ CLINICALLY USED INHALATION ANESTHETICS (Table 29-1)

■ Specific inhalation anesthetics

Cyclopropane

Cyclopropane is a gas that rapidly induces anesthesia accompanied by good analgesia and adequate muscle relaxation. The MAC is 9.2%. The major drawback is that cyclopropane is explosive and therefore hazardous to use without special precautions. Because of the hazard, cyclopropane is very rarely used today. Cyclopropane sensitizes the heart to catecholamines and cardiac arrhythmias may develop. Emergence from anesthesia is rapid because cyclopropane is poorly soluble in blood, but delirium is frequent in the absence of a narcotic analgesic. Nausea, vomiting, and headache are common after anesthesia with cyclopropane.

Diethyl ether

Diethyl ether is a volatile liquid that is very flammable and explosive. The MAC is 1.9%. A long time is required for induction and emergence when ether alone is used because ether is highly soluble in blood. In addition, ether is unpleasant to inhale because it has a noxious, pungent odor, irritates the respiratory tract, and stimulates secretions. An anticholinergic drug may be administered to minimize these secretions. The explosive hazard and the noxious, pungent odor account for the rare use of ether in modern surgery. Nevertheless, ether is still used in areas of the world where sophisticated equipment is unavailable for monitoring the patient. Ether has a wide margin of safety and has minimal effects on the cardiovascular system, factors that allow ether to be administered without sophisticated control of concentration. Ether also produces good analgesia and muscle relaxation, making additional medication unneeded.

Enflurane

Enflurane (Ethrane) is a halogenated hydrocarbon and a nonflammable liquid. The MAC is 1.7% and induction is fairly rapid. Enflurane is one of the stimulant anesthetics that produces muscle contractions and seizure-like brain wave patterns at high concentrations. Enflurane is usually administered with nitrous oxide to avoid using high concentrations of enflurane, which can cause central nervous system stimulation and cardiovascular depression. Enflurane causes a decrease in blood pressure resulting from a depressed cardiac output and a decreased peripheral resistance. Emergence is usually uneventful except for shivering. About 2.5% of enflurane is metabolized to release a low concentration of fluoride ion. The amount of fluoride ion is not harmful except for those patients with preexisting kidney damage.

TABLE 29-1. Properties of inhalation anesthetics

Drug	Physical properties	Onset	MAC	Cardiovascular effects	Muscle relaxation	Elimination	Other properties
Cyclopropane	Flammable gas	Very rapid	9.2%	Sensitizes heart to catecholamines	Good	Lungs	Good analgesia. Nausea, vomiting, headache, delirium on emergence.
Diethyl ether	Flammable liquid	Slow	1.92%	Minimal	Excellent	Lungs	Excellent analgesia. Nausea, vomiting on emergence. Secretions stimulated.
Enflurane (Ethrane)	Nonflammable liquid	Rapid	1.68%	Decreased blood pressure May sensitize heart to catecholamines	Good	Lungs 2% to 5% metablized by liver	Causes low body temperature, hypothermia, and shivering.
Halothane (Fluothane)	Nonflammable liquid	Rapid	0.77%	Decreased blood pressure Sensitizes heart to catecholamines	Fair	Lungs 20% metabolized by liver	Poor analgesia.
Isoflurane (Forane)	Nonflammable liquid	Rapid	1.3%	Minimal	Good	Lungs Little metabolism by liver	
Methoxyflurane (Penthrane)	Nonflammable liquid	Slow	0.16%	Decreased blood pressure	Good	Lungs 70% metabolized by liver	Excellent analgesia.
Nitrous oxide	Nonflammable gas	Very rapid	101%	Minimal	—	Lungs	Widely used with other drugs for anesthesia. Good analgesia.

Halothane

Halothane (Fluothane) is a nonflammable liquid halogenated hydrocarbon and currently is the most widely used of the volatile liquid anesthetics. The MAC is 0.77% and induction is fairly rapid. Postoperative nausea and vomiting are not a problem with halothane. Halothane is a direct myocardial depressant and causes a dose-dependent reduction in cardiac output with no change in heart rate, a combination of effects that lowers the blood pressure. Halothane also sensitizes the myocardium to exogenously administered catecholamines. This sensitization means that a sympathomimetic drug must be used cautiously during surgery to maintain blood pressure, since sympathomimetic drugs may precipitate arrhythmias. Catecholamines may be used topically, such as on the brain or in irrigation of the bladder, to stop bleeding. Halothane does not provide adequate muscle relaxation, and a separate muscle relaxant must be used.

Very rarely (1 out of 800,000 times) halothane is responsible for a fatal hepatitis. Current theory is that free radical metabolites, which are very reactive compounds, may be produced by the liver and damage liver cells.

Isoflurane

Isoflurane (Forane) is a chemical isomer of enflurane, but unlike enflurane, isoflurane is a depressant anesthetic like halothane. The MAC is 1.3%. Induction is smooth and rapid and muscle relaxation adequate. The heart is not sensitized to catecholamines, but the blood pressure does fall resulting from a decrease in the peripheral resistance of blood vessels. Only a tiny proportion (0.25%) of isofluranc is metabolized. Isoflurane is a new anesthetic that many anesthesiologists feel will become widely used in the future.

Methoxyflurane

Methoxyflurane (Penthrane) is a nonflammable liquid halogenated hydrocarbon. It produces an analgesia adequate for dentistry and obstetrics. The MAC is 0.16%. Methoxyflurane depresses the cardiovascular system but does not sensitize the heart to catecholamines. The methoxyflurane that is not exhaled is metabolized extensively (70%) by the liver to fluoride ion. Prolonged anesthesia with methoxyflurane may result in a high-output renal failure because in the presence of the fluoride ion the kidney loses its concentrating ability so that the urine volume is high. This renal failure is usually reversible.

Nitrous oxide

Nitrous oxide is a nonexplosive gas that is still widely used for anesthesia. The major limitation of nitrous oxide is that the maximum concentration allowable, 65% to 70% N_2O and 30% to 35% O_2, does not produce surgical anesthesia because the MAC is 101%. Nevertheless, nitrous oxide produces good analgesia and is used for this purpose in dental and obstetrical procedures. In addition, nitrous oxide is widely used with other anesthetics to produce surgical anesthesia. The effect of nitrous oxide is additive with other anesthetics so that a 50% MAC concentration of nitrous oxide and a 50% MAC concentration of another inhalation anesthetic will produce surgical anesthesia. In addition, nitrous oxide is widely used as one component of *balanced anesthesia* in which a narcotic analgesic, a skeletal muscle relaxant, and nitrous oxide are used together to produce surgical anesthesia.

Nitrous oxide has been shown to increase the incidence of spontaneous abortions in women and to decrease spermatogenesis in men who work in operating rooms. Scavenging equipment must now be used in the operating room to remove nitrous oxide. Nitrous oxide is very much (34 times) more soluble than nitrogen in the blood so that pockets of trapped gas in the patient will expand as nitrogen leaves and is replaced by larger amounts of nitrous oxide. Locations where trapped gas is common include a blocked middle ear, pneumothorax, loops of intestine, lung, renal cysts, and in the skull following a pneumoencephalogram. These conditions represent contraindications for nitrous oxide, since the large increases in pressure or volumes that may result following nitrous oxide administration may produce serious damage.

■ CHARACTERISTICS OF INTRAVENOUS ANESTHETICS

The intravenous anesthetics include the ultrashort-acting barbiturates: thiopental (Pentothal), methohexital (Brevital), and thiamylal sodium (Surital); two benzodiazepines: diazepam (Valium) and flunitrazepam (Rohypnol); and ketamine (Ketaject). Only ketamine is a true anesthetic, abolishing the perception of and reaction to pain. The barbiturates and benzodiazepines do not abolish reflex to pain even when they are administered in doses large enough to render the patient unconscious. These drugs are used primarily as induction agents to bypass stage II of anesthesia. The advantage of the intravenous agents is that they are effective seconds after administration.

It may seem paradoxical that an intravenous anesthetic would be so short acting when it must be metabolized to be excreted. The explanation is that the intravenous anesthetics are very lipid soluble. They are initially distributed to the brain, liver, and kidneys, the organs with the largest blood flow, but after a while the drug is *redistributed* to body fat and skeletal muscle, which are less well perfused. This redistribution lowers the circulating concentration to that which no longer maintains anesthesia. This redistribution is responsible for the short duration of action. Metabolism of the drug proceeds as the drug passes through the liver.

■ CLINICALLY USED INTRAVENOUS ANESTHETICS (Table 29-2)

■ Barbiturates

Thiopental, methohexital, and thiamylal

Thiopental (Pentothal), methohexital (Brevital) and thiamylal (Surital) are all ultrashort-acting barbiturates used primarily to induce anesthesia. Loss of consciousness occurs within 60 seconds of injection. Thiopental or thiamylal are effective as the sole anesthetic for about 15 minutes. Methohexital is even shorter acting. Barbiturates provide no analgesia and can cause excitement or delirium in the presence of pain in an awake patient. Changes in blood pressure or cardiac output are not common unless the injection is made rapidly. Respiration is markedly depressed and yawning, coughing, or laryngospasm may occur. Methohexital can cause hiccups.

Solutions of barbiturates should be injected only into veins. Arterial injections can cause inflammation and clotting. The solution will damage tissue if it leaks around the injection site and can lead to gangrene.

■ Benzodiazepines

Diazepam

Diazepam (Valium) is a benzodiazepine used occasionally as an induction agent but more frequently to sedate patients undergoing cardioversion or endoscopic or dental procedures. Intravenous diazepam takes about 60 seconds to become effective. Sedation, sleep, and amnesia are achieved with little depression of cardiovascular or respiratory functions. Unlike the barbiturates, diazepam is metabolized to active products and has a long duration of action. See Chapter 24 for a further discussion of diazepam.

Flunitrazepam

Flunitrazepam (Rohypnol) is a benzodiazepine that is more potent than diazepam so that a smaller dose is needed. Otherwise flunitrazepam is similar to diazepam.

■ Ketamine

Ketamine

Ketamine (Ketaject, Ketalar) is neither a barbiturate nor a benzodiazepine. Unlike those two drug classes, ketamine produces a cataleptic anesthesia in which the patient appears to be awake but neither responds to pain nor remembers the procedure. This is sometimes referred to as *dissociative anesthesia*. Also ketamine is not a controlled substance so it is readily available in emergency rooms. Ketamine is rapidly effective when administered intramuscularly as well as when administered intravenously. By itself ketamine provides anesthesia for 5 to 10 minutes when given intravenously and for 10 to 20 minutes when given intramuscularly.

Ketamine enhances muscle tone and increases blood pressure, heart rate, and respiratory secretions. The major side effect is seen in the recovery period when patients may experience vivid, unpleasant dreams or hallucinations. Adults are more prone than children to these experiences. Ketamine may also cause vomiting and shivering. Ketamine is related chemically to phencyclidine (PCP), an illicit hallucinogen.

Ketamine should be used cautiously in patients with convulsive disorders, psychosis, mild hypertension, or who are undergoing eye surgery and is contraindicated for patients with coronary artery disease, severe hypertension, stroke, or treated hypothyroidism.

TABLE 29-2. Injectable drugs for anesthesia

Generic name	Trade name	Dosage and administration	Comments
BARBITURATES			
Methohexital sodium	Brevital Sodium	INTRAVENOUS: *Adults*—for induction, 5 to 12 ml of 1% solution no faster than 1 ml every 5 sec. Maintenance, 2 to 4 ml of 1% solution as required.	Methohexital has the shortest duration of action (5 to 7 min) of the barbiturates. Some patients develop hiccups after rapid injection of methohexital. Schedule IV substance.
Thiamylal sodium	Surital	INTRAVENOUS: *Adults*—for induction, 2 to 4 ml of 2.5% solution every 30 to 40 sec, with maximum dose 3 to 5 mg/kg body weight. Maintenance, 2 to 4 ml of 2.5% solution as required.	Duration of action about 15 min. Schedule III substance.
Thiopental sodium	Pentothal	INTRAVENOUS: *Adults*—for induction, 50 to 100 mg (2 to 4 ml) in 2.5% solution every 30 to 40 sec or 3 to 5 mg/kg body weight. Maintenance, 2 to 4 ml of 2.5% solution as required. *Children*—3 to 5 mg/kg body weight as described for adults.	Duration of action about 15 min. May cause yawning, coughing, or laryngospasm. Schedule III substance.
BENZODIAZEPINES			
Diazepam	Valium	INTRAVENOUS: *Adults*—0.1 to 1.0 mg/kg body weight to induce sleep. Basal sedation requires only 5 to 30 mg, so 2.5 to 5 mg is injected every 30 sec until a light sleep or slurred speech is produced.	Do not mix with other liquids. A local anesthetic may be required for intravenous injection.
Flunitrazepam	Rohypnol	INTRAVENOUS: *Adults*—for induction, 36 to 50 μg/kg body weight over a period of 20 to 40 sec. Maintenance, 10 μg/kg as needed.	Used for induction of anesthesia. Also used to produce sedation, sleep, and amnesia for procedures such as endoscopy.
MISCELLANEOUS			
Ketamine	Ketaject Ketalar	INTRAVENOUS: *Adults and children*—1 to 4.5 mg/kg over a period of 60 sec, ½ of initial dose used for maintenance as needed. INTRAMUSCULAR: *Adults and children*—6.5 to 13 mg/kg body weight, ½ of initial dose for maintenance as needed.	Produces a cataleptic anesthesia with good analgesia. Not a scheduled drug.
Fentanyl citrate	Sublimaze	INTRAVENOUS: *Adults and children over 2 yr*—0.002 to 0.003 mg/kg in divided doses over a period of 6 to 8 min. Maintenance, 0.05 to 0.1 mg every 30 to 60 min. Onset: 1 to 2 min.	A potent, short-acting narcotic analgesic. Used with droperidol and nitrous oxide for neuroleptic anesthesia and with nitrous oxide for balanced anesthesia.
Droperidol	Inapsine	INTRAVENOUS: *Adults and children over 2 yr*—0.15 mg/kg body weight. Onset: 10 to 15 min. Duration: 3 to 6 hr.	An antipsychotic drug. Used with fentanyl citrate and nitrous oxide to produce neuroleptanesthesia. May cause extrapyramidal symptoms.

■ BALANCED ANESTHESIA

Since no one anesthetic drug has all the properties required for surgical anesthesia, one widely used combination of agents is called *balanced anesthesia*. This refers to a combination of a narcotic analgesic, nitrous oxide, and a skeletal muscle relaxant. Anesthesia is induced, generally with a short-acting barbiturate or occasionally with diazepam or other agents, and then the narcotic analgesic, nitrous oxide, and skeletal muscle relaxant are administered. Respiration must be controlled because the narcotic analgesics are potent respiratory depressants and the patients are usually paralyzed by a skeletal muscle relaxant. Nitrous oxide is effective at a 60% concentration because of its synergism with the narcotic analgesic. The skeletal muscle relaxant is necessary because neither the narcotic analgesic nor the nitrous oxide provides the muscular relaxation necessary for surgery. The choice of the narcotic analgesic is determined by the anticipated length of surgery. Fentanyl (Sublimaze) is a short-acting narcotic analgesic the use of which is largely confined to surgery. Meperidine (Demerol) is widely used for longer surgeries. Morphine is used as an alternate to meperidine and is also preferred for cardiac and poor-risk patients.

The advantage of balanced anesthesia is that the cardiovascular system is neither depressed nor sensitized to catecholamines. Respiration is depressed, but controlled ventilation is readily available. The incidence of postoperative nausea, vomiting, and pain is low.

■ NEUROLEPTANESTHESIA

Neuroleptanesthesia refers to the combination of droperidol (Inapsine), an antipsychotic drug of the butyrophenone class; a narcotic analgesic (usually fentanyl); and nitrous oxide. A skeletal muscle relaxant may be used if needed. A fixed combination of the narcotic analgesic fentanyl and droperidol is available as Innovar. Nitrous oxide produces the loss of consciousness and if nitrous oxide is discontinued, the patient becomes conscious but in an altered state of awareness. Neuroleptanesthesia is useful for aged and poor-risk patients and for such procedures as bronchoscopy and carotid arteriography. Innovar alone greatly facilitates intubations in patients who are awake.

Side effects of neuroleptanalgesia or neuroleptanesthesia are hypotension, a slow heart rate (bradycardia), and respiratory depression. The action of droperidol persists for 3 to 6 hours, whereas the analgesic effect of fentanyl persists for only 30 minutes. Droperidol has adrenergic-receptor blocking, antifibrillatory, antiemetic, and anticonvulsant actions. About 1% of patients receiving droperidol may have extrapyramidal muscle movements (Chapter 25) as long as 12 hours after administration of the drug. These movements may be controlled by administration of atropine or benztropine (Chapter 32).

■ THE NURSING PROCESS

■ Assessment

The need for general anesthesia is determined by the physician, the patient, and the nurse anesthetist or anesthesiologist after assessment of the physical condition and consideration of the procedure to be performed. Subjective and objective data to include in the assessment are the vital signs, chest x-ray films, laboratory data, and studies specific to known medical problems, for instance, coagulation studies in patients with liver disease or pulmonary function studies in patients with severe chronic obstructive pulmonary disease. The patient's age, previous experience with anesthesia, preference, and the location and type of surgery will all be considered.

■ Management

The actual delivery of general anesthesia is beyond the scope of this book and requires knowledge and facility with management of the respiratory and cardiovascular system, multiple drugs, and the immobilized unconscious patient. For further information, consult appropriate textbooks of nursing medicine and anesthesiology.

■ Evaluation

The ideal general anesthetic produces loss of pain sensation, total relaxation, is excreted quickly, and leaves the patient with little or no residual effects as discussed in the text. No anesthetic achieves the ideal. The patient who has received general anesthesia needs careful frequent evaluation of vital signs, the respiratory and cardiovascular status, the level of consciousness, and the ability to handle secretions. If nausea and/or vomiting occur, it should be treated not only for patient comfort but also for prevention of fluid loss, fluid and electrolyte imbalance, and other possible side effects. Unusual or rare side effects should be treated if they occur (e.g., psychological disturbances with ketamine). As the patient is recovering from anesthesia the level of pain experienced should be assessed. Observations relating to the surgery should be made, including the condition and drainage of wound, the presence of pulses distal to the site of surgery, and whatever is appropriate for the surgical procedure performed. For additional specific information, see the patient care implications section.

■ PATIENT CARE IMPLICATIONS

General anesthesia

1. It is beyond the scope of this text to discuss the actual administration of general anesthesia. For this information, please refer to appropriate textbooks.
2. Preoperative medications are an integral part of the planned anesthesia, and care should be taken to administer them as ordered and on time.
3. Preparation for surgery should include teaching the patient and family about the surgical procedure and what to expect postoperatively; patient practice of any exercises or activities that will be required postoperatively (such as coughing); an opportunity for the patient to discuss questions and concerns about anesthesia with the anesthesiologist or nurse anesthetist; a visit to the intensive care unit if possible and appropriate; and time for the patient to express concerns and questions and to obtain answers, reassurance, and emotional support.
4. Frequently expressed fears by patients who are to have surgery include the following:
   a. That they will not be completely asleep when surgery is begun and will "feel the surgery"
   b. That the anesthetics will cause them to talk and reveal personal information about themselves

   Anticipate these and other questions and answer them if possible or refer them to the nurse anesthetist or anesthesiologist.
5. The patient should be taught how to cough preoperatively and told that it will be necessary to do this regularly and frequently postoperatively to prevent respiratory complications.

Postoperative

1. Vital signs (temperature, pulse, respirations, and blood pressure) should be monitored frequently during the immediate postoperative period. With the exception of the temperature, this may mean every 5 minutes, decreasing in frequency to every 15 to 30 minutes as the patient becomes more alert and the overall condition improves.
2. Patients should be kept on their sides or supervised carefully until awake to prevent aspiration if vomiting should occur. Some drugs are more prone to producing vomiting during the emergence phase than others (see text). In some instances it is necessary to medicate with an antiemetic. Suctioning equipment should always be at the bedside.
3. Often patients are brought to the recovery room still intubated from surgery, and the endotracheal tube is removed in the recovery room. Regardless of whether the patient is intubated or not, the respiratory function must be monitored closely in terms of rate, depth, and ability to handle secretions. After major surgery, measurement of arterial blood gases may be necessary to assist in the respiratory management. Suctioning equipment should be at the bedside, and ventilatory support equipment should be available.
4. Each patient should be evaluated individually in deciding how soon to medicate a patient for pain in the immediate postoperative period (the first 2 to 4 hours after surgery). The evaluation involves considering such parameters as the patient's blood pressure, pulse, respirations, anesthetic agent, length of anesthesia, level of consciousness, and the effects the analgesic may have on these parameters. Often the decision is made to medicate the patient for pain the first time using one fourth to one half of the ordered dose of analgesic. Note that the decision to give a reduced dose should be made only with the approval of the physician. It is specifically recommended that when Innovar is used (see text) the first dose of postoperative analgesic be a small dose.
5. Siderails should be kept up on postoperative patients during the first day after surgery and longer if necessary. Supervise and assist with ambulation until the patient is clearly alert and steady while standing and vital signs are stable.
6. Unless specifically contraindicated, postoperative patients should be assisted to breathe deeply and to cough several times every 2 hours. In addition, other treatments such as blow bottles or *I*ntermittent *P*ositive *P*ressure *B*reathing (IPPB) may be ordered to prevent pulmonary complications, and these should be administered as ordered. For specific instructions on how to assist patients with these measures, refer to a fundamentals of nursing textbook.
7. Effects of anesthesia persist even after the patient appears to be alert and awake. If it is necessary to give instructions about activity, diet, or medications (as it might be in the outpatient or day surgery setting), they should be given both verbally and in writing to the patient and reviewed with family members if present.
8. Patients who have a severe reaction or response to any anesthetic should be cautioned to carry with them the name of the particular agent and, if surgery is ever again needed, to inform the anesthesiologist of the previous agent used and the poor response.
9. See the patient care implications section for narcotic analgesics in Chapter 28. Patient ability to perform required postoperative activities will be increased if patients are adequately medicated for pain.

Ketamine (Ketaject)

1. Psychic disturbances are relatively common and include unpleasant dreams, emergence delirium, irrational behavior, disorientation, and hallucinations. The occurrence of these side effects may be lessened by providing the patient with a quiet wake-up period, perhaps in the quietest corner of the recovery room. Excessive stimulation should be avoided, although vital signs must still be monitored.
2. If psychic side effects occur, provide calm reassurance and reorientation to the patient. Rarely a small hypnotic dose of a short-acting barbiturate may be needed to help terminate a severe reaction. If side effects occur, the patient should not be left unattended. If the patient is returned to the patient care unit from the recovery room, the room should be kept dimly lit and noise and stimulation kept to a minimum. Inform family members of the probable cause of behavior and enlist their aid in patient reorientation and reassurance.

■ SUMMARY

Anesthesia is the abolition of the perception of pain and the reaction to painful stimuli. General anesthesia depends on the disruption of the reticular activating system. Traditionally, four stages of general anesthesia have been described with Stage III being that of surgical anesthesia.

Inhalation anesthetics are believed to alter the lipid structure of the cell membrane rather than to occupy membrane receptors. The effective concentration of inhalation anesthetics is determined by the partial pressure of the gas, whereas the solubility of the gas in the blood determines how long the induction and recovery periods are. Major factors determining the choice of inhalation anesthetics are the cardiovascular effects produced and the flammability of the anesthetic. Production of analgesia and muscle relaxation may require the administration of supplemental drugs specific for these effects.

Nitrous oxide and halothane (Fluothane) are the most widely used inhalation anesthetics. Isoflurane (Forane) is a new inhalation anesthetic. Methoxyflurane (Penthrane) is used mainly for its analgesic property in obstetrics and dental practice. Enflurane (Ethrane) is a stimulant anesthetic. The use of diethyl ether and cyclopropane is essentially obsolete because of their high flammability.

The ultrashort-acting barbiturates (thiopental [Pentothal], methohexital [Brevital], and thiamylal [Surital]) and the benzodiazepines diazepam (Valium) and flunitrazepam (Rohypnol) are given intravenously to render the patient unconscious or mentally uninvolved in such procedures as induction of general anesthesia, cardioversion, endoscopy, or tooth extractions.

Ketamine is a true anesthetic that can be administered intravenously or intramuscularly.

Selected combinations of drugs are used to produce surgical anesthesia. Balanced anesthesia refers to the administration of a narcotic analgesic, a skeletal muscle relaxant, and nitrous oxide for general anesthesia after induction with an ultrashort-acting barbiturate or diazepam. Neuroleptanesthesia refers to the combination of the antipsychotic-type drug droperidol (Inapsine), the short-acting narcotic analgesic fentanyl (Sublimaze), and nitrous oxide. Innovar is a combination product containing droperidol and fentanyl.

■ STUDY QUESTIONS

1. How are general anesthetics believed to work?
2. What are the four stages of anesthesia under the scheme treating general anesthesia as pure central nervous system depression?
3. How does Winter's scheme for describing general anesthesia differ from the scheme treating general anesthesia as pure central nervous system depression?
4. What are the properties of an ideal anesthetic?
5. What measurement determines the effective concentration of an inhalation anesthetic? How does this differ from the concentration based on total solubility?
6. What is MAC?
7. What factors determine induction and emergence?
8. Why are cyclopropane and diethyl ether seldom used in the United States?
9. Which inhalation anesthetics are halogenated hydrocarbons?
10. Which inhalation anesthetics sensitize the heart to catecholamines?
11. Which inhalation anesthetics are metabolized to some degree?
12. Which inhalation anesthetics lower blood pressure during surgery?
13. What factor limits the use of nitrous oxide alone as an anesthetic? How is this limitation overcome?
14. What are the special hazards of nitrous oxide to the patient? To operating room personnel?
15. Which barbiturates are used as intravenous induction agents for anesthesia? How is their action effectively terminated?
16. Which benzodiazepines are used as intravenous induction agents for anesthesia?
17. What is the nature of anesthesia with ketamine?
18. Describe ''balanced anesthesia.''
19. Describe neuroleptanesthesia.

■ SUGGESTED READINGS

Bortnowski, P.M.: Psychic disturbances traced to ketamine anesthesia, Nurses' Drug Alert **2**(12):141, 1978.

Brown, B.R., Jr.: Clinical significance of the biotransformation of inhalation anesthetics, Resident and Staff Physician **24**(4):72, 1978.

Clark, R.B.: Anesthesia in obstetrics. I. General, Postgraduate Medicine **53**(4):158, 1973.

Garfield, J.M.: Psychologic problems in anesthesia, American Family Physician **10**(2):60, 1974.

Pilon, R.N.: Anesthesia for uncomplicated obstetric delivery, American Family Physician **9**(1):113, 1974.

Price, H.L.: Neuroleptic agents in anesthesia, American Family Physician **8**(4):222, 1973.

Risser, N.L.: Preoperative and postoperative care to prevent pulmonary complications, Heart and Lung **9**(1):57, 1980.

Salanitre, E., and Rackow, H.: Considerations in neonatal anesthesia, AORN Journal **25:**879, 1977.

Schmidt, K.F.: Premedication for anesthesia, American Family Physician **10**(4):113, 1974.

Smith, B.J.: Safeguarding your patient after anesthesia, Nursing '78 **8**(10):52, 1978.

White, M.J., and Wolf-Wilets, V.C.: Memory loss following halothane anesthesia, AORN Journal **26:**1053, 1977.

Winter, W.: Effects of drugs on the electrical activity of the brain: anesthetics, Annual Review of Pharmacology and Toxicology **16:** 413, 1976.

30 Local anesthetics

■ BACKGROUND

Cocaine was the first local anesthetic used clinically following the observation in the late 1880's that when cocaine was administered orally to patients, their tongues and throats became numb. The main use of cocaine as a local anesthetic was to desensitize the cornea to allow local surgery on the eye without using a general anesthetic. Cocaine quickly became recognized as an abused drug and was replaced by procaine (Novocain) in 1905. Today lidocaine (Xylocaine), introduced in the 1940's, is the most versatile and widely used local anesthetic. There are more than 20 local anesthetics available, but they vary in their suitability for different applications.

■ MECHANISM OF ACTION

Local anesthesia is achieved by drugs that reversibly inhibit nerve conduction. A local anesthetic is administered at the desired site of action, and the inhibition of nerve conduction persists until the drug diffuses away and enters the circulation for subsequent degradation and excretion. All neurons in the area of administration, whether pain, motor, or autonomic neurons, are affected, so in addition to the loss of pain, there is a loss of sensory, motor, and autonomic activities. The size of the nerve fiber determines its sensitivity to local anesthetics with the smaller fibers being the most sensitive. Since sensory fibers are smaller than motor fibers, a loss of sensation precedes the loss of motor activity and, conversely, motor activity is regained before sensory function.

Chemically, most local anesthetics are weak bases, being secondary or tertiary amines. This means that under physiological conditions most of the molecules carry a positive charge and are not very lipid soluble. However, it is the uncharged form that diffuses across the nerve membrane and then reequilibrates to both charged and uncharged forms. Within the neuron it is the positively charged form that blocks nerve conduction. The positively charged form displaces calcium bound to the inner membrane and thereby prevents the inward flow of sodium ions. Since the action potential is generated by the influx of sodium ions, the local anesthetic depresses the action potential so that it is not propagated. The resting potential of neurons is not affected by local anesthetics.

■ SIDE EFFECTS AND ADVERSE REACTIONS

The factor limiting the safety of local anesthetics is that they eventually enter the systemic circulation and can affect other organs. The relative safety of procaine and chloroprocaine is due to their rapid hydrolysis in the plasma by pseudocholinesterases. Other local anesthetics are slowly degraded by the liver and have a longer plasma half-life.

Although cocaine is unique in causing euphoria, all local anesthetics act as central nervous system stimulants if absorbed systemically, producing symptoms such as anxiety, a tingling feeling (paresthesia), tremors, and ringing in the ears (tinnitus). This central nervous system stimulation may ultimately result in convulsions. Intravenous diazepam (Valium) in 2.5-mg increments or small doses of an ultrashort-acting barbiturate such as thiopental (Pentothal), thiamylal (Surital), or methohexital (Brevital) are used to stop these convulsions.

A high plasma concentration of a local anesthetic causes central nervous system depression, with or without prior symptoms of central nervous system stimulation. This depression of central nervous system function is serious, due to loss of vasomotor control, and results in profound hypotension, respiratory depression, and coma.

In addition to the central nervous system effects, the direct cardiovascular effects of local anesthetics are important. Local anesthetics cause direct vasodilation, which increases blood flow and so favors the removal of the drug. For this reason epinephrine is sometimes added to the local anesthetic because epinephrine will cause vasoconstriction and prolong the time the local anesthetic remains at the site of injection. Cocaine is unique among the local anesthetics in being a potent vasoconstrictor. Prolonged abuse of cocaine by insufflation (sniffing into the nose) can cause loss of the nasal septum because of tissue death following ischemia (insufficient blood flow).

Local anesthetics are cardiac depressants. Lidocaine is used to depress cardiac arrhythmias (Chapter 16).

Local anesthetics that are esters (chloroprocaine, procaine, and tetracaine) can give rise to an allergic response. Anaphylaxis is rare and more commonly the topical use of a local anesthetic with an ester bond leads to a skin rash (contact dermatitis).

■ CLINICAL USES

In general local anesthetics can be divided into those applied topically to provide surface anesthesia and those injected into an area to produce local anesthesia. Only lidocaine (Xylocaine), dibucaine (Nupercaine), and tetracaine (Pontocaine) are used both topically and by injection.

■ Local anesthetics for surface anesthesia

Those local anesthetics applied as drops, sprays, lotions, creams, or ointments are listed in Table 30-1. Distinction is made between those drugs safely applied to the eyes, those applied to the skin, and those applied to mucosal areas. Only tetracaine (Pontocaine) is suitable for application to all three types of sites.

Most of the drugs listed for surface anesthesia are effective when applied to the skin. These drugs are poorly soluble so there is little systemic absorption when they are applied to the skin for the relief of itching or the pain of mild burns. The main potential toxicity of local anesthetics applied to the skin is the development of allergy, usually a contact dermatitis. Since there are several chemical classes represented by local anesthetics, a drug from a different chemical group can be substituted if an allergy develops.

The mucosal membranes of the nose, mouth, and throat (bronchotracheal mucosa) and of the urethra, rectum, and vagina are highly vascular and allow ready absorption of the local anesthetic into systemic circulation. Application of excessive amounts of local anesthetics to mucosal surfaces is the most common cause of systemic toxicity with local anesthetics. A local anesthetic is commonly used to eliminate the gagging reflex when inserting an endotracheal tube or to limit the discomfort of endoscopic procedures. The lowest concentration possible of the local anesthetic should be used on mucosal surfaces to avoid systemic toxicity, and the total amount of drug used should be recorded and matched against recommended total doses.

TABLE 30-1. Local anesthetics for surface anesthesia

Generic name	Trade name	Eye*	Mucous membranes†	Skin	Comments
Benoxinate hydrochloride	Dorsacaine	+	0	0	Applied topically to eye to anesthetize cornea and conjunctiva.
Benzocaine	Americaine	0	0	+	Widely used. Included in many nonprescription preparations for the relief of sunburn, itching, and mild burns. Long-acting and poorly absorbed.
Butamben picrate	Butesin Picrate	0	0	+	Nonprescription ointment for relief of itching and burning.
Cocaine hydrochloride		+	+	0	Schedule II drug. Medically used in ear, nose, and throat procedures where vasoconstriction and shrinking of mucous membranes are desired. Ophthalmic preparations anesthetize cornea and conjunctiva.
Cyclomethycaine sulfate	Surfacaine	0	+‡	+	Nonprescription drug used as a cream, ointment, or jelly on skin. Prescription drug for use on genitourinary areas.
Dibucaine hydrochloride	Nupercaine Hydrochloride	0	0	+	Nonprescription skin ointment or cream.
Dimethisoquin hydrochloride	Quotane Hydrochloride	0	0	+	Nonprescription ointment. Do not apply more than 4 times daily.
Diperodon	Diothane	0	0	+	Nonprescription ointment for surface anesthesia.
Dyclonine Hydrochloride	Dyclone	0	+	+	Used to suppress the gag reflex and to lessen the discomfort of genitourinal endoscopy. Will be precipitated by the iodine of contrast media used in pyelography and should not be used.
Hexylcaine hydrochloride	Cyclaine	0	+	0	Used to provide surface anesthesia for bronchoscopy, endotracheal intubation, gastroscopy, and genitourinary procedures.
Lidocaine	Xylocaine	0	+	+	Widely used for topical anesthesia in ear, nose, and throat procedures, upper digestive tract procedures, and genitourinary procedures. Rapid onset and intermediate duration. Not irritating and low incidence of hypersensitivity.
Lidocaine hydrochloride	Xylocaine Hydrochloride	0	+	+	
Piperocaine hydrochloride	Metycaine Hydrochloride	0	+	0	Primarily used to provide surface anesthesia in nose, larynx, upper gastrointestinal, and genitourinary procedures.
Pramoxine hydrochloride	Tronothane Hydrochloride	0	+‡	+	Nonprescription cream or ointment primarily used to relieve pain of itching, burns, and hemorrhoids.
Proparacaine hydrochloride	Ophthaine Hydrochloride	+	0	0	Applied topically to the eye to anesthetize the cornea and conjunctiva.
Tetracaine hydrochloride	Pontocaine Hydrochloride	+	+	+	Topically, the onset is 5 min and duration is 45 min. Usual topical dose is 20 mg, maximum, 50 mg because of toxicity and slow degradation. Ophthalmic preparations are dilute solutions for instillation.

*+ indicates suitable site for application; 0 indicates site not suitable for application.
†Mucous membranes include the bronchotracheal mucosa and the mucosa of the urethra, rectum, and vagina.
‡Not for application to the bronchotracheal mucosa.

TABLE 30-2. Local anesthetics for injection

Generic name	Trade name	Local infiltration or nerve block or epidural block*	Spinal block (subarachnoid)	Duration†	Comments
Bupivacaine	Marcaine	+	Investigational	Long‡	Provides long-acting epidural anesthesia in labor with no reported effects on fetus. Maximal dose, 200 mg.
Chloroprocaine hydrochloride	Nesacaine	+	Investigational	Short	Little systemic toxicity because of rapid hydrolysis in the plasma. No effects reported on fetus after epidural anesthesia in mother. Maximal dose, 800 mg.
Dibucaine	Nupercaine	0	+	Long	The most potent and toxic of the local anesthetics. Onset can take 15 min. Available in hyperbaric (heavy), isobaric, and hypobaric (light) solutions. Total dose, 2.5 to 10 mg, depending on use.
Etidocaine	Duranest	+	0	Long	Highly lipid soluble. Onset for epidural block, 5 min. Profound muscle relaxation is desirable for abdominal surgery but not for labor.
Lidocaine	Xylocaine	+	+	Intermediate	Widely used local anesthetic. Maximum dose, 300 mg (4.5 mg/kg). Can cause drowsiness, fatigue, and amnesia.
Mepivacaine	Carbocaine	+	0	Intermediate	Chemically related to lidocaine. Maximum dose, 400 mg (7 mg/kg).
Prilocaine	Citanest Hydrochloride	+	0	Intermediate	Maximum dose, 600 mg (8 mg/kg). Useful for outpatient surgery because of the low incidence of drowsiness or fatigue as side effects. Metabolites can cause methemoglobinemia.
Procaine hydrochloride	Novocain	+	+	Short	Noted for its safety because of its rapid hydrolysis in the plasma. Maximum dose, 600 mg (10 mg/kg). Duration of epidural block is unreliable.
Tetracaine	Pontocaine Hydrochloride	0	+	Long	The most widely used drug for spinal anesthesia. Onset, 5 min. Dose for spinal anesthesia, 2 to 15 mg. Available in hyperbaric (heavy), isobaric, and hypobaric (light) solutions.

*+ indicates suitable use; 0 indicates use not suitable.
†Duration without epinephrine: short, 1 hr; intermediate, 2 hr; long, 3 hr (approximations).
‡Duration of bupivacaine in nerve block is 6 to 13 hr.

FIG. 30-1

The sites for injection of local anesthetic to achieve spinal, epidural, and caudal anesthesia. The degree of anesthesia achieved and special techniques used are described in detail in the text.

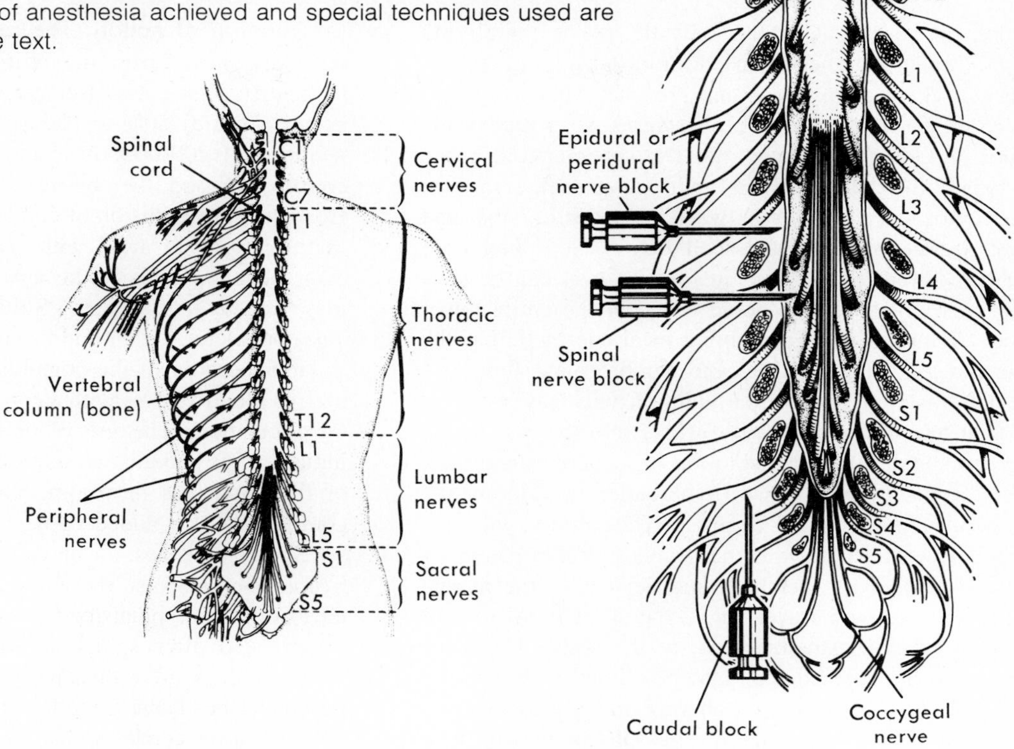

■ Local anesthetics used by injection

The local anesthetics used by injection are listed in Table 30-2. The potency and the duration of action increase together with the lipid solubility of the drug. The onset of anesthesia is determined by the concentration of drug and the size of the nerve. Before infiltrating an area with a local anesthetic, the syringe should first be aspirated to ensure that a blood vessel has not been entered. This is because the concentration of drug is high and could prove fatal if injected systemically.

The area affected by a local anesthetic depends on how and where it is injected. The anesthesia produced is described by the technique of injection: infiltration, nerve block, epidural, and spinal anesthesia. These techniques will be described with their potential for producing toxic side effects.

Infiltration anesthesia refers to the superficial application of a local anesthetic. To suture a cut or to perform dental procedures, the local anesthetic is injected superficially in small amounts to block the small nerves and numb the area. To work on the scalp or to make an incision in the skin, the anesthetic is infused around the area. Small incisions require only a small volume and a low concentration of drug so there is little toxicity associated with these uses. However, systemic toxicity from local anesthetics is frequently seen in the emergency room where large cuts are infiltrated with local anesthetic.

Nerve block anesthesia refers to the injection of a local anesthetic along a nerve before it reaches the site of operation. The volume and concentration of a local anesthetic for a nerve block must be larger than in infiltration anesthesia to penetrate the larger nerve.

The most extensive field of local anesthesia is achieved by applying the local anesthetic around the nerve roots near the spinal cord to produce *epidural anesthesia* or, alternatively, *spinal anesthesia*. As shown in Fig. 30-1, the spinal cord proper ends at the lumbar region. The spinal cord is surrounded by three membranes: first the pia mater, then the arachnoid, and finally the outer membrane, the dura mater. These membranes extend below the spinal cord proper to form a sack in the lumbar and sacral region. The dura mater and arachnoid membranes are close together, but there is a space, the subarachnoid space, between the arachnoid and pia mater. The cerebrospinal fluid fills the subarachnoid space throughout the spinal cord.

For *epidural* (or *peridural*) *anesthesia,* the local anesthetic is administered outside of the dura mater, as indicated in Fig. 30-1, so that the nerve roots are blocked at the point after they emerge from the dura mater. The extent of anesthesia depends on the volume and concentration of local anesthetic used. *Caudal (sacral) anesthesia* is another form of epidural anesthesia and is achieved by administering the local anesthetic epidurally at the base of the spine as indicated in Fig. 30-1. The extent of anesthesia affects only the pelvic region and legs. Caudal anesthesia is used for obstetrics and for surgery on the rectum, anus, and prostate gland.

Spinal (subarachnoid) anesthesia is achieved by injecting local anesthetic into the subarachnoid space between the arachnoid and pia mater membranes in the lumbar area, usually between the second lumbar and first sacral vertebrae and well below the spinal cord proper. From the diagram in Fig. 30-1, it can be seen that this will block the nerve roots for the entire lower body. If the solution containing local anesthetic has the same density (isobaric) as the cerebrospinal fluid and is administered slowly, the solution will stay where it is injected and only slowly diffuse into the rest of the cerebrospinal fluid. The solution of local anesthetic can also be made more dense (hyperbaric) by diluting the local anesthetic into 5% dextrose. The solution will then move downward (toward the ground). If the patient is on a tilt bed with feet high and head low, the hyperbaric solution will travel "up" the spinal cord toward the head and anesthetize more of the body. The solution of local anesthetic can also be diluted with distilled water to be less dense (hypobaric). In the patient positioned on the tilt bed as before, this solution would move to the end of the dura mater and anesthetize only the lower part of the body. The procedures employing hypobaric and hyperbaric solutions of local anesthetic require skill in positioning the patient. If the level of anesthesia is adjusted to block more of the spinal cord than just the lumbar and sacral regions, there is danger of paralyzing the intercostal and phrenic nerves, thereby paralyzing spontaneous respiration.

If the patient is seated when the local anesthetic is administered as a low spinal anesthetic, only those nerves affecting the parts of the body that would be in contact with a saddle are affected, hence the name *saddle block*. This procedure is used principally in obstetrics for vaginal delivery.

With spinal anesthesia the patient is awake, breathing and cardiovascular function are not immediately affected, and there is good muscle relaxation. These are advantages for patients with heart and lung disease or for elderly persons. However, the sympathetic fibers to the blood vessels are blocked so that vasodilation with hypotension is a frequent side effect of spinal anesthesia. Spinal anesthesia is therefore considered hazardous for abdominal surgery in poor-risk patients because of the potential for this sudden vasodilation and hypotension. Spinal anesthesia is widely used in obstetrics, particularly for cesarean sections.

Duration of action. The rate at which local anesthetic is removed from the infiltrated area depends largely on the degree of vascularization. The duration can be increased by 50% to 100% with the inclusion of epinephrine, 1:200,000, or phenylephrine to cause vasoconstriction and thereby restrict systemic absorption. However, the inclusion of epinephrine is contraindicated for infiltration of areas with end arteries (fingers, toes, ears, nose, and penis) because the resultant ischemia may lead to tissue death. Similarly, the addition of a vasoconstrictor is contraindicated in epidural anesthesia in labor because of the potential vasoconstriction of the uterine blood vessels with a resultant decrease in placental circulation. The use of epinephrine is also contraindicated for patients with severe cardiovascular disease or thyrotoxicosis in whom cardiac function would be compromised by added vasoconstrictors.

Spinal anesthesia can cause a variable degree of hypotension because the neurons controlling vasomotor tone are in the spinal tract. A severe headache may be experienced after spinal anesthesia and may last for hours or days after the anesthesia has worn off. This postspinal headache is believed to reflect a drop in the pressure of the cerebrospinal fluid caused by a leak at the point where the dura mater was penetrated. The incidence of a spinal headache is reduced when patients are kept flat on their backs and instructed not to raise their heads for 12 hours following spinal anesthesia. This minimizes the hydrostatic pressure of the cerebrospinal fluid on the head.

■ THE NURSING PROCESS

■ Assessment

Patients requiring local anesthetics will be seen in a variety of situations. These patients may need minor surgery, dental work, suturing of small injuries, or may require spinal anesthesia for major surgery. The decision to use a local anesthetic depends on the patient's condition, age, the procedure to be performed, the possible need of the patient to be awake, the patient's preference, and the patient's previous experience with various anesthetics. Basic assessment data would include the vital signs and temperature, history of allergies, response to previous surgery, and overall condition.

■ Management

Except for topical application, local anesthetics are usually administered by the physician, the nurse anesthetist, or the anesthesiologist. For minor or brief procedures such as suturing or some dental work, careful observation of the patient may be sufficient. For longer procedures or when spinal anesthesia is used, it is necessary to monitor the vital signs and other parameters of patient function. With spinal anesthesia there should be careful positioning of the lower extremities. It may be appropriate to insert a Foley catheter to allow urinary output. The level of consciousness should be monitored. Since allergic responses are possible when local anesthetics are used by any route, there should always be epinephrine readily available and equipment for possible resuscitation should anaphylaxsis occur.

■ Evaluation

Local anesthetics are effective if the procedure can be completed without pain, if there are no side effects, and if there is no damage to the patient due to anesthesia. All of the anesthetics require time to wear off, and specific nursing care depends on the area that has been anesthetized. For example, if the throat has been anesthetized for a bronchoscopy or similar procedure, part of the follow-up will include evaluation of the ability to swallow, positioning of the patient on the side to reduce the possibility of aspiration, restricting oral intake until the patient can swallow, and, occasionally, keeping a suction machine at the bedside. Following spinal anesthesia the patient should be kept flat for 12 to 24 hours. The position of the lower extremities should be checked by the nurse to prevent pressure areas, and the patient should be kept in bed until sensation returns to the lower extremities. The fluid intake and output should be checked and the vital signs monitored.

If the patient is still under the effects of the local anesthetic at discharge, the patient should be able to explain any restrictions in activity or diet to be followed until the anesthesia wears off in addition to any restrictions due to the surgical problem itself. If analgesic medications have been prescribed for use after anesthesia wears off, the patient should be able to explain correctly their use (Chapter 28). Finally, in those instances in which local anesthetics are to be used on an outpatient basis, the patient should be able to explain how to use the medication, with what frequency, and what to do if the medication proves to be ineffective. For further information, see the patient care implications section at the end of this chapter.

■ PATIENT CARE IMPLICATIONS

1. Before any local anesthetic is used, patients should be questioned about possible allergies to local anesthetics. Remember, to many people "Novocain" is the term applied to all local anesthetics, regardless of the actual preparation.
2. To monitor the systemic effects of local anesthetics, monitor the blood pressure and pulse. If spinal anesthesia is being used, monitor the respirations also.
3. The routine for monitoring vital signs in the recovery room should be the same regardless of the type of anesthesia used.

4. Following spinal anesthesia, the patient should be kept flat for the specified number of hours (usually 12). Thus the patient should be transferred flat from the transport stretcher to the bed. Usually a thin pillow can be used by the patient without increasing the chance of headache. Even with excellent postoperative care, some patients will develop "spinal" headaches.
5. Patients who have had spinal anesthesia may have difficulty voiding or feeling the need to void until the anesthesia has completely worn off. If the patient has not voided within 8 to 12 hours after surgery, notify the physician.
6. Patients who have received spinal anesthesia should be assisted when getting up the first time.
7. Keep the siderail up on all patients who have received any form of spinal anesthesia until it is clear that the patient's sensation has returned in the lower extremities.
8. The patient who has had spinal anesthesia should be positioned carefully in the bed because there will be no sensation in the lower extremities to warn the patient of wrinkles, tight sheets, or other irritations to the skin.
9. Application of heat or cold to areas numb from local or spinal anesthesia should be done with extreme caution as the patient will be unable to indicate if there is skin irritation or burning. If it is necessary to apply heat or cold, the skin should be well shielded from the heat or cold source by layers of padding, the temperature of the heat source should be checked frequently, and the patient should be checked every 15 minutes.
10. If some form of local anesthesia is being used for delivery, be certain to monitor not only the mother but the baby. Monitor fetal heart tones every 5 to 15 minutes. The mother's sensation of uterine contractions may be absent or altered, and she may need additional instructions to assist with the delivery. For more complete information about delivery with each type of anesthesia, see a textbook of obstetrics.
11. Although serious systemic reactions are rare with local anesthetics, epinephrine, antihistamines, and resuscitation equipment should be available whereever local anesthetics are used.
12. Remember that the patient in the operating or delivery room who is receiving local anesthesia may be drowsy from preoperative medications but will usually be alert and able to understand conversation in the room. Conversation and noise should be kept to a minimum as some patients find excessive conversation overstimulating. Care should be taken to avoid discussing other patients, pathology reports, or complications as these topics might alarm the patient.
13. Patients should be cautioned to use surface anesthetics as instructed and not to increase the frequency of application or to use the preparation on surfaces for which it was not designed.
14. Instruct patients to report any rash or skin irritation that occurs as a result of local anesthetic application.
15. Pain is a protective body mechanism. After a local anesthetic has been used, the body is not able to perceive pain in the anesthetized area, and injury may occur. For this reason it is important to instruct patients carefully about the extent to which they may use an anesthetized area until the effects of the local anesthesia wear off. For example, a dental patient might be instructed not to chew and to avoid extremely hot or cold liquids until the anesthesia has worn off. A patient who has had local anesthesia to a joint might be instructed to abstain from using the joint for a certain number of hours or until the anesthesia has worn off.

■ SUMMARY

Local anesthetics are drugs that penetrate the nerve membrane and prevent sodium influx, a mechanism which blocks the development and propagation of an action potential. Systemic absorption of a local anesthetic produces toxic effects initially characteristic of central nervous system stimulation (anxiety, tingling, tremors, ringing in the ears) and finally characteristic of central nervous system depression (hypotension, respiratory depression, coma). Local anesthetics are vasodilators, except for cocaine which is unique in being a vasoconstrictor. Local anesthetics depress cardiac excitation, and lidocaine is used to depress cardiac arrhythmias.

The site of administration determines the extent of anesthesia:

1. Surface anesthesia for the eyes, skin, and mucosal areas
2. Infiltration anesthesia for superficial numbing (dental procedures and skin sutures)
3. Nerve block anesthesia for numbing regions of the body
4. Epidural anesthesia (blocking major nerve roots exiting from the base of the spinal cord at a site outside of the dura mater) and spinal anesthesia (blocking major nerve roots at a site within the subarachnoid space) to anesthetize the lower part of the body for delivery and for surgery

Most local anesthetics are safely used for only certain of these routes of administration. The larger the nerve to be blocked, the more local anesthetic is required. All nerves, motor and autonomic as well as pain neurons, are anesthetized. The duration of action can be increased by the inclusion of a vasoconstrictor (epinephrine or phenylephrine) to slow systemic absorption of the injected local anesthetic.

Allergic skin reactions are the most frequent side effect of surface anesthetics. Hypotension may accompany spinal anesthesia because of the blockade of neurons within the spinal cord controlling vasomotor tone. A ''spinal'' headache is a common aftereffect of spinal anesthesia.

■ STUDY QUESTIONS

1. What is the mechanism of action of local anesthetics?
2. What property of procaine and chloroprocaine makes them relatively safe?
3. What are the toxic effects of systemic absorption of local anesthetics?
4. Which are the three types of surfaces to which local anesthetics are applied?
5. Describe the areas of anesthesia achieved by infiltration, nerve block, epidural, and spinal anesthesia.
6. What are the special hazards associated with spinal anesthesia?
7. How is the duration of local anesthetics prolonged?

■ SUGGESTED READINGS

Baida, M.R.: Nursing care in the use of local anesthetics, AORN Journal **28:**855, 1978.

Covino, B.G.: Local anesthesia (second of two parts), New England Journal of Medicine **286:**1035, 1972.

Cwik, J., Dunlevy, J.H., Greenberg, B.L., Kelly, A.J., Moore, L.T., and Smith, B.E.: The right local agent by the right route, Patient Care **9:**22, Feb. 1, 1975.

Dahle, J.S.: Caring for the patient with local anesthesia, AORN Journal **27:**985, 1978.

Floyd, C.C.: Drugs for childbirth: your guide to their benefit and risks, RN **49**(5):41, 1977.

Grad, R.K., and Woodside, J.: Obstetrical analgesics and anesthesia: methods of relief for the patient in labor, American Journal of Nursing **77:**242, 1977.

Marx, G.F.: Analgesia and anesthesia for labor and delivery, AANA Journal **47:**537, 1979.

Maternal anesthesia and newborn behavior, Briefs **43**(2):28, 1979.

Wheeler, A.S., and James, F.M.: Anesthesia for complicated obstetrics, AANA Journal **47:**300, 1979.

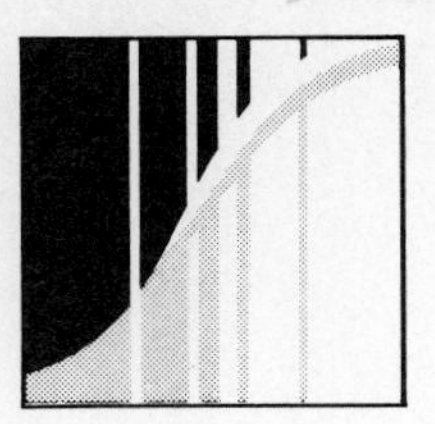

VIII DRUGS USED TO CONTROL DISORDERS OF CENTRAL MUSCLE CONTROL

Section VIII, Drugs used to control disorders of central muscle control, covers anticonvulsants as well as drugs to control involuntary muscle movements. Chapter 31, **Anticonvulsants,** reviews the new classification of seizures. The anticonvulsants are presented by drug class but are also referenced for their role in controlling specific seizure patterns. Chapter 32, **Central Motor Control: Drugs for Parkinsonism and Centrally Acting Skeletal Muscle Relaxants,** covers drugs to treat disorders of central motor control in two sections. The first section presents the drug classes used to treat parkinsonism and discusses the step therapy to control the symptoms of the progressive disease of parkinsonism as well as the role of these drugs in treating the drug-induced parkinsonian symptoms. The second section of Chapter 32 presents drugs to control spasticity as well as drugs acting centrally to relieve local muscle spasms.

31 Anticonvulsants

Epilepsy: seizure patterns

■ CAUSES OF EPILEPSY

Epilepsy is a neurological disorder characterized by a *recurrent* pattern of abnormal neuronal discharges within the brain, resulting in a sudden loss or disturbance of consciousness, sometimes in association with motor activity, sensory phenomena, or inappropriate behavior. Between 1% and 2% of the population is estimated to have epilepsy. The cause of epilepsy may be unknown (idiopathic) or may be traced to a known brain lesion. In general, epilepsy appearing in childhood or adolescence is likely to be idiopathic, whereas epilepsy appearing in adulthood is likely to relate to a definable cause such as a head injury, stroke, or brain tumor.

An appropriate choice of drugs, taken on a long-term basis, can control the seizures of epilepsy in about 80% of the patients. The choice of drugs depends on a careful diagnosis of the seizure pattern, which ideally is made from the observation of a seizure and the recording of the brain wave pattern with an electroencephalogram (EEG) during the seizure. The diagnosis is critical to the selection of a drug or drugs, since different seizure patterns are controlled by different drugs. Other causes of seizures must be ruled out, since seizures may be secondary to an organic disorder such as a brain tumor, poisoning, fever, hypoglycemia, and hypocalcemia. An overdose of certain drugs, for example, local anesthetics and ketamine, causes seizures. Abrupt withdrawal of some drugs such as the barbiturates and most other sedative-hypnotic drugs including alcohol can precipitate seizures.

■ CATEGORIES OF EPILEPSY

Epilepsy is now most frequently described by the classification published by the International League Against Epilepsy in 1970. This classification is presented in Table 31-1. The purpose of this classification is to describe the seizure pattern by the area of brain involved.

■ Partial seizures and generalized seizures

Partial seizures and generalized seizures are the two major categories of epilepsy. Partial seizures are those arising from a focal lesion of the brain in which the abnormal discharge of cells involves a limited area of the brain. The location of the lesion determines the type of seizure observed: motor, cognitive, behavioral, or sensory. Consciousness is usually not lost, but the patient may not remember seizure episodes when cognitive or behavioral function is involved. Focal seizures and psychomotor seizures are two examples of partial seizures that will be discussed more fully. Generalized seizures result from the discharge of cells over both side of the brain. Grand mal seizures, petit mal seizures, infantile spasms, and myoclonus are examples of generalized seizures which will be described more fully.

Grand mal epilepsy. Grand mal or general tonic-clonic epilepsy involves the contraction of all skeletal muscles. Before the seizure begins, the patient may experience an *aura*. An aura is a sensation peculiar for that patient, which can be a visual disturbance or a certain dizziness or numbness that warns the patient of an impending seizure. The patient then suddenly loses consciousness and may utter a cry as the diaphragm contracts and expels air from the lungs. The seizure consists of tonic (sustained) contractions and/or clonic (intermittent) contractions of the muscles. The patient may become incontinent. When the contractions cease, the patient regains consciousness but is usually confused and drowsy and lapses into prolonged sleep (postictal depression).

Petit mal or absence epilepsy. Petit mal or absence epilepsy occurs mainly in children 4 to 12 years old. The child suddenly loses consciousness for a few seconds although body tone is seldom lost and consciousness is regained with no confusion. The appearance is

TABLE 31-1. International classification of seizures

Class	Specific signs and symptoms
Generalized seizures: without focal onset, symmetrical on both brain hemispheres. Consciousness is lost unless otherwise indicated.	1. Tonic-clonic seizures (grand mal). 2. Tonic seizures: sustained contraction of a large muscle group. 3. Clonic seizures: arrhythmic contractions of parts of the body. 4. Absence seizures (petit mal): brief loss of consciousness, 3 spikes per second EEG. 5. Bilateral massive epileptic myoclonus (consciousness is usually not altered), isolated clonic jerks. 6. Infantile spasms: muscle spasms, bizarre EEG. 7. Atonic seizures: loss of postural tone with sagging of the head (head drop) or falling down. 8. Akinetic seizures: complete relaxation of all muscles.
Partial seizures: focal seizures	1. Elementary symptoms, consciousness is not lost. a. Motor symptoms (jacksonian). b. Sensory (hallucinations—visual, auditory, taste) or somatosensory (tingling) symptoms. c. Autonomic symptoms. d. Compound forms. 2. Complex symptoms, consciousness impaired (temporal lobe or psychomotor epilepsy). a. Cognitive symptoms: confusion, memory distorted. b. Affective symptoms: bizarre behavior. c. Psychosensory symptoms: automatisms—repetitive, purposeless behaviors.
Unilateral seizures: only one half of brain involved.	
Unclassified: incomplete data.	

one of inattention or daydreaming and may be accompanied by slight blinking or hand movements. The attacks usually occur several times a day. The EEG shows a three-per-second spike wave pattern. Petit mal epilepsy does not generally continue into adulthood, but many patients with petit mal epilepsy subsequently develop other types of epilepsy, particularly grand mal epilepsy. For this reason, many physicians treat children with petit mal epilepsy prophylactically for grand mal epilepsy in addition to treating the petit mal epilepsy. There is some evidence that this prophylactic treatment reduces the incidence of subsequent grand mal epilepsy.

Infantile spasms. Infantile spasms denote a major generalized seizure that occurs in the first year of life. The seizure consists of a sudden, transient, repetitive contraction of the limbs and trunk. There is a sudden shocklike jerk accompanied by a sharp cry. The legs are extended, and the arms are carried forward in front of the head. These spasms may occur hundreds of times a day and are believed to originate from a congenital malformation or neonatal injury and to reflect an immature nervous system. If the seizures persist after 1 year of age, the seizure pattern changes, most commonly to a petit mal (absence) seizure, a myoclonic seizure, or a "head drop" seizure in which consciousness is lost for 10 to 15 minutes, accompanied by a loss of muscle tone in the neck.

Myoclonus epilepsy. Myoclonus epilepsy is a generalized seizure pattern that develops secondarily to anoxic brain damage (intentional myoclonus) or as a genetic disorder (progressive myoclonic epilepsy). Intentional myoclonus is a neurological symptom consisting of sudden involuntary contractions of skeletal muscles, which are aggravated by purposeful activity (hence the term *intentional*) as well as by visual, auditory, tactile and emotional activity. The genetic disorder, progressive myoclonic epilepsy, is a particular form of intentional myoclonus that appears in childhood and becomes progressively worse. When untreated, the genetic disease leads to death after 15 to 20 years.

Psychomotor or temporal lobe epilepsy. Psychomotor or temporal lobe epilepsy has complex symptoms that include an aura, automatism, and motor seizures, independently or in combination. These seizures usually last about 5 minutes. The patient will remember the aura, but not the automatism or motor seizure. The automatism may consist of chewing or swallowing motions, tempermental changes, confusion, feelings of unreality, or unexplained, bizarre behavior. A detailed neurological examination may be required to differentiate psychomotor epilepsy from psychotic mental illness.

TABLE 31-2. Drug choice by seizure type

Seizure type	First-choice drugs*	Additional drugs for second-choice drugs†	Refractory cases
General: tonic-clonic (grand mal) Partial: cortical focal (including jacksonian)	Alone or in combination: 1. Phenytoin (Dilantin)—adults 2. Phenobarbital (Luminal)—children 3. Carbamazepine (Tegretol)	1. Other barbiturates: primidone (Mysoline) or mephobarbital (Mebaral) 2. Valproic acid (Depakene)	1. Acetazolamide (Diamox)
General: absence (petit mal)	Alone 1. Ethosuximide (Zarontin) 2. Valproic acid (Depakene)	1. Other succinimides: methsuximide (Celontin) or phensuximide (Milontin) 2. Benzodiazepines: diazepam (Valium) or clonazepam (Clonopin)	1. Trimethadione (Tridione) 2. Acetazolamide (Diamox)
General: myoclonus (intentional or progressive)	1. Valproic acid (Depakene)	1. Clonazepam (Clonopin) 2. 1,5,-Hydroxytryptophan and carbidopa (experimental)	1. Ethosuximide (Zarontin) 2. Diazepam (Valium)
General: infantile spasms	1. ACTH	1. Clonazepam (Clonopin)	
Partial: complex (temporal lobe, psychomotor)	1. Carbamazepine (Tegretol)	1. Primidone (Mysoline) 2. Phenytoin (Dilantin)	1. Phensuximide (Milontin)
Status epilepticus: continuous tonic-clonic	1. Intravenous diazepam (Valium) 2. Intravenous phenytoin sodium (Dilantin) 3. Intravenous phenobarbital sodium (Luminal Sodium)	1. Rectal paraldehyde 2. Intravenous amobarbital sodium (Amytal Sodium)	1. Lidocaine (Xylocaine)

*First-choice drugs are those which are generally effective for most patients with the least incidence of toxic effects.
†Second-choice drugs are those which are sometimes effective when the first-choice drugs are not effective alone or which are associated with a higher incidence of side effects.

Focal seizures. Focal seizures are not associated with a loss of consciousness. Focal sensory seizures may be visual, such as flashes of light; tactile, such as a feeling of numbness or tingling; or motor. Focal motor seizures of the jacksonian type begin with clonic seizures of a few muscles on half of the face or in one extremity; the seizures then progress *(march)* to include more body musculature (e.g., finger, hand, arm).

Status epilepticus. Status epilepticus refers to seizures that last 30 minutes or longer or to seizures that are repeated for 30 minutes or longer and during which consciousness is not regained. Status epilepticus of the generalized tonic-clonic type is a medical emergency. In about 80% of patients with status epilepticus, the seizures are secondary to a disease, frequently associated with a low blood concentration of calcium or glucose, or the seizures are secondary to withdrawal from drugs such as the barbiturates or other sedative-hypnotic drugs. The immediate goals are to establish an airway, to stop the seizures, and then to identify the cause of the seizures.

■ DRUGS TO CONTROL SEIZURES

■ General principles for drug therapy of epilepsy

Several drugs are available for control of epileptic seizures. The drug choice depends on the diagnosis of the seizure patterns and on the tolerance and response of the patient to the drug prescribed. The drugs most frequently effective for various seizure patterns are listed in Table 31-2. Table 31-3 lists the dosage information for these drugs.

Mechanism of action. The molecular mechanism by which anticonvulsant drugs act is not understood. In general terms, these drugs depress the excitability of neurons, particularly those which fire inappropriately to initiate the seizure, and thereby prevent the spread of seizure discharges. Presumably the mechanisms will be found to modify the ionic movements of sodium, potassium, or calcium across the nerve membrane associated with the action potential or to modify the release or uptake of neurotransmitters.

TABLE 31-3. Anticonvulsant drugs

Generic name	Trade name	Dosage and administration	Comments
LONG-ACTING BARBITURATES			
Phenobarbital	Luminal	ORAL: *Adults*—50 to 100 mg 2 to 3 times daily. *Children*—15 to 50 mg 2 to 3 times daily.	May begin at twice usual dose for the first 4 days to raise plasma concentration rapidly. Multiple daily doses are to minimize sedation. Effective serum concentration, 15 to 40 μg/ml. In addition to its use for epileptic seizures, phenobarbital is used prophylactically for febrile seizures in children.
	Luminal Sodium	INTRAMUSCULAR, INTRAVENOUS (SLOW): *Adults*—200 to 320 mg, can repeat after 6 hr. INTRAMUSCULAR: *Children*—3 to 5 mg/kg body weight.	For status epilepticus. Sodium salt must be used for injection.
Mephobarbital	Mebaral	ORAL: *Adults*—400 to 600 mg daily in divided doses. *Children*—over 5 yr; 32 to 64 mg given 3 to 4 times daily; under 5 yr, 16 to 32 mg given 3 to 4 times daily.	Mephobarbital is metabolized to phenobarbital.
Primidione	Mysoline	ORAL: *Adults*—250 mg daily at bedtime or up to 2 Gm daily in divided doses. *Children*—over 8 yr, as for adults; under 8 yr, ½ adult dosage.	Effective serum concentrations, 5 to 10 μg/ml.
HYDANTOINS			
Phenytoin	Dilantin	ORAL: *Adults*—300 mg daily in 3 doses. Maintenance dose, 300 to 600 mg daily. *Children*—5 mg/kg daily in 2 to 3 doses. Maximum dose, 300 mg daily.	May be given once a day to improve compliance. Effective serum concentration, 10 to 20 μg/ml. Brand name should be specified because of varying bioavailability among brands.
Mephenytoin	Mesantoin	ORAL: *Adults*—200 to 600 mg daily. *Children*—100 to 400 mg daily.	
Ethotoin	Peganone	ORAL: *Adults*—1000 mg daily increased gradually to 2000 to 3000 mg in 4 to 6 divided doses. *Children*—500 to 1000 mg in divided doses.	
SUCCINIMIDES			
Ethosuximide	Zarontin	ORAL: *Adults*—500 mg daily increased gradually every 4 to 7 days to control seizures. *Children*—over 6 yr, as for adults; 3 to 6 yr, 250 mg daily increased gradually to control seizures.	Effective serum concentration, 40 to 80 μg/ml.
Methsuximide	Celontin	ORAL: 300 mg daily for 1 wk, increased weekly by 300 mg to control seizures to a maximum dose of 1200 mg daily.	
Phensuximide	Milontin	ORAL: 500 to 1000 mg 2 to 3 times daily.	

TABLE 31-3. Anticonvulsant drugs—cont'd

Generic name	Trade name	Dosage and administration	Comments
OXAZOLIDINEDIONES			
Trimethadione	Tridione	ORAL: *Adults*—900 mg daily divided into 3 to 4 doses, can increase by 300 mg daily every 7 days to control seizures; maximum, 2400 mg daily. *Children*—40 mg/kg body weight daily divided into 3 to 4 doses.	No longer widely used because of serious side effects and high teratogenic potential. Effective serum concentration of dimethadione (active metabolite), 700 μg/ml or higher.
BENZODIAZEPINES			
Diazepam	Valium	INTRAVENOUSLY, to terminate status epilepticus: *Adults*—5 to 10 mg (no faster than 5 mg/min, use a large vein). Can repeat every 10 to 15 min to a maximum dose of 30 mg. *Children*—30 days to 5 yr, 0.2 to 0.5 mg slowly every 2 to 5 min, maximum 5 mg; over 5 yr, 1 mg slowly every 2 to 5 min, maximum 10 mg.	See Chapter 24 for use as an antianxiety drug. Rarely used orally as an anticonvulsant agent. Do not mix or dilute into intravenous fluids.
Clonazepam	Clonopin	ORAL: *Adults*—1.5 mg daily in 3 doses, increase every 3 days by 0.5 to 1 mg to control seizures; maximum total dose, 20 mg daily. *Children*—Infants to 10 yr, 0.01 to 0.03 mg/kg body weight, increased by 0.25 to 0.5 mg every 3 days to control seizures to a maximum of 0.2 mg/kg daily.	Effective therapeutic plasma concentrations, 5 to 70 ng/ml.
MISCELLANEOUS			
Acetazolamide	Diamox	ORAL: *Adults and children*—8 to 30 mg/kg body weight in divided doses.	A weak diuretic. Tolerance usually develops.
Adrenocorticotropic hormone (ACTH)		INTRAMUSCULAR: *Infants*—10 units daily, increase by 5 units every 5 days up to 60 units for 6 to 7 wk.	If ACTH is ineffective, diazepam, 3 mg/lb, is added. If ACTH is effective in 2 wk, may switch to cortisone, 3 mg/lb, as an alternative to increasing ACTH. Cortisone is brought down by 1 mg/lb over 3 wk.
Carbamazepine	Tegretol	ORAL: *Adults and children over 12 yr*, 200 mg twice on day 1, increase by 200 mg daily to control seizures; maximum dose, 1000 mg (less than 15 yr) or 1200 mg (over 15 yr). Doses are taken every 6 to 8 hr.	Take medication with meals to avoid gastrointestinal distress. Effective therapeutic plasma concentrations, 4 to 12 μg/ml.
Lidocaine hydrochloride	Xylocaine Hydrochloride	INTRAVENOUS: *Adults*—to terminate status epilepticus: Infuse 1 to 3 mg/min to terminate seizures.	A last resort for terminating status epilepticus. If given in excess, lidocaine itself can induce convulsion.

Continued.

TABLE 31-3. Anticonvulsant drugs—cont'd

Generic name	Trade name	Dosage and administration	Comments
Paraldehyde		INTRAMUSCULAR, INTRAVENOUS, to terminate status epilepticus: *Adults or children*—0.15 ml/kg body weight. Solution must be diluted. RECTAL: *Children*—0.3 ml/kg body weight diluted 1:1 in olive oil or milk.	A last resort for terminating status epilepticus.
Valproic acid	Depakene	ORAL: *Adults and children*—15 mg/kg body weight daily in divided doses. Can be increased by 5 to 10 mg/kg daily every 7 days to control seizures, up to 60 mg/kg daily.	The newest anticonvulsant in the United States. Clinical potential still to be explored, but drug effective in controlling myoclonic epilepsy refractory to most other anticonvulsant drugs. Effective serum concentrations reported to be 50 to 100 μg/ml.

Because the specific mechanisms underlying seizure activity are not understood, the development of better drugs for controlling seizures is a matter of screening drugs using animal models that incompletely parallel human seizure disorders. Three new drugs for treatment of epilepsy were approved by the Food and Drug Administration (FDA) in the 1970's: carbamazepine (Tegretol), clonazepam (Clonopin), and valproic acid (Depakene).

Drug administration. The drug of choice is started out in small doses to allow the patient to develop a tolerance to the drowsiness and motor incoordination (ataxia) associated with most of the anticonvulsant drugs. (The exception is phenytoin [Dilantin], which is initially given in a high "loading" dose.) The drug dose is increased until the seizures are stopped or until toxic effects of the drug appear. If the drug has been partially effective in controlling seizures, a second drug may be added. If the first drug tried has not been effective, the patient is switched to a different drug.

Since the most common cause of drug failure is the failure of the patient to take the prescribed drugs, the plasma concentration of drug may be determined before deciding that the drug per se is ineffective. Patients must be warned not to discontinue medication when the seizures are under control or the side effects are disturbing. The sudden discontinuance of medication greatly increases the incidence of seizures. Blood and urine analyses are often routinely carried out because many of the anticonvulsant drugs infrequently produce blood dyscrasias and/or renal damage.

Many patients with epilepsy will require drug therapy throughout their lives to control seizures. However, some patients with epilepsy may be able to discontinue medication. These patients are those reaching adulthood after treatment from childhood for petit mal epilepsy and those patients who have had several seizure-free years. If the EEG of such a patient appears normal, medication can be gradually discontinued. Seizures recur in ¼ to ½ of such patients.

Therapy and pregnancy. Women with epilepsy who wish to have children need to be advised that their offspring carry a two- to three-fold greater risk for congenital defects, particularly when the mother is taking phenytoin (Dilantin) or phenobarbital (Luminal). In the absence of any medication the fetus is still at greater than normal risk because of anoxia during seizures. Pregnancies during which the woman is taking trimethadione (Tridione) are associated with an 80% incidence of spontaneous abortions or birth defects. If possible, a woman taking trimethadione should be switched to ethosuximide (Zarontin) before becoming pregnant.

Long-acting barbiturates

Phenobarbital

Phenobarbital (Luminal) has been widely used for 60 years and is a drug of choice in the treatment of grand mal and focal motor epilepsy. Phenobarbital is also used for treatment of withdrawal from barbiturates or alcohol. Phenobarbital is cross-tolerant with alcohol and other barbiturates but requires only once-a-day administration because of its long plasma half-life of 4 days. Because of this long plasma half-life, 14 days are required to reach constant serum concentrations of this drug. Phenobarbital is sometimes given intravenously to stop the seizures of status epilepticus, but the degree of respiratory depression can be profound.

The main side effects of the barbiturates are sedation

and drowsiness at the beginning of treatment, but tolerance usually develops to these effects. In the elderly and in children a paradoxical excitement may be seen that impairs learning ability in the children. Phenobarbital does increase the incidence of congenital malformations in the fetus but not to the degree associated with phenytoin and trimethadione. Phenobarbital induces liver microsomal enzymes and can thereby speed its own metabolism as well as the metabolism of other drugs. The sudden rather than gradual withdrawal of the drug can precipitate convulsions. Barbiturates are contraindicated for patients with the metabolic disorder called *porphyria* and for patients who are depressed and might consider suicide.

Mephobarbital

Mephobarbital (Mebaral) is metabolized by the liver to phenobarbital, so there is no advantage to substituting mephobarbital for phenobarbital.

Primidone

Primidone (Mysoline) is a deoxybarbiturate that is metabolized to phenobarbital and phenylethylmalonamide. Primidone can therefore substitute for phenobarbital in the treatment of grand mal and focal motor seizures, but in addition is effective in treating temporal lobe (psychomotor) epilepsy.

■ Hydantoins

Phenytoin

Phenytoin (Dilantin), formerly called diphenylhydantoin, is a drug of choice in controlling grand mal and focal motor epilepsy in adults and is occasionally used in treating psychomotor epilepsy.

Pharmacokinetics. Phenytoin has a plasma half-life of 24 hours, so it takes 4 days to reach steady plasma levels when initiating therapy. To decrease this time, the initial dose is sometimes given as a loading dose at three times the usual daily dose. At serum concentrations much above therapeutic concentrations, the capacity of the liver to metabolize phenytoin is saturated so that plasma concentrations decrease very slowly. Phenytoin is irregularly absorbed from the intestine. Since the absorption depends on the formulation, it is best to stay with a particular brand of phenytoin.

Phenytoin should not be given intramuscularly or subcutaneously because it is highly irritating and can precipitate in the tissue. The sodium salt can be administered intravenously but too rapid an administration can produce severe hypotension and cardiac arrest. Sodium phenytoin is administered intravenously to control status epilepticus either alone or after intravenous diazepam has controlled the seizures. Intravenous sodium phenytoin is also used to control some cardiac arrhythmias (Chapter 16).

Adverse effects. Effective serum concentrations are 10 to 20 μg/ml, and side effects are seen at higher serum concentrations: at greater than 20 μg/ml, involuntary movement of the eyeballs (nystagmus) are seen; at greater than 30 μg/ml, incoordination (ataxia) and slurred speech are observed. Tremors and nervousness or drowsiness and fatigue may be side effects of higher serum concentrations. However, an acute overdose of phenytoin is seldom fatal. Persistance of these side effects requires reducing the dose or switching to another drug, usually phenobarbital.

About 20% of patients taking phenytoin have an overgrowth of the gums (gingival hyperplasia), which is particularly severe in children. Occasionally, a folic acid or vitamin D deficiency can be produced because phenytoin interferes with the normal metabolism of these compounds. Phenytoin can also cause an allergic rash that can be mistaken for measles or infectious mononucleosis. Phenytoin also makes a case of acne worse, which is especially bothersome to teenagers, and can increase growth of body hair (hirsutism), which is undesirable in women. Mention has been made of the higher incidence of congenital malformations in infants of mothers taking phenytoin. These infants are also at risk for hemorrhage and coagulation deficiencies at birth that can be corrected with vitamin K.

Drug interactions. Several important drug interactions are noted with phenytoin. Phenobarbital can increase the metabolism of phenytoin in some individuals by inducing liver microsomal enzymes, but in other individuals phenobarbital decreases the rate of phenytoin metabolism by competing with phenytoin for the degrading enzymes. Dicumarol, the oral anticoagulant, and carbamazepine, the anticonvulsant, decrease the metabolism of phenytoin by competing with the enzymes for degradation. Valproic acid, the anticonvulsant, displaces bound phenytoin from protein to increase the free concentration of phenytoin while decreasing the total concentration of phenytoin because more free phenytoin is available for metabolism. Phenytoin enhances the rate of estrogen metabolism, which can decrease the effectiveness of some birth control pills.

Other anticonvulsant drugs related to phenytoin are *mephenytoin (Mesantoin)* and *ethotoin (Peganone).* Mephenytoin is associated with a high incidence of agranulocytosis and aplastic anemia. Ethotoin is not widely used, although it does not seem to cause gingival hyperplasia, hairiness, or incoordination.

■ Succinimides

Ethosuximide

Ethosuximide (Zarontin) is a drug of choice for controlling absence (petit mal) seizures and may be effective in treating myoclonic seizures. The plasma half-life of ethosuximide is 30 hours in children and 60 hours in adults. The effective serum concentration is 40 to 80 μg/ml, but serum concentrations of up to 160 μg/ml can be tolerated without excessive toxicity. Side effects include dizziness, drowsiness, and gastrointestinal irritation. Blood counts are performed routinely because of the occasional occurrence of agranulocytosis.

Related drugs are *phensuximide (Milontin),* which is sometimes effective in treating psychomotor epilepsy, and *methsuximide (Celontin).*

■ Oxazolidinediones

Trimethadione

Trimethadione (Tridione) was the first drug found to be effective in controlling absence seizures (petit mal epilepsy), but this drug is now a third-choice drug for absence seizures because of the high incidence of serious side effects.

Trimethadione can produce a serious allergic dermatitis, kidney and liver damage, agranulocytosis, and aplastic anemia. Blood counts and urinalysis are done routinely with trimethadione therapy. In adults, trimethadione frequently produces an intolerance to light (photophobia). The 80% incidence of spontaneous abortions or congenital anomalies in infants of mothers taking trimethadione has been mentioned.

The other anticonvulsant of the oxazolidinedione class, *paramethadione (Paradione)* is no longer used because of its toxicity.

■ Benzodiazepines

Diazepam and clonazepam

Diazepam (Valium) and clonazepam (Clonopin) are used as anticonvulsant drugs. Diazepam, administered intravenously, is the drug of choice for terminating the clonic-tonic seizures of status epilepticus and is sometimes used to terminate the seizures of eclampsia. Oral diazepam is occasionally used with other anticonvulsants to control myoclonic seizures, akinetic (head drop) seizures, and absence (petit mal) seizures. The main side effects are drowsiness, dizziness, and ataxia. Respiratory depression must be watched during intravenous administration. However, overall diazepam is a safe drug. The major use of diazepam is as an antianxiety drug (Chapter 24).

Clonazepam is one of the new anticonvulsants and was approved for use by the FDA in 1976. Clonazepam is effective in controlling absence (petit mal) seizures, myoclonic seizures, and infantile spasms. Tolerance can develop to clonazepam, and seizures recur in about one third of treated patients. The effectiveness of clonazepam in controlling tonic-clonic (grand mal) seizures and temporal lobe (psychomotor) seizures is being tested but is probably not sufficient.

The plasma half-life of clonazepam is 20 to 40 hours. Clonazepam is metabolized in the liver to a compound that probably has little anticonvulsant activity.

Neurological side effects are commonly seen during therapy with clonazepam and include drowsiness, incoordination (ataxia), and personality changes. Children treated with clonazepam may become hyperactive, irritable, aggressive, violent, or disobedient. Slurred speech, tremors, abnormal eye movements, dizziness, and confusion may also be noticed. These effects are dose related and may subside with time or on lowering the dose. Increased salivation and increased bronchial secretions sometimes occur and create respiratory problems in children.

■ Miscellaneous drugs

Adrenocorticotropic hormone (ACTH)

ACTH is the treatment of choice for infantile spasms. If daily administration for 20 days is effective, the course of treatment is repeated after 2 to 4 weeks or glucocorticoids (usually prednisone) are given. The action of ACTH is to stimulate the adrenal cortex to synthesize glucocorticoids (Chapter 35). Presumably the effectiveness of ACTH in treating infantile spasms is related to this endocrine action.

Acetazolamide

Acetazolamide (Diamox) is used alone or with other drugs in treating petit mal epilepsy. The mechanism of action is the inhibition of the enzyme carbonic anhydrase in the brain, which results in an altered ratio of intracellular to extracellular sodium. Acetazolamide is also a weak diuretic. Side effects of acetazolamide include loss of appetite, drowsiness, confusion, and a tingling feeling. The usefulness of acetazolamide is limited by the frequent development of tolerance to its anticonvulsant action.

Carbamazepine

Carbamazepine (Tegretol) is one of the new anticonvulsant drugs approved by the FDA in 1974. It is particularly effective in controlling the seizures of temporal lobe (psychomotor) epilepsy and clonic-tonic (grand mal) seizures. The plasma half-life is 12 hours, so the drug must be given in divided doses. Carbamazepine is metabolized by the liver, and one of the metabolites has anticonvulsant activity. Absorption from the gastrointestinal tract is slow and can be improved if the drug is taken at meals.

Carbamazepine is chemically related to the tricyclic antidepressants, and a positive side effect is the increased alertness and improvement of mood in patients taking the drug. The side effects most frequently experienced are drowsiness, dizziness, incoordination (ataxia), visual disturbances (particularly double vision), and gastrointestinal upset. Carbamazepine infrequently causes rashes, liver damage, and bone marrow depression, which require discontinuance of the drug. Blood counts should be made frequently in the early course of treatment and occasionally thereafter.

The drug interactions encountered with carbamazepine include a decreased plasma concentration in the presence of other anticonvulsants, presumably because the other agents induce drug-metabolizing enzymes in the liver. Propoxyphene napsylate (Darvon napsylate) dramatically increases plasma concentrations of carbamazepine, probably by competing for metabolizing enzymes.

Lidocaine hydrochloride

Lidocaine hydrochloride (Xylocaine hydrochloride) is another drug used as a last resort to terminate status epilepticus. Lidocaine is a local anesthetic (Chapter 30) and can itself induce convulsions at high doses. Lidocaine can also depress the heart, an effect that is utilized in treating some cardiac arrhythmias (Chapter 16).

Paraldehyde

Paraldehyde is a sedative-hypnotic drug that is seldom used today because of its objectionable odor and chemical instability on storage. When other drugs are ineffective in terminating status epilepticus, paraldehyde may be tried. An advantage is that administration may be intramuscular, intravenous, or rectal. However, when given intravenously, it must be diluted and administered slowly not only to avoid producing severe coughing, which can result from bronchopulmonary irritation, but also to avoid irritating the veins, which can result in thrombophlebitis. Use of paraldehyde is contraindicated in patients with pulmonary disease, because the drug aggravates bronchopulmonary disease, and in patients with liver disease, because paraldehyde is metabolized by the liver.

Valproic acid

Valproic acid (Depakene) was approved for use as an anticonvulsant in 1978 in response to public pressure. In Europe, valproic acid had been dramatically shown to be effective in controlling the seizures of progressive myoclonus, a particularly disabling type of epilepsy in children for which there had previously been no effective treatment. In addition, valproic acid is effective in treating other types of general seizures: absence (petit mal) and tonic-clonic (grand mal) seizures. Since the plasma half-life of valproic acid is only 8 to 12 hours, the drug is administered 3 or 4 times per day.

Valproic acid is an analogue of the inhibitory central neurotransmitter, gamma aminobutyric acid (GABA), which inhibits neuronal activity. One mechanism by which valproic acid may act is to increase the concentration of this inhibitory neurotransmitter.

Side effects. The most frequent side effect experienced with valproic acid is gastrointestinal distress. Sedation is marked at the beginning of treatment unless the doses are gradually raised. An overdose has been reported to produce coma but with uneventful recovery. The incidence of liver damage among patients taking valproic acid is being examined in light of some reports of liver failure.

Drug interactions. Drug interactions with valproic acid include its decreased plasma concentration in the presence of other anticonvulsants that induce liver microsomal enzymes: phenobarbital, primidone, phenytoin, and carbamazepine. Phenytoin can also raise the concentration of free plasma valproic acid by displacing the fraction bound to plasma proteins.

■ THE NURSING PROCESS FOR ANTICONVULSANT DRUGS

■ Assessment

With a few exceptions, most patients using the drugs in this chapter will be the ones who have had a seizure, and it is usually safe to assume that once the correct drugs and dosages have been chosen for a patient, the drugs will be needed on a long-term basis. Patients who have had a seizure will be monitored carefully for the possible effects of the seizure and for possible later seizures. In relation to drug therapy, a baseline patient assessment should be done with special emphasis on areas known to be affected by the drugs that will be used. For example, since phenytoin causes gingival hyperplasia frequently, a baseline assessment of the mouth, teeth, and gums should be done and recorded at the start of phenytoin therapy.

■ Management

Drug dosages are adjusted until the seizures are controlled or until toxic effects are noted. The nurse should monitor the general condition of the patient with an emphasis on known drug side effects. For example, monitoring the amount of sedation produced by phenobarbital would provide important information toward determining the most effective dose. Serum levels of the prescribed drugs may be monitored. If the patient is continuing to have seizures, the nurse should observe the type and duration of seizures and continue nursing measures to prevent injury, such as padding siderails or supervising ambulation. See a textbook of nursing for additional information. Referring the patient on discharge to the health department for follow-up care may be helpful, as may referral to social service or vocational rehabilitation if appropriate.

■ Evaluation

Ideally anticonvulsants would halt the seizures and thus there would be no side effects resulting from drug therapy. Often this is not possible. Although seizure activity may be controlled, the long-term therapy and combinations of drugs sometimes needed often produce at least a few side effects. It is then necessary for the health care team to decide which side effects cannot be permitted and which can be treated or tolerated. The nurse should evaluate the patient regularly through observation, should reassess known problem areas (e.g., the mouth with phenytoin therapy), and should make appropriate referrals. For instance, if phenytoin is causing a problem with acne, but the decision is made that the anticonvulsant must be continued, referral to a dermatologist may be appropriate.

On discharge, the patient or parent should be able to name the drugs being taken and to state how to take them correctly, including the dose, the time of day, and the correct preparation of the dose; to explain the side effects that may occur, which need to be reported immediately, how to treat or prevent those which are more likely to occur, and what to do if a dose is missed. The patient should be able to state the importance of wearing a medical identification tag or bracelet. For additional information, see the patient care implications section at the end of this chapter.

■ PATIENT CARE IMPLICATIONS

General guidelines for patients receiving anticonvulsants

1. Women of childbearing age may wish to consider using birth control measures while on anticonvulsant therapy. If a woman desires to conceive, she should discuss her plans with her physician so that she can obtain current information about the risks associated with each drug.
2. Instruct patients to continue taking anticonvulsants as ordered, even after they have been seizure free for a period of time. Point out that they are seizure free because they are taking the ordered medications. Suddenly discontinuing anticonvulsants increases the chances of having more seizures.

3. Patients on long-term anticonvulsant therapy should be encouraged to wear a medical identification tag or bracelet. In addition, suggest that they carry in their wallets a card listing current drugs and dosages and keep this listing current.
4. Encourage patients to return for follow-up visits, at which time discussion and evaluation of any side effects can occur. In addition, routine blood work to monitor for hepatic, renal, or hematopoietic effects can be done.
5. Remind patients to keep all health care providers informed of all medications being taken.
6. Referral to appropriate agencies for assistance and follow-up should be done. Such agencies might include the local visiting nurse association, vocational rehabilitation, or the Epilepsy Foundation of America, 1828 L Street, Washington, D.C. 20036.
7. Patients should avoid the use of alcohol unless permitted in small amounts by the physician. Alcohol can alter the seizure threshold in some patients and causes central nervous system depression.
8. The care of a patient during a seizure is beyond the scope of this text. Please refer to general texts of pediatric or medical-surgical nursing or to appropriate journal articles.

Long-acting barbiturates and primidione

1. The major troubling side effect is drowsiness; with continued therapy, this will usually begin to diminish. Caution patients to avoid activities for which mental alertness is essential, for example, driving or operating machinery. Other side effects include rash, gastrointestinal upset, nausea, and vomiting.
2. Signs of intoxication or overdose include slurred speech, ataxia, and vertigo. If these signs occur, instruct the patient and family to notify the physician; a reduction in dosage is probably necessary.
3. The barbiturates may lower the blood levels of oral anticoagulants, resulting in insufficient anticoagulation and perhaps a need for an increase in dosage.
4. Intravenous phenobarbital: If using powder, dilute as instructed. Desired dose of solution should be further diluted to a volume of 10 ml. Administer slowly, 60 mg per minute. In patients with status epilepticus or grand mal seizures, it may not be possible to monitor the blood pressure. Be alert for hypotension and respiratory depression.
5. Observe patients for respiratory depression for 30 to 60 minutes after intramuscular injections.
6. Caution patients to keep these and all medications out of reach of children.
7. See also Chapter 24.

Hydantoins

1. The preferred route of administration for phenytoin is the oral route. The capsule preparation manufactured by Parke-Davis has been approved for once-a-day dosing if desired instead of divided doses. Once-a-day administration may result in better patient compliance; consult the physician.
2. It is important that patients continue to take the same brand of phenytoin. Switching brands may result in alterations in absorption and metabolism.
3. An oral suspension of phenytoin is available. Instruct patients and parents of children to shake the bottle vigorously before preparing each dose. Without adequate resuspension the patient may be underdosed with the liquid near the top of the bottle and overdosed as the contents of the bottle near the bottom are used.
4. Patients should be taught to use meticulous oral hygiene while taking hydantoins, including regular brushing and flossing. Sometimes children will be more interested in regular brushing if there is an electric toothbrush available. Even with good oral hygiene, some patients will still develop gingival hyperplasia. Regular dental care should be stressed and patients instructed to tell the dentist that phenytoin is being used.
5. Toxicity and overdose can be observed by the alert parent, family member, or health care provider. Signs include ataxia, nystagmus, and slurred speech. If these occur, notify the physician.
6. Intravenous phenytoin: The drug should be reconstituted only with the diluent provided by the manufacturer. The drug is incompatible with other drugs and intravenous fluids, so it should not be mixed. The drug is administered by slow intravenous push (bolus) at a rate not exceeding 50 mg per minute. Given via this route, the drug can cause hypotension and cardiac arrest. If at all possible, the patient should be attached to a cardiac monitor during intravenous administration.
7. Remember that even if phenytoin is being used for its anticonvulsant effects, it still has the same cardiac effects as discussed in Chapter 16.
8. There are a variety of side effects with phenytoin: nausea, vomiting, hirsutism, acne, rash, dizziness, insomnia, and headache. Instruct the patient to report side effects to the physician.
9. Phenytoin is best taken with meals, a snack, or milk to reduce gastric irritation.
10. Phenytoin may cause hyperglycemia. Diabetics should monitor urine glucose levels carefully; an increase in insulin dosage may be necessary.

11. Megaloblastic anemia, a result of a folic acid deficiency caused by long-term phenytoin use, may occur. Symptoms develop slowly and include easy fatigability, weakness, fainting, and headache, although the first sign may be alteration in routine blood work. Treatment is with folic acid therapy.
12. Symptoms of other blood dyscrasias (thrombocytopenia, agranulocytosis, pancytopenia) include fatigue, pallor, easy bruising or bleeding, fever, and sore throat.
13. Some patients experience drowsiness with the hydantoins, especially with mephenytoin. If drowsiness occurs, caution the patient to avoid activities requiring mental alertness (driving, operating machinery) until the drowsiness diminishes, as it may with continued therapy.
14. Review the drug interactions discussed in the text.

Succinimides

1. Symptoms of agranulocytosis include fatigue, pallor, fever, and sore throat. Instruct the patient to report these or any unusual symptoms immediately.
2. Drowsiness may occur but will usually diminish with continued use. If it occurs, patients should be instructed to avoid situations requiring mental alertness (driving, operating machinery). If severe, it may be necessary to reduce the dose.
3. Other side effects include anorexia, nausea, vomiting, diarrhea, rash, gum hypertrophy, and hirsutism. Patients should be instructed to use meticulous oral hygiene, including brushing and flossing, and to continue regular dental checkups. Taking the medications with meals may reduce gastric irritation.
4. Psychiatric disturbances have been reported but are seen more often in patients with a history of psychological problems; these disturbances include inability to concentrate, aggressiveness, paranoid psychosis, depression, and attempted suicide. Patients and family should be instructed to report any changes in personality or behavior.

Diazepam

1. Diazepam is discussed at length in Chapter 24.
2. For intravenous use in status epilepticus:
   a. The drug should not be mixed with infusion fluids or other drugs in a syringe.
   b. Administer at a rate not exceeding 5 mg per minute and even more slowly in children.
   c. Hypotension, respiratory depression, apnea, and bradycardia may occur. Monitor vital signs.
   d. It may be appropriate to have the patient attached to a cardiac monitor if large doses are being used, although this may be impossible or of limited value during a seizure.
   e. Resuscitation equipment should be available.

Clonazepam

1. Clonazepam is a central nervous system depressant so it may cause drowsiness. Caution patients to avoid activities requiring mental alertness (e.g., driving, operating machinery).
2. The use of other central nervous system depressants (drugs and alcohol) should be avoided by the patient taking clonazepam.
3. Because clonazepam may cause an increase in salivation and hypersecretion in the upper respiratory passages and depresses respirations, it should be used with caution in patients with chronic respiratory disease or in small children.
4. Behavior problems may occur as a side effect of therapy. Reported problems include confusion, depression, hallucinations, hysteria, psychosis, increased libido, and attempted suicide. As mentioned in the text, children may become irritable, aggressive, hyperactive, violent, or disobedient. Report behavioral and personality changes to the physician.
5. Neurological side effects include ataxia, abnormal eye movements, headache, nystagmus, slurred speech, and vertigo. A wide variety of other side effects have been reported. Caution patients or parents of children to report any unusual sign or symptom.

Acetazolamide

Acetazolamide is discussed in Chapter 14.

Adrenocorticotropic hormone (ACTH)

ACTH is discussed in Chapter 35.

Carbamazepine

1. Instruct the patient to report any rash, fever, sore throat, bruising, or bleeding because these signs may indicate hematopoietic reactions.
2. Side effects include drowsiness, dizziness, ataxia, visual disturbances, and gastrointestinal disturbances. Caution patients to avoid activities requiring coordination and mental alertness if side effects begin to occur.
3. Patients should take carbamazepine with meals because it may improve absorption and reduce gastrointestinal side effects.
4. Propoxyphene napsylate (Darvon-N) should be avoided by patients taking carbamazepine.
5. This drug is also used in the treatment of trigeminal neuralgia (tic dololoureux).
6. Because of the wide variety of side effects, patients should be monitored frequently with blood work and appropriate investigation of specific complaints. It is recommended that serum concentrations be used to assist in determining the correct dose for a patient. Therapeutic levels for adults should fall between 4 and 12 μg/ml.

Paraldehyde

1. Paraldehyde decomposes readily. Use only fresh, previously unopened containers, and always check the expiration date before using.
2. Paraldehyde reacts with some plastics, so it should be measured with glass syringes or containers.
3. This drug can be given via the intramuscular route but should be well diluted with sodium chloride, and care should be taken to avoid injection into any peripheral nerves. There will be pain at the injection site.
4. Intravenous paraldehyde can be extremely dangerous. Dilute as instructed in the manufacturer's literature and administer slowly, 1 ml of diluted medication per minute. Monitor vital signs.
5. For rectal instillation, the drug should be diluted in 2 volumes of olive oil to prevent irritation to the mucosa. Administer as for a retention enema. It is difficult to control the amount or rate of absorption via this route.
6. For oral administration, dilute the liquid form in juice or milk to avoid gastrointestinal irritation. Capsules are available.
7. The drug imparts a characteristic odor to the patient's breath.
8. Paraldehyde is partly excreted via the lungs, and the drug may cause coughing and an increase in bronchial secretions. Especially during intravenous administration, patients should be placed on their sides, and suctioning equipment should be available in the event secretions would be excessive.

Valproic acid

1. A variety of side effects can occur, including drowsiness, central nervous system stimulation, and excitement, but these side effects may be influenced by other anticonvulsants or drugs the patient is taking. After initiating therapy with valproic acid it is often possible to reduce the dose of or eliminate the need for some of the other drugs the patient is receiving.
2. Patients should be instructed to avoid activities requiring mental alertness (e.g., driving, operating machinery) until it is known that valproic acid will not make them drowsy or dizzy.
3. Because valproic acid is partly excreted as a ketone-containing metabolite, the urine test for ketones may be falsely positive. Patients with diabetes mellitus should be warned of this side effect.
4. Valproic acid may prolong the bleeding time, although this seems to be a greater problem when the patient is taking other drugs affecting coagulation. Instruct patients to report any bleeding, bruising, or petechiae. Patients should avoid the use of aspirin unless it is cleared by the physician.
5. Because of the possibility of drug interactions, it will often be necessary to monitor the serum concentrations of all the drugs the patient is receiving for several weeks after the initiation of therapy with valproic acid. In addition, blood tests to evaluate liver function should be performed frequently, especially during the first 6 months of therapy.
6. Instruct the patient to report any unusual sign or symptom.
7. Taking valproic acid with meals may reduce gastric irritation.
8. The capsule form should be swallowed whole and not chewed to avoid irritation to the mouth and throat. There is a liquid preparation available for those who cannot swallow capsules.
9. Tremor and transient alopecia (hair loss) may occur.

■ SUMMARY

Epilepsy is a neurogenic disorder in which certain neurons in the brain discharge abnormally to produce seizures. The site of the neurons involved determines the type of seizure experienced. As summarized in Table 31-1, the seizure pattern is recurrent and may be partial (jacksonian, psychomotor) or generalized (grand mal, petit mal, myoclonus, infantile spasms) seizures. Most seizures can be controlled by drugs, and Table 31-2 indicates which drugs are used for which seizure types.

The key anticonvulsant drug classes and their characteristics include the following:

1. Long-acting barbiturates. Phenobarbital is used to control grand mal and focal motor epilepsy in adults. Phenobarbital is generally well tolerated, and drowsiness is experienced mainly at the start of therapy. Phenobarbital induces liver microsomal enzymes and thereby speeds the metabolism of many drugs. Mephobarbital is metabolized to phenobarbital. Primidone is a related drug used to treat psychomotor epilepsy.
2. Hydantoins. Phenytoin is used to control grand mal epilepsy, especially in children, and focal motor and psychomotor epilepsy. Nystagmus, ataxia, and slurred speech are common side effects that may be controlled if the dose can be lowered. Gingival hyperplasia occurs in about 20% of patients. Important drug interactions are seen with phenobarbital, dicumarol, carbamazepine, valproic acid, and estrogens. Mephenytoin and ethotoin are not widely used.
3. Succinimides. Ethosuximide is effective in treating absence (petit mal) seizures and myoclonus. Blood counts are made to monitor for agranulocytosis. Phensuximide is used for treating psychomotor epilepsy.

4. Oxazolidinediones. Trimethadione is only rarely used for absence (petit mal) seizures because of a high incidence of serious side effects: allergic dermatitis, kidney and liver damage, agranulocytosis, and aplastic anemia.
5. Benzodiazepines. Diazepam is used principally as an intravenous medication to terminate status epilepticus. Clonazepam is a new anticonvulsant for absence (petit mal) and myoclonic seizures and infantile spasms. Personality changes (hyperactivity, aggressive behavior) or slurred speech, confusion, and abnormal eye movements are sometimes seen in children treated with clonazepam. These symptoms can usually be controlled by lowering the dose.
6. Carbamazepine. Carbamazepine is effective in treating psychomotor and grand mal epilepsy. Side effects of carbamazepine include drowsiness, ataxia, double vision, and gastrointestinal upset. Blood counts are required to monitor for bone marrow depression.
7. Valproic acid. Valproic acid is a new anticonvulsant effective in treating progressive myoclonus that had previously resisted therapy. Gastrointestinal distress is an occasional side effect, and the incidence of liver damage is being examined.
8. Other drugs. Acetazolamide is a carbonic anhydrase inhibitor used in treating absence (petit mal) seizures. Paraldehyde and lidocaine are drugs of last resort to terminate status epilepticus. Adrenocorticotropic hormone (ACTH) is used to treat infantile spasms.

■ STUDY QUESTIONS

1. Define epilepsy and list some of the known causes. What other conditions can precipitate seizures?
2. Describe grand mal, absence (petit mal), myoclonal, psychomotor, and focal seizures and infantile spasms. List the drug of choice for treating each type of epilepsy.
3. What is status epilepticus and how is it treated?
4. What considerations need to be made in beginning drug administration to control epilepsy?
5. Which are the long-acting barbiturates used in treating epilepsy? What are the side effects?
6. What are the adverse effects and drug interactions of phenytoin?
7. What are the adverse effects of the succinimides?
8. Why is trimethadione no longer widely used to treat absence (petit mal) seizures?
9. Which benzodiazepines are used as anticonvulsants? For which seizure types are they effective?
10. What are the uses and side effects of carbamazepine?
11. Why is valproic acid a valuable anticonvulsant?
12. Describe the use of acetazolamide, paraldehyde, lidocaine, and adrenocorticotropic hormone (ACTH) as anticonvulsants.

■ SUGGESTED READINGS

Chee, C.M.: Symposium on central nervous system disorders in children. Seizure disorders, Nursing Clinics of North America **15**(3):71, 1980.

Cloyd, J.C., Gumnit, R.J., and McLain, L.W., Jr.: Status epilepticus: the role of intravenous phenytoin, Journal of the American Medical Association **244:**1479, 1980.

Coping with neurologic problems proficiently, Nursing skillbook, Horsham, Pa., 1979, Intermed Communications.

Coughlin, M.K.: The child with epilepsy. Teaching children about their seizures and medications, MCN **4**(3):161, 1979.

Cutler, P., Mackey, R.W., McMasters, R.E., and Liske, E.: Therapeutics seminar: a practical guide to convulsions, Hospital Physician **9**(10):32, 1973.

Davis, J.E., and Mason, C.B.: Neurologic critical care, New York, 1979, D. Van Nostrand Co.

Dreifuss, F.E.: Use of anticonvulsant drugs, Journal of the American Medical Association **241:**607, 1979.

Farley, J.N.: The child with epilepsy. Valproic acid for children with uncontrolled epilepsy, MCN **4**(3):163, 1979.

Feldman, R.G.: Patients with epilepsy, American Family Physician **12**(4):135, 1975.

Forman, P.M.: Therapy of seizures in children, American Family Physician **10**(3):144, 1974.

Goldfrank, L., and Bresnitz, E.: Phenytoin—uses and toxicity in anticonvulsant therapy, Hospital Physician **14**(11):47, 1978.

Hawken, M., and Ozuna, J.: Practical aspects of anticonvulsant therapy, American Journal of Nursing **79:**1062, 1979.

Koch-Weser, J., and Browne, T.R.: Drug therapy: clonazepam, New England Journal of Medicine **299:**812, 1978.

Krall, R.L., Penry, J.K., Kupferberg, H.J., and Swinyard, E.A.: Antiepileptic drug development. I. History and a program for progress, Epilepsia **19:**393, 1978.

Krall, R.L., Penry, J.K., White, B.G., Kupferberg, H.J., and Swinyard, E.A.: Antiepileptic drug development. II. Anticonvulsant drug screening, Epilepsia **19:**409, 1978.

Livingston, S., and Pruce, I.: Petit mal epilepsy, American Family Physician **17**(1):107, 1978.

Livingston, S., Pauli, L.L., Pruce, I., and Kramer, I.I.: Phenobarbital versus phenytoin for grand mal epilepsy, American Family Physician **22**(2):123, 1980.

Lovely, M.P.: Identification and treatment of status epilepticus, Journal of Neurosurgical Nursing **12**(6):93, 1980.

Massey, E.W., Folger, W.N., and Riley, T.L.: Managing the epileptic patient, Postgraduate Medicine **67**(2):134, 1980.

Millichap, J.G.: Drug therapy: drug treatment of convulsive disorders, New England Journal of Medicine **286:**464, 1972.

Penry, J.K.: Are you using the "new" antiepileptic? Patient Care **12:**23, July 15, 1978.

Pippenger, C.E., and Sharkey, P.: Guide to the use of phenytoin in epilepsy, Nurses' Drug Alert **3**(6):73, 1979.

Spitz, P.: Kids in crisis. Common emergencies—correct actions to take, Nursing '78 **8**(4):26, 1978.

Swanson, P.D.: Anticonvulsant therapy: approaches to some common clinical problems, Postgraduate Medicine **65**(3):147, 1979.

Swift, N.: Helping patients live with seizures, Nursing '78 **8**(6):24, 1978.

Wiley, L.: The stigma of epilepsy, Nursing '74 **4**(1):36, 1974.

32 Central motor control: drugs for parkinsonism and centrally acting skeletal muscle relaxants

■ THE NEUROPHARMACOLOGY OF PARKINSON'S DISEASE

■ Characteristics of Parkinson's disease

Parkinson's disease is a movement disorder characterized by rigidity, akinesia, and tremor. *Rigidity* means that the muscle tone is greatly increased but reflex activity is not. When a limb is passively forced through flexor or extensor movements, the muscular resistance alternately increases and decreases to give a cogwheel effect. *Akinesia* (no motion) refers to the difficulty the patient has in initiating any movement. The face even has a masklike fixed expression devoid of emotion. Early in the course of Parkinson's disease the difficulty in initiating movement is not as marked and is termed *bradykinesia* (slow motion). The tremor of Parkinson's disease is seen mostly in the limbs at rest and decreases with movement of the limbs.

Roles of acetylcholine and dopamine. The insight to the neurochemical defect in Parkinson's disease is the classic example of our growing knowledge of the role of neurotransmitters in controlling given functions within the complex central nervous system. For many years anticholinergic drugs such as atropine had been used to decrease the tremor characteristics of Parkinson's disease. Acetylcholine therefore seemed important in accounting for some of the symptoms seen in Parkinson's disease. When the antipsychotic drugs (major tranquilizers) were introduced in the 1950's, symptoms indistinguishable from Parkinson's disease began to appear in patients treated with these drugs. It is now known that this is because these drugs block receptors for the central nervous system neurotransmitter dopamine. Subsequently, patients with Parkinson's disease were shown to have degeneration of crucial dopaminergic neurons projecting to certain of the basal ganglia of the extrapyramidal system in the brain. This system is responsible for maintaining motor coordination at the central nervous system level.

The present understanding of Parkinson's disease is that it represents a deficiency in the neurotransmitter dopamine in certain basal ganglia. Dopamine from these neuronal tracts is believed to exert an inhibitory influence on cholinergic neurons of the extrapyramidal system controlling muscle tone. When dopamine is lacking, muscle tone increases because of the unopposed action of acetylcholine, resulting in muscular rigidity, inhibition of spontaneous movements, and tremor. The lack of dopamine is secondary to a progressive degeneration of specific dopaminergic neurons. This degeneration can occur because of encephalitis, carbon monoxide poisoning, manganese poisoning, a cerebral vascular accident, or more commonly, unknown causes. This degeneration cannot be arrested. Drugs will only alleviate the symptoms for a few years.

The current rationale for the pharmacological treatment of Parkinson's disease is to make the motor symptoms less severe by blocking the excessive action of acetylcholine and/or by replenishing the dopamine to return the balance of excitatory acetylcholine action and inhibitory dopamine action toward normal.

Drug-induced parkinsonism. Certain drugs can also cause symptoms of Parkinson's disease. Reserpine (Serpasil), which depletes neuronal stores of dopamine as well as of norepinephrine, and the antipsychotic drugs, which block dopamine receptors, are the most common cause of drug-induced parkinsonism. Since the symptoms are dependent on the presence of the drug, lowering the dosage or discontinuing the drug will eliminate the symptoms.

■ Anticholinergic drugs to treat parkinsonism (Table 32-1)

Early in the course of Parkinson's disease an anticholinergic drug is frequently given to lessen rigidity, bradykinesia, and tremor. Atropine and scopolamine, the classic anticholinergic drugs, were used for treatment of the symptoms of Parkinson's disease for many years. The anticholinergic drugs used today are synthetic drugs that are centrally active and produce fewer peripheral side effects. These drugs include *cycrimine (Pagitane), procyclidine (Kemadrin), trihexyphenidyl* (*Tremin* and others), *benztropine (Cogentin), biperiden (Akineton),* and *ethopropazine (Parsidol).* An anticholinergic drug is also the drug of choice to treat extrapyramidal reac-

TABLE 32-1. Drugs for treating parkinsonism

Generic name	Trade name	Dosage and administration	Comments
ANTICHOLINERGICS			
Benztropine mesylate	Cogentin	ORAL: *Adults*—0.5 to 1 mg at bedtime initially. Increased gradually to 4 to 6 mg if required. For drug-induced extrapyramidal reactions: ORAL, INTRAMUSCULAR, INTRAVENOUS: *Adults*—1 to 4 mg 1 to 2 times daily. For an acute dystonic reaction: ORAL, INTRAVENOUS: *Adults*—2 mg IV, then 1 to 2 mg orally twice daily.	To treat Parkinson's disease and drug-induced extrapyramidal reactions. Particularly effective in reversing an acute dystonic reaction to an antipsychotic drug.
Biperiden	Akineton	ORAL: *Adults*—2 mg 3 times daily. May increase dose up to 20 mg daily if required. For drug-induced extrapyramidal reactions: ORAL: *Adults*—2 mg 1 to 3 times daily. INTRAMUSCULAR: *Adults*—2 mg repeated as often as every 30 min but no more than 4 doses in 24 hours. *Children*—0.04 mg/kg as often as every 30 min but no more than 4 doses in 24 hours.	To treat Parkinson's disease and drug-induced extrapyramidal reactions.
Cycrimine hydrochloride	Pagitane Hydrochloride	ORAL: *Adults*—1.25 mg 3 times daily. May be increased to 12.5 to 20 mg daily if required.	To treat Parkinson's disease.
Ethopropazine	Parsidol	ORAL: *Adults*—50 mg 1 to 2 times daily initially. Mild to moderate cases require 100 to 400 mg daily. Severe cases may require 500 to 600 mg daily.	To treat Parkinson's disease. A phenothiazine with only anticholinergic effects and devoid of antidopaminergic effects.
Procyclidine hydrochloride	Kemadrin	ORAL: *Adults*—5 mg twice daily. Up to 20 to 30 mg daily if required. For drug-induced extrapyramidal reactions: ORAL: *Adults*—2 to 2.5 mg 3 times daily. Increased to 10 to 20 mg daily if required.	To treat Parkinson's disease and drug-induced extrapyramidal reactions.
Trihexyphenidyl hydrochloride	Antitrem Artane Hexyphen Pipanol HCl Tremin	ORAL: *Adults*—2 mg 2 to 3 times daily. Increased to 15 to 20 mg daily (usually) or 40 to 50 mg daily (rarely) to control symptoms. For drug-induced parkinsonism: ORAL: *Adults*—1 mg initially. Subsequent doses are increased if symptoms do not decrease. Usual daily dose is 5 to 15 mg.	To treat Parkinson's disease and drug-induced extrapyramidal reactions.
ANTIHISTAMINES			
Chlorphenoxamine hydrochloride	Phenoxene	ORAL: *Adults*—50 mg 3 times daily. Increased to 100 mg 2 to 4 times daily if required.	To treat Parkinson's disease.

TABLE 32-1. Drugs for treating parkinsonism—cont'd

Generic name	Trade name	Dosage and administration	Comments
Diphenhydramine hydrochloride	Benadryl	ORAL: *Adults*—25 mg 3 times daily. Increased to 50 mg 4 times daily if required. For drug-induced extrapyramidal reactions: INTRAMUSCULAR, INTRAVENOUS: *Adults*—10 to 50 mg with maximum daily dose of 400 mg. *Children*—intramuscular 5 mg/kg daily. Maximum, 300 mg in 24 hr.	To treat Parkinson's disease and drug-induced extrapyramidal reactions. Marked sedative effects.
Orphenadrine	Disipal	ORAL: *Adults*—50 mg 3 times daily; up to 250 mg if required.	To treat Parkinson's disease.
OTHER DRUGS TO TREAT PARKINSONISM			
Amantadine	Symmetrel	ORAL: *Adults*—100 mg daily after breakfast for 5 to 7 days. An additional 100 mg may be added after lunch.	To treat Parkinson's disease. An antiviral agent. Side effects are similar to anticholinergic effects.
Levodopa	Dopar Larodopa	ORAL: *Adults*—initially 300 to 1000 mg daily in 3 to 7 doses during waking hours with food. Increase dosage 100 to 500 mg every 2 to 3 days or more until desired control is achieved. Usually requires 4 to 6 Gm and 6 to 8 weeks to achieve control. After several months to 1 year the dosage may be lowered.	To treat Parkinson's disease.
Carbidopa-levodopa	Sinemet	ORAL: *Adults*—Initial daily dose of Sinemet should be ¼ of the levodopa daily dose. Sinemet should be administered 8 hours after the last levodopa dose and is given in 3 to 4 doses daily. Patients not previously receiving levodopa are started with 10:100 mg (carbidopa:levodopa) 3 times daily, and the dosage is gradually increased as required.	To treat Parkinson's disease. Ratio of levodopa to carbidopa is 10:1. Carbidopa inhibits the degradation of dopamine outside the central nervous system.

tions arising from the antipsychotic drugs: akathisia, acute dystonia, and parkinsonism. Tardive dyskinesia is not reversed by anticholinergic drugs. These extrapyramidal reactions are described in Chapter 25.

Administration and side effects. The dosage of the anticholinergic drugs must be started low and increased gradually to overcome side effects and to individualize the dose. The common side effects of the anticholinergic drugs are the classic effects of dry mouth, constipation, urinary retention, and blurred vision. Common mental effects include an impairment of recent memory, confusion, insomnia, and restlessness. Mental effects can become serious with the development of agitation, disorientation, delirium, paranoid reactions, or hallucinations. Mental problems are more common with those elderly patients who have preexisting mental disturbances. Patients who have prior histories of glaucoma (particularly narrow-angle glaucoma) or some type of urinary or intestinal obstruction or tachycardia are not good candidates since anticholinergic drugs can aggravate any of these conditions. Characteristic actions of anticholinergic drugs are discussed in detail in Chapter 7.

■ Antihistaminic drugs to treat parkinsonism (Table 32-1)

Those antihistaminic drugs that have pronounced anticholinergic effects may be substituted for anticholinergic drugs. Three antihistaminic drugs are sometimes used to treat the symptoms of parkinsonisn: *chlorphenoxamine (Phenoxene), diphenhydramine (Benadryl)* and *orphenadrine (Disipal)*. Compared to the anticholinergic drugs, these antihistamines have milder though similar side effects and are less potent. The effectiveness of the antihistamines in treating the symptoms of parkinsonism is attributed to their anticholinergic effect. Antihistamines also have a sedative effect. Antihistamines are discussed in detail in Chapter 21.

■ Other drugs to treat parkinsonism

(Table 32-1)

Amantadine (Symmetrel)

Amantadine is an antiviral agent that has also been found effective in reducing the severity of symptoms of Parkinson's disease when used either alone or with an anticholinergic or antihistaminic drug. Amantadine promotes the release of dopamine from the central neurons, an action unrelated to its antiviral action.

Amantadine is often used as a first drug to control the symptoms of parkinsonism. Amantidine has the advantages of being effective when administered as a single daily dose and of having few side effects. Side effects that are sometimes seen include dizziness, nervousness, inability to concentrate, ataxia, slurred speech, insomnia, lethargy, blurred vision, dryness of the mouth, gastrointestinal upset, and rash. Amantadine may also be used with anticholinergic drugs or with levodopa because amantadine enhances the effectiveness of these other drugs and allows a reduction of their dosage.

Levodopa (Dopar, Larodopa)

Mechanism of action. When the drugs just mentioned can no longer adequately relieve the symptoms of Parkinson's disease, levodopa is administered. Levodopa therapy does not stop the progression of Parkinson's disease, but the drug does relieve the symptoms and dramatically improves the ability of patients to function. Levodopa is the chemical precursor of dopamine, and unlike dopamine, levodopa readily crosses the blood-brain barrier. Levodopa is converted to dopamine by the enzyme dopa decarboxylase. About 75% of a dose of levodopa is converted to dopamine in the periphery rather than in the brain, however, and the high plasma concentration of dopamine is responsible for the nausea and cardiac effects attending levodopa therapy.

Administration. Levodopa is taken orally, and the peak effect is seen 1 to 2 hours later. The dosage is adjusted up or down gradually every 2 to 3 days to lessen the incidence of nausea and to avoid precipitating side effects.

Emetic side effect. Dopamine is the neurotransmitter for the chemoreceptor trigger zone of the medulla and thereby produces nausea, vomiting, and anorexia. To produce tolerance to this emetic action, levodopa therapy must be initiated by starting with low doses that are gradually increased. A snack high in protein also helps to prevent nausea. Antiemetics from the phenothiazine class should not be used, since they will block the therapeutic action of dopamine. Trimethobenzamide (Tigan) may be taken early in the morning to control nausea.

Cardiovascular side effects. Another side effect sometimes seen at the start of levodopa therapy is orthostatic hypotension. The mechanism is not known but is believed to be a central nervous system effect rather than a peripheral effect. This hypotension tends to decrease with time. An increase in heart rate and force of contraction may also be apparent at the start of levodopa therapy. These cardiac actions are caused by the direct action of dopamine on the heart. Cardiac arrhythmias may develop and must then be controlled by appropriate medication.

Other side effects. Additional effects of levodopa therapy may include an assortment of gastrointestinal effects, including bleeding, difficulty in swallowing, and a burning sensation of the tongue. Respiratory effects such as cough, hoarseness, and disturbed breathing may appear. Because of these side effects levodopa therapy is used cautiously for patients with a history of heart disease, asthma, emphysema, or peptic ulcer. Problems in urination from incontinence to retention may arise.

Blurred vision or dilated pupils may be caused by levodopa therapy. Levodopa therapy is not considered for patients with narrow-angle glaucoma and only with careful monitoring for patients with chronic (wide-angle) glaucoma. Hepatic, hematopoietic, cardiovascular, and renal function tests are performed periodically on patients receiving long-term levodopa therapy. This is because many laboratory test values are high for patients receiving levodopa therapy and only careful monitoring can determine whether there is a real problem or not. Hematocrit and white blood cell counts may be lowered by levodopa therapy, but therapy is discontinued only when abnormally low counts are found. Therapy is not initiated in patients with blood disorders.

Additional effects commonly noted after the start of levodopa therapy include an increased alertness, sense of well-being, and an increased sex drive. All these effects are attributed to behavioral roles of dopamine in the brain. Further mental changes may occur with prolonged levodopa therapy. Most frequently seen are euphoria, restlessness, anxiety, irritability, hyperactivity, insomnia, and vivid dreams. Patients may occasionally become paranoid and experience psychotic episodes or become depressed, with or without suicidal tendencies. These mental changes are usually reversed with a lowering of the dosage.

Side effects after prolonged therapy. After prolonged therapy with levodopa, abnormal involuntary movements (dyskinesia) alternating with a sudden lapse in symptom control (the "on-off" phenomenon) may appear. The dyskinesia usually comprises abnormal involuntary movements of the mouth, tongue, face, and/or neck. Dyskinesia usually appears 1 to 2 hours after the

■ THE NURSING PROCESS FOR DRUGS TO TREAT PARKINSON'S DISEASE

■ Assessment

None of the drugs used to treat Parkinson's disease can cure this disease. Drug therapy will often be withheld until the patient and/or the physician feel that the symptoms of the disease are troublesome to the patient. The drugs used are associated with side effects. Obtain a general baseline patient assessment, including the vital signs, joint movement, amount of tremor, affect and objective signs of the disease, and ability to ambulate and perform activities of daily living. Because this is often a disease of the elderly, also obtain a baseline view of other known health problems such as hypertension, diabetes, and cardiovascular or renal disease.

■ Management

The drugs are prescribed sequentially with anticholinergic or antihistamine drugs being used before levodopa or carbidopa. The nurse should look for the presence of side effects and treat these when possible. The patient should be included in the discussion of the goals of therapy. Occasionally patients will find that the side effects resulting from a drug are worse than if the disease were left untreated, at least at some stages in the progression of the disease. There should be improvement in the symptoms of the disease to outweigh the discomfort of the side effects. In preparing the patient for discharge, the patient needs instruction about the drugs prescribed as well as referral to social service, vocational rehabilitation, visiting nurse, and other agencies. The patient having difficulty with specific activities of daily living should be assisted to find new ways to perform these activities.

The nurse should observe the patient for the side effects of the drugs or for aggravation of preexisting conditions. For example, amantadine has precipitated congestive heart failure. In patients with a history of congestive heart failure, the nurse should check the weight and blood pressure and auscultate the lungs on a regular basis.

■ Evaluation

Evaluation of the therapeutic effectiveness involves both the subjective and objective improvement of the patient in comparison to the number and severity of side effects present. The symptoms of the disease should be evaluated on a regular basis for progression of the disease and the patient's overall functioning monitored. Family members in frequent contact with the patient may also be helpful in providing data. Before discharge and at regular intervals during therapy the patient should be evaluated for the ability to explain the drug, its dose, and how to take the drug correctly; the expected goals of therapy; and the side effects that occur, how to treat them, and which ones require that the physician be notified. The patient should also be able to explain any necessary dietary or vitamin restrictions. For additional specific information, see the patient care implications section at the end of this chapter.

---

last dose of levodopa and represents a mild levodopa toxicity. There can also be "end-of-the-dose" akinesia. This means that the akinesia appears just before a new dose is to be taken and can usually be avoided by increasing the frequency of levodopa administration.

Carbidopa-levodopa (Sinemet)

Carbidopa inhibits the conversion of levodopa to dopamine. Since carbidopa cannot enter the central nervous system, only the peripheral conversion is inhibited. This means that levodopa is converted to dopamine only in the brain so that the presence of carbidopa lowers the dose of levodopa required by 75%. Since the emetic effects of levodopa reflect peripheral dopamine concentrations, the incidence of nausea and vomiting are much reduced with carbidopa-levodopa combination. Carbidopa is available only in a fixed ratio combination with levodopa.

■ Experimental drugs for the treatment of Parkinson's disease

Currently under study are two different drugs for the treatment of Parkinson's disease. One drug is *bromocriptine (Parlodel),* a drug that mimics the action of dopamine in the brain. Bromocriptine is currently approved in the United States only to inhibit prolactin secretion (Chapter 37), an action normally mediated by dopamine.

Another experimental drug is *deprenyl,* an inhibitor of the enzyme monoamine oxidase B that degrades dopamine in the brain. Since dopamine is not rapidly degraded in the presence of deprenyl, it is hoped that deprenyl will improve response to levodopa in patients with Parkinson's disease.

■ CENTRALLY ACTING SKELETAL MUSCLE RELAXANTS

■ Drugs to treat spasticity (Table 32-2)

Spasticity results from the loss of inhibitory tone in the polysynaptic pathways in the spinal cord so that fine control of motor activity is lost. Since the inhibitory tone is controlled largely by neural pathways from the brain, spasticity is seen in patients in whom these inhibitory pathways have been disrupted through spinal cord injury, strokes, multiple sclerosis, or cerebral palsy. The patient with spasticity will have exaggerated reflexes (spinal spasticity) or inappropriate posture (cerebral spasticity).

Three drugs have been found effective in relieving some cases of spasticity: *diazepam (Valium), baclofen (Lioresal),* and *dantrolene (Dantrium).* Diazepam and baclofen are believed to act within the spinal cord to restore some inhibitory tone, but dantrolene is unique in acting within the muscle itself.

Diazepam

Diazepam (Valium) is a benzodiazepine commonly prescribed as an antianxiety drug (Chapter 24). Although the action of diazepam as an antianxiety drug results from depression of the reticular activating system, diazepam also enhances inhibitory descending pathways in the spinal cord governing muscular activity apparently by enhancing the activity of the inhibitory neurotransmitter gamma aminobutyric acid (GABA). Diazepam is effective both in relieving spasticity associated with spinal cord injury, multiple sclerosis, and cerebral injury and in treating muscle spasms (see next section). Relatively high doses of diazepam are required to relieve muscle hyperactivity, and drowsiness and incoordination may be prominent side effects.

Baclofen

Baclofen (Lioresal) is an analogue of the inhibitory neurotransmitter gamma aminobutyric acid (GABA) and although the effect elicited is that desired of a GABA agonist, this mechanism of action cannot be demonstrated in the laboratory. Baclofen is most effective in relieving spasticity secondary to spinal cord injury and is less effective in relieving spasticity secondary to brain damage. Side effects include drowsiness, incoordination, and occasional gastrointestinal upset.

Dantrolene

Dantrolene (Dantrium) is not a centrally acting skeletal muscle relaxant but instead affects the muscle directly by interfering with the intracellular release of calcium necessary to initiate contraction. At therapeutic doses this effect is limited to skeletal muscle and is not seen in the heart or smooth muscle. Dantrolene will cause muscular weakness and can worsen the overall condition if the patient has marginal strength already. Dantrolene is most useful for the patient for whom spasticity causes pain, discomfort, or limits functional rehabilitation. In addition to the spasticity secondary to spinal cord injury, dantrolene can be effective in relieving the spasticity of stroke, cerebral palsy, or multiple sclerosis for which the other drugs have limited effectiveness.

The major limitation to the use of dantrolene is liver damage. Baseline liver function studies are made before therapy starts and regular liver function studies are performed throughout therapy. The drug is discontinued if no relief of spasticity is achieved in 6 weeks.

■ Muscle spasms and their treatment (Table 32-2)

Muscle spasms are local muscle contractions initiated by muscle or tendon injury and inflammation. Muscle spasms occur in conditions such as sprains, bursitis, arthritis, and lower back pain. The primary treatment of muscle spasms includes analgesics, antiinflammatory drugs, immobilization of the affected part, if possible, and physical therapy. If relief is not achieved through these means, a centrally acting skeletal muscle relaxant may be added. Although the mechanism postulated for the centrally acting skeletal muscle relaxants is depression of the polysynaptic pathways in the spinal cord modulating muscle tone, the drugs used as centrally acting skeletal muscle relaxants are related to various antianxiety drugs. Since anxiety itself will make a muscle spasm worse, treatment of the anxiety that accompanies a muscle spasm may be the more important mechanism of action.

The centrally acting skeletal muscle relaxants commonly prescribed to treat muscle spasms are listed in Table 32-2 and include *carisoprodol (Rela, Soma), chlorphenesin (Maolate), chlorzoxazone (Paraflex), cyclobenzaprine (Flexeril), diazepam (Valium), methocarbamol (Delaxin and others),* and *orphenadrine (Norflex and others).* With the exception of cyclobenzaprine, these drugs are similar to sedative-hypnotic or antianxiety drugs with respect to side effects, drug interactions, and drug dependency (Chapter 24). For these reasons,

TABLE 32-2. Centrally acting skeletal muscle relaxants

Generic name	Trade name	Dosage and administration	Comments
DRUGS TO TREAT SPASTICITY			
Baclofen	Lioresal	ORAL: *Adults*—Begin with 5 mg 3 times daily. Increase by 5 mg 3 times daily every 3 days as required. Maximum daily dose is 80 mg.	Diminishes reflex responses by decreasing transmission in the spinal cord.
Dantrolene	Dantrium	ORAL: *Adults*—25 mg 1 to 2 times daily. Increase to 25 mg 3 to 4 times daily, then 50 to 100 mg 4 times daily as required. Increments are made every 4 to 7 days.	Acts peripherally to inhibit calcium release within the muscle.
Diazepam	Valium	ORAL: *Adults*—2 to 10 mg 4 times daily. *Children*—0.12 to 0.8 mg/kg body weight daily divided into 3 or 4 doses. INTRAVENOUS: *Adults*—2 to 10 mg injected no faster than 5 mg (1 ml) per min. Do not mix or dilute with other solutions, drugs, or intravenous fluids. *Children*—0.04 to 0.2 mg/kg body weight with a maximum of 0.6 mg/kg in an 8 hr period.	A benzodiazepine that is also used for the treatment of spasticity or muscle spasm.
DRUGS TO TREAT MUSCLE SPASMS			
Carisoprodol	Rela Soma	ORAL: *Adults*—350 mg 4 times daily.	Related to meprobamate. May cause drowsiness.
Chlorphenesin	Maolate	ORAL: *Adults*—800 mg 3 times daily. Can decrease to 400 mg 4 times daily as improvement is noted.	May cause drowsiness and dizziness.
Chlorzoxazone	Paraflex	ORAL: *Adults*—250 to 750 mg 3 or 4 times daily. *Children*—20 mg/kg body weight in 3 to 4 divided doses.	May cause drowsiness. Watch for signs of liver damage (rare).
Cyclobenzaprine	Flexeril	ORAL: *Adults*—10 mg 3 times daily up to a maximum total dose of 60 mg.	Related to the tricyclic antidepressants. Does not cause drug dependence but may cause changes in the liver.
Diazepam	Valium	See Drugs to treat spasticity	
Methocarbamol	Delaxin Robamol Robaxin Romethocarb Spenaxin	ORAL: *Adults*—1.5 to 2 Gm 4 times daily for 2 to 3 days. Decrease to 1 Gm 4 times daily for maintenance. INTRAMUSCULAR: *Adults*—500 mg every 8 hr, alternating between the gluteal muscles. INTRAVENOUS: *Adults*—1 to 3 Gm daily for a maximum of 3 days. Inject no faster than 300 mg (3 ml) per min.	Not recommended for patients with epilepsy. Do not administer parenterally to patients with impaired renal function because the drug vehicle may worsen kidney function.
Orphenadrine	Flexon Neocyten Norflex Tega-Flex X-Otag	ORAL: *Adults*—100 mg twice daily. INTRAMUSCULAR, INTRAVENOUS: *Adults*—60 mg twice daily.	Anticholinergic effects are common side effects. Not for patients with glaucoma, myasthenia gravis, tachycardia, or urinary retention.

■ THE NURSING PROCESS FOR CENTRALLY ACTING SKELETAL MUSCLE RELAXANTS

■ Assessment

Muscle spasticity is seen in multiple sclerosis, in spinal cord injury or disease, and in a few other situations. Less severe muscle spasm is seen after orthopedic trauma and/or surgery and with some musculoskeletal diseases. In the case of severe spasticity, the spasticity is often clearly visible at all times or occurs in response to stimulation. Some kinds of spasticity are localized with a specific muscle group such as spasticity associated with severe low back pain. In general nursing situations, diazepam will be used most often; dantrolene is reserved for use when no other drug will work and/or when spasticity is moderate to severe.

The baseline data should include a general patient assessment with an additional focus on the spasticity, including such parameters as the degree of spasticity, the aggravating factors, the associated pain, the degree to which the spasticity interferes with the activities of daily living or the activities that could increase independence. If dantrolene is to be used, baseline liver fuction studies should be obtained.

■ Management

During the adjustment of drug dosage, the nurse should monitor the patient for both the drug effectiveness and the presence of side effects. Often weeks of therapy may be needed before a lessening of spasticity occurs. These drugs may also be used with other therapies, including traction, physical therapy, exercises, bed rest, and application of heat. If drowsiness occurs, appropriate measures to provide for the patient's safety should be employed, including keeping the side rails up and supervising ambulation. Liver function studies should be monitored with dantrolene therapy.

■ Evaluation

The goal of therapy is to decrease spasticity, but this does not always occur. At regular intervals, the nurse should evaluate the continuing degree of spasticity. Not all side effects that may occur are undesirable, so decisions related to them should be individualized. For example, a patient who is drowsy when receiving short-term diazepam therapy may be better able to tolerate enforced bed rest because of the drowsiness. Before discharge the patient should be able to explain the drugs and how to take them correctly, the side effects that may occur and which ones require notification of the physician, how to perform additional therapies that should be used, such as application of heat and exercises, and when to return for additional help. For specific information, see the patient care implications section at the end of this chapter.

---

short-term therapy rather than long-term therapy is the rule. Cyclobenzaprine is related to the tricyclic antidepressants and does not cause drug dependence or alter sleep patterns.

Drowsiness and dizziness are common side effects of all the centrally acting skeletal muscle relaxants, and they should not be combined with alcohol or other drugs that depress the central nervous system.

■ PATIENT CARE IMPLICATIONS

General guidelines for patients receiving drugs for Parkinson's disease

1. Patients should not suddenly discontinue their drugs for Parkinson's disease.
2. Parkinson's disease is usually a disease of older adults. If, however, a premenopausal woman should have Parkinson's disease, she should consider the use of birth control meaures during therapy with the antiparkinsonism drugs.
3. Patients and family members should be taught about the side effects of these drugs because it may often be the family who notices side effects before the patient does.

4. Some elderly patients become confused easily. For these patients it may be necessary to have family members supervise the taking of medications to avoid accidental overdoses.

Anticholinergic drugs

1. Review the side effects discussed in the text.
2. Because anticholinergic drugs can cause drowsiness, patients should be cautioned to avoid activities requiring mental alertness such as driving or operating machinery.
3. Monitor the blood pressure and pulse every 4 hours when patients are being started on therapy, when dosages are being changed, or when other medications are added. It may take several days for the effects of the drug to be fully manifested because the drugs have cumulative action.
4. Because of possible drowsiness and hypotension, patients should be cautioned to rise slowly and to call for assistance as needed. At night, hospitalized patients should be assisted when up.
5. Instruct patients to report any gastrointestinal problems such as constipation or abdominal pain. Although rare, fatal paralytic ileus has occurred. If constipation is a chronic problem, encourage the patient to increase fluid intake to 2500 to 3000 ml per day, to increase the bulk intake, to modify the diet to include foods that may have a laxative effect (e.g., prunes, juices, coffee, hot chocolate), and to increase exercise and ambulation. It may be necessary to prescribe stool softeners on a regular basis.
6. Anticholinergic drugs may produce anhidrosis (inability to sweat), resulting in intolerance to heat and rarely, hyperthermia. Caution patients to limit strenuous activities, especially in hot weather, and to take frequent rest periods to cool off.
7. Patients should be routinely screened for the presence of glaucoma. Anticholinergic drugs are contraindicated in closed-angle glaucoma.
8. Urinary retention can be a problem, especially in patients with prostatic hypertrophy or immobility. Measuring the intake of fluids and output of urine may be appropriate.
9. Nausea and dry mouth can be a problem. When severe it may be necessary to reduce the dosage. Sometimes altering the times the medications are given can help decrease these side effects. Taking the medications just before meals may help with the dry mouth, unless this produces nausea. Taking the drug after meals may prevent nausea, in which case giving some mints, hard candies, or chewing gum may help to make the dry mouth more tolerable. Some patients may find the use of a commercially prepared saliva substitute to be helpful.
10. Psychiatric problems (e.g., confusion, euphoria, disturbed behavior, agitation) may occur. If severe, the drug should be stopped for a few days and resumed at a lower dosage.
11. Patients with a known history of cardiac arrhythmias should be watched carefully because the anticholinergics may aggravate the cardiac problems.
12. Parenteral administration. The anticholinergic drugs are supplied in solution. Administer as ordered for intramuscular use. For intravenous use, administer slowly over several minutes, monitoring pulse and blood pressure.

Antihistamines

Antihistamines are discussed in Chapter 21.

Phenothiazines

Phenothiazines are discussed in Chapter 25.

Amantadine

1. Review the side effects discussed in the text.
2. Patients with a history of seizures should be observed closely because there may be a chance of increased seizure activity.
3. Amantadine has precipitated congestive heart failure. Patients with a history of this condition should be observed carefully when being started on amantadine. Weigh daily, monitor the blood pressure, check for increasing fluid retention in dependent areas, auscultate the lungs for fluid, and observe the neck veins for venous distention.
4. Because amantadine can cause drowsiness and blurred vision, patients should be cautioned to avoid activities requiring mental alertness (e.g., driving, operating machinery).
5. During periods of dosage adjustment or when new drugs are added to the medical regimen, patients should have their blood pressure checked every 4 hours; hypotension is a known side effect. Caution patients to rise slowly. If dizziness or lightheadedness occurs, the patient should sit down. It may be necessary to supervise ambulation, especially at night.

Levodopa

1. Levodopa and antidepressants that are monoamine oxidase (MAO) inhibitors should not be given concurrently; MAO inhibitors should be discontinued at least 2 weeks before administering levodopa. Levodopa is contraindicated for patients with closed-angle glaucoma, with a history of melanoma, or for patients with suspicious undiagnosed skin lesions.

2. Patients with a history of cardiovascular disease, myocardial infarction, or arrhythmia should be observed carefully for signs of cardiac irregularity or arrhythmia. If possible, these patients should be in a cardiac monitoring setting during periods of initiating therapy or changing the dose.
3. Observe patients with a history of peptic ulcer disease for signs of reactivation of the disease such as abdominal pain or occult blood in the stools.
4. Because levodopa can cause hypotension, the blood pressure should be monitored every 4 hours during periods of dosage adjustment or when other drugs are added to the regimen. Caution patients to move slowly from supine to sitting or standing positions, to sit down if dizziness or lightheadedness occurs, and to call for assistance if needed. It may be necessary to supervise ambulation, especially at night. Sometimes wearing elastic stockings may be helpful; consult the physician.
5. A variety of personality changes can occur: confusion, hallucinations, delusions, agitation, euphoria, depression, and suicidal tendencies. Observe patients carefully for signs of personality or behavior change, and ask the patient and family to report any symptoms.
6. Pyridoxine hydrochloride (vitamin B_6) reverses the effects of levodopa; therefore vitamin mixtures containing this vitamin should be avoided. Caution patients not to take over-the-counter vitamin preparations without first checking with the physician.
7. Warn patients that several weeks of therapy may be necessary before full results can be seen.
8. The urine, saliva, and perspiration may become darker while patients are receiving levodopa therapy. Other effects of the drug that are rare but that may cause concern are a bitter taste in the mouth, hot flashes, and foul body odor.
9. Gastrointestinal side effects may be decreased by taking levodopa with meals or milk. If nausea is severe, it may be necessary for the patient to take an antiemetic. Gastrointestinal symptoms often diminish with prolonged therapy. Because of the disease and the drug side effects, the patient with Parkinson's disease may be poorly nourished. Allow the patient plenty of time to eat and weigh the patient weekly.
10. Urinary retention can be a problem if the patient is immobilized or has a history of urinary retention or prostatic hypertrophy. Monitor the fluid intake and the urinary output.
11. There are many side effects that have been attributed to levodopa therapy. Patients receiving this drug need individualized titration of the dose and careful evaluation. Any patient complaint or unusual signs or symptoms should be carefully assessed.
12. If therapy must be interrupted for prolonged periods, it may be necessary to resume the drug at a lower dose and progressively increase the dose until the desired dose is again reached.

Carbidopa-levodopa combination

1. When starting the carbidopa-levodopa combination, levodopa alone should have been discontinued at least 8 hours previously.
2. Gastrointestinal side effects are usually much less severe with the combination product than with levodopa alone.
3. Pyridoxine (vitamin B_6) is not contraindicated with the combination product.

Baclofen

1. Because baclofen may cause drowsiness, patients should be cautioned to avoid activities requiring mental alertness (e.g., driving, operating machinery) until the effects of the drug are known.
2. Patients taking baclofen should be instructed to avoid alcohol and other central nervous system depressants (e.g., tranquilizers, narcotic analgesics, hypnotics, sedatives) because their action may potentiate the central nervous system depressant action of the baclofen.
3. The drug should be administered cautiously to patients with a history of seizures because a loss of seizure control has been reported.
4. The major side effects of the drug are identified in the text. There are, however, many side effects that have only rarely been reported or that in part may be due to the patient's underlying disease. Instruct the patient to report any unusual signs or symptoms so that the cause can be determined.
5. The use of baclofen may cause the following alterations in blood tests: increased SGOT, increased alkaline phosphatase, and elevated blood sugar levels.
6. Caution patients with diabetes mellitus to monitor their urine sugar concentration carefully. In some cases it may be necessary to increase the dose of insulin or oral hypoglycemic agent while the patient is receiving baclofen.
7. Abrupt withdrawal of baclofen may cause hallucinations. Caution patients to discontinue use of this drug only on the advice of the physician.
8. This drug should only be used during lactation or pregnancy when the benefit clearly outweighs the risk. Consult the physician.

Dantrolene

1. Because of the risk of serious hepatitis, patients receiving dantrolene sodium should be cautioned to report any jaundice, yellowing of sclera, right upper quadrant abdominal pain, nausea, or fever. In addi-

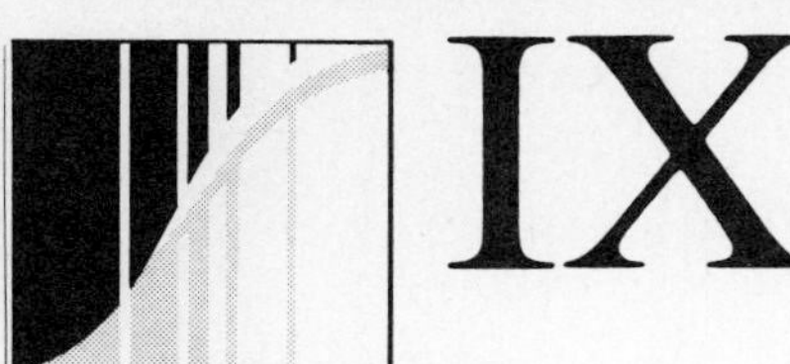

IX DRUGS AFFECTING THE ENDOCRINE SYSTEMS

This section is designed to present the pharmacology of the endocrine systems. Chapter 33, **Introduction to Endocrinology,** defines the terms that must be mastered before the material in the subsequent chapters can be understood. This chapter also describes the concepts involved in treating endocrine diseases or in using hormones in therapy of other diseases. Understanding this material facilitates the comprehension of many of the nursing assessments and actions described later in other chapters.

Chapters 34 through 39 cover specific endocrine systems. In these chapters the pertinent physiology of the endocrine system is first reviewed. Where appropriate, specific endocrine diseases are described so that discussion of the therapy of these diseases becomes more rational. Three classes of agents are described in these chapters: natural hormones, synthetic forms of hormones, and nonhormonal drugs affecting the endocrine system. The purpose of therapy with each of these agents is clearly defined. Diagnostic tests are also described so that the student may understand the information that must be considered during the assessment of the patient.

Some of the agents discussed in this section have significant medical uses outside of endocrinology. For example, the synthetic adrenal steroids (Chapter 35) are widely used as antiinflammatory agents. We have chosen to discuss these drugs in this section because students find it easier to understand the actions of the synthetic drugs if their similarity to the natural hormones is stressed. For similar reasons, the anabolic steroids are considered in this section along with the androgens (Chapter 38).

33 Introduction to endocrinology

This introduction to endocrinology is intended to define important terms, introduce the classes of hormones, and illustrate the concept of hormonal regulation of body processes. Detailed consideration of the properties of individual hormones is presented in subsequent chapters.

■ PROPERTIES OF HORMONES

A *hormone* is a substance produced by a particular cell type, which acts on other cells in the body to produce a physiological or biochemical response. Traditionally hormones have been considered to be compounds that are synthesized by a specific cell type, are released into the circulation, and act on target tissues elsewhere in the body. An example is thyrotropin (TSH), which is synthesized in the adenohypophysis, released into the systemic circulation, taken up by the thyroid gland, and there stimulates the production of thyroid hormones (Chapter 36).

Organs producing hormones that enter systemic circulation are the *endocrine glands*—pancreas, adrenal glands, thyroid gland, parathyroid glands, testes, ovaries, neurohypophysis, and adenohypophysis. The neurohypophysis and adenohypophysis comprise the pituitary gland. Those tissues affected by the hormones from the endocrine glands are designated *target tissues*. For example, the target tissue of thyrotropin secreted by the adenohypophysis is the thyroid gland. No other tissue in the body responds to thyrotropin.

Some compounds that have been called hormones act strictly locally, producing their effect at or near the site where they are synthesized. Examples of such compounds are acetylcholine, which is synthesized, acts, and is destroyed at the nerve terminal, and prostaglandins, which are formed from membrane fatty acids at the sites of prostaglandin action. Acetylcholine has been considered in Chapter 7, and prostaglandins will be considered in terms of their action on the uterus in Chapter 37. These locally acting substances are not further considered in this chapter.

Hormones may be divided into two classes on the basis of their chemical composition. One class is the *steroid hormones,* which are derived from cholesterol. This class of hormones includes the hormones of the adrenal gland (cortisol, cortisone, aldosterone, corticosterone, and others) and the hormones of the sex glands (androgens, estrogens, and progestins). Many of these steroid compounds have been synthesized by organic chemists so their production for medicinal purposes does not depend entirely on isolating them from such natural sources as bovine or porcine adrenal glands obtained as by-products of the meat-packing industry. Some of the clinically useful steroids, however, are obtained from natural sources because the steroids are present in such high concentrations and are so easily extracted as to make the procedure economically feasible. An example of such a preparation is Premarin, a mixture of conjugated estrogens extracted from the urine of pregnant mares. In addition to their relative abundance in natural sources and the ease with which they may be chemically modified or completely synthesized by pharmaceutical manufacturers, the steroids have another characteristic that makes them convenient medicinal agents—many, although not all, may be taken orally.

The second class of hormones is comprised of hormones formed from amino acids. There are two subclasses within this group: (1) amino acid derivatives and (2) proteins. Examples of the first subclass are thyroxine and triiodothyronine, the iodinated tyrosine derivatives produced in the thyroid gland, and the catecholamines produced in various tissues from the amino acid tyrosine. The second subclass includes both peptides and proteins. Peptides and proteins are distinguished arbitrarily by difference in size, with peptides containing fewer amino acids than proteins. Chemically, peptides and proteins are similar in that both are formed by the peptide bond linking carboxyl and amino groups of adjacent amino acids. Examples of peptide hormones are the releasing factors produced in the hypothalamus, including thyrotropin-releasing hormone (TRH) composed of three amino acids and the neurohypophyseal hormones oxytocin and vasopressin, which are each composed of eight amino acids. Examples of protein hormones within this second sublcass include insulin with 51 amino acids and a molecular weight of 6000 and follicle-stimulating hormone with a molecular weight of 41,000.

The active forms of many of the protein hormones

are derived from larger protein molecules called *prohormones*. For example, insulin is originally synthesized as part of a prohormone containing at least 86 amino acids. Cleavage of 35 amino acids from this larger, inactive precursor molecule releases active insulin.

The peptide and protein hormones in general are present in very small quantities in natural sources. This fact makes their isolation and purification very difficult. For example, insulin, the protein hormone most often used medically is prepared by pharmaceutical manufacturers in large quantities from either beef or pork pancreas glands by tedious and expensive extraction procedures. In contrast growth hormone, a protein hormone used to treat a rare endocrine disease, is relatively easily extracted from anterior pituitary tissue (adenohypophysis), but the only form that is active in human beings is the growth hormone from primate sources. The supply of this hormone is therefore restricted by the limited supply of source material. The only growth hormone presently approved for human use comes from human anterior pituitary glands obtained postmortem.

A new and fascinating method for producing human hormones has recently become possible as a result of *genetic engineering*. Genetic engineering involves taking the genes from one species and inserting them into an unrelated species, thereby creating new characteristics in the recipient. The human genes for insulin, growth hormone, and other hormones have been inserted into certain bacteria. These altered bacteria may then be grown on a large scale in fermentation tanks and will produce large quantities of the human hormone. Insulin produced in this way is now in clinical trial. This technique is potentially applicable to a wide variety of hormones and may overcome the problem of limited supply of clinically useful hormones.

The protein and peptide hormones are somewhat inconvenient for the patient to use. Although thyroxine and triiodothyronine may be taken by mouth, none of the larger peptides and proteins survive the action of digestive juices in the stomach and intestine. For this reason peptides and proteins must be administered by injection. Even when given parenterally, these compounds may not be effective, for the patient may suffer an allergic, foreign protein reaction or develop resistance due to the production of antibodies directed at the foreign protein.

■ USES OF HORMONES

The hormones discussed in this section are used clinically in one of three ways: (1) as diagnostic agents, (2) in replacement therapy, or (3) as pharmacological agents.

The most common *diagnostic use* of hormones is to assess the function of the target organ of the administered hormone. For example, adrenocorticotropin may be administered to test the ability of the adrenal gland to produce steroids. Another adenohypophyseal hormone, thyrotropin, is administered to test the capacity of the thyroid gland for synthesizing thyroid hormones.

Replacement therapy is aimed at restoring normal levels of hormones, which, for one reason or another, a patient's body no longer produces. Physiological doses are used in an attempt to maintain normal hormone levels without producing toxic effects from hormone excesses. The use of thyroxine to treat hypothyroidism and of cortisol to treat Addison's disease (chronic adrenal insufficiency) are examples of replacement therapy.

The use of hormones as *pharmacological agents*, with administered doses far in excess of those required to produce physiological levels, makes use of some function of the compound other than the one seen at physiological concentrations. For example, adrenal corticosteroids may be given in large doses to suppress inflammatory responses in certain diseases. This antiinflammatory effect is not obvious at physiological concentrations of the steroid.

■ REGULATION OF HORMONE ACTION

Hormones are potent agents capable of producing profound effects on metabolism. It is imperative for healthy functioning of the body that these compounds act only where they are needed and when they are needed and that they be present at the proper concentrations. The time of appearance and the blood concentration of a hormone may be regulated by controlling its rate of synthesis, its rate of release from storage sites, its rate of degradation, and its rate of clearance from the body. A number of hormones are stored after synthesis and released from storage sites only when the proper stimulus is received. Examples are thyroxine and triiodothyronine stored in complex with thyroglobulin in the thyroid gland and insulin, which is stored in granules within the beta cell of the pancreas. In both these cases, when the endocrine gland is stimulated to release hormone, it is the stored hormone that is first released. Then if required, newly synthesized hormone is released into the bloodstream.

Regulation of synthesis and release of many hormones involves the interaction of the central nervous system with the endocrine glands. For example, the hypothalamus in the brain controls the hypophysis or pituitary gland, which in turn regulates the production of hormones by ovaries, testes, and thyroid and adrenal glands. This system is the negative feedback regulation discussed in detail in the next chapter.

Hormones disappear from the bloodstream when they are taken up by various organs or when they are degraded by enzymes in the bloodstream. The kidney is the site of degradation and/or excretion for a number of hormones, including most of the steroids. Both the

■ THE NURSING PROCESS

The specific considerations of endocrine-related drugs will be covered in the remaining chapters within this section. The following presentation illustrates how the general concepts presented in this chapter can guide the nurse through the nursing process.

■ Assessment

The nurse should identify which endocrine system is involved in the patient's condition and consider what other systems may be affected by the primary condition. For example, pituitary disease may influence multiple organ systems and may require therapy at several levels. The nurse may be required to understand the various testing methods used to diagnose the loss of normal endocrine regulation.

■ Management

In identifying goals of therapy, the nurse should distinguish between replacement therapy and other forms of endocrine therapy. In replacement therapy the goal is to restore normal levels of a hormone in the patient's body, thereby restoring normal function of the endocrine system. In other types of therapy the goal may be to suppress overfunction of an endocrine tissue, control the symptoms of excess hormone levels, or affect a nonendocrine tissue with high levels of hormones. By working with the physician, the nurse should be able to define the goal of therapy for a particular patient. The nurse may then begin teaching the patient about the endocrine condition and the effects of the medications being used.

■ Evaluation

Evaluating the patient requires that the nurse be thoroughly aware of the expected actions of the endocrine-related drugs and be able to recognize the side effects these agents may produce.

---

kidney and the liver degrade insulin. Vasopressin, in contrast, is very rapidly destroyed by enzymes in the bloodstream. The half-life of vasopressin, that is, the time required for half of the injected dose to disappear from the blood, is approximately 15 minutes. Other hormones persist for much longer periods. For example, the thyroid hormone thyroxine has a plasma half-time around 7 days. How rapidly a hormone is lost from the body is of clinical importance in selecting doses and dosage schedules when these hormones are administered to patients. Knowledge of the elimination half-time is also helpful in dealing with toxic reactions whose duration may be related to the persistence of the compound in the body.

Controlling the location of action of a certain hormone is accomplished in the body in one of two ways. The first localization mechanism is simply to restrict the distribution of the hormone. Examples are the *releasing factors* synthesized in the hypothalamus and released into local portal veins carrying the hormones directly to the target organ (the adenohypophysis) and not into the general circulation.

A second mechanism localizes the effect of generally released hormones. These hormones interact with specific *receptors,* which are found only in their target tissues. The specific receptor is required for hormone activity. For example, progesterone receptors are found primarily in tissues of the female reproductive tract but not in most other organs. Therefore, even though progesterone is released into the general circulation, it acts only on those tissues possessing receptors.

The receptors for hormones may be within cells. For example, steroids and thyroid hormones affect target cells by interacting with intracellular receptors. The steroid hormones are bound by soluble receptors, which transport the hormones through the cytoplasm of the cell and into the cell nucleus. The final effect of the hormone is produced by this action within the cell nucleus. The mechanisms of action of the thyroid hormones seem similar, although the details of receptor binding within the cell are not as well established. Thyroid hormones do, however, bind to specific sites within cell nuclei and alter protein synthesis in that cell.

In contrast to the receptors for steroids and thyroid hormones, receptors for peptide and protein hormones exist on the external surface of cell membranes. The peptide and protein hormones therefore need not enter the cell to become effective. One mechanism by which these externally bound hormones act is by releasing an internal regulator, or second messenger. For example, parathyroid hormone binds to a receptor on the surface of certain kidney cells. This receptor is associated with an enzyme called *adenylate cyclase* so that when parathyroid hormone binds to the receptor, adenylate cyclase is stimulated to release cyclic AMP within the cell. Cyclic AMP is the second messenger that actually alters the internal processes of the cell. Vasopressin acts in a similar way on other cells within the kidney. Not all hormone receptors on the cell surface membrane are linked to adenylate cyclase and the second messenger cyclic AMP. For example, the multiple metabolic changes produced by insulin within target cells do not depend on cyclic AMP.

The response of a target cell to a hormone is dependent on the number and availability of hormone receptors. Regulating the number of receptors is, therefore, another mechanism by which the body can maintain metabolic balance. An example of this type of regulation is found in obese persons with a high food intake. These persons have chronically high insulin concentrations in the bloodstream. To protect itself from the metabolic effects of this high amount of insulin, the body eliminates a certain percentage of the insulin receptors on cells. This loss of insulin receptors (called *down-regulation*) lowers the responsiveness of the cell to insulin.

Understanding the role of receptors in fulfilling the metabolic role of hormones allows a clearer understanding of endocrine diseases and how they are classified. It should now be obvious that an endocrine deficiency can arise either from a lack of hormone or from a lack of receptor, which enables the tissue to respond to the hormone. An example is the disease called *diabetes insipidus,* which may be produced either by a lack of antidiuretic hormone (ADH) or by a lack of receptors in the kidney that can respond to ADH. Likewise, *diabetes mellitus* can be characterized by the lack of insulin in the bloodstream, or by high levels of insulin in the bloodstream but lower than normal numbers of active insulin receptors on cells.

The material in this chapter was designed to introduce general concepts underlying the action of the endocrine system. Subsequent chapters examine the specific function of each gland and the effects of related drugs.

■ SUMMARY

Hormones are substances that are produced by certain cells within the body but that act on other cells to produce a physiological response. The organs that release hormones which are transported throughout the body are the endocrine glands. The tissues directly and specifically affected by the hormones from the endocrine gland are called *target tissues*. Chemically, hormones can be classified as steroids, amino acid derivatives, or peptides and proteins.

Hormones are commonly used as diagnostic agents to test the function of a target organ. Hormones are also given as replacement therapy to restore normal amounts of hormone, which a particular patient may lack. Finally hormones may be given as pharmacological agents, usually at doses higher than those used in replacement therapy.

The amount of hormone present in the body may be regulated by controlling the rate of synthesis and the rate of degradation of the hormone. Regulating the site of action of a hormone is accomplished by restricted distribution of the hormone or by means of specific receptors for the hormone on target cells. Hormone receptors may be intracellular or may exist on the external surface of the cell membrane. Hormones that act on intracellular receptors are themselves transported within the cell to produce metabolic effects. Hormones acting on receptors on the cell surface do not necessarily enter the cell and may produce internal effects by means of the second messenger, cyclic AMP, or by other cyclic AMP–independent mechanisms. Responses to hormones can be regulated by altering the number of receptors in target tissues.

■ STUDY QUESTIONS

1. What is a hormone?
2. What is a target tissue?
3. Describe the two major chemical types of hormones.
4. What is a prohormone?
5. Name three ways in which large amounts of hormones may be obtained for clinical use.
6. What are the three primary clinical uses of hormones?
7. Describe how the amount of hormone in the body may be regulated.
8. How may the site of action of a hormone be restricted?
9. In what ways may the actions of hormones be terminated?
10. What is a releasing factor?
11. What are the two main types of hormone receptors? How do these receptors differ in the way they interact with hormones?
12. Describe the two general types of endocrine deficiency diseases.

■ SUGGESTED READINGS

Anthony, C.P., and Thibodeau, G.A.: Textbook of anatomy and Physiology, ed. 10, St. Louis, 1979, The C.V. Mosby Co.

Blecher, M.: Cell-surface receptors in health and disease, Clinical Chemistry **25:**11, 1979.

Guillemin, R.: New endocrinology of the brain, Prospectives in Biology and Medicine **22:**S74, 1979.

Marx, J.L.: Hormones and their effects in the aging body, Science **206:**805, 1979.

Pollet, R.J., and Levey, G.S.: Principles of membrane receptor physiology and their application to clinical medicine, Annals of Internal Medicine **92:**663, 1980.

Rubenstein, E.: Diseases caused by impaired communication among cells, Scientific American **242**(3):102, 1980.

34 Drugs affecting the pituitary gland

The pituitary gland, or hypophysis, lies in the sella turcica, a bony cavity at the base of the brain. Although the gland weighs less than a gram, it nevertheless is of major importance in regulating the entire endocrine system, controlling normal growth, and regulating water balance.

The pituitary gland in humans is divided into two portions with very different tissue compositions and embryological origins (Fig. 34-1). These two regions are the anterior pituitary, or adenohypophysis, and the posterior pituitary, or neurohypophysis. The structure and function of each of these tissues, the function and regulation of the various hormones produced, and the pathological states resulting from abnormalities in hormone production are considered in this chapter.

■ THE NEUROHYPOPHYSIS

The neurohypophysis, or posterior pituitary, is composed of nerve fibers embryologically derived from the hypothalamus. Intimate contact between the central nervous system and the neurohypophysis is maintained by the nerve fibers that run from the hypothalamus through the hypophyseal stalk to the neurohypophysis (Fig. 34-1).

Two octapeptide hormones closely related in structure are known to be released by the neurohypophysis. These hormones are antidiuretic hormone and oxytocin. Both oxytocin and antidiuretic hormone are synthesized in the hypothalamus and are transported in secretion granules down the axons running between the hypothalamus and the neurohypophysis. The granules accumulate at the nerve fiber terminals and are stored in the neurohypophysis where their release into the systemic circulation is regulated by nerve impulses originating in the hypothalamus. Damage to the hypophyseal stalk impairs transport of the secretory granules to the neurohypophysis and interferes with the appropriate release of the hormones into the circulation.

■ Neurohypophyseal hormones

Antidiuretic hormone

Mechanism of action. Antidiuretic hormone (ADH), also called *vasopressin,* has as its primary target tissue the renal tubular epithelium (Table 34-1). ADH increases the permeability of certain sections of the renal tubule to water, allowing water to be reabsorbed from the tubule and returned to the bloodstream. This is the mechanism by which normal kidneys concentrate the urine.

Regulation of secretion. The regulation of antidiuretic hormone secretion is largely by means of hypothalamic monitoring of the plasma osmolarity (concentration of solute molecules that increase osmotic pressure). Therefore when the blood increases in effective osmotic pressure, reflecting dehydration, the osmoreceptors of the hypothalamus respond by stimulating the neurohypophysis to secrete ADH, which in turn causes the kidney to conserve body water and prevent or slow further dehydration. This recovery from dehydration is further aided by the concomitant stimulation of the thirst center, leading to increased intake of fluids. Reduction in the effective plasma volume produced by hemorrhage or reduced cardiac output will also stimulate ADH release and promote antidiuresis.

In addition to these physiological controls, certain drugs may also influence ADH secretion. Acetylcholine, nicotine, morphine, barbiturates, and bradykinin have been shown to cause release of ADH in normal subjects. Ethanol and phenytoin, on the other hand, are thought to promote diuresis by inhibiting ADH release.

Effects of ADH deficiency. When ADH is markedly reduced or absent due to destruction of the hypothalamic region responsible for its synthesis or due to separation of the hypophyseal stalk above the median eminence (Fig. 34-1), urinary concentration is impossible and copious amounts of dilute sugar-free urine are produced. This condition is called *diabetes insipidus* and is not to

FIG. 34-1
Anatomy of the pituitary gland.

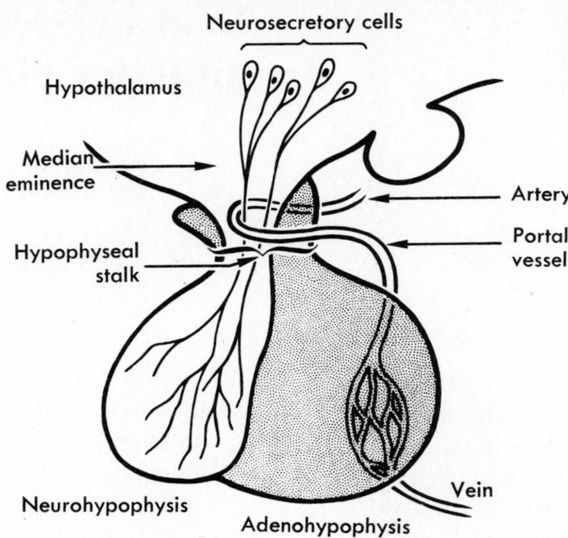

TABLE 34-1. Neurohypophyseal hormones

Descriptive name	Other names	Target tissue	Target tissue response
Antidiuretic hormone	ADH	Renal tubule epithelium	Increased water permeability
	Vasopressin	Smooth muscle in blood vessels	Vasoconstriction
		Smooth muscle of gastrointestinal tract	Contraction, increasing gastrointestinal motility
Oxytocin	—	Uterine smooth muscle	Increased uterine contractions
		Breast myoepithelium	Milk letdown

be confused with the disease diabetes mellitus arising from the inability to utilize blood glucose or release insulin. Diabetes insipidus is not in itself a life-threatening condition unless severe electrolyte imbalances develop. So long as the patient has a fully functional thirst center and can balance the excessive fluid losses with high fluid intakes, severe imbalances do not frequently occur. However, in situations in which a person is unconscious and unable to take in adequate quantities of fluids, severe dehydration may set in before the condition is noticed. For this reason, in patients with traumatic head injuries or surgery to the hypothalamic region of the brain it is critically important for health care personnel to monitor urinary specific gravity and blood sodium levels, along with fluid intake and urinary volumes, to detect excessive diuresis and resultant dehydration.

In many patients with trauma to the hypothalamus or the hypophyseal stalk, the resultant diabetes insipidus may be transitory. In patients whose condition is chronic, reversal of symptoms can be achieved in one of two ways: replacement therapy with a form of ADH or therapy with pharmacological agents that relieve the symptoms of the disease.

ADH preparations used in replacement therapy. Since ADH is a peptide hormone, it cannot be administered orally, and all replacement therapy with ADH involves the administration of the hormone parenterally or intranasally (Table 34-2).

Vasopressin (Pitressin), an aqueous preparation of purified ADH, is not routinely used for therapy since the half-life of ADH in the blood is quite short. This preparation is infused intravenously for short-term management of unconscious patients. The duration of action of vasopressin may be extended by slowing absorption. *Lypressin,* a synthetic form of ADH that is sprayed onto the mucous membranes of the nasal passages, is usually administered four times daily. This preparation has largely replaced *posterior pituitary extract,* which was also administered as a snuff but which tended to irritate nasal passages and produce unwanted effects caused by proteins other than ADH that were present in the extract.

A new synthetic vasopressin for intranasal adminis-

TABLE 34-2. Clinical summary of drugs used to treat diabetes insipidus

Generic name	Trade name	Drug class	Adminis-tration	Properties	Uses	Side effects
Desmopressin acetate	DDAVP	Synthetic derivative of neurohypophy-seal hormone	Nasal	Peptide with longer serum half-life than vasopressin; increases renal reabsorption of water.	Replacement therapy in diabetes insipidus.	Vasoconstriction; smooth muscle contraction.
Lypressin	Diapid	Synthetic derivative of neurohypophy-seal hormone	Nasal	Peptide with short serum half-life increases renal reabsorption of water.	Replacement therapy in diabetes insipidus.	Vasoconstriction; smooth muscle contraction.
Posterior pitu-itary extract	Pituitrin	Neurohypophyseal hormone	Parenteral or nasal	Peptide with short serum half-life; contains ADH and oxytocin; in-creases renal reabsorption of water.	Rarely used; contains vasopressin and oxy-tocin. (See Chapter 37.)	Vasoconstriction; smooth muscle contraction.
Vasopressin	Pitressin	Neurohypophyseal hormone	Parenteral	Peptide with short serum half-life; increases renal reabsorption of water.	Test ADH response of kidney. Short-term maintenance of unconscious patient.	Vasoconstriction; smooth muscle contraction.
Vasopressin tannate in oil	Pitressin Tannate in oil	Neurohypophyseal hormone	Intramus-cular depot	Peptide derivative slowly absorbed; increases renal reabsorption of water.	Replacement therapy in diabetes insipidus.	Vasoconstriction; smooth muscle contraction
Chlorothiazide	Diuril	Thiazide diuretic	Oral	Promotes sodium, chloride excretion.	Control of diuresis in diabetes insipidus.	Hyponatremia; hypo-kalemia.
Chlorpro-pamide	Diabinese	Sulfonylurea oral hypoglycemic agent	Oral	Increases vasopressin action in the kidney.	Control of diuresis in diabetes insipidus.	Hypoglycemia.
Clofibrate	Atromid S	Hypolipidemic agent	Oral	Increases vasopressin action in the kidney.	Control of diuresis in diabetes insipidus.	Nausea; weakness and muscle cramps.

tration recently has become available. This drug, *desmopressin acetate (DDAVP),* is a chemically altered form of vasopressin, differing from the natural hormone by having a longer serum half-life, a more potent antidiuretic effect, and less pressor activity. Desmopressin acetate need only be administered once or twice daily in contrast to other ADH preparations. In theory side effects due to the pressor action of vasopressin should be less of a problem with this vasopressin derivative.

Long-term control of diabetes insipidus may also be achieved with *vasopressin tannate* in peanut oil, which is given as an intramuscular depot injection. With this preparation patients have reported normal concentration of the urine for up to 48 hours following injection. Patients should be warned not to repeat the injection until the diuresis recurs. Overdoses of ADH may produce water intoxication characterized by hyponatremia and excessive water retention with sodium loss via the kidney.

In the past ADH has been used as a pressor agent but it is not now recommended for that use. In fact its vasoconstrictor action prevents its safe use for patients with vascular disease or coronary artery disease. Even small doses may cause difficulty to a patient prone to angina attacks. Occasionally this vasoconstrictor action is used to help control massive gastrointestinal bleeding.

ADH also possesses the ability to promote activity of the smooth muscle of the intestinal tract. During routine therapy of diabetes insipidus, the action of ADH on intestinal smooth muscle may result in nausea, belching, and cramps.

Other drugs used to treat diabetes insipidus

Three types of agents other than ADH preparations have been used to treat diabetes insipidus (Table 34-2). Paradoxically, *thiazide diuretics* (Chapter 14) are effective in some cases. The effectiveness of these convenient oral agents is apparently based on their blockade of electrolyte reabsorption, resulting initially in increased sodium and water excretion. The kidney responds to this change by reabsorbing more water by mechanisms that do not depend on ADH. Moderate salt restriction enhances the action of these drugs in many patients. The most common side effect of this class of drugs is potassium depletion, which in the extreme may induce cardiac arrhythmias, as well as impair neuromuscular functions and the normal functions of the gastrointestinal tract and the kidney.

Another agent used to treat diabetes insipidus is *chlorpropamide,* a sulfonylurea used as an oral hypoglycemic agent in the treatment of diabetes mellitus (Chapter 39). This drug, used alone or in combination with a thiazide diuretic, is usually effective in reducing urine volumes. The major potential toxicity is hypoglycemia. When chlorpropamide is used to treat diabetes insipidus, the action sought is a direct sensitization of the kidney to vasopressin so that lower than normal levels of vasopressin cause near normal water reabsorption. The drug is apparently not effective in patients who produce no vasopressin at all. There is some evidence that chlorpropamide may also stimulate the pituitary to release vasopressin.

Clofibrate, an oral agent used to reduce serum triglyceride levels (Chapter 18), may also be effective in diabetes insipidus and may be used alone or in combination with a thiazide diuretic. The drug may produce nausea or, rarely, muscle cramps and weakness. Clofibrate appears to act on the kidney in a manner similar to chlorpropamide.

The symptoms of diabetes insipidus may also be produced if the neurohypophysis is producing normal amounts of ADH but the kidney is unresponsive or responds poorly to ADH. This syndrome, called *nephrogenic diabetes insipidus,* may be treated by the thiazide diuretics but is, of course, resistant to therapy by ADH. Although nephrogenic diabetes insipidus may arise as a genetic disease, it may also be induced by certain drugs such as lithium used in treating mental disease and demeclocycline, a tetracycline antibiotic.

Oxytocin

The second hormone released by the neurohypophysis is oxytocin. The major target organs of this octapeptide hormone are breast myoepithelium and the smooth muscle of the uterus, especially during the second and third stages of labor. Oxytocin is discussed in detail in Chapter 37, so its uses will not be discussed at this point. Suffice it to say that oxytocin speeds delivery of the fetus by promoting uterine contractions during the last stages of labor when the cervix is fully dilated. A second important function of oxytocin is causing milk ejection by stimulating contraction of the myoepithelium of the alveoli of the breast.

The regulation of oxytocin release is a particularly good example of the close interaction of the central nervous system with pituitary function. It has been shown that suckling by the infant induces afferent nerve impulses from the breast to the brain, which cause new oxytocin to be synthesized and stored hormone to be released. A similar reflex loop may operate in parturition when dilation of the cervix is thought to stimulate synthesis and release of oxytocin.

No specific syndrome resulting from abnormalities in oxytocin function has been described.

■ THE ADENOHYPOPHYSIS

The adenohypophysis, or anterior pituitary, constitutes approximately 75% by weight of the total pituitary

TABLE 34-3. Adenohypophyseal hormones

Descriptive name	Other names	Hypothalamic releasing factor	Target tissue	Target tissue response
Adrenocorticotropic hormone	ACTH Corticotropin	Corticotropin-releasing factor (CRF)	Adrenal cortex Pigment cells of skin	Increased steroid synthesis Increased pigmentation
Follicle-stimulating hormone	FSH	Gonadotropin-releasing hormone (GnRH); FSH-releasing hormone (FRH or FSH-RH)	Ovary Seminiferous tubules	Increased estrogen production Maturation
Growth hormone	GH Somatotropin STH	Somatotropin or growth hormone-releasing factor (SRF or GRF); somatostatin or somatotropin-release inhibitory factor (SRIF)	Whole body	Increased anabolism, cell size, cell numbers
Lipotropin	—	Corticotropin-releasing factor (CRF)	Unknown	Unknown
Luteinizing hormone or interstitial cell-stimulating hormone	ICSH LH	Gonadotropin-releasing hormone (GnRH); luteinizing hormone-releasing factor or hormone (LRF, LRH, LHRF, or LHRH)	Ovary Leydig cells	Ovulation; formation of corpus luteum Increased androgen synthesis
Prolactin	LTH Luteotropic hormone	Prolactin-inhibiting factor (PIF); prolactin-releasing factor (PRF)	Breast	Milk formation
Thyroid-stimulating hormone	Thyrotropin TSH	Thyrotropin-releasing hormone or factor (TRH or TRF)	Thyroid gland	Increased T_3, T_4 synthesis

gland and is rightfully considered to be the master gland of the entire endocrine system. The adenohypophysis secretes seven known hormones, most of which directly stimulate secretion by the adrenal glands, the thyroid gland, and the reproductive organs (Table 34-3). Recent evidence suggests that other factors which regulate central nervous system function are also released from the adenohypophysis. These are the beta lipotropin family of peptides, including endorphins and enkephalins (Chapter 28).

Although the adenohypophysis is true secretory tissue and synthesizes as well as releases its hormones, control of those secretions still lies in the brain. Small polypeptides, called *neurohormones,* are synthesized in the median eminence of the hypothalamus and released into the portal venous system (Fig. 34-1), which carries them directly to the adenohypophysis. In the adenohypophysis these neurohormones, which may be *releasing hormones* or *inhibitory hormones,* act on the specific target cell to stimulate or inhibit the synthesis and release of the proper hormone.

■ Adenohypophyseal hormones

Growth hormone

Mechanism of action. Growth hormone is the only one of the adenohypophyseal hormones to exert effects on the whole body rather than on specific target organs or tissues. Growth hormone controls the length of the long bones of the skeleton, which determine adult stature. In addition, the hormone is a potent anabolic agent, which acts on many tissues of the body to increase cell size and cell numbers. This anabolic action is the result of changes produced in protein, carbohydrate, and fat metabolism. The hormone increases the rate of amino acid transport into cells and elevates the cellular rate of protein synthesis. Growth hormone also possesses an antiinsulin effect, which tends to decrease glucose uptake and carbohydrate utilization thereby elevating liver glycogen and blood glucose levels. Finally growth hormone increases the mobilization of fats for energy, which is manifested by a rise in blood levels of free fatty acids.

Many of these actions of growth hormone are mediated by proteins called *somatomedins*. Growth hormone stimulates the production of somatomedins by the liver. The somatomedins then act on various body tissues to change metabolism.

Effects of growth hormone deficiency. Damage to the hypophysis may cause that gland to produce insufficient quantities of hypophyseal hormones. This condition is called *panhypopituitarism*. Adults suffering from this syndrome may require replacement therapy with thyroid hormones, adrenal steroids, and appropriate sex steroids. Children with panhypopituitarism may, in addition, suffer growth stunting due to a lack of growth hormone.

Distinguishing among the various causes of short stature in children has been very difficult in the past but is more reliable now, since a sensitive radioimmunoassay for detecting blood levels of growth hormone is available. True pituitary dwarfism, once diagnosed, can be treated successfully with growth hormone preparations (Asellacrin, Crescormon) derived from either human or other primate sources. Because of its protein nature and the limited supply, growth hormone for clinical use is expensive and relatively rare (Chapter 33). In those cases of pituitary dwarfism that have been treated, the child or adolescent with stunted growth typically shows an immediate increase in growth and may increase a foot or more in height over a period of several years treatment. Ultimately, the patients develop resistance to the protein and growth tapers off.

Many of the actions of growth hormone antagonize those of insulin and in predisposed individuals prolonged treatment with growth hormone may precipitate diabetes mellitus. For this reason patients receiving growth hormone are monitored to detect elevated blood glucose levels or altered glucose tolerance. In patients with established diabetes, destruction of the pituitary gland with loss of growth hormone causes diabetic adults to require less insulin.

Regulation of secretion of growth hormone. The secretion of growth hormone is regulated by two factors from the hypothalamus, one stimulating release and one inhibiting release. The releasing factor has not been fully studied. The inhibitory factor is a peptide called *somatostatin*. In addition to regulating growth hormone release, somatostatin may also influence thyroid-stimulating hormone (TSH) and adrenocorticotropic hormone release from the pituitary gland. Somatostatin is found in other tissues such as gut and pancreas (Chapter 39) and may play different regulatory roles in those tissues.

Effects of excess growth hormone. Acromegaly and gigantism are two of the most striking endocrinopathies. Both conditions are produced by excess growth hormone, but the age of onset causes marked differences in the manifestations of the disease. Excessive growth hormone from an early age produces the rare condition of gigantism. In these individuals growth may be rapid. Growth rates of 3.5 inches per year have been reported. One pituitary giant on record was 8 feet 11 inches tall.

If the onset of excessive growth hormone production is delayed until after puberty, that is, after the plates of the long bones have joined and normal skeletal growth has halted, acromegaly results. In this condition only those tissues still able to grow and expand respond to growth hormone, with the result that malproportions occur. Typically, the bones of the fingers flare at the end and the fingers thicken to produce a spatula-like appearance. Bones and cartilage of the face also grow and thicken, producing coarse features and a massive lower jaw.

Both gigantism and acromegaly are related to the presence of pituitary neoplasms, which secrete the excessive amounts of growth hormone. Consequently, therapy is usually aimed at destruction or removal of the tumor. Successful treatment results in the arrest of the progressive symptoms of the disease but does not erase the existing deformations.

Gonadotropic hormones

Mechanism of action. The gonadotropic hormones of the adenohypophysis are follicle-stimulating hormone, luteinizing hormone, and prolactin. Follicle-stimulating hormone and luteinizing hormone regulate maturation and function of the male and female sexual organs. In women prolactin stimulates milk formation in the estrogen- and progestin-primed breast.

In the maturing male follicle-stimulating hormone causes the maturation of the seminiferous tubules. Luteinizing hormone, which is sometimes called *interstitial cell–stimulating hormone* in the male, increases the numbers of testicular interstitial cells and stimulates their secretion of androgens. These androgens are the male steroid hormones that complete the process of maturation, leading to the production of viable sperm and to the development of the secondary male sexual characteristics.

In the maturing female follicle-stimulating hormone and luteinizing hormone begin to be produced in greater quantities at puberty and stimulate ovarian estrogen production. Estrogens, which are the female steroid hormones, cause the development of the female secondary sex characteristics.

Regulation of gonadotropin secretion in adult females. In addition to their role in development, follicle-stimulating hormone and luteinizing hormone control the menstrual cycle in the mature female (Fig. 34-2). The regulation of this function involves the hypothalamus, the adenohypophysis, the ovaries, and the endometrium or uterine lining. The first event in the cycle is the rise in the concentration of follicle-stimulating hormone in the bloodstream. In response, in the ovary one of the hundreds of primordial follicles begins to develop. As the follicle matures under the influence of follicle-stimulating hormone, it begins to produce increasing amounts of estrogens, which greatly increase the adenohypophyseal secretion of luteinizing hormone. It is the surge of luteinizing hormone at midcycle that is the pri-

FIG. 34-2

Pituitary regulation of the menstrual cycle. Changes in circulating hormone levels are correlated with ovarian follicle and endometrial alterations. Details of site of synthesis and site of action for each hormone are in the text. (Redrawn from Segal, S.J.: Sci. Am. Sept., 1974, p. 58. With permission of W.H. Freeman and Co.)

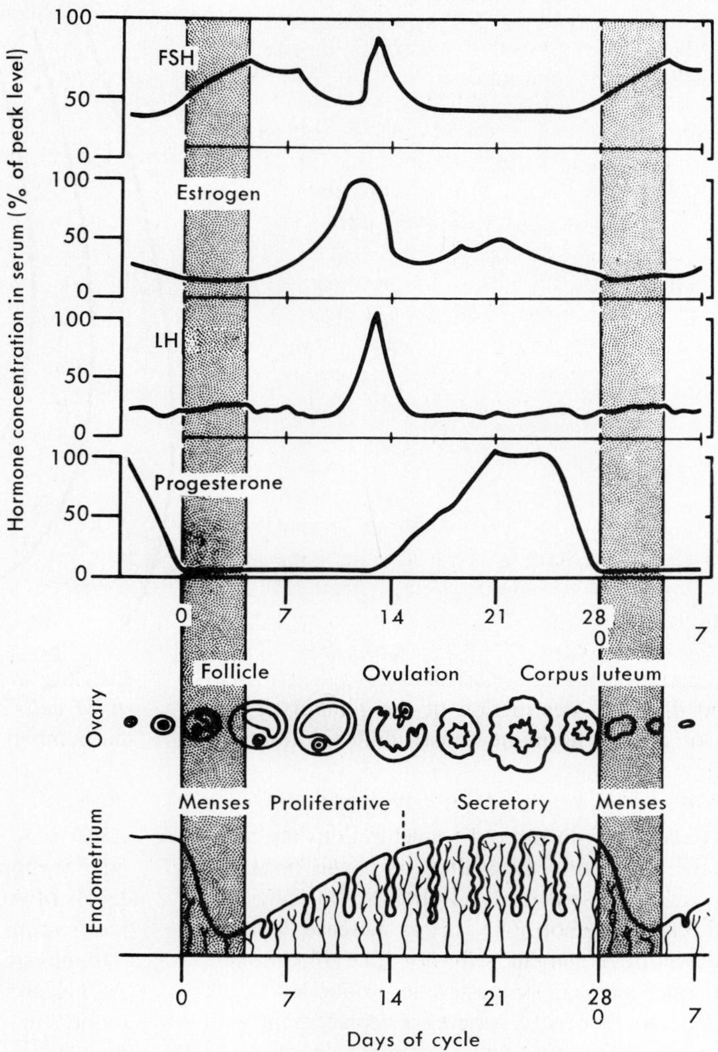

mary trigger for ovulation, the release of the ovum from the mature follicle.

In the second half of the menstrual cycle, luteinizing hormone causes the follicle from which the ovum was released to develop into a thickened, secretory tissue called a *corpus luteum,* which secretes large quantities of progesterone, another of the female steroid hormones. By day 21 of the cycle the large quantities of circulating estrogen and progesterone inhibit the secretion of follicle-stimulating hormone and luteinizing hormone from the adenohypophysis (Fig. 34-2), and the corpus luteum begins to involute. Steroid hormone production falls rapidly as the corpus luteum fails and brings about the final stage in the cycle—the collapse of the endometrial lining.

During the menses the entire inner surface of the uterus is denuded as the endometrium rapidly collapses to about 65% of its former thickness. About 70 ml of blood and serum is lost along with necrotic and dissolving tissue during a typical menstrual period. Normally this blood does not clot due to the presence in the fluid of fibrinolysin, an enzyme that digests the fibrin matrix on which blood clots form. In spite of the seemingly favorable environment for bacterial growth, the uterus during menstruation is resistant to infection. A contributing factor to this resistance is the presence of great numbers of leukocytes in the menstrual fluid.

Effects of gonadotropin deficiency. Alterations in hypophyseal or ovarian function can upset this finely balanced regulatory sequence we have just described. Throughout childhood, pituitary secretion of follicle-stimulating hormone and luteinizing hormone is very

FIG. 34-3

Regulation of hormone synthesis by negative feedback loops. Each arrow indicates the hormone, its source, and its target tissue. The hypothalamic synthesis of individual releasing factors is suppressed by high blood concentrations of the appropriate final hormone. For example, cortisol suppresses CRF synthesis and release, thereby blocking further cortisol synthesis. Other loops are similarly regulated.

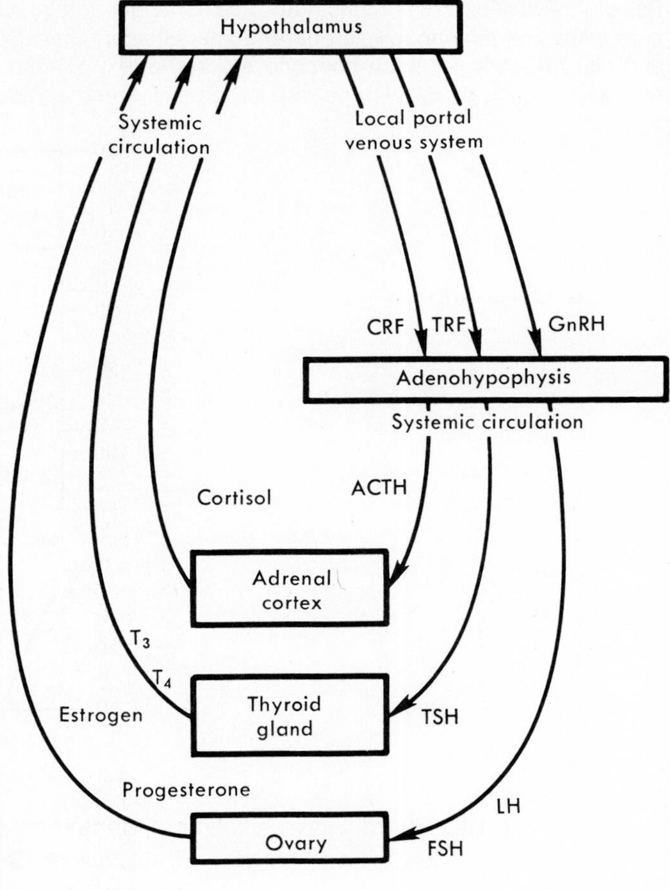

low, and circulating sex steroid concentrations are quite low as well. At puberty the adenohypophysis normally greatly increases its secretion of follicle stimulating hormone and luteinizing hormone. If this increase does not occur, sexual development will not take place since androgen, estrogen, and progesterone production is not induced. Therapy for these patients is replacement with the target tissue hormones—the convenient, inexpensive steroids discussed in Chapters 37 and 38 rather than the peptide hormones of the adenohypophysis that are not only difficult to obtain in large quantities but also must be given parenterally and may cause foreign protein reactions.

Adrenocorticotropic hormone (ACTH) and lipotropin

Mechanism of action. When ACTH is released by the adenohypophysis, it stimulates the adrenal cortex to synthesize and release cortisol, a major adrenocortical steroid hormone, as well as other glucocorticoids and minor amounts of sex steroids (Chapter 35).

Regulation of secretion of ACTH. Cortisol blood levels are monitored by the hypothalamus, which adjusts the rate of release of corticotropic-releasing factor (CRF) into the hypophyseal portal venous system to the adenohypophysis, thereby controlling the systemic levels of ACTH. When cortisol levels become too high, the hypothalamus reduces CRF release. The adenohypophysis, lacking appropriate stimulation, reduces ACTH production and blood levels of the peptide hormone fall. The adrenal cortical production of cortisol then falls due to the lowered ACTH levels. Blood levels of the adrenal steroid are thereby prevented from exceeding an upper limit. Conversely, when cortisol levels in the blood fall too low, the hypothalamus normally prevents a dangerously low level from developing. CRF is released in large amounts into the hypophyseal portal venous system, the adenohypophysis in response releases ACTH, and the adrenal cortex in response to ACTH elevates cortisol production. This intricate regulatory sequence is an example of a negative feedback loop, a regulatory mechanism in which the end product of a reaction sequence inhibits the operation of the sequence, thereby keeping the concentration of the product between certain limits (Fig. 34-3).

Lipotropin is mentioned in connection with ACTH, since both peptides are produced by a single cell type in the adenohypophysis and both seem to be derived

■ THE NURSING PROCESS

■ Assessment

In most cases patients with problems with the pituitary hormones will have had chronic excesses or deficiencies of the hormones before the diagnosis is made. There may be few objective signs of a problem, as with prolactin deficiency, or major changes, as with growth hormone overproduction. When an endocrine problem is suspected, the nurse should make a thorough examination to obtain baseline data, paying particular attention to those subjective and objective changes that the patient may indicate have occurred over an extended period.

■ Management

The management of pituitary problems may be pharmacological, surgical, or both. In most cases of drug treatment the therapy will be long term and improvement slow. The nurse should monitor the patient for expected side effects of the drugs. With the help of the physician, the nurse should determine the best objective measures of improvement and monitor them (e.g., fluid intake and output, laboratory values). Before the patient is discharged, the nurse should begin the teaching and emotional support needed to help the patient move to self-management and should help the patient develop reasonable goals of therapy.

■ Evaluation

In general drug therapy is successful if the hormonal balance is returned more closely to normal, and the patient has no serious side effects and can manage the self-therapy alone. Before discharge the nurse should ascertain that the patient is able to explain why the prescribed drugs are necessary, how to administer them correctly, signs of overdosage or underdosage, side effects that might occur, and which ones should be reported immediately. If a patient does not have a medical identification tag or bracelet before leaving the hospital, the patient should state the need to obtain one. Preexisting medical conditions may be altered by the drugs (e.g., diabetes, angina pectoris), and the patient should be able to explain what the effect of the drugs will be on these preexisting conditions and how to manage them. For further information, see the patient care implications section at the end of this chapter.

---

from a single prohormone. The function of lipotropin is not completely established, but a portion of the lipotropin molecule is identical to beta endorphin. Beta endorphin is one of the newly discovered natural peptides that produces whole body analgesia (Chapter 28). These peptides may be derived from lipotropin.

Thyroid-stimulating hormone

Negative feedback regulation applies not only to the adrenal cortex and the ovary, but also to the thyroid gland (Fig. 34-3). We will discuss thyroid-stimulating hormone (TSH) in detail in Chapter 36.

■ PATIENT CARE IMPLICATIONS

Diabetes insipidus

1. Diabetes insipidus may develop subsequent to traumatic head injuries or surgery to the hypothalamic region of the brain. It is therefore critically important for the health personnel to monitor fluid intake, urine output, urine specific gravity, and blood sodium levels in these patients to detect excessive diuresis and resultant dehydration. In diabetes insipidus the urine is characteristically light in color, produced in large quantities often exceeding measured fluid intake, and of low specific gravity, 1.000 to 1.005 (normal usually being 1.010 to 1.030). The diagnosis is often first made by the observant nurse.
2. Excessive urine production may also occur in diabetes mellitus due to glycosuria. Careful monitoring of urine and blood glucose levels will distinguish this patient from one with diabetes insipidus.
3. To administer vasopressin tannate in oil (Pitressin Tannate in oil), the following procedure is used:
   a. Heat the unopened vial in warm water for several minutes to decrease the viscosity of the peanut oil.
   b. Vigorously shake the ampule to resuspend the medication, which is usually an inconspicuous film on the side of the vial. Resuspension is adequate when no particles of medication remain

on the bottom or sides of the vial. Failure to shake sufficiently will result in inaccurate dosage and erratic absorption.

c. The correct dose should be drawn up into a syringe fitted with a large bore (19 to 21 gauge), 1½ inch needle, and administered intramuscularly immediately before the oil cools too much.

d. Inject the medication with slow, even pressure on the plunger. Attempts to inject too rapidly can cause pressure to increase within the syringe so that the needle and syringe separate and the medication is spilled.

e. Appropriate injection sites would include the buttocks, thigh, or ventrogluteal site. The oil base, which allows slow absorption, can produce palpable lumps at injection sites. For this reason, injection sites should be rotated and the deltoid muscle avoided.

f. Oil-based medications should never be given intravenously.

4. Because the aqueous preparation and the oil-based preparation of vasopressin have similar trade names, the nurse should clearly understand which preparation has been ordered and question an inappropriate order. For example, *Pitressin* (the aqueous preparation) would be appropriate to achieve rapid control of diabetes insipidus, but it would be an inappropriate drug for long-term management of the discharged patient.
5. Patients may require special help in learning to administer the nasal powders or the solutions that are snuffed into the nose. A severe cold, allergies, or nasal surgery might make the nasal mucous membrane route of administration inappropriate. These patients may require temporary control with injectable forms of vasopressin.
6. Patients taking medications via the nasal route will usually find that no significant increase in drug level occurs if more than two sprays per nostril are needed. It is usually of more benefit to increase the frequency of dosing rather than to increase the number of sprays per nostril.
7. Patients with known or suspected vascular disease should be carefully monitored when therapy with vasopressin or related drugs is begun. Patients with angina may find that they have more heart pain while taking this drug.
8. Overdoses of vasopressin may produce water intoxication characterized by hyponatremia (low blood sodium) and excessive water retention with sodium loss via the kidney. Patients should therefore be instructed not to repeat their dosage until diuresis recurs.
9. Patients with diabetes insipidus will usually find that it is not necessary to measure their urinary output to monitor the disease at home; increased frequency of urination will usually signal loss of control.
10. The nurse must be fully familiar with the side effects of the drugs the patient receives for diabetes insipidus. The nurse must recognize that gastrointestinal complaints may signal too high a dose of vasopressin and that weakness and fatigue in a patient receiving chlorpropamide may signal a hypoglycemic reaction to that drug.
11. After pituitary surgery, even for removal of the pituitary gland, diabetes insipidus may be only temporary.
12. Patients with diabetes insipidus should wear a medical identification tag or bracelet indicating their diagnosis.

Growth hormone

1. Treatment with growth hormone (Asellacrin, Crescormon) should be reserved for patients in whom growth hormone deficiency is clearly demonstrated.
2. Growth hormone should be prescribed only when epiphyses have not yet closed and significant short stature is present.
3. The drug is administered intramuscularly three times a week. Injection sites should be rotated.
4. Growth hormone should be used cautiously if there is progression of any underlying intracranial lesion.
5. Treatment with growth hormone can precipitate hypothyroidism.
6. Growth hormone has a potential diabetogenic effect. Monitor urine sugar concentration, and teach the patient or family to test the urine for sugar at home. Insulin may be required during the course of therapy; see Chapter 39 for a discussion of the management of diabetes mellitus.
7. In diabetic adults destruction of the pituitary gland with loss of growth hormone may cause the patient to require less insulin.
8. During therapy with growth hormone, parents should be instructed to keep weekly weight and height charts and to report any excessive gain in either area, according to parameters outlined by the physician.

Panhypopituitarism

1. The patient who loses all or nearly all pituitary function due to trauma, surgery, or disease must be treated with replacement hormonal therapy to survive. Treatment with exogenous forms of cortisol usually substitutes for ACTH loss. Thyroid hormones usually replace TSH. Except in the child, growth hormone is not replaced. ADH may only need tempo-

rary replacement, as it is synthesized in the hypothalamus. Lipotropin is not replaced. The gonadotropic hormones, follicle-stimulating hormone, luteinizing hormone, and prolactin are rarely used in replacement therapy. More often the estrogens or androgens (Chapters 37 and 38) are used to help the patient maintain his or her own sexual identity. In the female it is difficult to recreate the monthly cyclic surges of these hormones, so this may not be attempted unless requested by the patient; thus the female is sterile. Oxytocin is not usually replaced unless the woman has been able to conceive and the hormone would be needed to assist with labor and delivery. For information on individual hormones, see Chapters 34 to 38.
2. Patients should wear a medical identification tag indicating what replacement therapy they are receiving.

■ SUMMARY

The pituitary gland, or hypophysis, is composed of two distinct regions. The anterior pituitary, or adenohypophysis, is composed of true secretory tissue, which both synthesizes and releases seven known peptide hormones. The posterior pituitary, or neurohypophysis, is composed of neural tissue, which stores and releases two peptide hormones. These peptide hormones, antidiuretic hormone (ADH) and oxytocin, are synthesized in the hypothalamus and transported to the neurohypophysis through the pituitary stalk.

ADH increases the permeability of parts of the renal tubule to water, allowing water to be reabsorbed and returned to the bloodstream. ADH is released from the neurohypophysis in response to increasing osmolarity of the plasma, an indicator of dehydration. Lowered plasma volume also stimulates release of the hormone. Loss of ADH results in diabetes insipidus, a disease characterized by production of excessive amounts of dilute, sugar-free urine. This condition may be treated by replacing the missing ADH, or the symptoms may be controlled directly. Drugs such as thiazide diuretics, chlorpropamide, and clofibrate may alter kidney function and/or increase intrinsic ADH activity sufficiently to control diuresis in these patients.

Oxytocin is also released by the neurohypophysis. Oxytocin causes contraction of the smooth muscle of the breast and uterus, facilitating delivery of the fetus and milk letdown in the nursing mother.

Synthesis of the hormones of the adenohypophysis is controlled in the hypothalamus by means of neurohormones, which function as releasing or inhibiting hormones in the pituitary gland. Growth hormone, synthesized and released by the adenohypophysis, causes the synthesis of somatomedins in the liver, which act on many tissues to produce characteristic anabolic changes. Persons lacking growth hormone fail to achieve normal adult height. These patients may receive growth hormone as replacement therapy.

The gonadotropic hormones produced by the adenohypophysis are follicle-stimulating hormone, luteinizing hormone, and prolactin. These hormones affect growth and development of the sexual organs in males and females and also regulate the monthly ovarian cycle in adult females. Gonadotropin deficiency prevents normal sexual development and function. Replacement therapy usually is carried out with the specific steroids such as androgens and estrogens rather than with the protein hormones of the adenohypophysis.

Adrenocorticotropic hormone (ACTH) and beta lipotropin are derived from a single prohormone in the adenohypophysis. The target tissue of ACTH is the adrenal gland, which responds to ACTH by synthesizing cortisol. Control of secretion of ACTH is through a negative feedback loop involving cortisol from the adrenal gland and corticotropin-releasing factor from the hypothalamus. ACTH, as a protein, is inconvenient for use in replacement therapy, although ACTH can cause the release of cortisol and other steroids from the adrenal gland. Lipotropin may be a precursor for the endorphins, peptides that produce whole body analgesia.

■ STUDY QUESTIONS

1. What are the two divisions of the pituitary gland, or hypophysis?
2. What is the nature of neurohypophyseal tissue?
3. What hormones are released by the neurohypophysis?
4. Where are the hormones released by the neurohypophysis actually synthesized?
5. What is the target tissue of antidiuretic hormone (ADH)?
6. What is the mechanism of action of ADH?
7. What physiological conditions stimulate the release of ADH?
8. What is diabetes insipidus?
9. What two types of therapy may be used to treat diabetes insipidus?
10. Compare and contrast the route of administration and duration of action of vasopressin and vasopressin tannate in oil.
11. What advantage does nasal administration of vasopressin preparations such as lypressin have over intramuscular use of vasopressin itself?
12. What advantage does desmopressin acetate (DDAVP) have over other vasopressin preparations administered nasally?
13. What are the side effects associated with vasopressin use?
14. What drugs other than vasopressin derivatives have been used to control the symptoms of diabetes insipidus?
15. What is the mechanism of action by which thiazide diuretics control diuresis in diabetes insipidus?
16. What is the mechanism of action of chlorpropamide and clofibrate in treating diabetes insipidus?

17. What are the target tissues of oxytocin?
18. How is the secretion of oxytocin controlled?
19. What hormones are secreted by the adenohypophysis?
20. Where are the hormones secreted by the adenohypophysis actually synthesized?
21. What are neurohormones and where are they synthesized?
22. What are the target tissues of growth hormone?
23. What are the anabolic effects of growth hormone?
24. What are the antiinsulin effects of growth hormone?
25. What are somatomedins?
26. What is the effect of growth hormone deficiency?
27. What is the treatment of growth hormone deficiency?
28. Why is replacement therapy with growth hormone rarely carried out?
29. What is the effect of excess growth hormone?
30. What is the difference between gigantism and acromegaly?
31. What are the gonadotropic hormones?
32. What are the target tissues of follicle-stimulating hormone?
33. What are the target tissues of luteinizing hormone?
34. What are the target tissues of prolactin?
35. What roles do follicle-stimulating hormone and luteinizing hormone play in causing the development and release of a mature ovum from the ovary?
36. What are the effects of gonadotropin deficiency?
37. What is the target tissue for adrenocorticotropic hormone (ACTH)?
38. How is the concentration of ACTH in the bloodstream regulated?
39. What is the role of beta lipotropin?
40. What are the endorphins?

■ SUGGESTED READINGS

Comunas, C.: Transphenoidal hypophysectomy, American Journal of Nursing **80:**1820, 1980.

Cryer, P.E.: The hypothalamus and pituitary. In Diagnostic endocrinology, Oxford, 1976, Oxford University Press.

Fairchild, R.S.: Diabetes insipidus: a review, Critical Care Quarterly **3**(Sept.):111, 1980.

Guillemin, R.: Beta-lipotropin and endorphins: implications of current knowledge, Hospital Practice **13**(11):53, 1978.

Hershman, J.M.: Pituitary disease. In Endocrine pathophysiology: a patient-oriented approach, Philadelphia, 1977, Lea & Febiger.

Hobdell, E.F.: Growing up without growing: the child with growth hormone deficiency, American Journal of Maternal Child Nursing **2**(5):298, 1977.

Krieger, D.T., and Liotta, A.S.: Pituitary hormones in brain: where, how, and why? Science **205:**366, 1979.

Newsome, H.H., Jr.: Vasopressin: deficiency, excess, and the syndrome of inappropriate antidiuretic hormone secretion, Nephron **23:**126, 1979.

Rush, D.R., and Hamburger, S.C.: Drugs used in endocrine metabolic emergencies, Critical Care Quarterly **3**(Sept.):1, 1980.

Schally, A.V.: Aspects of hypothalamic regulation of the pituitary gland, Science **202:**18, 1978.

Wachter-Shikora, N.: ACTH. A review of anatomy, physiology, and structure related to neuroendocrine effects, Journal of Neurosurgical Nursing **11**(2):105, 1979.

Zusman, R.M., Keiser, H.R., and Handler, J.S.: A hypothesis for the molecular mechanism of action of chlorpropamide in the treatment of diabetes mellitus and diabetes insipidus, Federation Proceedings **36:**2728, 1977.

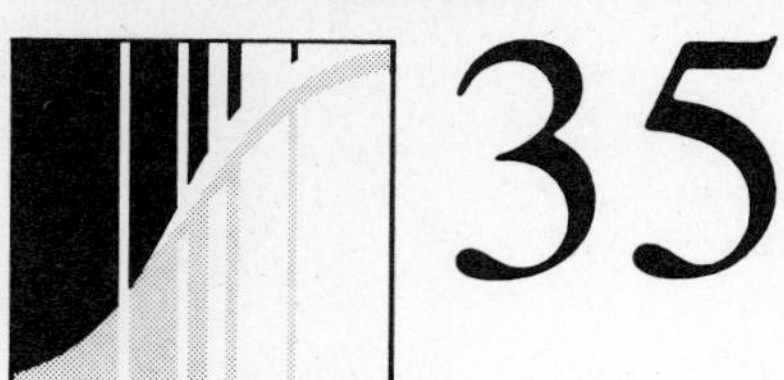

35 Drugs affecting the adrenal gland

In humans the adrenal gland is divided into two distinct functional units: the adrenal medulla and the adrenal cortex. These two regions of the gland differ in embryological origin and type of cells composing the tissue, as well as in hormones produced. The structure and function of these regions of the adrenal gland, the regulation of synthesis of the various hormones produced, and the pathological states arising from abnormalities in hormone production are discussed in this chapter. The widespread clinical uses of several of these hormones and their derivatives in diagnosis and therapy are also considered.

■ THE ADRENAL CORTEX

The adrenal cortex is composed of lipid-rich secretory tissue embryologically derived from coelomic epithelium. Three distinct layers within the cortex may be distinguished on the basis of histology. These regions differ not only in cellular arrangement, but also in the major steroid hormone produced and in the regulation of steroid synthesis (Fig. 35-1).

■ Adrenal steroids and their actions

Mineralocorticoid synthesis and actions. The outer layer, or zona glomerulosa, is the site of conversion of the precursor cholesterol to the mineralocorticoids. These steroids act on the kidney, causing the retention of sodium and associated water, while promoting potassium loss. Regulation of mineralocorticoid synthesis is primarily through the renin-angiotensin system (Fig. 35-2). The regulatory trigger for this feedback system is in the kidney where lowered blood sodium levels or lowered intravascular volume cause the release of renin into the bloodstream. Renin is an enzyme, which in the bloodstream converts angiotensinogen, a protein from the liver, to angiotensin I. Another enzyme found in the bloodstream and the lung rapidly converts angiotensin I to angiotensin II. Angiotensin II in turn stimulates the adrenal cortical zona glomerulosa to secrete the mineralocorticoids, especially aldosterone. The end result of this regulatory loop is that the mineralocorticoids released into the bloodstream slow the further loss of sodium and water through the kidneys. When sodium and water retention exceeds certain limits, the plasma volume becomes expanded and renin release is decreased. When the concentration of renin falls, the production of angiotensin II slows, aldosterone secretion by the adrenal gland falls, and the kidneys begin to rid the body of accumulated sodium.

Glucocorticoid synthesis. The inner two layers of the adrenal cortex convert cholesterol to the glucocorticoids and the sex steroids (primarily androgens and progestins). The synthesis of these steroids is regulated by the pituitary gland and the hypothalamus via the negative feedback loop described in the preceding chapter. Cortisol is the major glucocorticoid produced, and it is also the key to the regulation of steroid synthesis in the zona fasciculata and zona reticularis. Low levels of cortisol in the bloodstream stimulate and high levels suppress total steroid synthesis by respectively raising and lowering ACTH release from the pituitary gland.

Glucocorticoid action. The glucocorticoids produce potent and varied effects on metabolism. The primary metabolic effect is stimulation of gluconeogenesis (the formation of new glucose) by actions on the liver and peripheral tissues. In striated muscle, glucocorticoids mobilize amino acids from muscle protein. The result is an increase in circulating levels of amino acids and an overall depletion of muscle protein, which ultimately is expressed as a negative nitrogen balance (more nitrogen is excreted than is taken in the diet). In the liver glucocorticoids increase the activities of enzymes that convert amino acids to glucose. Much of this excess glucose is then stored in the liver as glycogen. In addition, amino acids are the ultimate source of precursors for fat synthesis, which is also increased in the presence of glucocorticoids.

Glucocorticoids have multiple direct actions in the body. They maintain water diuresis by antagonizing the effects of antidiuretic hormone in the kidney, lower the threshold for electrical excitation in the brain, and reduce the amount of new bone synthesis. In addition, the glucocorticoids affect the immune system by suppressing the activity of lymphoid tissue and by reduc-

FIG. 35-1

Regions of the adrenal gland. Each of the histologically distinguishable zones of the adrenal gland synthesizes specific hormones and is controlled by specific regulators as shown. The medulla forms the center of the adrenal gland and is actually thicker than shown in the cross-section.

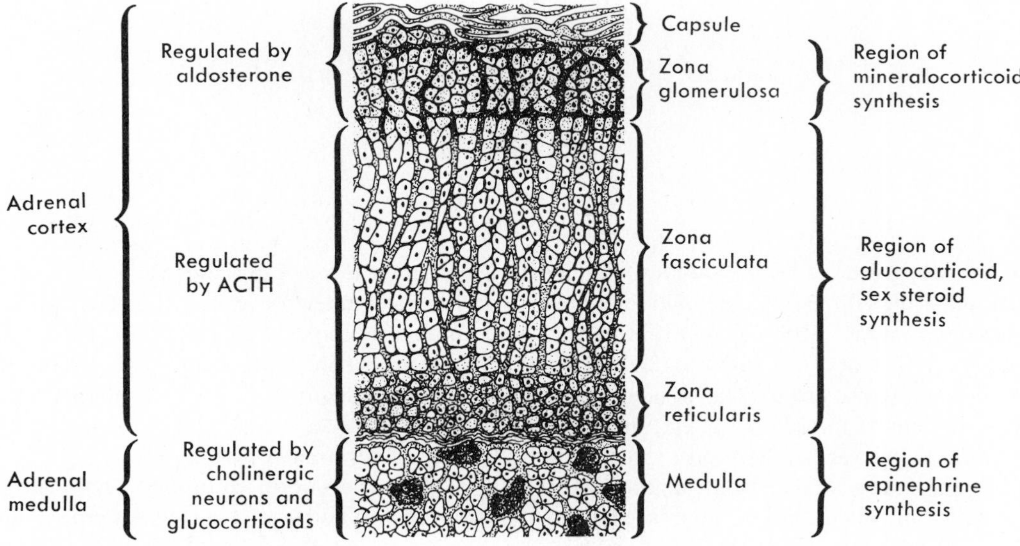

ing the numbers of circulating lymphocytes. These steroids also reduce inflammatory processes through multiple mechanisms, an action that has several useful therapeutic applications.

In addition to the direct effects mentioned, glucocorticoids have so-called permissive activities that allow the body to deal successfully with stress or trauma. For example, cortisol sensitizes the arterioles to norepinephrine, allowing the catecholamine to increase blood pressure. In the liver, cortisol must be present before epinephrine and glucagon can stimulate hydrolysis (breakdown) of liver glycogen to glucose, releasing the sugar to serve as energy source for peripheral muscle.

■ Abnormalities of adrenal hormone production

Adrenal insufficiency. Failure of the adrenal cortex is life-threatening. If the failure is sudden, as might be the case following adrenal injury or thrombosis, death may occur within hours. Early symptoms of *acute adrenal insufficiency* include confusion, restlessness, and nausea with vomiting. Circulatory collapse rapidly follows, and the patient enters deep shock and dies, perhaps even before the diagnosis is made.

If synthesis of glucocorticoids is reduced but not halted altogether, a patient may not be in immediate danger of circulatory collapse and death in the absence of stress or trauma but he or she may still suffer from inadequate amounts of the glucocorticoids. This *chronic primary adrenal insufficiency* is called *Addison's disease*. The symptoms include weakness, weight loss, dehydration, hypotension, hypoglycemia, and anemia. Most patients with chronic adrenal insufficiency also display increased pigmentation of the skin. This unusual or excessive tanning is due to a direct effect on melanin-containing skin cells by the chronic excess of ACTH, which is secreted by the pituitary gland in response to the elevated corticotropin release factor (CRF) induced by chronically low blood levels of cortisol.

Symptoms quite similar to Addison's disease are produced when the adenohypophysis is diseased or destroyed and no longer produces adequate ACTH. Without ACTH the zona reticularis and zona fasciculata do not synthesize cortisol and over a period of time these adrenal tissues atrophy. This condition is called *secondary adrenal insufficiency*. One characteristic that frequently visibly distinguishes these patients from those with Addison's disease is the absence of excessive pigmentation in the former. In secondary adrenal insufficiency the pituitary gland does not release large quantities of ACTH and the skin is not darkened.

Excessive glucocorticoids. Overproduction of cortisol, a condition called *Cushing's syndrome*, may be induced by a variety of factors. Some patients have high cortisol production due to tumors of the adrenal cortex, which may synthesize massive amounts of the steroid. Other patients have high cortisol synthesis because of increased ACTH release into the bloodstream, which keeps the zona fasciculata and zona reticularis maximally stimulated to produce the glucocorticoids. Excess

FIG. 35-2

The negative feedback loop regulating mineralocorticoid synthesis and release.
The kidney is the key to regulating the synthesis and release of aldosterone, the primary natural mineralocorticoid. Renin is released from the juxtaglomerular cells of the kidney to set the cascade in motion, and it is the kidney that is the ultimate target of aldosterone. The expanded plasma volume, which results when the kidney retains sodium ion (Na^+) and water, is the regulator that halts renin release.

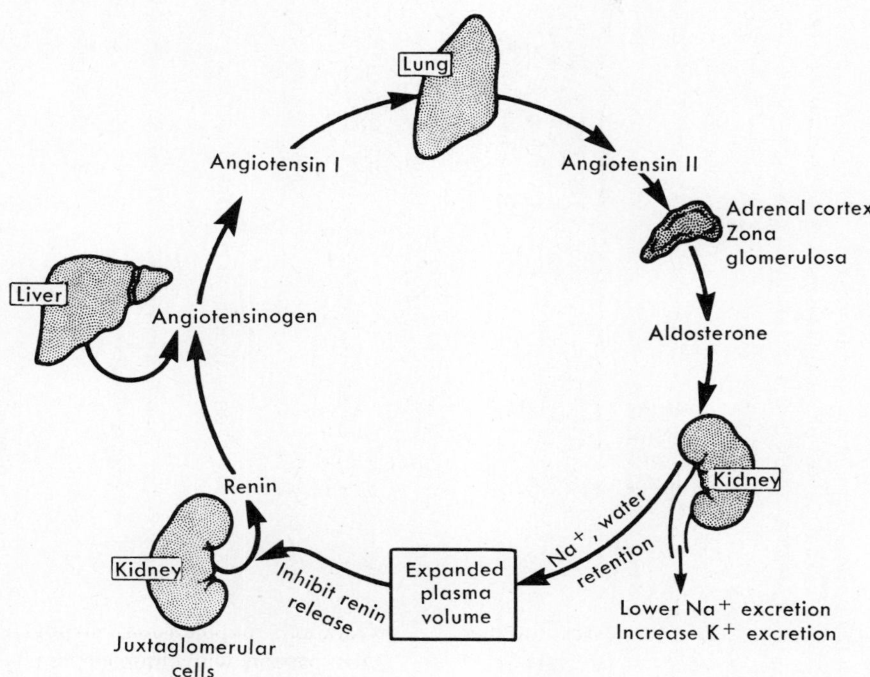

ACTH usually comes from a tumor of the pituitary gland, but occasionally the ACTH comes from some unusual source such as a lung tumor, which would not ordinarily be expected to synthesize ACTH. Most commonly, however, Cushing's syndrome is caused by administration of glucocorticoids as drugs.

The symptoms of Cushing's syndrome can be predicted from the metabolic actions of cortisol. Certain fat stores, especially those on the face and shoulders are increased as a result of cortisol stimulation of fat synthesis. The extremities may be weak and in more advanced cases may be thin due to the muscle wasting effects of the hormone. The skin is fragile and easily bruised due to protein breakdown in that tissue. Examination of the skin on the trunk of the body may reveal striae, or stretch marks, over areas where fat deposition is most pronounced. Many patients also have superficial fungal infections of the skin, related in part to the fragility of the skin and in part to the reduced host immune response caused by the excess steroid. Bone thinning occurs due to the changes in calcium metabolism; compression fractures of the spine may occur relatively easily. Diabetes may be precipitated due to the increased insulin demand caused by excess cortisol. Hypertension is very common in these patients and atherosclerosis may occur. Mood changes are also common and may be extreme. Psychosis may be precipitated.

Hyperaldosteronism. Certain tumors of the adrenal gland produce excessive amounts of aldosterone, or less commonly, one of the other mineralocorticoids. In these patients two types of symptoms appear: those associated with hypertension and those associated with hypokalemia (low blood potassium concentration). Hypertension is produced by the sodium and water retention arising from excess aldosterone acting on the kidney, whereas the muscle weakness associated with hypokalemia is a result of the potassium-wasting action of the steroid in the kidney. Treatment ultimately involves surgical removal of the tumor.

Secondary sexual abnormalities. The sex steroids produced in the adrenal cortex are of minor importance in normal circumstances, the output of the adrenal gland being small compared to that of the gonads. Under certain conditions, however, sex steroid overproduction in the adrenal gland may produce a devastating endocrine imbalance. For example, a female bearing an androgen-producing tumor of the adrenal gland may undergo masculinization including suppression of the menstrual

TABLE 35-1. Comparison of activity of natural and synthetic adrenal steroids

Generic name	Drug class	Duration of action (hr)	Activity relative to cortisol		Major use	Major toxicity
			Anti-inflammatory	Sodium-retaining		
Cortisol	Glucocorticoid (natural)	<12	1.0	1.0	Replacement therapy in adrenal insufficiency; as an antiinflammatory agent in a wide variety of nonendocrine diseases	Overdosage produces symptoms of Cushing's disease; abrupt withdrawal produces symptoms of adrenal insufficiency
Cortisone	Glucocorticoid (natural)	<12	0.8	0.9	Antiinflammatory agent	As for cortisol
Corticosterone	Glucocorticoid (natural)	—	0.3	15.0	Not used clinically	High sodium-retaining effects relative to its potency as antiinflammatory agent
Betamethasone	Glucocorticoid (synthetic)	>48	25.0	0	As cortisol	Overdosage produces cortisol-like effects on fat, protein, and carbohydrate metabolism but relatively few effects on sodium retention
Dexamethasone	Glucocorticoid (synthetic)	>48	30.0	0	As cortisol	As for betamethasone
Prednisolone	Glucocorticoid (synthetic)	12 to 36	4.0	0.8	As cortisol	As for cortisol
Prednisone	Glucocorticoid (synthetic)	12 to 36	3.5	0.8	As cortisol, when oral dosage is desired	As for cortisol
Methylprednisolone	Glucocorticoid (synthetic)	12 to 36	5.0	0	As cortisol, when oral or parenteral dosage is desired	As for betamethasone
Triamcinolone	Glucocorticoid (synthetic)	12 to 36	5.0	0	As cortisol	As for betamethasone; has high muscle-wasting activity
Aldosterone	Mineralocorticoid (natural)	—	0.2	>250	Not used clinically	
Desoxycorticosterone	Mineralocorticoid (synthetic)	24	0	100	Replacement therapy in adrenal insufficiency; therapy in adrenal disease causing salt loss	Overdosage produces symptoms of excess salt and water retention with potassium loss
Fludrocortisone	Mineralocorticoid (synthetic)	24	ca 1.0	ca 100	As desoxycorticosterone	As for desoxycorticosterone

cycle and the development of secondary male sex characteristics. A male with an estrogen-producing tumor may develop breast tenderness and enlargement with loss of libido. A child may show precocious sexual development.

■ Pharmacology of adrenal steroids and related compounds

Major actions of adrenal steroids. Three major activities of the adrenal steroids may be identified: (1) metabolic effects on carbohydrate, protein, and fat metabolism; (2) antiinflammatory and immunosuppressive activity; and (3) sodium-retaining activity associated with potassium loss. The first two activities listed are classified as glucocorticoid actions and the third as a mineralocorticoid action. The natural adrenal steroids, cortisol, cortisone, and corticosterone, possess both glucocorticoid and mineralocorticoid activity (Table 35-1). Treatment with one of the natural adrenal steroids therefore results in all these associated effects, although one usually predominates. For example, cortisol in the high doses required for antiinflammatory action may cause progressive protein loss from skin and muscle associated with increased protein catabolism and may produce excessive sodium retention and potassium loss, a mineralocorticoid effect. To simplify treatment and reduce the incidence of unwanted side effects, chemists began modifying the structure of the steroid molecule with some success. For example, four major glucocorticoids that are essentially free of mineralocorticoid activity have now been synthesized: betamethasone, dexamethasone, methylprednisolone, and triamcinolone. These synthetic glucocorticoids have the additional advantage of having potent antiinflammatory effects at lower doses than the naturally occurring glucocorticoids.

Duration and mechanism of action. The duration of action of the various adrenal steroids are listed in Table 35-1. For this class of drugs the duration of action is not the same as the plasma half-life of the drug. The duration of action refers to the length of time adrenal suppression is detectable following a single dose of the steroid. For example, the drug prednisone suppresses adrenal function for up to 36 hours following a single dose, but the plasma half-life of this drug is only about 2.5 hours. This discrepancy may be explained in part by the mechanism of action of the steroid hormones. To produce their effects the steroids must pass through the membranes of target cells, bind to soluble receptors in the cell cytoplasm, and be transported to the nucleus of the cell. Once in the nucleus the steroid induces changes in RNA and protein synthesis, which may ultimately be expressed as some change in the function of the target cell. There may be a considerable time lag between the uptake of the steroid into the cell and the appearance of the effect in the target cell. Further time may elapse before the effect is terminated and the steroid destroyed.

Preparations for various routes or sites of administration. The steroids most commonly used clinically are listed in Table 35-2. Forty-nine preparations are listed by brand name in this table, but other brand names may be encountered, since the list presented is by no means exhaustive. The various generic drugs listed in Table 35-2 are subdivided as to chemical form available. For example, cortisol is available in the natural form and also as the acetate, sodium phosphate, or sodium succinate ester. Each chemical form of the generic drug is further subdivided into preparations available for administration by various routes. Steroid preparations exist for nearly every route of administration employed clinically.

The various steroid forms shown in Table 35-2 have differing pharmacological properties. For example, most of the steroid preparations available for parenteral use are suspensions, since the natural steroids and many of their derivatives are not very water soluble. These suspensions must never be given intravenously. When given intramuscularly, they may not be very rapidly absorbed, again due to the low water solubility of the compounds. Therefore, in an emergency such as acute adrenal insufficiency, one of the water-soluble derivatives must be used. Cortisol is available in two water-soluble forms, the sodium phosphate and sodium succinate. The sodium phosphates of dexamethasone and prednisolone and the sodium succinates of prednisolone and methylprednisolone are the only other water-soluble forms suitable for intravenous use.

The topical preparations are used primarily for the control of various dermatological conditions. Since the steroids are applied directly to the skin, a therapeutic dose may be achieved at the site where action is desired. Since the total dose of steroid is relatively small and the drugs are not well absorbed through the skin, systemic actions of the steroids are usually avoided. Absorption of a significant dose is possible with chronic, heavy application to wide areas of the skin or with rectal applications, also considered a topical route.

Certain steroid forms have been promoted primarily because of specific enhancement of topical activity. For example, betamethasone valerate is much more active topically than is betamethasone itself. Likewise, the acetonide derivative of triamcinolone is superior to the parent compound as a topical agent.

The ophthalmic preparations are special forms for topical application to the eye. Relatively high doses of steroids may be achieved in the eye, ordinarily with low absorption into systemic circulation. With chronic use of high doses, some drug may pass into the body and cause toxic effects. Toxicity is also possible in the eye

TABLE 35-2. Glucocorticoids and mineralocorticoids in clinical use

Generic name	Trade name	Chemical form	Administration
Cortisol (also called hydrocortisone)	Cort-Dome Cortef Cortril Heb-Cort Hydrocortone Others	—	ORAL: Tablets PARENTERAL: Suspension TOPICAL: Cream, lotion, ointment, enema OPHTHALMIC: Suspension
	Cortril-A Cortef Acetate Hydrocortone Acetate	Acetate	PARENTERAL: Suspension TOPICAL: Cream, lotion, ointment, rectal foam, suppositories OPHTHALMIC: Suspension, ointment
	Hydrocortone phosphate	Sodium phosphate	PARENTERAL: Solution
	Solu-Cortef	Sodium succinate	PARENTERAL: Solution
Cortisone	Cortone Acetate	Acetate	ORAL: Tablets PARENTERAL: Suspension
Betamethasone	Celestone	—	ORAL: Tablets, syrup
	Celestone Soluspan	Sodium phosphate	PARENTERAL: Suspension
	Benisone Flurobate	Benzoate	TOPICAL: Cream, gel, lotion
	Valisone	Valerate	TOPICAL: Cream, lotion, ointment, aerosol
Dexamethasone	Decadron Deronil Gamma-corten	—	ORAL: Tablets, elixir TOPICAL: Cream, gel, aerosol OPHTHALMIC: Suspension
	Hexadrol, Others Decadron L.A.	Acetate	PARENTERAL: Suspension
	Decadron Phosphate Hexadrol Phosphate	Sodium phosphate	PARENTERAL: Solution TOPICAL: Cream, aerosol for nasal application OPHTHALMIC: Solution, ointment
Prednisolone	Delta-Cortef Paracortol Others	—	ORAL: Tablets TOPICAL: Cream, aerosol
	Meticortelone Acetate Neo-Delta-Cortef Others	Acetate	PARENTERAL: Suspension OPHTHALMIC: Suspension, ointment
	Hydeltrasol P.S.P. IV Others	Sodium phosphate	PARENTERAL: Solution OPHTHALMIC: Solution, ointment
	Meticortelone Soluble	Sodium succinate	PARENTERAL: Solution
	Hydeltra-T.B.A.	Tebutate	PARENTERAL: Suspension
Prednisone	Delta-Dome Meticorten Others	—	ORAL: Tablets
Methylprednisolone	Medrol Wyacort	—	ORAL: Tablets
	Depo-Medrol Medrol Acetate	Acetate	PARENTERAL: Suspension
	Solu-Medrol	Sodium succinate	PARENTERAL: Solution

TABLE 35-2. Glucocorticoids and mineralocorticoids in clinical use—cont'd

Generic name	Trade name	Chemical form	Administration
Triamcinolone	Aristocort Kenacort	—	ORAL: Tablets
	Aristocort A Kenalog	Acetonide	PARENTERAL: Suspension TOPICAL: Cream, lotion, ointment, foam, spray, paste
	Aristocort Diacetate Kenacort Diacetate	Diacetate	ORAL: Syrup PARENTERAL: Suspension
	Aristospan	Hexacetonide	PARENTERAL: Suspension
Desoxycorticosterone	Doca Acetate Percorten Acetate	Acetate	ORAL: Tablets for buccal absorption PARENTERAL: Oil solution, pellet for implantation
	Percorten pivalate	Pivalate	PARENTERAL: Suspension
Fludrocortisone	Florinef Acetate	Acetate	ORAL: Tablets

itself. Certain patients with a genetic predisposition toward glaucoma will show increased intraocular pressure following the use of an ophthalmic steroid preparation. For most patients the intraocular pressure returns to normal when the drug is discontinued, but a few patients have been reported to develop glaucoma that did not respond to medication and required surgery. Another common adverse reaction to steroids is the development of secondary infections in the eye. These infections are commonly viral or fungal and may be dormant conditions, which are activated when host defenses are suppressed by steroids. The use of steroids in injured eyes may allow a new infection to develop.

Adrenal suppression. Patients should not be abruptly withdrawn from long-term steroid therapy. All adrenal steroids suppress the normal function of the hypothalamus, adenohypophysis, and adrenal gland in the patient. If exogenous steroids are withdrawn suddenly, patients may die of acute adrenal insufficiency, since their own adrenal glands cannot immediately produce the required steroids. This type of reaction is most likely in patients receiving relatively high doses for long periods. It may require 6 to 9 months for the natural negative feedback loop that regulates adrenal steroid synthesis to regain normal function after long-term steroid therapy, apparently because atrophy of the tissues occurs to some extent. Schedules for gradual withdrawal from steroids are available and must be followed faithfully, with dosage adjusted only to relieve symptoms of adrenal insufficiency if they develop during withdrawal.

To minimize hypothalamic-pituitary-adrenal suppression during long-term therapy with a glucocorticoid, many physicians prefer an *alternate day treatment schedule,* once an effective dosage has been established. The patient is given a single large dose of the steroid in the early morning of the treatment day. This regimen mimics the normal daily cycle, in which glucocorticoid levels are high in the morning and decrease throughout the day. On the next day no drug is given. The intermediate-acting steroids commonly employed in this regimen suppress the hypothalamic-pituitary-adrenal system for only about 12 to 36 hours (Table 35-1). Therefore, on the day no drug is given, the normal regulatory mechanisms recover and the patient's adrenal gland produces glucocorticoids. Most patients complain of some discomfort on the drug-free day, but these complaints must be weighed against the benefits of maintaining adrenal function. Not all diseases will be adequately controlled by this regimen, so frequent assessment is necessary.

Drug-induced Cushing's syndrome. In all of the steroid derivatives so far produced, increased antiinflammatory action has also been associated with increases in the metabolic effects characteristic of glucocorticoids. Therefore, any of the compounds with glucocorticoid activity, if given in high enough doses, will produce Cushing's syndrome. This toxicity is one of the most common reactions seen with glucocorticoid therapy (Table 35-1). Indeed, in most endocrine clinics many more patients are seen with Cushing's syndrome produced by drugs than with any other form of the disease. For these patients the steroid dose should be reduced if allowed by the severity of the condition being treated. Even when the condition being treated is not considered life-threatening, dose reduction may be difficult, since many patients tolerate the symptoms of steroid overdose

TABLE 35-3. Summary of toxic reactions to long-term glucocorticoid therapy with pharmacological doses

Toxic reaction	**Cause**	**Comments**
Impaired glucose tolerance and/or hyperglycemia	Gluconeogenic action of glucocorticoids	If diabetes develops, it is usually mild and reversible.
Fat deposition on trunk of body increased as are plasma triglyceride levels	Stimulation of lipid synthesis by glucocorticoids	Changes in lipid metabolism produce classic Cushing-type signs of moon face and truncal obesity.
Muscle weakness or muscle wasting	Stimulation of protein breakdown by glucocorticoids	This side effect is more pronounced with fluoride derivatives of glucocorticoids, for example, triamcinolone.
Peptic ulcer or intestinal perforation	Direct irritation and/or protein-wasting effects of glucocorticoids	It is not entirely clear whether steroids induce these conditions or whether they merely mask the symptoms and allow the condition to progress to a serious stage before diagnosis.
Pancreatitis	Not known but may involve effects on lipid metabolism	Glucocorticoids may mask symptoms of disease in early stages.
Growth inhibition	Glucocorticoid inhibition of growth hormone action	Glucocorticoids should be given with caution to children; doses below those producing growth inhibition should be used if possible.
Mood changes or psychoses	Not known	All patients receiving glucocorticoids should be closely observed for altered mood or behavior, especially patients with a past history of this type of disorder.
Osteoporosis or bone fractures	Glucocorticoids alter several aspects of calcium metabolism, which increase bone resorption	This side effect is noted especially in patients with arthritis, in postmenopausal women, or persons with low calcium intake.
Sodium retention and potassium loss	Mineralocorticoid activity associated with some glucocorticoids	Newer, synthetic glucocorticoids minimize these effects.
Increased susceptibility to infection	Glucocorticoid inhibition of immune system	Infections are more difficult to eradicate in these patients even with good antibiotic therapy.
Glaucoma	Glucocorticoids interfere with normal aqueous outflow from eye and elevate intraocular pressure	The risk is especially great in genetically predisposed patients or diabetics.
Cataracts	Not known	Topical or systemic therapy has been implicated.

better than the symptoms of the inflammatory disease being treated, although the drug overdose may be medically more dangerous.

Toxic reactions. Toxic reactions to antiinflammatory doses of the glucocorticoids resemble the symptoms of naturally occurring Cushing's syndrome but are not identical. For example, peptic ulcer is a rather common finding in a person receiving high doses of steroids but is relatively rare in Cushing's syndrome that is not drug induced. Other common symptoms of glucocorticoid toxicity are listed in Table 35-3. These reactions occur following long-term administration of the glucocorticoids. Large doses given for a short time to control acute allergic responses or other acute conditions are not usually associated with any significant signs of toxicity. For these purposes a large dose might be given on day 1, with the dose halved for each of the succeeding 3 or 4 days and then stopped before toxic reactions develop.

Drug interactions. The effects of many drugs are altered in patients receiving the glucocorticoids. Steroids may increase the excretion of salicylates in the kidney and make it necessary to increase salicylate dosage in a patient receiving both drugs. In other instances glucocorticoids may directly affect the action of a drug. Certain coumarin anticoagulants are less effective when steroids are present. In some cases drugs may have an unexpected effect in patients receiving glucocorticoids. For example, a safe level of anesthetic given to produce general anesthesia may cause dangerous hypotension in a patient receiving long-term steroid therapy due to suppression of the adrenal cortex.

One of the most common drug interactions involves liver metabolism of drugs. Steroids, barbiturates, phenytoin, and many other drugs are all inactivated by the same liver microsomal enzyme system. These enzymes have the capacity to be induced, that is, more enzymes may be formed when certain drugs are chronically available in the bloodstream. The effect of enzyme induction is to speed up drug metabolism, not only for the drug that induced the enzymes but also for any other drug metabolized by these enzymes. For example, phenobarbital may precipitate a worsening of asthma being treated with glucocorticoids by increasing the destruction of the steroid in the liver. The same effect may be seen if an asthmatic who is receiving long-term steroid therapy has an asthmatic crisis. Ordinarily a dose of 100 mg of hydrocortisone is effective in treating an acute asthma attack. However, in the patient who has been receiving long-term therapy with glucocorticoids, 300 to 1000 mg of hydrocortisone may be required to achieve the same effect, again presumably due to the liver's increased ability to destroy the hormone.

■ Clinical uses of adrenal steroids and their derivatives

The adrenal steroids are used clinically primarily in one of two ways: (1) at physiological doses in replacement therapy for endocrine diseases such as pituitary deficiency or adrenal hypofunction or (2) at pharmacological doses in the therapy of various nonendocrine diseases.

Replacement therapy. When used in replacement therapy, the doses of these drugs are relatively low, being intended only to replace the body's normal amounts of the hormone. Examples of replacement therapy include the use of cortisol to treat Addison's disease or to treat secondary adrenal insufficiency. Since the normal daily production of cortisol is about 15 to 25 mg, the daily replacement dose would be designed to achieve approximately the level of activity produced by that amount of cortisol. Table 35-1 shows the relationship of the activities of the various agents to the activity of cortisol. Wide variations in dosage exist, however, since stress and a number of other factors affect the steroid requirement. Each patient is an individual whose dosage must be adjusted to his or her needs and monitored to assure continued success of the therapy. Usual replacement doses slightly exceed normal daily production of steroids but would not be expected to cause Cushing's syndrome.

Treatment for some forms of adrenal insufficiency must include not only glucocorticoids but also mineralocorticoids. Two synthetic mineralocorticoids are available: desoxycorticosterone and fludrocortisone. Desoxycorticosterone is not as potent a mineralocorticoid as the natural hormone aldosterone, but it is more easily produced by chemists and has the advantage of possessing very little glucocorticoid activity. However, it is not active when given by the oral route. Fludrocortisone is an orally absorbed mineralocorticoid. For some patients, successful treatment of adrenal insufficiency is obtained with cortisol or cortisone, natural glucocorticoids with sufficient mineralocorticoid activity to maintain sodium balance in many individuals. Other patients, however, may require additional supplementation with a mineralocorticoid.

Antiinflammatory therapy. When used in pharmacological doses in therapy the antiinflammatory action of the glucocorticoid is the primary action sought. The level of steroid at the site of action must be maintained at a level much higher than normally would be found at that site to achieve the antiinflammatory effect. In some cases this goal may be achieved by topical or local application of the steroid; in other cases the steroids must be administered systemically.

TABLE 35-4. Nonendocrine conditions effectively treated with glucocorticoids (FDA designation)

Condition	Treatment regimen	Rationale
ALLERGIC STATES		
Bronchial asthma Serum sickness	Systemic steroids used to control acute episodes unresponsive to conventional therapy.	Glucocorticoids block histamine-induced and other inflammatory responses. In asthma glucocorticoids may enhance effects of sympathomimetic agents.
Contact dermatitis	Topical therapy as required. Systemic therapy rarely justified.	
COLLAGEN DISEASES		
Systemic lupus erythematosus Acute rheumatic carditis	Systemic steroids to control acute episodes or lower doses for maintenance. Topical steroids to control dermatological manifestations of lupus erythematosus.	Glucocorticoids antagonize autoimmune responses causing tissue damage in these diseases.
DERMATOLOGICAL DISEASES		
Seborrheic dermatitis Mycosis fungoides Pemphigus Severe erythema multiforme Severe psoriasis	Topical therapy as needed. Some skin lesions may require injection at the site. Systemic therapy may be employed when symptoms are widespread or especially severe.	Glucocorticoids have antiinflammatory and antimitotic actions that control symptoms.
EDEMATOUS STATES		
Nephrotic syndrome Cerebral edema	Systemic steroids for short periods to control acute episodes; used with other treatment.	Therapy empirical.
HEMATOLOGICAL DISORDERS		
Autoimmune hemolytic anemia Thrombocytopenia	Systemic steroids in large doses for acute disease; lower doses for maintaining remission.	Glucocorticoids antagonize autoimmune processes destroying blood cells.
NEOPLASTIC DISEASES		
Leukemias Lymphomas	Systemic steroids along with other antineoplastic agents produce remissions and palliation of symptoms.	Glucocorticoids have antilymphocytic action, which aids in destroying tumors of these tissues.
OPHTHALMIC DISEASES		
Allergic conjunctivitis Allergic corneal marginal ulcers Chorioretinitis Iritis and iridocyclitis Keratitis Optic neuritis	Superficial conditions may be treated with steroids applied directly to the eye. Diseases of the internal structures of the eye may require systemic therapy.	Glucocorticoid antiinflammatory action reduces permanent eye damage as well as controls acute symptoms.
RHEUMATIC DISORDERS		
Acute and subacute bursitis Acute nonspecific tenosynovitis Acute gouty arthritis Ankylosing spondylitis Psoriatic arthritis Rheumatoid arthritis	Intraarticular injection may be required for selected cases. Modest oral doses minimize side effects while providing relief for many patients.	Glucocorticoid inhibition of inflammatory and autoimmune processes relieves symptoms of disease.
RESPIRATORY DISEASES		
Pulmonary tuberculosis Symptomatic sarcoidosis	Systemic steroids may give symptomatic relief to certain patients.	Glucocorticoid antiinflammatory action may relieve symptoms of disease but no long-term benefit is demonstrable.

TABLE 35-5. Nonendocrine conditions for which glucocorticoid treatment is "probably" effective (FDA designation)

Condition	Treatment regimen
ALLERGIC STATES	
Urticaria	Systemic steroids when disease not adequately controlled by conventional methods
DENTAL CONDITIONS	
Postoperative inflammatory reactions	Local application
EDEMATOUS STATES	
Cirrhosis of the liver with ascites	Systemic steroids in conjunction with diuretics
Congestive heart failure	
GASTROINTESTINAL DISEASES	
Ulcerative colitis	Systemic steroids may aid in short-term recovery but do not change the long-term prognosis
Regional enteritis	
Intractable sprue	
RESPIRATORY DISEASES	
Pulmonary emphysema with bronchial edema	Systemic steroids in conjunction with other therapy or after other therapy has failed
Interstitial pulmonary fibrosis	

Other clinical uses. Steroids in one form or another have been used to treat a seemingly endless list of conditions. Whether these treatments are helpful or not is frequently difficult to evaluate and requires large-scale clinical testing with careful comparison of the results for treated patients with those of untreated or placebo-treated individuals. Table 35-4 lists 30 nonendocrine diseases in which glucocorticoid therapy was listed as effective, based on an FDA evaluation of information supplied by the National Academy of Sciences and National Research Council. Not all forms of these diseases will respond to steroids, but the drugs may prove useful to most patients at some stage of their disease. Specific notes concerning the treatment regimen employed are also included in Table 35-4. Table 35-5 lists the same information for diseases in which glucocorticoid therapy has not been rigorously proven to be effective. Nevertheless, the glucocorticoids are frequently used clinically to treat these conditions.

■ Compounds used in diagnosing adrenal disorders

Adrenocorticotropic hormone

Adrenocorticotropic hormone (ACTH, corticotropin) was discussed in Chapter 34 as part of the natural feedback regulatory cycle controlling adrenal function. ACTH directly stimulates the adrenal cortex to synthesize adrenal steroids. This action can be used diagnostically to distinguish between primary adrenal insufficiency (Addison's disease) and secondary adrenal insufficiency resulting from pituitary dysfunction (Table 35-6). Normal adrenal glands respond to ACTH by synthesizing and releasing cortisol into the bloodstream where it may be measured. In Addison's disease the adrenal gland cannot respond to ACTH, and no excess cortisol is produced. In patients with low pituitary function, the adrenal gland may be suppressed and respond less rapidly to ACTH than does a normal gland.

ACTH has in the past been used to treat adrenal insufficiency or other diseases responding to glucocorticoids. The rationale for this therapy was that adrenal function was maintained and that a natural balance of steroids was produced. However, ACTH therapy in practice was not as reliable or convenient as steroid therapy. ACTH must be injected since it is a peptide, whereas oral glucocorticoids are available. In addition, the response of the adrenal gland to ACTH was not easily predictable, making dosage adjustment unreliable. Finally, many patients developed antibodies to ACTH and became unresponsive to the drug. For these reasons and others ACTH is no longer widely used in therapy.

Dexamethasone

The highly potent synthetic glucocorticoid dexamethasone is also used diagnostically to test steroid suppression of cortisol synthesis. Relatively small doses of dexamethasone given over 2 days inhibit cortisol production in a normal person and, to a lesser extent, in a person with pituitary-induced Cushing's syndrome. Ordinarily, tumor production of cortisol is unaffected.

Metyrapone

Metyrapone (Metopirone) blocks cortisol synthesis in the adrenal gland and may be used to test the ability of the pituitary gland to increase ACTH release. Before the metyrapone test is run, it should be demonstrated that the patient's adrenal gland will respond to ACTH. While metyrapone is being administered, cortisol synthesis falls dramatically. In normal persons the fall in blood cortisol level stimulates the hypothalamus and in turn the pituitary gland, with the result that ACTH is released into the bloodstream. Under the influence of ACTH, early steps in steroid synthesis proceed but metyrapone

TABLE 35-6. Clinical summary of agents used in diagnosis of adrenal gland dysfunction

Generic name	Trade name	Dosage and administration	Comments
Adrenocorticotropic hormone	ACTH Acthar Corticotropin	INTRAMUSCULAR, SUBCUTANEOUS: 20 units 4 times daily. INTRAVENOUS: 25 to 40 units in 500 ml of dextrose or saline infused over 8 hr.	Adrenocorticotropic hormone is used to determine if the adrenal gland can respond to normal regulation. The side effects are those expected of adrenal steroids and allergic reactions.
Adrenocorticotropic hormone	ACTH gel Corticotropin Gel Cortigel Cortrophin Zinc H. P. Acthar Gel	INTRAMUSCULAR REPOSITORY: 40 to 80 units every 24 to 72 hr.	As above.
Cosyntropin	Cortrosyn	INTRAMUSCULAR, INTRAVENOUS: *Adults*—0.25 mg single dose. *Children under 2 yr*—0.125 mg single dose.	Synthetic form of ACTH used for diagnostic purposes only. Less allergenic than ACTH.
Metyrapone	Metopirone	ORAL: 750 mg every 4 hr for 6 doses. INTRAVENOUS: 30 mg/kg infused over a 4 hr period.	Metyrapone is used to determine if ACTH levels rise appropriately when the adrenal gland lowers cortisol production. Metyrapone blocks cortisol production, leading to appearance of cortisol precursors in urine if ACTH is present. The drug may induce acute adrenal insufficiency in some patients.

prevents cortisol from being formed in normal amounts. Therefore, the steroid precursors accumulate and are excreted in the urine. If no precursors accumulate under these conditions, it is concluded that the pituitary gland failed to produce ACTH. If the metyrapone test is administered to a person with adrenal insufficiency, there is a danger of precipitating an adrenal crisis, since in these patients metyrapone may virtually stop cortisol synthesis.

THE ADRENAL MEDULLA

The adrenal medulla arises from neuroectodermal tissue during embryonic life and remains intimately associated with the autonomic nervous system at maturity. The cells (pheochromocytes or chromaffin cells) are capable of synthesizing catecholamines by the same series of reactions found in nerve terminals and release catecholamines into the bloodstream in response to sympathetic cholinergic presynaptic neurons. One major difference between the synthetic pathways is that nerve terminals form norepinephrine as the final product, whereas the adrenal medulla converts norepinephrine to epinephrine. The enzyme for this final conversion is induced by adrenal steroids, indicating that the anatomical proximity of the disparate tissues of the cortex and medulla may have functional importance.

The hormones of the adrenal medulla are not essential to survival, but they are useful in adapting to stress. Epinephrine produces widespread effects throughout the body, mediated by the beta and alpha adrenergic receptors. The actions of epinephrine are discussed in Chapter 8, and the clinical uses of epinephrine are discussed in Chapter 12.

■ THE NURSING PROCESS

■ Assessment

Problems associated with the hormones manufactured in the adrenal gland result from too much or too little of the specific hormones. The nurse obtains the same data base in either case, although the results of a measurement may be excessively high or low, depending on the direction of the imbalance. Thus too little cortisol causes hypotension; too much causes hypertension. If an adrenal problem is suspected, a complete patient assessment is needed. The nurse should monitor temperature, pulse, respirations, blood pressure, and weight and should check the blood and urine for glucose. The body and skin should be carefully observed, noting color and character of the skin, distribution of body mass (fat and muscles), and the presence of bruises, or petechiae, and the condition of hair and nails. The nurse should determine the time of onset of these problems if appropriate.

■ Management

Depending on the problem, the treatment is surgical, pharmacological, or both. It is important to remember that adrenal cortical steroids are one of the most frequently used groups of drugs in present-day medicine and may also be prescribed as a temporary adjunct to treatment, even though hormonal insufficiency has not been demonstrated. Regardless of the reason for prescribing the adrenal corticosteroids, the nurse should monitor the blood pressure, weight, serum electrolyte levels, and sugar concentration in the blood and urine. Remember that wound healing may be slowed, that infection may be masked, and that improvement in the appetite and the sense of well-being may be due to drug therapy. Drug-induced diabetes may require treatment with insulin. The nurse should monitor the effect of the steroids on other medical conditions (e.g., diabetes).

In planning for discharge the nurse should determine with the physician the discharge dose and schedule of drugs and begin teaching the patient. Most patients have heard of steroids, but many will know only the negative qualities of the drugs before teaching has begun.

■ Evaluation

Ideally, treatment with adrenal corticosteroids would result in improvement in the patient's condition, with only desirable side effects occurring (e.g., increased sense of well-being). Even with physiological doses, however, undesired side effects such as weight gain and hyperglycemia may occur. With pharmacological doses, especially those prescribed on a long-term basis, side effects will always occur. Before discharge to self-management the patient should be able to explain why the drug has been prescribed, the desired goals of therapy, how to take the drug correctly (e.g., daily or alternate day therapy), and side effects that may occur. The patient should be able to explain additional therapies needed because of the drugs, such as antacid therapy or dietary restrictions such as a low sodium diet. The nurse should be certain that the patient can explain special circumstances requiring contact with the physician, such as nausea and vomiting preventing taking the drug, illnesses that might necessitate a dosage increase, or effects of the drug on other medical problems (e.g., diabetes requiring an increase in insulin dose to control). Patients must understand the need not to discontinue or decrease the dose without physician approval and, if receiving long-term therapy, the need to obtain and wear a medical identification tag or bracelet. Finally the patient should be able to explain what parameters, if any, should be monitored at home, such as the weight, blood pressure, or urine glucose concentration.

■ PATIENT CARE IMPLICATIONS

Remember that most steroids have both glucocorticoid and mineralocorticoid functions, although one usually predominates. Refer to the text of the chapter in addition to the following.

Long-term glucocorticoid administration

1. Most side effects of glucocorticoid administration will not be a problem when the course of therapy is less than 7 to 10 days.
2. Monitor the urine sugar levels of patients receiving steroids. Even in previously nondiabetic individuals, insulin may be required to reduce hyperglycemia. The need for insulin will decrease as the dose of steroids is reduced. Known diabetics will need specific guidelines regarding changes in insulin dosage based on urine sugar levels.
3. To decrease the possibility of peptic ulceration:
   a. Suggest that the patient take oral steroids with meals.
   b. Some physicians prescribe four to six daily doses of antacids when patients are receiving steroids, with or without concomitant use of cimetidine (Tagamet).
   c. Small, more frequent meals during the day may reduce gastric irritation.
   d. Monitor stools for occult blood.
   e. Instruct the patient to inspect stools and report any change or the formation of dark, tarry stools.
   f. Monitor the vomitus of the hospitalized patient for occult blood. Teach the outpatient to report bloody vomitus or the appearance of coffee-ground–like emesis.
   g. Caution the patient to avoid aspirin unless otherwise prescribed for the medical problem.
   h. Note that the gastric ulceration can also occur in patients receiving parenteral steroids.
4. If osteoporosis has developed, fractures of bones may occur with no apparent unusual stress; the patient may report having heard the bone crack while sitting, turning, or moving. Caution the patient to report any musculoskeletal pain and to avoid any strenuous activities such as contact sports, heavy physical labor, or heavy housecleaning. The immobilized patient must be moved and turned very carefully to avoid fractures.
5. Bruising may occur very easily. Caution the patient to avoid strenuous activities if bruising is a problem.
6. Caution the arthritic patient not to overuse joints that may feel better after systemic or intraarticular steroids.
7. Monitor blood pressure regularly.
8. Weigh the patient regularly.
9. Caution patients to avoid the company of individuals with active infections, even a common cold.
10. Patients receiving steroids on a long-term basis, especially those who might also be receiving other immunosuppressive drugs, should be taught the importance of reporting immediately any fever, cough, sore throat, chest congestion, signs of urinary tract infection, or any other infection so that treatment can be started at once. Any delay in healing should be reported to the physician.
11. In addition to regular medical follow-up, the patient receiving steroids on a long-term basis should have regular follow-up every 3 to 6 months with an ophthalmologist to help detect increased intraocular pressure and cataract formation.
12. The patient should be taught the importance of taking the prescribed steroid every day, as ordered. If the patient is sick and unable to take the medication, the physician should be notified. For some patients, especially those with known adrenal insufficiency, it may be appropriate to teach self-administration of parenteral steroids for those times when the patient cannot take an oral dose. Consult with the physician.
13. Explain to the patient why it is necessary to taper the dose of steroids when the decision has been made to reduce or stop long-term therapy.
14. The patient receiving long-term steroid therapy should wear a medical identification tag or bracelet.
15. For patients with a history of previous tuberculosis or positive TB test, isoniazid or other antituberculosis drug may be prescribed while they are receiving steroids.
16. Steroids are not advised during pregnancy unless the drugs are being taken in replacement therapy or for a life-threatening condition. Consult with the physician.
17. Instruct the patient to advise other physicians and dentists providing treatment that he or she is receiving steroid therapy. Allergy skin testing while the patient is receiving steroids may be not accurate. Smallpox vaccination should be avoided.
18. Various dietary adjustments may be necessary or helpful: increased intake of potassium-rich foods, decreased intake of sodium, and increased protein intake. Consult with the patient, physician, and dietician, and instruct the patient about the needed modifications.
19. Increased stress may result in a need for an increased dose in steroids. Instruct the patient to report any feeling of increased malaise, weakness, or other unusual signs during or following periods of intense stress.

20. Additional side effects include menstrual irregularities, hirsutism, increased appetite (this may be desirable in some patients, for example, those with cancer), euphoria, increased sense of well-being (again, often desirable), depression, and acne. Most will clear or diminish when steroids are discontinued.
21. Read vials carefully; there are a limited number of steroids safe for intravenous administration.
22. Patients receiving glucocorticoids as replacement therapy for adrenal insufficiency should be reassured that the doses of medication they are receiving are not expected to cause symptoms like those of Cushing's syndrome.

Long-term mineralocorticoid administration

1. Review the side effects associated with glucocorticoid administration.
2. The major mineralocorticoid-related problems are associated with sodium retention and electrolyte imbalance. Monitor and record the weight daily or every other day; monitor the blood pressure daily initially, tapering to less often after therapy is adjusted. Patients may need to learn to keep these measurements themselves after discharge. Monitor carefully any patient in whom sodium retention or fluid overload might be a problem, including those with cardiovascular disease, hypertension, seizures, peripheral vascular disease, and arteriosclerosis.
3. Consult with the physician, patient, and dietitian, determine an appropriately restricted low sodium diet, and teach the patient about the diet and its importance.
4. Potassium deficit often accompanies sodium retention. Symptoms include anorexia, drowsiness, muscle weakness and cramping, nausea, polyuria, postural hypotension, and mental depression. The patient may require potassium replacement therapy and should also be instructed to increase the intake of potassium-rich foods: orange juice and citrus fruits, bananas, whole grains, leafy vegetables, avocados. Teach the patient to report any signs of potassium depletion.
5. The patient should wear a medical identification tag or bracelet.
6. Instruct the patient to keep other physicians and dentists informed that he or she is receiving drug therapy.
7. For a discussion of subcutaneous implantation of drugs, see the patient care implications section in Chapter 38.
8. For a discussion of intramuscular administration of oil-based preparations, see the patient care implications section in Chapter 34 under vasopressin tannate in oil.

■ SUMMARY

The adrenal cortex is composed of three distinct layers, which differ in the major steroids produced and in the regulation of steroid synthesis. Mineralocorticoids are synthesized in the outer layer in a process regulated by the renin-angiotensin system. Mineralocorticoids cause the retention of salt and water by the kidney. Glucocorticoids are synthesized by the inner layers of the adrenal cortex in a process regulated by the pituitary gland and the hypothalamus. Glucocorticoids stimulate gluconeogenesis and mobilize amino acids from muscle protein.

Acute or chronic adrenal insufficiency is treated by replacement therapy with the adrenal steroids. The doses used are adjusted to supply the amount of hormone that would normally be synthesized by the adrenal gland. These doses should not cause Cushing's syndrome in which excess amounts of the glucocorticoids produce excess protein breakdown, increased fat deposition, weakness of the extremities, calcium loss from bone, and hypertension.

Glucocorticoids may be used at higher than replacement dosages to take advantage of the antiinflammatory and immunosuppressive actions of these drugs. Naturally occurring glucocorticoids also have mineralocorticoid activity, which will appear during high dose therapy. The synthetic glucocorticoids betamethasone, dexamethasone, methylprednisolone, and triamcinolone have less mineralocorticoid activity. Higher doses used in this type of therapy for nonendocrine diseases may produce toxic signs similar to those seen in Cushing's syndrome. Patients should not be withdrawn abruptly from long-term high dose therapy, since the chronically high glucocorticoid concentrations in the bloodstream of these patients will have suppressed adrenal function. Alternate day therapy may minimize adrenal gland suppression but may be inadequate to control some disease processes.

Most of the steroid preparations are insoluble suspensions of the drug, but a few water-soluble derivatives are available. These water-soluble phosphates and succinates are more useful in an emergency when rapidly absorbed preparations are required. Topical preparations are available for use in dermatological conditions. Betamethasone valerate and triamcinolone acetonide are most useful as topical agents. Special preparations for use in the eye are also available.

ACTH is used primarily in diagnosing the ability of the adrenal gland to respond to normal regulatory influences. Dexamethasone may be used in a diagnostic procedure to test the ability of cortisol production to be suppressed by excess glucocorticoid. Metyrapone blocks glucocorticoid synthesis in the adrenal gland and may be used to test the ability of the system to respond to the stimulus of lowered cortisol.

The adrenal medulla is closely associated with the autonomic nervous system. The medulla synthesizes and releases epinephrine, a catecholamine that helps the organism adapt to stress.

■ STUDY QUESTIONS

1. What are the two functional units of the adrenal gland?
2. What are mineralocorticoids?
3. In which part of the adrenal cortex are mineralocorticoids synthesized?
4. What hormones regulate mineralocorticoid synthesis?
5. Where are glucocorticoids synthesized?
6. What are the main effects of glucocorticoids on metabolism?
7. What is the result of untreated acute adrenal insufficiency?
8. What is Addison's disease?
9. What is secondary adrenal insufficiency?
10. What is Cushing's syndrome?
11. What are the symptoms of Cushing's syndrome?
12. What is the effect of overproduction of mineralocorticoids?
13. What are the three major activities or actions of adrenal steroids?
14. What is the effect of chronic overdosage with glucocorticoids?
15. Why should steroid therapy not be stopped suddenly in a patient who has been receiving long-term therapy?
16. What are the advantages and disadvantages of alternate day therapy?
17. What are the two major clinical uses of adrenal steroids?
18. What is the aim of replacement therapy in treating adrenal insufficiency?
19. Which are the mineralocorticoids available for clinical use?
20. Which are the water-soluble glucocorticoid preparations, and when are they preferred over the suspensions?
21. Which steroids are particularly effective as topical agents?
22. What drug interactions occur commonly with adrenal steroids?
23. How is ACTH used in diagnosis?
24. Why is ACTH not commonly used in replacement therapy?
25. How is metyrapone used in diagnosis?
26. What hormone is released by the adrenal medulla?

■ SUGGESTED READINGS

Burry, H.C.: Use and abuse of corticosteroids in rheumatic diseases, Drugs **19:**447, 1980.

Comunas, C.: Transphenoidal hypophysectomy, American Journal of Nursing **80:**1820, 1980.

Cryer, P.E.: Diagnostic endocrinology, Oxford, 1976, Oxford University Press.

Harvey, S.: Drugs in metabolic emergencies, burns and drug accidents, Nurses' Drug Alert (special issue) **2**(Dec.):145, 1978.

Hershman, J.M.: Endocrine pathophysiology: a patient-oriented approach, Philadelphia, 1977, Lea & Febiger.

Katkis, J.V., and Pitts, L.H.: Complications associated with use of megadose corticosteroids in head-injured adults, Journal of Neurosurgical Nursing **12**(Sept.):166, 1980.

Lancour, J.: ADH and aldosterone: how to recognize their effects, Nursing '78 **8**(9):36, 1978.

LoDolce, D., and Clancey, J.: Alternate programs of steroid administration for patients on long-term therapy, Journal of Neurosurgical Nursing **12**(Dec.):187, 1980.

Miller, J.A., and Munro, D.D.: Topical corticosteroids: clinical pharmacology and therapeutic use, Drugs **19:**119, 1980.

Newton, D.W., Nichols, A.O., and Newton, M.: You can minimize the hazards of corticosteroids, Nursing '77 **7**(6):26, 1977.

Rush, D.R., and Hamburger, S.C.: Drugs used in endocrine metabolic emergencies, Critical Care Quarterly **3**(Sept.):1, 1980.

Schimke, R.N.: Adrenal insufficiency, Critical Care Quarterly **3**(Sept.): 19, 1980.

Swartz, S.L., and Dluhy, R.G.: Corticosteroids: clinical pharmacology and therapeutic use, Drugs **16:**238, 1978.

36 Drugs affecting the thyroid and parathyroid glands

The thyroid gland in humans is a richly vascularized, horseshoe shaped structure lying across the trachea in the region of the larynx (Fig. 36-1). The gland contains at least two cell types differing in function and embryological origin. These are the follicular cells, derived from endoderm at the base of the tongue, and the parafollicular cells, derived from ultimobranchial bodies. A third endocrine tissue closely associated with the thyroid is found in the parathyroid glands. These small bodies normally lie behind the lobes of the thyroid but rarely may be found within the thyroid itself.

The function of each of these tissues, the hormones produced, and the medications commonly employed in the diagnosis and treatment of disease states associated with deficient or excessive thyroid or parathyroid function will be described in this chapter.

Follicular cells of the thyroid

The function of the follicular cells of the thyroid is to regulate the basal metabolic rate (BMR) in the body, mainly by altering oxidative processes in target tissues. The iodine-containing hormones, thyroxine (T_4) and triiodothyronine (T_3), released by the follicular cells into the general circulation, establish the metabolic rates for most body tissues. Regulation of thyroid hormone levels in the bloodstream is accomplished in part by the negative feedback system described in Chapter 34. Thyroid-stimulating hormone (TSH) from the anterior pituitary stimulates each of the steps in thyroid hormone synthesis described in the next section.

■ Synthesis of thyroid hormones

The first step in synthesizing the iodine-containing thyroid hormones is *iodine uptake* by the follicular cell (Fig. 36-2). Since iodide ion levels in the bloodstream are relatively low, the follicular cell must actually concentrate iodine to carry out the synthetic reactions required. In the normal human body the concentration of iodide ion in the thyroid is 30 to 40 times that found in plasma.

In the second step in thyroid hormone synthesis, *iodide ion activation* is catalyzed by the peroxidase enzyme formed in follicular cells. This activation step takes place on the surface of the microvilli, which protrude into the colloid filling the thyroid follicle (Fig. 36-2).

Once activated, iodine may be attached to thyroglobulin in a process called *organification* (Fig. 36-2). Thyroglobulin, a large protein synthesized in the follicular cell and extruded into the follicle, is the major protein component of the colloid. Most of the iodine atoms are attached to tyrosine molecules contained within the peptide chains of thyroglobulin. The tyrosine may contain one (3-monoiodotyrosine or MIT) or two (3,5-diiodotyrosine or DIT) atoms of iodine.

Following iodination, some of the tyrosine molecules may undergo a *coupling reaction* in which two molecules of DIT combine to produce one molecule of thyro-

FIG. 36-1
Anatomical location of thyroid and parathyroid glands.

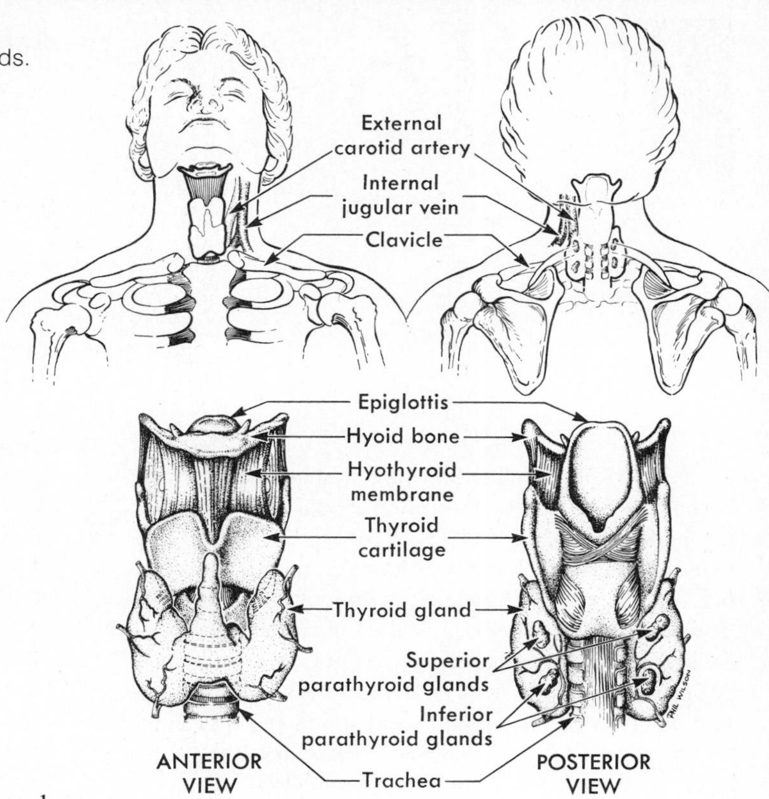

globulin-bound T_4. Coupling may also occur between 1 molecule each of DIT and MIT to yield 1 molecule of T_3. These coupling reactions are also believed to be catalyzed by the peroxidase enzyme from the follicular cell (Fig. 36-2).

Thyroglobulin serves primarily as a storage depot for thyroid hormones and the precursors MIT and DIT. In normal humans, each molecule of thyroglobulin contains about 6 molecules of MIT, 5 molecules of DIT, and 2 molecules of T_4. Less T_3 is stored. A single molecule of T_3 occurs in about 1 out of 3 molecules of thyroglobulin. Normal thyroids thus contain within the thyroglobulin of the follicles a 30-day supply of T_3 and T_4 and a 20-day supply of iodine stored as MIT and DIT.

When release of the thyroid hormones is required, TSH stimulates the microvilli of the follicular cells to take droplets of colloid into the cell (Fig. 36-2). Once inside the cell, the colloid droplets fuse with lysosomes to form vesicles called *phagolysosomes*. The low pH and the protein-digesting enzymes from the lysosomes allow proteolysis (digestion) of the thyroglobulin to amino acids. During proteolysis, T_3, T_4, MIT, and DIT are released into the cell. T_3 and T_4 are transported to the cell surface and released into the bloodstream. In contrast, MIT and DIT are retained within the cell, and the iodine they contain is reclaimed for use in new hormone synthesis. This iodine salvage is an important function. Patients who lack the salvage pathway lose excessive iodide ion in the urine and ultimately fail to produce sufficient thyroid hormones. This syndrome is a rare cause of hypothyroidism.

■ Disposition of thyroid hormones

Once in the bloodstream the thyroid hormones are rapidly and almost completely bound to plasma proteins. Most of the hormones are bound to a special alpha globulin called thyroid-binding globulin (TBG). A less important carrier is prealbumin. Very little thyroid hormone is bound to plasma albumin in normal man, since the thyroid hormones are so tightly bound to TBG. However, the amount of thyroid hormone that may be bound to TBG is limited. TBG can bind about 2.5 times more hormone than it ordinarily carries. When that limit is reached, the excess hormone is bound to albumin and prealbumin. Although these proteins are less avid carriers than TBG, they have nearly unlimited capacity for the hormones. In normal humans, 99.96% of T_4 in the bloodstream is bound to protein. Therefore only 0.04% of the total T_4 in the bloodstream may be considered active. T_3 is less firmly bound; 0.4% of the T_3 in the bloodstream is unbound and therefore active.

The relative distribution of T_3 and T_4 differs within the body. T_4 is much more abundant than T_3 in the thyroid and in the bloodstream. However, T_3 is less tightly bound to plasma proteins than T_4. More importantly, T_4 is rapidly converted to T_3 in most tissues. Therefore

FIG. 36-2

Synthesis of T_3 and T_4 by follicular cells within the thyroid gland. A single follicular cell is depicted. The base of the cell is intimately in contact with the bloodstream, and the apex of the cell is in contact with colloid. Cells of this type surround areas of colloid to form thyroid follicles. The parafollicular cells of the thyroid gland, discussed later in the chapter, do not directly contact colloid.

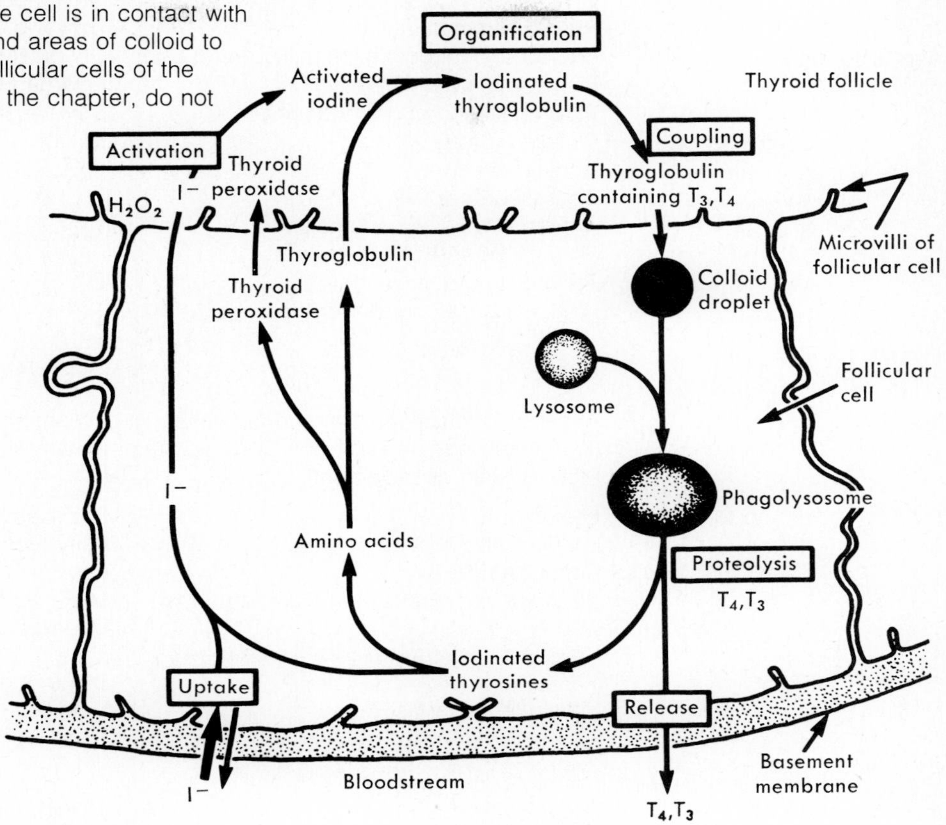

the most abundant form of thyroid hormone in target cells is T_3. For this reason, T_3 may be considered to be the most important thyroid hormone.

T_3 and T_4 are metabolized by the liver to glucuronide and sulfate derivatives, which then are eliminated in the bile. In humans no significant reuptake of the hormones occurs from the gut, that is, there is no enterohepatic circulation of these compounds. Other hormone destruction occurs in the target tissues of the body where the hormones are deiodinated and transformed to inactive products.

■ HYPOTHYROIDISM

Hypothyroidism occurs whenever the body's production of thyroid hormones is insufficient to meet the body's demands. Mild hormone deficiencies produce minimal disease with vague symptoms, sometimes making the condition difficult to diagnose. Untreated patients ultimately may develop a myriad of characteristic signs and symptoms related to the slowing of metabolic rates and changes in the central nervous system (Table 36-1). The severe form of the disease is called *myxedema*.

Hypothyroidism may develop in the fetus when a pregnant woman receives antithyroid drugs. However, the most common cause of hypothyroidism in newborns is an embryological or genetic defect in the fetus that arrests thyroid development or prevents its function. A child lacking adequate thyroid function during fetal development may appear nearly normal at birth, since much of fetal development can proceed in the absence of fetal thyroid hormones. However, if the disease is not detected very soon after birth, irreversible brain damage and a host of associated physical signs will develop. Congenital hypothyroidism is called *cretinism* (Table 36-1).

TABLE 36-1. Signs and symptoms of thyroid disorders

Condition	Symptoms	Physical appearance
Hypothyroidism, adult onset (also called myxedema and Gull's disease)	Diminished vigor and muscle weakness Reduced mental acuity Emotional changes, especially depression Memory impairment Slow relaxation of deep tendon reflexes Muscle cramps Constipation Decreased appetite Abnormal menses in females Slow pulse and enlarged heart Tendency to gain weight Lowered basal metabolic rate	Puffy face and eyes Thin and coarse hair and eyebrows Dry, scaly, cold, and slightly yellow skin Enlarged tongue Slow, husky speech Dull or slow-witted appearance
Hypothyroidism, congenital (cretinism)		
At birth	Absence of distal femoral and proximal tibial epiphyses Slowed brain development	Essentially normal Slightly longer and heavier than normal
At 3 mo with no treatment	Lethargy Feeding difficulty Constipation Neonatal jaundice lasting beyond normal period Respiratory distress Hoarse cry Intermittent cyanosis	Enlarged tongue Puffy face Poor muscle tone Thick neck Depressed nasal bridge with broad, flat nose Distended abdomen Umbilical hernia Short legs
Hyperthyroidism (also called thyrotoxicosis or Graves' disease)	Cardiac arrhythmia Enlarged thyroid gland Rapid pulse rate Increased basal metabolic rate Muscle weakness and wasting Fine tremor Heat intolerance Weight loss in most patients	Restlessness or nervousness Abrupt actions and speech Warm, moist palms Loosening of fingernails from nail beds Bulging eyes with sclera visible all around iris White, unpigmented patches on the skin (vitiligo)

Hypothyroidism that develops after the neonatal period but before puberty is called *juvenile hypothyroidism*. The most prominent early sign of juvenile hypothyroidism is growth stunting. If not appropriately treated, juvenile hypothyroid patients will not only suffer arrested growth but also other signs and symptoms associated with adult forms of the disease.

■ Diagnosis of hypothyroidism

Hypothyroidism may be accurately diagnosed by the judicious use of a combination of the thyroid function tests summarized in Table 36-2. An understanding of these tests requires an understanding of normal thyroid physiology, which was discussed earlier in this chapter, as well as an understanding of the negative feedback regulation of the thyroid (Chapter 34).

In *primary hypothyroidism* the thyroid gland itself is defective. The diagnosis of primary hypothyroidism requires establishing that a patient has lower than normal thyroid hormone levels and elevated levels of TSH in the bloodstream. Of the many tests available, TSH determinations are the most widely used. Free thyroxine (FT_4) levels are lower than normal in 80% to 90% of hypothyroid patients tested, but this test is technically

TABLE 36-2. Common tests used to evaluate thyroid function

Test	Procedure	Diagnostic use	Normal values	Comments
Serum T_4	*Total* serum T_4 is measured by competitive protein binding test or radioimmunoassay.	To distinguish hyperthyroid or hypothyroid conditions from euthyroid state.	5 to 12 μg/100 ml serum.	Conditions that elevate thyroid-binding globulin (TBG) levels, such as pregnancy or estrogen administration, also elevate total serum T_4 levels. Lowered TBG levels in cirrhosis or nephrotic syndrome also lower total serum T_4 levels. In both cases, free hormone levels are usually normal, and the patients are functionally euthyroid.
Free thyroxine (FT_4)	Calculated from percent of radioactive T_4 remaining free when added to patient's serum.	To distinguish hyperthyroid or hypothyroid conditions from euthyroid state.	1 to 2.5 ng/100 ml (0.001 to 0.0025 μg/100 ml).	Normal values may vary greatly from laboratory to laboratory. This test is rarely used.
T_3 uptake (T_3U) or resin T_3 uptake (RT_3U)	Test measures the degree of saturation of patient's TBG with endogenous thyroid hormones.	To distinguish hyperthyroid or hypothyroid conditions from euthyroid state.	25% to 45%, or 0.82 to 1.35 when expressed as a ratio of T_3U to normal.	Hyperthyroidism elevates the ratio; hypothyroidism lowers the ratio. Levels of TBG and T_4 in the patient's blood affect the test more than do T_3 values.
Serum T_3	*Total* serum T_3 is measured by specific radioimmunoassay.	To distinguish hyperthyroid conditions from euthyroid state.	0.08 to 0.20 μg/100 ml.	Test is not useful for hypothyroidism, since T_3 may be relatively more abundant than T_4 in hypothyroidism.
Protein-bound iodine (PBI)	Measures *total* protein-bound iodine in the blood.	To distinguish hyperthyroid or hypothyroid conditions from euthyroid state.	6 to 13 μg/100 ml.	Measures all protein-bound iodine in blood. Ordinarily 80% to 90% of this value is T_4, but this percentage may change in certain conditions. Since other available tests are more accurate, the use of PBI is declining.

Continued.

TABLE 36-2. Common tests used to evaluate thyroid function—cont'd

Test	Procedure	Diagnostic use	Normal values	Comments
Serum TSH	Serum TSH is measured by specific radioimmunoassay.	To distinguish hypothyroid conditions from euthyroid state; to distinguish primary from secondary hypothyroidism.	0.5 to 5 μU/ml.	Hypothyroidism caused by thyroid failure (primary) will show elevated TSH levels; hypothyroidism caused by pituitary failure (secondary) will show little or no TSH.
Thyroid-releasing hormone test (TRH test)	Synthetic TRH (500 μg) is given IV, causing a peak release of TSH 30 min later in patients with normal pituitary glands	To distinguish hypothyroidism caused by pituitary failure from other forms of hypothyroidism.	Peak concentrations of TSH produced in normal patients are 5 to 35 μU/ml serum.	No rise is usually observed in serum TSH in hyperthyroid patients.
Thyroid uptake of radioiodine	Radioactivity in the thyroid measured 4, 6, and 24 hr after administration of tracer dose of radioactive iodine.	To distinguish hyperthyroid and hypothyroid conditions from euthyroid state.	Normal glands take up 10% to 35% of tracer dose in 24 hr.	This test may be affected by the dietary intake of iodine, by the administration of iodine-containing medications, or by the use of antithyroid drugs.
TSH test	Bovine TSH is given IM, after which serum T_4 or radioiodine uptake is measured.	To distinguish primary from secondary hypothyroidism.	A normal thyroid gland responds by increasing iodine uptake and T_4 release.	This test is rarely used where TSH levels may be measured.
Thyroid suppression tests	T_3 (75 μg) is given daily for 7 days. Radioiodine uptake by the thyroid gland is measured before and after the test.	To distinguish hyperthyroid conditions from euthyroid state.	Uptake is 50% or less of the pretest uptake.	This test may be dangerous for elderly patients, weakened patients, or patients with heart disease.

difficult to perform and is actually used at few medical centers. Serum T_4, T_3 uptake or protein-bound iodine (PBI) may also be measured, although each of these tests may be affected by conditions unrelated to thyroid disease that change the serum concentration of TBG (Table 36-2). Measurements of PBI are not commonly performed today, since other more accurate tests of thyroid function are available.

The thyroidal uptake of iodine is also lowered in hypothyroidism. However, this test is seldom useful in diagnosing the disease, since thyroidal uptake of iodine is affected by the patient's intake of iodine, whether as part of the diet or as a constituent of medications that are received. The patient may not be aware that iodine is being taken. For example, potassium iodide, used as an expectorant, is a common constituent of many asthma medications.

By far the most common form of hypothyroidism is primary hypothyroidism. The exact cause of this disease is usually not known for a particular patient, although in some cases it can be concluded that disease or chemical exposure led to thyroid failure. Hypothyroidism may also arise from insufficient pituitary function. If the pituitary fails to release adequate TSH, insufficient thyroid hormone will be synthesized and *secondary hypothyroidism* develops. Occasionally a patient with damage to the hypothalamus will fail to produce TRH (thyrotropin-releasing hormone), which is required to stimulate TSH production in the pituitary (Chapter 34). This latter condition in which TRH production is impaired is called *tertiary hypothyroidism*.

Secondary and tertiary hypothyroidism may be distinguished from primary hypothyroidism by measuring TSH. Whereas in primary hypothyroidism TSH is elevated by the natural action of the negative feedback system attempting to elevate thyroid hormone levels, TSH levels are low or undetectable in the other two forms of hypothyroidism. If the TSH assay is not available, a TSH test may be performed in which injected TSH is expected to stimulate T_4 formation and release in secondary or tertiary hypothyroidism but not in primary hypothyroidism (Table 36-2).

Secondary and tertiary hypothyroidism may be distinguished from each other by application of the TRH test, which measures the ability of the pituitary gland to respond to its normal regulatory hormone (Table 36-2). If TSH rises after TRH administration, the implication is that the hypothalamus is defective and both the anterior pituitary and the thyroid would be capable of normal function if properly stimulated.

■ Treatment of hypothyroidism

Treatment of hypothyroidism requires replacement therapy with the thyroid hormones. The aim of therapy is to produce the euthyroid state (normal thyroid hormone levels). A number of preparations containing either natural or synthetic forms of the hormones are available from various manufacturers (Table 36-3). Selection of one or the other of these oral agents is largely a matter of preference for the physician. The only appropriate clinical use of these thyroid hormones is to treat thyroid deficiency. They should never be employed in weight loss programs.

Thyroid U.S.P.

Thyroid U.S.P. is a defatted extract of whole thyroid glands. It contains T_4 and T_3 in the natural ratio of 2.5 to 1. The iodine content of these preparations is regulated by law in the United States. Although thyroid hormone activity is not directly standardized in these products, many physicians have found them to be quite constant in potency, especially when fresh, dry preparations are compared. Considerable potency may be lost on long storage or if the powder is allowed to become moist.

Thyroglobulin

Thyroglobulin is also prepared from whole thyroid glands and like thyroid extract contains T_4 and T_3 in the ratio 2.5 to 1. This preparation is more expensive than thyroid U.S.P. Some physicians prefer thyroglobulin because it is directly standardized for thyroid hormone activity rather than for total iodine content.

Levothyroxine sodium

Levothyroxine sodium is a pure synthetic form of the natural thyroid hormone thyroxine, or T_4. It therefore has the properties of T_4 previously outlined: high affinity for binding to serum proteins, long half-life in the bloodstream, and conversion to T_3 by peripheral tissues.

Liothyronine sodium

Liothyronine sodium is a pure synthetic form of the natural thyroid hormone triiodothyronine, or T_3. It therefore has the properties previously outlined for T_3: shorter half-life in the bloodstream than T_4, greater potency than T_4, and conversion to inactive products in peripheral tissues. In addition, T_3 seems to be better absorbed from the gut than does T_4.

Liotrix

Liotrix is a thyroid preparation that contains both pure synthetic T_4 and T_3 in the ratio of 4 to 1. This mixture was designed to produce normal thyroid function tests when therapy was adequate. In contrast, note that if T_3 is given alone, a patient may be clinically euthy-

TABLE 36-3. Drugs used in the diagnosis or treatment of hypothyroidism

Generic name	Trade name	Dosage and administration	Properties	Comments
NATURAL THYROID HORMONES				
Thyroid U.S.P.	Delcoid Thyrar Thyrocrine Thyro-Teric	ORAL: *Adults*—120 to 180 mg daily for maintenance. Initial doses 15 mg daily. Double the dose every 2 wk until appropriate maintenance dose is reached.	Impure mixture of thyroid components that includes T_3 and T_4.	Replacement therapy for hypothyroidism. Overdose produces symptoms of hyperthyroidism. Too large a dose at onset of therapy may cause vascular occlusion, especially in patients with arteriosclerosis.
Thyroglobulin	Proloid	ORAL: *Adults*—120 to 180 mg daily for maintenance. Initial doses are small and are gradually increased to maintenance levels.	Contains T_3 and T_4, as well as other iodine-containing compounds.	Replacement therapy for hypothyroidism. Overdose produces the same symptoms as seen with thyroid U.S.P.
SYNTHETIC THYROID HORMONES				
Levothyroxine sodium	Cytolen Levoid Levothyroid Synthroid Sodium	ORAL: *Adults*—150 to 200 μg daily for maintenance. Initial doses are small and are gradually increased to maintenance levels. *Children over 1 yr*—3 to 5 μg/kg daily. INTRAVENOUS: *Adults*—0.5 mg with mannitol (Synthroid) or without (Levoid).	Chemically pure form of T_4.	Replacement therapy for hypothyroidism. Intravenous form for myxedemic coma. Peak effect occurs 9 days after start of therapy; serum half-life about 11 days.
Liothyronine sodium	Cytomel	ORAL: *Adults*—25 to 75 μg daily for maintenance. Initial doses should be low and gradually increased to maintenance levels.	Chemically pure form of T_3.	Replacement therapy for hypothyroidism. Peak effect occurs in 2 days; serum half-life 4 to 6 days.
Liotrix	Euthroid Thyrolar	ORAL: *Adults*—30 μg T_4 with 7.5 μg T_3 or 25 μg T_4 with 6.25 μg T_3. Doses may be gradually increased as needed.	Chemically pure T_4 and T_3 combined in a ratio of 4:1.	Replacement therapy for hypothyroidism.
ADENOHYPOPHYSEAL HORMONE				
Thyroid-stimulating hormone (TSH)	Thytropar	INTRAMUSCULAR, SUBCUTANEOUS: 10 IU once or twice daily.	Extract of bovine anterior pituitary contains natural peptide, TSH.	Diagnostic agent to establish hypothyroidism. May cause release of thyroid hormones that can precipitate adrenal crisis in patient with secondary adrenal insufficiency. May also cause cardiovascular symptoms and rare allergic reactions.
Protirelin (thyrotropin-releasing hormone, TRH)	Relefact TRH Thypinone	INTRAVENOUS: *Adults*—400 to 500 μg.	Synthetic preparation of natural hypothalamic tripeptide hormone.	Diagnostic agent to differentiate pituitary-induced hypothyroidism from other types of hypothyroidism. May transiently produce nausea, facial flushing, hypertension, and an urge to micturate.

FIG. 36-3

Time-course of thyroid hormone effects. The patient in each of the tests received a single oral dose of the medication indicated. The doses T_3 and T_4 administered are equimolar (equivalent numbers of molecules).

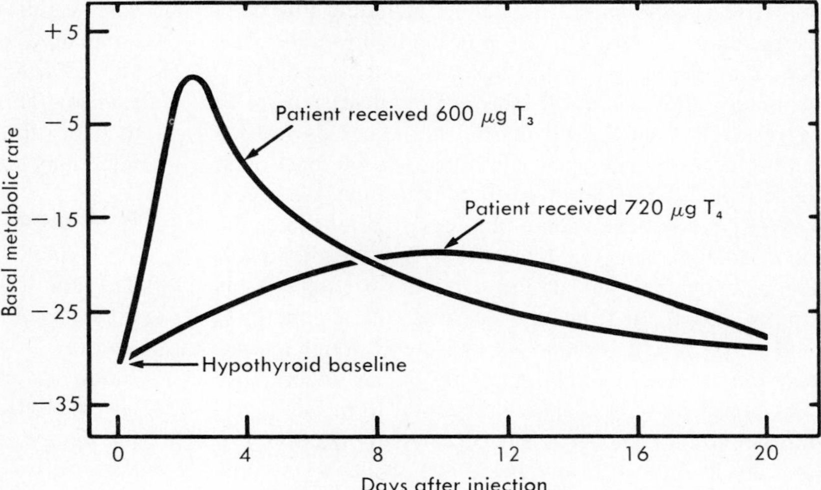

roid, but since T_3 is not converted to T_4, any diagnostic test based on T_4 will likely give low values. In theory these mixtures containing 4 to 1 ratios of T_4 to T_3 bring T_3, T_4, and PBI all within normal range during therapy. There is no firm evidence that this treatment has any clinically apparent advantage to the patient over any other treatment regimen.

Relative potency of agents used to treat hypothyroidism

One obvious difference among the preparations just discussed is their relative potencies. In terms of biological activity, 60 mg of thyroid U.S.P. = 60 mg thyroglobulin = 1 mg or less of levothyroxine = 0.025 mg of liothyronine = liotrix tablets containing 0.06 mg T_4 + 0.015 mg T_3 or 0.05 mg T_4 + 0.0125 mg T_3. A wide range of tablet sizes is available in each of these preparations so that a dosage may be easily adjusted to the patient's particular need.

■ Absorption, distribution, and excretion of hormones used to treat hypothyroidism

The protein-binding properties of the thyroid hormones explain some of the clinically important differences between these agents. T_4, being more highly protein bound, leaves the bloodstream more slowly than does T_3. Therefore the onset of action for T_4 is about 2 days, whereas T_3 effects may be expected within 6 hours of administration (Fig. 36-3). Moreover, T_4, which is bound to plasma protein, is less available for elimination, excretion, or tissue biotransformation than is the more freely available T_3. Therefore T_4 persists longer in the body than does T_3. The effects of a single equimolar dose (same number of molecules) of T_3 and T_4 are shown in Fig. 36-3, in which the basal metabolic rate was followed as an indicator of thyroid hormone action in these hypothyroid subjects. When patients are switched from T_4 to T_3, or vice versa, consideration must be made for these different time courses. For example, a patient being switched from a preparation containing primarily T_4 to T_3 alone might suffer from excessive thyroid hormone action if started immediately on full T_3 doses after T_4 administration was terminated. Therefore patients are given small doses of T_3 after T_4 is stopped, and the dose of T_3 is gradually raised as necessary to maintain the euthyroid state.

In a newly diagnosed hypothyroid patient, thyroid medications are begun at very low doses and increased at varying intervals until the euthyroid state is achieved. Thyroid U.S.P. and levothyroxine doses are doubled roughly every 2 weeks, but liothyronine doses are doubled weekly until adequate control is achieved. These gradually increasing doses are justified, since a sudden return to adequate thyroid hormone levels produces acute stress on several body systems. One common and dangerous example observed occasionally even with low doses is the production of angina pectoris, coronary occlusion, or stroke in elderly or predisposed patients. Another difficulty some patients may experience is a relative adrenal insufficiency. This latter difficulty arises primarily in patients with inadequate pituitary function who suffer from both secondary hypothyroidism and secondary adrenal insufficiency. If thyroid hormone therapy is begun in these patients without also restoring adequate glucocorticoid levels, the patients may suffer a dangerous adrenal crisis.

Severe hypothyroidism may ultimately result in the grave condition called *myxedemic coma*. In this condition patients possess most of the clinical features of hypothyroidism shown in Table 36-1, including low body temperature as a result of the profoundly lowered metabolic rate, depressed central nervous system, and hypoventilation. Patients at this stage of the disease must be aggressively treated with thyroid hormones as well as with glucocorticoids and other supportive measures. Since rapid replacement with thyroid hormones is necessary in these patients, some physicians prefer to use the more rapidly acting T_3. However, T_3 is not readily available commercially in an injectable form. Since T_3 is rapidly absorbed from the gastrointestinal tract, T_3 tablets may be crushed and administered through a nasogastric tube. Alternatively, some physicians prefer to use the commercially available T_4 injection form that is administered intravenously. It is occasionally necessary to use catecholamines to combat the shocklike symptoms found in myxedemic coma. Patients so treated are especially at risk of suffering cardiac arrhythmias, since both the catecholamines and the thyroid hormones have the potential of causing this dangerous side effect.

Elimination of the thyroid hormones used in replacement therapy is the same as for the normal hormones, the major routes being biliary excretion and tissue metabolism of the compounds.

■ HYPERTHYROIDISM

Hyperthyroidism occurs whenever excess thyroid hormones are released into the circulation. The disease may range from very mild forms displaying few of the symptoms shown in Table 36-1 to a severe condition called *thyroid storm,* in which death may result from an uncontrolled rise in body temperature and vascular collapse. Increased thyroid hormone production may result from hyperfunction of the entire gland or from the excessive output of one or more small nodules within the thyroid. A rare cause of hyperthyroidism is excess TSH either from the pituitary gland or from a tumor.

Several terms are in use to describe various forms of hyperthyroidism. Basically hyperthyroidism may occur with or without thyroid nodules. The disease without nodules is the most common form of hyperthyroidism and is referred to as *toxic diffuse goiter, thyrotoxicosis,* or *Graves' disease* (or rarely *Basedow's* or *Parry's disease*). Many patients with this disease display exophthalmus (bulging eyes). This symptom and the fact that many patients also have enlarged thyroid glands gives rise to another common name for this condition: *exophthalmic goiter*. Toxic nodular goiter produces the same general symptoms as Graves' disease except that eye symptoms are rare in the nodular form.

Hyperthyroidism is rare in children and is most common in adults in the third or fourth decade of life. Women are much more frequently afflicted than are men, the reasons for which are not clear. Moreover, Graves' disease seems to be precipitated in women by puberty, pregnancy, or menopause. A condition called *subacute thyroiditis* can produce a reversible form of hyperthyroidism. This condition seems to appear sometime after recovery from viral diseases and may be caused by the infectious process.

■ Diagnosis of hyperthyroidism

Hyperthyroidism is characterized by elevated serum T_4, serum T_3, free T_4, and free T_3 levels in most patients. Therefore the diagnostic tests that directly measure one of these parameters are most commonly used: serum T_4 and serum T_3 testing. The T_3 resin uptake test may also be used, since hyperthyroidism increases the degree of TBG saturation with thyroid hormones. Radioactive iodine uptake may also be measured and is useful in distinguishing between various forms of hyperthyroidism. Obviously these diagnostic tests form part of a larger clinical picture. Much information is gained by determining the size of the thyroid by palpation, the presence or absence of nodules in the thyroid, and the results of a thyroid scan to measure the pattern of radioactive iodine concentration in the gland.

Diagnosis of Graves' disease has been aided by the realization that the disease has an immunological basis. In this condition the thyroid is chronically overstimulated by a group of immunoglobulins that supplant TSH as the regulator of thyroid function. These immunoglobulins are found in the sera of nearly all patients with Graves' disease, and the amounts of the immunoglobulins correlate with the severity of the hyperthyroidism observed in the patient.

■ Treatment of hyperthyroidism

Hyperthyroidism is most commonly controlled with drugs or with radioactive iodine. The drugs used to treat hyperthyroidism fall into two main classes: drugs that control the symptoms of hyperthyroidism and drugs that lower the production of T_3 and T_4 by the thyroid.

Propranolol

Propranolol, a drug previously discussed as a beta adrenergic blocking agent (Chapter 13), represents the class of drugs that control the symptoms of hyperthyroidism but produce no change in thyroid hormone levels. Propranolol is effective because some of the most dangerous and disturbing symptoms of hyperthyroidism are produced in part by excessive sensitivity of certain tissues to catecholamines when thyroid hormone levels are high. By blocking the catecholamine effects, the symptoms of palpitation, tremor, sweating, proximal

■ THE NURSING PROCESS FOR THYROID DISORDERS

■ Assessment

The nursing process in diseases of the thyroid gland is the same, regardless of whether the problem is hyperthyroidism or hypothyroidism. In most cases the original problem develops insidiously. The nurse should obtain a complete assessment of the patient, including temperature, pulse, respiration, blood pressure, weight, history of changes in weight, level of energy, mood, subjective feeling, and response to temperature. The height of children should be checked. Questioning the family members may be helpful to determine onset of symptoms. The nurse should also check thyroid function test results and the glucose content of urine and blood.

■ Management

The goal of therapy is to restore normal or near-normal functioning of the thyroid gland or to exogenously replace the thyroid hormones to normal levels. During the dosage-adjustment phase the nurse should monitor the temperature, pulse, respiration, blood pressure, weight, height of children, and glucose content of urine and blood. The patient should be questioned about subjective reaction to therapy. If weight reduction is an additional goal of therapy, referral and/or diet teaching should be done. If radioactive iodine is used, hospital procedures for the handling of radioactive materials should be followed.

■ Evaluation

It is difficult to determine the effectiveness of therapy for weeks or months after the drugs have been started. Before discharge, patients should be able to explain the action of the drug and how to take the prescribed dose. Other parameters the patient should monitor and record at home include pulse, weight, and height. The nurse should explain the side effects that may occur and what to do about them, adjustments needed in the treatment of other medical problems (for example, changes in insulin dose or anticoagulant dose), the need for continuing the medication, and the need to wear an identification tag or bracelet. With radioactive iodine, the patient will not be on long-term drug therapy but should be able to explain what symptoms should be reported to the physician. For further specific guidelines, see the patient care implications section at the end of this chapter.

---

muscle weakness, mental agitation, and cardiac arrhythmias are reduced. One advantage of propranolol therapy is that clinical improvement is seen rapidly. With many other drugs used for hyperthyroidism, relief of symptoms may be greatly delayed. Propranolol may be used to prepare a hyperthyroid patient for surgery.

Thioamides

The thioamides represent the class of drugs that inhibit the synthesis of thyroid hormones. Although the exact mechanism of action of these compounds is not agreed on, they are known to inhibit each step in synthesis except iodine uptake (Fig. 36-2), and they are thought to preferentially inhibit the peroxidase-catalyzed reactions (coupling and organification). Since these compounds are primarily enzyme inhibitors, they do not directly destroy thyroid tissue but only prevent its excessive action.

Thioamide action is immediate on the thyroid gland, and reduced hormone synthesis can be demonstrated within hours. Observable clinical response to the drugs, however, does not appear for days or weeks, the period required for stored thyroid hormones to be depleted. Patients may be maintained on one of the thioamides for months, providing the hyperthyroidism is well-controlled during that time. Usually after about a year, the thioamide is withdrawn and thyroid function is reevaluated. Many patients remain euthyroid after the thioamides are discontinued. For this 15% to 50% of all patients treated, no further therapy may ever be required.

Thioamides are rapidly absorbed following oral administration and are concentrated in the thyroid. The drugs are also distributed to other tissues and cross the placenta to enter the fetus. Thioamides appear in the milk of nursing mothers. The thioamides are metabolized and excreted in the urine.

TABLE 36-4. Drugs used in the treatment of hyperthyroidism

Generic name	Trade name	Dosage and administration	Properties	Comments
THIOAMIDES				
Propylthiouracil (PTU)		ORAL: *Adults*—50 to 300 mg daily. Initial doses range from 300 to 600 mg daily.	Inhibits thyroid hormone synthesis but not release.	Used to lower thyroid hormone levels. Clinical improvement of hyperthyroid is delayed. Agranulocytosis may occur in 1.4% of patients during first 2 mo of therapy; skin rashes occur in roughly 3% of patients.
Methimazole	Tapazole	ORAL: *Adults*—5 to 20 mg daily. Initial doses range from 30 to 60 mg daily.	Inhibits thyroid hormone synthesis but not release.	Drug is similar to PTU.
MONOVALENT CATION				
Lithium carbonate		Not established. Doses of 900 mg daily for manic states depress thyroid function in some patients.	Inhibits synthesis and release of thyroid hormones by a mechanism different from thioamides.	When used for treatment of manic states, side effects include nausea and vomiting, twitching muscles, and central nervous system changes. Severe intoxication causes convulsions, coma, and death.
BETA ADRENERGIC BLOCKER				
Propranolol hydrochloride	Inderal	ORAL: *Adults*—40 to 160 mg daily in divided doses. INTRAVENOUS: *Adults*—5 mg or less administered at 1 mg/min or more slowly.	Controls symptoms of hyperthyroidism but does not lower T_3 and T_4 levels.	Controls palpitations, tremor, sweating, proximal muscle weakness, and cardiac symptoms of hyperthyroidism by competitively blocking beta adrenergic receptors. Bronchospasm may occur in asthmatics; may precipitate frank heart failure in patient with heart function maintained by sympathetic tone.
IODINE				
Potassium or sodium iodide	Strong Iodine Solution Lugol's Solution	ORAL: *Adults*—0.1 to 0.3 ml 3 times daily. INTRAVENOUS: *Adults*—250 to 500 mg daily for thyrotoxic crisis.	Produces short-term inhibition of thyroid hormone synthesis by direct action on the thyroid.	Used as presurgical medication to reduce the size of the thyroid gland after thioamide therapy. Used with thioamide and propranolol for hyperthyroid crisis. May produce iodism.
RADIOACTIVE IODINE				
^{131}I or ^{125}I as NaI		ORAL: *Adults*—4 to 10 mCi as a single dose for Graves' disease. For thyroid carcinoma, single doses of up to 150 mCi may be used. Smaller doses are used for diagnostic purposes (Table 36-2).	These radionuclides are concentrated in the thyroid and release radiation, which destroys thyroid tissue.	Used to destroy thyroid tissue without surgery for control of Graves' disease or thyroid carcinoma. Hypothyroidism ultimately develops in most patients.

TABLE 36-5. Miscellaneous compounds affecting the thyroid gland

Chemical	Use or occurrence	Action on the thyroid
Complex anions—thiocyanate	Formerly used as an antihypertensive; also formed in the body during digestion of foods such as cabbage	Blocks iodine concentration in the thyroid gland
Aniline derivatives—aminosalicylic acid	Used in long-term treatment of tuberculosis	May produce hypothyroidism and goiter following long-term use
Sulfonamides—sulfathiazole, sulfadiazine	Used as antibacterial agents	Suppress thyroid function, but not at doses routinely used in humans
Polyhydric phenols—phloroglucinol, hexylresorcinol, resorcinol	Used in ointments intended for treatment of skin lesions	Suppress thyroid function; absorption of the compounds may be increased when they are applied to abraded skin for long periods
Miscellaneous agents		
Goitrin	Found in plants of the mustard family and in turnips	Causes goiter
Aminotriazole	Used as an herbicide	Suppresses thyroid function
Phenylbutazone	Clinically used antiinflammatory agent	Weak antithyroid action not significant in humans
Thiopental	Clinically used sedative-hypnotic	Weak antithyroid action not significant in humans
Dimercaprol	Used to treat poisoning by heavy metals	Antithyroid action seen in humans

Two thioamides are currently in use in the United States (Table 36-4). These drugs differ from one another primarily in potency and in the incidence of toxic reactions. One of these drugs, propylthiouracil, also inhibits the conversion of T_4 to T_3 in peripheral tissues.

Perchlorate

Perchlorate, available as the sodium or potassium salt, competitively inhibits iodine uptake by the thyroid gland. Although in theory perchlorate could be used like the thionamides in long-term therapy, it is rarely so used today because of relatively dangerous toxic reactions produced (aplastic anemia).

Lithium carbonate

Lithium carbonate may be used as an antithyroid drug because the monovalent cation Li^+ inhibits thyroid hormone release and synthesis. Lithium is presently used in the treatment of maniac-depressive disease, and its use in thyroid disease is being explored.

Iodine

Iodine is the oldest of the antithyroid preparations currently in use. Although iodine is the required starting material for the synthesis of the thyroid hormones, high concentrations of iodine suppress the continued uptake of iodine and the synthesis of thyroid hormones in the thyroid gland. Suppression of hormone synthesis is by no means complete with iodine administration, and many patients return to the hyperthyroid state even with continued administration of high iodine doses. Iodine is seldom used today for long-term suppression of the hyperactive thyroid gland. The most common current usage of iodine is to prepare a hyperthyroid patient for surgery. Iodine not only suppresses thyroid function, but also reduces the vascularization of the gland. By these two mechanisms, iodine reduces the surgical risk to the hyperthyroid patient. Iodine pretreatment is especially important for the hyperthyroid patient who has received thioamide therapy, since those drugs increase the vascularization of the thyroid gland. Iodine may also be used as part of the emergency therapy for hyperthyroid crisis. When used for emergency therapy, iodine is administered intravenously after one of the thioamides has been given.

Radioactive iodine

Radioactive iodine is also used in the treatment of hyperthyroidism as well as in diagnosis. This therapy depends on the ability of the radioactive iodine to be concentrated in the thyroid gland, where it then destroys surrounding tissue by emitting low-energy radiation. The doses of actual iodine in this therapy are small. The use of radioactive iodine allows the thyroid to be functionally destroyed without resorting to surgery. Nearly all patients treated with radioactive iodine ultimately become hypothyroid and require treatment with thyroid hormones. The incidence of hypothyroidism is about 10% of treated patients during the first year after therapy and about 3% per year thereafter. Because of the likelihood of hypothyroidism, patients should be urged to return periodically for thyroid evaluation.

Incidental antithyroid compounds

Many compounds in our chemical-rich environment have antithyroid effects. None of these compounds has found clinical usefulness as an antithyroid drug, although some are used clinically for other purposes. Some of the compounds listed in Table 36-5 occasionally appear in the food chain of man and may be responsible for rare chemical-induced hypothyroidism.

Parafollicular cells of the thyroid

The parafollicular cells, which constitute about 10% to 20% of the total number of thyroid cells, synthesize the peptide hormone called *calcitonin*. In animals calcitonin is thought to prevent blood calcium levels from exceeding the normal range after meals; the physiological role of calcitonin in humans has not been resolved. Nevertheless, calcitonin does have demonstrable effects when administered exogenously. Calcitonin prevents the loss of calcium from bone, augments the urinary excretion of calcium and phosphate, and blocks the absorption of calcium from the small intestine.

Calcitonin has been used therapeutically in man to treat Paget's disease, in which excessive bone resorption leads to thinned and fragile bones. The preparation most often used clinically in humans is a synthetic form of salmon calcitonin (Table 36-6). Salmon calcitonin is used because it is the most potent of the naturally occurring forms of the hormone. The dose is 50 to 100 units given intramuscularly or subcutaneously. Some patients suffer nausea and vomiting, facial flushing, and occasional inflammatory reactions at the injection site. Since the hormone is a peptide and it is administered in a gelatin solution, allergic reactions may occur.

The parathyroid glands

■ Actions of parathyroid hormone

The parathyroid glands in humans synthesize parathyroid hormone, a peptide whose major function is to maintain blood calcium levels above the critical threshold required for body function. In many ways parathyroid hormone acts exactly opposite to calcitonin. For example, parathyroid hormone increases reabsorption of calcium from bones, lowers renal excretion of calcium, and along with vitamin D increases calcium absorption from the intestine. The overall interaction of parathyroid hormone, calcitonin, and vitamin D allows the body to maintain blood calcium levels within a very narrow margin. This close control of calcium levels is required because very small increases or decreases in blood calcium levels can profoundly alter many cellular functions.

Hyperparathyroidism. Hyperparathyroidism (excess parathyroid hormone) usually arises as a result of excess secretion of parathyroid hormone from a tumor. Many patients with this condition show decreases in bone calcification as a result of the action of parathyroid hormone. High amounts of calcium are excreted by these patients, and renal stones are common. No specific inhibitors of parathyroid release are available for clinical use; thus therapy consists primarily of surgery to remove the source of excess parathyroid hormone synthesis. Calcitonin may temporarily control hypercalcemia in hyperparathyroidism.

Hypoparathyroidism. Hypoparathyroidism (insufficient parathyroid hormone) usually results following thyroid or parathyroid surgery, but idiopathic (unknown cause) forms of the disease exist. Whatever the cause, hypoparathyroidism is associated with low blood calcium levels (hypocalcemia). This electrolyte imbalance produces symptoms such as paresthesia, muscle spasms, tetany, and convulsions. In theory, parathyroid hormone could be used to raise blood calcium levels in conditions where blood levels are abnormally low; however, administration of one of the forms of vitamin D with or without calcium is the preferred treatment.

Several forms of vitamin D are available for clinical use. Vitamin D_3, or cholecalciferol, is normally formed in skin by the irradiation of 7-dehydrocholesterol. Vitamin D_3 is equivalent in humans to vitamin D_2, or ergocalciferol. Both drugs are available in orally administered forms suitable for convenient, long-term therapy. Calcitriol (1,25-dihydroxycholecalciferol) is the most active vitamin D derivative and represents the final active metabolite of the vitamin in humans. Although very effective, this drug form is expensive. Since adequate treatment is possible for most conditions with other

TABLE 36-6. Clinical summary of agents used to alter calcium metabolism

Generic name	Trade name	Dosage and administration	Clinical use
Calcitonin	Calcimar	INTRAMUSCULAR, SUBCUTANEOUS: 100 units daily or higher if required.	To lower hypercalcemia in hyperparathyroidism or vitamin D intoxication; to control Paget's disease (excessive bone remodeling).
Parathyroid hormone		INTRAVENOUS: 200 units.	Diagnosis of pseudohypoparathyroidism.
Vitamin D			
Calcitriol	Rocaltrol	ORAL: 0.5 to 1 μg daily.	Treatment of rickets, pseudohypoparathyroidism.
Cholecalciferol		ORAL: dose equivalent to 400 units or higher.	Treatment of rickets, hypoparathyroidism.
Dihydrotachysterol	Hytakerol	ORAL: dose equivalent to 400 units or higher.	Treatment of rickets, hypoparathyroidism.
Ergocalciferol	Drisdol Geltabs	ORAL: dose equivalent to 400 units or higher.	Treatment of rickets, hypoparathyroidism.

■ THE NURSING PROCESS FOR PARATHYROID DISORDERS

■ Assessment

Disorders involving only the parathyroid gland are unusual. Hypoparathyroidism is seen most often in patients who have had accidental removal or destruction of the parathyroid glands during thyroid surgery or other surgical procedures. As mentioned in the text, hyperparathyroidism is most often seen with tumors of the parathyroid gland. In these cases the nurse should do a total patient assessment and monitor the patient's vital signs and serum calcium levels. Symptoms of hypoparathyroidism would be those of paresthesia, muscle spasms, tetany, and convulsions.

■ Management

The plan of therapy is to return serum calcium levels to the normal range and to treat any underlying patient condition. The nurse should continue to monitor the vital signs, to measure the serum calcium levels, and to check for progression or regression of any symptoms discovered during the initial assessment. If calcitonin is being prescribed for outpatient use, the patient should be instructed in the correct procedure for subcutaneous drug administration.

■ Evaluation

Therapy for parathyroid disorders is successful if the serum calcium level can be maintained within the normal range and the patient suffers no side effects resulting from therapy. Before discharge, the patient should be able to explain how and why to take the prescribed drugs, to demonstrate any special administration techniques, and to explain what symptoms should warrant notification of the physician. The patient should be able to state the need to wear a medical identification tag or bracelet. For additional specific information, see the patient care implications section at the end of this chapter.

forms of the vitamin, calcitriol is reserved for those rare patients who respond only to this drug form.

Pseudohypoparathyroidism is a condition in which the kidney, bone, and intestine do not respond to parathyroid hormone in the normal way. Parathyroid hormone is occasionally used in the diagnosis of this condition. Some of these patients respond to treatment with calcitriol.

■ Pharmacology of vitamin D

Vitamin D, a lipid-soluble substance, is adequately absorbed following oral administration. The vitamin is transported in the bloodstream by a specific alpha globulin. Depending on exactly what form of the vitamin is administered, a variety of biotransformations is possible. The liver converts vitamin D_3 to the more active 25-hydroxyvitamin D_3. The kidney converts 24-hydroxyvitamin D_3 to 1,25-dihydroxyvitamin D_3, the most active metabolite of the vitamin. Most of the vitamin D metabolites are excreted in the bile. Excess or deficiency of vitamin D produces symptoms that are primarily those expected of high or low blood calcium concentrations.

■ PATIENT CARE IMPLICATIONS

Hypothyroidism

1. Replacement therapy for hypothyroidism is usually begun with low doses of medication, and the doses are increased in strength over several weeks until the desired result is achieved.
2. Signs and symptoms of excessive thyroid medication are the same as for hyperthyroidism (Table 36-1). The easiest way to monitor the effect of thyroid medication is to take the pulse. A pulse rate greater than 100 beats per minute in an adult may indicate overdosage with thyroid medication. In some hospitals it is required that the pulse be taken daily before thyroid medication is administered; if the adult's pulse exceeds 100 beats per minute, the dose is not given and the physician is notified.
3. In planning the discharge of a patient recently begun on thyroid medication, it may be appropriate to teach the patient to take his own pulse and to report rates over a certain limit determined after consultation with the physician. Parents of a hypothyroid child should also be taught to take the child's pulse, although the upper limits of a normal pulse rate vary depending on the child's age. In addition, hypothyroid children should have their height measured regularly as another parameter reflecting normal thyroid function.
4. The patient needs to understand that thyroid medication may need to be continued for life; it should not be discontinued once the patient feels better.
5. Occasionally what appears to be a treatment failure may result from the use of old thyroid medication that has lost potency because of lengthy or improper shelf storage. The medication should be kept dry and remain in a light-resistant container if so supplied.
6. Use of thyroid preparations to treat obesity in the absence of hypothyroidism is inappropriate.
7. Occasionally thyroid medication is prescribed to the euthyroid individual with an enlarged thyroid. The exogenous thyroid will permit the thyroid gland to return to normal size (this may not work if the gland has been enlarged many years).
8. Treatment of congenital hypothyroidism (cretinism) should be begun and maintained as soon as the diagnosis is made. Treatment will not, however, reverse any mental retardation that has already occurred. Many states now require that newborns be tested for adequate thyroid hormone levels.
9. Thyroid medications increase the action of anticoagulants; patients receiving both may need their dose of anticoagulants reduced.
10. Thyroid medications may enhance the toxic effects of digitalis preparations.
11. Diabetic patients who are started on thyroid medication may need an increase in their dose of insulin or oral hypoglycemic agent because the thyroid medications can produce hyperglycemia.
12. Adrenal insufficiency should be corrected before beginning thyroid medication. Patients already taking adrenal steroids may need their dosages readjusted.
13. Patients undergoing neurosurgery for pituitary tumors or destruction of the pituitary gland for pain control or other reasons will be evaluated 2 to 3 weeks after surgery for thyroid function, and may require thyroid replacement therapy if pituitary thyroid stimulating hormone (TSH) is lost.
14. Patients on long-term thyroid medication should wear a medical identification tag or bracelet indicating the nature of their problem.

Hyperthyroidism

1. Long-standing exophthalmus may not improve in appearance even after treatment for hyperthyroidism has begun.
2. Because of the danger of agranulocytosis when taking the thioamides, patients should be taught to report to their physician any sore throat, fever, or rash. Other reported side effects of these drugs include nausea, vomiting, dizziness, and drowsiness.
3. The thioamides can be cautiously given to a pregnant woman, although as a woman approaches term the physician will monitor her closely and may discontinue the medication or add a thyroid preparation to prevent hypothyroidism in the infant. The drugs are excreted in breast milk so mothers taking one of the thioamides should not breast-feed.
4. Signs of overdosage with the thioamides are those of hypothyroidism (Table 36-1). The easily monitored signs include the pulse rate, weight changes, and facial edema. Signs develop slowly.
5. Propylthiouracil can produce hypoprothrombinemia. Caution the patient to report excessive bruising, purpura, or unexplained or excessive bleeding.
6. Oral anticoagulants may be potentiated by propylthiouracil, necessitating a reduction in the dosage of anticoagulant.
7. Lugol's solution or any iodide solution is foul tasting and should be well diluted in juice, milk, or beverage of the patient's preference. In addition, it may stain the teeth, so it should be taken through a straw.
8. Signs of iodism (excessive iodide) include metallic taste in the mouth, sneezing, swollen and tender thyroid gland, vomiting, and bloody diarrhea. Concomitant excessive use of over-the-counter preparations containing iodine (e.g., asthma or cough preparations) may contribute to iodism.
9. Although the radiation dose of radioactive iodine is not high, those preparing the preparation should be careful not to spill the mixture on themselves or countertops. Rubber gloves should be worn.
10. Side effects (other than eventual hypothyroidism) are rare with radioactive iodine but include soreness over the thyroid gland and in rare cases difficulty swallowing and breathing because of gland enlargement.
11. To prevent damage to the infant, radioactive iodine should not be taken by pregnant women or nursing mothers.
12. Emergency treatment of thyroid crisis might include intravenous sodium iodide, which is given after an antithyroid drug has been administered. The ordered dose of iodine (usually 1 to 2 Gm) should be diluted in at least 100 ml of normal saline solution, 5% dextrose in saline solution or water, or Ringer's solution. Administer slowly over 30 minutes. Discard any cloudy or colored solution or one containing particulate matter. Sodium iodide is contraindicated in persons with known iodine sensitivity. There is no specific antidote; treatment of a sensitivity reaction is supportive.
13. Thyroid surgery carries with it the possible side effect of accidental removal or destruction of the parathyroid glands. Signs of hypoparathyroidism include hypocalcemia, muscle twitching, muscle spasm, numbness and tingling of fingers and toes, and tetany; Chvostek's and Trousseau's signs are positive. Treatment for acute hypocalcemia is usually with a 10% solution of calcium gluconate intravenously. The drug can be given diluted or undiluted but should be given slowly because of potential cardiac effects; it will also increase digitalis toxicity. Calcium gluconate should be readily available to those caring for patients undergoing thyroid surgery.

Calcitonin

1. Calcitonin may be used in treatment of Paget's disease or other cases of hyperparathyroidism.
2. Calcitonin is protein in nature and may cause an allergic response. Epinephrine, antihistamines, glucocorticoids, and equipment for possible resuscitation should be available in settings where calcitonin is used.
3. Monitor the serum calcium and serum alkaline phosphotase levels to chart progress of the underlying condition.
4. Calcitonin is administered via subcutaneous or intramuscular routes. For outpatient therapy, the subcutaneous route is preferred. In preparation for discharge, the patient should be able to demonstrate sterile technique in preparing and administering the dose and should be able to explain the need for rotation of sites.
5. The major side effects associated with therapy, other than major alterations in calcium balance, are nausea and local irritation resulting from the injection.

Vitamin D

1. Side effects associated with vitamin D therapy are minimal once the dose has been adjusted to the needs of the patient.
2. Monitor the serum calcium level on a regular basis.
3. Other side effects that may occur include drowsiness, gastrointestinal complaints, and hypertension. Encourage the patient to report the appearance of any new signs or symptoms.

■ SUMMARY

The follicular cells of the thyroid gland regulate the basal metabolic rate in the body by releasing the hormones thyroxine and triiodothyronine. These hormones are formed from iodine and tyrosine in the thyroid gland and stored in thyroglobulin in the thyroid follicles. When released into the bloodstream, the thyroid hormones are bound to thyroid-binding globulin. Thyroxine is very tightly bound, whereas triiodothyronine is less firmly bound and therefore more able to penetrate tissues. Target cells may convert thyroxine to triiodothyronine. These hormones are metabolized by the liver and excreted in the bile as well as being broken down at other sites in the body.

Adult hypothyroidism (myxedema) produces characteristic signs of slowed metabolic rates. In addition, congenital hypothyroidism may produce mental retardation, and juvenile hypothyroidism may produce growth stunting. All forms of hypothyroidism require replacement therapy with thyroid hormones. Preparations of varying potency and purity are available, but all are capable of adequately replacing thyroid hormone. Preparations containing only thyroxine have a slower onset of action and a longer duration of action than preparations containing only triiodothyronine. Therapy with these agents should be started at low doses and gradually increased to avoid excessive stress to the patient. Angina pectoris and other cardiac or cardiovascular symptoms may be produced.

Hyperthyroidism may be produced by generalized overactivity of the thyroid gland such as that of Graves' disease or by overproduction of thyroid hormones by nodules or tumors of the thyroid gland. Temporary hyperthyroidism can be produced by subacute thyroiditis. Hyperthyroidism may be treated by controlling the symptoms of the disease or by actually lowering the amounts of thyroid hormones circulating in the body. Propranolol, a beta adrenergic blocking agent, controls the symptoms of hyperthyroidism by blocking catecholamine effects on heart, muscle, and other tissues. This drug is effective because many of the symptoms of hyperthyroidism result from oversensitivity of tissues to catecholamines in the presence of high levels of thyroid hormones. Propranolol rapidly controls the palpitation, tremor, muscle weakness, and cardiac arrhythmias that may be associated with hyperthyroidism. Thioamides block synthesis of thyroid hormones and therefore can control hyperthyroidism. However, since the thyroid gland stores a large amount of hormone, the clinical effect of the thioamides is not apparent until these stored hormones are depleted—a matter of several days. Radioactive iodine may be used to slow thyroid hormone synthesis, since the isotope will be concentrated in thyroid tissue and destroy a portion of the hyperactive gland.

The parafollicular cells of the thyroid produce the peptide hormone calcitonin. Calcitonin can prevent the loss of calcium from bone, augment the urinary excretion of calcium and phosphate, and block the absorption of calcium from the intestine. The hormone has been used therapeutically in humans to treat Paget's disease.

The parathyroid glands produce the peptide parathyroid hormone. Parathyroid hormone antagonizes many of the actions of calcitonin, increasing calcium reabsorption from bones, lowering renal excretion of calcium, and increasing calcium absorption from the intestine. This latter effect is produced through the action of vitamin D. Overproduction of parathyroid hormone results in high calcium excretion, frequently producing renal stones. Hypoparathyroidism produces low blood levels of calcium and hence paresthesia, muscle spasms, tetany, and convulsions. Treatment is with a preparation of vitamin D with or without calcium supplements. Vitamin D increases the absorption of calcium and elevates the blood concentration of this ion.

■ STUDY QUESTIONS

1. What is the function of the follicular cells of the thyroid gland?
2. What are the hormones produced by the follicular cells of the thyroid gland?
3. What is the function of thyroid-stimulating hormone (TSH) and where is it produced?
4. What are the steps in thyroid hormone synthesis?
5. How much T_3 and T_4 is stored in the thyroid gland?
6. What is the function of thyroglobulin?
7. How are the thyroid hormones transported in the bloodstream?
8. How are the thyroid hormones eliminated from the body?
9. Which of the thyroid hormones is found most abundantly in target cells?
10. What are the characteristic signs of hypothyroidism?
11. What different symptoms are produced when hypothyroidism develops immediately after birth or later in childhood, as opposed to during adult life?
12. In primary hypothyroidism, how do the blood concentrations of TSH and thyroid hormones differ from normal?
13. What is secondary hypothyroidism?
14. What is tertiary hypothyroidism?
15. What is the treatment for all forms of hypothyroidism?
16. Which of the available preparations of thyroid hormones is the most potent?
17. How do T_3 and T_4 differ in onset and duration of action?
18. What side effects may occur with replacement therapy of thyroid hormones?
19. Which thyroid hormone is available as an injectable preparation?
20. Why would the administration of T_3 by nasogastric tube sometimes be preferred over injection of T_4 in the treatment of myxedemic coma?
21. What is Graves' disease?
22. What is subacute thyroiditis?
23. What is the cause of Graves' disease?

24. What general classes of drugs are used to treat hyperthyroidism?
25. To what class of drugs does propranolol belong and why is it useful in treating hyperthyroidism?
26. What is the mechanism of action of the thioamides?
27. How are the thiomides distributed in the body?
28. How may radioactive iodine be used in the treatment of hyperthyroidism?
29. What is the function of the parafollicular cells of the thyroid?
30. What metabolic effects does calcitonin have?
31. What is the function of the parathyroid glands?
32. What are the metabolic effects of parathyroid hormone?
33. What are the symptoms of hypoparathyroidism?
34. How is hypoparathyroidism treated?
35. Which of the metabolites of vitamin D is the most active?
36. What is the metabolic function of vitamin D?
37. What is the fate of vitamin D in the body?

■ SUGGESTED READINGS

Arney, G.K., Kudzma, D.J., and Mazzaferri, E.: A practical guide to thyroid disorders, Hospital Physician **11**(2):30, 1975.

Cobb, W.E., and Jackson, I.M.D.: Management of hypothyroidism, Drug Therapy Reviews **2:**377, 1979.

Hallal, J.C.: Thyroid disorders, American Journal of Nursing **77:** 417, 1977.

Harvey, S.: Drugs in metabolic emergencies, burns, and drug accidents, Nurses' Drug Alert **2:**145, Dec., 1978.

Jackson, I.M.D.: Management of thyrotoxicosis, Drug Therapy Reviews **1:**144, 1977.

McConahey, W.M.: Hypothyroidism, Hospital Medicine **11**(4):98, 1975.

Neelon, F.A.: Nail changes in thyroid disease, Drug Therapy **10**(11): 153, 1980.

Ordering and evaluating thyroid tests, Patient Care **8**(3):29, 1974.

Rush, D.R., and Hamburger, S.C.: Drugs used in endocrine metabolic emergencies, Critical Care Quarterly **3:**1, Sept., 1980.

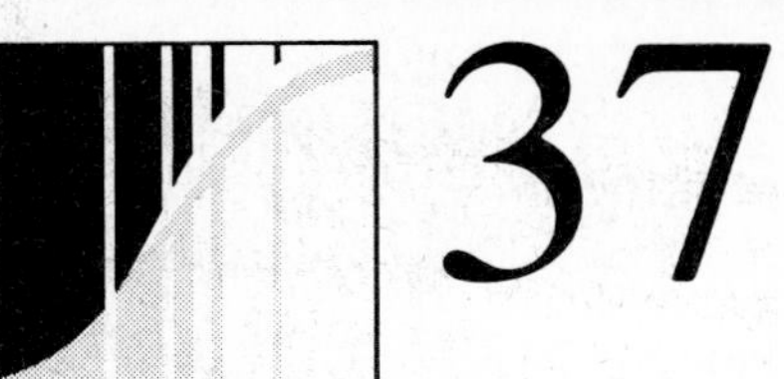

37 Drugs acting on the female reproductive system

Female reproductive function is dependent on a complex, exquisitely regulated interaction of endocrine tissues. The negative feedback loop regulating the menstrual cycle involves the hypothalamus, the anterior pituitary, and the ovaries (Chapter 34). The actions of the natural female hormones, the clinical uses of synthetic and natural drugs affecting the female reproductive system, the endocrine control of pregnancy, and drugs used during childbirth and the postpartum period are discussed in this chapter.

■ HORMONES INVOLVED IN FEMALE REPRODUCTION

■ Sources of hormones involved in female reproduction

The major hormones involved in developing and maintaining female reproductive capacity include examples of all the chemical classes of hormones. The hypothalamus supplies gonadotropin-releasing hormone (GnRH), which acts directly on the anterior pituitary, stimulating synthesis and release of follicle-stimulating hormone (FSH) and luteinizing hormone (LH). In addition, the central nervous system neurotransmitter dopamine is the inhibitory factor that regulates the release of prolactin from the anterior pituitary. FSH, LH, and prolactin are the major gonadotropins in human beings. Each of these hormones has a different primary target tissue. FSH stimulates the ovarian cells, which form the follicle and nurture the maturing ovum. Under the influence of FSH these cells synthesize the potent steroid estrogen estradiol. LH acts primarily on the mature follicle to cause release of the ovum. Prolactin stimulates breast tissue to allow milk production. Prolactin may also affect the ovary, but details of how the hormone acts in this tissue are lacking.

The major steroid hormones regulating female reproduction are estrogens and progestins. Estrogens are compounds that stimulate female reproductive tissues; progestins are compounds that specifically stimulate the uterine lining. Estrogens are produced primarily in the FSH-stimulated cells of the ovarian follicle. Progesterone, the most important progestin, is synthesized in the cells remaining in the follicle after the expulsion of the ovum. This tissue is called the corpus luteum.

All the steroids produced in the ovary are derived from cholesterol. Progestins are formed first and are the precursors of androgens. Androgens, the steroid hormones capable of producing masculinization, are primarily precursors for estrogen synthesis in females. Androstenedione is the androgen precursor of estrone, a major circulating estrogen that is formed mostly in peripheral tissues and not in the ovary. Estradiol, which is the most abundant circulating estrogen, is formed in the ovary.

■ Hormones affecting development of the female reproductive system

At birth the ovary is already in an advanced stage of development and contains between 2 and 4 million oocytes (cells that will form ova). The primordial follicles containing oocytes are not quiescent during the prepubertal years, but undergo a process called *atresia* in which oocytes are destroyed and follicles resorbed. At menarche (when menstrual cycles begin during puberty) an estimated 400,000 oocytes remain. Even after ovulation is initiated, atresia continues and is responsible for the destruction of over 99% of the follicles present in the ovary.

As puberty begins, the immature ovaries are stimulated by the increasing amounts of pituitary gonadotropins. As a result, estrogen synthesis is promoted and estrogen levels in the bloodstream rise. The primary function of estrogens during early puberty is to promote development of the female reproductive system. The uterus and fallopian tubes are enlarged to adult proportions. The vagina is enlarged, and the vaginal epithelium is thickened and strengthened. In the breast, estrogen promotes proliferation of stromal tissue as well as the ductile tissue, which will allow milk formation and make it available to the suckling infant. The secondary sexual characteristics of the female are also dependent on estrogens. These hormones promote the increased deposition of fat, especially in the breasts and hips. Without estrogens, the typical contours of the female body do not develop.

Estrogens are also involved in the growth spurt that is characteristic of puberty. Along with other hormones, estrogen causes the retention of calcium and phosphorus and thereby promotes bone growth. However, estrogens also induce closure of the epiphyses. When this closure occurs, no further increase in height takes place.

■ Hormones affecting ovulation

The process of ovulation requires the proper functioning of the hypothalamus, anterior pituitary, and ovary in the negative feedback loop described in Chapter 34. Both FSH and LH are required to act on the developing follicle before a mature ovum may be released to begin its journey down the fallopian tube to the uterus. Estrogen synthesis is required both for its action on the follicle and for its ability to trigger the midcycle surge of LH from the anterior pituitary.

■ Hormones affecting endometrial function

The uterus is composed of smooth muscle (myometrium) and glandular epithelium (endometrium). The endometrium, which exists to nourish and to support the ovum during development, is controlled primarily by estrogens and progestins. Estrogens promote the proliferation of the endometrium during the first half of the menstrual cycle before ovulation occurs. Progesterone, which is formed in the corpus luteum of the ovary during the second half of the menstrual cycle, acts on both the endometrium and the myometrium. Progesterone reduces the activity of the myometrium and prevents muscular contractions. Progesterone promotes the development of the secretory capacity of the endometrium. Actions on these two tissues aid in establishing the environment in which the fertilized ovum may successfully implant and begin fetal development. Once implantation of the ovum has actually occurred, progesterone continues to alter the endometrium, ultimately changing the tissue so that a second implantation becomes impossible.

■ Hormones in pregnancy

Pregnancy obviously requires that a mature ovum be released from the ovary at the appropriate time, that the ovum be successfully fertilized within about 2 days of its release, and that the ovum be able to implant itself within the endometrium and begin to draw nourishment to support the early stages of development. The most important hormone during these first days and weeks of pregnancy is progesterone. Without adequate progesterone, the endometrium will be sloughed and the fertilized ovum will be lost. Luteal progesterone continues to be produced for about the first 10 weeks of pregnancy. Control of progesterone synthesis is exercised by cells of the fetus, which will develop into the placenta. A few days after implantation of the ovum in the endometrium, these fetal cells begin to produce a hormone called *human chorionic gonadotropin* (HCG), which takes over control of the corpus luteum and maintains its production of progesterone. By the fifth week of pregnancy the placenta has developed to the stage where it begins to synthesize progesterone directly. Placental progesterone production increases during the remainder of the pregnancy, while progesterone production in the corpus luteum virtually disappears.

The continuing high progesterone levels during pregnancy are thought to aid in maintaining the pregnancy by suppressing myometrial contractions. At the end of pregnancy, progesterone levels begin to decrease, allowing the uterus to begin to produce hormones called prostaglandins. Prostaglandins, which are formed from fatty acids within cell membranes, are capable of stimulating powerful uterine contractions. Although the exact role of prostaglandins in normal childbirth is not yet established, it is known that the contractions produced by prostaglandins are sufficiently strong to bring about the expulsion of the fetus from the uterus.

Oxytocin, a hormone produced by the posterior pituitary, is also capable of inducing uterine contractions. The uterus increases in sensitivity to oxytocin at term and during the puerperium (period immediately following birth). Oxytocin also acts on breast tissue, where it stimulates the myoepithelium of the breast and promotes milk letdown. Suckling the infants sets off a reflex action in which oxytocin release is stimulated. Central nervous system control of this process is clearly demonstrated by the fact that for some women the mere sight of the infant is sufficient to induce oxytocin release and milk letdown. Oxytocin action is responsible for the improved uterine muscle tone in nursing mothers and for the more rapid return of the uterus to the pregravid size in these women.

■ PHARMACOLOGICAL AGENTS AFFECTING FEMALE SEXUAL FUNCTION

Many of the conditions of the female reproductive tract for which women seek medical aid may be successfully treated by replacement therapy. The most common conditions are those that arise as a result of estrogen deficiency. A lack of estrogen during puberty will prevent normal growth and sexual development; menarche may not occur. This endocrine malfunction is only one of a number of abnormalities that may be responsible for amenorrhea (no menstrual cycles). After the menopause, the gradual decline in estrogen levels may be responsible for a host of symptoms, including vasomotor symptoms (hot flashes, sweating), osteoporosis (bone loss), and atrophy of vaginal and urethral tissue.

TABLE 37-1. Pharmacological therapy of dysfunctions of the female reproductive system

Clinical condition	Treatment	Rationale
Amenorrhea	Cyclic estrogen-progestin or menotropins	Estrogens are required to promote secondary sex characteristics. Other hormonal support may be required for full fertility. Depending on the cause of the amenorrhea, surgery or other therapy may be required.
Menopause		
Vasomotor symptoms	Estrogens	Hot flashes and sweating are relieved by estrogens.
Osteoporosis	Estrogens	Loss of calcium may be temporarily halted but not reversed.
Atrophy of vaginal and urethral tissue	Estrogens	Estrogen support is needed to maintain tissue tone.
Dysfunctional uterine bleeding	Estrogen and progestin	Combination stops bleeding; drug withdrawal induces endometrial sloughing.
Luteal phase defect (infertility)	Progestins	Infertility resulting from inadequate synthesis of progesterone from the corpus luteum may be treated by progestin early in the pregnancy.
Postpartum breast engorgement	Estrogens or estrogen-androgen combinations	Used to suppress lactation, these agents probably block prolactin effects in the breast.
Metastatic breast carcinoma	Estrogens, androgens, or progestins	Tumors show differing sensitivities to these hormones.
Metastatic endometrial carcinoma	Progestins	Natural suppressive effect of progestins on the endometrium is retained in some of these tumors.
Galactorrhea	Bromocriptine	Suppresses prolactin release, thereby preventing the excessive stimulation of breast secretary tissue.
Dysmenorrhea	Oral contraceptives	Suppression of ovulation gives relief to many but by no means all patients.
Pelvic endometriosis	Estrogen and progestin Danazol	Suppresses proliferation of endometrial tissue. This experimental agent inhibits gonadotropins, thereby preventing proliferation of endometrial tissue.
Habitual and threatened abortions	Estrogens	Therapy is not clear. Diethylstilbestrol and progestins, used in the past, are now known to alter the fetus and are no longer used.
Anovulation (infertility)	Clomiphene citrate, menotropins, or HCG	Ovulatory failure may be overcome by proper use of agents that promote gonadotropin release (clomiphene) or supply them directly (menotropins). HCG acts as LH to trigger release of the ovum.

There are other medical problems of the female reproductive system that cannot definitely be ascribed to a specific hormone deficiency. Nevertheless, many of these conditions respond to hormones used for some pharmacological action rather than as replacement therapy. Examples of such conditions include dysfunctional uterine bleeding, dysmenorrhea (menstrual cramps), pelvic endometriosis, luteal phase defects, postpartum breast engorgement, and breast or endometrial carcinomas. The rationale for therapy for these conditions is listed in Table 37-1.

Estrogen doses used in the clinical setting vary depending on the nature of the condition being treated. When used in replacement therapy, estrogen doses tend to be low. Higher doses are used to treat conditions such as advanced breast cancer. A drug handbook or the pharmacy should be consulted for the actual dose of a specific preparation used to treat a specific condition.

TABLE 37-2. Estrogens used in the clinic

Generic name	Trade name	Chemical form	Administration	Duration of action
Estradiol	Estrace Estradiol		Aqueous suspension or oil for intramuscular injection Tablets for oral use	3 to 7 days 1 day (oral)
	Depo-estradiol cypionate Depogen Duraestrin Span-F	Cypionate	Oil solution for intramuscular injection	2 to 3 wk
	Ardefem Delestrogen Estate Span-Est Valergen	Valerate	Oil solution for intramuscular injection	2 to 3 wk
Estrone	Gravigen Theelin A.T.V. Estrovag Theelin		Aqueous suspension or oil solution for intramuscular injection Vaginal suppository	3 to 7 days 1 day
	Ogen	Piperazine sulfate	Tablets for oral use Vaginal cream	1 day 1 day
	Duogen-RP Femspan Mer-Estrone Spanestrin "P" Theelin R-P Tri-Estrin	Combination of water-soluble and water-insoluble forms	Aqueous suspension for intramuscular injection	3 to 7 days
	Amnestrogen Conjutabs Estratab Evex Femogen Menest SK-estrogens	Esterified estrogens (sulfates)	Tablets for oral use	1 day
	Centrogen Estrogenic Substances Hormonin Menagen Urestrin	Mixtures (also called estrogenic substance)	Aqueous suspension or oil solution for intramuscular injection Capsules or tablets for oral use	3 to 7 days 1 day

Continued.

TABLE 37-2. Estrogens used in the clinic—cont'd

Generic name	Trade name	Chemical form	Administration	Duration of action
	Co-Estro Estrogenic Substances, conjugated Genisis Premarin Feminone	Conjugated estrogens	Tablets for oral use Vaginal creams	8 to 24 hr 1 day
Ethinyl estradiol	Estinyl		Tablets for oral use	8 to 24 hr
Diethylstilbestrol (DES)	Dicorvin Diethylstilbestrol Stilbestrol	Nonsteroid	Tablets for oral use	1 day
	Stilphostrol	Diphosphate	Tablets for oral use	1 day
	Sold under generic name	Dipropionate	Tablets for oral use	1 day
Dienestrol	Dienestrol DV	Nonsteroid	Tablets for oral use Vaginal creams and suppositories	1 day 1 day
Hexestrol	Sold under generic name	Nonsteroid	Tablets for oral use	1 day
Methallenestril	Vallestril	Nonsteroid	Tablets for oral use	1 day
Chlorotrianisene	TACE	Nonsteroid	Capsules for oral use	1 day

Estrogens

Absorption and excretion. Estrogens of various types are available in the United States (Table 37-2). The two naturally occurring steroid estrogens used in the clinical are estradiol and estrone. As steroids, these compounds are not water soluble, but they are soluble in oil. In the case of estradiol, a slower absorption and longer duration of action may be achieved by using either the cypionate or the valerate ester of the natural steroid. Estradiol is orally absorbed if the drug crystals are reduced to particles 1 to 3 μm in diameter.

Estrone is not well absorbed orally in its natural form but may be used orally if it is converted to the piperazine sulfate. Estrone is also the major component of a variety of estrogen mixtures described as esterified estrogens, estrogenic substance, or conjugated estrogens. These mixtures, which are isolated from such sources as the urine of pregnant mares, are relatively cheap and effective for many purposes, and all can be taken orally, making them a convenient drug form for many patients.

Synthetic estrogens such as ethinyl estradiol are also available. Ethinyl estradiol is more potent than naturally occurring estrogens. This drug used orally has a relatively short duration of action but does persist in the body longer than any of the natural estrogens.

Nonsteroid estrogens are all oral agents. The best-known of these drugs is *diethylstilbestrol* (DES). DES, which was discovered in 1938, was once widely used to prevent spontaneous abortions. Recently it was noticed that the children who were in utero at the time of DES treatment may have suffered from the effects of the drug. As adults, female offspring have an increased incidence of vaginal adenosis and adenocarcinoma; male offspring may be more prone to develop epididymal cysts. DES has also been used as a growth stimulant in the cattle industry. Although the FDA required cattle to be taken off the drug several weeks before slaughter, some DES has nevertheless entered the human food chain. The FDA halted the use of DES as an additive for cattle feed in 1977. DES is still available for clinical use and has been used as estrogen replacement therapy or any other use for which estrogens are approved. DES is being investigated for use as a postcoital contraceptive (''the morning-after pill'').

Natural estrogens do not persist long in the body, since they are rapidly metabolized by the liver and excreted by the kidney. Ethinyl estradiol is less rapidly metabolized and is therefore longer acting than natural estrogens. Nonsteroidal estrogens are not metabolized rapidly and also persist longer than natural estrogens.

Toxicity. Side effects of estrogens include overreactions of certain reproductive tissues to the hormones. Breast tenderness is reported by many women receiving estrogens. The endometrium is stimulated to proliferate by estrogens, and there is some evidence that estrogens

TABLE 37-3. Estrogens in fixed combinations with other drugs

Estrogen	Trade name	Other active ingredients	Administration
Estradiol	Test-Estrin	Testosterone (androgen)	Aqueous suspension for intramuscular injection Tablets for buccal absorption
Estradiol cypionate	Depo-Testadiol Duratestrin Estratest Mal-O-Fem Cyp Spenduo	Testosterone cypionate (androgen)	Oil solution for intramuscular injection
Estradiol valerate	Deladumone Mal-O-Fem L.A. Testradiol-90/4	Testosterone enanthate (androgen)	Oil solution for intramuscular injection
Estrone	Cormone Mal-O-Fem Testagen	Testosterone (androgen)	Aqueous suspension for intramuscular injection
Ethinyl estradiol	Halodrin Gynetone	Fluoxymesterone (androgen) Methyltestosterone (androgen)	Tablets for oral use Tablets for oral use
Conjugated estrogens	Milprem PMB	Meprobamate (antidepressant)	Tablets for oral use
	Mediatric	Methyltestosterone, methamphetamine, vitamin, and mineral supplements (androgen, central nervous system stimulant)	Tablets, capsules, or liquid for oral use
Esterified estrogens	Menrium	Chlordiazepoxide (antidepressant)	Tablets for oral use
	Estratest ZESTe M.T.	Methyltestosterone (androgen)	Tablets for oral use
Estrogenic substances	Cyclogesterin	Progesterone (progestin)*	Oil solution for intramuscular injection

*For other fixed combinations of estrogens and progestins, see Table 37-6.

may increase the risk of endometrial cancer. There is no evidence that estrogens increase the risk for breast cancer.

Estrogens are frequently associated with acute adverse reactions such as nausea, vomiting, anorexia, and mild diarrhea. Malaise, depression, or excessive irritability are also related to estrogen therapy in some women. Estrogens promote salt and water retention and may therefore produce edema in some patients. Atherosclerosis is a definite risk for patients receiving estrogens, especially if they have other high-risk factors, such as smoking. Hypertension has been associated with estrogen use.

As mentioned earlier, estrogens may be used as replacement therapy or in pharmacological doses for a variety of dysfunctions of the female reproductive tract.

Uses. Estrogens are also available in fixed combinations with a variety of other drugs (Table 37-3). Some of these combinations are intended for a specific medical purpose, such as the combination of estrogens with antidepressants or sedatives that are intended for use in treating severe reactions during menopause. However, to a certain degree these combinations violate pharmacological principles. The main objection to fixed combinations is that dosage adjustment for best effectiveness of both drugs becomes impossible in some patients. For example, some women may be extremely sensitive to the androgen in a fixed estrogen-androgen combination. To reduce the androgen level, it would be necessary to administer less of the medication, but that would also reduce the estrogen dose. The overall result may be that the effectiveness of one of the drugs is lost or diminished.

Estrogens are also combined with vitamin supplements, central nervous system stimulants, minerals, and a host of other agents. Most of these combinations have

TABLE 37-4. Clinically used progestins

Generic name	Trade name	Chemical form	Administration	Duration of action
Dydrogesterone	Duphaston Gynorest		Tablets for oral use	Short; 2 to 4 doses daily
Hydroxyprogesterone	Corlutin L.A. Delalutin Gesterol L.A. Hyproval-P.A.	Caproate	Oil solution for intramuscular injection	9 to 17 days
Medroxyprogesterone	Amen Depo-Provera Provera	Acetate	Aqueous suspension for intramuscular injection Tablets for oral use	Doses repeated daily
Megestrol	Megace	Acetate	Tablets for oral use	Short; 4 doses daily
Norethindrone	Norlutin		Tablets for oral use	Doses repeated daily
	Norlutate	Acetate	Tablets for oral use	Doses repeated daily
Progesterone	Gesterol Lipo-Lutin Profac-O Progelan		Aqueous suspension or oil solution for intramuscular injection	Doses repeated daily

no place in medical practice. Some of the preparations are sold for external use as creams and lotions to prevent aging of the skin. There is no evidence that beneficial effects are produced by such uses of estrogens.

The most important estrogen combinations are those with progestins, which are discussed in the section on oral contraceptive drugs. These combinations are available with so many different ratios of estrogen to progestin that adjustment for individual patient needs is possible.

Progestins

Absorption and excretion. Progestins available for use medically include the natural steroid hormone progesterone as well as synthetic derivatives of that compound (Table 37-4). Although progesterone itself is not useful orally, many of the derivatives are conveniently and effectively administered by that route. Injections of progesterone are painful and may produce local inflammation.

Progesterone and other progestins are rapidly metabolized by the liver and eliminated in the urine.

Toxicity. Adverse reactions to the progestins may involve a number of organ systems in addition to the organs of reproduction. Some of these reactions are similar to those seen with estrogens: edema, breast tenderness and swelling, gastrointestinal disturbances, depression, and weight change. Other reactions include changes in menstrual blood flow, midcycle spotting or breakthrough bleeding, cholestatic jaundice, and rashes. Many of the progestins have some androgenic activity and may cause masculinization of female fetuses. Because of this danger, the use of progestins as a test for pregnancy is no longer recommended. Patients with a history of thromboembolic disorders or thrombophlebitis should not be treated with progestins.

Uses. Progestins are used clinically for their effects on the endometrium. High doses of progestins suppress bleeding of the endometrium, and withdrawal of the drug induces sloughing of the tissue. Lower doses of progestins induce changes in the endometrium and cervical mucus that prevent pregnancy. This use of progestins is discussed in the section on pharmacological contraception.

TABLE 37-5. Agents used to increase female fertility

Generic name	Trade name	Classification	Mechanism of action	Administration
Clomiphene citrate	Clomid	Nonsteroid stimulator of ovulation	Ovulation is stimulated, probably by hypothalamic mechanisms.	Tablets for oral use
Human chorionic gonadotropin (HCG)	Antruitrin-S A.P.L. Follutein	Placental hormone related to LH	Ovulation is stimulated by an action resembling that of LH.	Intramuscular injection
Menotropins	Pergonal	Human menopausal gonadotropins (urinary)	FSH and LH in the preparations stimulate the ovary	Intramuscular injection

■ Agents that restore female fertility

Loss of fertility in a woman may be a result of any one of a large number of causes. Therapy depends in part on evaluating the reason for the infertility. In some women the pituitary and the ovary seem normal, but the proper stimulus to activate follicular development is not transmitted. For these women, *clomiphene citrate* may be effective (Table 37-5). This drug seems to activate the pituitary by hypothalamic mechanisms, and ovarian stimulation is thereby achieved. Stimulation of several follicles in the ovaries may be induced by clomiphene, and multiple births have occurred.

In women whose pituitary is unable to supply sufficient gonadotropins to properly stimulate the ovary, infertility may also occur. For these women, *menotropins* may be prescribed. This mixture of compounds extracted from the urine of postmenopausal women contains FSH and LH in approximately equal amounts. When LH action alone is required, *HCG* may be prescribed. HCG is chemically related to LH and possesses many of the same physiological actions, including the ability to stimulate ovulation.

Bromocriptine is a chemical relative of the ergot alkaloids, which are used as oxytocin agents. Bromocriptine, however, is clinically useful because of its ability to inhibit prolactin secretion. Bromocriptine is approved in the United States to control galactorrhea (spontaneous milk production) caused by excessive prolactin secretion, usually from functional tumors. Amenorrhea (no menstrual cycles) and infertility are also produced when prolactin secretion is excessive. Bromocriptine suppression of prolactin secretion reverses these symptoms, and fertility becomes possible. The use of bromocriptine specifically to restore fertility is not yet officially approved in the United States.

■ Pharmacological contraception

Reversible sterility induced by pharmacological agents has been a possibility since the late 1950's when the oral contraceptive agents became available. The agents in use today contain either a combination of estrogen and a progestin or a progestin alone. The effectiveness of these agents is very high. Most reports give estimates of less than 1 failure in 200 woman years of use for the combined estrogen-progestin agents. This pregnancy rate is in contrast to rates of 1 failure per 25 to 50 woman years for mechanical devices such as IUDS, diaphragms, and condoms.

The estrogen-progestin combinations are known to suppress ovulation, and it was on this basis that they were first suggested as contraceptives. In addition, these drugs induce changes in the cervical mucus, which makes it difficult for sperm to enter the uterus. Changes also occur in the endometrium that make implantation difficult even if fertilization occurs. The preparations containing progestins alone alter the cervical mucus and the endometrium in the same manner as the combination products, but they do not suppress ovulation. The effectiveness of the agents containing only progestins is less than that of the combined preparations.

To achieve contraception and to mimic the normal menstrual cycle, the oral contraceptives are usually taken for 20 or 21 consecutive days. The increased estrogen and progestin levels produced suppress the hypothalamus and the pituitary so that no LH is released at the time when ovulation would normally occur. This is the mechanism by which ovulation is suppressed. During the 7 days when hormones are not administered, the endometrium involutes and sloughs off, primarily as a result of loss of progestin activity. This withdrawal period prevents excessive proliferation of the endometrium.

The progestins used in oral contraceptives are synthetic derivatives of natural compounds. Progesterone, a natural progestin, is used in an intrauterine device. This device is not to be confused with the more common

TABLE 37-6. Oral contraceptives

Progestin	Estrogen	Progestin/ estrogen ratio	Trade name
Ethynodiol diacetate	Mestranol	1 mg:100 μg	Ovulen
	Ethinyl estradiol	1 mg:50 μg	Demulen
Norethindrone	Mestranol	10 mg:60 μg	Norinyl
		2 mg:100 μg	Ortho-Novum
		1 mg:80 μg	
		1 mg:50 μg	
	Ethinyl estradiol	1 mg:50 μg	Brevicon
		0.5 mg:35 μg	Modicon
		0.4 mg:35 μg	Ovcon
Norethindrone acetate	Ethinyl estradiol	2.5 mg:50 μg	Loestrin
		1.5 mg:30 μg	Norlestrin
		1.0 mg:50 μg	Zorane
		1.0 mg:20 μg	
Norethynodrel	Mestranol	9.85 mg:150 μg	Enovid
		5.0 mg:75μg	
		2.5 mg:100 μg	
Norgestrel	Ethinyl estradiol	0.5 mg:50 μg	Lo/Ovral
		0.3 mg:30 μg	Ovral
Norethindrone	None	0.35 mg	Micronor Nor-QD
Norgestrel	None	0.075 mg	Ovrette

intrauterine devices (IUDs) that contain no hormonal agents. The progesterone-releasing IUD was developed to administer the fertility-controlling drug directly to the target tissue. The very small amounts of progesterone released are retained within the reproductive tract rather than being systemically absorbed. The effectiveness of this device is dependent both on the purely mechanical effects of the IUD and on the pharmacological effects of the progesterone.

Toxicity. The oral contraceptive agents available in the United States are shown in Table 37-6. Some of these agents, such as Enovid and Ovulen, are considered to be estrogen dominant. Estrogen excess in a patient may be associated with nausea, bloating, breast fullness, edema, hypertension, and cervical discharges. These symptoms may suggest that the patient be tried on a preparation with less estrogen. Agents such as Loestrin, Ovral, and Lo/Ovral are predominantly progestin-like in their action. Progestin excess in a patient taking oral contraceptives may produce hair loss, hirsutism, oily scalp, acne, increased appetite and weight gain, tiredness and depression, breast regression, and reduced menstrual blood flow. By changing the contraceptive preparation prescribed, the physician may finally be able to achieve the proper balance of estrogen and progestin so that the adverse effects listed are minimized.

Oral contraceptives are among the most widely used drugs today. Throughout the world, 50 million or more women rely on these agents for the prevention of pregnancy. The oral contraceptives are without doubt highly effective, but questions about the safety of these agents have been raised. In particular, the incidence of unexpected serious or fatal medical conditions has been studied in the relatively healthy, normal women who receive oral contraceptives. Risk of certain serious medical conditions can now be shown to be increased in oral contraceptive users when they are compared to similar women who do not take these drugs (Table 37-7).

As with any medication, the oral contraceptives must be considered in terms of the risk-to-benefit ratio. Of first importance may be how much value the patient places on almost complete protection against unwanted pregnancy. Women who desire this high level of control should next consider the safety factors of the medication. Many of the dangerous complications, such as stroke and thromboembolitic diseases, are rare even among oral contraceptives users. The risk of these complications is greater than the risk among nonusers of oral contraceptives, but much lower than the risk of these complications during pregnancy. Also to be considered are the other predisposing risk factors, such as smoking, obesity, and hypertension. The combination of oral contra-

TABLE 37-7. Adverse reactions noted in users of oral contraceptives

Adverse reaction	Relation to oral contraceptives	Comments
Thromboembolitic diseases	Risk increased 2- to 7-fold in users over nonusers. Incidence about 100/100,000 woman years; fatalities 2/100,000 woman years.	Obesity, family history of thromboembolitic disorders, immobility, and/or group A blood type may increase risk. Group O blood type women have lower risk. May be related to estrogen dosage.
Cerebrovascular disease		
Thrombotic stroke	Risk increased 3.1 to 6-fold. Incidence about 25/100,000 woman years; fatalities 0.5/100,000 woman years.	Hypertension increases the risk.
Hemorrhagic stroke	Risk increased at least 2-fold. Incidence about 10/100,000 woman years.	Hypertension and heavy smoking are strong risk factors.
Coronary artery disease	Actual increased risk with pill use alone is not established.	Synergistic increase in risk if oral contraceptives are used by heavy smokers.
Hypertension	Between 1% and 5% of patients show an increase in blood pressure. Clinical hypertension is more rare.	Risk is increased by age, obesity, and parity.
Gallbladder disease	Risk increased an estimated 2-fold.	Risk may be related to the dose of progestin.
Liver disease	20% to 50% of patients show reduced liver function. Incidence 10/100,000 woman years for jaundice. Tumors are exceedingly rare.	Reversible. Dangerous for patients with preexisting liver disease (hepatitis, cholestasis). Liver tumors may be related specifically to mestranol.
Carbohydrate metabolism	Most patients show reduced glucose tolerance	Important only in prediabetics who may become insulin dependent.
Lipid metabolism	Most patients have increased serum triglyceride levels.	Reversible effect; relationship to coronary artery disease in these patients is unknown.
Chloasma	3% to 4% of patients treated.	Increased sensitivity to sunlight also occurs. Reversible.
Headaches	Variable reports with no clear conclusion.	Migraines and headaches have been reported to be increased, decreased, or unchanged. Appearance of chronic headache may presage stroke.
Visual disturbances	Often mentioned but not yet causally linked to oral contraceptive use.	Temporary blindness, blind spots, and changes in field of vision have been mentioned.
Emotional state	Variable reports with no clear conclusion.	No evidence that oral contraceptives significantly increase depression.
Endometrial cancer	No increased risk when combined estrogen-progestin agents used.	Risk is increased by estrogens alone but reduced by progestins.
Cervical cancer	No relationship established.	Frequency of coitus and number of sexual partners more important risk factors.
Breast cancer	No relationship established.	Benign breast tumors are actually improved.
Permanent infertility	No relationship established.	Most patients quickly return to fertility when oral contraceptives are discontinued.
Outcome of later pregnancies	No increased risk to mother or fetus has been demonstrated.	Data are for pregnancies begun after oral contraceptives have been discontinued.

ceptives with these conditions leads to unacceptable risk for many patients. All women receiving oral contraceptives should be urged to stop smoking.

Some medical conditions are actually improved or the symptoms are ameliorated by oral contraceptives. Many patients report a reduction in menstrual disorders and especially in dysmenorrhea. Menstrual blood flow is usually reduced, and anemia is prevented or lessened in many women. Benign breast tumors are improved in a time-dependent fashion by oral contraceptive therapy.

Current medical information suggests that oral contraceptives are safe drugs when used in relatively young women in whom other risk factors are minimized. The most prudent course of action seems to be to carefully select patients before administering oral contraceptives. Women with a history of hypertension or thromboembolitic diseases probably should not receive the drugs. Women who elect to receive oral contraceptives should be given thorough physical examinations yearly. The dose of estrogen and progestin should be the lowest dose that achieves contraception and prevents unwanted side effects such as breakthrough bleeding. Careful history taking may reveal symptoms that the patient has not linked to oral contraceptive use. Migraine headaches, dizziness, and visual disturbances are frequently not related by the patient to oral contraceptive use and may not be mentioned spontaneously. However, breakthrough bleeding, excessive cervical mucus formation, breast tenderness, and other changes in the reproductive tract are usually quickly connected to oral contraceptive use by the patient. These latter symptoms are usually more annoying than serious. However, severe headaches or visual disturbances are frequently early signs of impending stroke, and such symptoms may be sufficient cause to discontinue the medications.

■ DRUGS USED DURING CHILDBIRTH AND POSTPARTUM CARE

■ Physiology of childbirth

To understand the pharmacological management of labor and delivery, an understanding of the physiological processes involved is necessary. During stage I of parturition, uterine contractions begin to increase in frequency and intensity and the cervix begins to dilate. In stage II, uterine contractions occur at the rate of about 1 every 2 minutes. The cervix is fully dilated, and the uterine contractions bring about the delivery of the infant. During stage III labor, the frequency of the contractions decreases, and the placenta separates from the uterus and is expelled. Uterine contractions continue for a period of hours to days, with the frequency and intensity of the contractions diminishing with time.

When contractions occur during labor and delivery, the myometrium compresses the major blood vessels supplying oxygen to the infant. The result is that during a contraction, the baby is relatively anoxic. When the uterus relaxes between contractions, this condition is quickly rectified. If the uterus is overstimulated and fails to relax sufficiently between contractions, the result may be prolonged fetal anoxia that may harm the infant. Induction of labor with one of the oxytocic drugs carries with it the risk of producing this condition. Therefore all patients in whom labor is being induced should receive continuous care, and fetal monitoring should be done where possible. Oxytocin is the drug of choice to induce or stimulate labor, since that drug seems to allow the uterus to relax between contractions. The ergot alkaloids and other oxytocic drugs tend to increase the overall tone of the myometrium as well as increase the strength of contraction and therefore have a greater risk of producing fetal anoxia.

The uterine contractions that occur after delivery have two beneficial effects on the mother. First, they are responsible for the expulsion of the afterbirth and produce a general cleansing of the uterus. Second, these contractions aid in controlling postpartum bleeding by clamping the vessels that were ruptured by the birth process. If bleeding is a problem at this stage, the physician may use one of the agents with a longer and more continuous action, such as one of the ergot alkaloids. The ergot alkaloid preparations are also the only oxytocic drugs that may be effectively administered orally.

■ Oxytocic drugs

Oxytocic drugs are those that induce contraction of the myometrium (Table 37-8). The drug class is named for the natural posterior pituitary hormone oxytocin. The uterus is relatively insensitive to the action of oxytocin until labor has actually started. No clear role of oxytocin in regulating unassisted, normal labor has been established.

TABLE 37-8. Clinical summary of oxytocic drugs

Generic name	Trade name	Dosage and administration	Medical use	Comments
POSTERIOR PITUITARY HORMONE				
Oxytocin	Pitocin	INTRAVENOUS: 10 milliunits/ml infused at 1 to 2 milliunits/min, gradually increased up to about 10 milliunits/min.	Induction or stimulation of labor.	Stimulates uterine contraction with relaxation between contractions. Fetal or maternal cardiac arrhythmias, acute hypertension, nausea, and water intoxication may occur. Overdose may produce uterine hypertonicity with fetal and/or maternal injury.
		INTRAVENOUS: 20 to 40 milliunits/ml infused at 40 milliunits/min.	Control of uterine atony and/or bleeding.	As above.
		INTRAMUSCULAR: 3 to 10 units (0.3 to 1 ml) postpartum.	Control of uterine atony and/or bleeding.	As above.
	Pitocin Citrate	BUCCAL: 200 units/30 min initially. Dose increased every hour up to 600 units/30 min.	Induction or stimulation of labor.	Variable absorption. Rapid termination when buccal tablet removed.
	Syntocinon	NASAL: 1 spray of 40 units/ml solution before nursing.	Aids in breast feeding by stimulating milk letdown.	Also causes nasal vasoconstriction. Onset of action is within 2 or 3 min, and duration of action is short.
ERGOT ALKALOIDS				
Ergonovine maleate	Ergotrate Maleate	ORAL: 0.2 to 0.4 mg 2 to 4 times daily for 2 days. INTRAMUSCULAR: 0.2 mg repeated in 2 to 4 hr if needed. INTRAVENOUS: 0.2 mg as emergency medication.	Control of postpartum bleeding.	May cause nausea and vomiting. Hypertensive episodes are especially likely when vasopressors or spinal anesthesia is also used.
Methylergonovine maleate	Methergine	ORAL, INTRAMUSCULAR, INTRAVENOUS: As for ergonovine maleate.	As for ergonovine maleate.	May cause nausea and vomiting, transient hypertension, headache, dizziness, palpitation, or chest pain.
PROSTAGLANDINS				
Dinoprost tromethamine	Prostin F2 alpha	INTRAUTERINE: 40 mg slowly infused. Second dose of 10 or 20 mg may be given 6 hr later if needed.	Abortion in second trimester.	Stimulates uterine contractions. Vasomotor disturbances, cardiac arrhythmias, hyperventilation, and chest pain are possible.
Dinoprostone	Prostin E2	VAGINAL: 20 mg suppositories inserted every 3 to 5 hr until abortion ensues.	Abortion in second trimester.	Stimulates uterine contractions. Gastrointestinal symptoms are common; cardiovascular symptoms are possible.

Another class of natural hormones, the *prostaglandins,* is involved in regulating myometrial activity. These derivatives of fatty acids are rapidly formed in their target tissues and very rapidly degraded without persisting in the bloodstream for any appreciable time. In the uterus these hormones induce very powerful myometrial contractions. Recent research has suggested that prostaglandins, especially the E and F series (PGE_2 and $PGF_{2\alpha}$), may play a role in the natural induction of labor. Prostaglandin levels rise in the amniotic fluid and other pelvic reproductive tissues as term draws near. This increasing concentration of prostaglandins has been suggested to be the stimulus causing Braxton-Hicks contractions, the mild myometrial contractions occurring during the last few weeks of pregnancy.

The prostaglandins have been investigated for use in the induction of labor. Although more research remains to be done, the results suggest that these drugs elevate uterine muscle tone and may be dangerous for the infant. The drugs are potent stimulators of the myometrium, however, and have been successfully used to produce abortion during the second trimester of pregnancy when the uterus is resistant to oxytocin. Systemic side effects of these drugs can be serious, and the most comfortable and safest route of administration may well be by transabdominal instillation into the amniotic fluid. Administered in this fashion, the drug stays primarily within the uterus and persists in action for some hours.

Compounds other than oxytocin and prostaglandins have been discovered to be powerful oxytocics. One of the most clinically useful of these types of drugs are the *ergot alkaloid* derivatives (Table 37-8). The ergot alkaloids are compounds produced by fungal contaminants of rye and other cereal grains. These fungal products have been known as poisons since the Middle Ages when it was noted that people who ate grain contaminated with this fungus suffered from dry gangrene. This extreme reaction is caused by the potent vasoconstrictive effect of the ergot alkaloids. Blood flow to the limbs may be so severely reduced that the tissues die and the limbs eventually fall away with little or no bleeding produced. In addition, pregnant women who ate the affected grain were noted to enter an abrupt and devastating labor that expelled fetuses at any stage of development. Today it is not this crude mixture of ergot alkaloids that is useful in the clinic but rather derivatives of one or another of the compounds.

■ Uterine relaxants

Specific uterine relaxation in cases of hypertonicity or premature labor is not yet possible. Nevertheless, several types of compounds will produce uterine relaxation along with other reactions. For example, premature labor is sometimes treated with agents that stimulate beta-2 adrenergic receptors, since stimulation of these receptors in the uterus causes relaxation of the myometrium. Agonists of beta-2 adrenergic receptors cause side effects throughout the body, however, as a result of beta stimulation in other tissues.

The best beta-2 adrenergic agonist for use in halting premature labor at present appears to be ritodrine. This new agent effectively relaxes the myometrium but also has effects on the peripheral vasculature and other tissues. The heart is sensitive to stimulation with ritodrine, suggesting that the drug is also an agonist with some activity on beta-1 adrenergic receptors. Ritodrine is usually administered intravenously when premature labor begins. When contractions have been controlled for 12 to 24 hours, the patient may be started on oral ritodrine, and the intravenous infusion may be discontinued. The major side effects noted with this drug have been heart palpitations, nausea, vomiting, trembling, flushing, and headache. These effects appear transient and rarely cause termination of therapy. Patients should be observed for undue tachycardia or signs of cardiac distress. The fetal heart is also stimulated by ritodrine. Ritodrine increases the work load of the mother's heart and is contraindicated in patients with preexisting cardiac disease. The primary indication for ritodrine is to halt spontaneous labor when it appears after the twentieth week of pregnancy and before the thirty-sixth week of pregnancy. Spontaneous labor beginning before the twentieth week of pregnancy is frequently associated with a defective fetus and is not usually interrupted.

Central nervous system depressants may halt premature labor. Ethanol, which in addition to being a central nervous system depressant is also an inhibitor of oxytocin release, has been used to halt premature labor successfully. The levels required to relax the uterus are sufficient to produce acute alcohol intoxication. Controlled clinical trials have suggested ritodrine is more effective and less toxic.

General anesthetics may also relax the uterus. Ether has been used in the past for this purpose, although halothane is the more widely used agent today. In addition to central nervous system effects, these agents may act directly on the myometrium and may also slow catecholamine release from the adrenal gland, thereby reducing endogenous stimulators of myometrial activity.

Progesterone is the natural steroidal compound that normally functions in the body as a uterine relaxant. However, the use of this compound or one of the other progestins is not recommended in cases of uterine hypertonicity during delivery, since the hormone may not reach the uterus in sufficient quantities to relax the uterus quickly and effectively. Use of progesterone during earlier stages of pregnancy is not recommended because progesterone may have undesirable effects on the developing fetus.

■ THE NURSING PROCESS

■ Assessment

Drugs acting on the female reproductive system are used as replacement therapy, to cause or inhibit ovulation and conception, to aid in pregnancy or labor, and to treat hormonally sensitive tumors. The nurse should obtain a complete patient assessment with a focus on the problem being addressed by the drug. Include in the data base the temperature, pulse, respiration, blood pressure, weight, description of the menstrual cycle in the female, assessment of breasts (male and female), and condition of skin. In the pregnant woman a history of previous pregnancies and deliveries and assessment of the fetus should be done (e.g., fetal heart tones, position).

■ Management

Because of controversies surrounding the use of some of these drugs, the patient should be fully informed of possible side effects and benefits before therapy is begun. The nurse should continue to monitor the pulse, blood pressure, and weight. The patient activities needed to help ensure success should be explained in detail. For example, alternate birth control measures during the first month of birth control pill therapy, temperature charts to monitor possible ovulation, and saving urine specimens to measure hormone or drug excretion need thorough explanation. With oxytocics, the mother and fetus should be monitored closely, and the use of an intravenous infusion monitoring device should be considered. The calcium levels in the patient being treated for cancer should be followed. Except for the oxytocics, most of these drugs will be taken on an outpatient basis, and side effects will not occur until well into the course of therapy.

■ Evaluation

Success of drug therapy occurs if the desired outcome is seen and the patient has no or few side effects. Thus if pregnancy is prevented and the woman has no side effects of drug therapy, then therapy with birth control pills has been successful. Note, though, that with long-term drug therapy, the possibility of side effects is always present.

Before discharge the patient should be able to explain why and how to take the drug, possible side effects that might occur, which side effects require immediate medical attention, and the risks associated with therapy.

■ PATIENT CARE IMPLICATIONS

Estrogens, progestins, or combinations, including birth control pills

1. Encourage patients receiving these drugs to continue with regular health care follow-up, to take their medications only as ordered, and to report any unexplained signs or symptoms.
2. Refer to Table 37-7. Question women carefully for family or patient history of obesity, cardiovascular disease, thromboembolic disease, hypertension, and diabetes. Patients should stop smoking when taking estrogens, progestins, or combinations of these two.
3. Monitor the patient's weight weekly and blood pressure at regular intervals. Patients with conditions that can be aggravated by fluid retention should be especially careful when taking these medications. Use of diuretics and/or a sodium-restricted diet may help. Patients with a history of seizures may find that fluid restriction increases the incidence of seizures.
4. Patients with diabetes mellitus may find that their glucose balance is altered while taking these drugs and may require changes in insulin dosage.
5. Side effects may include nausea or vomiting, but these often subside after 1 to 2 months of therapy.
6. As discussed in the text, visual changes can occur. Teach the patient to report immediately any headaches, blurring, diplopia, loss of vision, or other visual problems. Patients wearing corrective lenses may find that reexamination is needed with a change in refraction required.

7. Teach the patient to report any change in skin color or color of sclera, because these may indicate liver damage.
8. The effects of these hormonal agents on the body continue for several months, even after therapy has been discontinued. Teach patients to report to all physicians, pathologists, and dentists that they are or have been on some form of hormonal therapy or birth control pills.
9. Taking estrogens, progestins, or birth control pills predisposes to candidal vaginal infections. Instruct the patient to report vaginal discharge or itching.
10. Overdosage with vaginal creams and suppositories is possible. Instruct patients to use these forms of medications only as directed and to report any unanticipated signs or symptoms.
11. Estrogens can be used to treat prostate cancer and some forms of breast cancer. In the male, estrogen therapy may produce gynecomastia, reduced libido, cessation of spermatogenesis, and testicular atrophy. Reassure the male that female characteristics will usually disappear after therapy is stopped. The cancer patient with metastasis to bone may develop severe hypercalcemia after starting estrogen therapy. Instruct the patient to report the appearance of the following symptoms: thirst, polyuria, anorexia, nausea, vomiting, constipation, and lethargy. Coma may eventually develop. In some instances it may be necessary to stop estrogen therapy, at least temporarily, to lower the concentration of calcium in the blood.
12. Because of the increased incidence of thrombophlebitis associated with estrogens and progestins, women with a history of thromboembolic disorders should not take these drugs. In addition, patients should be instructed to report leg pain, sudden onset of chest pain, shortness of breath, coughing up blood, headache, dizziness, changes in vision or speech, or weakness or numbness of an arm or leg.
13. Taking estrogen, whether alone or in combination, will usually result in clearing of acne, although initially the acne may worsen. In rare individuals, estrogens will cause acne to worsen. After discontinuing estrogen therapy, some women may experience several months of rebound worsening of acne.
14. The effects of progestins may be reduced when the patient is taking phenobarbital or phenylbutazone or increased when the patient is also taking phenothiazines. The effects of estrogen may be reduced when the patient is also taking rifampin, barbiturates, phenylbutazone, phenytoin, or ampicillin.
15. Estrogen therapy, like birth control pills, is often cyclic to prevent continuous hormonal stimulation of the body. The schedule is frequently to take the medication for 3 weeks and stop for 1 week, or to take the estrogen for the first 21 days of the month and to omit the medication for the rest of the month, then resume the estrogen on the first of each month. Before discharging the patient, ascertain that she can correctly repeat her dosage schedule.
16. Estrogen therapy has been associated with a reported increased incidence of gallbladder disease and benign liver tumors. The patient should report any persistent or unexplained abdominal discomfort.
17. If a single birth control pill is missed, the patient should take the missed dose as soon as she remembers. If 2 consecutive pills are missed, the patient should double up on each of the next 2 days, then resume her regular schedule but use additional birth control measures until she completes that cycle. If 3 or more consecutive tablets are missed, the patient should stop the pills for 7 days after the first missed tablet, then begin a new cycle of tablets. She should also use additional contraceptive measures from the time the missed tablets are noticed until 7 days after the new course of therapy is started.
18. Birth control pills, estrogens, and progestins are all contraindicated during pregnancy. If the patient misses two consecutive periods while on birth control pills, she should stop the pills and see her physician to rule out pregnancy.
19. Anovulation and amenorrhea may persist for as long as 6 months after birth control therapy has been discontinued.
20. If a woman discontinues birth control tablets for the purpose of becoming pregnant, it has been recommended that she use an alternate form of birth control for 2 months after stopping the pills to ensure more complete excretion of the hormonal agents before conceiving and thus reduce the potential effects of the medications on the fetus.
21. The "mini-pill," the oral contraceptive containing only progestins, should be taken daily, all year long, even if the patient is menstruating.
22. If elective surgery is planned, it may be desirable to stop birth control pills at least a month before surgery. Check with the physician.
23. Some progestins are prescribed to treat hormonal imbalance and not to prevent ovulation. Instruct the patient that conception can occur. It is possible to accurately monitor basal body temperature to help determine ovulation in cases of amenorrhea being treated with progestins.
24. Some estrogen preparations are available as pellets for subcutaneous implantation. When administered via this route, they are effective for about 3 months. For a discussion of this route of administration, see

the patient care implications section in Chapter 38.

25. Oil-based solutions may be cloudy if they have been stored in the refrigerator. Let the preparation warm to room temperature before administering; it should then be clear. For a discussion of intramuscular administration of oil-based preparations see the patient care implications section in chapter 34 under the discussion of vasopressin tannate in oil.
26. Roll vials of aqueous suspensions between both hands for several minutes before administering to resuspend the medication.
27. Estradurin may be very uncomfortable when administered intramuscularly; concomitant use of a local anesthetic may be indicated. See literature supplied by the manufacturer and check with the physician.

Human chorionic gonadotropin (HCG)

1. Side effects include headache, depression, edema, gynecomastia, irritability, precocious puberty in young males, and pain at the injection site. Severe ovarian hyperstimulation can require hospitalization.
2. When a couple is using HCG for ovulatory stimulation, they should be instructed to monitor the woman's basal body temperature, character of vaginal secretions, or collect 24-hour urine specimens for urinary estrogen excretion. The couple should have sexual intercourse daily or every other day, beginning on the day before HCG is administered until one or more of the parameters just listed indicates that ovulation has occurred.
3. HCG is used to treat cryptorchidism in boys; if there is no anatomical obstruction, administration of HCG will cause the testes to descend.
4. The usual dilution of HCG is 1000 units/ml; the average dose is 5000 to 10,000 units IM. Divide the dose so that no volume larger than 5 ml is administered per injection site. The drug should be given intramuscularly.

Clomiphene

1. Side effects include hot flashes, breast tenderness and engorgement, cyclic ovarian pain, and nausea, but these rarely require cessation of therapy and subside after the drug is discontinued. If visual problems occur, they should be reported immediately; the drug will usually be discontinued.
2. The dose is individualized for the patient. The usual starting dose is 25 to 50 mg per day, starting on the fifth day of the menstrual cycle and continuing for 5 days. The basal body temperature and other parameters are monitored to ascertain if ovulation occurs during that cycle. If ovulation has not occurred and the patient has suffered no serious side effects, the dose is increased monthly. The usual daily dose rarely exceeds 100 mg, although some patients require doses as high as 150 to 200 mg per day.
3. The incidence of multiple births may be as high as 7% to 10%.

Menotropins

1. Side effects caused by ovarian stimulation result in ovarian enlargement, abdominal discomfort, flatulence, nausea, vomiting, and diarrhea. Severe ovarian stimulation can result in increased weight, ascites, pleural effusion, oliguria, and hypotension, and may require hospitalization. If significant ovarian stimulation occurs, the couple should refrain from intercourse during that cycle and contact the physician.
2. Menotropins are rarely given alone because they stimulate only follicular growth and maturation; usually HCG is also administered. The couple should be informed that the incidence of multiple births may be as high as 17% to 53%. An increased incidence of abortion has also been reported.
3. When menotropins are administered, monitoring of urinary estrogen secretion is often done. If the 24-hour level of urinary estrogen exceeds 150 μg, the drug is withheld. The actual dose is based on individual response. For additional information see the leaflet supplied by the manufacturer.

Danazol

1. Danazol, used to treat endometriosis, induces atrophy of the endometrium and amenorrhea; when the drug is stopped, ovulation and menstruation usually begin again within a month. The drug is a weak androgen with no estrogenic activity.
2. Side effects include weight gain, reduction in breast size, acne, hirsutism, severe fluid retention, and monilial vaginitis.
3. The usual course of therapy is for 6 months or longer. The endometriosis tends to recur after therapy is completed, but it may take years for this to occur.
4. This medication is expensive. A 200 mg dose costs around $1, and the average daily dose is 800 mg.

Oxytocics

1. Oxytocic drugs should be used only in the hospital or where a physician is immediately available.
2. Oxytocic drugs are contraindicated in a variety of situations, including any time that hyperstimulation of the uterus would be dangerous, for example, the first stage of labor, malpresentation of the fetus, previous cesarean section or uterine surgery, fetal distress, or when hypertension is contraindicated, for example, severe toxemia, preexisting hypertension, or cardiovascular disease.

3. Monitor the mother's blood pressure and the fetal pulse rate, and carry out electronic fetal monitoring when possible during intravenous oxytocic administration. Have available drugs to counteract a hypertensive crisis.
4. Buccal tablets are available for use, but the dose and rate of absorption are difficult to control.
5. The use of this drug for treatment of cystic breast disease is being investigated. For this problem, the daily dose is 200 to 400 mg. If treatment is successful, breast discomfort usually ceases 4 to 6 weeks after therapy is started. In the lower dose (200 mg) amenorrhea may not be produced, but it may appear at the higher doses. The drug should not be used during pregnancy. Additional information will become available as further research is done.

■ SUMMARY

The hormones involved in female reproduction are gonadotropin-releasing hormone (GnRH) from the hypothalamus; follicle-stimulating hormone (FSH), luteinizing hormone (LH), and prolactin from the anterior pituitary; and estrogens and progestins from the ovary. GnRH stimulates the release of FSH and LH from the pituitary. FSH stimulates estrogen production in the ovary. LH is the major signal for ovulation and progesterone production. Prolactin stimulates milk production in the breast. Estrogens cause development of the primary and secondary sexual characteristics of the female. Progestins maintain endometrial function during the last half of the menstrual cycle and during pregnancy. Human chorionic gonadotropin maintains production of progestins from the corpus luteum during early pregnancy. Oxytocin from the posterior pituitary stimulates uterine contractions in the late stages of labor and postpartum, and stimulates milk letdown in the breast.

Estrogens may be used in replacement therapy when estrogen production is low or absent. These drugs are also used in pharmacological doses for a variety of other conditions of the female reproductive tract. The natural estrogens are rapidly metabolized by the liver and are thus short-acting agents. The synthetic steroidal estrogens and the nonsteroidal estrogens are less readily metabolized and are therefore longer acting agents. Side effects of estrogens include overreactions of certain reproductive tissues, such as breast tenderness and endometrial proliferation. These drugs also cause nausea, vomiting, anorexia, malaise, irritability, water and salt retention, atherosclerosis, and hypertension.

Progestins are used in the clinic for their effects on the endometrium. Although progesterone, the naturally occurring compound, is not well absorbed orally, the synthetic derivatives are well absorbed. Progestins may cause edema, midcycle bleeding, and cholestatic jaundice and may increase the likelihood of thromboembolic disorders.

Female infertility of certain types can be reversed with pharmacological agents. Menotropins contain FSH and LH, which may restore fertility in a patient lacking normal pituitary mechanisms. Clomiphene citrate activates the pituitary by hypothalmic mechanisms, thereby ultimately stimulating the ovaries.

Temporary infertility can be induced with estrogen-progestin combinations or with progestins alone. The combination of agents suppresses LH and prevents ovulation. The agents containing only progestins do not block ovulation, but the progestins change the properties of the endometrium and cervix so that fertilization and implantation are impaired. The oral contraceptive agents may cause side effects such as those mentioned for estrogens and progestins. The risk of stroke and thromboembolitic disease is increased in patients using oral contraceptives, especially if the patient is obese or hypertensive or if the patient smokes.

Oxytocic drugs are used to speed delivery in an uncomplicated birth. These drugs must be used with care to prevent the excessive stimulation of uterine contractions that can cause anoxia in the fetus. Oxytocin is rapidly degraded and must be administered intravenously for best control. The ergot alkaloids may be used orally as well as parenterally and have a longer duration of action than does oxytocin. Prostaglandins also promote uterine contractions, but to date these drugs have been used primarily for producing abortions early in pregnancy when the uterus is resistant to oxytocin.

Uterine relaxation can be produced by stimulation of the beta-2 receptors of the uterine muscle, by central nervous system depressants, and by the direct action of progestins. Ritodrine is an agonist for beta-2 receptors that is effective in halting premature labor. Ethanol has also been used for this purpose, since the drug is a central nervous system depressant and also inhibits the release of oxytocin. General anesthetics also produce a degree of uterine relaxation. Progesterone is the natural hormone believed to relax the uterus during pregnancy, but the pharmacodynamics of the drug do not allow it to be used as a pharmacological agent to halt labor.

■ STUDY QUESTIONS

1. What are the gonadotropic hormones?
2. How are the synthesis and release of FSH, LH, and prolactin regulated?
3. What are the major steroid hormones affecting the female reproductive tract?
4. What is the chemical precursor of estrogens and progestins?
5. What are the functions of estrogens during puberty?
6. What hormones regulate the process of ovulation in the mature female?
7. What effect do estrogens have on the endometrium in adult females?
8. What effects does progesterone have on the endometrium and myometrium?
9. What is the function of progesterone in pregnancy?
10. What is the role of human chorionic gonadotropin (HCG) in pregnancy?
11. How do the steroidal estrogens differ from the nonsteroidal estrogens in duration of action and route of excretion from the body?
12. What types of side effects and toxic reactions are seen with the chronic use of estrogens?
13. Why are many of the fixed combinations of estrogens with other compounds of limited medical use?
14. What side effects are characteristic of pharmacological use of the progestins?
15. What is the mechanism of action of clomiphene citrate and what is its medical use?
16. What hormones are contained within the preparations known as menotropins?
17. What is the mechanism of action of bromocriptine and how is this drug currently used in the clinic?
18. What agents are used to produce pharmacological contraception?
19. What is the mechanism of action of the oral contraceptive agents?
20. What toxic reactions have been associated with the oral contraceptive agents?
21. What side effects occur with use of the oral contraceptives?
22. How do oxytocin and prostaglandins differ in their ability to stimulate uterine contractions?
23. What are the ergot alkaloids?
24. How does the administration and effect of the ergot alkaloids differ from that of oxytocin?
25. What three classes of drugs have the potential for relaxing the musculature of the uterus?
26. What is the mechanism of action of ritodrine?
27. What is the mechanism of action of ethanol used to control premature labor?

■ SUGGESTED READINGS

Barden, T., Peter, J., and Merkatz, I.: Ritodrine hydrochloride: a betamimetic agent for use in pre-term labor. I. Pharmacology, clinical history, administration, side effects, and safety, Obstetrics and Gynecology **56:**1, 1980.

Blake, J.P., Collinge, D.A., McNulty, H., Leach, F.N., and Grant, E.J.: Drugs in pregnancy. Weighing the risks, Patient Care **14**(10): 22, 1980.

Bressler, R., and Durand, J.L.: A guide to prescribing oral contraceptives, Drug Therapy **9**(7):79, 1979.

Bressler, R., and Durand, J.L.: Oral contraceptive risks: a realistic appraisal, Drug Therapy **9**(10):81, 1979.

Decker, E.L., Greenblatt, R.B., and Nelson, R.M.: When oral contraceptives talk back, Patient Care **9:**104, Oct. 1, 1975.

Drug therapy and the nursing mother, Patient Care **14**(11):59, 1980.

Greenberger, P., and Patterson, R.: Safety of therapy for allergic symptoms during pregnancy, Annals of Internal Medicine **89:**234, 1978.

Hill, R.M., and Stern, L.: Drugs in pregnancy: effects on the fetus and newborn, Drugs **17:**182, 1979.

Jones, D.E.D., and Halbert, D.R.: Oral contraceptives: clinical problems and choices, American Family Physician **11**(10):115, 1975.

Judd, S.J.: Bromocriptine: a new advance. Rational therapy for some common disorders in obstetrics and gynaecology, Drugs **16:**167, 1978.

Kay, C.R.: Oral contraceptives—the clinical perspective. In Garattini, S., and Berendes, H.W., editors: Pharmacology of steroid contraceptive drugs, New York, 1977, Raven Press.

Krantz, K., Millerick, J.D., Rosenwaks, Z., and Seegar-Jones, G.: Quelling severe menstrual cramps, Patient Care **12:**198, April 15, 1978.

McQueen, E.G.: Hormonal steroid contraceptives: a further review of adverse reactions, Drugs **16:**322, 1978.

Nordin, B.E.C.: Treatment of postmenopausal osteoporosis, Drugs **18:**484, 1979.

Tyler, L.B., and Michaels, R.M.: Estrogen for contraception and menopause, Nurses' Drug Alert (special issue) **1:**169, Dec., 1977.

Weir, R.J.: When the pill causes a rise in blood pressure, Drugs **16:**522, 1978.

Yen, S.S.C.: Neuroendocrine regulation of the menstrual cycle, Hospital Practice **14**(3):83, 1979.

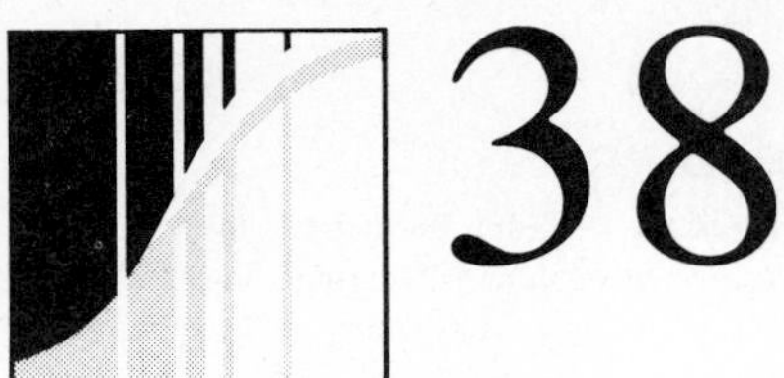

38 Drugs acting on the male reproductive system

The major reproductive hormones in men are steroids, which are synthesized primarily in the testes and to a lesser extent in the adrenal gland. Within the testes the status of interstitial or Leydig cells and the seminiferous tubular cells is most important for determining male sexual potential. The Leydig cells synthesize testosterone, the major masculinizing steroid hormone. The seminiferous tubules contain the germ cells that in the adult male produce functional sperm. The endocrine control of male sexual development and function, the actions of natural male hormones, and the clinical uses of synthetic and natural drugs acting on the male reproductive system are discussed in this chapter.

■ PITUITARY REGULATION OF REPRODUCTIVE POTENTIAL IN THE MALE

In the adult male sexual function is dependent on the proper interaction of the hypothalamus, anterior pituitary, and the testes. Regulation of testicular function is by a negative feedback loop similar to others previously mentioned. The primary hormones in this cycle are testosterone from the testes, interstitial cell–stimulating hormone (ICSH; also called *luteinizing hormone* [*LH*]) and follicle cell–stimulating hormone (FSH) from the anterior pituitary and gonadotropin-releasing hormone (GnRH; also called LHRH, LHRF, and FSH-RH) from the hypothalamus. When testosterone levels in the blood are low, GnRH is released from the hypothalamus to enter the anterior pituitary through the portal venous system. Under the influence of GnRH, both ICSH and FSH are released from the pituitary gland into the general circulation where they may act on testicular tissues.

The action of these regulatory hormones is slightly different during the three stages of life in which they act. During fetal development Leydig cells develop in the embryonic testis as a result of stimulation with the maternal hormone, human chorionic gonadotropin (HCG). These embryonic cells produce the small amounts of testosterone that are necessary for the development of the male external genitalia; without testosterone, genetically male infants will be born with female genitalia. After birth these Leydig cells regress, since the stimulus of HCG is no longer available.

The second period of life when these regulatory processes are most important is during puberty. In childhood very low concentrations of gonadotropins are found in the blood. With the onset of puberty the pituitary gland begins to synthesize and release greater quantities of the gonadotropins ICSH and FSH. The target organ for ICSH in the male is the Leydig cell where ICSH stimulates testosterone production. FSH acts directly on the cells of the seminiferous tubule and associated cells to prepare that tissue for spermatogenesis. This process cannot be completed unless testosterone from the Leydig cells is also present. With both FSH and testosterone acting on the seminiferous tubules, mature sperm can be produced. Testosterone acts not only within the testes but also throughout the body at this stage of life. These actions are discussed in the next section.

The third period of life to be considered is the period of sexual maturity. During this period ICSH continues to be important in the maintenance of sexual function, since ICSH is still required for the synthesis of testosterone. Testosterone is required for the maintenance of spermatogenesis.

A third hormone of the anterior pituitary is involved in male sexual function. This hormone is prolactin. The mechanisms by which prolactin release in males is regulated are not completely understood. However, men with pituitary tumors that secrete large quantities of prolactin often have decreased libidos and low concentrations of ICSH, FSH, and testosterone in their bloodstream. Prolactin seems to suppress synthesis and release of ICSH and FSH from the pituitary gland and may directly interfere with the actions of these hormones on the testes.

■ ANDROGENIC STEROIDS

■ The role of naturally occurring steroids

The major steroid affecting male sexual function is testosterone. This hormone is synthesized both in the Leydig cells of the testes and in the adrenal cortex. The action of testosterone in the testes has already been mentioned, but that is only part of the action of the hormone. Testosterone is a potent androgen (a substance that stimulates growth of the organs of the male reproductive tract). Testosterone is responsible for the enlargement and maturation of the penis, scrotum, seminal vesicles, prostate gland, and other accessory tissues of the male reproductive tract. These actions constitute the primary sexual effects on the male.

Testosterone is also the major hormone responsible for the development of the secondary sexual characteristics of the male. It is the increased testosterone level during puberty that stimulates the growth of facial hair as well as pubic hair and hair on chest and armpits. Sustained levels of testosterone trigger the onset of baldness in genetically predisposed males. The other dramatic changes that occur in the pubertal male are also related to the increased testosterone levels: lowering of the voice due to thickening of the vocal cords; stimulation of sebaceous glands of the skin; and stimulation of the libido. Psychologists working with primates other than man have even related aggression to high testosterone levels.

In addition to these primary and secondary sexual effects, testosterone also has profound effects on metabolism. Androgens are anabolic, that is, they stimulate synthetic rather than degradative processes. Testosterone increases nitrogen retention and protein formation, as well as increasing overall metabolic rate. This anabolic action is responsible for the increase in muscle mass associated with puberty and the distribution of this mass in the male pattern. In addition, calcium is retained and the size and strength of bone is enhanced. Blood-forming cells are also affected so that more red blood cells may be formed.

Although testosterone is the major circulating androgen in human males, it is not the only metabolically important androgen. There is evidence that testosterone is transformed within many target cells to dihydrotestosterone, which is a more potent androgen than testosterone itself. Small amounts of another androgen, androstenedione, may also affect various tissues of the body.

Both testosterone and androstenedione are close chemical relatives of the estrogens (steroid hormones that have feminizing effects). Some tissues such as brain, breast tissue, and the testes themselves can convert androgens to estrogens. Low estrogen concentrations are therefore found in the blood of normal adult males. These estrogens have no obvious influence on normal men, but under certain circumstances the concentrations of estrogen may increase and produce pathological signs such as breast development.

■ The use of androgens in replacement therapy

Androgenic drugs are primarily used in replacement therapy for patients who have reduced endogenous androgen production. For some patients the loss of androgens occurs early and prevents the normal changes of puberty. Androgen loss after puberty may cause a loss in libido or sexual desire or cause mild feminizing tendencies. Aging males produce less testosterone than younger men and may suffer from loss of sexual drive. Some older men suffer more severe symptoms suggestive of a male climateric or male menopause. All these conditions as well as others related to specific malfunctions of the male sexual organs may be treated with testosterone or one of the other androgenic compounds. For these patients with reduced natural testosterone production, this treatment constitutes replacement therapy.

Certain forms of impotence and feminization in the male do not respond well to replacement therapy with androgenic steroids. One type of patient unresponsive to androgens has very high blood levels of prolactin. As noted earlier, prolactin may interfere with the production and function of ICSH and FSH, lowering testosterone production. Bromocriptine, a drug that blocks prolactin synthesis, lowers prolactin levels in these patients, increases testosterone as well as ICSH and FSH levels, and restores sexual potence. Bromocriptine is available in the United States but officially is recommended only for the control of galactorrhea in females (Chapter 37).

Testosterone in its natural form is not water soluble and is therefore used as an aqueous suspension suitable only for intramuscular injection (Table 38-1). In this form the drug has a short duration of action and produces somewhat erratic clinical responses. Testosterone can be absorbed from the gastrointestinal tract. However, this route of administration does not produce clinically useful testosterone concentrations in the bloodstream, since the steroid absorbed from the intestine passes directly into the portal circulation and enters the liver before it circulates to the rest of the body. The liver is capable of very rapidly inactivating testosterone by converting it to a glucuronide or to sulfated derivatives. For long-term replacement therapy, pellets of free testosterone can be implanted subcutaneously. These pellets slowly release testosterone into the circulation over a period of several months. Although these pellets are convenient for the patient, they do result in less flexible control of the symptoms than can be achieved with more frequent injections.

Testosterone esters are much more useful than tes-

TABLE 38-1. Clinical summary of androgens

Generic name	Trade name	Drug form and dosage	Duration of action	Major clinical uses	Adverse reactions
NATURAL HORMONE					
Testosterone	Histerone Malogen Neo-Hombreol-F Testaqua Testoject	INTRAMUSCULAR: *Adults*—aqueous suspension for intramuscular use only. Doses range from 25 to 200 mg.	Relatively short. Doses must be repeated 2 to 5 times per week.	Replacement therapy in androgen deficiency (male climacteric, eunuchism, certain types of impotence). Relieve postpartum breast engorgement (3 to 4 days of therapy).	Masculinization in females. Precocious sexual development and premature closure of the epiphyses in children. Excessive sexual stimulation (short-term) or inhibition of testicular function (long-term) in males.
	Oreton	SUBCUTANEOUS: *Adults*—pellet for implantation, 150 to 450 mg.	3 to 4 months due to slow absorption.	Replacement therapy in androgen deficiency (male climacteric, eunuchism, impotence of certain types).	As for testosterone, aqueous suspension.
TESTOSTERONE ESTERS					
Testosterone enanthate	Delatestryl Span-Test Testate	INTRAMUSCULAR: *Adults*—oil solution for deep injection into gluteal muscle, 100-400 mg.	3 to 4 weeks.	As for testosterone cypionate.	As for testosterone, aqueous suspension.
Testosterone cypionate	Depo-Testosterone Duratest Malogen CYP	INTRAMUSCULAR: *Adults*—oil solution for deep injection into gluteal muscle, 100 to 400 mg.	3 to 4 weeks.	Replacement therapy in androgen deficiency (male climacteric, eunuchism, castration, oligospermia).	As for testosterone, aqueous suspension.
Testosterone propionate	Malotrone-P Neo-Hombreol	INTRAMUSCULAR: *Adults*—oil suspension for intramuscular use only. Doses range from 25 to 100 mg.	Relatively short. Doses must be repeated 2 to 5 times per week.	As for testosterone, aqueous suspension.	As for testosterone, aqueous suspension.

ORAL ANDROGENS					
Fluoxymesterone	Halotestin Ora-Testryl	ORAL: *Adults*—tablets for oral administration. 2 to 10 mg (male); 10 to 30 mg (female).	Short. Doses must be repeated daily.	Replacement therapy in androgen deficiency (eunuchism, male climacteric, certain forms of impotence). Relieve postpartum breast engorgement (4 to 5 days of therapy). Treatment of sensitive breast carcinomas.	As for testosterone, aqueous suspension. Nausea and vomiting, diarrhea, peptic ulcer–like symptoms. May increase sensitivity to anticoagulants. Hepatotoxicity, including jaundice.
Methyltestosterone	Android Metandren Oreton Methyl Testred	ORAL: *Adults*—tablets or capsules. 10 to 40 mg (male); 80 to 200 mg (female).	Short. Doses must be repeated daily.	Replacement therapy in androgen deficiency (eunuchism, male climacteric, postpubertal cryptorchidism). Relieve postpartum breast engorgement (3 to 4 days of therapy). Treatment of sensitive breast carcinomas.	As for testosterone, aqueous suspension. Nausea and vomiting, diarrhea, peptic ulcer–like symptoms. May increase sensitivity to anticoagulants. Hepatotoxicity, including jaundice.
BUCCAL AGENTS					
Methyltestosterone	Android-Muguets Metandren linguets Oreton Methyl	ORAL: *Adults*—tablets for buccal administration. 5 to 20 mg (male); 40 to 100 mg (female).	Short. Doses must be repeated daily.	As for oral methyltestosterone.	As for testosterone, aqueous suspension. May increase sensitivity to anticoagulants. Hepatotoxicity, including jaundice.
Testosterone propionate	Oreton propionate	ORAL: *Adults*—tablets for buccal administration. 10 to 20 mg (male); 40 to 100 mg (female).	Short. Doses must be repeated daily.	As for oral methyltestosterone.	As for testosterone, aqueous suspension.

tosterone itself for producing sustained androgenic effects. Two preparations commonly employed clinically are *testosterone enanthate* and *testosterone cypionate* (Table 38-1). Both of these are supplied as suspensions in oil, which when injected intramuscularly are slowly absorbed and therefore effective for 3 to 4 weeks. This increased convenience for the patient is at the cost of less flexibility in control. Another testosterone ester, *testosterone propionate,* has a short duration of action more like that of testosterone itself.

Orally absorbed androgens have been developed. Two of these compounds are *methyltestosterone* and *fluoxymesterone*. These compounds are effective orally, since they are resistant to the action of liver enzymes that degrade testosterone. Unfortunately these compounds are also associated with liver toxicity of various types, including cholestatic jaundice.

Tablets of methyltestosterone and testosterone propionate are available for buccal administration. Absorption through the mucous membranes of the mouth may be more effective than oral administration, since buccally absorbed materials do not directly enter portal circulation and therefore are circulated to the rest of the body before they enter the liver.

■ ANABOLIC STEROIDS

In addition to androgenic properties, the natural male steroids also possess anabolic properties that may be useful in certain clinical situations (Table 38-2). For example, these drugs may be used to treat conditions for which increased nitrogen retention and protein formation are desirable. Accordingly, these drugs are used to alleviate the catabolic state produced by corticosteroid therapy. Patients who have suffered extensive burns or other trauma may benefit from the action of the anabolic steroids. These drugs may also be effective when bone loss is a problem, since anabolic steroids increase bone deposition. Anabolic hormone effects on red blood cell formation make these drugs valuable in the treatment of certain forms of anemia.

Steroid chemists have long labored to separate the androgenic action from the anabolic action of these compounds with limited success. A few anabolic compounds are on the market that have relatively low androgenic potency. However, all anabolic steroids do possess androgenic properties to some degree. Although these androgenic effects may be indistinguishable in normal males, they may become painfully obvious when the compounds are used to treat women or children. Patients receiving these compounds may develop an increased libido. Males may develop priapism (continuous erection). Females should be especially watched for androgen-induced changes such as inappropriate hair development, voice changes, or personality alterations. Children, if they receive these compounds at all, should be watched very closely for precocious sexual development. These compounds, while promoting bone growth in children, also promote fusion of the epiphyses, which permanently halts skeletal growth. Therefore full adult height may actually be diminished, although a growth spurt may be attained when the drugs are first given. For this reason as well as because of the effects on sexual development, these drugs are less than ideal for therapy in children.

TABLE 38-2. Clinical summary of anabolic steroids

Generic name	Trade name	Drug form and dosage	Duration of action	Major clinical uses	Adverse reactions
Ethylestrenol	Maxibolin	ORAL: *Adults*—tablets or elixir, 4 to 16 mg daily.	Short. Doses must be repeated daily.	To produce weight gain following traumatic injury, chronic disease, or long-term corticosteroid therapy. Control symptoms of osteoporosis and certain anemias.	Virilism is possible, especially in women and children. Premature epiphyseal closure may be produced in children, resulting in diminished adult height. Hepatotoxicity.
Methandrostenolone	Dianabol	ORAL: *Adults*—tablets, 2.5 to 5 mg daily.	Short. Doses must be repeated daily.	As for ethylestrenol. Also used for growth stimulation in children and pituitary dwarves.	As for ethylestrenol.
Methandriol	Anabol Methabolic Probolik Steribolic	INTRAMUSCULAR: *Adults*—aqueous suspension (Anabol) or oil solution for intramuscular injection.	Relatively long. 50 to 100 mg once or twice weekly; 10 to 40 mg daily.	Osteoporosis.	Androgenic effects, especially in children.
Nandrolone decanoate	Deca-Durabolin	INTRAMUSCULAR: *Adults*—oil solution for deep intramuscular injection, 50 to 100 mg.	Long. Repeat doses every 3 to 4 weeks.	Refractory anemias, metastatic breast cancer, weight gain, osteoporosis. High doses may be required to treat anemias.	Virilism is possible, especially in women and children. Premature epiphyseal closure may be produced in children, resulting in diminished adult height.
Nandrolone phenpropionate	Durabolin	INTRAMUSCULAR: *Adults*—oil solution for deep intramuscular injection, 25 to 50 mg.	Long. Repeat doses every 2 to 4 weeks.	As for nandrolone decanoate.	As for nandrolone decanoate.
Oxandrolone	Anavar	ORAL: *Adults*—tablets, 5 to 10 mg daily.	Short. Repeat doses daily.	Weight gain or relief of bone pain in osteoporosis.	As for ethylestrenol.
Oxymetholone	Adroyd Anadrol	ORAL: *Adults*—tablets, 5 to 10 mg daily.	Short. Repeat doses daily.	Osteoporosis and anemias.	As for ethylestrenol.
Stanozolol	Winstrol	ORAL: *Adults*—tablets, 6 mg daily.	Short. Doses are taken with meals.	Aplastic anemia and osteoporosis.	As for ethylestrenol. Therapy should be intermittent.

■ THE NURSING PROCESS

■ Assessment

Patients usually receive these drugs for reversing insufficient androgen production, for treatment of a hormonally sensitive tumor, or for the anabolic effects of the drugs in a condition such as severe trauma or burns. A complete patient assessment should be done prior to the initiation of drug therapy. Include in the data base the vital signs, blood pressure, weight, serum calcium level, height, and glucose content of the urine and blood. In addition, the nurse should focus part of the patient assessment on the presenting problem. For example, in treatment of reduced androgen production, an assessment of the secondary sexual characteristics of the patient should be included. In the patient receiving androgen therapy for its anabolic effects, a careful assessment of the nutritional needs, level of mobility, and food and fluid intake and output would also be appropriate.

■ Management

As with many hormones, the effects of the drugs acting on the male reproductive system will not be seen for several weeks after the initiation of therapy in most cases. As therapy is started, the nurse should monitor the vital signs and other data mentioned in assessment. In anticipating the patient's discharge, the nurse should review possible and probable side effects with the patient. For example, the female receiving androgen therapy for hormonally sensitive tumors will in most cases develop some secondary male sexual characteristics such as deepening of the voice and clitoral enlargement. These changes should be reviewed in detail with the patient at the beginning of therapy. For patients receiving steroids for their anabolic effects, referral to the hospital or community dietitian may also be helpful.

■ Evaluation

As with all drugs, the goal is to produce the desired effect but without causing side effects. In replacement therapy for insufficient androgen production, the expected outcome would be increased height and weight and development of secondary sexual characteristics in the male. Ideally this improvement would occur without the development of side effects such as priapism. In doses used to treat female patients with hormonally sensitive cancers, the development of male characteristics almost always occurs. Before discharge the patient should be able to explain how and why to take the drugs, anticipated side effects, side effects that require immediate notification of the physician (e.g., symptoms of hypercalcemia in the cancer patient), how to treat side effects that may be troublesome but are not serious, and what parameters should be measured on a regular basis at home to monitor the effectiveness of the drug. For example, the height and weight of a young male receiving androgens as replacement therapy should be monitored. For additional specific guidelines, see the patient care implications section at the end of this chapter.

■ PATIENT CARE IMPLICATIONS

1. Androgens are contraindicated in pregnancy and lactation and should be used with caution in women of childbearing age because of the potential danger of masculinizing the fetus.
2. Androgens are contraindicated in males with cancer of the breast or prostate gland and should be used with caution in men with benign prostatic hypertrophy.
3. Androgens should be used with caution in patients with existing medical conditions that could be aggravated by fluid retention: hypertension, cardiovascular disease, and renal disease.
4. To monitor fluid retention, weigh patients daily; then taper to weighing patients weekly; monitor blood pressure. A sodium-restricted diet and/or diuretics may help reduce fluid retention.

5. Oily skin and acne can be a distressing side effect, especially for teenagers. Teach the patient to maintain good hygiene.
6. Gastric irritation associated with oral androgens can be reduced by taking the medication with meals.
7. Hypercalcemia is a potentially serious side effect of androgen therapy that can occur in the immobilized patient and in women being treated for breast cancer. Symptoms include thirst, polyuria, anorexia, nausea, vomiting, constipation, lethargy, and eventually coma. Women who have a hormonally sensitive breast cancer and associated metastasis to bone may have a significant rise in calcium concentrations in the blood at the start of androgen therapy. Review the symptoms with susceptible patients, and instruct them to report the appearance of any of the symptoms. It may be necessary to stop the androgen therapy, at least temporarily, and to reduce the serum calcium concentrations.
8. The effectiveness of anabolic steroids in burned, traumatized, or immobilized patients will be enhanced by the concomitant use of a diet high in calories, protein, vitamins, and minerals. Regular physical therapy should be continued to help reduce demineralization of bone.
9. Because androgens can enhance the effect of anticoagulants, teach patients taking both drugs to report any signs of bruising, petechiae, or unexplained bleeding.
10. Virilization in females can be particularly upsetting. Older women in particular may find an increased libido to be disconcerting. Teach patients to report changes in menses, hirsutism, balding, voice changes, clitoral enlargement, or any other unusual sign or symptom. Some changes may reverse after discontinuing the drug. Virilization is usually dose related, but some females are very sensitive even to low doses. At the high doses used to treat breast cancer, virilization can be expected, so the patient should be taught to anticipate it. If the androgen therapy for breast cancer is felt to be producing positive results, the physician may not want to discontinue the therapy even if some virilization is occurring.
11. Teach patients receiving oral androgens to report pruritus, jaundice, changes in skin color or color of sclera. These may be signs of liver dysfunction, an occasional side effect.
12. Androgens have a sustained effect on the body and may produce alterations in laboratory studies up to several weeks after the drug is discontinued. Instruct patients to report to their physicians that they have been taking androgens even if they are not presently taking them.
13. Androgens may decrease the fasting blood sugar concentration or predispose to hypoglycemia. In the diabetic this may necessitate a reduction in insulin dose.
14. Androgens can cause increased circulating levels of oxyphenbutazone or phenylbutazone; reduction in the dosage of these two drugs may be necessary.
15. In children anabolic steroids may be used to treat pituitary dwarfism when growth hormone is not available. This therapy is not without risk, since many times the children are prepubertal. Therapy for these children is usually preceded by careful evaluation, including x-ray films of the wrist and hand to determine the degree of bone maturation. X-ray films will be continued throughout the period of drug therapy, since the drugs produce bone maturation that precedes linear growth. In addition to regular x-ray films, drug therapy will usually be on an intermittent basis, again to prevent too early bone maturation. It is especially important to question young children tactfully about side effects: priapism, erections, clitoral enlargement, and others signs of precocious puberty.
16. Anabolic steroids can cause an increase in muscle mass but do not enhance intrinsic athletic ability.
17. For a discussion of how to administer intramuscular oil-based suspensions, refer to the discussion of vasopressin tannate in oil, Chapter 34.
18. Buccal tablets should be placed in the mouth between the upper or lower gum and the cheek and allowed to dissolve. While the tablet is in place, the patient should refrain from eating, drinking, chewing, or smoking. The patient should rotate sites with each administration. The patient should be encouraged to maintain good oral hygiene and to report any oral irritation.
19. Pellets for subcutaneous implantation can be inserted surgically or with a specially designed injector. Either procedure can be done easily in the physician's office, but aseptic technique must be maintained. Usual sites of insertion are the infrascapular area or along the posterior axillary line. Two or more pellets may be inserted at one time, although not necessarily into the same subcutaneous pouch. The drug will be slowly absorbed from the pellets for up to 4 to 6 months. Sloughing of the pellet can occur and should be reported to the physician; it often indicates placement too superficially or lack of aseptic technique. Because the dosage of subcutaneous pellets cannot be easily regulated, proper dosage for the patient is usually determined by oral medication before a switch is made to subcutaneous. For additional information, see the information supplied by the manufacturer with the medication.

■ SUMMARY

Male sexual development and function are regulated by hormones produced in the hypothalamus (gonadotropin-releasing hormone [GnRH]), the anterior pituitary (interstitial cell–stimulating hormone [ICSH] and follicle-stimulating hormone [FSH]), and the testes (androgenic steroids). Development of male genitalia during fetal life requires the presence of small amounts of androgen, which is produced in response to maternal chorionic gonadotropin (HCG). Development of primary and secondary sexual characteristics at puberty depends on proper concentrations of GnRH, ICSH, FSH, and androgens. In the adult male, maintenance of sexual function requires that adequate concentrations of androgens be maintained.

The most plentiful natural androgen is the steroid testosterone. Other androgens such a dihydrotestosterone and androstenedione may also be formed. These steroids are all formed in the testes and in lesser amounts in the adrenal glands of normal males. Androgen deficiency can cause loss of libido, or sexual desire, and may ultimately cause loss of some secondary male sex characteristics. Replacement therapy with androgens can reverse these changes and control most of the symptoms of androgen deficiency.

Testosterone may be injected intramuscularly as an aqueous suspension but has a very short duration of action. The steroid may be implanted under the skin as pellets that release testosterone slowly over a period of months. However, sustained androgenic effects are best achieved by intramuscular injection of long-acting testosterone esters, testosterone enanthate and testosterone cypionate. Orally administered androgens such as methyltestosterone and fluoxymesterone are also useful for long-term therapy in androgen deficiency, but these agents have a higher incidence of liver damage than other androgens. Buccal absorption of methyltestosterone and testosterone propionate is useful, since this route of administration bypasses the portal circulation to the liver where testosterone is rapidly degraded.

Natural androgens are also anabolic hormones. Synthetic androgen derivatives are available, which minimize the androgenic properties of the compounds and maximize the anabolic properties. These drugs may be used in clinical situations in which increased nitrogen retention and protein formation are desirable. These anabolic steroids retain enough androgenic activity to cause masculinization in sensitive females and precocious sexual development in some children.

■ STUDY QUESTIONS

1. What three organs produce hormones that affect male sexual development and function?
2. What is the function of gonadotropin-releasing hormone (GnRH) in the adult male?
3. What is the function of interstitial cell–stimulating hormone (ICSH) in the adult male?
4. What is the function of follicle-stimulating hormone (FSH) in the adult male?
5. What is the function of testosterone during fetal development in males?
6. How do ICSH, FSH, and testosterone actions convert the immature, prepubertal male genitalia to the fully functional adult form?
7. What is the primary natural androgenic steroid?
8. What are the primary sexual characteristics of the male?
9. What are the secondary sexual characteristics of the male?
10. What effect does testosterone have on metabolism?
11. Name two naturally occurring androgens besides testosterone.
12. Are estrogens found in normal males?
13. What is the most common clinical use of androgen steroids?
14. Why is testosterone not administered by the oral route?
15. What advantages do testosterone esters such as testosterone enanthate have over testosterone itself for long-term replacement therapy of androgen deficiency?
16. What two androgenic steroids are well absorbed orally?
17. What disadvantages do the orally administered androgenic steroids possess compared to other androgenic agents?
18. What is the advantage of administering testosterone by the buccal route rather than by the oral route?
19. What is the major effect of the anabolic steroids?
20. What side effect is frequently associated with anabolic steroids?

■ SUGGESTED READINGS

Anthony, C.P., and Thibodeau, G.A.: The male reproductive system. In Textbook of anatomy and physiology, ed. 10, St. Louis, 1979, The C.V. Mosby Co.

Cole, N.J.: Drugs that influence sexual expression, Consultant **20**(12): 280, 1980.

Hershman, J.M.: Sexual differentiation and development. In Endocrine pathophysiology: a patient oriented approach, Philadelphia, 1977, Lea & Febiger.

Hershman, J.M.: Male reproductive abnormalities. In Endocrine pathophysiology: a patient oriented approach, Philadelphia, 1977, Lea & Febiger.

Mills, L.C.: Drug-induced impotence, American Family Physician **12**(2):104, 1975.

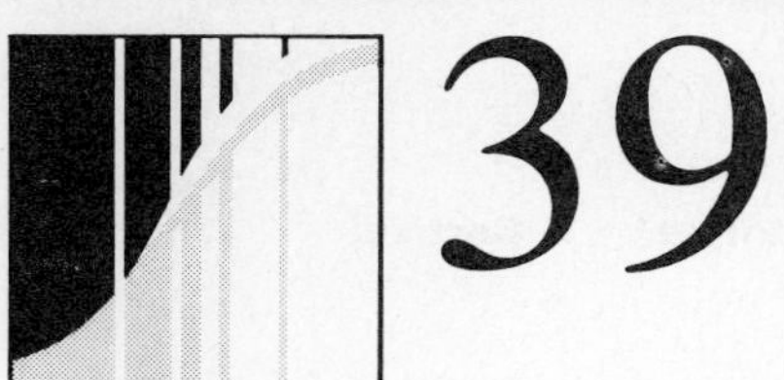

39 Drugs to treat diabetes mellitus

Within the tissue of the pancreas, an exocrine gland that supplies digestive juices to the small intestine, lie discrete clusters of cells whose functions are very different from most pancreatic cells. These cell clusters, called the islets of Langerhans, contain several types of endocrine cells. Three of these cell types release peptide hormones that affect glucose metabolism: A (alpha) cells, which synthesize and release the peptide hormone glucagon; B (beta) cells, which synthesize and release insulin; and D cells, which synthesize somatostatin. This chapter includes an examination of the function of the islet cells, a description of diabetes mellitus, and a description of the drugs used in the diagnosis and control of that disease.

■ NORMAL HORMONAL REGULATION OF METABOLISM

■ Glucose metabolism

One of the rules of metabolic regulation is that the body seldom relies on a single mechanism to control an important physiological function. This rule applies especially well to the processes by which the body regulates glucose utilization. The major hormone regulating glucose metabolism is insulin, a peptide hormone synthesized in the beta cells of the pancreas. Insulin stimulates glucose uptake in fat and muscle cells and the conversion in the liver of glucose to the storage carbohydrate glycogen. But insulin does not work alone, and its metabolic actions must always be considered in relation to the actions of other hormones. For example, the elevated blood glucose level following a meal stimulates insulin release from the pancreas. Blood glucose levels are thereby lowered, since insulin stimulates both the burning of glucose for energy in fat and muscle cells and the storage of glucose in the liver. But as blood glucose levels fall in response to insulin, glucagon release from the alpha cells of the pancreas is stimulated. Glucagon in many ways directly opposes the action of insulin in glucose metabolism. Glucagon stimulates the liver to break down glycogen and amino acids so that glucose is released into the blood. Glucagon also inhibits the uptake of glucose by muscle and fat cells. By balancing the action of these two hormones, the body protects itself from hyperglycemia (high blood glucose) on the one hand and hypoglycemia (low blood glucose) on the other hand.

However, even the concept of metabolic balance achieved with two antagonistic hormones does not adequately describe glucose regulation. For example, somatostatin (Chapter 34) released from D cells inhibits release of both insulin and glucagon from islet cells. Other hormones antagonize the peripheral effects of insulin. Cortisol (an adrenocortical glucocorticoid) and epinephrine (a catecholamine from the adrenal medulla), which are elevated during stress, antagonize the actions of insulin in muscle or fat cells (Table 39-1). The overall action of these two hormones is to increase blood glucose levels. Growth hormone (Chapter 34) also increases blood glucose, primarily by lowering glucose uptake in muscle cells.

■ Fat and protein metabolism

Although insulin is most frequently considered as a regulator of glucose metabolism, it is also important in regulating fat and protein metabolism. Insulin directly stimulates the synthesis of storage lipid within the fat cell, blocks the breakdown and release of stored lipid, and promotes protein synthesis both by stimulating amino acid uptake and by directly stimulating protein synthetic processes. As in carbohydrate metabolism, the action of insulin in regulating fat and protein metabolism is opposed by other hormones. For example, epinephrine, glucagon, cortisol, and growth hormone all stimulate fat breakdown in fat cells, thereby directly opposing the action of insulin in that tissue. These hormones therefore tend to raise the blood content of free fatty acids and other breakdown products of lipids. In addition, glucagon and cortisol block protein synthesis in direct opposition to insulin action. Growth hormone differs in this regard from the other insulin-opposing hormones in that growth hormone directly stimulates protein synthesis in many tissues of the body.

An understanding of this delicate balance of hormonal actions is important to appreciate the origin of some of the metabolic derangements that occur in diabetes mellitus.

TABLE 39-1. Metabolic actions of insulin and insulin-opposing hormones

Tissue and metabolic process	Insulin	Glucagon	Epinephrine	Cortisol	Growth hormone
LIVER					
Glycogen formation	Increase	Decrease	Decrease	Increase	—
Glucose formation from amino acids	Decrease	Increase	—	Increase	Decrease
Glucose formation from glycogen	Decrease	Increase	Increase	—	—
SKELETAL MUSCLE					
Glucose uptake or utilization	Increase	Decrease	Decrease	Decrease	Decrease
Amino acid uptake	Increase	—	—	—	Increase
Protein synthesis	Increase	Decrease	—	Decrease	Increase
Glucose release from glycogen	Decrease	Increase	Increase	—	—
FAT CELLS					
Synthesis of storage lipid	Increase	Decrease	Decrease	Decrease	Decrease
Release of free fatty acids from stored lipid	Decrease	Increase	Increase	Increase	Increase
BLOOD					
Glucose level	Decrease	Increase	Increase	Increase	Increase
Free fatty acid level	Decrease	Increase	Increase	Increase	Increase

■ DIABETES MELLITUS

■ Types of disease and causes

In diabetes mellitus, insulin action is lost. If all insulin production ceases, the disease is referred to as *juvenile-onset diabetes mellitus*. Another term for this form of the disease is *insulin-dependent diabetes*. If insulin production continues but is insufficient to meet the body's demands, the disease is referred to as *adult-onset diabetes mellitus*, or *noninsulin-dependent diabetes mellitus (NIDDM)*. Most diabetics are of this type. As the names imply, diabetes characterized by no insulin production is primarily a disease of the young, although it may in fact occur later in life as well. Adult-onset diabetes is usually a disease of persons over age 40 and the obese. Diabetes in these patients may involve insulin resistance, in that insulin concentrations in the blood may be normal but insulin receptor concentrations on target cells are reduced, making the tissues unresponsive to insulin.

The exact cause of diabetes mellitus has not been established. There may in fact be several ways in which the disease may arise or at least several factors that contribute to its development. Heredity may play a role in some types of diabetes, especially the adult-onset type (NIDDM). However, it has never been proven that heredity alone determines who will or who will not develop the disease. For example, in older individuals there is a clear linkage between obesity and adult onset diabetes mellitus.

Viral infections have been implicated in juvenile-onset diabetes (insulin-dependent diabetes), partly through epidemiological evidence linking viral epidemics to unexpected increases in new cases of juvenile-onset diabetes. Viruses can produce diabetes in laboratory animals, and at least one case is now on record in which viruses were isolated from the pancreas of a child who died during the acute onset of diabetes mellitus. The viruses from this child produced diabetes in experimental animals.

■ Metabolic derangements in diabetes mellitus

Significant metabolic derangements occur when insulin action is lost in diabetes mellitus. Without insulin, less glucose is utilized in muscle and fat cells, and more glucose is released into the circulation by the liver. Muscle cells, starved for energy sources, break down protein and release amino acids into the bloodstream. The liver converts a portion of these amino acids into glucose and returns the sugar to the bloodstream. All these processes contribute to the persistent elevated levels of glucose in the blood. When glucose levels in the bloodstream exceed a certain threshold (about 160 mg/dl), glucose begins to leak through the kidney and appear in the urine.

The most common early symptoms of diabetes mellitus can readily be seen to be a direct result of osmotic and metabolic changes just mentioned. Patients frequently first note a feeling of constant fatigue as energy production in body cells is impaired. An increased frequency of urination (polyuria), often first noticed at night, occurs due to the excess sugar in the urine that produces an osmotic diuresis (i.e., more water must be excreted to carry out the high concentration of sugar). As urine output increases, most patients develop excessive thirst (polydipsia), which results from the body's efforts to maintain normal hydration in the face of excessive fluid losses through the kidney. Some patients develop perineal infections, made likely by the presence of glucose in the urine.

The alterations in metabolism produced by insulin deficiency and the relative excess of catabolic hormones (catecholamines and steroids) ultimately result in greater than normal protein and fat breakdown. The protein is metabolized to amino acids and then to glucose, while the fats are converted to free fatty acids and then to ketone bodies that are released into the circulation. These excess amounts of metabolic breakdown products may cause the patient to become ketotic or acidotic. The potential for ketoacidosis is a serious acute complication of diabetes mellitus, and ketoacidotic coma is associated with mortalities of 3% to 30%. Mortality is highest when treatment is delayed. Ketoacidosis is primarily seen in juvenile-onset diabetics who have little or no endogenous insulin production. These patients are sometimes referred to as *ketosis-prone diabetics*. Adult-onset diabetics, who produce enough insulin to suppress lipid breakdown, are resistant to ketosis.

Any diabetic may become comatose as a result of dehydration. As the plasma becomes hyperosmolar (higher solute concentration than blood), water is pulled from body tissues and severe water and electrolyte imbalances occur. Patients in this type of hyperosmolar coma are as a rule older diabetics and have an even higher mortality than the patients in ketoacidotic coma.

■ Long-term complications of diabetes mellitus

Pathological changes in blood vessels, nerves, and kidneys occur in diabetics. Blood vessel defects are observed in the retina where hemorrhages may destroy sight. Other vessels may be similarly affected, although those changes are not so easily observed in the early stages of the disease; at later stages, circulation to the limbs may be grossly impaired. The kidney is another organ in which pathological changes occur, at first affecting glomerular filtration rate, then progressing to glomerulosclerosis with thickening of the capillary basement membranes. Nephrotic syndrome with protein loss through the kidney and frank kidney failure are late complications of diabetes. Nerve function is impaired so that late in the disease there may be loss of feeling in the limbs or other portions of the body. Sexual impotence is common among diabetic men.

Evidence from research laboratories suggests that many of the late pathological changes that occur in diabetics may be delayed or reduced in severity by strict control of the blood sugar level from the earliest possible time after the appearance of the diabetes. Clinical observations suggest strict control is especially useful in the young diabetic. No correlation between patient welfare and degree of diabetic control can yet be proven in milder, adult-onset forms of diabetes.

■ Diagnosis of diabetes mellitus

Diabetes mellitus is diagnosed by applying one of the following procedures.

Fasting blood sugar (FBS) is determined by obtaining a few milliliters of blood from an individual after a 12-hour fast and measuring the glucose content by any one of a number of methods approved for use in clinical laboratories. Most conveniently, the blood is taken in the early morning. The range of normal fasting plasma sugar values is 60 to 100 mg/dl for venous blood. A value above 120 mg/dl in a truly fasting individual suggests the diagnosis of diabetes mellitus. Values between 100 and 120 mg/dl may require further evaluation of the patient.

Glucosuria (glucose in the urine) is conveniently tested in screening programs with commercially available pretreated test strips (Dextrostix), which develop a particular color when exposed to urine containing glucose. Glucose does not routinely appear in the urine of nondiabetics since a blood sugar level of about 160 mg/dl is required before the normal kidney allows glucose to spill into the urine. Some diabetics spill glucose into the urine at lower blood glucose concentrations, possibly as a result of impaired kidney function.

The *oral glucose tolerance test (OGTT)* detects not only those persons who are overtly diabetic but also those persons who may progress to clinical diabetes in the future. The test consists of administering 50 to 100 Gm of glucose orally. Blood samples are then taken at hourly or 30-minute intervals, and the glucose levels in the plasma are compared to the value obtained from a sample taken immediately before the glucose was administered. In a normal person, plasma glucose levels rise in response to this acute glucose load and immediately trigger the release of insulin from the beta cells of the pancreas. As a result of the circulating insulin, glucose levels begin to fall within an hour or so after the

FIG. 39-1

Typical oral glucose tolerance tests for normal and diabetic patients. This test is performed preferably in ambulatory patients in the morning before breaking the overnight fast. The oral glucose load is usually about 75 Gm given in solution. Blood is drawn at appropriate intervals (before glucose and 60, 90, 120, and 180 minutes after) and analyzed for glucose.

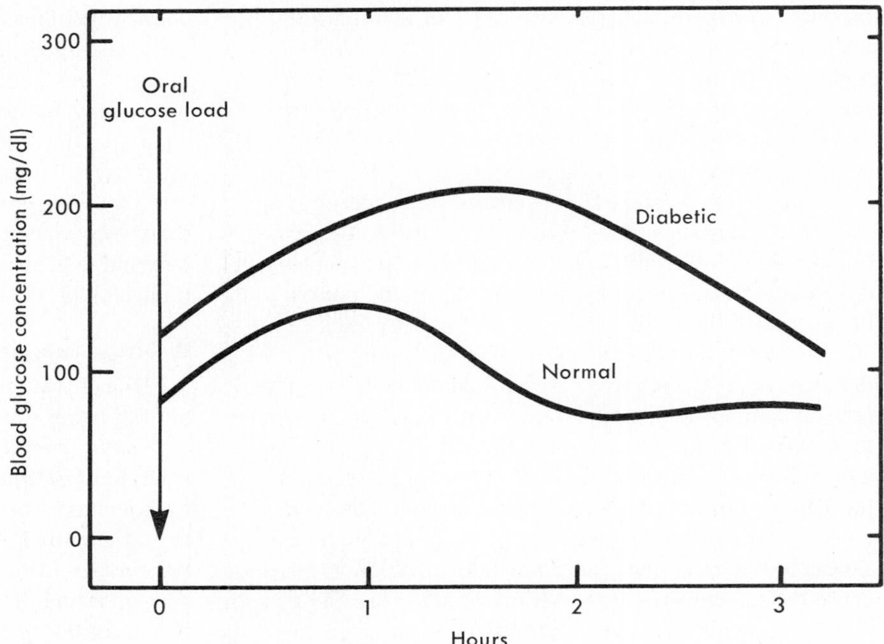

glucose load is administered and return to normal by 2 hours (Fig. 39-1). In contrast the plasma glucose levels of the diabetic fall more slowly than that of the normal person, since insulin is not released to aid in the disposition of the glucose load. Plasma glucose levels in the diabetic remain over 200 mg/dl of plasma 2 hours after the glucose load.

■ TREATMENT OF DIABETES MELLITUS

■ Insulin therapy

Mechanism of action. Insulin is used for treatment of diabetes when presumably there are no functional B cells in the islets left to respond to glucose levels. Such treatment constitutes replacement therapy. The administered insulin restores the ability of cells to utilize glucose as energy source and corrects many metabolic derangements of diabetes mellitus.

Absorption and fate. Insulin must be administered by injection, since it is a protein and would therefore be digested and destroyed in the gastrointestinal tract. In its natural form, insulin is relatively soluble in water and is rather quickly absorbed from subcutaneous injection sites. This property is reflected in the pharmacological behavior of regular insulin for injection (Table 39-2), which is rapidly absorbed, has its peak effect within 2 to 4 hours, and is no longer active after approximately 8 hours. The longer acting insulin preparations are prepared by crystallizing insulin in the presence of zinc to form slowly dissolving crystals or in the presence of protein (either protamine or globin) to form slowly dissolving complexes. These preparations differ from regular insulin and from each other in onset and duration of action primarily because of differences in absorption from the site of injection. The health care professional must be familiar with the properties of the major insulin products. It is by proper use of these various insulin forms that control can be adjusted to fit the life-style and metabolic demands of individual patients. Diabetics must become proficient not only in the techniques of storing, preparing, and injecting their insulin but they also must be taught the proper testing procedures. Moreover, they must understand the onset and duration of action of the insulin preparations they are receiving to avoid complications.

As an example of the many patterns of dosage that may be successfully employed, consider the following hypothetical case. A juvenile-onset diabetic who has been maintained on a single dose of lente insulin before breakfast each morning has begun to show hyperglycemia by the next morning. To overcome this problem, the physician split the insulin dose, giving 80% of the daily dose in the morning and the remainder before sup-

TABLE 39-2. Properties of insulin preparations

				Pharmacokinetic properties		
Generic name	**Trade name**	**Classification**	**Description**	**Onset of action**	**Peak action**	**Duration of action**
Insulin injection	Regular insulin	Rapidly acting insulin	Clear solution containing no zinc or modifying agents; intravenous or subcutaneous injection.	Within 1 hr	2 to 4 hr	6 to 8 hr
Prompt insulin zinc suspension	Semilente Iletin Semilente Insulin	Rapidly acting insulin	Cloudy suspension of amorphous insulin precipitated with zinc to slow absorption; subcutaneous only.	1.5 to 2 hr	4 to 7 hr	12 to 16 hr
Globin zinc insulin injection		Intermediate acting insulin	Clear solution; globin-bound insulin is slowly absorbed from injection site; subcutaneous only.	2 to 4 hr	10 to 14 hr	14 to 22 hr
Isophane insulin suspension	NPH Iletin NPH insulin	Intermediate acting insulin	Cloudy suspension of insulin complexed with protamine to slow absorption; subcutaneous only.	1 to 2 hr	10 to 16 hr	18 to 30 hr
Insulin zinc suspension	Lente Iletin Lente Insulin	Intermediate acting insulin	Cloudy suspension containing 30% Semilente insulin and 70% Ultralente insulin; subcutaneous only.	1 to 2 hr	10 to 16 hr	18 to 30 hr
Protamine zinc insulin	Protamine Zinc Insulin Protamine Zinc Iletin PZI	Long acting insulin	Cloudy when well mixed; suspension of insulin complexed with more protamine than NPH insulin; subcutaneous only.	6 to 8 hr	14 to 24 hr	24 to 36 hr or longer
Extended insulin zinc suspension	Ultralente Iletin Ultralente Insulin	Long acting insulin	Cloudy when well mixed; large complexes of insulin with zinc to slow absorption; no protein modifiers; subcutaneous only.	5 to 8 hr	16 to 18 hr	24 to 36 hr or longer

TABLE 39-3. Differential diagnosis of diabetic coma and hypoglycemic reactions

Clinical data	Diabetic coma	Hypoglycemic reactions
Symptoms	Thirst Abdominal pain Nausea and vomiting Headache Constipation Shortness of breath (Kussmaul breathing)	Nervousness Hunger Sweating Weakness Stupor Convulsions
Signs	Facial flushing Air hunger Soft eyeballs Normal or absent reflexes Acetone breath	Pallor Shallow respiration Normal eyeballs Babinski's reflex may be seen
Urine glucose	Positive	Negative or low
Urine acetone	Positive	Negative
Blood glucose	High (above 250 mg/dl)	Low (below 60 mg/dl)
Blood CO_2	Low	Normal
Precipitating factors	Untreated diabetes Infection or disease appearing in a previously controlled diabetic High degree of emotional or psychological stress	Insulin overdosage Skipping meals Excessive exercise before meals
History	Onset of symptoms usually occurs over a period of days	Onset of symptoms is somewhat related to the type of medication used; regular insulin overdose produces symptoms more rapidly than the longer acting insulins or oral agents

per. The rationale for this therapy is simple. Lente insulin injected at around 7:00 AM will be reaching its peak effect around dinner time. The small dose administered before supper helps to protect the patient from developing hyperglycemia overnight.

Many individualized schemes for insulin dosage may be devised for particular patients. Nevertheless, in all cases the principle is the same: doses of insulin must be timed so that the patient is protected from hyperglycemia and from hypoglycemia during peak periods of insulin action.

Side effects of insulin therapy. Insulin therapy is associated with two major acute side effects. If insulin therapy is inadequate, the diabetic may go into a coma resulting from the uncontrolled metabolic derangements discussed earlier. Blood sugar concentration is high and ketoacidosis or hyperosmolar coma may result. On the other hand, if inadvertent insulin overdosage occurs or if a patient does not eat or overexercises, the patient may lapse into coma resulting from a hypoglycemic reaction. It is critical for the health care professional to be able to differentiate between these two conditions. The distinguishing symptoms are outlined in Table 39-3. Treatment of hypoglycemia consists of elevating blood glucose level by oral administration of sugar in conscious patients or by glucagon injection or glucose intravenous infusion in unconscious patients. Treatment of diabetic coma requires insulin administration to lower blood sugar concentration and reduce ketone body formation.

Allergic reactions to insulin may occur. Local allergic reactions usually do not require treatment. Systemic allergic responses to insulin are more rare. Severe allergic reactions may usually be prevented in a sensitive patient by using a more highly purified insulin preparation (single component insulin) or by using insulin derived from a single animal species. For example, a patient sensitive to the standard preparations containing both porcine and bovine insulin may only be allergic to one form and may be able to take the insulin from the other species without allergic symptoms.

Many patients receiving insulin therapy have insulin antibodies in their bloodstream. These antibodies may contribute to insulin resistance in some patients.

Insulin may also cause subcutaneous fat near injection sites to atrophy. This lipoatrophy leads to the formation of hollows or depressions in the skin. Careful rotation of injection sites minimizes this effect. Lipoatrophy may be less common with the highly purified insulin preparations.

■ Oral hypoglycemic agents

Sulfonylureas

Mechanism of action. The major class of oral hypoglycemic agents is the sulfonylurea group. The sulfonylureas are useful only for those patients who produce some insulin on their own, that is, adult-onset diabetics. Clinical studies of adult-onset diabetics have shown many of these patients may have low, normal, or even above normal insulin levels in their bloodstream. The cells of many of these patients, however, have lower than normal numbers of insulin *receptors*. As mentioned in Chapter 33, a receptor is required for the action of hormones. Therefore in this type of adult-onset diabetic, insulin action is lost not because insulin is missing, but because insulin receptors are diminished.

Sulfonylureas have long been considered effective by virtue of their ability to stimulate insulin release from the pancreas. Sulfonylureas may also act on insulin-responsive tissues elsewhere in the body. In patients who respond to sulfonylureas, insulin receptors increase in number, whereas those patients who failed to respond showed no change in insulin receptors. The result of this increase in insulin receptors would be to render the available circulating insulin more effective, that is, to increase glucose uptake by tissues.

The effectiveness of sulfonylureas in obese, non-insulin-dependent diabetics is enhanced by caloric restriction and weight loss. This dietary manipulation also tends to increase the number of insulin receptors on target cells.

Absorption and fate. The sulfonylureas are chemically related compounds that differ from one another primarily in onset and duration of action (Table 39-4). The onset and duration of action of these drugs is strongly influenced by their metabolic fate in the body. For example, *tolbutamide* is relatively short acting, since it is quickly converted in the body to an inactive product. In contrast, *acetohexamide* and *tolazamide* must be converted in the body to active products before they become effective. Hence they are intermediate in action. *Chlorpropamide* is the longest acting member of the class and is tightly bound to plasma protein. This drug is not extensively metabolized by the body at all, being excreted unchanged in the urine.

Two new sulfonylureas have been widely tested in the United States. These drugs are *glyburide (Glibenclamide; Micronase)* and *glipizide (Glucotrol)*. Although not yet released for general use in the United States, these drugs have been widely used in Europe.

Side effects. Side effects of sulfonylurea therapy include gastrointestinal distress and neurological symptoms such as muscle weakness and paresthesias. Liver function tests may be altered and mild hematopoietic toxicity may be seen in some patients. Frank allergy to the drugs occurs in some patients, with skin reactions being more common than the more dangerous forms of allergic response. The incidence of these types of reactions is reported to be less than 5% of patients treated.

Hypoglycemia is an ever present danger with the sulfonylureas and may be caused by drug overdose, drug interaction, altered drug metabolism, or the patient failing to eat. Sulfonylureas should not be used when renal or liver function is inadequate; normal function of those organs is required for metabolism and elimination of the sulfonylureas (Table 39-4). Elderly patients also occasionally show excessive hypoglycemic reactions to these drugs.

The use of sulfonylureas in the treatment of diabetes mellitus has recently become controversial. Some clinical studies seem to show that treatment with sulfonylureas is no more effective than dietary therapy alone. Other studies have suggested that the toxicity of the sulfonylureas is higher than previously expected. Although these questions are far from resolved, some treatment centers avoid the use of these compounds and control mild adult-onset diabetes (nonketotic) with diet and exercise alone or, if necessary, combine diet and exercise with low doses of insulin. Even when the sulfonylureas are used, it is clear that careful attention to the diet is required for best results.

Drug interactions. The sulfonylureas are implicated in certain drug interactions that can have serious consequences to the patient (Table 39-4). The major interactions occur with ethyl alcohol, phenylbutazone, sulfonamides, and salicylates. Patients receiving sulfonylureas should routinely avoid alcohol. Several interactions between alcohol and sulfonylureas are possible. Some patients receiving sulfonylureas develop an "Antabuse or disulfiram reaction" when they ingest alcohol. The most striking symptoms of this reaction are an unpleasant flushing and severe headache. Other patients on sulfonylureas become hypoglycemic when they ingest alcohol, probably because ethanol itself is a hypoglycemic agent in some people.

Hypoglycemia can result when any one of a number of drugs are given to a patient taking sulfonylureas, the most important of which are the antiinflammatory agents, phenylbutazone and salicylates, and sulfonamide antibiotics. These three drugs are all tightly bound to plasma protein and may displace sulfonylureas and thereby elevate blood concentrations of free sulfonylurea. Since the free drug is the active form, the result is an enhancement of the hypoglycemic effect of the sulfonylurea. In addition to this mechanism, phenylbutazone may block excretion of the active metabolite of acetohexamide, an action that also tends to increase hypoglycemia. Sulfonamides may inhibit the metabolic breakdown of tolbutamide and thereby enhance its hypoglycemic action.

TABLE 39-4. Properties of the oral antidiabetic agents

Generic name	Trade name	Dosage range	Duration of action	Metabolic fate	Drugs that enhance hypoglycemia produced by antidiabetic agent	Drugs that interfere with hypoglycemic action of antidiabetic agent
Tolbutamide	Orinase	0.5 to 3 Gm daily, divided doses.	6 to 12 hr	Well absorbed from gastrointestinal tract. Strongly bound to serum proteins. Metabolized in liver to an inactive compound.	Phenylbutazone, certain sulfonamides, salicylates, ethyl alcohol, anabolic steroids, chloramphenicol, guanethidine.	Phenytoin, mephenytoin, thiazide diuretics, phenothiazines.
Acetohexamide	Dymelor	0.25 to 1.5 Gm daily, as a single or divided dose.	12 to 24 hr	Rapidly absorbed from gastrointestinal tract. Converted by the liver to an active metabolite, which appears in the blood later and stays longer than the parent compound. Active metabolite excreted via the kidney.	Ethyl alcohol, guanethidine, salicylates.	Phenothiazines.
Tolazamide	Tolinase	0.1 to 0.75 Gm daily; single dose for lower range, divided dose for higher range.	12 to 24 hr	Slowly absorbed from gastrointestinal tract. Bound to serum proteins. Converted by the liver to several active metabolites, which are excreted via the kidney.	Ethyl alcohol, guanethidine, salicylates, anabolic steroids.	Thiazide diuretics, mephenytoin, phenothiazines, phenytoin.
Chlorpropamide	Diabinese	0.1 to 0.5 Gm daily, single dose.	Up to 60 hr	Rapidly absorbed from gastrointestinal tract. Strongly bound to serum proteins. Excreted unchanged through the kidney.	Ethyl alcohol, anabolic steroids, chloramphenicol, guanethidine, salicylates, certain sulfonamides.	Thiazide diuretics, phenytoin, mephenytoin, phenothiazines.

■ THE NURSING PROCESS

■ Assessment

Patients are diagnosed with diabetes mellitus because they appear with the classic triad of symptoms (polyphagia, polydipsia, and polyuria) or because through evaluation of another medical condition they are found to have elevated glucose concentrations in the blood or urine. Diabetes occurs in all age-groups. Baseline assessment data of the diabetic would include all of the usual assessment data with emphasis on the vital signs, weight, blood glucose and urine glucose concentrations and any signs indicating the possible development of long-term effects, such as the development of ulcers on the lower extremities. In addition, the nurse should carefully assess the condition of skin and nails and note the presence of any unusual sign or symptom.

■ Management

The complete management of the diabetic patient is beyond the scope of this book. In relation to drug therapy, the nurse should monitor the glucose in blood and urine, look for the presence of ketones in the urine, and, depending on the patient's condition, examine other appropriate laboratory work such as electrolytes or arterial blood gases. Planning for discharge should be done as soon as the patient is diagnosed. The patient will require extensive teaching about such aspects of diabetes as the need for good foot care and dietary restrictions. The nurse should teach the diabetic about the medications that have been prescribed and their method of administration and how to test the urine as an indication of success of therapy. Appropriate referrals should be made at this time to such departments as the hospital or community dietitian and the local visiting nurse association. In addition, the patient may be referred to the local diabetes association.

■ Evaluation

Ideally treatment with drugs in diabetes mellitus would cause the patient to have normal blood glucose levels at all times and would prevent the known long-term effects of this disease. Thus far, however, it is not possible to produce this degree of control. Patient age, motivation, and willingness to follow prescribed regimens are only a few factors that influence the overall success of therapy for diabetes mellitus. Before discharge for self-management, the patient being treated with drugs for this disease should be able to explain why the drugs are prescribed and should be able to demonstrate how to administer insulin or other medications correctly. The nurse should be certain the patient can explain the symptoms of hyperglycemia and hypoglycemia and how to treat them and can explain other prescribed aspects of care such as foot care, dietary restrictions, and any limitations in activity that have been prescribed. The patient should be able to demonstrate how to accurately test the urine for glucose and ketones and be able to state what to do based on the information obtained from this test. The nurse should be certain the patient understands what symptoms should cause the patient to seek medical attention. The patient should be able to explain why it is appropriate to wear a medical indentification tag or bracelet at all times indicating that the patient is diabetic. For more complete information about this disease, see appropriate nursing textbooks. For further information about insulin and the oral hypoglycemic agents, see the patient care implications section at the end of this chapter.

■ Diet therapy

Mechanism of action. Obesity or, more specifically, excessive caloric intake, tends to reduce the number of insulin receptors. An understanding of this disease mechanism helps in appreciating the rationale for dietary control of diabetes: reduced caloric intake allows the number of insulin receptors to increase and makes the available insulin more effective. Dietary restriction may lower insulin requirements in obese diabetics and, in many cases, may be the only form of therapy required. The effectiveness of sulfonylureas in obese noninsulin-dependent diabetics is enhanced by caloric restriction and weight loss.

Careful dietary control is important for all diabetics. Successful long-term treatment of the condition frequently involves counseling by a dietitian and supportive follow-up for the rest of the patient's life.

■ PATIENT CARE IMPLICATIONS

Diabetes mellitus

1. Each diabetic should be taught the signs and symptoms of hyperglycemia and hypoglycemia (Table 39-3).
2. The patient should be able to explain the appropriate action to take in the event of hyperglycemia or hypoglycemia. Mild hypoglycemia is usually controlled by drinking a glass of orange juice or ginger ale or eating a few pieces of hard candy. Mild hyperglycemia may require an increase in the insulin dose, but this should be done only with the advice of the physician. Poor dietary control is the most frequently observed cause for hyperglycemia.
3. To manage their diabetes more easily, all diabetics should clearly understand the antidiabetic medications they receive. This knowledge should include onset, peak, and duration of action of their individual medications, as well as side effects.
4. Certain conditions predispose a patient to hypoglycemia (Table 39-3). In addition to those conditions listed in Table 39-3, the following conditions may precipitate hypoglycemia in some patients: stress, starting or stopping another medication, and menstruation. Exercise may significantly lower the required insulin dosage in a diabetic.
5. Drugs that may cause hypoglycemia in the diabetic include ethanol, anabolic steroids, guanethidine, monoamine oxidase inhibitors, salicylates, acetaminophen, propranolol, phenylbutazone, isoniazid, and certain antineoplastic agents.
6. Certain conditions predispose a patient to hyperglycemia (Table 39-3). In addition to those conditions listed in Table 39-3, the following conditions may precipitate hyperglycemia in some patients: excessive food intake, surgery, starting or stopping other medications, and menstruation.
7. Drugs that may cause or contribute to hyperglycemia in the diabetic include ethanol, corticosteroids, oral contraceptives, glucagon, acetazolamide, salicylates, phenothiazines, diazoxide, phenytoin, furosemide, chlorthalidone, lithium carbonate, growth hormone, and thyroid hormone.
8. In pregnancy, insulin requirements change. The woman may need less insulin in the first trimester but will usually need more insulin during the second and third trimesters.
9. An unusual problem occasionally encountered with insulin-dependent diabetics is the Somogyi effect, which is rebound hyperglycemia that occurs several hours after the insulin is administered. The treatment may require manipulation of the diet and the insulin dose. For more information, see the Suggested Readings.
10. Diabetics may find that minor illnesses such as colds, diarrhea, or vomiting may throw their diabetes out of control. If a diabetic is ill, cannot eat, or is otherwise unable to maintain a regular routine, the physician should be contacted for guidance.
11. Diabetics should avoid alcoholic beverages or use them in moderation, being careful to consider the caloric content of these beverages in diet planning.

Insulin

1. Insulin can be safely stored for about 1 month at room temperature, but for longer periods of time it should be refrigerated. Most hospitals, pharmacies, and patients keep their insulin refrigerated; it should not be frozen.
2. Insulin should not be administered cold but allowed to warm to room temperature. Cold insulin alters anticipated rates of absorption, causes more local reaction, and is thought to promote lipodystrophy at injection sites.
3. Inspect each vial of insulin before using. Note that regular insulin and globin zinc insulin should be crystal clear; all other forms of insulin will be cloudy.
4. Gently rotate each vial of insulin for at least 1 minute between both hands before drawing up the dose. This helps to resuspend the modified insulin preparations and will help to warm the medication. Vigorous shaking will promote foaming and bubbles in the solution and should be avoided.
5. Careful, accurate measuring of the ordered dose is essential. In many hospitals it is accepted practice that each time insulin is administered, the person preparing the medication has a professional colleague (R.N., L.P.N.) double-check to see that the correct dose of the correct type of insulin has been prepared.
6. Syringes designed for insulin should be used. These

customarily are 1 ml in volume for use with U100 insulin (U100 insulin contains 100 units of insulin/ml). For patients taking very small amounts of insulin, usually less than 35 units, there are syringes available that have clearer, more accurate markings for small doses of insulin. There are also available 2 ml insulin syringes for patients requiring greater than 100 units of insulin. Tuberculin syringes are not recommended for use with insulin because of the inaccurate dosage that can occur resulting from the dead space in the hub of the needle and the tip of the syringe.

7. Two kinds of insulin can be mixed in the same syringe within the following guidelines: Regular insulin can be mixed with any other kind of insulin. The lente insulins can be mixed with each other but should not be mixed with other insulins except regular insulin. Mixtures of the lentes, Regular insulin with NPH insulin, or Regular insulin with a lente insulin are stable at least 2 to 3 months. A mixture of Regular insulin with Protamine Zinc insulin (PZI) is not stable and should be administered immediately after preparation.
8. The procedure for mixing two insulins in the same syringe is as follows:
   a. With the syringe, inject air, in the amount equivalent to the dose to be drawn up, into the vial of modified insulin. Remove syringe.
   b. Inject the correct amount of air into the vial of Regular insulin; then withdraw the correct dose. Eliminate any air bubbles in the syringe.
   c. Return to the vial of modified insulin and withdraw the correct dose. If an error occurs, discard the syringe and begin again.

   Remember: The Regular insulin (unmodified) is always aspirated into the syringe first.
9. Insulin is administered subcutaneously. Acceptable sites for insulin injection include the upper arms, back, outer thighs, abdomen (avoiding the navel and midline tissue), and buttocks, although some experts feel the buttocks contain too much fatty tissue.
10. Any correct method for administering a subcutaneous medication may be used for insulin administrations, but some experts feel that the following method results in best absorption with fewest side effects:
    a. Clean skin with alcohol. Let alcohol evaporate.
    b. Pinch up the skin at the injection site.
    c. Insert the needle at a 20- to 45-degree angle at the base of the pinched skin. Aspirate for blood.
    d. Inject the insulin into the "space" between the fat and the muscle.
    e. Withdraw the needle. Apply pressure to the site if needed to stop bleeding. Do not rub the area.

    Note that the obese individual may require a needle longer than the ⅝-inch needle supplied with the insulin syringe. Rarely would an individual require a needle shorter than ⅝ inch.
11. Local reactions to insulin injection are not uncommon and may include itching, a reddened area, or excessive discomfort at the injection site. The reactions usually will clear on their own in 2 to 3 weeks, although some individuals may require oral antihistamines to decrease discomfort. Sometimes the irritation is due to not allowing the alcohol to dry before giving the injection; reevaluate the patient's injection technique.
12. Systemic reactions to insulin are rare, but when they occur they often result from reaction to the animal source of the insulin: beef, pork, or mixed beef and pork. The reaction should be treated symptomatically and an alternate source of insulin tried.
13. Hypertrophy (thickening) of the skin and lipodystrophy (dimpling) at injection sites were once thought to be unavoidable complications of insulin use. Today it is thought that these two problems often represent careless injection technique or repeated use of the same injection site. From the time the first insulin injection is given to a patient, a record of site use should be kept and sites rotated. The patient should be taught why sites must be rotated and how to keep a record of sites used. No individual injection site should be used more often than every 6 or 7 weeks.
14. Intravenous insulin is one of the drugs used in the treatment of diabetic coma. Note that only regular insulin (unmodified) is safe for intravenous administration. Intravenous insulin is incompatible with many other intravenous solutions and is unstable at a pH range outside 3.0 to 3.5. Check with the pharmacy before administering if questions occur.
15. Glucagon may be given to counteract an overdose of insulin, but the action of glucagon depends on the patient having sufficient glycogen stored in the liver to break down to glucose. Some physicians prefer to use glucose directly.

Urine testing

1. Many times the insulin dose is calculated on the basis of the urine test. Whenever possible, a double-voided specimen should be used, since this type specimen more accurately reflects blood glucose values near the time when insulin dosage is due. For a double-voided specimen the following procedure should be followed:
   a. The patient should urinate 45 to 60 minutes before the dose of insulin is due. This specimen may be discarded *unless* the physician orders it to

be tested or for some reason it is anticipated that the patient will not be able to obtain a second specimen before the insulin dose is due. Such reasons might include the patient's age, ability to understand, or general medical condition.

b. The patient may drink water.

c. A second urine specimen is obtained just before the insulin dose is due. The specimen is tested and the insulin dose is based on the result of the second specimen.

A single-void specimen is usually adequate for routine monitoring and when no insulin dose is to be calculated on the result. In addition, it may not be necessary for the patient to obtain double-voided specimens after discharge; check with the physician so that correct discharge teaching can be done.

2. There are two major types of urine sugar tests: cupric sulfate reagents and glucose oxidase reagents. In the former, many types of sugar (i.e., galactose, fructose, lactose, glucose) in the urine can cause a positive reaction. Cupric sulfate reagents are the basis for Benedict's test, Clinitest, and Diastix. Because these tests also measure lactose in the urine, they may be inappropriate for women in the third trimester of pregnancy or during lactation. Glucose oxidase reagents are specific for glucose and are the basis for Tes-Tape, Clinistix, and the sugar test portion of Uristix, Labstix, and Bili-Labstix.
3. Results from one type of urine test should not be compared to another because they vary in sensitivity and what they measure (see the preceding discussion). For discharge planning, the physician, nurse, and patient should choose a type of urine test. The patient should learn well how to use that test and not switch to others.
4. Many drugs can influence the result of the urine test, producing false positive or false negative results. If there is any question about the influence of a drug on the urine test, try another test, consult with the pharmacy, or notify the physician.
5. The presence of ketones in the urine is an important indicator of the diabetic's degree of control. During hospitalization the urine should always be tested for ketones when tested for sugar. At the time of discharge, the physician may indicate that the patient need only test for ketones at home if the urine sugar exceeds a certain level. The diabetic patient needs to be able to perform this test accurately and to identify when to test for ketones if not with each specimen. In addition, patients should know what to do if they begin to spill ketones (e.g., increase the insulin, notify the physician); clarify with the physician before discharge.

Discharge planning and teaching, insulin-dependent diabetes

1. Whenever possible, and depending on the age and condition of the patient, self-injection of insulin after discharge is preferred; it implies better acceptance of the diagnosis and promotes patient independence. As soon as it has been definitely decided by the physician that the patient will require insulin after discharge, the teaching about insulin and injections should be begun.
2. Choice of the type of syringe for use by the patient should be influenced by the patient's age, financial situation, visual acuity, manual dexterity, and preference. In any case, the patient should be able to draw up the required dose accurately, eliminate air bubbles, correctly identify injection sites, and administer the drug using correct and sterile technique.
3. If patients choose disposable needles and syringes, they should be taught proper disposal of the used syringe and needle. Recent studies have indicated that disposable syringe-needle units can be reused up to a total of 3 or 4 injections without a significant increase in infection (Greenough et al., 1979; Hodge et al., 1980). The limiting factor as perceived by patients was dulling of the needle. Reuse of disposable syringes could result in a significant savings for patients. Consult the physician.
4. If patients choose glass syringes, they should be given specific instructions on how to care for these syringes.
5. Whenever possible, at least one other family member should be taught how to give insulin injections. That individual can then give the injections to the back or buttocks of the diabetic, which are sites an individual cannot usually reach.
6. For visually or physically handicapped patients who are having difficulty drawing up the correct dose, some aids are available. Special syringes can be purchased that can be preset to allow only the desired dose to be aspirated. It may be easier for the patient to have a visiting nurse or family member draw up a week's supply of insulin into individual syringes and to store them in the refrigerator. Automatic injectors and needle guides are also available. Local pharmacies, the American Diabetes Association, or the American Foundation for the Blind, Inc., 15 West 16 St., New York, N.Y. 10011, may be of assistance.
7. It is appropriate for insulin-dependent diabetics to have their insulin technique and rotation schedule reevaluated on each admission to the hospital.

8. Diabetics who engage in active sports may find that the thigh and arm as injection sites should be avoided on days when heavy exercise is anticipated. Strenuous muscle use may result in rapid release of the insulin with resulting hypoglycemia. Heavy exercise also has a hypoglycemic effect independent of insulin.
9. Patients should be taught never to run out of insulin or syringes. If they do, they should markedly decrease their food intake and drink plenty of sugar-free beverages. The needed insulin or syringes should be obtained and used as soon as possible.
10. The patient and family should understand that hard candy, orange juice, or sugar cubes should always be available in the event of a hypoglycemic reaction. Some patients may wish to carry Glutol, Glutorea, Instant Glucose, or another commercial preparation with them. These jellylike products can be absorbed through the oral mucosa so they can be used when the patient is not alert or able to swallow. Of course, for severe hypoglycemic reactions the patient should be taken to the physician or emergency room whether or not the commercial glucose preparation is used.
11. In addition to information about their medications, diabetics should be well-informed about diet, foot care, prevention of complications, and all other aspects of the disease.
12. At least one family member should also receive training in recognizing the complications of diabetes and know the proper action to take. For example, restlessness and diaphoresis (sweating) in the sleeping diabetic may indicate hypoglycemia. These signs may be noticed by a family member.
13. Most diabetics can benefit from referral to a visiting nurse for extended follow-up.
14. Diabetics should be encouraged to wear a medical identification tag or bracelet indicating their diagnosis.
15. For additional information, patients can be referred to the American Diabetes Association, Inc., 18 East 48 St., New York, N.Y. 10017.
16. Travelling may necessitate adjusting the dosage of insulin or oral hypoglycemic agents. The physician should be consulted. While traveling the patient should carry sufficient insulin and syringes or sufficient oral hypoglycemic drugs for the expected duration of the trip and extra supplies in case of unexpected delays. Insulin should be protected from freezing in baggage compartments. A portion of the medication should be carried in hand luggage in case other luggage is lost or delayed.
17. Specific information concerning overseas travel can be obtained from the International Diabetes Foundation, 3-6 Alfred Place, London WC1, England.

Oral hypoglycemic agents

1. Diabetics requiring only oral hypoglycemic agents for control may find that appropriate weight reduction and adherence to the prescribed diet is all that is necessary to bring blood glucose levels back to normal and that in time the oral agents can be discontinued. For this reason it is essential that these patients be helped to understand the importance of their prescribed diet.
2. The major side effect of oral hypoglyemic agents is hypoglycemia, and this is frequently a problem with elderly patients. Nausea, vomiting, and skin rashes are usually transient. In rare cases, agranulocytosis is seen, so patients should be cautioned to report to their physician any sore throat, fever, or whenever they do not feel well.
3. Oral hypoglycemic agents are contraindicated during pregnancy.
4. Chlorpropamide may prolong the action of hypnotics and sedatives in some individuals.
5. Tolbutamide may potentiate the action of oral anticoagulants.
6. Patients should be taught to take their oral hypoglycemic agents as prescribed and not to ''catch up'' with missed doses. In addition, oral agents should not be taken at bedtime.
7. Patients being switched from insulin to oral agents or the reverse need to be carefully watched for hypoglycemia.
8. Individuals who can usually be managed on oral agents may requre insulin during times of illness, infection, hospitalization, or surgery.

■ SUMMARY

Insulin is the major hormone regulating glucose metabolism, stimulating uptake of glucose in fat and muscle cells and the conversion of glucose to glycogen in the liver. Glucagon opposes these actions of insulin. Somatostatin inhibits the release of insulin and glucagon from pancreatic islets. Other hormones such as cortisol, epinephrine, and growth hormone antagonize the action of insulin in muscle or fat cells. Insulin also stimulates lipid storage, blocks lipid breakdown, and promotes protein synthesis.

In diabetes mellitus, insulin action is lost. Insulin-dependent diabetics produce little or no insulin and the patients are mostly young and relatively lean. Noninsulin-dependent diabetics may produce insulin, but the amount is insufficient. These diabetics are usually obese older adults.

In diabetes mellitus, glucose utilization is impaired and the sugar accumulates in the bloodstream and is excreted in the urine. Excessively high glucose concentrations in the bloodstream can lead to hyperosmolar coma. Excessive fat and protein breakdown can produce ketoacidosis. Long-term complications of diabetes include pathological changes in blood vessels, nerves, and kidneys.

Insulin administration to patients with diabetes mellitus constitutes replacement therapy. Insulin restores the ability of cells to utilize glucose as an energy source and corrects many metabolic derangements of diabetes mellitus. Insulin must be injected, since it is a protein subject to digestion in the gastrointestinal tract. Regular insulin is water soluble, quickly absorbed from subcutaneous injection sites, and therefore relatively short acting. Longer acting insulin preparations are formed by creating relatively insoluble complexes of insulin with zinc (semilente, lente, and ultralente insulin) or proteins (globin zinc and NPH insulin) or both (protamine zinc insulin). Insulin administration must be timed to produce maximum hypoglycemic action during periods of food absorption. Insulin therapy is associated with two major acute side effects: hyperglycemia when insulin therapy is inadequate and hypoglycemia when insulin concentrations are larger than required. Insulin may also cause various allergic reactions and local subcutaneous fat atrophy at injection sites.

Sulfonylureas are oral hypoglycemic agents and are used only for patients with noninsulin-dependent diabetes. Sulfonylureas stimulate insulin release from the pancreas and increase the number of insulin receptors on target cells. The onset and duration of action of sulfonylureas depend on the metabolic transformations the drugs undergo, as well as the degree of plasma protein binding. Sulfonylureas may produce gastrointestinal distress, muscle weakness, paresthesias, allergies, and bone marrow toxicity. The most dangerous reaction is hypoglycemia. The effectiveness of sulfonylureas is greatest in obese, mild noninsulin-dependent diabetics, and the hypoglycemic effects are increased by dietary restriction. Patients taking sulfonylureas may suffer a disulfiram-like reaction to ethyl alcohol. Phenylbutazone, salicylates, and sulfonamides may increase effective concentrations of sulfonylureas in the bloodstream and thereby produce hypoglycemia.

■ STUDY QUESTIONS

1. What three peptide hormones from pancreatic islets affect glucose metabolism?
2. What effect does insulin have on glucose metabolism?
3. What effect does glucagon have on glucose metabolism?
4. What effect does somatostatin have on glucose metabolism?
5. What effects do cortisol, epinephrine, and growth hormone have on glucose metabolism?
6. What effect does insulin have on fat and protein metabolism?
7. What is diabetes mellitus?
8. What are the characteristics of insulin-dependent diabetes mellitus?
9. What are the characteristics of noninsulin-dependent diabetes mellitus?
10. What effect does diabetes mellitus have on glucose metabolism?
11. What effect does diabetes mellitus have on protein and fat metabolism?
12. What are the long-term complications of diabetes mellitus?
13. How is diabetes mellitus diagnosed?
14. How does insulin therapy relieve the symptoms of diabetes mellitus?
15. Why must insulin be injected?
16. What is the onset and duration of action of regular insulin?
17. What advantages do the insulin preparations containing relatively insoluble insulin complexes have over regular insulin?
18. Name the insulin preparations available.
19. What is the duration of action of each of the insulin preparations?
20. When does peak hypoglycemic action occur after a dose of Regular insulin? Semilente insulin? NPH insulin? Ultralente insulin? Protamine Zinc Insulin?
21. What are the two major acute side effects of insulin therapy?
22. What type of reactions may insulin produce at the site of injection?
23. What is the mechanism of action for the sulfonylureas as hypoglycemic agents?
24. What type of diabetic patient benefits from sulfonylurea therapy?
25. How are the sulfonylureas administered?
26. Which of the sulfonylureas is rapidly metabolized in the body?
27. Which sulfonylureas must be converted to active forms by the body to be effective?
28. Which is the longest-acting sulfonylurea?
29. What side effects occur with sulfonylureas?
30. Why does caloric restriction enhance sulfonylurea effectiveness?
31. What other drugs may enhance the hypoglycemic effect of sulfonylureas?
32. What reaction may be seen in patients receiving sulfonylureas who ingest ethyl alcohol?

■ SUGGESTED READINGS

Blevins, D.R.: The diabetic and nursing care, New York, 1979, McGraw Hill, Inc.

Boyles, V.A.: Injection aids for blind diabetics, American Journal of Nursing **77:**1456, Sept., 1977.

Breidahl, H.D.: What patients with diabetes want to know about their therapy, Drugs **19:**135, 1980.

Bressler, R.: Control of the blood glucose in diabetes mellitus: is it valuable? Is it feasible? Drugs **17:**461, 1979.

Ensinck, J.W., and Bierman, E.L.: Dietary management of diabetes mellitus, Annual Review of Medicine **30:**155, 1979.

Fonville, A.M.: Teaching patients to rotate injection sites, American Journal of Nursing **78:**880, May, 1978.

Gerich, J.E.: Somatostatin—another pancreatic islet hormone, Advances in Experimental Medicine and Biology **124:**63, 1979.

Greenough, A., Cockroft, P.M., and Bloom, A.: Disposable syringes for insulin injection, British Medical Journal **1:**1467, June 2, 1979.

Griffin, A.: How to prepare and inject insulin with one hand, Geriatric Nursing **1:**112, July-Aug., 1980.

Guthrie, D.W.: Exercise, diets and insulin for children with diabetes, Nursing '77 **7**(2):48, 1977.

Guthrie, D.W.: Helping the diabetic manage his self-care, Nursing '80 **10**(2):57, 1980.

Guthrie, D.W., and Guthrie, R.A.: Nursing management of diabetes mellitus, St. Louis, 1977, The C.V. Mosby Co.

Guthrie, D.W., and Guthrie, R.A.: Diabetic ketoacidosis: breaking the vicious cycle, Nursing '78 **8**(6):54, 1978.

Hagg, S.A.: Clinical use of oral hypoglycemic agents, Drug Therapy Reviews **1:**227, 1978.

Harvey, S.: Drugs in metabolic emergencies, burns, and drug accidents, Nurses Drug Alert (special issue) **2:**145, Dec., 1978.

Hodge, R.H., Krongaard, L., Sande, M.A., and Kaiser, D.L.: Multiple use of disposable syringe-needle units, Journal of the American Medical Association **244:**266, 1980.

Kiser, D.: The Somogyi effect, American Journal of Nursing **80:**236, 1980.

Landin, D.V.: Reporting urine test results: switch + to %, American Journal of Nursing **78:**878, 1978.

Lee, J.: Care and management of the adolescent diabetic, Pediatric Nursing **4:**42, May-June, 1978.

Managing diabetes properly, Nursing skillbook, Horsham, Pa., 1979, Intermed Communications, Inc.

McCarthy, J.: Somogyi effect: managing blood glucose rebound, Nursing '79 **9**(2):38, 1979.

Petrokas, J.C.: Common sense guidelines for controlling diabetes during illness, Nursing '77 **7**(12):36, 1977.

Rush, D.R., and Hamburger, S.C.: Drugs used in endocrine metabolic emergencies, Critical Care Quarterly **3:**1, Sept., 1980.

Seltzer, H.S.: Efficacy and safety of oral hypoglycemic agents, Annual Review of Medicine **31:**261, 1980.

Slater, N.L.: Insulin reactions versus ketoacidosis: guidelines for diagnosis and intervention, American Journal of Nursing **78:**875, May, 1978.

Taft, P.: Rational use of oral hypoglycemic drugs, Drugs **17:**134, 1979.

Wolfe, L.: Insulin: paving the way to a new life, Nursing '77 **7**(11): 38, 1977.

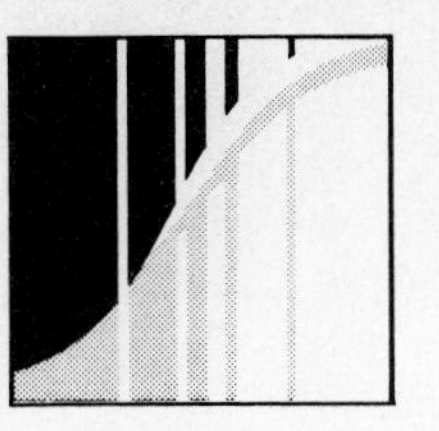
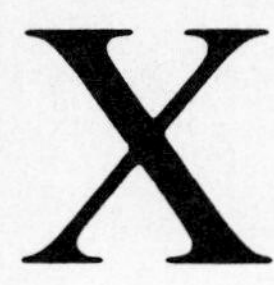

X ANTIINFECTIVE AND CHEMOTHERAPEUTIC AGENTS

This section discusses drugs that are effective by acting as selective poisons against certain organisms or types of cells. Chapter 40, **Introduction to the Use of Antiinfective Agents,** introduces the principle of selective toxicity that underlies all the information in the remaining chapters and focuses on the use of selective poisons to treat disease caused by bacteria or closely related microorganisms. Chapters 41 through 46 discuss specific antiinfective agents, grouping drugs into chapters on the basis of similar mechanisms of action (Chapters 41 to 43), similar toxic reactions and side effects (Chapter 44), and similar uses (Chapters 45 and 46).

Chapters 47 to 49 consider several types of drugs. Each of these chapters not only discusses specific drugs but also delineates the differences between therapy of diseases produced by viruses, fungi, or eucaryotic parasites from the therapy of bacterial disease.

Chapter 50, **Drugs to Treat Neoplastic Diseases,** presents the individual antineoplastic agents and the necessary information on the nature of neoplastic disease to make obvious the rationale behind the use of these agents. The mechanism of drug action is emphasized so that toxicity may be more readily understood. Understanding the mechanism of action allows the clinical properties of these drugs to be more easily appreciated and puts the nursing procedures into proper perspective.

40 Introduction to the use of antiinfective agents

In the preceding chapters the use of drugs that are intended to alter processes occurring naturally in the body was presented. For example, cardiotonic drugs alter existing patterns of ion flow in heart cells; the therapeutic goal of increasing contractility of the heart is achieved by this direct action of the drug. Similarly a direct action on normal physiological functions can be cited for each of the drugs discussed previously. In contrast, the drugs that will be considered in this section ideally do not directly affect any physiological process in the patient. The antiinfective agents may rightfully be considered to be selective poisons, for the goal of therapy with these drugs is to poison invading, pathogenic microorganisms without poisoning the patient in whom those microorganisms are causing disease.

This introductory chapter is intended to present concepts that are important in understanding antibiotic therapy. The microbiological principles that make antibiotic therapy effective will be reviewed, the general mechanisms by which these drugs act will be discussed, and the major problems associated with antimicrobial therapy will be presented. Specific drugs are discussed in subsequent chapters.

■ THE PRINCIPLE OF SELECTIVE TOXICITY

Although the microbial world was discovered by Anton Van Leeuwenhoek in 1676, the impact of these tiny organisms on human destiny was not appreciated until the last third of the nineteenth century. During this period, Louis Pasteur and Robert Koch, working in separate laboratories and on different microorganisms, clearly showed that bacteria could cause human disease. Once this fundamental fact was appreciated, two subsequent developments became almost inevitable. The first of these developments was that microbiologists and physicians began to classify human diseases in terms of the organism that produced the disease. By the early part of the twentieth century, the microorganisms that cause cholera, typhoid, bubonic plague, gonorrhea, leprosy, malaria, syphilis, and a host of other diseases were isolated and identified.

The second inevitable consequence of this new knowledge was that therapy of microbially induced diseases was put on a more rational basis. The first attempts at controlling diseases caused by microorganisms involved immunization. This form of therapy allowed certain diseases to be prevented. However, immunization was neither effective for all diseases nor was this therapy effective once the disease was established in the patient. Chemists, therefore, began to explore the possibility of finding agents that could eradicate invading pathogens in a living patient. A leader in this area was Paul Ehrlich who in 1912 introduced Salvarsan, a drug specifically useful for treating syphilis. Salvarsan and a related drug, Neosalvarsan, established the validity of the principle of selective toxicity. In 1935 a synthetic agent was discovered that could cure streptococcal infections, and in 1939 development was begun on an extract of culture fluid from the mold *Penicillium*. These discoveries marked the beginnings of the sulfonamides and penicillin. From that day to now, the search for more effective antimicrobial agents has not ceased. As subsequent chapters will illustrate, that search has been extraordinarily fruitful.

■ THE MICROBIOLOGICAL BASIS FOR SELECTIVE TOXICITY

There are many similarities in the chemical processes of all life forms on this planet. Nucleic acids (DNA and RNA) carry the genetic information for all living things, and all use the same code to translate DNA and RNA into proteins. Proteins, or enzymes, carry out all the metabolic transformations required for life. Some important differences in chemical or molecular organization do exist among living things. Based on these differences, life forms may be divided into two major categories: procaryotes and eucaryotes. Procaryotic cells are those in which the genetic material exists free within the cell protoplasm, whereas eucaryotic cells contain membrane-bounded nuclei in which the genetic material is stored. Other distinguishing characteristics exist. For example, procaryotes possess cell walls composed in part of peptidoglycan, a complex molecule containing amino acids and sugars. Eucaryotic cells from multicelled organisms usually contain no cell wall at all but only a cell membrane. Single-celled eucaryotic organisms such as algae and fungi may possess complex, rigid cell walls, but these walls do not contain peptidoglycan.

Procaryotes and eucaryotes also differ in certain internal functions. For example, the ribosomes in eucaryotes are larger than those in procaryotes, and the two forms differ in their response to certain chemicals (Chapters 42 to 44). Likewise, folic acid metabolism may differ in the two types of organisms. Many procaryotes cannot utilize folic acid from the environment but must synthesize the vitamin from simpler starting materials. In contrast, eucaryotes cannot synthesize folic acid but must absorb it from the diet.

The structural and metabolic differences just cited between procaryotes and eucaryotes form the basis for selective toxicity. Selective toxicity is defined as the selective poisoning of an invading, disease-causing organism using an agent that has no effect on the person in whom the disease exists.

An ideal antimicrobial agent would have no effect at all on the patient being treated and would destroy all the pathogens within that patient's body. However, no real drug yet approaches that ideal case, and every antiinfective agent we will discuss causes some direct effect on the human host. We must therefore consider some way to evaluate the degree of selective toxicity that may be achieved with a drug. One way to evaluate selective toxicity is by means of the therapeutic index (Chapter 2). The therapeutic index (TI) is defined as the ratio of the dose of a certain drug that kills 50% of the test animals to the dose of that drug that is effective in 50% of the animals ($TI = LD_{50}/ED_{50}$). A drug that is relatively nontoxic may be given in very large doses before animals are killed. If the drug is also potent, it may require rather small doses to achieve the desired clinical effect, which in this case would be cure of the infection. Such a drug as just described would have a large therapeutic index and would be considered to be a drug that displayed good selective toxicity, that is, it attacked the pathogen at doses well below those that were dangerous to the host. In contrast, a drug with a low therapeutic index would not have good selective toxicity. A drug with a therapeutic index of 1 would be equally toxic to the bacteria and to the patient.

The therapeutic index is obviously derived from studies performed on laboratory animals. It is sometimes difficult to correlate animal studies with the clinical effectiveness of a drug. For this reason, other indices of selective toxicity have been used to indicate clinical experience with a drug. For example, the *safety margin* of a drug is defined as the percentage increase above the standard therapeutic dose that may be required to produce serious toxic reactions in a certain percentage of patients. This evaluation is based entirely on clinical experience. It will be noted that a drug with a large therapeutic index and a wide safety margin is a drug that may be given to patients in larger than normal doses without causing significant toxicity in most patients. To illustrate this principle, consider the antibiotics cephaloridine and penicillin G. Cephaloridine must be given in carefully controlled doses because the drug can damage the kidneys if the concentration of the drug in the bloodstream becomes too high. Cephaloridine has a low therapeutic index and a narrow safety margin. Increasing the dose by 50% may cause significant toxicity (Chapter 41). In contrast, penicillin G, which was the first clinically useful penicillin, is a drug with a very wide safety margin and a high therapeutic index. As will be seen in the next chapter, direct toxicity with this drug is very low, and doses three or four times the standard dose may be administered with very little risk of toxic reactions in most patients.

■ MECHANISMS BY WHICH ANTIBIOTICS ACHIEVE SELECTIVE TOXICITY

Most of the antibiotics we will consider act in one of five ways on microorganisms. Antibiotics inhibit cell wall formation, block protein synthesis, disrupt cell membranes, interfere with nucleic acid synthesis, or prevent synthesis of folic acid. Each of these mechanisms of action exploits a biochemical difference between eucaryotic and procaryotic cells.

In addition to categorizing antibiotics in terms of specific mechanisms, antibiotics may be broadly categorized as bacteriostatic or bacteriocidal drugs. The term *bacteriocidal* refers to drugs that directly kill the bacterial cell. For example, by interfering with cell wall synthesis, several antibiotics cause the bacterial cell literally to explode as the osmotic forces generated within the cytoplasm can no longer be contained by the defective cell wall. Likewise, antibiotics that disrupt the bacterial cell membrane allow the cytoplasmic contents of the cell to leak out and the cell dies.

Bacteriostatic drugs, on the other hand, may not directly kill the bacterial cell but rather halt the cell's growth and reproduction. With bacteriostatic drugs, it may be possible to remove the bacteria from exposure to the drug and have the bacteria resume growth. If bacterial death is not caused directly, then how may these drugs achieve a cure? The key to this question is that the host's immune system must attack, immobilize, and eliminate the pathogens for therapy with bacteriostatic drugs to achieve a long-term cure. In theory cures can be effected with bacteriocidal drugs independent of the immune system. In fact such cures are not easily achieved, and it is fair to say that any cure of bacterial disease in normal persons is strongly dependent on immunological factors. In immunosuppressed patients, cures of bacterial infections are much more difficult to achieve even with appropriately prescribed bacteriocidal drugs.

To classify a drug as exclusively bacteriocidal or bacteriostatic is, in a sense, misleading. Many antibiotics may be either bacteriostatic or bacteriocidal depending on dose, site of infection, and the causative organism. For example, consider sulfonamides, which prevent folic acid synthesis in sensitive bacteria. These drugs might be considered bacteriostatic for a systemic infection but because of the high drug concentration achieved in urine may be bacteriocidal in the urine. Other examples would be cases in which two types of microorganisms differed greatly in sensitivity to a certain antibiotic. For the more sensitive organism, the serum and tissue levels achievable with normal dosage may be sufficient for bacteriocidal action, whereas the more resistant organism may simply suffer growth inhibition, that is, a bacteriostatic effect, at that same antibiotic concentration.

Based on this discussion, the term *antimicrobial spectrum* may be defined. By antimicrobial spectrum we refer to the type of microorganisms against which a particular drug is effective. Listed in Table 40-1 are commonly encountered pathogenic microorganisms grouped according to criteria established by microbiologists. A drug that is effective against only a few of these organisms would be considered narrow spectrum. An example would be penicillin G, which is primarily effective against gram-positive bacteria. In contrast, a drug that could be used against several groups of organisms would be classified as broad spectrum. An example would be tetracycline, which is effective against gram-

TABLE 40-1. Microbial pathogens of humans

Organisms	**Common diseases produced**
Viruses	
Influenza	Flu; upper respiratory tract infections
Herpes simplex	Skin, eye, brain infections
Chlamydia	Psittacosis; eye, genital infections
Rickettsia	Typhus; Q fever; Rocky Mountain spotted fever
Spirochetes	Syphilis; yaws
Eubacteria, gram negative	
Haemophilus	Meningitis
Escherichia	Urinary tract infections
Proteus	Urinary tract infections
Klebsiella	Urinary tract infections; pneumonia
Pseudomonas	Urinary tract infections; meningitis
Neisseria	Meningitis; gonorrhea
Salmonella	Typhoid; gastroenteritis
Shigella	Dysentery
Eubacteria, gram positive	
Staphylococcus	Soft tissue infections
Streptococcus	Upper respiratory tract infections
Mycobacteria	Tuberculosis; leprosy
Actinomycetes	Organ lesions and abscesses
Fungi	
Candida	Minor skin, mild respiratory, but severe systemic infections
Cryptococcus	
Histoplasma	
Blastomyces	

positive and gram-negative bacteria, as well as against *Rickettsia* and *Chlamydia*.

In the past it was thought desirable to have very broad spectrum antibiotics that could be used without regard to identifying the causative organism in an infection. Current practice argues against such reasoning, and there are today numerous examples of drugs that are primarily used for only one type of bacterial infection. This type of therapy is made possible by the very reliable microbiological techniques now available for identification of microorganisms.

Intimately related to the concept of the antimicrobial spectrum are the terms *minimum inhibitory concentration (MIC)* and *minimum bacteriocidal concentration (MBC)*. For each antibiotic and microorganism it is possible to determine in the laboratory the amount of that drug required to halt the growth of the organism and the amount required to kill the organism being tested. The concentrations are the lowest ones at which growth inhibition or cell death can be observed. A consideration of these figures as well as a determination of safe blood levels for an antibiotic are involved in determining an effective therapeutic regimen. For example, a blood concentration above the MBC is desirable but whether that concentration can be achieved will depend on the pharmacological properties governing drug absorption and elimination as well as the threshold for toxicity produced by the drug in the host.

■ MICROBIAL RESISTANCE TO ANTIBIOTICS

As we have already discussed, not all microorganisms are sensitive to all antibiotics. Resistance to antibiotics may be classified as *inherent* or *acquired*. Inherent resistance to an antibiotic is unrelated to prior exposure of the microbe to the drug. For example, the first time a culture of *Pseudomonas aeruginosa* was ever exposed to penicillin G, it was found to be resistant, that is, penicillin resistance was an inherent quality of the microorganism. In contrast, acquired resistance refers to resistance that is dependent on prior exposure of the microbe to the drug. For example, when penicillin G was first tested against *Staphylococcus aureus*, the organism was exquisitely sensitive. If the organism was exposed to sublethal doses of the drug for long periods of time, however, more and more penicillin-resistant microbes began to appear. The end result is that the entire population of a strain of *S. aureus* can be converted from penicillin sensitivity to penicillin resistance by continuous low level exposure to the drug, which allows genetic variants displaying penicillin resistance to proliferate. This phenomenon is called *acquired resistance*. Not only can acquired resistance be demonstrated in the laboratory, but it also occurs clinically. Again *S. aureus* is a good example, since strains isolated from clinical infections during the 1940's were almost always penicillin sensitive, whereas today clinically isolated *S. aureus* strains are mostly penicillin resistant.

Plasmids are small, circular pieces of DNA found separate from the chromosome in bacteria. Many of the genes for antibiotic resistance reside on plasmids. Since plasmids may be rapidly passed between bacterial cells, antibiotic resistance can rapidly spread through an entire bacterial population. This mechanism for acquired resistance usually results in serious therapeutic difficulty, since resistance to several antibiotics may occur simultaneously.

The precise mechanisms by which microorganisms achieve resistance to an antibiotic may be divided into three categories. The first of these mechanisms is actual destruction of the antibiotic by the microorganism. This process usually involves enzymes that chemically alter and thereby inactivate the antibiotic. Examples of this process include penicillinase, which destroys penicillin, and the acetylase, phosphorylases, and adenylating enzymes that inactivate the aminoglycoside antibiotics.

A second mechanism by which bacteria may achieve antibiotic resistance is by reducing the uptake of the drug into the bacterial cell. Many antibiotics freely enter and in some cases are concentrated within bacterial cells. By blocking this uptake, resistance may be achieved. An example of this type of resistance is seen with tetracyclines, which can be shown to freely enter sensitive bacteria but not resistant strains.

The third mechanism for resistance involves a mutation or an alteration in the target of the antibiotic in the microorganism. For example, erythromycin inhibits protein synthesis by binding to certain sites on the bacterial ribosome. Certain resistant microorganisms form altered ribosomes that do not bind erythromycin and are therefore resistant to the inhibitory action of that drug. Some types of streptomycin resistance may occur by similar means.

■ FACTORS THAT AFFECT THE OUTCOME OF ANTIBIOTIC THERAPY

In antibiotic therapy the first step is the proper identification of the microorganism causing the disease. In some infections the symptoms are sufficiently clear-cut to allow accurate diagnosis with a physical examination only. In other cases, actual culturing must be done to identify the organism. In some institutions nursing personnel are trained to take specimens for culture, whereas in others laboratory personnel or physicians perform this function.

The second step in treatment is the selection of the proper antibiotic, a process that obviously depends on a knowledge of the pathogen involved. This decision may be based entirely on clinical experience or may be aided by antibiotic sensitivity testing carried out in the microbiology laboratory on the pathogen isolated from the patient.

Even when the proper drug has been selected, several factors may influence the effectiveness of therapy. One of these factors is the site of infection. For example, meningitis is difficult to treat partly because many of the antibiotics available do not penetrate the blood-brain barrier very well, making an effective drug concentration at the infection site difficult to achieve. Similarly, many abscesses or soft tissue infections are not easily treated, since the areas of infections are poorly perfused and many drugs tend not to penetrate well into these areas. Healing is frequently hastened by surgical drainage.

Other drugs the patient is receiving may influence the outcome of antibiotic therapy. Immunosuppressant drugs are good examples of agents that limit antibiotic effectiveness by depressing immune mechanisms. Large doses of glucocorticoids cause significant immunosuppression. Other specific interactions may occur and will be mentioned with individual drug classes in subsequent chapters.

Finally the clinical status of the patient can alter the outcome of antibiotic therapy. In particular, kidney function is very important to consider, since many of the available antibiotics are excreted by the kidney. If kidney function is impaired, drugs eliminated through the kidney may accumulate. Likewise, liver disease may cause accumulation of drugs that are eliminated primarily by liver mechanisms. Patients with insufficiencies in either of these organ systems must be closely watched for signs of drug toxicity, and these signs may occur at lower doses than would be expected in normal persons.

■ PROBLEMS IN ANTIBIOTIC THERAPY

Direct drug toxicity is observed with many classes of antibiotics. Each antibiotic should be considered for its potential toxicity to the patient when it is administered. These direct toxic effects are frequently highly characteristic. For example, any aminoglycoside antibiotic can cause kidney damage and loss of hearing or loss of equilibrium. Therefore when these drugs are given, the patient should be closely observed for these characteristic toxic signs. Even very safe drugs may occasionally cause direct toxic reactions, an example being penicillin effects on the central nervous system. Nursing personnel should be alert for these signs. Many of these direct toxic reactions to antibiotics are dose dependent and would be expected to be more frequent and serious when high doses of the drugs are given or when drug accumulation occurs in patients with renal or hepatic impairment.

Allergies occur frequently with several antibiotics. The best examples are the penicillins, which can produce allergic reactions ranging from simple rashes to anaphylactic shock. Allergies occur in patients who have previously been exposed to the antibiotic, either in the medical setting or in the environment. Although in theory animals intended for immediate slaughter may not be treated with antibiotics also used in humans, in fact meat has on occasion contained sufficient quantities of antibiotics to sensitize some people who consumed the meat.

Suprainfections are infections that arise during antibiotic therapy. Suprainfections by definition involve microorganisms that are resistant to the antibiotic originally used. For this reason, these infections are often serious and difficult to treat. Such infections are more common with broad spectrum antibiotics than narrow spectrum ones. This observation is apparently based on the fact that broad spectrum antibiotics eliminate much more of the natural bacterial flora and upset the ecological controls that normally keep the resistant pathogens in check. With the tetracyclines, for example, yeasts such as *Candida* are frequently involved in suprainfections.

■ Misuses of antibiotics

Antibiotics are commonly misunderstood and misused by the lay public. One of the most common misconceptions concerning this class of drugs is that antibiotics will cure any type of infectious disease, including those caused by viruses. In fact we do not have effective drugs to treat minor viral infections such as colds. As will be discussed in Chapter 48, very few drugs are available for use in viral infections of any kind, and certainly none of the commonly employed antibiotics can be effectively used for viral diseases.

Many infectious diseases resolve quickly once appropriate antibiotics are administered. For this reason, it is tempting for patients to discontinue medication much earlier than the physician planned, namely as soon as the patient feels better. This practice is dangerous for several reasons. One is that the antibiotics with bacteriostatic action inhibit growth of bacteria but the cells remain viable, at least until the immune system can eliminate them. Therefore if therapy is discontinued too early, these organisms may again proliferate and a relapse may occur. Not only does this event prolong recovery for the patient, but it may also make the disease more difficult to treat. If we consider that the organisms most resistant to the drugs being used are the ones that will probably survive longest, we can appreciate that these resistant organisms may cause the relapse. Therapy may therefore be difficult, since some degree of drug resistance has occurred.

One of the excuses frequently given when patients discontinue antibiotic therapy early is that they wish to have the medication on hand in case they ever need it again. This practice is dangerous not only for the reasons just discussed but also because this reasoning assumes the patient will be able to accurately diagnose future illnesses. Self-medication with old, unused antibiotic prescriptions may delay proper medical attention and prolong or worsen the patient's disease. Once medication has been started, culture results become relatively unreliable and proper diagnosis may be impossible. For these reasons, patients should be discouraged from saving old antibiotics to take them "just until I can get to the doctor."

Finally, it should be recalled that many drugs require special storage conditions and do not remain active for very long when exposed to the warm, humid environment of most bathroom medicine cabinets. Drugs stored for weeks or months under such conditions may be inactive or may be converted to forms that are in fact more toxic. Penicillin in solution, for example, tends to form polymers that have been implicated in an increased incidence of anaphylactic episodes. Tetracyclines tend to be light-sensitive and break down to toxic compounds.

Any drug that remains in the household may be a

THE NURSING PROCESS

Assessment

Patients requiring drugs for antiinfective therapy usually have some sign of infection. These signs of infection usually include such things as fever, purulent drainage, elevation of the white blood cell count, and signs of inflammation such as redness, swelling, or tenderness. Occasionally, infections are diagnosed because of a positive culture even though the patient is asymptomatic as in the case of some urinary tract infections. Infections can occur in patients of any age, both inpatients and outpatients. Some infections would be self-limiting if left untreated. Some infections cause few symptoms, whereas others can cause debilitating symptoms and eventually death. The data base for a patient with a known or suspected infection would include a thorough total patient assessment. In addition, emphasis should be placed on the temperature and vital signs, subjective and objective evaluation of any area that is thought to be infected, results of culture and sensitivity testing, other appropriate laboratory work such as complete blood counts that might indicate elevated white blood cell counts, history of exposure to infecting organisms, and assessment of preexisting medical conditions.

Management

Once the decision is made to treat with one or more antiinfective agents, the nurse should then obtain additional data for the data base about particular organs or areas that might be affected by the prescribed antibiotics. For example, an assessment of the patient's hearing should be done before starting antibiotics that may cause ototoxicity; assessment of renal function should be done before starting antibiotics that are known to cause nephrotoxicity. In addition, the health care team members should remember that certain antibiotics when used together are more prone to cause toxicity to certain organs in the body. During the management phase the nurse should monitor the temperature and vital signs. Appropriate laboratory work such as blood counts, liver function tests, and renal function tests should be done to monitor for the desired effects and possible side effects of the drugs. Regular monitoring of the patient's subjective and objective signs of infections should also be done. Other therapies may be needed to help control the infectious process such as application of warm moist soaks, debridement of infected areas, and special wound-cleaning procedures. Adequate nutritional and fluid intakes should be maintained, and it may be appropriate to measure intake and output. Other drugs may be prescribed to assist in providing patient comfort such as antipyretics for fever and bladder analgesics for severe urinary tract infections. The nurse should check for known side effects of antibiotic therapy such as monilial overgrowth of the oral cavity or the vagina. The nurse should carefully evaluate the appearance of new symptoms that may or may not indicate a potentially serious reaction to the antibiotic. For example, diarrhea that occurs in the patient being treated with ampicillin may be a troublesome but not too serious side effect; diarrhea that appears in the patient being treated with clindamycin may indicate a serious side effect to this drug and may warrant discontinuing the medication. Because some antiinfective agents are known to cause allergic responses more often than other categories of drugs, there should always be available appropriate drugs and equipment for resuscitation should an acute allergic response occur.

Continued.

■ THE NURSING PROCESS—cont'd

■ Evaluation

The goal of therapy with antiinfective agents is to help the body eliminate the infection without causing side effects in the patient. Frequently this is exactly what happens, and many patients take antibiotics with no reported side effects. Occasionally side effects persist after therapy is discontinued or occur days to weeks after therapy has stopped. In preparation for discharge the patient should be able to explain why and how to take the drug ordered, the necessity of continuing the course of therapy for as long as prescribed, side effects that may occur, side effects that should cause the patient to notify the physician immediately, symptoms that would indicate that the medication is not effective (e.g., continuing fever or discomfort persisting 3 to 4 days after the start of therapy), recommended guidelines about diet and fluids that have been prescribed, and the importance of not sharing antiinfective agents with other individuals for whom the drug has not been prescribed. For additional information about specific kinds and locations of infections, the student should refer to appropriate textbooks. For specific information about individual antiinfective agents, see the remaining chapters in this text and the patient care implications section at the end of this chapter.

---

hazard to children. Proper use and disposal of drugs is important to protect children from accidental poisoning. In addition, as will be seen in subsequent chapters, very young children may be much more sensitive to certain antibiotics than adults and for this reason antibiotics should never be given to children without first consulting a physician.

■ PATIENT CARE IMPLICATIONS

1. Before administering any antiinfective agent, question the patient carefully about history of allergy. Remember that not all patients who develop an allergic response will have had a previous history of allergy and not all patients are reliable historians. It may be necessary to phrase questions in terms the patient can understand. For example, the question, "Are there any medicines that you should not take and why?" may elicit a different response than, "Are you allergic to penicillin or the cephalosporins?" If there is a question of allergy, the physician should be notified before the dose is given. The patient's health record should be clearly marked if there is a history of allergies. In some hospitals patients with allergies wear a second specially marked or colored identification bracelet indicating the nature of their allergies.
2. All patients receiving antinfectives should be observed carefully for possible allergic response. Epinephrine, antihistamines, steroids, oxygen, and resuscitation equipment should be readily available. An anaphylactic response is an acute emergency; if a physician is not on the premises at all times, it may be appropriate to have as part of the institution's policies and procedures written medical orders for management of an acute allergic response.
3. Persons with a known severe allergy to any medication should be encouraged to wear a medical identification tag or bracelet indicating their allergies.
4. Health care personnel with a known sensitivity to a specific antiinfective agent should avoid preparing or administering that drug or related drugs or should wear gloves while doing so.
5. Within each class of antiinfectives, there may be many preparations available. Health care personnel should read orders and labels carefully, should never substitute one preparation for another without physician approval, and should question any order that seems incorrect.
6. Patients being discharged who are taking antiinfective agents should be taught all the necessary information. This would include why they are receiving the drug, how to take it correctly (with meals, before meals, frequency), possible side effects to watch for and what to do if they appear, how long to continue the medication, how to store the medication (room temperature, refrigerator), how to prepare the correct dose (e.g., to shake the bottle vigorously, how to use a medicine dropper, what size teaspoon), what to do with any unused portion at the completion of the prescribed course of therapy, and the necessity of continuing treatment for the prescribed length of time. In some situations it may be appropriate to have the patient or family member demonstrate how to administer a dose so

that accuracy can be monitored (e.g., mothers of small infants or an elderly person with limited eyesight who might be taking a suspension form).

7. The use of some antibiotics during pregnancy is clearly contraindicated (e.g., tetracycline); others should be used only when the benefit clearly outweighs possible risks. Women of childbearing age should be questioned about the possibility of being pregnant before antiinfectives are prescribed. Many antibiotics are excreted in breast milk, so lactating mothers should consult with their physicians before continuing to breast-feed if antiinfectives have been prescribed.
8. Suprainfections (overgrowth by nonsusceptible organisms) can be a problem for any patient receiving antiinfectives. Common sites include the mouth, vagina, anus, and gastrointestinal tract. Good hygiene will help the patient feel more comfortable. Diarrhea, a common side effect of many agents, can at times be a symptom of suprainfection in the bowel. Patients should be instructed to report the appearance of any new symptom.
9. Most antinfectives, except tablets and capsules, once reconstituted, should be stored in the refrigerator to maintain potency, but the recommended storage time varies from drug to drug (see manufacturer's literature). Date all dilutions when prepared, do not use undated reconstituted medications, and observe expiration dates recommended by the manufacturer.
10. Reconstituted preparations should be mixed well before preparing an ordered dose. Shake oral suspensions well; agitate small bottles of parenteral solutions between two hands.
11. Rotate sites of intramuscular injections. It may be necessary to divide doses into two or more separate injections if the total volume is large. In the adult, 2.5 to 3 ml is the largest volume that should be administered to any single site, although up to 5 ml may rarely be given in the gluteus maximus. In children, the volume of the dose, the size of the child, and the ability of the child to cooperate should be taken into consideration. However, the gluteus maximus site should be avoided in infants and small children, the anterolateral aspect of the thigh being the preferred injection site. In any age patient, the larger the volume of the medication, the more uncomfortable the injection site will be. Sometimes the physician will indicate that the ordered dose is to be given via two or more injections.
12. In addition to the volume of medication contributing to discomfort at the injection site, many of the antiinfectives themselves are known to cause pain at the injection site, an example being the cephalosporins. Patients may prefer not to receive painful injections in the deltoid muscle if that site can be avoided. In young children, the deltoid muscle may not be developed enough for intramuscular injections.
13. It is especially important to aspirate before injecting intramuscular preparations of antiinfectives to avoid inadvertent injections into the vascular system.
14. As with all drugs, parents should be reminded to keep medications out of the reach of children to preven poisoning and overdose. Many of the antiinfectives come in forms designed to taste good, such as syrups and chewable tablets.
15. Instruct patients taking antiinfectives to avoid the use of nonprescription medications unless they first consult their physicians. Patients should keep all health care personnel informed of all medications they are taking.

■ SUMMARY

Successful therapy of diseases caused by pathogenic microorganisms depends on the use of selectively toxic agents, that is, agents that have no effect on the patient yet destroy the pathogenic microorganisms causing the disease. Selective toxicity of a drug is measured by the therapeutic index or the safety margin. Drugs that are highly toxic to pathogenic microorganisms but relatively nontoxic to the host have a high therapeutic index and a wide safety margin. Good selective toxicity is achieved by using drugs that antagonize a process in the microorganism that is absent or insensitive in humans. Resistance to various antibiotics is an inherent property of certain microorganisms. The antimicrobial spectrum of an antibiotic describes the array of microorganisms that are sensitive to the drug. Microorganisms may also acquire resistance to antibiotics. Acquired resistance results from a genetic change in the organism that causes the formation of enzymes to inactivate the antibiotic, blocks the uptake of the antibiotic, or alters the biochemical target of the antibiotic in the microbial cell. The success of antibiotic therapy depends on the use of the proper antibiotic for the particular pathogen causing the disease. In addition, the site of the infection, other drugs the patient may be receiving, as well as the clinical status of the patient may influence the outcome of antibiotic therapy. Improper patient compliance may also compromise therapy. Discontinuing antibiotics before the prescribed dose has been taken increases the risk of relapse and suprainfection. Use of old prescriptions of antibiotics held from previous illnesses risks creating additional toxicity from outdated or degraded drugs and may interfere with proper diagnosis should medical attention be sought after the drugs are taken.

■ STUDY QUESTIONS

1. What is the principle of selective toxicity?
2. Why is selective toxicity possible to achieve?
3. How is selective toxicity achieved?
4. How is selective toxicity measured?
5. What is the difference between a bacteriostatic and a bacteriocidal drug?
6. What is the antimicrobial spectrum of a drug?
7. Define the terms *minimum inhibitory concentration (MIC)* and *minimum bacteriocidal concentration (MBC)*.
8. What is the difference between inherent and acquired resistance?
9. What are the three types of mechanisms by which microorganisms become resistant to antibiotics?
10. Name five factors that influence the outcome of antibiotic therapy.
11. What are the three general types of problems that may arise during antibiotic therapy?
12. What are some of the common misuses of antibiotics?
13. What are the dangers associated with premature cessation of antibiotic therapy?
14. What are two of the dangers associated with saving left-over antibiotics in the home?

■ SUGGESTED READINGS

Bint, A.J., and Burtt, I.: Adverse antibiotic drug interactions, Drugs **20:**57, 1980.

Carruthers, M.M.: Antimicrobial therapy. In Youmans, G.P., Paterson, P.Y., and Sommers, H.M.: The biologic and clinical basis of infectious diseases, ed. 2, Philadelphia, 1980, W.B. Saunders Co.

DuPont, H.L.: Infection control. Rational antibiotic therapy, Topics in Clinical Nursing **1:**45, July, 1979.

Gahart, B.L.: Intravenous medications, a handbook for nurses and other allied health personnel, ed. 2, St. Louis, 1977, The C.V. Mosby Co.

Gilbert, W., and Villa-Komaroff, L.: Useful proteins from recombinant bacteria, Scientific American **242**(4):74, 1980.

Hermans, P.E.: General principles of antimicrobial therapy, Mayo Clinic Proceedings **52:**603, 1977.

How to use intravenous antibiotics, Nurses' Drug Alert (special issue) **1:**89, June, 1977.

McCabe, W.R.: Factors involved in the selection of an antimicrobial agent in clinical practice. In Bondi, A., Bartola, J.T., and Prier, J.E., editors: The clinical laboratory as an aid in chemotherapy of infectious disease, Baltimore, 1977, University Park Press.

Novick, R.P.: Plasmids, Scientific American **243**(6):102, 1980.

Robinson, L.A., and Whitacre, N.F.: Intravenous administration of antibiotics in children, Pediatric Nursing **3:**21, May-June, 1977.

Rose, H.D., and Wang, R.I.H.: General principles for the selection and use of antimicrobial agents. In Wang, R.I.H.: Practical drug therapy, Philadelphia, 1979, J.B. Lippincott Co.

Smith, A.L.: Microbes. Role in disease. In Smith, A.L.: Principles of microbiology, ed. 8, St. Louis, 1977, The C.V. Mosby Co.

Young, F.E., and Robertson, R.G.: Problem of development of resistant organisms: monitoring their emergence and study of mechanism of resistance. In Bondi, A., Bartola, J.T., and Prier, J.E., editors: The clinical laboratory as an aid in chemotherapy of infectious disease, Baltimore, 1977, University Park Press.

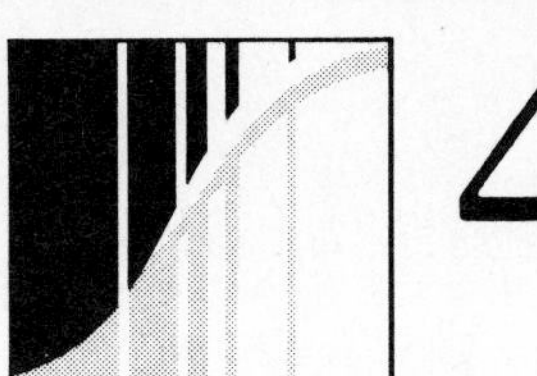

41 Antibiotics: penicillins and cephalosporins

This chapter is intended as an introduction to the most widely used family of antibiotics in medical practice today. These are the beta-lactam antibiotics, of which penicillins and cephalosporins are the most important representatives. This chapter first discusses the properties common to all members of this family of antibiotics and then considers the special features of individual agents.

■ PROPERTIES COMMON TO ALL PENICILLINS AND CEPHALOSPORINS

■ Mechanism of action and bacterial resistance

Penicillins and cephalosporins are irreversible inhibitors of a bacterial enzyme called *transpeptidase*. The function of this enzyme in bacterial cells is to cross-link parallel strands of cell wall material called *peptidoglycan*. When cross-linking occurs, peptidoglycan becomes very rigid and is an effective cell wall. When cross-linking is blocked by penicillin or cephalosporin, cell wall synthesis continues without cross-linking. Ultimately, the unreinforced strands that are formed are unable to resist the osmotic forces within the bacterial cell. The bacterium may literally explode. Since the exposed bacteria may be directly killed, the beta-lactam antibiotics are classified as bacteriocidal drugs. However, even at doses below those required to kill bacteria, penicillins and cephalosporins may be effective in some circumstances. Minimal disruption of the bacterial cell wall by these drugs may make the bacterium more liable to elimination by the immune system of the host.

Penicillins and cephalosporins do not destroy existing bacterial cell wall. Rather these drugs prevent formation of new, intact cell wall. For this reason penicillins and cephalosporins are most effective against actively growing bacteria.

Resistance to penicillins and cephalosporins develops in microorganisms. The mechanism for resistance involves enzymes called *beta-lactamases*. These enzymes are usually referred to as penicillinases or cephalosporinases, depending on which type of drug the enzyme is most effective against. These enzymes destroy the penicillin or cephalosporin nucleus (Fig. 41-1), rendering the drug inactive. Some organisms possess these enzymes as part of their normal metabolic makeup and are therefore intrinsically resistant to beta-lactam antibiotics. Other organisms may acquire the enzyme and thus be converted from antibiotic sensitivity to resistance. Clinically important examples of acquired penicillin resistance are *Staphylococcus aureus* and *Neisseria gonorrhoeae*. Although 25 years ago both organisms could routinely be considered to be sensitive to penicillin G, today significant resistance to penicillin G exists for both organisms. In some hospitals upwards of 90% of *S. aureus* strains are resistant.

■ Excretion

Penicillins and cephalosporins are excreted by the kidney, primarily by active secretion. For all the penicillins except nafcillin and for all the cephalosporins, the kidney is the main route of excretion. The secondary route of excretion is usually through the bile.

■ Toxicity of the penicillins and cephalosporins

Allergies are the most common adverse reaction to the penicillins. Many patients experience skin rashes or urticaria, but anaphylaxis is a much more dangerous allergic response. Whereas allergic rashes and drug fevers usually appear after several days of therapy, the onset of anaphylaxis is nearly always within 10 minutes. Injections of penicillin are responsible for most anaphylactic episodes, but any form of exposure to penicillin may produce anaphylaxis in sensitive individuals.

A patient beginning penicillin therapy should be asked to remain in the clinic for about 30 minutes after a penicillin injection so that if anaphylaxis develops, medical help will be immediately available. In the event that anaphylaxis occurs, the first action of medical personnel should be to administer subcutaneous epinephrine. Anaphylaxis involves profound vasomotor collapse, and there may be laryngeal edema to further complicate resuscitation efforts. Steroids may be required, as well as a tracheostomy and oxygen under positive pressure. All of these emergency supplies should be readily at hand in any clinical setting where antibiotics are administered.

Some physicians perform a skin test before administering penicillins to try to identify patients allergic to penicillins. It is estimated that 3% to 5% of the population at large is allergic to penicillin; about 10% of those who have previously received penicillin in a medical setting may be allergic. It is very important that patients about to receive penicillin be asked if they have ever been given penicillin before and if they have ever had a rash or other allergic symptom during penicillin therapy. This type of information, while necessary, is somewhat unreliable in the sense that many patients who report allergy to penicillin in the past do not experience allergic reactions when reexposed to the drug. In part this may be because the original reaction was not a true penicillin allergy. Ampicillin, for example, may cause a benign macular eruption rather than a urticarial reaction. This toxic rash is not a sign of allergy but may be reported as an allergy by the patient. Another explanation for apparent changes in sensitivity to penicillins is that some patients are allergic to contaminants which were present in early penicillin preparations but which are absent from the more purified modern penicillin preparations.

Some patients who report no previous allergies to penicillin and some patients who claim never to have received penicillin may nevertheless experience an allergic response when they receive the drug. In some cases the patient might be unaware of what drug was prescribed and will therefore not be a reliable source of information. Although it is a rare occurrence, some persons have become sensitized by being exposed to penicillin in the environment or in the food chain. For example, animals destined for human food use can be treated with penicillins by the feed lot owner, although a sufficient length of time should be allowed before slaughter so that the drug can be removed from the animal's system.

Cephalosporins like penicillins are good allergens, and many patients suffer allergic reactions to the drugs. Rashes are most common, but anaphylaxis is possible. Many patients who are allergic to penicillins are also allergic to cephalosporins and vice versa.

Direct drug toxicity with penicillin is very low. Truly massive doses have been given with no ill effect. The tissue most sensitive to direct effects is the central nervous system. Intrathecal injection (into the subarachnoid space or cerebrospinal fluid) may produce convulsions. Convulsions also occur occasionally in patients given high doses intramuscularly or intravenously, especially if the patient has some renal impairment and tends to accumulate the drug. A relatively high concentration in the cerebrospinal fluid must be achieved before convulsions occur. For example, this complication might occur in an elderly patient being treated for a serious infection such as streptococcal endocarditis. This patient might receive 25 to 40 million units of penicillin daily to maintain continuous bacteriocidal drug concentrations. Whereas normal persons can readily eliminate these large amounts of drug through their kidneys, elderly persons may have diminished renal function. Therefore drug accumulation may occur, and penicillin may begin to enter the central nervous system. The first sign may be loss of consciousness or myoclonic movements. Generalized seizures may follow.

Another group of patients with reduced ability to excrete penicillin are newborn infants. Because of their reduced ability to eliminate the drug, neonates receive carefully adjusted penicillin doses based on their body weight and reduced clearance of penicillin.

Cephalosporins are also excreted primarily by the kidney and like the penicillins may therefore accumulate in the patients with impaired renal function. Hence cephalosporin dosage may be reduced when renal function is lower than normal.

Oral penicillin preparations cause gastrointestinal distress in some patients. Reactions include irritation and inflammation of the upper gastrointestinal tract, nausea, vomiting, and diarrhea. Orally administered cephalosporins may also cause gastric irritation, nausea, and vomiting.

Several of the penicillin and cephalosporin preparations on the market contain sufficient sodium or potassium to alter electrolyte balance in some patients. For example, one million units of penicillin G and penicillin V may contain 1.5 mEq of potassium. Given in high enough doses for long enough periods, potassium intoxication and cardiac arrhythmias may occur. Carbenicillin and some preparations of penicillin G contain high concentrations of sodium, which may cause difficulties in patients with preexisting cardiac or renal difficulties.

Penicillins and cephalosporins require some care in handling and diluting for intramuscular or intravenous therapy. Many penicillins require properly buffered solutions for best stability, and for this reason not all penicillins are compatible with common intravenous fluids. Medical personnel should check the penicillin package insert or refer to the pharmacist before adding penicillins to any intravenous fluid.

Probenecid is a drug sometimes used with penicillins to increase the effective duration of action of the penicillins by slowing excretion of penicillin in the kidney. Probenecid itself may cause toxic reactions difficult to distinguish from a penicillin reaction. For example, probenecid may produce chills, fever, and rash as well as gastrointestinal irritation and anemia. Probenecid also blocks cephalosporin excretion in the kidney.

FIG. 41-1

Structure of penicillin G. All the penicillin antibiotics contain the penicillin nucleus shown. Any chemical disruption of the nucleus, such as that produced by acid or penicillinase, results in loss of antibiotic activity. The ionizable hydrogen may be replaced with sodium or potassium ion without effect on drug activity. Alterations of the side chain of penicillin affect the acid stability, penicillinase resistance, and antimicrobial spectrum of the drug. The penicillins in use in the clinic differ from one another in their side chain structures. Cephalosporins contain a slightly different nucleus and side chains than penicillins.

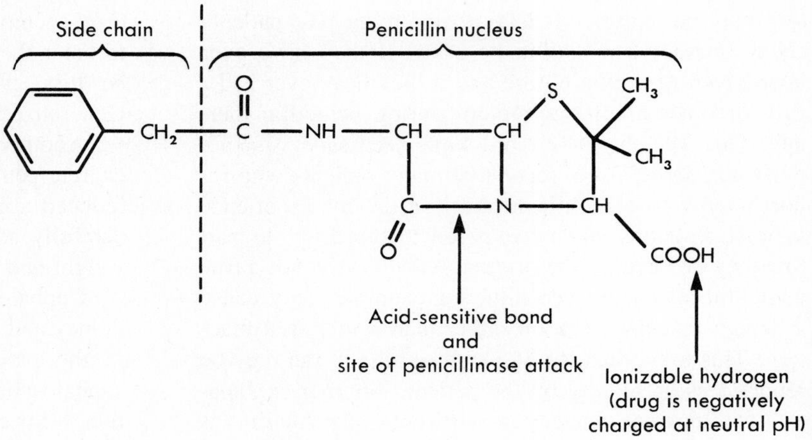

Side chain
Penicillin nucleus
Acid-sensitive bond and site of penicillinase attack
Ionizable hydrogen (drug is negatively charged at neutral pH)

FIG. 41-2

Serum concentration and urinary excretion of an intramuscular dose of penicillin G. Penicillin G is efficiently and rapidly absorbed following intramuscular injections. Peak plasma concentrations of the drug appear 20 to 30 minutes after injection. Penicillin G is actively secreted in the renal tubule, accounting for the very rapid elimination half-time of about 20 to 30 minutes. Most of the drug dose ends up in the urine as the active form of the drug.

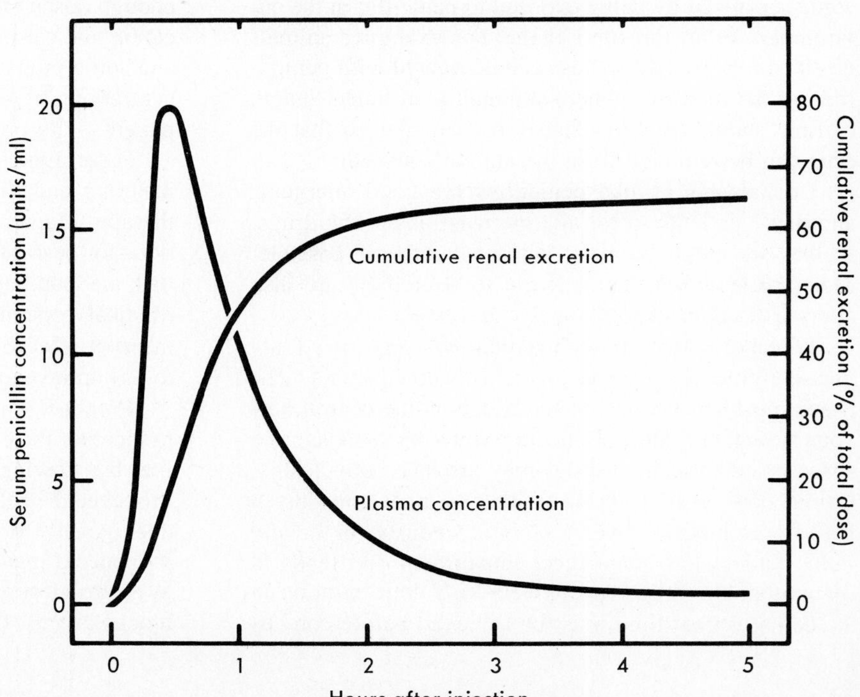

■ PROPERTIES OF INDIVIDUAL PENICILLINS

Penicillin G

Absorption. Penicillin G was the first penicillin to be used clinically with success. This drug is one of several so-called natural penicillins, being formed spontaneously by the *Penicillium* mold and released into the culture fluid. Of these naturally occurring compounds, penicillin G has the most potent antibacterial action. The structure of penicillin G is shown in Fig. 41-1. One of the main points to consider about the structure of penicillins is that the side chain portion of the molecule is variable. All the other types of penicillins we will consider are formed by changing the side chain and leaving the nucleus intact. The second point to be emphasized is that the penicillin nucleus must remain intact to retain antibacterial activity. As pointed out in Fig. 41-1, at least one bond in the nucleus is sensitive to acid, a fact that explains the lability of penicillin G in the stomach. Approximately 30% of an orally administered dose is actually absorbed, the rest being destroyed in the stomach or retained in the intestine and destroyed by bacteria in the large bowel. Because of the incomplete and somewhat variable absorption of penicillin G by this route, oral doses of penicillin G are higher than those commonly used intramuscularly or intravenously. Food interferes with the absorption of oral doses of penicillin G, so the drug should be given 1 hour before or 2 hours after meals.

Penicillin G is rapidly and completely absorbed following intramuscular injection (Fig. 41-2). Serum concentrations reach a peak within 20 to 30 minutes of the injection. Unfortunately, this peak concentration persists for only a very short time, primarily because the kidney so efficiently removes penicillin from the bloodstream. Within 2 to 3 hours after intramuscular injection about 60% of the penicillin dose has appeared in the urine. The drug in the urine is unchanged and still possesses antibacterial activity. Penicillin enters the urine by a process called *active secretion* in the renal tubule. This process involves a specific transport system for which several drugs may compete. Physicians may take advantage of this trait by using a drug such as probenecid to block penicillin excretion, thereby increasing the peak penicillin concentration in the serum and increasing its effective duration.

Distribution. Penicillin G is generally well-distributed throughout many body tissues with high concentrations being found in blood, liver, kidney, and bile. Virtually no drug is found in brain or cerebrospinal fluid in normal persons. If the meninges are inflamed, as in meningitis, penicillin can penetrate into the central nervous system in significant amounts.

Uses. Penicillin G is a narrow spectrum antibiotic.

TABLE 41-1. Antimicrobial spectrum of penicillin G

Organism	Typical infections
GRAM-POSITIVE BACTERIA	
Streptococcus, selected strains	Upper respiratory infections, endocarditis, bacteremia
Streptococcus pneumoniae	Abscesses, bronchitis, meningitis, pneumonia, bacteremia
Staphylococcus aureus	Skin and soft tissue infections, bronchitis, endocarditis, otitis, pneumonia, meningitis, bacteremia
Bacillus anthracis	Anthrax
Corynebacterium diphtherium	Diphtheria
Clostridium tetani	Tetanus
Clostridium perfringens	Gas gangrene
GRAM-NEGATIVE BACTERIA	
Neisseria gonorrhoeae	Gonorrhea
Meningococcus	Meningitis
SPIROCHETE	
Treponema pallidum	Syphilis

The organisms against which it is effective are summarized in Table 41-1. Most of the sensitive organisms are gram-positive bacteria. These bacteria are characterized by thick, peptidoglycan-rich cell walls, which react with the gram stain. Some of these gram-positive organisms, such as *S. aureus, Streptococcus* species, and *Streptococcus pneumoniae,* cause rather common infections of the upper respiratory tract and soft tissues, as well as more serious infections. Other rare gram-positive organisms, such as the ones which cause anthrax, gas gangrene, tetanus, and diphtheria, are also sensitive to penicillin. Among gram-negative organisms, clinically significant sensitivity to penicillin G is seen only with *N. meningitidis* (meningococcus) and *N. gonorrhoeae* (gonococcus). Other common gram-negative organisms normally found in the bowel and those frequently responsible for urinary tract infections are clinically resistant to penicillin G. In the laboratory some of these gram-negative bacteria can be affected by very high doses of penicillin G, but these high drug levels cannot routinely be achieved in patients. Although penicillin G is not effective against common pathogens in routine urinary tract infections, it is very effective against syphilis and gonorrhea. Syphilis, caused by a spirochete, and gonorrhea, caused by *N. gonorrhoeae,* may frequently be effectively treated by single dose penicillin therapy.

TABLE 41-2. Common dosages of representative penicillins

Generic name	Trade name	Dosage and administration
BIOSYNTHESIZED PENICILLINS		
Penicillin G	Pentids Pfizerpen Others	ORAL: *Adults*—200,000 to 500,000 units every 6 to 8 hr. *Children*—25,000 to 90,000 units/kg per day in 3 to 6 doses. INTRAMUSCULAR: *Adults*—300,000 to 1.2 million units in divided doses. *Children*—50,000 to 250,000 units/kg daily divided among 6 doses. INTRAVENOUS: *Adults and children*—As for intramuscular. Higher doses have been used for severe infections.
Penicillin V	Pen-Vee-K V-Cillin Veetids	ORAL: *Adults*—125 to 500 mg every 4 to 6 hr. *Children*—25 to 50 mg/kg daily in divided doses.
REPOSITORY PENICILLINS		
Benzathine penicillin G	Bicillin	INTRAMUSCULAR: *Adults*—600,000 to 1.2 million units every 2 to 4 weeks. *Children*—50,000 units/kg once.
Procaine penicillin G	Crysticillin Duracillin Wycillin	INTRAMUSCULAR: *Adults*—300,000 to 1.2 million units every 12 to 24 hr. (Uncomplicated gonorrhea, 4.8 million units in 1 dose divided between two sites.) *Children*—50,000 units/kg once daily.
PENICILLINASE-RESISTANT PENICILLINS		
Cloxacillin	Cloxapen Tegopen	ORAL: *Adults*—0.5 to 1 Gm every 4 to 6 hr. *Infants*—50 to 100 mg/kg daily divided into 4 doses.
Dicloxacillin	Dycill Dynapen	ORAL: *Adults*—0.25 to 1 Gm every 4 to 6 hr. *Children*—25 to 100 mg/kg daily divided into 4 doses.
Methicillin	Celbenin Staphcillin	INTRAMUSCULAR: *Adults*—1 Gm every 4 to 6 hr. *Children*—100 to 200 mg/kg per day in 4 to 6 doses. INTRAVENOUS: *Adults*—1 to 2 Gm every 4 to 6 hr. *Children*—as for intramuscular.
Nafcillin	Nafcil Unipen	ORAL: *Adults*—0.25 to 1 Gm every 4 to 6 hr. *Children*—50 to 100 mg/kg daily divided into 4 doses. INTRAMUSCULAR: *Adults*—500 mg every 4 to 6 hr. *Children*—150 mg/kg daily divided into 4 doses. INTRAVENOUS: *Adults*—0.5 to 1 Gm every 4 hr. *Children*—150 mg/kg daily divided into 4 doses.
Oxacillin	Bactocill Prostaphlin	ORAL: *Adults*—0.5 to 1 Gm every 4 to 6 hr. *Children*—50 to 100 mg/kg daily divided into 4 doses. INTRAMUSCULAR: *Adults*—0.25 to 1 Gm every 4 to 6 hr. *Children*—50 to 100 mg/kg daily divided into 4 to 6 doses. INTRAVENOUS: As for intramuscular.
BROAD SPECTRUM PENICILLINS		
Amoxicillin	Amoxil Larotid Polymox Trimox	ORAL: *Adults*—250 to 500 mg every 8 hr. *Infants*—20 to 40 mg/kg daily divided into 3 doses.
Ampicillin	Amcill Omnipen Polycillin Principen	ORAL: *Adults*—250 to 500 mg every 6 hr. *Infants*—50 to 100 mg/kg daily divided into 4 doses. INTRAMUSCULAR: *Adults*—as for oral. *Infants*—100 to 200 mg/kg daily divided into 4 doses. INTRAVENOUS: *Adults*—as for oral. *Infants*—as for intramuscular.

TABLE 41-2. Common dosages of representative penicillins—cont'd

Generic name	Trade name	Dosage and administration
ANTI-PSEUDOMONAS PENICILLINS		
Carbenicillin	Geopen	INTRAMUSCULAR: *Adults*—1 to 2 Gm every 6 hr. *Children*—50 to 200 mg/kg daily divided into 4 to 6 doses. INTRAVENOUS: *Adults and children*—as for intramuscular.
Carbenicillin indanyl ester	Geocillin	ORAL: *Adults*—382 to 764 mg (1 or 2 tablets) every 6 hr.
Ticarcillin	Ticar	INTRAMUSCULAR: *Adults*—1 Gm every 6 hr. *Children*—50 to 100 mg/kg daily divided into 3 or 4 doses. INTRAVENOUS: *Adults and children*—200 to 300 mg/kg per day in 4 to 6 doses.

Repository penicillins: procaine penicillin G and benzathine penicillin G

Absorption. One of the disadvantages of penicillin G is its very short duration of action. The repository penicillins were designed to slow absorption from intramuscular injection sites and thereby prolong the duration of action of penicillin. Along with slower absorption comes a lower peak serum concentration (Chapter 2). Once the drug is absorbed from the depot sites, it is hydrolyzed to release penicillin G, which is the active form of the drug.

The repository penicillins are procaine penicillin G and benzathine penicillin G. Procaine penicillin G reaches its peak serum concentration 3 to 4 hours after injection, and significant serum concentrations may persist for up to 48 hours. With a single dose of 300,000 units of aqueous penicillin G, peak serum levels for penicillin may reach 6 to 8 units/ml, whereas for procaine penicillin G at that same dose, the peak concentration will only be 1 to 2 units/ml. Benzathine penicillin G is even more slowly absorbed and reaches it maximal concentration around 8 hours after injection. This concentration decreases very slowly and significant serum levels are observed for 2 weeks or longer. A common adult dose of 1.2 million units produces peak serum levels of only 0.1 to 0.3 units/ml (Table 41-2).

Toxicity. The repository penicillins are intended only for deep muscular injections. Both preparations are stabilized suspensions of relatively insoluble forms of penicillin and contain up to about 2% weight/volume of emulsifying agents in addition to buffers. Such preparations should never be given intravenously. Care must be taken on intramuscular injection to prevent the accidental entry of these preparations into blood vessels, since occlusion of the blood vessel may result.

Uses. The repository penicillins are not appropriate for very serious infections where high serum concentrations of drug are required. Rather these drugs are appropriate to maintain modest serum levels for relatively long periods of time. These conditions would occur when very sensitive organisms were involved in mild to moderately serious infections or when prophylaxis was required.

Procaine penicillin G is associated with central nervous system toxicity produced by procaine. After injection, procaine may be released in significant amounts into the bloodstream and may produce anxiety, lowered blood pressure, respiratory depression, and convulsions. These central nervous system reactions to procaine are usually transient, lasting less than 1 hour.

Phenoxy penicillins: penicillin V

Absorption. Attempts to improve the oral absorption of penicillin G have led to the development of phenoxy derivatives of penicillin. The best-known member of this class is phenoxymethyl penicillin, or penicillin V. The phenoxy penicillins are more acid stable and therefore more efficiently absorbed from the gastrointestinal tract than penicillin G but are all less potent antibacterial agents than penicillin G.

Uses. The uses of penicillin V are restricted to those circumstances in which oral antibiotic therapy is appropriate. Mild to moderately serious infections caused by penicillin-sensitive organisms may be treated with penicillin V. Penicillin V may also be used in prophylaxis, being especially useful in patients who have had rheumatic fever. In these patients penicillin V prophylaxis may prevent recurrent streptococcal infections, which could lead to heart or kidney damage.

Other than being better absorbed orally, penicillin V resembles penicillin G. Penicillin V has the same antimicrobial spectrum, same pattern of distribution and excretion, and same toxicity as penicillin G. Like orally administered penicillin G, penicillin V should be given 1 hour before or 2 hours after meals, since food can interfere with absorption.

Penicillinase-resistant penicillins: methicillin

Absorption. Methicillin is not acid stable and must therefore be administered parenterally.

Toxicity. Methicillin is an unusual penicillin in that it can cause significant blood dyscrasias as well as interstitial nephritis. These reactions are uncommon for other penicillins. Methicillin is also unusual in that resistance to the drug does not involve penicillinase but rather some sort of bacterial cell tolerance to the antibiotic. When methicillin resistance occurs, the organism also becomes resistant to penicillin G, cephalosporins, other penicillinase-resistant penicillins, and other antibiotics as well.

Uses. Methicillin was the first penicillin developed to be resistant to attack by penicillinase. This important breakthrough in pharmaceutical development allowed penicillin therapy of penicillinase-producing staphylococcal infections. Methicillin is best used only in treatment of infections in which penicillinase is produced by the pathogenic organism; in all other penicillin-sensitive infections penicillin G is preferred, since penicillin G is more potent than methicillin.

Acid-stable, penicillinase-resistant penicillins: nafcillin, oxacillin, cloxacillin, and dicloxacillin

Absorption and excretion. This group combines two of the most useful features of penicillin derivatives: acid stability, which allows oral dosage, and resistance to penicillinase, which allows the drugs to be used against many penicillin G–resistant organisms. One member of this group, nafcillin, is unique among all the penicillins in that it is excreted primarily in the bile. All other penicillins are excreted primarily by the kidney. Although nafcillin is occasionally used orally, it is not as well absorbed as the other members of this class—oxacillin, cloxacillin, and dicloxacillin. With these latter drugs oral absorption can be approximately doubled by fasting. These drugs are all more potent than methicillin but less potent than penicillin G.

Uses. The primary use of this group of drugs is in initial therapy when a penicillinase-producing organism is suspected. If the infection is later demonstrated by culture results to be caused by a nonpenicillinase-producing organism, the patient may frequently be switched to penicillin V or penicillin G. One of the dangers in too common use of these drugs is that the unusual drug tolerance type of resistance may develop in more and more bacterial populations. As we discussed for methicillin, this type of resistance then affects all beta-lactam antibiotics and makes the resistant organism quite dangerous and difficult to eradicate.

Broad spectrum penicillins: ampicillin and amoxicillin

Absorption. Ampicillin is acid stable and may be used orally; however, amoxicillin is better absorbed by that route and may produce blood levels twice those of ampicillin following an equivalent oral dose. Amoxicillin is currently available only for oral use.

Uses. All the penicillins discussed to this point have relatively narrow antimicrobial spectra, being primarily useful against gram-positive organisms. The development of ampicillin and amoxicillin significantly broadened the penicillin spectrum to include several common gram-negative pathogens. Ampicillin apparently penetrates gram-negative cell walls better than does penicillin G and is therefore more effective against these organisms than penicillin G. Ampicillin is not resistant to penicillinase and so may not be effective against *S. aureus* resistant to penicillin G.

Anti-*Pseudomonas* penicillins: carbenicillin and ticarcillin

Absorption. These drugs must be administered parenterally and are ideally used only when *Pseudomonas* infection is suspected. For carbenicillin, an indanyl ester is available, which allows the drug to be used orally. However, indanyl carbenicillin does not produce high enough serum levels of carbenicillin to make the drug effective for most infections. Therefore indanyl carbenicillin is reserved for use in urinary tract infections, since the drug does accumulate to high concentrations in the urine following oral dosage.

Uses. One pathogenic organism that is not sensitive to ampicillin or amoxicillin is *Pseudomonas aeruginosa*. This gram-negative bacterium is responsible for certain urinary tract infections, bacteremias, and infections in burn patients and is unusually resistant to many antibiotics. For this reason drugs were developed specifically for use against this organism. Two of these drugs are the penicillins carbenicillin and ticarcillin.

Carbenicillin or ticarcillin may be used with gentamicin (Chapter 44) for the treatment of severe *Pseudomonas* infections. Gentamicin must never be directly mixed in the syringe or intravenous bottle with carbenicillin or ticarcillin, since these penicillins inactivate gentamicin.

■ CEPHALOSPORINS

Absorption. Most cephalosporins are used parenterally (Table 41-3), being well absorbed from intramuscular sites. Ordinary daily doses range from 1 to 6 Gm for adults but may go up to 12 Gm in certain circumstances. The elimination half-times of all these drugs are about twice as long as that of penicillin G and are roughly equivalent to those of ampicillin or the penicillinase-resistant penicillins.

TABLE 41-3. Common dosages of representative cephalosporins

Generic name	Trade name	Dosage and administration	Comments
Cefaclor	Ceclor	ORAL: *Adults*—1 to 4 Gm daily. *Children*—20 to 40 mg/kg not to exceed 1 Gm daily.	Used primarily as alternate for penicillins.
Cefamandole	Mandol	INTRAMUSCULAR, INTRAVENOUS: *Adults*—500 mg to 1 Gm every 4 to 6 hr. *Children*—50 to 100 mg/kg daily divided into 4 to 6 doses.	Broader spectrum of activity toward gram-negative bacteria.
Cefazolin	Ancef Kefzol	INTRAMUSCULAR, INTRAVENOUS: *Adults*—250 mg every 8 hr up to 1 Gm per 6 hr. *Children*—25 to 50 mg/kg total daily dose in 3 or 4 divided doses.	Slightly better action against gram-negative bacteria than cephalothin.
Cefoxitin	Mefoxitin	INTRAMUSCULAR, INTRAVENOUS: *Adults*—total daily dose normally 3 to 8 Gm given in 3 or 4 equal doses. *Children*—50 to 150 mg/kg daily divided into 4 to 6 doses.	Intramuscular injection painful.
Cephalexin	Keflex	ORAL: *Adults*—1 to 4 Gm daily. *Children*—25 to 50 mg/kg total daily dose divided into 4 doses.	Similar to oral cephradine.
Cephaloridine	Loridine	INTRAMUSCULAR, INTRAVENOUS: *Adults*—daily dose must not exceed 4 Gm. *Children*—30 to 50 mg/kg total daily dose in 3 divided doses.	Nephrotoxicity is common.
Cephalothin	Keflin	INTRAVENOUS: *Adults*—1 Gm every 3 to 6 hr. *Children*—80 to 160 mg/kg total daily dose.	Intramuscular injections are too painful to be tolerated.
Cephapirin	Cefadyl	INTRAVENOUS: *Adults*—500 mg every 6 hr up to 1 Gm per 4 hr. *Children*—40 to 80 mg/kg total daily dose.	Similar to cephalothin.
Cephradine	Anspor Velosef	ORAL, INTRAMUSCULAR, INTRAVENOUS: *Adults*—1 to 4 Gm total daily dose. *Children*—50 to 100 mg/kg divided into 4 daily doses.	Intramuscular injection painful.

Several cephalosporins are currently available for oral use (Table 41-3). These preparations are well absorbed and produce effective serum concentrations of antibiotic. Absorption of cephalosporins from the gastrointestinal tract is slowed by food in the stomach, but about the same amount of drug is ultimately absorbed as in a fasting patient. Ordinary adult doses for oral cephalosporins are from 1 to 4 Gm daily given in four doses.

Distribution. Cephalosporins are distributed in the body in a manner similar to penicillins except that cephalosporins do not penetrate the central nervous system well enough to be used in meningitis. These drugs are excreted by the kidney and are highly concentrated in the urine, making them useful in treating several common types of urinary tract infections.

Toxicity. Many of the cephalosporins produce pain at the injection site. When given intravenously the drugs cause phlebitis or thrombophlebitis and pain along the affected vein. Orally administered cephalosporins may cause gastric irritation, nausea, and vomiting.

Renal damage is a special danger with *cephaloridine*. This drug accumulates in renal tubular cells and produces renal tubular necrosis, which may destroy kidney function. Since this effect on the kidney is dose dependent, it is recommended that no more than 4 Gm per day be administered. Interstitial nephritis has occasionally been observed with cephalosporins.

The danger of synergistic nephrotoxicity should be considered when cephaloridine is given with other nephrotoxic agents such as the antibiotics gentamicin, kanamycin, and polymyxin or the diuretics furosemide and ethacrynic acid.

■ THE NURSING PROCESS

The student should refer to the nursing process section in Chapter 40 for general guidelines on the nursing process with antibiotic therapy. The additional material below relates specifically to the beta-lactam antibiotics, penicillins and cephalosporins.

■ Assessment

Penicillins and cephalosporins are prescribed for patients with many types of infections. Assessment of the patient should be carried out with emphasis on the organ in which the infection is thought to be present, if the infection is a localized one. Other clinical signs of infection should be monitored. The nurse should pay special attention to subjective data which suggest that the patient may have a history of allergy either to penicillins or to other agents. Since penicillins and cephalosporins are excreted mostly by the kidney, the nurse should assess renal function.

■ Management

Once the decision is made to administer penicillins or cephalosporins, the nurse should determine that emergency supplies are at hand to treat an anaphylactic reaction, should one occur. The patient should be closely observed for at least 20 to 30 minutes after the medication is administered. If the patient will continue to receive these antibiotics on an outpatient basis, the nurse should instruct the patient in the proper timing of doses and the need to continue therapy for the prescribed length of time. The nurse should also inform the patient about side effects such as rashes or gastrointestinal distress and teach the patient that these reactions may necessitate contacting the physician.

■ Evaluation

Penicillins and cephalosporins seldom cause long-term side effects and are usually very effective in treating common infections. Patients should show rapid objective and subjective improvement for most infections treated with these agents. The patient should demonstrate the ability to judge improvement in the infection and should be able to tell the nurse what reactions might be expected to the medications and when it would be appropriate to call the physician.

Uses. The primary usefulness of these drugs is based on the differences in the antimicrobial spectra of penicillins and cephalosporins. Cephalosporins resemble ampicillin in their effectiveness against gram-negative bacteria. Unlike ampicillin, however, cephalosporins resist the action of staphylococcal penicillinase and can be used when the organism is resistant to penicillin G. Until very recently all the cephalosporins could be considered quite similar in their antimicrobial spectra. However, three cephalosporins with somewhat extended spectra have recently appeared on the market. *Cefamandole* and *cefaclor* may be effective against ampicillin-resistant *Haemophilus influenzae,* an organism that frequently causes ear infections especially in children. *Cefoxitin* is more active against gram-negative bacteria than other cephalosporins but is less effective against gram-positive organisms.

■ PATIENT CARE IMPLICATIONS

1. Diabetic patients should be cautioned to rely on glucose oxidase methods (Clinistix or Tes-Tape) for urine testing while receiving penicillins or cephalosporins. These drugs can cause false positive results with Clinitest tablets (Fehling's or Benedict's reagent), which could lead to insulin overdose.
2. Routine laboratory work to monitor renal, hepatic, and hematopoietic function should be done on patients receiving penicillin or cephalosporins. Although abnormalities can occur in any patient, renal toxicity is more likely to occur in elderly persons, in very young infants, in those receiving high dose therapy, in those also receiving other nephrotoxic drugs or loop diuretics, and in patients with known decreased renal function.

TABLE 41-4. Guide for rate of direct infusion for penicillins and cephalosporins

Drug	Recommended dilution*	Rate of administration
Ampicillin	500 mg in at least 5 ml diluent	500 mg per min
Carbenicillin	1 Gm reconstituted drug in at least 5 ml diluent	1 Gm per 5 min
Methicillin	500 mg reconstituted drug in at least 25 ml diluent	10 ml per min
Nafcillin	Desired amount of drug in 15 to 30 ml diluent	500 mg per 5 to 10 min
Ticarcillin	1 Gm in at least 4 ml diluent, then further diluted to 1 Gm/10 ml	1 Gm per 5 min
Oxacillin	1 Gm/10 ml diluent	1 ml per min
Cephalothin	1 Gm/10 ml diluent	1 Gm per 5 min
Cephapirin	1 Gm/10 ml diluent	1 Gm per 5 min
Cefazolin	1 Gm/10 ml diluent	1 Gm per 5 min
Cephaloridine	1 Gm/10 ml diluent	1 Gm per 4 min
Cephradine	1 Gm/10 ml diluent	1 Gm per 5 min
Cefamandole	1 Gm/10 ml diluent	1 Gm per 5 min
Cefoxitin	1 or 2 Gm/10 ml diluent	1 or 2 Gm per 5 min

*For information about appropriate diluents, preparations for constant infusion, compatibilities with infusion fluids, storage conditions, and other questions consult the pharmacist and the manufacturer's information. Because the cephalosporins are so irritating to the vein, it is preferable, when possible, to dilute these drugs more than is indicated in the table.

3. Penicillins and cephalosporins vary considerably in the amount of sodium or potassium contained in individual products. Although this may cause no problem in most patients, it can be of concern in patients with renal or cardiovascular problems or in those receiving high doses. Consult the literature provided by the manufacturer for information about any specific drug. Monitor the patient's electrolyte levels.
4. The penicillins, with the exception of amoxicillin, should be taken 1 hour before meals or 2 hours after meals. The cephalosporins can be taken with meals, although absorption may be faster if taken on an empty stomach.
5. Penicillin products containing procaine, benzathine, or a combination of these should never be given intravenously. Administer intramuscularly using the gluteus maximus or vastus lateralis of an adult and the vastus lateralis of an infant or small child. Occasionally patients are sensitive to procaine; symptoms include anxiety, confusion, agitation, fear of impending death, and convulsions.
6. Many intramuscular preparations of penicillin are thick and require steady, even pressure on the plunger to prevent the needle from clogging.
7. Platelet dysfunction with resulting bleeding tendencies has been reported with several of the penicillins, including methicillin, carbenicillin, ticarcillin, and penicillin itself. This reaction may be more common in uremic patients.
8. The cephalosporins cause pain at intramuscular injection sites and frequently contribute to thrombophlebitis when given intravenously. This latter problem can be lessened by administering the drug slowly, diluting it well, and rotating insertion sites every 24 to 48 hours.
9. For instructions about reconstitution of penicillins and cephalosporins for parenteral use, refer to the medication vials and the manufacturer's accompanying literature. Table 41-4 is a guide to the appropriate rate of infusion for direct infusion of these agents (''IV push'' rate). Note that too rapid infusion of direct infusion penicillins may contribute to the development of seizures.

■ SUMMARY

Penicillins and cephalosporins are both beta-lactam antibiotics and share many common properties. Penicillins and cephalosporins inhibit cell wall biosynthesis in actively growing bacteria, are inactivated by bacterial enzymes, and are excreted primarily by the kidney. Direct drug toxicity from these antibiotics is relatively low, with allergic reactions being the most common unwanted effect produced by these drugs. Oral forms of penicillins and cephalosporins may cause various forms of gastrointestinal distress. Many of the penicillin and cephalosporin preparations on the market contain sufficient sodium or potassium to alter electrolyte balance in some patients. Many of these drugs are unstable in solution and must be diluted with care for intramuscular or intravenous use.

Penicillin G is the most potent penicillin against many gram-positive bacteria. The disadvantages of this drug are rapid excretion, narrow antimicrobial spectrum, variable oral absorption, and sensitivity to *Staphylococcus aureus* penicillinase. Procaine penicillin G and benzathine penicillin G are long-acting repository forms of penicillin G and are suitable only for intramuscular administration. These preparations differ from penicillin G itself only in having a long duration of action as a result of slowed absorption from injection sites. Penicillin V differs from penicillin G in being more acid stable and therefore more reliably absorbed orally than penicillin G. The penicillins developed for resistance to *S. aureus* penicillinase include methicillin, an agent used only parenterally, and nafcillin, an agent unique among the penicillins in being excreted primarily in bile. Penicillinase-resistant penicillins that are well absorbed orally include oxacillin, cloxacillin, and dicloxacillin. Bacterial resistance does develop against these penicillinase-resistant drugs, but the mechanism involves cell tolerance to the antibiotic rather than destruction of it. Penicillins with an extended spectrum toward gram-negative bacteria include ampicillin and amoxicillin. Both agents are used orally, although amoxicillin is the better absorbed of the two. Carbenicillin and ticarcillin are currently listed as anti-*Pseudomonas* penicillins and are used only parenterally.

Cephalosporins differ from penicillins in having a slightly extended spectrum against gram-negative microorganisms and in being resistant to *S. aureus* penicillinase.

■ STUDY QUESTIONS

1. What is the mechanism of action of penicillins and cephalosporins?
2. What is the effect of beta-lactam antibiotics on existing bacterial cell wall?
3. How do most bacteria gain resistance toward beta-lactam antibiotics?
4. What is the mechanism of excretion for most penicillins and cephalosporins?
5. What is the most common toxic reaction to penicillins and cephalosporins?
6. What is the purpose of skin tests for penicillin allergies?
7. What is the effect of penicillin on the central nervous system?
8. Name two groups of patients most at risk of accumulating penicillins given at normal doses.
9. What type of patient would be most at risk from the potassium and sodium contained in many penicillin and cephalosporin preparations?
10. Why is probenecid sometimes administered with penicillin G?
11. What is the effect of destroying the penicillin nucleus?
12. What is the effect of altering the penicillin side chain structure?
13. Why is penicillin G absorbed erratically from the gastrointestinal tract?
14. When does the peak concentration of penicillin G appear in the bloodstream following an intramuscular dose of the drug?
15. What is the elimination half-time for penicillin G in normal patients?
16. How does the penetration of penicillin G into the cerebrospinal fluid differ in normal patients and in persons with meningitis?
17. Name three groups of microorganisms that are sensitive to penicillin G.
18. Why do procaine penicillin G and benzathine penicillin G have longer durations of action than penicillin G itself?
19. By what route must the repository penicillins be administered?
20. Which would produce a higher serum concentration of antibiotic, one million units of penicillin G or one million units of procaine penicillin G?
21. What advantage does penicillin V possess over penicillin G?
22. Why would methicillin be useful in treating infections due to penicillinase-producing *Staphylococcus aureus?*
23. How do bacteria become resistant to methicillin?
24. What is the route of excretion of nafcillin?
25. What advantages do oxacillin, cloxacillin, and dicloxacillin possess over methicillin?

26. How does the antimicrobial spectrum of ampicillin and amoxicillin differ from that of penicillin G?
27. What advantage does amoxicillin possess over ampicillin?
28. Infections caused by what pathogen are appropriately treated with carbenicillin or ticarcillin?
29. How does indanyl carbenicillin differ from carbenicillin?
30. Why are cephalosporins not useful in treating meningitis?
31. What is the most common reaction expected from most cephalosporins when the drugs are administered intravenously?
32. How does the antimicrobial spectrum of the cephalosporins differ from that of penicillin G?
33. What is the special toxicity associated with the drug cephaloridine?

■ SUGGESTED READINGS

Asper, R., and Schwartz, A.R.: The newer penicillins, American Family Physician **11**(1):134, 1975.

Barza, M.: Antimicrobial spectrum, pharmacology, and therapeutic use of antibiotics. II. Penicillins, Drug Therapy Reviews **2:**90, 1979.

Barza, M., and Miao, P.V.M.: Antimicrobial spectrum, pharmacology, and therapeutic use of antibiotics. III. Cephalosporins, Drug Therapy Reviews **2:**114, 1979.

Cortez, L.M., Craig, C.P., Eickhoff, T., Hemmerlein, A., Rahal, J.J., Jr., Talley, J.H., and Wientzen, R.L.: Penicillins: which, when, how, why? Patient Care **14**(2):14, 1980.

How to use intravenous antibiotics, Nurses' Drug Alert, special issue **1:**89, June, 1977.

Penicillin in '77: still a threat to many patients, Nurses' Drug Alert **1:**34, Feb., 1977.

Rodman, M.J.: Anti-infectives you administer. I. The penicillins, RN **40:**73, March, 1977.

Thompson, R.L.: The cephalosporins, Mayo Clinic Proceedings **52:** 625, 1977.

Wagner, K.F., and Counts, G.W.: The penicillins and cephalosporins: choosing among the newer agents, Postgraduate Medicine **64**(3): 109, 1978.

Weinstein, A.J.: The cephalosporins: activity and clinical use, Drugs **20:**137, 1980.

Wilkowske, C.J.: The penicillins, Mayo Clinic Proceedings **52:**616, 1977.

Williams, T.W., Jr.: An up-to-date look at the penicillins, Consultant **20**(4):27, 1980.

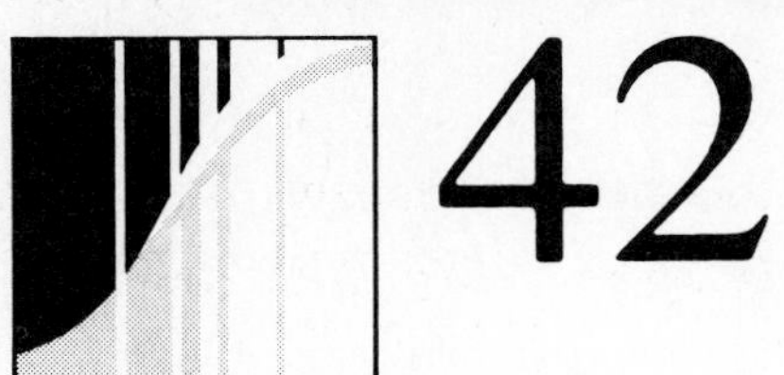

42 Antibiotics: erythromycin, clindamycin, and miscellaneous penicillin substitutes

In this chapter several antibiotics are introduced with antimicrobial spectra similar to narrow spectrum penicillins. Because of this property, these drugs are sometimes grouped together as penicillin substitutes. The mechanisms of action of these drugs, modes of bacterial resistance, absorption properties, drug distribution and excretion, as well as the unique toxic reactions these drugs may induce will be considered.

■ ERYTHROMYCIN

■ Mechanism of action and bacterial resistance

Erythromycin binds to bacterial ribosomes and thereby prevents bacterial protein synthesis. At low concentrations of erythromycin, this effect is bacteriostatic, but at high concentrations the drug may be bacteriocidal.

Bacteria become resistant to erythromycin by one of two mechanisms. Gram-negative organisms seem to be relatively impermeable to erythromycin and are therefore intrinsically resistant. Cell wall–deficient forms of these bacteria (L-forms) are permeable to erythromycin and are highly sensitive to the drug. Gram-positive organisms acquire resistance to erythromycin by chemically altering their ribosomes so that the ribosomes no longer bind erythromycin and, hence, protein synthesis is not inhibited. This ribosomal alteration is catalyzed by an enzyme that is synthesized from genes carried on a bacterial plasmid. Plasmids are discrete circular molecules of DNA that exist separate from the bacterial chromosome (Chapter 40). These plasmids can be transferred directly from one bacterial cell to another. Therefore resistance to erythromycin may spread rapidly throughout a bacterial population.

■ Absorption

Erythromycin is sensitive to acid and may therefore be extensively degraded in the stomach. For this reason erythromycin base is formulated with acid-resistant coatings so that the drug will pass intact through the stomach and be dissolved and absorbed in the small intestine. This tactic is based on the knowledge that the pH of the duodenum is near neutrality (Chapter 2).

Certain salts of erythromycin are used clinically primarily because of their increased resistance to acid and better oral absorption. These compounds are the stearate, ethylsuccinate, and estolate esters of erythromycin (Table 42-1). Erythromycin stearate and erythromycin ethylsuccinate are absorbed more rapidly and more completely from the gastrointestinal tract than erythromycin base. Free erythromycin is apparently absorbed from the duodenum with these agents following hydrolysis of the esters. With erythromycin estolate, much better oral absorption of drug is achieved and serum levels may be four times higher than can be achieved with other forms of erythromycin. However, with erythromycin estolate both free erythromycin and the ester are absorbed. Most of the drug in the serum is actually the ester, and controversy exists as to whether this form of the drug has biological activity. Many physician prefer the erythromycin estolate because of the high tissue and blood levels and note that many tissues and many bacteria can hydrolyze the ester form of the drug to release free erythromycin at the infection site.

Food may interfere with the oral absorption of most erythromycin preparations. Erythromycin estolate is the exception and is apparently well-absorbed even when food is present.

Erythromycin is available as the ethylsuccinate for intramuscular injection (Table 42-1). This preparation is not water soluble and must not therefore be accidentally injected into a vein. The drug suspension may be extremely viscous if it has been refrigerated, and the vial should be warmed in the hands to make the drug easier to withdraw. Intramuscular administration of erythromycin is avoided if at all possible because injections are extremely painful. In addition, many patients develop sterile abscesses or local tissue necrosis at the injection site. The doses that may be tolerated by the intramuscular route are too low to be effective for serious infections.

Erythromycin is available as the lactobionate or the gluceptate for intravenous injection (Table 42-1). These water-soluble products may be diluted with Sterile Water for Injection but should not be diluted in sterile water

TABLE 42-1. Clinical summary of erythromycins

Generic name	Trade name	Drug form	Dosage and administration
Erythromycin base	E-Mycin Ilotycin Robimycin RP-Mycin	Enteric or film-coated tablets	ORAL: *Adults*—250 mg 4 times per day (15 to 20 mg/kg per day). *Children*—30 to 50 mg/kg per day in 3 or 4 doses. *Patients with very severe infections*—up to 4 Gm per day.
Erythromycin stearate	Bristamycin Erypar Erythrocin Stearate Ethril Pfizer-E SK-Erythromycin	Film-coated tablets	ORAL: *Adults and children*—as for erythromycin base.
Erythromycin estolate	Ilosone	Tablets, capsules, suspension, chewable tablets	ORAL: *Adults and children*—as for erythromycin base.
Erythromycin ethylsuccinate	E.E.S. Pediamycin	Drops, suspension, chewable tablets	ORAL: *Adults*—400 mg 4 times per day. *Children*—Doses adjusted proportional to weight and severity of infection.
	Erythrocin Ethyl Succinate-IM Pediamycin	Solution containing 2% butyl aminobenzoate, polyethylene glycol, and benzyl alcohol	INTRAMUSCULAR: *Adults*—100 mg 3 to 6 times daily (5 to 8 mg/kg per day). Change to oral route as soon as possible.
Erythromycin lactobionate	Erythrocin Lactobionate-IV	Solution containing benzyl alcohol	INTRAVENOUS: *Adults*—15 to 20 mg/kg per day, preferably by continuous infusion; intervals between doses for intermittent therapy should be 6 hr or less. Doses of up to 4 Gm per day may be used for very severe infections.
Erythromycin gluceptate	Ilotycin Gluceptate-IV		

containing preservatives. Erythromycin lactobionate or erythromycin gluceptate may be rapidly inactivated if added to fluids below pH 5.5. This sensitivity to extremes of pH makes erythromycin incompatible in solution with a number of other drugs. Before adding erythromycin to any other drug solution, compatibility of the agents should be verified with the pharmacist. Erythromycin lactobionate and erythromycin gluceptate should be infused slowly into the vein to avoid pain.

■ Distribution and excretion

Erythromycin readily enters body tissues, and tissue concentrations of the drug may persist well beyond the time when drug can be detected in the serum. Erythromycin is especially concentrated in the liver and spleen. Erythromycin enters fluids of the middle ear and pleural fluids but not cerebrospinal fluid unless the meninges are inflamed. Erythromycin does cross the placenta, but fetal blood levels are less than 20% of maternal blood levels. Erythromycin also enters breast milk, with approximately 0.1% of the daily dose of the drug appearing in that fluid.

The liver is the major excretory organ for erythromycin. A large percentage of orally administered erythromycin is concentrated in bile and excreted in the feces. Some reabsorption of the drug from the intestine occurs in a process called *enterohepatic circulation* (Chapter 2). Another significant proportion of erythromycin is apparently inactivated in the liver. Less than 10% of orally administered erythromycin appears as active drug in the urine. With intravenous dosage, about 15% of the dose appears in the urine. Because of the relative importance of the liver and the kidney in drug excretion, patients with renal insufficiency might be expected to receive normal doses of erythromycin, whereas a patient with hepatic insufficiency might require reduced drug doses.

■ Toxicity

The most common patient complaint with oral erythromycin is some form of gastrointestinal difficulty. Abdominal discomfort and cramping are dose-related reactions to these drugs. At normal doses nausea, vomiting, and diarrhea are apparently less frequent than with oral penicillins or tetracyclines.

Allergic reactions to erythromycin have occurred, although these are rare. Reactions ranging from urticaria to anaphylaxis have been noted.

Rarely patients who receive more than 4 Gm of erythromycin lactiobionate per day have experienced hearing loss.

The most significant toxicity to erythromycin occurs with erythromycin estolate. This drug damages the liver, either by direct drug toxicity or by an immune reaction. This reaction, called *cholestatic hepatitis,* usually appears 10 to 12 days after therapy is begun but may appear earlier in patients previously exposed to the drug. These patients may experience severe abdominal pain, liver enlargement, fever, and jaundice. When the drug is discontinued, these symptoms rapidly disappear in most patients. Permanent liver damage has not been reported with these drugs.

■ Uses

Erythromycin has a similar antimicrobial spectrum to penicillin G but is chemically unrelated to penicillins and is not cross-allergenic with them. Therefore erythromycin is a very useful penicillin substitute in patients allergic to penicillins. In addition, since penicillins and erythromycin act by entirely different mechanisms, bacteria that become resistant to one of these drugs are still sensitive to the other.

There are a few conditions for which erythromycin is the first drug of choice. One of these is atypical pneumonias, such as Legionnaire's disease. Erythromycin may also be preferred over penicillin G for diphtheria, since erythromycin effectively eradicates the diphtheria carrier state. Another instance in which erythromycin may be exceedingly useful is in relapsing urinary tract infections. In this condition the relapse is frequently caused by L-forms of gram-negative organisms such as *Escherichia coli* or *Proteus mirabilis*. These L-forms lack cell wall and are therefore resistant to penicillins. The L-form bacteria remain latent during penicillin therapy, revert to normal, and again produce disease when penicillin therapy is stopped. Since erythromycin penetrates these L-forms and blocks protein synthesis, the infection may be eradicated.

Clinical studies suggest that pregnant women have variable absorption of oral erythromycin, and many of these women do not achieve effective serum concentrations of the drug. Because of this lack of effect and because erythromycin can accumulate over long periods in fetal livers, the drug is not usually recommended during pregnancy.

■ CLINDAMYCIN AND LINCOMYCIN

■ Mechanism of action and bacterial resistance

Clindamycin and lincomycin inhibit the action of bacterial ribosomes in a way analogous to erythromycin. These drugs halt bacterial protein synthesis and may be bacteriostatic or bacteriocidal depending on drug concentrations. Bacterial resistance to lincomycin and clindamycin apparently develops in several ways. Some organisms may become impermeable to the drugs. Others alter the ribosome so that it does not bind lincomycin or clindamycin. With this latter mechanism, organisms may become resistant to both the lincomycins and erythromycin. In practice, most clinically observed resistance to clindamycin and lincomycin develops slowly and in a gradual, stepwise manner.

■ Absorption

Lincomycin may be administered by oral, intramuscular, or intravenous routes (Table 42-2). When given orally, peak serum concentrations of lincomycin occur about 4 hours after the dose is administered. Food significantly hinders lincomycin absorption and results in serum levels much lower than those observed in the fasting state. For this reason the drug should be administered between meals so that no food is taken for 1 to 2 hours before and 1 to 2 hours after the drug.

In contrast to lincomycin, clindamycin absorption is not significantly impaired by the presence of food. Clindamycin is more rapidly absorbed orally than is lincomycin and produces higher blood concentrations at least during the first few hours of therapy. Clindamycin palmitate is also available as flavored granules to be used in suspension for oral administration. The palmitate is apparently rapidly removed to release active clindamycin.

Lincomycin or clindamycin-2-phosphate may be injected intramuscularly (Table 42-2). Clinical reports suggest that local pain following injection may be a problem with clindamycin-2-phosphate but has rarely been reported for lincomycin. Absorption of drug by this route is good, but serum peaks being achieved 30 to 60 minutes after injection. These two drugs are also suitable for intravenous use. By this route clindamycin-2-phosphate produces pain and phlebitis, whereas this reaction has not been observed with lincomycin. Clindamycin-2-phosphate is inactive as an antibiotic but is rapidly converted to clindamycin in the body.

■ Distribution and excretion

Clindamycin and lincomycin are well-distributed to most body tissues with the exception of the central nervous system. Lincomycin does not appear in the cerebrospinal fluid of normal patients but may enter the central

TABLE 42-2. Clinical summary of lincomycin and clindamycin

Generic name	Trade name	Drug form	Dosage and administration
Clindamycin	Cleocin	Capsules (hydrochloride hydrate)	ORAL: *Adults*—150 to 450 mg 4 times daily.
Clindamycin palmitate	Cleocin Pediatric	Granules in suspension	ORAL: *Children*—8 to 25 mg/kg per day in 3 or 4 doses for children over 10 kg. Smaller children should receive no more than 37.5 mg 3 times daily.
Clindamycin phosphate	Cleocin Phosphate	Solution with benzyl alcohol, disodium edetate, and/or hydrochloric acid or sodium hydroxide	INTRAMUSCULAR, INTRAVENOUS: *Adults*—0.6 Gm to an upper limit of 4.8 Gm per day (no more than 0.6 Gm per injection site IM). *Children over 1 month*—15 to 40 mg/kg daily in 3 or 4 doses.
Lincomycin	Lincocin	Capsules, syrup	ORAL: *Adults*—500 mg 3 or 4 times daily. *Children over 1 month*—30 to 60 mg/kg per day in 3 or 4 divided doses.
		Solution with 0.9% benzyl alcohol	INTRAMUSCULAR: *Adults*—600 mg once or twice daily. *Children over 1 month*—10 mg/kg once or twice daily.
		Solution with 0.9% benzyl alcohol	INTRAVENOUS: *Adults*—600 mg to 1 Gm 2 or 3 times daily; 8 Gm is the upper limit for daily doses. *Children over 1 month*—10 mg/kg once or twice daily.

nervous system when the meninges are inflamed by infection. Clindamycin does not appear in the cerebrospinal fluid even when meningitis is present. Both lincomycin and clindamycin appear in the milk of lactating females treated with these drugs.

Both clindamycin and lincomycin are extensively biodegraded in the body. The liver is the primary site of biotransformation with these drugs. Less than 20% of the total drug administered shows up as active antibiotic in the urine or feces. For this reason, these drugs are used at normal dosages in patients with renal insufficiency or renal failure. Neither lincomycin nor clindamycin are removed from the body by hemodialysis.

■ Toxicity

The most serious reaction to lincomycin or clindamycin is colitis. Symptoms range from mild diarrhea to a severe, life-threatening condition called *pseudomembranous colitis*. Any increase in frequency of bowel movements or softness of the stools may be reason to discontinue the drug, especially in elderly patients. Significant diarrhea should prompt discontinuation of the drug and may be relieved by that therapy alone. The appearance of blood or mucus in the stool may be a sign of severe colitis.

Pseudomembranous colitis is caused by a toxin produced by *Clostridium difficile*. Overgrowth of this organism in the bowel can occur as a result of antibiotic perturbation of the bacterial flora in the bowel. This suprainfection and its associated colitis may be specifically treated with vancomycin. Fluid and electrolyte replacement and other supportive therapy may also be required. Agents that slow peristaltic action may actually worsen the condition or prolong it. For this reason, opiates or diphenoxylate with atropine are not appropriate for use in these patients.

In addition to colitis, clindamycin and lincomycin may produce gastrointestinal irritation ranging from nausea and vomiting to glossitis and stomatitis.

Allergies to clindamycin and lincomycin do occur and range from mild rashes to drug fever and anaphylactic shock. These reactions may occur in any patient but are more common in those with other allergies. The appearance of any allergic response is cause for discontinuing the drug.

Some reports suggest blood dyscrasias and liver dysfunction occur during lincomycin or clindamycin therapy. A direct cause-and-effect relationship between the drugs and these reactions has not been demonstrated.

Lincomycin administered intravenously has produced hypotension in a few patients. Cardiopulmonary arrest has occurred. These reactions are apparently related to a too rapid intravenous injection. Lincomycin should be administered in an intravenous solution, no more concentrated than 1 Gm/100 ml at a rate no more rapid than 100 ml per hour.

■ Drug interactions

Lincomycin is incompatible in solution with the antibiotics novobiocin and kanamycin. Clindamycin is incompatible with aminophylline, ampicillin, barbiturates, calcium gluconate, magnesium sulfate, and phenytoin.

Both clindamycin and lincomycin have neuromuscular blocking properties. For this reason, these drugs may enhance the action of various neuromuscular blocking agents.

The absorption of oral doses of lincomycin may be decreased by food and other agents. The use of kaolin-pectin antidiarrheal agents given at the time oral lincomycin is ingested markedly lowers the serum concentrations of lincomycin.

■ Uses

Clindamycin and lincomycin have antimicrobial spectra similar to penicillin G or erythromycin, being primarily effective against gram-positive organisms. Lincomycin and clindamycin are not as effective as penicillin against *Neisseria gonorrhoeae* or other gram-negative cocci. Clindamycin is effective against a number of anaerobic organisms, particularly *Bacteroides fragilis*. Infections caused by these organisms are a major indication for clindamycin use.

The dangers of severe colitis have largely restricted the use of clindamycin and lincomycin to cases in which patients are allergic to safer drugs or the pathogenic organism is demonstrated by the microbiology laboratory to be sensitive to these agents. Clindamycin is more effective and less toxic than lincomycin and is much more commonly used.

■ VANCOMYCIN

■ Mechanism of action and bacterial resistance

Vancomycin prevents synthesis of bacterial cell walls by blocking peptidoglycan strand formation. This site of action is different from the sites sensitive to penicillin and other antibiotics interfering with cell wall synthesis.

Resistance to vancomycin is relatively uncommon and tends to develop slowly. As the drug is used clinically, it is a rapidly bacteriocidal agent. This fact may partially explain the low incidence of bacterial resistance to vancomycin.

■ Absorption

Vancomycin is a complex glycopeptide that may be positively or negatively charged, depending on the pH. Therefore vancomycin does not easily cross biological membranes and is not absorbed significantly following oral administration (Table 42-3). Vancomycin is most commonly administered intravenously by intermittent infusion. For this purpose 500 mg of vancomycin may be dissolved in 10 ml of sterile water and then added to 100 to 200 ml of 0.9% sodium chloride injection or 5% dextrose in water for infusion over a 20 to 30 minute period. This regimen may be repeated every 6 hours.

Vancomycin may rarely be given by mouth for intestinal infections. Bacteriocidal concentrations of the drug are not obtained in the systemic circulation under this circumstance.

■ Distribution and excretion

Vancomycin is well-distributed throughout the body and reaches clinically effective concentrations in various body fluid compartments such as pericardial, synovial, and pleural fluids. Vancomycin does not penetrate into normal cerebrospinal fluid but does enter the central nervous system when the meninges are inflamed.

The kidney is the major excretory organ for vancomycin. The drug appears in very high concentrations in the urine and is in the active form when excreted.

Vancomycin elimination by nonkidney routes is very limited. Therefore, in any patients with renal insufficiency, vancomycin may tend to accumulate unless drug doses are reduced to compensate for loss of excretory efficiency. In patients with no kidney function, vancomycin is commonly administered only once in the interval between dialysis. Less frequent intervals may be required for individual anephric patients. Vancomycin is not cleared from the body by hemodialysis.

■ Toxicity

Vancomycin causes deafness in some patients, especially when serum concentrations exceed 80 μg/ml serum. Since patients with impaired renal function and elderly patients will be more likely than normal persons to show drug accumulation, these patients should be very closely watched for tinnitus (ringing in the ears) or hearing loss. Some patients have apparently regained some hearing acuity when vancomycin was discontinued. Other clinics report hearing loss may continue even after the drug is stopped.

Nephrotoxicity may occur with vancomycin. Bloody urine and protein in the urine have occasionally been noted. Allergies manifested by urticarial rashes may also occur.

Intravenous infusion of vancomycin has produced nausea, flushing, and itching of the skin. These reactions are more likely when undiluted vancomycin is dripped directly into a running intravenous line rather than being properly diluted beforehand. If vancomycin inadvertently enters muscle or skin around the intravenous site, local tissue necrosis may develop.

TABLE 42-3. Clinical summary of miscellaneous penicillin substitutes

Generic name	Trade name	Drug form	Dosage and administration
Vancomycin	Vancocin	Powder	ORAL: As for intravenous. Note this route is for intestinal infections only.
		Powder to be reconstituted with sterile water	INTRAVENOUS: *Adults*—500 mg 4 times daily. *Children*—40 mg/kg per day in divided doses.
Bacitracin		Solution	INTRAMUSCULAR: *Infants*—over 2.5 kg, 1000 units/kg per day in 2 or 3 doses; infants below 2.5 kg, 900 units/kg per day in 2 or 3 doses.
		Ointment for ophthalmic or skin application	TOPICAL: *Adults and children*—ointments contain 500 units of antibiotic/Gm. Application may be every 3 hr or less frequently, depending on the infection.
Novobiocin	Albamycin	Capsules, syrup	ORAL: *Adults*—250 to 500 mg 4 times daily. *Children*—15 to 45 mg/kg per day.
		Solution	INTRAMUSCULAR: *Adults*—500 mg twice daily. *Children*—15 to 30 mg/kg per day in 2 doses.
		Solution	INTRAVENOUS: As for intramuscular.
Spectinomycin	Trobicin	Solution	INTRAMUSCULAR: *Adults*—2 to 4 Gm in a single dose.

■ Drug interactions

Vancomycin is compatible with many common intravenous fluids. The major consideration in combining vancomycin use with another drug should be to avoid administering another ototoxic drug such as streptomycin. The combined use of the two ototoxic drugs may produce additive toxic effects and severely impair hearing.

■ Uses

Vancomycin is primarily effective against gram-positive organisms and most commonly used in staphylococcal or streptococcal infections. Since the drug is chemically unrelated to penicillins and has a different mechanism of action, it is effective against organisms that are resistant to penicillins, including methicillin-resistant staphylococci. Since vancomycin and penicillin are not cross-allergenic, vancomycin is very useful for therapy in patients allergic to penicillins. Vancomycin also has special utility in treating antibiotic-induced colitis, which arises from a suprainfection with *Clostridium difficile* in the bowel.

■ BACITRACIN

■ Mechanism of action and bacterial resistance

Bacitracin blocks the regeneration of a lipid carrier that transports cell wall material through the bacterial cell membrane. This site of action is different from that of penicillins or other antibiotics that inhibit cell wall formation. In addition to this action, the drug interferes with bacterial cell membrane function.

Inherent resistance to bacitracin exists in gram-negative organisms, but acquired resistance among the gram-positive organisms is uncommon. Organisms resistant to bacitracin are not necessarily resistant to other antibiotics.

■ Absorption, distribution, and excretion

Bacitracin is well-absorbed from intramuscular injection sites and penetrates all body organs. The kidney eliminates the drug from the body, primarily by glomerular filtration.

The most common route of administration for bacitracin is by a topical route, either on the skin or in the eye (Table 42-3). When applied to the body surface or when used to lavage the peritoneal cavity, the drug seems not to be absorbed to any significant degree.

■ Toxicity

Bacitracin is extremely nephrotoxic. Glomerular and tubular necrosis have occurred. Protein may appear in the urine and azotemia (excess urea and other nitrogen-containing compounds in the blood) may develop. Because of the great risk of permanent kidney damage, bacitracin is not now used systemically except under very limited circumstances. Other less toxic drugs can usually be substituted. When used topically, the drug is practically nontoxic.

■ Uses

Bacitracin is effective against gram-positive bacteria, especially staphylococci.

THE NURSING PROCESS

The student should refer to Chapter 40 for general guidelines on the nursing process with antibiotic therapy. The following additional material relates specifically to the most commonly used penicillin substitutes: erythromycin, clindamycin, vancomycin, and spectinomycin.

Assessment

The penicillin substitutes are prescribed for many types of infections but are primarily narrow spectrum antibiotics similar in scope to penicillin G. A thorough assessment of the patient should be carried out with emphasis on the organ where the infection is thought to be present if the infection is a localized one. Other clinical signs of infection should be monitored.

Management

Once the decision is made to treat with one of the penicillin substitutes, the nurse should obtain additional data for the data base about particular organs or areas that might be affected by the prescribed antibiotic. For example, the nurse should pay special attention to liver function in patients receiving erythromycin or clindamycin, kidney function in patients receiving vancomycin and spectinomycin, and hearing acuity in patients receiving vancomycin. If the patient is to continue receiving the drug on an outpatient basis, the nurse should instruct the patient in the proper timing of the dosage and the need to continue the medication as prescribed. The nurse should inform the patient of specific signs of toxicity that might occur with a specific drug. A patient receiving clindamycin should be well-aware that diarrhea occurring during therapy should be immediately reported to the physician. Patients receiving erythromycin estolate should be informed of the signs of liver dysfunction that the drug might induce and should know to contact the physician if these signs arise.

Evaluation

Erythromycins and clindamycin seldom cause long-term side effects. Patients receiving these medications should be watched during and immediately after therapy for liver or gastrointestinal disturbances. Vancomycin can cause progressive hearing loss, and patients should be continuously evaluated for this problem. Spectinomycin is used for very short-term therapy of syphilis and is seldom associated with major toxicity. Outpatients should demonstrate the ability to judge improvement in the infection being treated and should be able to tell the nurse what reactions might be expected to the medications and when it would be appropriate to call the physician.

The most common use of bacitracin is as a topical ointment for superficial skin infections. The drug may be obtained alone or in combination with a variety of other antibiotics in a number of nonprescription preparations. Special formulations of bacitracin exist for use in the eye.

NOVOBIOCIN

Mechanism of action and bacterial resistance

Novobiocin has a mechanism of action distinct from other antimicrobial agents and inhibits several bacterial processes. Novobiocin is not cross-resistant with other antimicrobial agents. Bacterial resistance to novobiocin develops quickly during therapy.

Absorption, distribution, and excretion

Absorption of novobiocin is adequate from the gastrointestinal tract or from intramuscular injection sites (Table 42-3). Novobiocin may also be used intravenously. Novobiocin does not enter the normal central nervous system but may appear in cerebrospinal fluid when meningitis occurs.

Excretion of the drug is primarily via bile and feces. Little novobiocin is excreted by the kidney.

Toxicity

Novobiocin causes allergic skin reactions in a significant number of patients. More severe allergic reactions have occurred. Blood dyscrasias of various types have also been reported. Liver function tests and routine hematological testing is required in all patients receiving this drug.

Novobiocin may cause nausea, vomiting, diarrhea, and, occasionally, bloody stools.

■ Drug interactions

Novobiocin is incompatible with dextrose and should not be added to solutions containing dextrose. Novobiocin may also form insoluble precipitates with lincomycin, erythromycins, or aminoglycoside antibiotics.

■ Uses

The high toxicity of novobiocin, the narrow antimicrobial spectrum, and the availability of more effective and safer drugs have combined to virtually halt the clinical use of novobiocin. The drug is currently used only for *Staphylococcus aureus* infections shown to be sensitive to novobiocin and resistant to penicillins, cephalosporins, vancomycin, lincomycin, erythromycin, and tetracyclines. Novobiocin has occasionally been used orally for urinary tract infections caused by *Proteus* species that are resistant to other drugs tested. Because of the dangerous liver toxicity, novobiocin should not be used in neonates or very young children whose livers are immature.

■ SPECTINOMYCIN

■ Mechanism of action, bacterial resistance, and clinical use

Spectinomycin inhibits bacterial protein synthesis. Both gram-positive and gram-negative bacteria may be affected, but the ability of spectinomycin to inhibit *N. gonorrhoeae* is the basis for the clinical usefulness of the drug. On this basis it is classified as a penicillin substitute. Resistance to spectinomycin may occur.

■ Absorption, distribution, and excretion

Spectinomycin is administered by intramuscular injection in the treatment of gonorrhea (Table 42-3). Absorption is adequate to produce high serum concentrations of drug and to maintain those concentrations long enough after a single injection to eradicate *N. gonorrhoeae* from the infection site. Within 2 days, nearly all of the injected drug appears in active form in the urine.

■ Toxicity

Single doses of spectinomycin have caused nausea, chills and dizziness. Some patients report pain at the injection site, urticaria, or fever. Urine output may be diminished but renal damage has not been verified.

■ PATIENT CARE IMPLICATIONS

Review the patient care implications section in Chapter 40.

Erythromycin

1. Possible side effects include nausea, vomiting, rashes, urticaria, hearing loss, and hepatic toxicity. Caution patients to report any side effects, especially emphasizing the hearing loss and liver toxicity. Signs indicating possible liver dysfunction include right upper quadrant abdominal pain, jaundice, fever, and change in the color or consistency of stools.
2. Oral preparations should be taken on an empty stomach, either 1 hour before or 2 hours after eating. The exceptions are the estolate preparations, which can be taken with meals. Sometimes patients are instructed to take erythromycin preparations with meals to decrease gastric irritation and side effects, but this will result in reduced absorption.
3. Parenteral erythromycin: Both the lactobionate and gluceptate forms should be reconstituted with Sterile Water for Injection (without preservatives), then diluted further with solutions of appropriate pH and compatibility (see manufacturer's literature) to a concentration of 250 to 500 mg in 100 to 250 ml. Administer the diluted solution at a rate of 1 Gm over a period of 20 to 60 minutes. The rate should be slow enough to prevent pain in the vein.

Clindamycin and lincomycin

1. Side effects for both drugs include anorexia, nausea, vomiting, rash, and severe diarrhea, which has been fatal in some cases. Caution the patient about side effects, noting that any diarrhea should be reported to the physician immediately. Lincomycin can also cause tinnitus and vertigo.
2. Lincomycin should be taken on an empty stomach, either 1 hour before or 2 hours after eating. Clindamycin can safely be taken with meals.
3. Parenteral lincomycin:
   a. The drug is supplied in solution form, 300 mg/ml. The usual dose for adults is 600 mg (2 ml) intramuscularly. Pain at injection site is common.
   b. For intravenous use, the solution of medication should be further diluted in compatible solutions to a concentration not stronger than 1 Gm/100 ml (see literature). The rate of administration should not exceed 1 Gm per hour.
   c. Hypotension has occurred following parenteral administration. Caution the patient to remain lying down for a while after receiving the medication or supervise ambulation.
   d. Too rapid intravenous administration has caused cardiac arrest. The use of a microdrip infusion set

may be appropriate; establish the rate of infusion carefully. Check the patient frequently.

4. Parenteral clindamycin:
   a. The drug is supplied in a solution containing 150 mg/ml. A single intramuscular injection greater than 600 mg (4 ml) is not recommended.
   b. Pain, induration, and sterile abscesses at injection sites have occurred.
   c. For intravenous administration, further dilute the solution in 50 ml or more of appropriate diluent (see literature) and administer at a rate of 300 mg over a period of 10 minutes or longer. Administration of greater than 1200 mg over a period of 10 minutes is not recommended.
   d. Hypotension has occurred following parenteral administration. Caution the patient to remain lying down for a while after receiving the medication or supervise ambulation.

Vancomycin

1. Side effects include tinnitus, which may precede hearing loss, circumoral paresthesias, skin rash, fever, and hypotension. Evaluate patients frequently for hearing loss because it sometimes progresses even after the drug is discontinued. Nephrotoxicity may occur; evaluate the fluid intake and output, tell patients to report any changes in the appearance of urine, and monitor the blood urea nitrogen (BUN).
2. Parenteral vancomycin: Dilute the 500 mg of dry powder with 10 ml Sterile Water for Injection. Further dilute this solution with sodium chloride solution or 5% dextrose in water to make a final volume of 500 mg in 100 to 200 ml. Administer 500 mg over a period of 30 minutes. This drug is incompatible with many other drugs. For further information, consult the pharmacist or check the manufacturer's literature.

Bacitracin

1. This drug is used almost exclusively via the topical route and has very few side effects via this route. Caution the patient to apply only as directed and to report a rash or any other unexplained symptom.
2. Bacitracin ointment requires no prescription for purchase.
3. The parenteral route of administration is rarely used. Side effects from this route can include nausea, vomiting, rashes, pain at the injection site, and allergic reactions. In addition, the drug is very nephrotoxic; monitor the fluid intake and output, and force fluids during the course of therapy. See the manufacturer's literature for guides to proper dilution.

Spectinomycin

1. Spectinomycin can cause pain at the injection site, nausea, chills, fever, insomnia, rash, and oliguria. Alterations in laboratory results have also been noted, including a decrease in hemoglobin, hematocrit, and creatinine clearance and elevations of alkaline phosphatase, blood urea nitrogen (BUN), and serum glutamic pyruvic transaminase (SGPT).
2. The diluent is provided by the manufacturer, and the drug should be reconstituted as indicated on the vial. The manufacturer recommends the use of a 20-gauge needle for administration.

■ SUMMARY

Penicillin substitutes are antibiotics that have an antimicrobial spectrum similar to penicillin G and are frequently used in patients allergic to the penicillins or against organisms that have acquired resistance to penicillins.

Erythromycin is primarily used orally, with the esters of erythromycin being less acid-sensitive and better absorbed than erythromycin base. Erythromycin ethylsuccinate may be given intramuscularly but is usually avoided, since pain is severe and tolerated doses are low. Erythromycin lactobionate or gluceptate may be given intravenously but also causes pain. Erythromycin is excreted primarily by the liver. Erythromycin estolate may rarely produce cholestatic hepatitis. Allergies and hearing loss are rare reactions to erythromycins. The most common limiting toxicity with these drugs is gastrointestinal distress. Erythromycin has special utility in treating atypical pneumonias, infections resulting from bacterial L-forms, and diphtheria.

Clindamycin may be used orally or, when used as the phosphate, may be injected parenterally. Clindamycin does not enter the cerebrospinal fluid but is otherwise well-distributed to body tissues. The liver biodegrades the drug extensively and is the main route of elimination of clindamycin from the body. Clindamycin use can lead to a suprainfection of the bowel with *Clostridium difficile*. This organism produces a toxin that induces severe colitis. Diarrhea and the danger of this severe reaction limit the use of clindamycin.

Vancomycin is a parenteral agent well-distributed to most body tissues and fluids. The drug is excreted primarily by the kidney and may accumulate when kidney function is reduced. Vancomycin can produce deafness, nephrotoxicity, and an acute reaction on injection. Bacterial resistance to vancomycin is rare. One unique use of vancomycin is in treating antibiotic-induced colitis due to *C. difficile*.

Bacitracin is used primarily as a topical agent because it is too toxic toward the kidney for routine systemic use. Novobiocin is seldom used in modern clinical practice because it is toxic toward the liver and bone marrow and has no clinical advantage over safer drugs. Spectinomycin is used primarily in the treatment of gonorrhea when penicillin is inappropriate.

■ STUDY QUESTIONS

1. Why are erythromycin, clindamycin, vancomycin, bacitracin, novobiocin, and spectinomycin called *penicillin substitutes?*
2. What are two mechanisms that account for bacterial resistance to erythromycin?
3. What advantages do the esters of erythromycin possess over erythromycin base?
4. Which of the erythromycin esters is best absorbed orally and may be taken with meals?
5. Which forms of erythromycin can be used parenterally?
6. What property limits the parenteral use of erythromycin?
7. What is the major route of excretion of erythromycin?
8. What is the most common reaction to erythromycin?
9. What toxic reaction is unique to erythromycin estolate?
10. Name four clinical uses of erythromycin.
11. Bacterial resistance to clindamycin is associated with resistance to which other antibiotic?
12. How do clindamycin and lincomycin differ in oral absorption?
13. What form of clindamycin is appropriate for parenteral use?
14. How do clindamycin and lincomycin differ in their distribution to the central nervous system?
15. How is clindamycin eliminated from the body?
16. What is the limiting toxicity to clindamycin?
17. How is clindamycin-induced colitis best treated?
18. Why is bacterial resistance to vancomycin relatively rare?
19. By what route is vancomycin usually administered?
20. What is the major route of excretion of vancomycin?
21. What toxic reactions are most common with vancomycin?
22. Name three clinical uses for vancomycin.
23. By what route is bacitracin usually administered?
24. What toxicity is associated with the systemic use of bacitracin?
25. Why is the clinical use of novobiocin quite limited?
26. What is the primary clinical indication for spectinomycin?
27. What pharmacological property of spectinomycin makes this drug a useful replacement of penicillin in the treatment of gonorrhea?

■ SUGGESTED READINGS

Gallagher, N.D., and Goulston, S.J.M.: Antibiotic associated colitis: in search of a cause and treatment, Drugs **16:**385, 1978.

Geraci, J.E.: Vancomycin, Mayo Clinic Proceedings **52:**631, 1977.

How to use intravenous antibiotics, Nurses' Drug Alert (special issue) **1:**89, June, 1977.

Keighley, M.R.B.: Antibiotic-associated pseudomembranous colitis: pathogenesis and management, Drugs **20:**49, 1980.

Kucers, A., and Bennett, N. McK.: The use of antibiotics, ed. 3, London, 1979, William Heinemann Medical Books Ltd.

Rodman, M.J.: Anti-infectives you administer: alternatives to penicillin, RN **40:**77, April, 1977.

Wilson, W.R.: Tetracyclines, chloramphenicol, erythromycin, and clindamycin, Mayo Clinic Proceedings **52:**635, 1977.

43 Antibiotics: tetracyclines and chloramphenicol

In this chapter two antibiotics with very broad antimicrobial spectra, tetracyclines and chloramphenicol, are introduced. The tetracyclines are a large family of chemically related compounds, many of which are clinically useful. Chloramphenicol is unique in chemical structure, and no chemical relatives of this drug have been developed for clinical use.

■ TETRACYCLINES

■ Mechanism of action and bacterial resistance

The tetracyclines block bacterial growth by preventing ribosomes from binding messenger RNA, thereby preventing the initiation of protein synthesis. Members of this drug family are, therefore, bacteriostatic rather than bacteriocidal.

For tetracyclines to be effective, they must first be transported into the bacterial cell. Antibiotic uptake is accomplished by an energy-dependent transport system. Resistant bacteria lose the ability to transport tetracyclines into the bacterial cell, and the antibiotic does not come in contact with its intracellular target. Much of the observed tetracycline resistance involves a plasmid (Chapter 40), which is transmitted from bacterium to bacterium and may therefore spread rapidly throughout bacterial populations. For example, families of patients treated on a long-term basis with low doses of tetracyclines may show a conversion of the normal tetracycline-sensitive bacterial flora to tetracycline-resistant forms. Cross-resistance between the older tetracyclines is complete. The newer tetracyclines minocycline and doxycycline, however, are more lipid soluble than the older drugs and are transported into the bacterial cell by different mechanisms than the older drugs. These drugs may therefore penetrate into bacterial cells that do not concentrate the older tetracyclines. For example, strains of *Staphylococcus aureus* resistant to tetracycline do not accumulate tetracycline but do accumulate minocycline and are sensitive to it.

■ Absorption

Tetracyclines are primarily administered by the oral route (Table 43-1). Tetracyclines are frequently administered as the hydrochloride or the phosphate salt to increase solubility and thereby increase absorption. Most of the tetracycline that enters the circulation following an oral dose of the drug is absorbed from the stomach and the upper intestine.

Tetracyclines are variably absorbed from the gastrointestinal tract. Absorption is influenced by three factors: acid lability, water solubility, and lipid solubility. All the tetracyclines with the exception of doxycycline and minocycline are acid labile and are partly destroyed by stomach acid. Tetracyclines are not highly water soluble and this solubility may be further reduced by complex formation with metal ions or with solid material in the intestine. In these insoluble forms, the drugs are not absorbed but remain in the intestine and are excreted in the feces. Doxycycline and minocycline are the exceptions, being highly lipid soluble, and both drugs tend to pass freely through the gastrointestinal membranes and are much more completely and rapidly absorbed than most of the other tetracyclines.

Absorption of tetracyclines from intramuscular sites is generally poor and frequently causes local tissue irritation and pain at the injection site. Intramuscular use of tetracyclines is therefore limited.

Tetracyclines may be used intravenously in serious infections. Tetracycline, oxytetracycline, doxycycline, and minocycline all can be obtained in a form suitable for intravenous use. These drugs have a relatively low water solubility, however, and must be diluted extensively before use by this route. When used intravenously, tetracyclines may cause thrombophlebitis. Improper dilution of the drug or repeated infusion into the same vein increases the likelihood of thrombophlebitis.

■ Distribution and excretion

Tetracyclines are well distributed in most body tissues and fluids, appearing in liver, spleen, bone marrow, bile, and cerebrospinal fluid even in the absence of inflammation. The drugs pass the placental barrier and

TABLE 43-1. Clinical summary of tetracyclines

Generic name	Trade name	Dosage and administration
Tetracycline hydrochloride	Achromycin Bristacycline Cyclopar Panmycin Retet Robitet Sumycin Tetracyn	ORAL: *Adults*—1 to 2 Gm per day in 2 to 4 doses. *Children over 8 yr*—25 to 50 mg/kg per day.
	Achromycin IM Tetracyn IM	INTRAMUSCULAR: *Adults*—300 mg to 800 mg per day in divided doses. *Children over 8 yr*—15 to 25 mg/kg not to exceed 250 mg per dose.
	Achromycin IV Tetracyn IV	INTRAVENOUS: *Adults*—250 to 500 mg per day in 2 to 4 doses. *Children over 8 yr*—10 to 20 mg/kg per day in 2 doses.
Chlortetracycline hydrochloride	Aureomycin Aureomycin IV	ORAL: As for tetracycline INTRAVENOUS: As for tetracycline.
Oxytetracycline hydrochloride	Oxlopar Terramycin	ORAL: As for tetracycline.
	Terramycin IM Terramycin IV	INTRAMUSCULAR: As for tetracycline. INTRAVENOUS: As for tetracycline.
Methacycline hydrochloride	Rondomycin	ORAL: *Adults*—600 mg per day in 2 or 4 doses. *Children over 8 yr*—10 mg/kg per day in 4 doses.
Demeclocycline hydrochloride	Declomycin	ORAL: *Adults*—600 mg to 1 Gm per day in 4 doses. *Children over 8 yr*—6 to 12 mg/kg per day in 2 to 4 doses.
Doxycycline	Doxy-II Doxychel Doxycycline hyclate Vibramycin	ORAL: *Adults*—100 to 200 mg per day in 2 doses. *Children over 8 yr*—2 to 4 mg/kg per day in 2 doses.
	Vibramycin IV	INTRAVENOUS: As for oral.
Minocycline hydrochloride	Minocin Vectrin	ORAL: as for doxycycline.
	Minocin IV Vectrin IV	INTRAVENOUS: As for doxycycline.

enter fetal circulation in appreciable amounts. Tetracyclines also appear in the milk of nursing mothers.

Differences in lipid solubility among the tetracyclines affect the elimination of these drugs. The more polar or water-soluble drugs are eliminated through the kidney in greater amounts than are the lipid-soluble tetracyclines. All the tetracyclines enter the urine by passive glomerular filtration. However, the lipid-soluble drugs are more completely reabsorbed from the kidney tubule than drugs that are charged at the acid pH of the tubular fluid. This high degree of reabsorption is reflected in the longer elimination half-life for doxycycline and minocycline (*ca* 12 to 15 hours) than that of less lipid-soluble tetracyclines such as oxytetracycline, tetracycline, or chlortetracycline (*ca* 6 to 9 hours).

The second major route of elimination of the tetracyclines is by biliary excretion. The drugs are concentrated in the liver and bile and carried into the intestine where they may be reabsorbed by the process called *enterohepatic circulation*. The liver is also the site for biotransformation of several of the tetracyclines. In general the more lipid-soluble drugs penetrate the liver cells and are more extensively biotransformed. Minocycline is in particular extensively biotransformed. The high lipid solubility of doxycycline and its tendency to form insoluble complexes with intestinal solids account for an unusual mode of elimination for this drug. Doxycycline seems to diffuse directly into the intestine where the drug is sequestered by complex formation with fecal material. Because of this unusual mechanism for excretion, doxycycline does not accumulate during renal failure and may be safely used in such patients without dose adjustment.

■ Toxicity

Tetracyclines cause a wide variety of adverse reactions in patients. Perhaps the most common complaint with these drugs is gastrointestinal irritation. Many patients suffer nausea, vomiting, or pain with oral tetracyclines. Diarrhea may occur as a result of irritation by unabsorbed tetracycline remaining in the bowel. Diarrhea may also result from changes in the intestinal flora. Occasionally the effects of these broad-spectrum drugs on intestinal flora are so extensive that overgrowth of drug-resistant bacteria occurs. Staphylococcal enterocolitis may result and may be life-threatening, producing bloody diarrhea and extensive damage to the intestinal epithelium. Candida suprainfections of the throat, vagina, and bowel also occur occasionally.

Allergies to tetracyclines are uncommon. Urticaria, morbilliform rashes, and dermatitis have occurred, as well as more serious reactions such as asthma, angioedema, and anaphylaxis.

Tetracyclines are not completely specific for bacterial ribosomes and may inhibit mammalian protein synthesis to a small degree. This fact may explain the toxic effect tetracyclines have on various tissues. For example, kidney function may be impaired by tetracyclines, and the effects may be worse in a kidney already damaged by disease or trauma. Renal function should therefore be carefully watched in patients receiving these drugs. Likewise the liver is sensitive to tetracyclines. Hepatotoxicity may progress to jaundice, fatty liver, and death unless the drug is discontinued at the first sign of difficulty. Pregnant women are most sensitive to this complication and should rarely, if ever, be given tetracyclines. Elderly, extremely debilitated patients or patients recovering from extensive surgery or traumatic injuries may suffer metabolic derangement when given tetracyclines. These patients commonly show negative nitrogen balance. This reaction is thought to result from tetracycline inhibition of mammalian protein synthesis.

Tetracyclines also delay blood coagulation. The exact mechanism for this reaction is not known but may involve binding the calcium that is required in coagulation.

The ability of tetracyclines to bind calcium also leads to the deposition of these drugs in bones and teeth. In adults this binding produces little visible effect, but in children below 8 years of age the newly formed permanent teeth may be stained by the drug. This staining is irreversible. Binding of tetracyclines to bones may slow bone growth visibly in fetuses or very young children. Infants may also display an increase in intracranial pressure with bulging fontanelles when given tetracyclines.

Specific tetracyclines may cause unique adverse reactions. For example, minocycline can cause damage to vestibular function, thereby impairing balance. No other tetracyclines produce this effect, although other antibiotics do. Another specific reaction to a single tetracycline is the phototoxic effect of demeclocycline. All tetracyclines can be degraded to toxic products by exposure to light, but demeclocycline seems to be most effective in producing these reactions in the patient. The drug appears to be broken down by the action of ultraviolet light on the skin, and the toxic products released cause an intense sunburn reaction. Since tetracyclines other than demeclocycline have the potential of causing this reaction, it is prudent to suggest that patients receiving these drugs limit their exposure to direct sunlight, especially in subtropical or tropical climates.

Outdated tetracycline preparations have been implicated in occasional severe adverse reactions, apparently caused by toxic breakdown products of the drugs. A reaction called the *Fanconi syndrome* has been observed in which the patient loses amino acids, proteins, and sugar in the urine and suffers polyuria and polydipsia, acidosis, nausea, and vomiting. These reactions slowly disappear after the drug is discontinued. In other cases patients show symptoms reminiscent of systemic lupus erythematosus.

■ Drug interactions

Several tetracycline interactions with other drugs are the result of the ability of tetracyclines to form insoluble complexes with metal ions. For example, oral tetracyclines frequently cause gastric irritation, and for this reason patients may wish to take antacids along with the antibiotic. This practice should be discouraged, since common antacids include magnesium and aluminum salts, which complex with tetracyclines and prevent their absorption from the gastrointestinal tract. The antacids, therefore, reduce the antibacterial effect of the antibiotic. Likewise iron-containing preparations such as vitamin or mineral supplements may prevent tetracycline absorption. Milk and other dairy products are high in calcium and also impair tetracycline absorption. Sodium bicarbonate taken with a tetracycline tablet may impede tablet dissolution in the stomach and thereby reduce absorption of the drug.

Food in the stomach impairs absorption of oral tetracyclines, with the exception of doxycycline and minocycline. These lipid-soluble tetracyclines are absorbed well even in the presence of food or milk products in the stomach.

Several tetracyclines, but especially doxycycline and minocycline, are metabolized to some degree by the liver. Drugs such as barbiturates, which increase hepatic drug-metabolizing enzymes, shorten the duration of action of doxycycline and minocycline. This action may decrease the antibacterial effectiveness of these agents.

The bacteriostatic mechanism of action of tetracyclines leads to interactions with two different types of drugs: immunosuppressants and penicillins. Immunosuppressant drugs such as glucocorticoids depress the host defense mechanisms against bacterial infections. Since tetracyclines are bacteriostatic drugs, they depend on the patient's immune system to eliminate the pathogen. If this elimination cannot occur, the bacteria may overcome the inhibitory effects of the tetracycline and the effect of the drug is lost. Penicillins given with tetracyclines may be less effective than penicillin given alone. Penicillin is a bacteriocidal drug that is effective against actively growing bacteria. Tetracyclines inhibit bacterial growth, thereby making them resistant to the action of penicillin.

Tetracycline nephrotoxicity may become significant and dangerous when these antibiotics are given with other nephrotoxic agents. One example involves the anesthetic methoxyflurane (Penthrane). This anesthetic gas is itself nephrotoxic and when given to patients receiving tetracyclines may exacerbate kidney damage.

■ Uses (Table 43-1)

Tetracyclines are clinically important by virtue of the very wide antibacterial spectrum they display. Most gram-positive organisms are sensitive to tetracyclines; however, most infections due to these organisms are best treated by other agents because penicillins, cephalosporins, erythromycin, and clindamycin are equally or more effective against these organisms and are less toxic. Nevertheless, when laboratory results confirm the organism to be sensitive to tetracyclines, these drugs can be used for some gram-positive infections.

Gram-negative bacteria found in the bowel are usually sensitive to tetracyclines, but resistance does develop. *Serratia, Proteus,* and *Pseudomonas* strains are usually resistant.

Neisseria gonorrhoeae is sensitive to tetracyclines. Clinically, however, tetracyclines are used to treat gonorrhea only when penicillin is contraindicated.

Tetracyclines are clinically effective for a number of bacterial infections that are relatively rare in the United States: chancroid *(Haemophilus ducreyi),* rabbit fever or tularemia *(Francisella tularensis),* black plague *(Yersinia pestis),* brucellosis (*Brucella* species), and cholera *(Vibrio cholerae).*

Tetracyclines are highly effective for diseases caused by rickettsiae (tick fever, Rocky Mountain spotted fever, typhus, and Q fever), chlamydia (parrot fever or psittacosis, trachoma, lymphogranuloma venereum), and *Mycoplasma pneumoniae* (atypical or "walking" pneumonia).

Tetracyclines are useful in treating relapsing fever *(Borrelia recurrentis),* syphilis *(Treponema pallidum),* and yaws *(Treponema pertenue),* which are all diseases caused by spirochetes.

Tetracyclines may have a useful role in treating amebic dysentery. Minocycline in particular may be useful in nocardial infections.

Tetracyclines have been widely used in dermatology for the treatment of acne. Relatively low doses may be prescribed over long periods of time. Whereas this treatment is effective for many patients, questions arise as to long-term adverse effects of the drugs and to the contribution this practice makes to the development of tetracycline-resistant bacterial populations.

Pharmaceutical formulations of tetracyclines are quite varied. These antibiotics are available in 100 to 500 mg tablets or capsules, syrups for pediatric use, ophthalmic ointments or drops, and various forms for topical use.

■ CHLORAMPHENICOL

■ Mechanism of action and bacterial resistance

Chloramphenicol inhibits bacterial protein synthesis. The mechanism of action is different from that of tetracyclines in that chloramphenicol inhibits late rather than early steps in ribosomal function. Like tetracyclines, chloramphenicol is bacteriostatic rather than bacteriocidal.

Bacterial resistance to chloramphenicol nearly always involves destruction of the antibiotic by bacterial enzymes. These enzymes are not always present but may be induced by exposure of potentially resistant bacteria to sublethal doses of chloramphenicol. The genes required for synthesizing this enzyme are usually carried on small DNA molecules called *plasmids,* which may exist separately from the bulk of genetic material in the cell. Plasmids may be transmitted from bacteria to bacteria, and resistance to chloramphenicol may thereby be transmitted widely throughout bacterial populations.

■ Absorption, distribution, and excretion

Chloramphenicol is nearly completely absorbed from the gastrointestinal tract following oral administration. The peak serum concentration achieved by an oral dose is about the same as that produced by an equivalent dose given intravenously, although the attainment of the peak serum concentration is somewhat delayed with oral administration (Table 43-2). Intramuscular injection produces lower blood levels than oral administration and for this reason is not recommended. Seriously ill patients should receive chloramphenicol intravenously, since oral absorption may be impaired in these patients. The succinate form of chloramphenicol is used for intravenous administration only, whereas the parent drug, chloramphenicol, is used orally.

Chloramphenicol is very well distributed throughout body tissues and fluids. Significant and effective concentrations of the drug enter the eye, joint fluid (synovial), and pleural fluids. Unlike many other antibiotics, chloramphenicol enters the cerebrospinal fluid relatively easily, even when the meninges are not inflamed. Chloramphenicol also easily crosses the placenta and appears in human milk.

Most of the chloramphenicol in the body is inactivated in the liver. The drug is conjugated with glucuronic acid to form chloramphenicol glucuronide. This inactive drug form may be excreted in the kidney by tubular secretion, whereas unaltered chloramphenicol is excreted solely by glomerular filtration. The actual concentration of active chloramphenicol in the urine is high enough to be antibacterial, but the active chloramphenicol in the urine is only a small fraction of the total drug excreted by this route.

■ Toxicity

Chloramphenicol is a very effective antibiotic, but its clinical usefulness has been limited by its potential for bone marrow toxicity. A reversible form of bone marrow depression causes a reduction of reticulocytes and leukopenia. These symptoms usually resolve quickly when chloramphenicol is discontinued. Patients receiving chloramphenicol should have routine blood tests performed during therapy to detect early signs of this toxic reaction.

Chloramphenicol may also induce an irreversible bone marrow depression, which leads to aplastic anemia, a condition with a high mortality. This condition is usually characterized by pancytopenia (loss of all forms of blood cells), but in some cases one or more of the major blood cells will continue to be formed. Aplastic anemia, although rare, may appear weeks or months after chloramphenicol therapy. This time lag between drug administration and appearance of aplastic anemia complicates the accurate calculation of drug-associated risk, especially considering that most patients will have received more than one other drug during the interim between chloramphenicol therapy and development of aplastic anemia. Best estimates of the actual incidence suggest that roughly one out of 25,000 chloramphenicol-treated patients will develop aplastic anemia. Although this incidence is low, the frequently fatal outcome is sufficient cause to restrict the use of chloramphenicol to the treatment of very serious infections.

Less severe problems may also occur with chloramphenicol therapy. Allergies of various types may occur, as well as gastrointestinal irritation. Long-term therapy has been associated with neuritis, which may involve the optic nerve. Blindness has occurred in a few patients. Central nervous system symptoms are also seen in some patients: headache, mental confusion, depression, or delirium.

Patients with reduced liver function are at risk of severe toxic reactions due to drug accumulation. The liver normally converts over 90% of administered chloramphenicol, which is toxic, to the glucuronide, which is nontoxic. Therefore, any reduction in the liver's ability to detoxify the drug may result in accumulation of the toxic drug in the body, unless dosages are appropriately reduced. One group of patients especially at risk for this complication is newborn infants. Neonates have an immature liver, which lacks the enzyme to form the glucuronide. When these infants are given a weight-adjusted dosage based on adult doses, many develop a condition that has been called the *grey syndrome*. Drug accumulation proceeds without symptoms for 3 to 4 days, after which time the infant may develop abdominal distention, emesis, progressive pallid cyanosis, and irregular respiration. Vasomotor collapse and death may result in a high percentage of cases. Infants receiving smaller doses are less likely to develop these symptoms. If the early signs of this condition are noted by alert health care personnel and the drug is discontinued, most infants will recover.

■ Drug interactions

Chloramphenicol can inhibit drug-metabolizing enzymes of the liver. This property may lead to dangerous interactions with drugs that have two characteristic properties: (1) a relatively low therapeutic index and (2) a major route of elimination by microsomal enzymes of the liver. The three drugs that fall into this category are phenytoin, tolbutamide, and coumarin anticoagulants. When a patient who is receiving one of these drugs on a long-term basis is given chloramphenicol, these liver-metabolized drugs tend to accumulate. As a result well-controlled diabetics may become hypoglycemic, successfully anticoagulated patients may develop spontaneous bleeding, or controlled epileptics may develop phenytoin toxicity.

Since chloramphenicol is rarely used, these interactions are also rather rare. In the unusual case in which these drugs must be combined in the same patient, the early signs of drug interactions should be watched for.

■ THE NURSING PROCESS

The student should refer to the nursing process section in Chapter 40 for general guidelines on the nursing process with antibiotic therapy. The additional material below relates specifically to the broad spectrum antibiotics: tetracyclines and chloramphenicol.

■ Assessment

Tetracyclines may be prescribed for a very wide variety of infections, including bacterial and rickettsial diseases. Tetracyclines are not usually prescribed for pregnant patients or for children below the age of 8 years. Chloramphenicol is usually reserved for seriously ill patients, primarily those with typhoid fever or with bacteremia or meningitis due to a chloramphenicol-sensitive organism. A thorough assessment of the patient should be carried out with emphasis on the organ in which the infection is thought to be present, if the infection is a localized one, and on liver and kidney function. Other clinical signs of infection should be monitored.

■ Management

Once the decision is made to treat the patient with tetracyclines, the nurse should obtain additional data for the data base about kidney and liver function. Patients receiving chloramphenicol should be carefully checked for adequate liver function. The nurse should also question the patient about having received chloramphenicol in the past, since a history of treatment with the drug may predispose to the development of toxicity. The nurse should give special care to the proper timing of tetracycline doses, since the absorption of this drug from the gastrointestinal tract is so strongly influenced by the presence of food and other drugs. Most tetracyclines are best absorbed on an empty stomach. These drugs do cause gastrointestinal irritation, and the patient will need instruction on how to deal with this problem, since common remedies such as milk or nonprescription antacids greatly impair drug absorption. Patients receiving chloramphenicol should receive routine blood testing during and after therapy. The nurse should explain to the patient the need for this type of follow-up and encourage compliance.

■ Evaluation

Tetracyclines and chloramphenicol may cause reactions during and after therapy. Patients receiving tetracyclines not only should be evaluated for clearing of the infection being treated, but also should be observed for renal damage and signs of suprainfection. Candida suprainfections of the mouth, vagina, and bowel are relatively common with the use of tetracyclines. One of the tetracyclines, minocycline, can cause symptoms of vestibular damage. Chloramphenicol can cause blood dyscrasias, which appear long after the end of drug therapy. Patients should be watched for development of signs of blood abnormalities. Outpatients should demonstrate the ability to judge improvement in the infection being treated and should be able to tell the nurse what reactions might be expected with the medications and when it would be appropriate to call the physician.

TABLE 43-2. Clinical summary of chloramphenicol

Generic name	Trade name	Drug form	Dosage and administration	Comments
Chloramphenicol	Amphicol Chloromycetin Mychel	Tablets, capsules	ORAL: *Adults*—50 to 100 mg/kg per day in 4 doses. *Children*—25 mg/kg per day *or less,* depending on liver function.	Blood levels should ordinarily not exceed 20 μg/ml.
Chloramphenicol palmitate		Suspension	ORAL: *Children*—as for other oral forms.	This tasteless suspension is intended for pediatric use.
Chloramphenicol succinate		Solution	INTRAVENOUS: As for oral.	Should be administered as a 10% solution and injected slowly into the vein.

■ **Uses** (Table 43-2)

Because of dangerous toxic reactions, chloramphenicol is reserved for use only in serious infections. Chloramphenicol is the drug of choice for typhoid fever. In addition, life-threatening infections such as bacteremias or meningitis may be treated with chloramphenicol when the pathogen has been tested and proven sensitive to the drug. The antibacterial spectrum of chloramphenicol is quite similar to that of tetracyclines, being especially effective against gram-negative bacteria (except *Pseudomonas aeruginosa*), rickettsiae, and chlamydia.

■ PATIENT CARE IMPLICATIONS

Review the patient care implications section in Chapter 40.

Tetracyclines

1. Side effects of the tetracyclines include anorexia, nausea, vomiting, diarrhea, enterocolitis, and rashes. Superinfections can occur with patients receiving any antiinfective agents but may be more common with the tetracyclines. Rarely seen side effects include exacerbation of lupus erythematosus, bulging fontanelles in infants, and benign intracranial hypertension in adults.
2. Photosensitivity, manifested by an exaggerated sunburn reaction, is possible with all of the tetracyclines but is most common in patients receiving demeclocycline. Patients should be warned of this possible side effect, cautioned to report any skin changes, and encouraged to avoid exposure to the sun or to ultraviolet light while receiving therapy if possible.
3. Vertigo may occur in patients receiving minocycline. Patients should be warned of this possible side effect, instructed to report it if it occurs, and cautioned to avoid activities that might be dangerous should the vertigo occur: driving, operating dangerous equipment, and so on.
4. Tetracyclines should not be used during the last half of pregnancy or by children under 8 years of age because of permanent staining of teeth that can occur.
5. Kidney, liver, and hematopoietic function should be routinely monitored during tetracycline use. Health care personnel should monitor the patient's fluid intake and output and signs of liver dysfunction: jaundice, fever, and right upper quadrant abdominal pain.
6. Patients receiving anticoagulants for whom tetracyclines are also prescribed may require a reduction in anticoagulant dose during tetracycline therapy.
7. Minocycline and doxycycline may be given with foods or milk to minimize gastric irritation. All other tetracyclines should be taken on an empty stomach, at least 1 hour before or 2 hours after meals. Antacids, milk products, or vitamin and mineral products containing iron should not be administered simultaneously with tetracyclines, since these agents prevent absorption of the tetracyclines.
8. Patients should be cautioned to store tetracycline preparations properly in the container provided away from heat and light. Refrigerate, if indicated. The course of therapy should be completed as directed, and unused portions of medications should be discarded. Health care personnel should check for the expiration date before administering tetracyclines.
9. Intramuscular tetracycline can cause pain at the injection site. This is a rarely used route of administration. Follow directions for reconstitution in the manufacturer's literature.
10. Intravenous administration of the tetracyclines can cause thrombophlebitis. Proper dilution and slow administration minimize patient discomfort.
11. Intravenous tetracycline, chlortetracycline, and oxytetracycline: Dilute as instructed in the literature with appropriate fluids to a concentration not greater than 5 mg/ml. The rate of administration should not exceed 2 ml per minute.

12. Intravenous doxycycline: Refer to the manufacturer's literature for instructions about dilution. The recommended minimum infusion time for 100 mg or a solution containing 0.5 mg/ml is 1 hour. Concentrations below 0.1 mg/ml or greater than 1.0 mg/ml are not recommended.
13. Intravenous minocycline: The drug should be initially dissolved and then further diluted in appropriate fluids (see literature) to make a concentration of 100 to 200 mg/500 to 1000 ml. Administer at the ordered infusion rate.

Chloramphenicol

1. Because of the possibility of bone marrow depression, which may occur as a result of chloramphenicol therapy, blood work should be done prior to the initiation of therapy and at regular intervals during therapy. Studies should include hematocrit, differential, reticulocyte count, and leukocyte count. Since bone marrow depression often is not seen until several weeks or months after therapy, patients should also be taught to report any fever, sore throat, fatigue, bruising, or any unusual symptoms that might occur even after completion of therapy. Note that the bone marrow depression is a possible side effect with any route of administration.
2. Patients should be carefully questioned to determine whether they have ever received chloramphenicol before. The incidence of aplastic anemia seems to be higher among patients who have been exposed to the drug on more than one occasion.
3. Other side effects of therapy include allergic responses, gastrointestinal irritation, optic neuritis, headache, confusion, depression, and delirium.
4. Health care personnel working in newborn nurseries should be alert to the development of grey syndrome, a result of chloramphenicol therapy, which is seen in newborn infants up to 3 months old. Symptoms include abdominal distention, progressive pallid cyanosis, hypothermia, irregular respirations, and acute circulatory failure. It can be rapidly fatal. The syndrome usually occurs after 3 or 4 days of therapy. Note that chloramphenicol taken during labor or the last few days of pregnancy can also precipitate grey syndrome in the newborn infant.
5. Newborn infants, elderly persons, and those with decreased liver and kidney function are more at risk for toxic side effects; doses for these groups of patients should be based on blood concentrations of the drug.
6. Patients taking chloramphenicol who are also receiving phenytoin, tolbutamide, or coumarin anticoagulants are at risk for side effects due to increased serum concentrations of those three groups of drugs. It may be necessary to reduce the dose of those three drugs during chloramphenicol therapy. Review with patients the signs of toxicity of the three drugs as needed, and caution patients to report any of these signs if they appear.
7. Patients receiving chloramphenicol succinate may complain of a bitter taste, which lasts for a few minutes after the injection.
8. Intravenous chloramphenicol: Dissolve the dry powder as directed; then further dilute in Sterile Water for Injection or 5% Dextrose in Water to make a 10% concentration (100 mg/ml). Rate of administration should not exceed 100 mg per minute. If desired, the drug may be further diluted and administered over a period of 30 to 60 minutes as an intermittent infusion. For additional information see the manufacturer's literature or consult the pharmacist.

■ SUMMARY

Tetracyclines are bacteriostatic drugs that inhibit bacterial protein synthesis. Tetracyclines are primarily used as oral agents, but only doxycycline and minocycline are efficiently absorbed from the gastrointestinal tract. All other tetracyclines are sensitive to acid, tend to form insoluble complexes in the intestine, and are therefore incompletely absorbed. Tetracycline, oxytetracycline, doxycycline, and minocycline may be used intravenously but must be extensively diluted, since the drugs tend to cause thrombophlebitis. Intramuscular use of tetracycline is limited by poor absorption and local tissue irritation. The tetracyclines are well distributed in body fluids and tissues. The more polar tetracyclines are largely eliminated by the kidney, whereas the newer lipid-soluble tetracyclines (doxycycline and minocycline) are eliminated primarily in the bile or by direct intestinal adsorption. Tetracyclines frequently irritate the gastrointestinal tract following oral use and may extensively alter the bacterial flora of the intestine. Suprainfections in the mouth, vagina, and bowel may result from tetracycline therapy. These drugs may also damage the liver and kidneys as well as interfere with blood coagulation. Tetracyclines bind to calcium in bones and teeth and may discolor the teeth if administered to children during the years when teeth are forming. Tetracyclines in general and especially demeclocycline may cause phototoxic reactions. Minocycline may cause vestibular damage. Outdated tetracycline preparations may be more toxic than newly prepared drugs, since the breakdown products of tetracyclines are highly toxic. Tetracyclines are most useful in practice because of the very wide antimicrobial spectrum of this family of drugs.

Chloramphenicol has a similar mechanism of action and antimicrobial spectrum to the tetracyclines. Chloramphenicol is well absorbed orally and may be used intravenously in the succinate form. The drug penetrates the central nervous system efficiently. Most of the chloramphenicol administered is converted to inactive products by the liver and then eliminated by the kidney. Chloramphenicol may accumulate in patients with impaired liver function. Chloramphenicol may also produce various blood dyscrasias, the most serious being aplastic anemia. Aplastic anemia is a rare complication and occurs weeks to months after therapy, but it is a fatal drug reaction. The danger of this severe toxic reaction limits the clinical use of this otherwise very effective drug.

■ STUDY QUESTIONS

1. What is the mechanism of action of tetracycline antibiotics?
2. What is the mechanism by which bacteria become resistant to tetracyclines?
3. What factors influence the oral absorption of tetracycline antibiotics?
4. How does the absorption of minocycline and doxycycline differ from that of other tetracyclines?
5. What factors limit the intramuscular use of tetracyclines?
6. What precautions are necessary for using tetracyclines intravenously?
7. What are the three main routes of excretion for the tetracyclines?
8. Are minocycline and doxycycline eliminated in the same way as the other tetracyclines?
9. What are the main toxic reactions common to all tetracycline antibiotics?
10. What toxic reaction is especially associated with demeclocycline?
11. What toxic reaction is especially associated with minocycline?
12. What toxicity is associated with the use of outdated tetracycline preparations?
13. What is the effect of administering tetracyclines with antacids?
14. Why do immunosuppressant drugs interfere with the clinical effect of tetracyclines?
15. Why do tetracyclines interfere with the antimicrobial action of penicillins?
16. Name three groups of organisms against which the tetracyclines are effective.
17. What is the mechanism of action of chloramphenicol?
18. What is the mechanism by which bacteria become resistant to chloramphenicol?
19. Which routes of administration give the most rapid and complete absorption of chloramphenicol?
20. Does chloramphenicol efficiently enter the cerebrospinal fluid?
21. What is the primary route of elimination of chloramphenicol from the body?
22. What is the most dangerous toxic reaction associated with chloramphenicol?
23. What is the grey syndrome?
24. Name one clinical indication for chloramphenicol.

■ SUGGESTED READINGS

Barza, M., and Scheife, R.T.: Antimicrobial spectrum, pharmacology, and therapeutic use of antibiotics. I. Tetracyclines, Drug Therapy Reviews **2:**69, 1979.

How to use intravenous antibiotics, Nurses' Drug Alert (special issue), **1:**89, June, 1977.

Neuvonem, P.J.: Interactions with the absorption of tetracyclines, Drugs **11:**45, 1976.

Rodman, M.J.: Anti-infectives you administer: choosing the right drug for every job, RN **40:**73, May, 1977.

Wilson, W.R.: Tetracyclines, chloramphenicol, erythromycin, and clindamycin, Mayo Clinic Proceedings **52:**635, 1977.

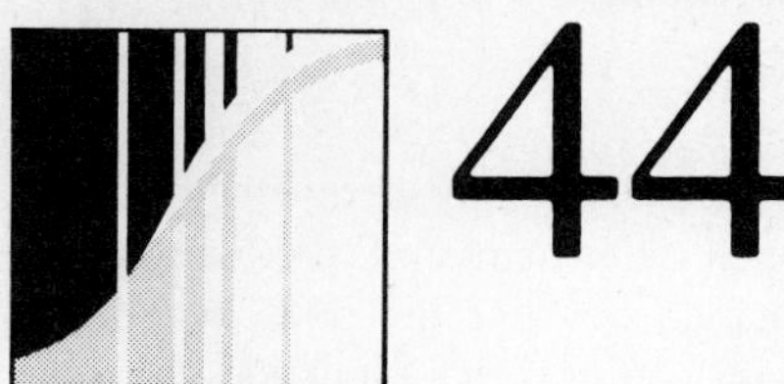

44 Antibiotics: aminoglycosides and polymyxins

In this chapter two groups of antibiotics with primary usefulness against gram-negative bacteria are introduced. The aminoglycosides are antibiotics composed of three or four amino sugars held together in glycosidic linkage. Great variability in structure is possible in these component sugars, and as a result several antibiotics of this type exist. Polymyxins are peptide antibiotics created by a spore-forming bacillus found in the soil. These two groups of drugs are considered together, since they have similar antimicrobial spectra and share certain toxic properties.

■ AMINOGLYCOSIDES

■ Mechanism of action and bacterial resistance

The aminoglycosides inhibit early steps in bacterial protein synthesis by binding to bacterial ribosomes. Under certain conditions bacterial protein synthesis may continue in the presence of aminoglycosides but with a greatly increased error rate. Defective proteins formed may damage the bacterial cell. Aminoglycosides also have a somewhat delayed effect on the bacterial cell membrane. Aminoglycosides are usually considered to be more bacteriocidal than many other antibiotics that inhibit bacterial protein synthesis.

Resistance to aminoglycosides occurs by one of three mechanisms: decreased antibiotic uptake, changes in antibiotic binding to the ribosome, and enzymatic destruction of the aminoglycosides. By far the most common mechanism for resistance involves antibiotic destruction. To understand this latter mechanism of bacterial resistance to aminoglycosides, two facts must be appreciated. First, many sites for enzymatic attack exist on the amino sugar components of aminoglycosides. Second, several different enzymes exist that modify the aminoglycosides by different mechanisms. The primary sites of attack are amino groups and hydroxyl groups on the sugars. Amino groups may be acetylated and hydroxyl groups may have a phosphate or an adenylate group added. Any of these substitutions may render the aminoglycoside inactive. At least nine separate enzymes catalyzing these reactions have been identified. Table 44-1 lists the clinically useful aminoglycosides and indicates how many of these degrading enzymes can attack an individual drug. As would be predicted, those drugs sensitive to fewer enzyme forms have a broader antimicrobial spectra.

TABLE 44-1. Sensitivity of clinically useful aminoglycoside antibiotics to antibiotic degrading enzymes from bacteria

Drug	Number of aminoglycoside degrading enzymes that inactivate the drug
Streptomycin	2
Neomycin	3
Kanamycin	4
Gentamicin	4
Tobramycin	4
Amikacin	1

Rarely bacterial resistance may result from reduced drug uptake. This mechanism has been observed especially for amikacin. An equally rare mechanism of resistance involves lowering drug binding to the ribosome. Occasional streptomycin-resistant strains arise by this mechanism.

■ Absorption

Aminoglycosides are polycationic molecules at physiological pH. As a result of being charged, these drugs do not penetrate mammalian membranes readily and are not absorbed orally. Therapy with aminoglycosides is therefore by intramuscular or intravenous routes and usually involves a hospitalized patient suffering from a moderate to severe infection. Absorption of aminoglycosides from intramuscular sites is rapid, and peak serum concentrations occur between 1 and 1.5 hours after injection.

■ Distribution and excretion

Aminoglycosides do not enter the central nervous system to any significant extent in normal persons. Some drug does appear in cerebrospinal fluid when meningitis is present. Aminoglycosides enter most other body fluids and tissues with the exception of bile. These drugs cross the placenta and achieve significant concentrations in the fetus.

Aminoglycosides are excreted by glomerular filtration in the kidney. Active drug is concentrated in the urine. Since the kidney is the primary site for elimination of these drugs, any reduction in renal function may lower the excretion sufficiently to cause aminoglycoside accumulation. The approximate half-time for elimination of these drugs is normally about 2 to 4 hours but in renal failure may be greatly prolonged. Excretion is also lower in neonates who have immature kidneys and in elderly patients whose renal function is diminished simply as a function of age.

■ Toxicity

The aminoglycosides show significant toxicity of three major types: eighth cranial nerve damage, renal toxicity, and neuromuscular blockade. Toxicity toward the eighth cranial nerve may be manifested by progressive hearing loss, loss of equilibrium control, or both. Hearing loss in some patients continues even after the drug is discontinued. Loss of equilibrium may be less obvious than hearing loss but can usually be revealed by appropriate tests. Nausea or dizziness may be a patient complaint that signals disturbance of equilibrium. Damage to the eighth cranial nerve is usually more severe when serum concentrations of aminoglycosides exceed 8 to 10 μg/ml. Total dose administered may also be a factor, since some patients treated over long periods may display these symptoms in spite of never having excessively high serum levels of the drug. Aminoglycosides may damage both tubules and glomeruli in the kidney, especially when high doses of the drugs are given. This toxic potential of aminoglycosides can cause a rapid clinical deterioration, since renal damage can cause drug accumulation and further toxicity to the kidney. This cycle of accumulation and increasing renal damage can destroy kidney function. Patients who accumulate the drug due to renal dysfunction are also more prone to eighth cranial nerve toxicity.

The third characteristic toxic reaction to aminoglycosides is neuromuscular blockade. This reaction is usually observed in surgical patients when an aminoglycoside is used to lavage the peritoneal cavity. Neuromuscular blockade in this case usually is manifested by respiratory paralysis, since the muscles of the chest involved in breathing are prevented from functioning. Some of the aminoglycosides produce a competitive neuromuscular blockade, which may be reversed by neostigmine. Others, such as kanamycin, produce a irreversible blockade, which neostigmine does not affect, although calcium may relieve the blockade in some cases. Patients who have recently received muscle relaxants are more prone to suffer neuromuscular blockade with aminoglycosides. Patients with myasthenia gravis are also more sensitive to this effect.

Toxic reactions caused by individual aminoglycosides are summarized in Table 44-2.

■ Drug interactions

The ototoxicity and nephrotoxicity of aminoglycoside antibiotics may be enhanced by a variety of agents. For example, if a patient who is receiving an aminoglycoside is also given a nephrotoxic drug such as cephaloridine (Loridine) or methoxyflurane (Penthrane), the risk of kidney damage in the patient is increased. Likewise ototoxic drugs such as ethacrynic acid may enhance ototoxicity in a patient receiving an aminoglycoside antibiotic.

All aminoglycoside antibiotics possess neuromuscular blocking activity. This section of aminoglycosides has led to enhanced effects from agents used for neuromuscular blocking action during surgery.

Gentamicin is frequently used with carbenicillin to treat *Pseudomonas aeruginosa* infections. Although these drugs may be used in the same patient, they should never be physically mixed, since carbenicillin chemically inactivates gentamicin in solution.

Aminoglycosides are many times more effective at the slightly alkaline pH of normal serum (pH 7.4) than at the acidic pH of normal urine (pH 5). Therefore, in the treatment of urinary tract infections with these drugs, a therapeutic advantage may be gained by alkalinizing the urine.

Neomycin when used orally causes mucosal alterations in the bowel, which may in extreme cases lead to malabsorption syndrome. Oral neomycin may also impair absorption of orally administered drugs. This potential interaction has been documented with penicillin V, digoxin, and vitamin B_{12}. If these drugs must be given to a patient receiving oral neomycin, extra care may need to be taken to assure that adequate amounts of the other orally administered medications are being absorbed.

■ Uses

The clinical use of these drugs is limited by their toxic potential. As a general rule the aminoglycosides are reserved for use in serious infections caused by gram-negative bacteria or by mycobacteria (Chapter 46). Individual drugs in this family differ in specific uses as a result of differences in relative toxicity and antibacterial

TABLE 44-2. Summary of toxicity observed with clinically useful aminoglycosides

Drug	Eighth cranial nerve toxicity		Renal toxicity	Neuromuscular blockade	Other toxicity
	Vestibular	**Hearing**			
Streptomycin	May affect 75% of patients receiving 2 Gm daily for 2 to 4 mo and 25% of patients receiving 1 Gm daily.	Loss usually partial but may be complete; affects 4% to 15% of patients receiving drug longer than 1 wk.	Not common unless high drug doses are used and the urine is acid.	May occur following peritoneal lavage; reversed by neostigmine and/or calcium.	Allergies: 5% of patients show exfoliate dermatitis. Irritation: tender, hot masses at intramuscular sites and fever are relatively common. Neurotoxicity: optic neuritis, peripheral neuritis occur rarely.
Neomycin	Not common.	Irreversible hearing loss progressing to complete deafness is common.	Reversible, progressive kidney toxicity causing an increase in blood urea.	Occurs following peritoneal lavage; usually reversed by neostigmine.	Suprainfection: oral use may lead to staphylococcal enterocolitis. Gastrointestinal: irritation and malabsorption syndrome may occur.
Kanamycin	Vertigo or other symptoms of vestibular damage affect about 7% of treated patients.	Up to 30% of treated patients suffer detectable hearing loss; fewer patients develop complete deafness.	Blood urea and creatinine may rise; hematuria and other signs of renal irritation may occur. Most signs of damage disappear when drug is discontinued.	Occurs following peritoneal lavage; usually not reversed by neostigmine and occasionally not reversed by calcium.	Neurotoxicity: headaches, paresthesias, tachycardia, blurring vision. Allergies: most commonly eosinophilia. Gastrointestinal: similar to neomycin but milder. Irritation: pain at injection site.
Gentamicin	About 2% of treated patients suffer permanent mild to severe vestibular damage.	Less frequent than vestibular damage and usually involves high tone hearing loss.	Acute renal failure has occurred. Blood urea and creatinine may rise; proteinuria may occur. Damage is usually but not always reversible.	May occur, but is less common than with above three aminoglycosides.	Allergies: macular skin eruptions, suprainfections. Oral use may induce *Candida* overgrowth in bowel.
Tobramycin	Not fully evaluated but may be less than for other aminoglycosides.		Not fully evaluated but expected.	Expected from animal studies.	Not fully evaluated.
Amikacin	Not fully evaluated but may be less than for other aminoglycosides.		Not fully evaluated but expected.	Expected from animal studies.	Not fully evaluated.

TABLE 44-3. Clinical uses of aminoglycoside antibiotics

Drug	Indications
Streptomycin	Used alone to treat tularemia (rabbit fever), plague (bubonic or black plague). Used in combination with other antibiotics to treat bacterial endocarditis (with penicillin G), tuberculosis (with isoniazid or other antituberculosis agents), brucellosis (with tetracyclines), *Listeria* infections (with ampicillin or penicillin G).
Neomycin	Oral use for reducing bacterial population in the bowel.
Kanamycin	Serious infections due to aerobic gram-negative bacteria other than *Pseudomonas*. Oral use to reduce bacterial population of the bowel.
Gentamicin	Serious infections due to aerobic gram-negative bacteria including *Pseudomonas aeruginosa*.
Tobramycin	Primarily for *P. aeruginosa* infections; may also substitute for gentamicin in other infections.
Amikacin	Primarily for *P. aeruginosa* infections caused by organisms resistant to other aminoglycosides.

activity. Table 44-3 lists the most important clinical uses of individual aminoglycosides. Streptomycin is most useful today in combination with other agents to treat infections in which strict bacteriocidal action is required for most effective therapy. Examples of these infections are bacterial endocarditis and tuberculosis (Chapter 46). Neomycin is too toxic for parenteral use but may be administered orally with the intent that the drug will remain in the bowel and lower the bacterial population. This effect may be useful prior to bowel surgery or in hepatic coma. Certain specific infections of the bowel may also respond to this therapy. Kanamycin may occasionally be used orally in a manner similar to neomycin; however, kanamycin is most useful for serious systemic infections. One difference between kanamycin, gentamicin, tobramycin, and amikacin is the different degrees of activity against *P. aeruginosa*. Amikacin and tobramycin are most effective against this pathogen. Gentamicin is usually effective against *Pseudomonas*, whereas kanamycin is not. Amikacin differs from gentamicin, kanamycin, and tobramycin in being less sensitive to common aminoglycoside degrading enzymes. Amikacin is therefore active against some bacterial strains that are resistant to other aminoglycosides.

Table 44-4 lists the common dosages for aminoglycosides employed in patients with normal renal function. When renal function is significantly impaired or is in question, it may be necessary to monitor serum levels of these drugs in order to prevent intoxication.

■ POLYMYXINS

■ Mechanism of action and bacterial resistance

Polymyxins alter the permeability of bacterial cell membranes, causing the loss of required small molecules and ions from the cell. This action is made possible by the combination of highly ionic groups along with lipid-soluble hydrocarbon chains all within the same molecule. The positively charged portion of the polymyxin molecule is attracted to the negatively charged surface of the bacterial membrane. Membrane disruption occurs then when the hydrocarbon chain portion of the polymyxin is inserted into the lipid-rich bacterial membrane. Bacterial cell death is an inevitable consequence of the loss of cell nutrients and cofactors required for energy production. Polymyxins are effective in either actively growing or static bacterial cells.

Polymyxins are of clinical interest because of their bacteriocidal action on gram-negative bacteria. With the exception of *Proteus, Neisseria,* and *Bacteroides,* most gram-negative organisms including *P. aeruginosa* are sensitive to the polymyxins. Gram-positive organisms are usually considered resistant to the polymyxins.

Clinical resistance to polymyxins has not increased since the drugs were first introduced into clinical practice in 1947. Organisms that are naturally resistant to these drugs apparently possess barriers which prevent polymyxin from contacting the cell membrane.

■ Absorption, distribution, and excretion

Polymyxins are not absorbed from the gastrointestinal tract, but effective systemic concentrations of the drugs can be achieved by parenteral administration (Table 44-5). Peak blood levels are ordinarily reached about 2 hours after intramuscular injection, but severe pain may result with this route of administration.

Intravenous administration of the polymyxins is by relatively slow infusion. These drugs should never be given rapidly by vein, since the resulting high blood levels can produce respiratory paralysis in some patients.

Polymyxins are bound to various tissues and persist at those sites for up to 3 days after therapy is stopped. These drugs do not penetrate joint or pleural fluids effectively and do not enter the cerebrospinal fluid to any useful degree. Significant concentrations of polymyxins

TABLE 44-4. Administration and dosage of aminoglycoside antibiotics

Generic name	Trade name	Dosage and administration
Streptomycin	Streptomycin	INTRAMUSCULAR, INTRAVENOUS: *Adults*—1 to 4 Gm daily in 2 or 3 doses (15 to 25 mg/kg daily). Elderly patients may require less drug. Lower doses are used for long-term treatment of mild tuberculosis. Intravenous route rarely used. *Children*—20 to 40 mg/kg daily in 2 doses.
Neomycin	Mycifradin Neobiotic Neomycin	ORAL: *Adults*—4 to 8 Gm daily in up to 6 doses. *Children*—50 to 100 mg/kg daily in 4 doses.
	Myciguent Neomycin	TOPICAL: *Adults and children*—Commonly used as 0.5% creams and ointments. Also used in numerous combinations with other antibiotics.
Kanamycin	Kantrex	ORAL: *Adults*—Up to 8 Gm daily in 4 to 6 doses. *Children and infants*—50 mg/kg daily in 4 to 6 doses. INTRAMUSCULAR, INTRAVENOUS, INTRAPERITONEAL: *Adults and children*—Not to exceed 15 mg/kg daily, given at 12 hr intervals.
Gentamicin	Garamycin	INTRAMUSCULAR, INTRAVENOUS: *Adults*—3 to 5 mg/kg daily in 3 doses. *Children*—6 to 7.5 mg/kg daily in 3 doses. *Neonates*—5 mg/kg daily in 3 doses.
Tobramycin	Nebcin	INTRAMUSCULAR, INTRAVENOUS: *Adults, children, infants*—3 to 5 mg/kg daily in 3 doses.
Amikacin	Amikin	INTRAMUSCULAR, INTRAVENOUS: *Adults, children, infants*—15 mg/kg daily in 2 or 3 doses. Do not exceed 1.5 Gm daily.

TABLE 44-5. Clinical summary of polymyxins

Generic name	Trade name	Dosage and administration	Clinical use
Colistin sulfate	Coly-Mycin S	ORAL: *Children and infants*—5 to 15 mg/kg daily in 3 doses. The oral form is not used for adults.	Reserve drug for treatment of *Pseudomonas aeruginosa*.
Colistimethate sodium (colistin methane sulfonate)	Coly-Mycin M	INTRAMUSCULAR, INTRAVENOUS: *Adults and children*—2.5 to 5 mg/kg daily in 2 to 4 doses up to 300 mg daily. Dosage must be reduced if renal impairment exists.	As for colistin sulfate.
Polymyxin B sulfate	Aerosporin	INTRAMUSCULAR: *Adults and children*—25,000 to 30,000 units/kg daily in 4 to 6 doses.	Not recommended due to extreme pain at injection site.
		INTRAVENOUS: *Adults and children*—15,000 to 25,000 units/kg daily by infusion in 300 to 500 ml 5% dextrose.	As for colistin sulfate.
		INTRATHECAL: *Adults*—50,000 units daily in single dose. *Children under 2 yr*—20,000 units in single daily dose.	Reserve drug for *Pseudomonas aeruginosa* meningitis.

do appear in fetuses when these drugs are administered to the mother.

Excretion of polymyxin is primarily by the kidney. For polymyxin B sulfate the excretion is delayed, beginning 12 hours after the first dose. Colistimethate sodium is more rapidly excreted. The serum half-life for polymyxins in the body is on the order of 2 to 3 hours in a patient with normal renal function.

A significant proportion of the polymyxin administered to patients is apparently inactivated by body tissues. This inactivation may vary in rate from patient to patient. For this reason, anuric patients may eliminate the drug with a half-life ranging from several hours to 2 or 3 days.

■ Toxicity

Since the detergent-like action of polymyxins on cell membranes is rather nonspecific, this family of drugs has a low therapeutic index. Significant neurotoxicity, nephrotoxicity, and neuromuscular blockade can be produced by these drugs.

Neuromuscular blockade is produced by a curare-like action of polymyxin at the neuromuscular junction. This effect is most often observed clinically as respiratory paralysis. The neuromuscular blockade produced by polymyxins differs from that produced by curare in that polymyxins produce noncompetitive blockade. Therefore the effects of polymyxins are not reversed by neostigmine. Calcium chloride may relieve the blockade in some patients.

Nephrotoxicity, manifested by decreased glomerular filtration rates and increased serum creatinine and BUN, occurs when polymyxin concentrations in the blood exceed recommended levels. Nephrotoxicity is usually reversible. However, patients in whom renal toxicity is not recognized may suffer a rapid deterioration in clinical status produced by the cycle of drug accumulation, increasing renal deterioration, further drug accumulation, and additional drug toxicity.

Neurotoxicity of polymyxins is manifested by symptoms of numbness, tingling of the extremities, generalized pruritus, and dizziness. Paresthesias are observed fairly commonly. At higher doses or in patients suffering drug accumulation, more severe symptoms may be observed. These symptoms include giddiness or mental confusion, slurring of speech, ataxia, convulsions, or coma. The signs of neurotoxicity usually disappear when polymyxins are discontinued.

■ Drug interactions

The most important clinical interaction of polymyxins occurs with muscle relaxing agents. In some patients, unexpected neuromuscular blockade and respiratory paralysis have occurred when the patient received both polymyxin and another antibiotic with curare-like action. Potential for this interaction exists with kanamycin, streptomycin, neomycin, and probably other aminoglycoside antibiotics as well.

The muscle relaxing agents used in conjunction with surgery are the drugs most commonly involved in drug interactions with polymyxins. These curariform muscle relaxants include ether, tubocurarine, succinylcholine, gallamine, decamethonium, and sodium citrate. Patients who are receiving or have recently received these drugs should be most carefully observed for respiratory paralysis if polymyxins must be administered.

■ Uses

Because of their relatively narrow antimicrobial spectrum and relatively high toxicity, the uses for these drugs are limited. They are reserved for use in serious infections caused by gram-negative organisms, especially *P. aeruginosa*. Specific uses of the individual members of this drug class are listed in Table 44-5.

Polymyxins are also used in various ointments and creams intended for topical application. For this purpose polymyxins are frequently combined with neomycin and bacitracin.

■ PATIENT CARE IMPLICATIONS

Review the patient care implications section in Chapter 40.

Aminoglycosides

1. Review Table 44-2 for summary of toxicity observed with aminoglycosides.
2. Signs of ototoxicity include tinnitus, roaring in ears, decreased hearing, feelings of fullness in the ears, nausea, dizziness, ataxia, and vertigo. A baseline audiometric test and periodic tests during the course of therapy should be done if practicable, and aminoglycoside therapy discontinued if there is a loss of high frequency perception. Newborn infants of mothers who received aminoglycosides during pregnancy or labor may suffer ototoxicity. Elderly persons and patients with preexisting tinnitus, vertigo, hearing loss, or who have previously received ototoxic drugs will need especially careful evaluations.
3. Signs of renal toxicity include oliguria and increasing urine specific gravity. There may be proteinuria, appearance of casts or cells in the urine, and increased creatinine clearance. Blood work indicative of possible renal toxicity would include increasing blood urea nitrogen (BUN), nonprotein nitrogen (NPN), serum creatinine, and elevated serum concentrations of the specific drug. The potential for renal toxicity is increased if other nephrotoxic drugs are given concomitantly (e.g., other aminoglyco-

■ THE NURSING PROCESS

The student should refer to Chapter 40 for general guidelines on the nursing process with antibiotic therapy. The additional material below relates specifically to the aminoglycosides and polymyxins.

■ Assessment

Aminoglycoside antibiotics are prescribed for a relatively limited number of indications, primarily in patients with moderate to severe infections (Table 44-3). Since the drugs are administered parenterally, the patient population is primarily in hospital. Polymyxins are not widely used to treat systemic infections, but when they are used it is in seriously ill patients with very specific diseases (Table 44-5). A full assessment of the patient should be carried out with emphasis on the organ where the infection is thought to be present, if the infection is a localized one. Other clinical signs of infection should be monitored. Renal function, hearing acuity, and vestibular function should be assessed carefully. Other medications the patient may be receiving should be noted.

■ Management

Once the decision is made to administer aminoglycosides or polymyxins, the nurse should gather the proper supplies for proper administration by the parenteral route chosen. The nurse should note whether the patient has received any other neuromuscular blocking agents or whether the patient has any other condition (such as myasthenia gravis), which would predispose the patient to respiratory paralysis. Equipment should be on hand to deal with respiratory paralysis if it occurs. The nurse should see that the medications are administered exactly at the times prescribed. If samples are being taken for the measurement of blood levels of these drugs, these samples must be taken exactly as ordered, since the timing is critical for proper interpretation of the information.

■ Evaluation

In the short term, the vital signs of the patient should be closely monitored, and evidence of objective and subjective recovery from serious illness should be noted. Hearing loss caused by aminoglycosides and polymyxins may progress during and after therapy. The nurse should continuously evaluate the patient for this symptom and for any loss of control of equilibrium as evidenced by difficulty in walking, staggering, or dizziness.

---

sides, some cephalosporins, the loop diuretics, cisplatin). Monitor the patient's fluid intake and output and keep the patient well hydrated.

4. Neuromuscular blockade caused by aminoglycoside therapy is most frequently seen in patients receiving other neuromuscular blocking agents during surgery and patients with myasthenia gravis or Parkinson's disease. Apnea has been reported after too rapid administration of an intravenous bolus. Monitor the respiratory rate of patients receiving aminoglycosides, especially those with myasthenia gravis or those during the early postoperative period. Administer intravenous aminoglycosides slowly.
5. Other side effects of aminoglycoside therapy include nausea, vomiting, drug fever, paresthesias, hypotension, and elevations of transaminase levels (SGOT, SGPT) and bilirubin.
6. Because of the possibility of vertigo or hypotension, patients should be cautioned not to rise suddenly from a supine position. It may be necessary to supervise ambulation.
7. Serum concentrations of a specific drug are frequently used to help regulate the dose. To interpret these levels correctly, blood is drawn at specific intervals before (trough level) and after (peak level) a dose of the drug is given. It is important to administer the drug on the prescribed schedule and to be familiar with the institution's procedures for blood sample collections for serum aminoglycoside levels so that errors are not made.

8. Oral neomycin impairs absorption of other oral drugs, such as penicillin V, digitalis preparations, and vitamin B_{12}. Patients receiving neomycin who are also receiving any of the three drugs should be regularly evaluated for the continuing effect of these medications.
9. Patients receiving oral aminoglycosides may absorb a relatively small amount of the drug from the gastrointestinal tract. In some sensitive patients the amount absorbed may be sufficient to cause renal or ototoxicity, so patients should be regularly evaluated.
10. With topical preparations of aminoglycosides, nephrotoxicity and ototoxicity are rare but possible side effects. Factors influencing the likelihood of toxicity would include the frequency of applications, the size of the area to which the preparation is being applied, whether the skin surface was intact, and the amount and kind of other ototoxic or nephrotoxic drugs the patient might be receiving concomitantly. Photosensitivity has been reported in patients using gentamicin topical preparations. Caution patients using gentamicin topical preparations to avoid direct exposure to the sun or ultraviolet light.
11. Pain at the injection site can accompany the intramuscular use of any aminoglycoside.
12. A separate form of gentamicin, without preservatives, is available for intrathecal administration.
13. The aminoglycosides are incompatible with other medications in the same syringe. For other incompatibilities, see the manufacturer's literature or consult the pharmacist.
14. *Intramuscular streptomycin:* Dilute the powder with 0.9% Sodium Chloride Injection or Sterile Water for Injection as directed on the vial.
15. *Intravenous kanamycin:* Dilute the prescribed dose in Normal Saline, 5% Normal Saline, or 5% Dextrose in Water to a concentration of 500 mg in 100 to 200 ml and administer over 1 hour.
16. *Intravenous gentamicin:* Dilute a single dose in 50 to 200 ml of Normal Saline or 5% Dextrose in Water. The concentration should not exceed 0.1% (1 mg/ml). Administer each dose over 1 to 2 hours.
17. *Intravenous tobramycin:* Dilute an adult dose in 50 to 100 ml of 5% Dextrose in Water or Normal Saline and administer over 20 minutes to 60 minutes. For pediatric doses, consult the literature.
18. *Intravenous amikacin:* Dilute 500 mg in 200 ml of Normal Saline or 5% Dextrose in Water and administer over 30 to 60 minutes. For pediatric doses, consult the literature.

Polymyxins

1. Patient care implications for the polymyxins in relation to nephrotoxicity and neuromuscular blockade are the same as those just given for the aminoglycosides.
2. Neurotoxic effects include itching, dizziness, numbness, confusion, slurring of speech, ataxia, convulsions, or coma. The likelihood of neurotoxic side effects occurring is increased when the polymyxins are given to patients with myasthenia gravis, those receiving other potentially neurotoxic drugs, those receiving neuromuscular blocking agents, or those receiving magnesium, quinidine, or quinine parenterally. If side effects occur, discontinue the drug and notify the physician.
3. Other side effects may include fever, gastrointestinal disturbances, and pain at intramuscular injection sites.
4. There are a variety of products containing polymyxin B in combination with other drugs. Examples include Neosporin and Neo-Polycin, both of which are ointments that contain polymyxin B, bacitracin, and neomycin.
5. *Parenteral colistimethate sodium*
   a. For intramuscular use, reconstitute with Sterile Water for Injection as directed on the vial.
   b. For intravenous use, it can be administered as reconstituted for intramuscular use and given as a bolus slowly over 3 to 5 minutes. It can also be further diluted with appropriate fluids (see literature) and administered over 1 to 2 hours.
6. *Polymyxin B sulfate*
   a. For intravenous use, dissolve 500,000 units of the drug in 300 to 500 ml of 5% Dextrose in Water. The rate of administration should not exceed 60 to 90 minutes.
   b. For intrathecal use, dissolve 500,000 units in 10 ml Sodium Chloride Injection to produce a concentration of 50,000 units per ml.

■ SUMMARY

Aminoglycoside antibiotics inhibit bacterial protein synthesis producing bacteriocidal as well as bacteriostatic effects. Bacterial resistance to aminoglycosides arises by decreased antibiotic uptake, decreased antibiotic binding to the ribosome, or enzymatic destruction of the antibiotic. The most common mode of resistance involves aminoglycoside destruction, which may be carried out by as many as nine different enzymes. Aminoglycosides are not absorbed orally but are rapidly and efficiently absorbed from intramuscular sites. Aminoglycosides do not enter the central nervous system very efficiently but are well distributed to most other tissues. The drugs are excreted almost exclusively by the kidney.

Aminoglycosides may damage the eighth cranial nerve controlling hearing and balance and may produce nephrotoxicity and neuromuscular blockade. Damage to the eighth cranial nerve and to the kidney is more extreme when aminoglycosides accumulate in the body or are used at too high a dose. Neuromuscular blockade is more likely in patients with preexisting impairment at the neuromuscular junction, that is, a patient with myasthenia gravis or a patient who has recently received a neuromuscular blocking agent in conjunction with surgery. Streptomycin is used in combination with penicillins to treat certain serious infections caused by gram-positive bacteria and in combination with other agents for the treatment of tuberculosis. Neomycin is too toxic for systemic use. Kanamycin may be used for serious infections due to gram-negative bacteria, but gentamicin, tobramycin, or amikacin must be used if the pathogen is *Pseudomonas aeruginosa*.

Polymyxins disrupt cell membranes of gram-negative bacteria, causing bacterial cell death. Resistance to polymyxins has not been observed. These drugs are not absorbed from the gastrointestinal tract. Intramuscular administration causes pain at the injection site. Intravenous infusion can produce respiratory paralysis if the rate of infusion is too rapid. These drugs do not penetrate to the cerebrospinal fluid from the bloodstream. Polymyxins are excreted by the kidney and are inactivated by body tissues. Polymyxins may produce neuromuscular blockade and nephrotoxicity. In addition, these drugs may produce neurotoxicity, including numbness, paresthesias, and tingling of the extremities. More serious central nervous system reactions may result with higher drug doses.

■ STUDY QUESTIONS

1. What is the mechanism of action of aminoglycoside antibiotics?
2. What are the three mechanisms by which bacteria gain resistance to aminoglycoside antibiotics?
3. What is the most common mechanism for bacterial resistance to aminoglycosides?
4. What routes of administration are appropriate for aminoglycosides?
5. What is the primary route of excretion of aminoglycosides?
6. What effect may aminoglycoside antibiotics have on the function of the eighth cranial nerve?
7. What effects do the aminoglycoside antibiotics have on the kidney?
8. What groups of patients might be more prone to aminoglycoside toxicity toward the eighth cranial nerve and the kidney?
9. What is the effect of aminoglycosides on the neuromuscular junction?
10. What groups of patients are most likely to develop respiratory paralysis following therapeutic use of aminoglycoside antibiotics?
11. What special precautions must be taken when gentamicin and carbenicillin are used in the same patient?
12. What drugs may be poorly absorbed when neomycin is used orally?
13. Name three clinical uses of streptomycin.
14. Name two clinical indications for neomycin.
15. How does the clinical indication for the use of kanamycin differ from the indications for gentamicin, tobramycin, and amikacin?
16. What is the mechanism of action of polymyxins?
17. By what routes are polymyxins best administered?
18. How is polymyxin eliminated from the body?
19. What are the three most common toxic reactions to polymyxins?
20. What patients are most at risk of neuromuscular blockade with polymyxins?

■ SUGGESTED READINGS

Aminoglycoside therapy, Nursing '80 **10**(2):82, 1980.

Barza, M., and Scheife, R.T.: Antimicrobial spectrum, pharmacology, and therapeutic use of antibiotics. IV. Aminoglycosides, Drug Therapy Reviews **2:**137, 1979.

Benn, R.A.V.: Treatment of infections due to *Pseudomonas aeruginosa,* The Medical Journal of Australia (special supplement) **2:** 9, 1977.

Brewer, N.S.: The aminoglycosides, Mayo Clinic Proceedings **52:** 675, 1977.

Brummett, R.E.: Drug-induced ototoxicity, Drugs **19:**412, 1980.

Dorff, G.J.: Avoiding aminoglycoside toxicity, Drug Therapy **8**(1): 153, 1978.

How to use intravenous antibiotics, Nurses' Drug Alert (special issue) **1:**89, June, 1977.

Keys, T.F., and Washington, J.A., II: Gentamicin-resistant *Pseudomonas aeruginosa:* Mayo clinic experience. 1970-1976, Mayo Clinic Proceedings **52:**797, 1977.

Kirby, W.M.M., Clarke, J.T., Libke, R.D., and Regamy, C.: Clinical pharmacology of amikacin and kanamycin, The Journal of Infectious Diseases **134:**S312, 1976.

Neu, H.C.: The pharmacology of newer aminoglycosides, with a consideration of the application to clinical situations, The Medical Journal of Australia (special supplement) **2:**13, 1977.

Rodman, M.J.: Anti-infectives you administer: choosing the right drug for every job, RN **40:**73, May, 1977.

Silverblatt, F.J.: Unraveling the mechanisms of aminoglycoside toxicity, Drug Therapy **9**(8):55, 1979.

Yoshikawa, T.T.: Proper use of aminoglycosides, American Family Physician **21**(5):125, 1980.

Yu, P.K.W., and Washington, J.A., II: Antimicrobial susceptibility of gentamicin-resistant *Pseudomonas aeruginosa,* Mayo Clinic Proceedings **52:**806, 1977.

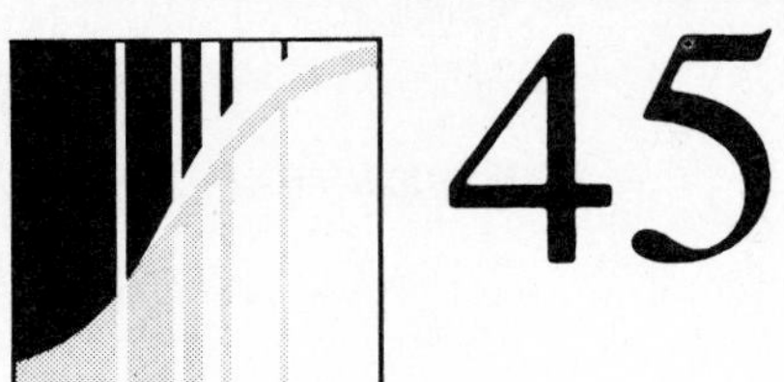

Antibiotics: sulfonamides, trimethoprim, furantoins, and nalidixic acid

In this chapter the sulfonamides, trimethoprim, nitrofurantoin, and nalidixic acid are considered. These four drugs or groups of drugs represent four separate chemical types of agents. Sulfonamides, nalidixic acid, and nitrofurantoin are considered together, since they all are most commonly used today in the treatment of urinary tract infections. Trimethoprim is considered with the sulfonamides by virtue of its similar mechanism of action and the fact that in the United States trimethoprim is most commonly administered in combination with a sulfonamide.

■ SULFONAMIDES AND TRIMETHOPRIM

■ Mechanism of action and bacterial resistance

Sulfonamides are metabolic inhibitors that block bacterial synthesis of folic acid, a vitamin required for the synthesis of amino acids and nucleic acids (Fig. 45-1). The metabolically active form of folic acid, tetrahydrofolic acid (THFA), is synthesized in bacteria by two enzymes working in sequence. The first enzyme, dihydrofolic acid synthetase, converts paraaminobenzoic acid (PABA) and other small molecules to dihydrofolic acid. The second enzyme, dihydrofolic acid reductase, forms THFA. The sulfonamides competitively inhibit the first enzyme in this sequence, dihydrofolic acid synthetase.

Sulfonamides are selectively toxic to organisms that must form folic acid from paraaminobenzoic acid and the other precursors. Fortunately, humans are not sensitive to this action, since we cannot synthesize folic acid but must absorb it pre-formed from our diet. Sulfonamides are primarily bacteriostatic against those organisms they affect.

Trimethoprim inhibits the second step in THFA synthesis, the enzyme dihydrofolic acid reductase. Trimethoprim therefore also prevents THFA formation in bacteria. Dihydrofolic acid reductase functions both in humans and in bacteria, since much of the vitamin in the mammalian diet is dihydrofolic acid. Therefore trimethoprim might be expected to be toxic to humans as well as to bacteria. This is not the case, however, since dihydrofolic acid reductase from humans is relatively resistant to the action of trimethoprim, and the drug may be given at doses that inhibit this enzyme in bacteria but not in humans.

Sulfonamides are potentially active against a wide range of gram-positive and gram-negative organisms as well as *Nocardia, Chlamydia,* and *Actinomyces*. Bacterial resistance to the sulfonamides has become widespread, however, and has reduced the clinical usefulness of these drugs. Some bacteria such as pneumococci acquire an altered dihydrofolic acid synthetase, which is less sensitive to sulfonamides. Overproduction of paraaminobenzoic acid is a common mechanism of resistance for several pathogens, including staphylococci, pneumococci, and gonococci. Since sulfonamides are only competitive inhibitors of paraaminobenzoic acid incorporation into folic acid, excess paraaminobenzoic acid will overcome the sulfonamide inhibition.

Trimethoprim has a similar spectrum of antimicrobial activity to that of the sulfonamides with the following exceptions: (1) trimethoprim is more active against the gram-negative bacteria *Proteus, Klebsiella,* and *Serratia;* (2) trimethoprim is not useful alone against *Chlamydia* or *Nocardia;* and (3) trimethoprim resistance has not yet become widespread. Until recently trimethoprim was used in the United States only in combination with a sulfonamide. A preparation of trimethoprim alone is now available for use in urinary tract infections.

■ Absorption, distribution, and excretion

Sulfonamide antibacterial agents with a wide variety of pharmacokinetic properties are available (Tables 45-1 to 45-3). Some of these drugs are not absorbed from the gastrointestinal tract and when used are intended to remain within the bowel and reduce the bacterial population therein. Some systemic absorption of these agents can occur through ulcerated regions of the bowel. Systemic absorption can likewise occur when sulfonamides are used on extensive areas of burned skin.

The sulfonamides used for treatment of systemic infections are all well absorbed from the gastrointestinal tract. Distribution of these drugs to body tissues is rather

FIG. 45-1

Synthesis of tetrahydrofolic acid (THFA) in bacteria and humans. THFA is a vitamin required for nucleic acid and amino acid synthesis. Many bacteria form this vitamin from paraaminobenzoic acid (PABA) and other small molecules. Two enzymes are involved in this synthesis: dihydrofolic acid synthetase and dihydrofolic acid reductase. Sulfonamides inhibit the first of these enzymes, thereby blocking THFA synthesis in bacteria. Mankind is immune from this action since preformed folate and dihydrofolic acid are taken in the diet.

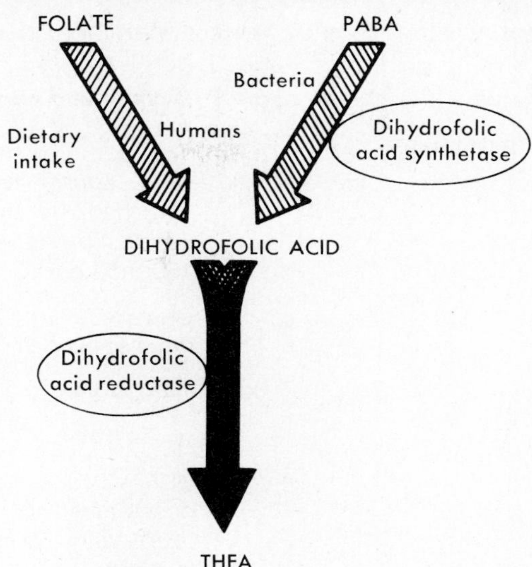

good, including to the brain. Concentrations of sulfonamides in cerebrospinal and other body fluids may approach that of serum. Sulfonamides also pass the placental barrier and enter fetuses.

Elimination of sulfonamides from the body involves both the liver and kidneys. The liver converts a portion of the sulfonamide in the bloodstream to an acetylated derivative, which is usually bacteriologically inactive. Both the acetylated and the free drug are eliminated in the kidney primarily by glomerular filtration. Protein binding in the bloodstream varies from less than 20% to more than 95% for various individual sulfonamides. The more highly protein-bound drugs are less available for glomerular filtration and persist longer in the body (Table 45-1). Tubular reabsorption is significant for some sulfonamides. Since absorbed sulfonamides are excreted by the kidney in part in the free, unacetylated form, the urine contains antibacterial activity. Excretion of the sulfonamides is favored by alkalinizing the urine. This procedure increases the solubility of these drugs in urine and also converts the drugs to a charged form that does not undergo renal tubular reabsorption.

The use of trimethoprim in fixed combination with sulfamethoxazole (Table 45-2) represents a clever exploitation of drug properties for good therapeutic effect. These drugs are administered in tablets containing the agents in the ratio of 1:5, trimethoprim:sulfamethoxazole. Both drugs are well absorbed from the gastrointestinal tract. Serum concentrations of the free drug not bound to serum proteins are usually in the ratio 1:20, trimethoprim:sulfamethoxazole. At this concentration ratio, the drugs have maximal antibacterial activity. The combination is actually synergistic, that is, more effective in combination than would be expected from the action of either drug alone. Synergistic action may result, since both drugs ultimately starve sensitive bacteria for THFA, but the drugs work on two different enzymes in the sequence of reactions leading to THFA. The sequential blockade of this metabolic pathway is much more effective than blockade of a single step by one drug at high concentrations.

Trimethoprim has synergistic effects with any of the systemically effective sulfonamides. Sulfamethoxazole was chosen for use in the fixed combination with trimethoprim because the kinetics of elimination of the two drugs are quite similar. Therefore use of this fixed combination does not lead to accumulation of one or the other of the drugs.

Trimethoprim penetrates body tissues better than sulfamethoxazole. Trimethoprim concentrations in breast milk, bile, prostatic fluid, vaginal fluids, liver, spleen, skin, and kidney actually may exceed plasma concentrations of the drug. Penetration into other tissues is adequate, including the central nervous system.

Trimethoprim appears in the urine at a concentration approximately 100 times the plasma concentration, most of the drug being in the active form. Sulfamethoxazole in the urine is mostly in the acetylated form, and the urine concentration is about five times the plasma concentration.

Sulfonamides are available in a number of fixed combinations (Table 45-2). Those combinations which contain only sulfonamides are formulated so that the amount of any one agent is well below the recommended dosage; dosage is calculated on total sulfonamide content. These formulations are designed to avoid sulfonamide insolubility in the urine of treated patients. Each drug in the combination dissolves independently of the others so that total sulfonamide concentration in the urine exceeds that possible with a single agent.

TABLE 45-1. Clinical summary of sulfonamides: single component formulations

Generic name	Trade name	Dosage and administration	Clinical use
SHORT-ACTING AGENTS			
Sulfachlorpyridazine	Nefrosul Sonilyn	ORAL: *Adults*—single loading dose of 2 to 4 Gm, then 2 to 4 Gm daily in 3 to 6 doses. *Children over 2 mo*—75 mg/kg to load, then 150 mg/kg daily in 4 to 6 doses.	Urinary tract infection.
Sulfacytine	Renoquid	ORAL: *Adults*—500 mg loading dose, then 250 mg 4 times daily. Not for children under 14 yr.	As for sulfachlorpyridazine.
Sulfadiazine		ORAL: As for sulfachlorpyridazine.	Urinary tract infections, rheumatic fever prophylaxis, nocardiosis.
		INTRAVENOUS: *Adults*—100 mg/kg daily in 4 doses after a 50 mg/kg loading dose. *Children over 2 mo*—50 mg/kg, then 100 mg/kg daily in 4 doses.	Meningitis due to susceptible meningococci.
Sulfamethoxazole	Gantanol	ORAL: *Adults*—single 2 Gm loading dose, then 1 Gm 2 or 3 times daily. *Children over 2 mo*—50 to 60 mg/kg loading dose, then 25 to 30 mg/kg twice daily.	Urinary tract infections.
Sulfamethizole	Microsul Sulfstat Forte Thiosulfil Urifon	ORAL: *Adults*—0.5 to 1 Gm, 3 or 4 times daily. *Children over 2 mo*—30 to 45 mg/kg daily in 4 doses.	Urinary tract infections.
Sulfisoxazole	Gantrisin Rosoxol SK-Soxazole Sulfalar	ORAL: *Adults*—2 to 4 Gm loading dose, then 4 to 8 Gm daily in 3 to 6 doses. *Children over 2 mo*—75 mg/kg loading dose, then 150 mg/kg daily in 4 to 6 doses.	Urinary tract infections, systemic infections, and meningitis due to sensitive organisms, nocardiosis.
	Gantrisin	INTRAMUSCULAR, INTRAVENOUS, SUBCUTANEOUS: *Adults*—50 mg/kg initial dose, then 100 mg/kg daily in 2 to 4 doses. *Children*—smaller volumes per injection site are used.	As for oral sulfisoxazole.
LONG-ACTING AGENTS			
Sulfameter	Sulla	ORAL: *Adults*—1.5 Gm loading dose, then single daily dose of 500 mg. Not for use in children under 12 yr.	Urinary tract infections.
Sulfamethoxy-pyridazine	Midicel	ORAL: *Adults*—1 Gm initially, then 500 mg in single daily dose. *Children*—30 mg/kg loading dose, then 15 mg/kg daily.	Urinary tract infections, upper respiratory tract infections, bacillary dysentery, soft tissue infections, rheumatic fever prophylaxis.
NONABSORBED AGENTS			
Phthalylsulfathiazole	Sulfathalidine	ORAL: *Adults and children*—50 to 100 mg/kg daily in 3 to 6 doses, not to exceed 8 Gm daily.	Possibly effective as adjunctive therapy for ulcerative colitis.
Sulfasalazine	Azulfidine SAS-500 Sulcolon	ORAL: *Adults*—3 to 4 Gm daily in divided doses. *Children*—40 to 60 mg/kg daily in 3 to 6 doses.	Treatment of ulcerative colitis.

TABLE 45-2. Clinical summary of sulfonamides: fixed combinations for oral use

Components of combination		Drug form	Trade name	Dosage	Clinical use
Sulfamethoxazole Trimethoprim	400 mg 80 mg	Tablet	Bactrim Septra	*Adults*—2 tablets every 12 hr. *Children*—8 mg/kg trimethoprim and 40 mg/kg sulfamethoxazole daily in 2 doses.	Urinary tract infections, otitis media, enteritis due to sensitive *Shigella*.
Sulfamerazine Sulfadiazine	250 mg 250 mg	Per 5 ml suspension	Sulfonamide Duplex	*Adults*—2 to 4 Gm total sulfonamide loading dose, then 2 to 4 Gm daily in 3 to 6 doses. *Children*—75 mg/kg to load, then 150 mg/kg daily in 4 to 6 doses.	Urinary tract infections.
Sulfamerazine Sulfadiazine Sulfamethazine	167 mg 167 mg 167 mg	Tablet or per 5 ml suspension	Neotrizine Quadetts Sulfaloid Triple Sulfa Trisulfapyrimidines	As for sulfamerazine, sulfadiazine combination.	As for sulfamerazine, sulfadiazine combination.
Sulfamerazine Sulfadiazine Sulfamethazine Sulfacetamide Sulfamethizole	100 mg 100 mg 100 mg 100 mg 100 mg	Tablet	Sul-V	As for sulfamerazine, sulfadiazine combination.	As for sulfamerazine, sulfadiazine combination.
Sulfamethoxazole Phenazopyridine	500 mg 100 mg	Tablet	Azo-Gantanol	*Adults*—4 tablets to load, then 2 tablets every 12 hr for 3 days.	Urinary tract infections only.
Sulfamethizole Phenazopyridine	250 or 500 mg 50 mg	Tablet	Azo Sulfstat Sul-A Thiosulfil-A Uremide	*Adults*—2 to 4 tablets 2 or 3 times daily. *Children*—30 to 45 mg of sulfamethizole per kg daily in 4 doses.	Urinary tract infections only.
Sulfisoxazole Phenazopyridine	500 mg 50 mg	Tablet	Azo-Gantrisin Azo-Soxazole Azosul Suldiazo	*Adults*—4 to 6 tablets to load, then 2 tablets every 12 hr for 3 days. *Children*—Dose as for sulfisoxazole alone.	Urinary tract infections only.

TABLE 45-3. Clinical summary of sulfonamides: topical agents

Generic name	Trade name	Application form	Clinical use	Comments
Mafenide acetate	Sulfamylon	Cream: 85 mg mafenide acetate/Gm.	Treatment of second and third degree burns.	Drug is effective against a broad spectrum of pathogens, including *Pseudomonas aeruginosa*. Drug may be absorbed through burned tissues.
Silver sulfadiazine	Silvadene	Cream: 10 mg/Gm	Treatment of second and third degree burns.	Drug is effective against a broad spectrum of pathogens, including *P. aeruginosa* and certain yeasts. Drug may be absorbed through burned tissues.
Sulfacetamide	Bleph Liquifilm Sulamyd Sulf-10	Solution: 10%, 15%, or 30% Ointment: 10%	Ophthalmic only. For conjunctivitis, corneal ulcer, trachoma.	Drug allergy may develop in sensitive patients.
Sulfisoxazole	Gantrisin Ophthalmic	Solution: 4% Ointment: 4%	Ophthalmic only. For conjunctivitis, corneal ulcer, trachoma.	Drug allergy may develop in sensitive patients.

Sulfonamides may be combined with phenazopyridine for the treatment of urinary tract infections (Table 45-2). The sulfonamide component supplies antibacterial activity while the phenazopyridine, which is excreted in the urine, exerts an analgesic effect upon the mucosa of the urinary tract. The added phenazopyridine therefore relieves the symptoms of pain, burning, and itching associated with the urinary tract infection.

■ Toxic reactions to sulfonamides

Sulfonamides induce allergic reactions in a significant proportion of patients receiving the drugs. The most common reactions are skin rashes and pruritus, but drug fever and other more serious reactions may occur. Anaphylaxis has been reported. Since sulfonamides are chemically related to the thiazide diuretics, acetazolamide, and oral hypoglycemic agents, a patient who becomes allergic to a sulfonamide may also become allergic to one or more of these agents.

Gastrointestinal disturbances also occur with the sulfonamides. In addition to nausea, vomiting, and diarrhea, pancreatitis, hepatitis, and stomatitis may occur.

Central nervous system alterations have been observed, including headache, ataxia, hallucinations, and convulsions.

Deaths from aplastic anemia and other blood dyscrasias, although rare, have been reported in connection with sulfonamide therapy. Sore throat, fever, or pallor may signal the onset of a serious blood dyscrasia.

Renal toxicity was of great concern with the sulfonamides in use before about 1960. Most of the renal damage associated with these older agents was produced by drug precipitation or crystallization in the urine. These drugs precipitated because of their low solubility in normal, acidic urine. The newer sulfonamides are much more soluble under these conditions, and drug precipitation is seldom a problem. However, patients should receive sufficient fluids to produce at least a liter of urine daily while receiving sulfonamides. Solubility of the sulfonamides in urine may be increased by alkalinizing the urine. Sulfamethizole and sulfasalazine produce a yellow-orange coloration in alkaline urine. This coloration, which may also be observed in skin, is not harmful.

Patients with preexisting renal or hepatic disease may be more prone to develop toxic reactions, since these organs are the primary means of removal of sulfonamides from the body. Patients with a known genetic deficiency of glucose-6-phosphate dehydrogenase are also more at risk from hemolytic anemia induced by sulfonamides. The highest frequency of glucose-6-phosphate dehydrogenase deficiency is observed among blacks and Mediterranean racial groups; patients from these groups should be watched with special care for signs of anemia.

Trimethoprim appears to be less toxic than the sulfonamides, although it may affect the bone marrow. When trimethoprim is used in combination with sulfamethoxazole, treated patients should be observed for all signs of sulfonamide toxicity.

■ Drug interactions with sulfonamides

Certain sulfonamides are highly bound to serum proteins and may therefore displace other drugs from protein binding sites. This displacement can occur with oral anticoagulants, sulfonylureas (oral hypoglycemic agents), and with the antineoplastic agent methotrexate.

Paraaminobenzoic acid may interfere with the action of sulfonamides. Procaine, a local anesthetic that is derived from paraaminobenzoic acid, may also block the action of sulfonamides on dihydrofolic acid synthetase (Fig. 45-1).

■ NITROFURANTOINS

■ Mechanism of action and bacterial resistance

Nitrofurantoin apparently works as an inhibitor of certain bacterial enzymes required for proper metabolism of sugar and perhaps other compounds. The drug is effective against a variety of gram-positive and gram-negative organisms, including most common pathogens of the urinary tract. *Pseudomonas* and *Proteus* species are, however, usually resistant. Development of resistance to nitrofurantoin during therapy is not a significant problem.

■ Absorption, distribution, and excretion

Many compounds that are effective antibacterial agents in the laboratory are ineffective when used to treat systemic infections in patients because of the unfavorable pharmacokinetics of the drugs. One example of such a compound is nitrofurantoin. Nitrofurantoin, in spite of being well absorbed from the small intestine in humans, never achieves satisfactory blood levels. Low blood levels result from a rapid excretion of the drug in the kidney. Removal of the drug from the system occurs so quickly that it fails to accumulate in the bloodstream. Therefore, in spite of the broad antibacterial spectrum of nitrofurantoin, it is ineffective against systemic infections. However, nitrofurantoin is concentrated in the kidney and achieves antibacterial concentrations in the urine. Nitrofurantoin in the renal tubule diffuses into kidney tissues so that the final concentration in the kidney is much greater than would be expected from the very low blood concentrations of the drug. These properties of nitrofurantoin make the drug effective against urinary tract infections.

TABLE 45-4. Clinical summary of nitrofurantoin, nalidixic acid, and oxolinic acid

Generic name	Trade name	Dosage and administration	Comments
Nitrofurantoin	Cyantin Furadantin Furalan Nitrex Sarodant	ORAL: *Adults*—50 to 100 mg 4 times daily. *Children*—5 to 7 mg/kg daily in 4 divided doses. The drug should not be given to children under 3 mo.	Gastric irritation may be minimized by administering the drug with food or milk.
Nitrofurantoin macrocrystals	Macrodantin	As for nitrofurantoin.	Large crystal size minimizes gastric irritation.
Nalidixic acid	NegGram	ORAL: *Adults*—1 Gm 4 times daily for 1 to 2 wk. Prolonged use may require cutting dosage back to 2 Gm or less daily. *Children under 12 yr*—55 mg/kg daily in 4 divided doses, initially. For long-term therapy the dose may be reduced to 33 mg/kg daily. *Children under 3 mo* should not receive this drug.	Emergence of resistant bacterial strains is a common cause of treatment failure with this drug.
Oxolinic acid	Utib I.D.	ORAL: *Adults*—750 mg twice daily for 2 wk. *Children and infants* should not receive this drug.	This drug is similar in action to nalidixic acid but seems to be more toxic.
Trimethoprim	Proloprim Trimpex	ORAL: *Adults*—100 mg every 12 hr. *Children*—the drug has not been extensively tested in children and is not recommended.	Blood changes can occur with this drug.

■ Toxic reactions

One of the more common reactions to nitrofurantoin is gastric irritation with anorexia, nausea, and emesis. This reaction is apparently lessened if the drug is administered as large crystals (Macrodantin, Table 45-4) rather than the original microcrystalline form. The large crystals are more slowly absorbed, but this does not interfere with clinical effectiveness.

Rashes, allergies, and reversible blood dyscrasias have been observed with nitrofurantoin. Hemolytic anemia similar to that seen with sulfonamides may also be seen with nitrofurantoin. Infants under 3 months of age have undeveloped enzyme systems that make them especially susceptible to hemolytic anemia induced by nitrofurantoin. Nitrofurantoin should be used with care in pregnant patients.

Oral suspensions of nitrofurantoin may stain the teeth. Nitrofurantoin also causes the urine to turn brown, but this is a harmless effect of the drug. An occasional patient may suffer hair loss while receiving the drug.

Peripheral neuropathy is one of the most serious toxic effects of nitrofurantoin. If detected early, the condition disappears following discontinuation of the drug. Damage may be permanent if the drug is continued after signs of peripheral neuropathy have developed. As with any drug that is excreted primarily by the kidney, nitrofurantoin may accumulate in patients with a degree of renal failure. These patients are more likely to suffer from significant side effects of nitrofurantoin therapy. Vitamin B deficiency, a common finding in alcoholics, may also predispose a patient to peripheral neuropathy. Diabetes mellitus, a disease that may itself cause peripheral neuropathies, may produce added risk of neural complications to the patient receiving nitrofurantoin.

Patients receiving nitrofurantoin for long periods should be observed for pneumonitis or pulmonary fibrosis, which may develop gradually or appear as an acute illness.

Nitrofurantoin is used in the clinic to treat certain types of urinary tract infections, especially when the causative organism is a sensitive strain of *Escherichia coli*.

■ NALIDIXIC ACID

■ Mechanism of action and bacterial resistance

Nalidixic acid exerts bacteriocidal action against a wide variety of gram-negative bacteria. The exact mechanism of action of the drug remains unknown, but it is known to interfere directly with DNA synthesis in susceptible bacteria. Resistance to the action of nalidixic acid is readily achieved, often appearing clinically during the first 48 hours of therapy. Resistance to nalidixic acid is apparently not carried on transferrable R factors and so is not directly passed between bacteria. Clinical relapse, therefore, is more likely to be produced by the proliferation of those bacteria that mutate to the drug-resistant form. Clinical resistance to nalidixic acid develops in as many as 15% of treated patients. Resistance to nalidixic acid confers cross-resistance only to oxolinic acid, another antibiotic that inhibits DNA synthesis by a mechanism similar to nalidixic acid. Cross-resistance to other antibiotics has not been observed.

■ Absorption, distribution, and excretion

Nalidixic acid rapidly enters the bloodstream following oral administration. Portal circulation carries the drug to the liver where the glucuronide and hydroxylated derivatives of the drug are formed. The hydroxylated form of nalidixic acid is biologically active and comprises a significant proportion of the active drug in the bloodstream and in the urine. Over 90% of the nalidixic acid in the bloodstream is bound to serum proteins. Little of the drug enters most body tissues. The only organ in which the drug concentration exceeds the plasma concentration is the kidney.

The kidney is the major organ of excretion for nalidixic acid. Peak levels of drug in the urine occur 3 to 4 hours after an oral dose and follow the peak plasma concentrations that occur 1 to 2 hours after ingestion of the drug. The active form of nalidixic acid and its glucuronides may accumulate in patients with renal failure. During liver failure, glucuronide formation is reduced and toxic amounts of the active forms of nalidixic acid may accumulate.

■ Toxic reactions

The most serious toxicity associated with the use of nalidixic acid is central nervous system toxicity. Symptoms include convulsions, mental instability, headache, dizziness, and visual disturbances. These complications are rare, and when they occur they usually involve high doses of the drug or unusual drug accumulation. Convulsions may be made more likely by a prior history of convulsive disorders. Elderly patients may be more sensitive to the confusion and central nervous system irritability that this drug produces, especially when cerebral arteriosclerosis exists.

Nalidixic acid causes rashes of various types in some patients. Most of these reactions are minor, but severe photosensitivity reactions can occur. Patients receiving nalidixic acid should be advised to limit exposure to the sun.

Hemolytic anemia and other blood dyscrasias may occur in patients treated with nalidixic acid. Newborn infants should not receive nalidixic acid because of their increased susceptibility to this type of reaction. Pregnant women should also avoid this drug during the first trimester of pregnancy.

Because nalidixic acid is tightly bound to serum proteins, it may displace other drugs from those proteins. The result may be increased toxic reactions due to the displaced drug. This type of drug interaction has been observed between nalidixic acid and coumarin anticoagulants.

The combination of nalidixic acid with other antibacterial agents is usually best avoided, since the combinations have somewhat unpredictable actions. For example, gentamicin seems to act synergistically with nalidixic acid in laboratory tests but combining nalidixic acid with tetracycline or with nitrofurantoin may actually be antagonistic, that is, the effect of the combination is less than that of either drug alone.

Nalidixic acid is used to treat urinary tract infections, since that is the only organ in which reliably high concentrations of the drug may be achieved. To minimize the appearance of resistant organisms, 1 Gm four times daily has been recommended in adults. For long-term therapy the daily total dose may be reduced (Table 45-4). A related drug, oxolinic acid, has been suggested to be more effective than nalidixic acid and to be effective with only 2 doses per day. However, oxolinic acid seems to cause more central nervous system disturbances than does nalidixic acid and therefore cannot be concluded to have any overall superiority to nalidixic acid. Oxolinic acid should not be substituted for nalidixic acid when resistance develops.

■ PATIENT CARE IMPLICATIONS

Review the patient care implications in Chapter 40.

Sulfonamides

1. Side effects may include nausea, vomiting, diarrhea, pancreatitis, hepatitis, and stomatitis. Central nervous system side effects include headache, ataxia, hallucinations, and convulsions. A variety of serious blood dyscrasias have been attributed to this group of drugs, so blood work (hematocrit, hemoglobin, differential) should be done prior to beginning therapy and periodically during therapy. Many blood dyscrasias, however, are first picked up by their symptoms. Caution the patient to report any pallor, fever, sore throat or mouth, fatigue, jaundice, bleeding, or unusual bruising. Finally, Stevens-Johnson syndrome, a rare but occasionally fatal skin disease, has occurred in patients taking sulfonamides. Instruct the patient to notify the physician if a rash appears.
2. The sulfonamides displace oral anticoagulants, oral hypoglycemics, and methotrexate from protein binding sites resulting in higher than desired serum levels of these drugs. Patients receiving oral anticoagulants should be alert to increased bleeding or bruising, whereas patients receiving oral hypo-

■ THE NURSING PROCESS

The student should refer to Chapter 40 for general guidelines on the nursing process with antibiotic therapy. The additional material below relates specifically to the sulfonamides, nitrofurantoins, and nalidixic acid.

■ Assessment

Nitrofurantoins and nalidixic acid are used exclusively for the treatment of urinary tract infections, and the sulfonamides are most commonly used in this way. Assessment of the patient should be carried out with emphasis on renal function. Other clinical signs of infection should be monitored as well. Objective data such as blood tests, history of allergies, and mental function should also be obtained.

■ Management

Nitrofurantoins, nalidixic acid, and sulfonamides are used to cure bacterial infections of the urinary tract. Progress of treatment may be monitored by clinical signs alone, such as relief of pain and itching or may be monitored by culturing the urine. The nurse should be certain that urine samples are appropriately collected to prevent trivial contamination, which renders the culture results meaningless. Blood tests may be required for patients receiving sulfonamides. All patients being treated for urinary tract infections should receive adequate fluids to maintain good urine flow. Patient teaching should include instruction on the signs of blood dyscrasias for those receiving sulfonamides, signs of pulmonary distress and peripheral neuropathy for those receiving nitrofurantoins, and signs of central nervous system distress in those receiving nalidixic acid. These side effects are usually sufficient cause for the physician to discontinue medication.

■ Evaluation

Nitrofurantoins, nalidixic acid, and sulfonamides are all capable of producing a cure of urinary tract infections. However, relapses or failure of therapy are not uncommon for several reasons. First, bacterial resistance may develop. This form of therapeutic failure is relatively common with nalidixic acid. Secondly, reinfections may occur frequently in some people. In some cases the reinfection may reflect inadequate hygiene, whereas in other cases the reinfection may reflect a defect within the urinary tract that impedes urine flow and promotes infections.

The nurse should make certain that the patient can explain how to take the prescribed medication and can point out which side effects are sufficient reasons to call the physician. The patient should also be capable of properly collecting urine for testing.

---

glycemics should be warned that they may have difficulty with hypoglycemia. Patients receiving methotrexate may have more trouble with drug-related side effects (Chapter 50).

3. The sulfonamides bear a chemical similarity to some other classes of drugs (certain goitrogens, diuretics, and oral hypoglycemic agents). Rarely, patients taking sulfonamides may develop or experience goiter production, diuresis, or hypoglycemia.
4. Patients receiving sulfonamides should be well hydrated, with an intake of 2000 to 2500 ml per day (for an adult) if possible.
5. Phenazopyridine will color urine orange-red. Any patients receiving a sulfonamide in combination with phenazopyridine (Table 45-2) should be so warned.
6. Azulfidine can also cause alopecia and reduced sperm count. It should be given in evenly divided doses throughout the 24 hours, with no period between doses, even at night, exceeding 8 hours. It should be given after meals when possible. It also causes an orange-yellow color to the skin and urine.
7. Patients receiving sulfamethizole should be warned that the drug can cause the urine and skin to be yellow-orange in color.
8. Sulfonamides may cause photosensitivity. Caution

patients to avoid exposure to the sun or ultraviolet light.

9. Both mafenide and silver sulfadiazine are used in the treatment of burns, although mafenide can cause pain and can contribute to electrolyte imbalance. Both creams should be applied with sterile gloves to the burned areas. Both work less effectively in the presence of pus, debris, and blood, so regular cleaning of the wounds is recommended. Dressings are not necessary, although patients may request them. Because the rate of absorption through the skin cannot be easily measured, it is recommended that routine serum sulfonamide levels be drawn to monitor for possible toxic levels.
10. Parenteral sulfisoxazole:
    a. For intramuscular use, dissolve as directed on the ampule with Sterile Water for Injection and administer. There may be pain at the injection site.
    b. For intravenous use, further dilute the dissolved drug to a 5% solution (e.g., combine a 5 ml ampule with 35 ml Sterile Water for Injection; only this diluent should be used). Administer slowly, about 1 ml per minute or through slow infusion. For further information, consult the manufacturer's literature or the pharmacist.

Nitrofurantoins

1. Side effects may include anorexia, nausea, vomiting, and gastrointestinal irritation. This latter problem may be reduced if the drug is taken with meals, but the use of antacids should be avoided. Rashes and allergic responses may also occur.
2. Occasionally, patients develop pulmonary complications that manifest as acute pneumonitis: cough, dyspnea, wheezing, fluid infiltration, or pulmonary edema. Caution the patient to report any of these signs immediately. With long-term therapy, the pulmonary sensitivity reaction may develop insidiously, with fatigue, malaise, cough, dyspnea, and changes on x-ray film, including pulmonary fibrosis.
3. Peripheral neuropathy can occur as a side effect. Symptoms include numbness, tingling, weakness, or other unusual feelings in the extremities. It may be more common in patients with renal impairment, diabetes, or vitamin B deficiency.
4. Warn the patients that oral suspensions may stain the teeth. To help prevent this, suspensions can be well diluted in milk or juices before taking.
5. Nitrofurantoins will turn the urine brown.
6. Patients should be kept well hydrated, with an intake of 2000 to 2500 ml per day (in the adult) if possible.

Nalidixic acid

1. Side effects include abdominal pain, diarrhea, fever, and rashes. Photosensitivity may occur, and patients should be cautioned to avoid exposure to the sun or ultraviolet light. Central nervous system side effects include mental confusion and instability, headache, dizziness, visual disturbances, and convulsions. Because of these central nervous system effects, the drug should be used cautiously in elderly persons and avoided if possible in persons with a history of convulsions. Finally, nalidixic acid has caused bulging fontanelles and papilledema in infants.
2. Patients taking oral anticoagulants should be alerted that while taking nalidixic acid they will be more prone to toxic effects of the anticoagulants. Caution them to be alert for bruising and bleeding.
3. Nalidixic acid may cause false positive reactions when urine is tested with Benedict's solution, Fehling's solution, or Clinitest tablets. While taking nalidixic acid, patients who must monitor urine sugar concentration should use Clinistix or Tes-Tape.
4. Resistance to nalidixic acid, when it occurs, does so within the first couple of days of therapy. Follow-up cultures should be done 2 or 3 days after starting therapy to check for sterility.
5. Patient should be kept well hydrated with a daily intake of 2000 to 2500 ml (in the adult) if possible.

■ SUMMARY

Sulfonamides are metabolic inhibitors that block bacterial synthesis of tetrahydrofolic acid (THFA), a vitamin required for the synthesis of amino acids and nucleic acids. Sulfonamides are effective against a wide range of gram-positive and gram-negative bacteria. Sulfonamides are available for topical use and for use as nonabsorbable oral agents. However, most sulfonamides are well absorbed orally and penetrate most body tissues, including the brain. Sulfonamides are acetylated by the liver and excreted by the kidneys. Since the drugs are present in a high concentration in an active form in the urine, the sulfonamides are very useful for urinary tract infections. Sulfonamides cause allergies, gastrointestinal distress, and blood dyscrasias. Patients receiving sulfonamides should receive 2000 to 2500 L of fluid daily to prevent urinary precipitation of the sulfonamides.

Trimethoprim blocks the conversion of dihydrofolic acid to THFA in bacteria. Trimethoprim produces synergistic antibacterial effects when used with sulfonamides and for that reason is most frequently used in fixed combination with sulfamethoxazole. Trimethoprim is well distributed to tissues and is excreted by the kidney, most of the drug remaining in the active form. Trimethoprim appears relatively nontoxic but may affect the bone marrow.

Nitrofurantoins are orally administered antibacterial agents that achieve effective concentrations only in the urine. Nitrofurantoin may irritate the gastrointestinal tract, especially when administered in the microcrystalline form. Rashes, allergies, and blood dyscrasias may also develop. Peripheral neuropathy and pneumonitis are associated with long-term use of nitrofurantoin.

Nalidixic acid is concentrated in the kidney following oral absorption. The drug is therefore useful in treating urinary tract infections, although early development of bacterial resistance is commonly encountered. Nalidixic acid may produce central nervous system toxicity, rashes, and blood dyscrasias.

■ STUDY QUESTIONS

1. What is the mechanism for the antibacterial effect of sulfonamides?
2. Why are sulfonamides not equally toxic to humans and bacteria?
3. What is the effect of paraaminobenzoic acid on sulfonamide action in bacterial cells?
4. By what routes may sulfonamides be administered?
5. Do sulfonamides enter the cerebrospinal fluid from the bloodstream?
6. What is the route of elimination of sulfonamides from the body?
7. What is the purpose of combining sulfonamides with phenazopyridine in the treatment of urinary tract infections?
8. What are the major toxic reactions to sulfonamides?
9. How has the renal toxicity of the sulfonamide preparations used clinically changed since the early 1940's?
10. What is the mechanism for the antibacterial effect of trimethoprim?
11. Why is trimethoprim not equally toxic to humans and bacteria?
12. Why are trimethoprim and sulfamethoxazole combined for the treatment of urinary tract infections and infections at other sites?
13. Why is nitrofurantoin not effective for systemic infections?
14. By what route is nitrofurantoin administered?
15. What reactions to nitrofurantoin are commonly encountered with short-term therapy?
16. What reactions to nitrofurantoin are associated with long-term therapy?
17. By what route is nalidixic acid administered?
18. What toxic reactions are commonly encountered with nalidixic acid?
19. What is the major clinical use of nalidixic acid?

■ SUGGESTED READINGS

Conklin, J.D.: The pharmacokinetics of nitrofurantoin and its related bioavailability, Antibiotic Chemotherapy **25**:233, 1978.

Keys, T.F.: Antimicrobials commonly used for urinary tract infection: sulfonamides, trimethoprim-sulfamethoxazole, nitrofurantoin, nalidixic acid, Mayo Clinic Proceedings **52**:680, 1977.

Kucers, A., and Bennett, N. McK.: The use of antibiotics, ed. 3, London, 1979, William Heinemann Medical Books, Ltd.

46 Drugs to treat tuberculosis and leprosy

Tuberculosis and leprosy are diseases produced by *Mycobacterium* infections. Both diseases have been known since ancient times and are among the earliest examples of diseases that were recognized as infectious. Tuberculosis, or the white plague, was a major cause of death in Europe and the Orient throughout the Middle Ages up until recent times. Leprosy, while less common, was greatly feared for the disfigurement it caused in its victims. This grim picture changed in the early 1940's when the first effective antituberculosis agent, streptomycin, was discovered. Around the same time a sulfone was discovered to be effective in controlling leprosy. With these and other more recently discovered agents, both diseases may now be effectively treated. In this chapter, the clinical features of *Mycobacterium* infections which make their treatment more difficult than that of most other bacterial diseases are considered. Second, the properties of the drugs used to treat these diseases and the ways in which they are employed are covered.

■ TREATMENT OF TUBERCULOSIS

■ Clinical features of tuberculosis

The disease referred to as tuberculosis is produced by *Mycobacterium tuberculosis,* or less commonly by other mycobacteria harbored by cattle or birds. Three features of *M. tuberculosis* are especially important to recall when considering how disease is produced in humans by these organisms. First, mycobacteria are strict aerobic organisms. This property decrees that the organism must live in an oxygen-rich environment and may explain the fact that the first site of infection in humans is usually along the alveoli of the lung. Second, mycobacteria induce activity of macrophages, causing these cellular immunity factors to phagocytize *M. tuberculosis*. Rather than helping prevent infection, this action actually may enhance survival and spread of the disease-causing organisms, since *M. tuberculosis* is resistant to the acids and enzymes that usually destroy bacteria within macrophages. *M. tuberculosis* actually reproduces within macrophages at a near-normal rate and may be carried by macrophages throughout the body. Third, mycobacteria are extremely slow-growing organisms, relative to other bacteria. The time required for the tubercle bacilli to reproduce is 10 to 12 hours, as compared to 20 to 30 minutes for other bacteria such as *Escherichia coli* or *Pseudomonas aeruginosa*. This slow growth contributes to the difficulty encountered in treating the disease, since it is during active growth that the organism is most susceptible to metabolic interference.

The disease produced by *M. tuberculosis* may pass through several phases. The initial or primary infection usually occurs in the lung as a result of inhaling droplets containing live *M. tuberculosis*. These infective aerosols are generated when a patient with an established active case of tuberculosis coughs or sneezes. Once in the alveoli, the *M. tuberculosis* is phagocytized and begins to multiply. Infected macrophages may remain in the lung, but a significant number enter the lymphatic system and a few enter the bloodstream and are carried throughout the body. In response to the increasing number of tubercle bacilli in the lung, a pneumonia-like condition may develop within a few weeks. This inflammatory response to the infection may continue for a few weeks, but in most people this process is ultimately halted by the delayed immune reaction provoked by the infection. This acquired cellular immunity results in an increased effectiveness of macrophages in destroying the *M. tuberculosis*. Lesions within the lung resolve as infective loci become calcified. Living tubercule bacilli no longer appear in sputum at this stage, and the disease is said to be inactive. Living *M. tuberculosis* remains within the body, however, for relapses may occur months or years after the initial infection. When relapse occurs, localized areas again become sites for active multiplication of tubercle bacilli. Local necrosis develops as the cellular immunity factors attempt to isolate the infection. Necrosis may spread as a result of this inflammatory response and may cause large cavities within the lungs or other tissues.

M. tuberculosis, like most other bacteria, has the ability to acquire resistance to drugs. Development of resistance is rather common when tuberculosis patients are treated with a single drug. To minimize this therapeutic complication, multiple drug therapy of tuberculosis is used. The rationale for this therapy is that since mutations are required for the development of resistance to a drug, if two drugs that have different mechanisms of action are administered then the organism must acquire two independent mutations to become resistant to both drugs. Since mutations are rare events, the likelihood of simultaneously acquiring two specific mutations is very small. The probability of developing resistance is further reduced by using three drugs with independent mechanisms of action.

The traditional method of chemotherapy for established tuberculosis has been to administer a combination of drugs for 2 years and perhaps longer. Patients so treated rapidly cease to be infectious, but chemotherapy must be continued for long periods to eliminate most of the dormant tubercle bacilli. Frequency of relapse seems inversely proportional to the duration of therapy. Recent clinical studies in Great Britain and Africa have suggested that shorter treatment periods may be employed if three drugs are used continuously for the first 2 months of therapy, followed by an additional 6 to 9 months with two of the drugs. Clinical trials are also being conducted with intermittent therapy in which drugs are administered twice weekly. Intermittent therapy at present seems best suited to patients who do not reliably take their medication without direct medical supervision. For these patients the drugs may be administered by a visiting nurse.

Many drugs are now available for antituberculosis therapy. These agents may be divided into two categories, depending in part on their potency and spectrum of activity and in part on their toxicity. The so-called first-line drugs are isoniazid, rifampin, streptomycin, ethambutol, and paraaminosalicylic acid (PAS). The second-line, or reserve, drugs are pyrazinamide, cycloserine, ethionamide, and capreomycin. The properties and proper uses of these drugs are considered in the following sections.

■ Properties of individual agents

Isoniazid

Clinical use. Isoniazid is considered to be the best antituberculosis drug now available. Isoniazid, also referred to as *INH,* is the most commonly used first-line drug and is the only antituberculosis agent used routinely for prophylaxis.

Mechanism of action. Although isoniazid is known to alter several metabolic processes in mycobacteria, it is not yet known which of these actions is critical for destruction of the microorganism in vivo. Isoniazid is a potent inhibitor of an enzyme involved in cell wall synthesis and also blocks pyridoxine (vitamin B_6) utilization in a number of intracellular enzymes. Nucleic acid synthesis is inhibited by isoniazid, but this effect seems secondary to other metabolic events.

Whatever the precise mechanism of action of isoniazid, mycobacteria possess the ability to rapidly acquire resistance to it. In very early clinical trials when isoniazid was used alone to treat active pulmonary tuberculosis, 11% of the patients carried isoniazid-resistant strains at the end of 1 month of therapy. At the end of the third month, 71% of these patients harbored isoniazid-resistant *Mycobacterium*. Observations such as these have led to the clinical practice of combining isoniazid therapy with the use of one or two other drugs. Combined drug therapy successfully suppresses the appearance of resistant organisms in most patients.

Isoniazid is used alone for prophylaxis. The drug is prescribed for persons exposed to tuberculosis or patients who have recently converted from negative to positive reactions in the skin test for tuberculosis. These latter patients usually have smaller numbers of *Mycobacterium* than would be found in an active, symptomatic case of tuberculosis, and for them the use of isoniazid alone is usually successful.

Isoniazid is most effective against *M. tuberculosis,* inhibiting the growth of over 90% of tested strains at a concentration of 0.2 mg/ml. Some evidence suggests that resistant strains of *M. tuberculosis* are less pathogenic than sensitive strains. For this reason isoniazid therapy may be continued even after isoniazid-resistant strains are cultured from the patient.

Mycobacterium kansasii, which rarely causes disease in humans, is less sensitive to isoniazid than is *M. tuberculosis*. Other mycobacteria are resistant to the drug.

Absorption, distribution, and excretion. Isoniazid is well absorbed following oral administration, achieving peak serum levels in 1 to 2 hours. The drug enters body tissues relatively efficiently, and bacteriostatic concentrations are found in most tissues, including pleural fluids and caseous exudates surrounding active loci of tuberculosis infections in the lung.

Isoniazid undergoes a number of metabolic conversions in the liver, most resulting in inactive drug, which is excreted primarily in the kidney. The major metabolite is an acetylated form of isoniazid. The rate of drug acetylation differs markedly among populations, and two genetically determined types may be distinguished. The so-called *rapid acetylators* inactivate isoniazid two to three times as rapidly as the *slow acetylators*. As would be expected, rapid acetylators have lower blood concentrations of active drug than slow acetylators. Nevertheless, both types of patients respond well to standard therapeutic doses administered once daily. Increasing the drug dose or the frequency of administration in slow acetylators is not wise, since these patients tend to accumulate the acetylated metabolite, which is hepatotoxic.

Slow acetylators comprise 45% to 65% of the Northern European and American white or black populations. Oriental and Eskimo populations contain predominantly "rapid acetylators."

Toxicity. Isoniazid is a relatively nontoxic drug. Nevertheless, as with any drug, untoward reactions can occur in a small percentage of treated patients. The most commonly encountered toxic reaction is peripheral neuropathy. Diabetics, alcoholics, and malnourished persons are more prone to this complication than the general population. At least some of these reactions are related to low pyridoxine (vitamin B_6) levels and may be prevented by administration of 5 mg of the vitamin daily. Peripheral neuropathies are more likely to occur in slow acetylators.

Hepatotoxicity is the most serious side effect associated with isoniazid. Fatalities due to liver failure have been noted, even among persons receiving the drug prophylactically. Hepatitis due to isoniazid is rare among patients under 20 years of age and occurs in patients aged 20 to 34 years at a rate of around 3 cases/1000 patients treated. After age 50, the incidence increases to 23 cases/1000 patients treated. Patients also have an increased risk of hepatitis if they are rapid acetylators of isoniazid, if they ingest ethanol daily, or if they also receive the drug rifampin. Liver function should be monitored in all patients receiving isoniazid and most carefully watched in those patients at high risk. Various other reactions have occasionally been reported with isoniazid, including allergies, blood dyscrasias, gastric distress, and metabolic acidosis.

Ethambutol

Clinical use. Ethambutol is an effective antituberculosis drug discovered in 1961. Ethambutol is chemically unrelated to other antituberculosis drugs or antibiotics and is apparently effective only against mycobacteria and no other bacteria, viruses, or fungi tested. Ethambutol has become a first-line drug in conventional antituberculosis therapy and is frequently used as one of the drugs in intermittent therapeutic programs.

Mechanism of action. The precise antibacterial action of ethambutol is unknown. The drug interferes with the formation of several cellular metabolites in the *Mycobacterium,* and death follows in about 24 hours. Nearly all strains of *M. tuberculosis* are sensitive to the drug. Nearly all strains of *M. avium* are resistant. Other mycobacteria have intermediate sensitivity to ethambutol.

Resistance to ethambutol will develop in vivo if the drug is used alone in therapy. Since ethambutol is chemically unrelated to other antituberculosis drugs and presumably has a different mechanism of action, ethambutol does not induce cross-resistance to other antituberculosis agents.

Absorption, distribution, and excretion. Ethambutol is administered orally and is well absorbed from the gastrointestinal tract in the presence or absence of food. Peak serum concentrations are observed 2 to 4 hours after the oral dose. Ethambutol is less extensively metabolized than isoniazid and up to 50% of the drug excreted in the urine is in the unaltered, active form. Up to 15% of the drug in the urine is in the form of a metabolite. Fecal concentrations of the drug represent unabsorbed material.

Ethambutol has been detected in cerebrospinal fluid following oral therapy, although the levels are below those found in plasma. The drug is also known to concentrate in erythrocytes.

Toxicity. Ethambutol has become a first-line antituberculosis drug because of its relatively wide spectrum of activity against *Mycobacterium* species and its relatively low toxicity. These advantages have outweighed the disadvantage that the drug is somewhat less potent than several other antituberculosis agents.

The most commonly reported toxic reaction to normal therapeutic doses of ethambutol is a visual disturbance. Some patients report changes in color vision, whereas others suffer a more prominent loss of visual acuity. These signs are cause to terminate ethambutol use. If the drug is discontinued when these visual signs appear, the changes are reversible, although full recovery may take months.

Other reactions to ethambutol appear rare. Allergic reactions have occasionally been reported. Peripheral neuritis is a rare complications, occurring with higher doses of ethambutol. Some reactions attributed to ethambutol may actually have been caused by other drugs administered concomitantly. Uric acid levels are reported elevated in patients receiving ethambutol, although evidence linking this action directly to ethambutol is scanty.

Rifampin

Clinical use. Rifampin, originally developed as an antibacterial drug, was observed to be effective against *Chlamydia,* some viruses, and mycobacteria. Rifampin is as potent as isoniazid against mycobacteria and has the broadest spectrum of activity of any antituberculosis agent against species of mycobacteria. These advantages have placed rifampin in the group of first-line antituberculosis agents. The disadvantages of the drug include its expense and its tendency to cause increased toxicity when administered intermittently. These disadvantages limit the usefulness of the drug at present to therapy in developed countries where small numbers of patients may be treated.

Mechanism of action. Rifampin inhibits DNA-dependent RNA polymerase in sensitive organisms. As a result of the action of the drug, gene transcription halts and protein synthesis is prevented. Metabolic activity in the *Mycobacterium* stops, and the cell ultimately dies or is eliminated by host defenses.

Resistance to rifampin can occur when the drug is used alone against *Mycobacterium*. Resistant strains have an altered DNA-dependent RNA polymerase that is no longer inhibited by the drug. Cross-resistance to other antituberculosis drugs does not occur.

Absorption, distribution, and excretion. Rifampin is absorbed orally in adequate amounts in the presence or absence of food. The slightly slower absorption observed in the presence of food is apparently not clinically important.

Rifampin is a relatively lipid-soluble agent. This property explains why rifampin is found in higher concentrations in body tissues than in serum. The lipid solubility of rifampin also explains the ability of this drug to penetrate white blood cells and attack *Mycobacterium* living therein. This ability to attack intracellular mycobacteria is unusual for antituberculosis drugs.

Roughly 40% of a dose of rifampin is excreted in the bile and a little less in the urine. Rifampin is also deacetylated by the liver, and the deacetylated metabolite is excreted via the bile into the feces.

Toxicity. Rifampin can cause a variety of mild reactions such as gastrointestinal upset and central nervous system disturbances. The drug also turns body fluids such as tears, sweat, saliva, and urine an orange-red color, which might be mistaken for blood. This coloration is harmless.

Liver abnormalities seem to be the most common reaction observed with rifampin. Mild abnormalities in liver function may return to normal without discontinuing the drug, but increases in alkaline phosphatase or the appearance of jaundice signals that the drug should be discontinued.

High doses of rifampin given intermittently may cause an immune reaction that is associated with a variety of symptoms. This flulike syndrome may progress from chills, fever, vomiting, diarrhea, and myalgia to acute renal failure. Deaths have occurred. Since these symptoms occur when therapy is restarted, patients should be advised not to miss doses of rifampin, especially if they are receiving relatively high doses. Some treatment centers have significantly lowered rifampin dosage for intermittent therapeutic programs and have reduced these immune reactions (Table 46-1).

Rifampin induces liver enzymes involved in drug and hormone metabolism in humans. This action of rifampin leads to the drug interactions listed in Table 46-1.

Rifampin also seems to be an immunosuppressant in humans, producing delayed effects on the immune system. The implication of this action on the clinical effectiveness of rifampin is unknown.

Streptomycin

Clinical use. The first of the antituberculosis drugs to be discovered, streptomycin is still a reliable first-line agent. Streptomycin is frequently used as part of a three-drug regimen for initial therapy (Table 46-1). Streptomycin is usually discontinued after the number of infective organisms has been strongly reduced, usually 2 to 4 months. The patient may continue to receive the remaining two drugs throughout the treatment period. Streptomycin has also been used as part of intermittent treatment programs where the drug is given two or three times a week for the first 2 months of therapy.

Mechanism of action. Streptomycin inhibits protein synthesis in sensitive bacteria and mycobacteria (Chapter 44). The drug is highly effective against most types of pathogenic mycobacteria with the exception of *M. avium*.

Resistance to streptomycin may develop when the drug is used alone. When streptomycin is used in combination with isoniazid or another first-line agent, development of resistance is minimized.

Absorption, distribution, and excretion. Streptomycin is not absorbed orally and must be administered by intramuscular injection for routine clinical use (Chapter 44). This property restricts the use of streptomycin to the hospital setting or to a well-supervised outpatient program. Because of the difficulties of daily injections, patients are frequently taken off streptomycin after 2 to 4 months of therapy, so long as bacteriological improvement is obvious. Therapy is continued in these cases with other antituberculosis drugs.

Streptomycin is well distributed in the body and may be used to treat tuberculosis meningitis and other forms of nonpulmonary tuberculosis.

The excretion of streptomycin has been discussed in Chapter 44.

Toxicity. Streptomycin has the potential to produce any toxic reaction seen with other aminoglycoside antibiotics (Chapter 44), but ototoxicity is the most commonly encountered reaction in tuberculosis patients. Careful attention to maintain dosage within safe limits (Table 46-1) will prevent the reaction in most patients. Patients with renal insufficiency, elderly patients, and patients receiving long-term streptomycin therapy are more prone to develop toxic reactions.

Para-aminosalicylic acid

Clinical use. Para-aminosalicylic acid (PAS) is an effective first-line antituberculosis drug, but the use of this agent has declined with the introduction of ethambutol and rifampin. PAS was in the past included in the standard three-drug regimen for tuberculosis in which streptomycin, isoniazid, and PAS were administered for 3 to 4 months. After active mycobacteria have disap-

TABLE 46-1. Summary of first-line antituberculosis drugs

Generic name	Trade name	Dosage and administration	Clinical use	Patient populations with increased risk of toxicity	Drug interactions
Isoniazid or isonicotinic acid hydrazide	Hyzyd Niconyl Nydrazid Rolazid Teebaconin Nydrazid	ORAL: *Adults*—300 mg daily maximum. *Children*—10 to 20 mg/kg daily.	In multidrug therapy for active tuberculosis. For prophylaxis: as above.	Patients also receiving rifampin have an increased risk of drug-induced hepatitis. Older patients have higher risk of drug-induced hepatitis. Vitamin B_6 depletion observed in alcoholics, malnourished patients, and diabetics increases the risk of peripheral neuropathies. Pregnant women or nursing mothers should be observed to see if isoniazid is harming the fetus or nursing infant. Liver or renal disease may impair disposition of isoniazid and increase its toxic effects.	Isoniazid decreases the metabolism of phenytoin and may lead to increased toxic reactions to the drug.
		INTRAMUSCULAR, INTRAVENOUS: As for oral.	As for oral in treatment of acute, active tuberculosis.		
Ethambutol	Myambutol	ORAL: *Adults*—15 mg/kg in a single daily dose. *Children under 13 yr* should not receive the drug.	In multidrug initial therapy of tuberculosis.	Patients with reduced renal function require reduced drug doses. Patients with preexisting visual defects may be difficult to evaluate for drug-induced visual changes. Pregnant women or nursing mothers should be observed to see if ethambutol is harming the fetus or nursing infant.	None yet reported.
		ORAL: *Adults*—25 mg/kg in a single daily dose for 2 mo, after which dose may be reduced to 15 mg/kg daily.	In multidrug treatment of tuberculosis.		
		ORAL: *Adults*—45 to 50 mg/kg twice weekly or 90 mg/kg once weekly.	In multidrug intermittent therapy of tuberculosis.		
Rifampin	Rifadin Rimactane	ORAL: *Adults*—600 mg daily in 1 dose. *Children*—10 to 20 mg/kg up to 600 mg daily.	In multidrug initial therapy or retreatment for pulmonary tuberculosis.	Patients with prior liver disease are more likely to suffer drug-induced hepatotoxicity. Pregnant women or nursing mothers should be observed to see if rifampin is harming the fetus or nursing infant.	Rifampin induces liver microsomal enzymes, thereby decreasing the effectiveness of coumarin anticoagulants, oral hypoglycemic agents, metha-

					done, and digitalis. Steroid breakdown may be accelerated, thereby decreasing the effectiveness of oral contraceptives or replacement doses of cortisol.
Streptomycin		INTRAMUSCULAR: *Adults*—1 Gm daily for 2 to 4 mo or longer. After initial therapy dosage may be reduced to 1 Gm 2 or 3 times weekly. *Children and elderly patients*—may require smaller doses.	In multidrug therapy for all forms of tuberculosis.	Patients with renal insufficiency are more prone to accumulate streptomycin and develop ototoxicity. Elderly patients are more sensitive to ototoxic effects of streptomycin.	Streptomycin may enhance actions of muscle relaxants.
Para-amino-salicylic acid (PAS)	Aminosalicylic Acid Teebacin Acid	ORAL: *Adults*—10 to 12 Gm daily in 3 or 4 doses. *Children*—200 to 300 mg/kg daily in 3 or 4 doses.	In multidrug therapy for active tuberculosis.	None yet reported.	None yet reported.
Aminosalicylate acid sodium salt (10.9% sodium)	P.A.S. Sodium Pamisyl Sodium Parasal Sodium Pasdium Teebacin	ORAL: *Adults*—12 to 15 Gm daily in 2 or 3 doses. *Children*—200 to 300 mg/kg daily in 3 or 4 doses.	In multidrug therapy for active tuberculosis.	Patients with active hypertension or other diseases in which sodium overload is undesirable.	None yet reported.
Aminosalicylate sodium and aminosalicylic acid (85% sodium salt)	Neopassalate	ORAL: *Adults*—14 to 17 Gm daily in 2 or 3 doses. *Children*—280 to 420 mg/kg daily in 3 or 4 doses.	In multidrug therapy for active tuberculosis.	Patients with active hypertension or other diseases in which sodium overload is undesirable.	None yet reported.
Aminosalicylate potassium (20% potassium)	Teebacin Kalium	ORAL: *Adults*—12.5 to 15 Gm daily in 2 or 3 doses. *Children*—250 to 375 mg/kg daily in 3 or 4 doses.	In multidrug therapy for active tuberculosis.	Patients with impaired renal function.	None yet reported.
Aminosalicylate calcium (12% calcium)	P.A.S. Calcium Teebacin Calcium	ORAL: As for aminosalicylate acid sodium salt.	As for aminosalicylate acid sodium salt.	Patients with a tendency to form renal stones, or who have hypercalcemia (high blood levels of calcium).	None yet reported.

TABLE 46-2. Summary of second-line antituberculosis drugs

Generic name	Trade name	Dosage and administration	Clinical use	Toxic reactions
Capreomycin	Capastat	INTRAMUSCULAR: *Adults*—15 to 20 mg/kg daily in single dose. Not recommended for children.	Retreatment of tuberculosis.	Nephrotoxicity; low blood potassium level; eighth cranial nerve toxicity.
Cycloserine	Seromycin	ORAL: *Adults*—15 mg/kg daily in 2 doses up to maximum daily dose of 1 Gm. Dosage not established for children.	Retreatment of tuberculosis; urinary tract tuberculosis.	Central nervous system toxicity, including psychotic reactions.
Ethionamide	Trecator S.C.	ORAL: *Adults*—0.5 to 1 Gm daily in 1 to 3 doses. Dosage not established for children.	Any form of tuberculosis when primary drugs are inappropriate.	Nausea and vomiting induced by central nervous system effects; liver toxicity.
Pyrizinamide		ORAL: *Adults*—20 to 35 mg/kg daily up to 3 Gm. Dosage not established for children.	Retreatment of tuberculosis.	Hepatotoxicity; increased blood concentrations of uric acid (hyperuricemia).

peared from sputum and other fluids, PAS and isoniazid were continued for another 2 years. Currently, treatment protocols are more likely to include ethambutol or rifampin than PAS. PAS does find usefulness in intermittent therapy of tuberculosis, as a second-line or reserve drug, and in mass chemotherapy programs in developing countries.

Mechanism of action. PAS inhibits mycobacterial growth by interfering with folic acid metabolism. The mechanism is probably similar to sulfonamide inhibition of bacterial growth. Mycobacteria can develop resistance to PAS, and the drug is never used alone in therapy. *M. tuberculosis* is usually sensitive to PAS, but other types of mycobacteria are generally resistant.

Absorption, distribution, and excretion. PAS is efficiently absorbed by the oral route and is well-distributed to most body tissues. PAS does not enter the cerebrospinal fluid in the absence of inflamed meninges. Excretion of the drug is primarily via the kidney, but PAS is also acetylated in the liver and inactivated.

Toxicity. PAS is not well-tolerated by most patients. Nearly all patients receiving the drug report gastrointestinal irritation of one form or another. Taking the drug with food or antacids prevents some but not all of the irritation produced by the large amount of drug contained in a normal dose (Table 46-1).

Various allergic symptoms have also been reported with PAS. Some reactions are relatively mild rashes, but exfoliative dermatitis has also been reported. Severe organ damage linked to allergic reactions to PAS also occurred, including hepatitis.

One source of toxic reactions to PAS is the ion carried with the drug. PAS is available as the free acid and as the sodium, potassium, or calcium salt. Each form of the drug has its own advantages and disadvantages for certain patients. For example, patients with hypertension would not tolerate the excess sodium contained in sodium PAS. Patients with increased blood calcium level or in whom renal stone formation is common should avoid the calcium salt of PAS. Since the daily dose of PAS is large, these ion effects may be more serious than with other drugs given in much smaller daily doses.

The low patient acceptance of PAS and the availability of better tolerated and more effective agents have combined to restrict the use of PAS.

■ Reserve drugs used in tuberculosis therapy

The major properties of the second-line, or reserve drugs, used to treat tuberculosis are summarized in Table 46-2. The wide use of these drugs is limited by various factors. As a group, the reserve drugs are more toxic than the first-line drugs. Moreover, many of the reserve drugs are not as potent as the more commonly used drugs. Nevertheless, these reserve agents are quite useful when strains of mycobacteria resistant to first-line drugs appear or when a patient develops intolerable toxic reactions to these first-line drugs.

■ THE NURSING PROCESS FOR DRUGS TO TREAT TUBERCULOSIS

■ Assessment

Antituberculosis drug therapy is used in patients who are diagnosed as having active tuberculosis or in patients whose tuberculosis skin tests convert from negative to positive. In some instances patients receiving high doses of adrenalcortical steroids may require antituberculosis therapy. In this latter group of patients, the concern is that the high doses of steroids will alter the patient's ability to resist infection from tuberculosis or will cause reactivation of earlier tubercular infections. Patients may present with a picture of chronic illness, may be seriously ill, or may be well in appearance and have been diagnosed only through conversion of the tuberculin skin test. The initial assessment needs to be based in part on the obvious condition of the patient. Certainly a thorough total patient assessment should be done, with an emphasis on subjective complaints the patient has, possible history of tuberculosis in the patient and family, and recent activities such as travel or moving that might have influenced exposure to the disease. Not all patients have the characteristic cough associated historically with tuberculosis. If a cough with sputum production exists, the sputum should be sent for culture and drug sensitivity testing. Tuberculosis can appear in other organs besides the lung (e.g., tuberculosis meningitis). Obviously the focus of the assessment would be different if the patient has a nontraditional form of tuberculosis.

■ Management

The diagnosis of tuberculosis still causes many health care professionals and patients to develop unnecessary anxiety and fear about this disease. As soon as the diagnosis is made it is important to begin patient education so that unreasonable fears can be calmed. If health care personnel are unsure of the local standards regarding care of tuberculosis patients, the local health department or hospital infection control department should be contacted. The hospitalized patient will be placed in isolation. It is beyond the scope of this book to go into detail about such procedures as isolation for the various forms of tuberculosis; refer to appropriate nursing textbooks for these procedures. It is important to remember that many tuberculosis patients are diagnosed and treated entirely on an outpatient basis. Because drug therapy for tuberculosis is chronic, usually lasting 2 years or longer, the management phase can be thought of as a long-term process. New cases of tuberculosis should be reported to the local health department so that they can follow up possible family and social contacts of the patient who has been diagnosed with this disease.

■ Evaluation

Success with antituberculosis therapy is manifested by a resolution of the disease. Many factors influence the success of therapy, such as patient motivation to continue the long-term course of therapy, actual patient compliance, and the incidence of side effects that occur with the drugs. In fact noncompliance is a major cause of treatment failures for tuberculosis. Before the patient begins self-management, the patient should be able to explain why and how to take the drugs ordered, possible side effects that can occur, ways to treat minor side effects such as nausea associated with taking the medication, and side effects that require notification of the physician. The patient should also be able to explain when and why return visits for evaluation of laboratory work and other patient data are scheduled and should be able to explain and demonstrate the measures to take to decrease the possibility of spreading the disease to others. If the patient has had a markedly positive skin test, the patient should be able to explain that skin tests in the future should be refused, and that follow-up should be made via x-ray film. If side effects have occurred with the drugs, such as peripheral neuropathy with isoniazid therapy, patients will receive appropriate additional pharmacological management. While not related directly to actions with the patient, it is important the health care personnel accept responsibility for having TB skin tests or chest x-ray films on a regular basis to diagnose possible exposure to tuberculosis. For further specific information, see the patient care implications section at the end of this chapter.

TABLE 46-3. Summary of drugs used to treat leprosy

Generic name	Trade name	Dosage and administration	Toxicity	Comments
Dapsone	Avlosulfon	ORAL: *Adults*—up to 100 mg daily. *Children*—1.4 mg/kg daily.	Mild, rare gastrointestinal disturbance.	Patients with glucose-6-phosphate dehydrogenase deficiency are more prone to hemolytic reactions and must receive reduced doses.
Clofazimine	Lamprene	ORAL: *Adults*—100 mg daily. (Investigational only.)	Gastrointestinal distress	Red drug imparts a dark red color to skin and other body tissues. This coloration is harmless.
Rifampin	Rifadin Rimactane	ORAL: *Adults*—600 mg daily.	Liver toxicity; abdominal distress.	Not yet approved for this use in the United States.
Sulfoxone sodium	Diasone Sodium	ORAL: *Adults*—330 mg daily.	As for dapsone.	A sulfone that is converted to dapsone in the body.

■ THE NURSING PROCESS FOR DRUGS TO TREAT LEPROSY

■ Assessment

In the United States the diagnosis of leprosy is very unusual. Baseline assessment data should include a thorough total patient assessment, with special emphasis on subjective and objective deviations from normal.

■ Management

Perhaps more than tuberculosis, the diagnosis of leprosy causes a great deal of fear and anxiety in patients. As soon as the diagnosis is made, referral to appropriate agencies for education and support should be made, and patient and family education should be begun. Appropriate agencies would include the local health department and the Center for Disease Control in Atlanta, Georgia. The ongoing management of the patient would include regular total patient assessment, with a focus on identifying possible toxic and side effects of the drugs being prescribed for this disease. Early in the management phase, instruction should be started about the drugs that will be used and their possible side effects.

■ Evaluation

Therapy for leprosy, as indicated in the text, is often continued for 5 years or longer. Before discharging the patient for self-management, the nurse should be certain that the patient is able to explain why and how to take the drugs prescribed, side effects which may occur, side effects which require notification of the physician, possible ways to treat more commonly seen side effects, and any additional measures which may be prescribed related to the actual stage of the disease as it was diagnosed. This disease needs to be reported to the local health department for family follow-up.

■ TREATMENT OF LEPROSY

Leprosy, like tuberculosis, is today primarily found in developing countries and rarely encountered in the United States or Great Britain. Also like tuberculosis, leprosy is a disease that is curable with appropriate drug therapy.

The primary drug used to treat leprosy is a sulfone called *dapsone*. Although other sulfone drugs are available, dapsone is the most reliable and least toxic. Patients require a minimum of 5 years of therapy; some must be treated for life. Long-term treatment is required because *Mycobacterium leprae,* the causative agent of leprosy, is a very slow-growing organism and may remain dormant for long periods in the human body.

Alternatives to the sulfones are slowly being introduced into therapeutic regimens for leprosy. One investigational drug is *clofazimine,* which seems as effective as dapsone. Moreover, strains of *M. leprae* that acquire resistance to dapsone remain sensitive to clofazimine. Rifampin has also been used in other countries for the treatment of leprosy and is apparently effective. This use of rifampin has not yet been approved in the United States.

Several studies are now underway evaluating a multidrug treatment schedule for leprosy. These studies have used sulfones, clofazimine, rifampin, and another drug used also for tuberculosis, ethionamide. Although this combination chemotherapy is rational, the clinical evaluation of effectiveness will take several years.

The properties of drugs used to treat leprosy are summarized in Table 46-3.

■ PATIENT CARE IMPLICATIONS

General guidelines on the care of patients with tuberculosis or leprosy

1. Patients who learn they have tuberculosis or leprosy are often upset at their diagnosis and need repeated comforting, teaching, and emotional support. The family should also be included in teaching sessions.
2. It is important that patients understand the need for long, continuous therapy with drugs for tuberculosis and leprosy. If patients fail to take their medications as ordered, individualized problem solving with the patient is often needed to help the patient cope with the diagnosis, the drugs, and the drug side effects.
3. Encourage patients to return for their routine follow-up visits, as blood work can be done to monitor for possible side effects of drug therapy, additional cultures can be done if needed, and the patient's overall condition can be monitored.
4. Working with patients who are diagnosed as having tuberculosis (pulmonary tuberculosis being the most common form) should cause little concern to health care practitioners. Patients should be started on drug therapy and instructed to cough or sneeze into disposable tissues and to dispose of tissues appropriately. With these precautions, there is little danger of contracting tuberculosis unless there is repeated prolonged contact with the patient. Of greater danger to health care personnel are undiagnosed patients with tuberculosis.
5. Referral to a visiting nurse association will be helpful.
6. For more information about these two diseases, consult an infection control nurse at a local hospital; the state, county, or city health department; or the Center for Disease Control in Atlanta, Georgia.
7. Practicing health care personnel should be tested for tuberculosis on a regular basis, at least annually or as frequently as the employing agency requires.
8. Review the patient care implications section in Chapter 44.
9. Review the information in Tables 46-1 to 46-3.

Isoniazid

1. Patients receiving isoniazid should be questioned about numbness, tingling, paresthesias, and feelings of heaviness in the arms and legs as this may indicate the development of peripheral neuropathy. Some physicians will choose to treat all patients who are taking isoniazid with pyridoxine prophylactically to prevent the peripheral neuropathy rather than waiting until symptoms develop.
2. Symptoms of hepatitis include fever, jaundice, right upper quadrant abdominal pain, and sometimes changes in the appearance of stools. Encourage the patient to report any unusual symptoms.
3. Phenytoin may be potentiated in patients taking isoniazid, so it may be necessary to monitor phenytoin blood concentrations and even to reduce the dosage while patients are taking isoniazid. Caution patients to be alert to signs of phenytoin toxicity (Chapter 31).
4. Patients should be encouraged to avoid the use of alcohol.
5. Taking isoniazid with meals may reduce gastric irritation.
6. A wide variety of side effects has been attributed to isoniazid therapy, but a causal relationship has not always been found. Encourage patients to return for routine follow-up and to report any symptoms that seem unusual. Appropriate assessment should be done of any patient complaint.
7. *Parenteral isoniazid:* Reconstitute the drug as directed on the vial. Pain may occur at the injection site following intramuscular administration. If the drug crystallizes in the vial, warm the solution to room temperature to redissolve.

Ethambutol

1. Encourage patients to report any visual changes they experience (examples might be changes in color vision, decreased acuity, decreased peripheral vision). Pretreatment ophthalmological examinations are probably indicated only in patients with cataracts, diabetic retinopathy, and optic neuritis, but careful questioning and assessment of visual ability should be done with all patients during follow-up visits.
2. General side effects include anorexia, nausea, vomiting, gastrointestinal upset, and abdominal pain. Taking ethambutol with meals may reduce gastric irritation.

Rifampin

1. Alert patient to the fact that body fluids (tears, sweat, feces, and urine) may turn orange-red while they are receiving therapy. Soft contact lenses may become permanently stained.
2. Liver abnormalities are the most common side effect of this drug. Symptoms that may indicate liver dysfunction include anorexia, malaise, jaundice, or a change in the stools. Instruct the patient to report any unusual feelings or symptoms.
3. Abdominal distress, aching in joints and muscles, and leg cramps are often reported after initiation of therapy but will usually disappear in a few weeks.
4. Encourage patients not to miss rifampin doses. An immunological reaction characterized by dyspnea, wheezing, purpura, thrombocytopenia, and anaphylactic-type reactions have occurred with intermittent therapy or when the drug has been resumed after a lapse of days or weeks.
5. Patients taking coumarin anticoagulants, methadone, oral hypoglycemic agents, digitalis, oral contraceptives, or replacement doses of corticosteroids may find the effectiveness of these drugs decreased, resulting in a need for a change in dosage. Persons relying on oral contraceptives for birth control may wish to use additional or alternate methods of birth control while receiving rifampin therapy.
6. Although taking rifampin with food may not be clinically significant in relation to the amount absorbed, it is recommended that rifampin be taken 1 hour before or 2 hours after a meal if it can be tolerated that way.

Streptomycin

This drug is discussed in Chapter 44.

Para-aminosalicylic acid

1. Gastrointestinal upset is a very common problem with PAS and is often the source of patient noncompliance. Encourage patients to take the drug with meals, antacids, or a snack. It is unpleasant to take; a 12 Gm per day adult dose requires consumption of 24 of the 500 mg tablets.
2. Because of the rare but serious side effect of exfoliative dermatitis, the patient should be cautioned to report immediately the appearance of any rash or skin changes.
3. Hepatic dysfunction may be manifested by malaise, jaundice, anorexia, change in stools, and fever. Instruct patients to report any unusual sign or symptom.
4. Patients receiving oral anticoagulants may require a change in dosage of their anticoagulant.
5. Discoloration of the tablets indicates deterioration, and the tablets should be discarded and a new supply obtained.
6. Because PAS is excreted primarily in the urine, patients should be encouraged to maintain a good intake (2000 to 2500 ml per day in the adult) to prevent crystalluria.

Dapsone

1. Complete blood counts should be done before initiating therapy with dapsone and at regular intervals during therapy. Drug-related blood dyscrasias can include agranulocytosis and aplastic anemia. Instruct the patient to report symptoms of malaise, fever, sore throat, jaundice, or purpura.
2. Dermatitis is a rare side effect but may be serious, as exfoliative dermatitis can ensue. The patient should be cautioned to report the appearance of any skin changes.
3. Peripheral neuropathy is a rare but definite complication that can occur. Patients should be instructed to report any tingling, heaviness, numbness, unusual sensations, or paresthesias that occur in the arms and legs.
4. General side effects include nausea, vomiting, abdominal pain, headache, vertigo, and tinnitus.

■ SUMMARY

The disease called tuberculosis is caused by four strains of *Mycobacterium*. Mycobacteria are slow-growing strict aerobes that resist the digestive action of macrophages. These properties of the organism make tuberculosis more difficult to treat than other bacterial infections. The disease is contagious only during active phases. Long dormant periods are common. Mycobacteria can develop resistance to antituberculosis drugs, causing therapeutic failures. To minimize this complication, multiple drug therapy is the rule.

Isoniazid may be used in combination with other drugs to treat tuberculosis or alone for prophylaxis in patients who have been exposed to the disease. Isoniazid inhibits cell wall biosynthesis and utilization of pyridoxine in mycobacteria. Isoniazid is well absorbed orally and is actively metabolized by the liver. Rapid acetylators and slow acetylators exist in most normal populations. Isoniazid is associated most prominently with hepatotoxicity, especially in older patients.

Ethambutol is an effective first-line drug; it is as well absorbed as isoniazid but less extensively metabolized. Ethambutol may cause visual disturbances, which are reversible if therapy is stopped when this reaction appears.

Rifampin inhibits DNA-dependent RNA polymerase in several strains of mycobacteria. This oral agent is relatively lipid soluble and may concentrate in body tissues. The drug is eliminated via the bile. Rifampin may produce a flulike syndrome leading to life-threatening complications, especially if the drug is used intermittently.

Streptomycin inhibits protein synthesis in mycobacteria as well as in other types of bacteria. The drug is used only by the intramuscular route and is therefore most frequently used in initial therapy as part of a two- or three-drug treatment program.

PAS inhibits folic acid metabolism in *Mycobacterium*. PAS is absorbed by the oral route and excreted by the kidney. PAS produced significant gastrointestinal toxicity in most patients. Other toxicity is related to allergic reactions to the drug and electrolyte imbalances produced by the high ion content of the PAS preparations.

Capreomycin, cycloserine, ethionamide, and pyrizinamide are considered second-line drugs for tuberculosis primarily because of lower activity and higher toxicity of these agents.

Leprosy, a very slowly developing disease produced by a strain of *Mycobacterium leprae*, is effectively treated with sulfones. The most effective of these agents is dapsone. Therapy must continue for several years to assure that the disease will be cured.

■ STUDY QUESTIONS

1. What organisms cause the disease called tuberculosis?
2. What properties of mycobacteria make control of tuberculosis more difficult than that of many other bacterial diseases?
3. Where is the initial site of tuberculosis infection?
4. During what phase of tuberculosis is the disease contagious?
5. Why is tuberculosis usually treated by multiple drug therapy?
6. What is the duration of therapy for tuberculosis?
7. What is the mechanism of action of isoniazid?
8. What is the outcome of using isoniazid alone to treat active tuberculosis?
9. When may isoniazid be used alone in therapy of tuberculosis?
10. How is isoniazid administered in tuberculosis therapy?
11. What is the fate of isoniazid in the body?
12. What toxicity is associated with isoniazid?
13. What is the mechanism of action of ethambutol?
14. How is ethambutol administered in tuberculosis therapy?
15. What toxicity is associated with ethambutol?
16. What is the mechanism of action of rifampin?
17. How is rifampin administered in tuberculosis therapy?
18. How may the timing of rifampin therapy influence the toxicity the drug produces?
19. What is the mechanism of action of streptomycin?
20. How is streptomycin administered?
21. What toxicity is associated with the use of streptomycin?
22. What is the mechanism of action of PAS?
23. How is PAS administered in tuberculosis therapy?
24. What toxicity is associated with the use of PAS?
25. Why are certain drugs classed as second-line drugs in tuberculosis therapy?
26. What drugs are most useful in treating leprosy?
27. How long must therapy continue for control of leprosy?

■ SUGGESTED READINGS

Iseman, M.D.: Tuberculosis—far from eradicated, Consultant **20**(12):157, 1980.

Modderman, E.S.: Dapsone, still the first choice in leprosy, Pharmacy International **1**(10):198, 1980.

Pinsker, K.L., and Koerner, S.K.: Chemotherapy of tuberculosis, Drug Therapy Reviews **1**:186, 1977.

47 Antifungal agents

Fungal diseases range from mild infections in localized areas of the skin to grave systemic infections. Diseases of various types may be produced by a wide range of fungi, and to a great extent the seriousness of the infection is determined by the nature of the infective organism. In this chapter some of the more common and some of the more serious fungal diseases are examined and the drugs that are used to control these specific infections are considered.

■ SELECTIVE TOXICITY IN THE TREATMENT OF FUNGAL DISEASES

Although the fungi that cause disease in humans are single-celled organisms, they are eucaryotes (Chapter 40) and therefore resemble humans more than bacteria in their biochemical properties. These biochemical similarities to humans present therapeutic problems. For instance, none of the antibiotics that inhibit bacterial protein synthesis affect that process in fungi. The ribosomes that form protein in fungi are very much like those from humans and are sensitive to the same drugs. Therefore selective toxicity cannot be achieved by this mechanism. Likewise fungi resist the action of sulfonamides as do mammalian cells. Moreover fungal cells do not contain a peptidoglycan cell wall, which renders them resistant to all antibiotics that block peptidoglycan synthesis (e.g., penicillins). For these reasons the antimicrobial agents considered in previous chapters are useless in treating fungal disease.

Design of new antifungal agents is limited by the number of known biochemical differences between fungal and mammalian cells. A few individual enzymes seem to possess different drug sensitivities in humans and fungi. However, the only systematically exploited difference between humans and fungi lies in the outer membranes of the two cell types. The cells of humans contain cholesterol in their membranes, whereas those of fungi contain ergosterol. This feature of membrane structure is the basis of action of the polyene antifungal drugs. Polyene antifungal agents have a greater affinity for ergosterol than for cholesterol and therefore somewhat selectively react with ergosterol from fungal cell membranes. This action destroys the integrity of the cell membrane, cytoplasmic components are lost, and the cell dies. However, the selectivity of these drugs is not so great as most drugs used for treating bacterial infections.

Fungal cells do possess many cell surface antigens, which ultimately provoke host immune responses. Most fungal infections resolve in this way, many times without the host ever being aware of an active disease. This pattern is especially common with the fungal diseases spread by breathing in spores from contaminated soil. Examples of diseases of this type are histoplasmosis, blastomycosis, coccidioidomycosis, cryptococcosis, and aspergillosis. Several of these diseases are concentrated in specific geographic areas. For example, coccidioidomycosis is most common, or endemic, in the southernmost portions of California, Nevada, Utah, Arizona, New Mexico, and Texas, whereas histoplasmosis is most common in the states bordering the Mississippi and Ohio rivers. Blastomycosis is common in isolated areas along the Mississippi and Ohio rivers, around the Great Lakes, the St. Lawrence river, and in the Carolinas.

Some fungal diseases are spread by contact with soil contaminated with bird droppings. Birds are not necessarily affected by these diseases, but they do frequently carry the organisms. Cryptococcosis frequently follows exposure to high concentrations of pigeon droppings. Histoplasmosis is associated with avian excreta such as chicken or starling droppings or bat guano.

Although pulmonary forms of the aforementioned diseases are usually mild and limited by effective development of immunity in the victim, in rare cases the fungus may become disseminated and invade other body tissues. A notorious example is the yeast *Cryptococcus neoformans,* which can cause meningitis as well as pulmonary disease and infections at many other sites. The disseminated, or systemic, fungal diseases are most likely to develop in patients whose immune system is depressed by disease or drug therapy, especially with glucocorticoids or immunosuppressant antineoplastic agents.

The yeast *Candida* may cause a range of infections from serious systemic disease to annoying mucous membrane infections. Since *Candida* is normally found on the skin and mucous membranes of healthy persons, the growth of *Candida* to cause disease usually represents an opportunistic infection. *Candida* infections are therefore most common in persons receiving broad-spectrum antibacterial drugs such as tetracyclines (suprainfections, Chapter 40) or in persons with suppressed immune systems.

Fungi whose growth is almost always restricted to the skin of humans are termed *dermatophytes*. These fungi cause the annoying infections commonly known as *ringworm* and *athlete's foot,* as well as several others. This group of infections is frequently referred to as *tinea*. Drugs used for these superficial infections are not the same as those employed for systemic fungal infections. Many of the drugs used topically are not absorbed extensively through the skin. Therefore much more toxic agents may be employed and selective toxicity is achieved against many dermatophytes.

■ DRUGS USED TO TREAT SYSTEMIC FUNGAL INFECTIONS

Amphotericin B

Mechanism of action. Amphotericin B is a polyene antifungal drug whose action depends on selectively damaging membranes containing ergosterol, that is, fungal membranes. Unfortunately, this membrane-disruptive effect is not entirely selective, and some of the cholesterol-containing membranes of mammalian cells are also damaged. Nevertheless, amphotericin B can be clinically useful in treating a broad spectrum of fungal diseases, including those caused by *Histoplasma, Blastomyces, Cryptococcus, Aspergillus,* and others. Amphotericin B may also be used to treat systemic *Candida* and *Coccidioides* infections.

Absorption, distribution, and excretion. Amphotericin B is not absorbed orally and must be administered intravenously, although the drug is irritating to vascular tissue and frequently causes phlebitis. The drug is lipid soluble and is administered as a colloidal suspension stabilized with small amounts of the detergent desoxycholate. Amphotericin B must be infused at a concentration of less than 0.1 mg/ml in a 5% dextrose solution. Higher drug concentrations will cause the precipitation of the drug in the intravenous solution and will endanger the patient.

Since amphotericin B has a high affinity for lipid, the drug tends to bind to tissues rather than remain in the bloodstream. The elimination half-life of the drug is about 12 hours following a single intravenous dose. During long-term therapy, only a fraction of the daily dose can be recovered in the urine or feces. The unrecovered drug is apparently held in tissues, since amphotericin B continues to appear in the urine for long periods after therapy is halted. The tissue binding properties and the relative water insolubility of amphotericin B prevent the drug from entering body fluids efficiently. For this reason, concentrations of the drug in the cerebrospinal fluid or in ocular fluid are rather low and may not be high enough to effectively eliminate infections at those sites. To overcome this problem, amphotericin B may be injected intrathecally (into the cerebrospinal fluid) for meningitis.

Toxicity. Most patients treated with amphotericin B are begun on low doses of the drug, and the dosage is increased as tolerance to the ensuing toxic reactions develop. Headache, fever, nausea, and vomiting may occur after the first few injections but usually subside as therapy continues. Renal damage progresses with length of therapy and may become irreversible when total doses of amphotericin B approach 4 Gm. Anemia also develops with time, as do a number of electrolyte disturbances including acidosis and hypokalemia (low blood potassium).

Amphotericin B therapy must be continued for long periods to create the possibility of a cure for disseminated fungal disease. No firm guidelines for therapy exist, although as a general rule, physicians try to limit the total drug dose to under 4 Gm. Even with doses approaching this limit, cures are not always obtained. For many patients therapy must be discontinued early because of toxic effects of the drug.

Flucytosine

Mechanism of action. Flucytosine is a pyrimidine analog which is apparently converted to the cytotoxic agent 5-fluorouracil in sensitive fungi. Since this metabolite is not freely formed in humans, a degree of selective toxicity is achieved. Unfortunately, a relatively narrow range of fungi are sensitive to the drug, including *Cryptococcus, Candida,* and a few other very rarely encountered pathogenic fungi. Intrinsic resistance to flucytosine may exist in a significant number of clinically encountered *Candida* strains, and resistance to the drug may be acquired by *Cryptococcus* during therapy. This pattern of resistance has limited the usefulness of flucytosine.

Absorption, distribution, and excretion. Flucytosine is a water-soluble drug that is well absorbed from the gastrointestinal tract and well distributed into body fluids. Drug concentration in cerebrospinal fluid may be 50% to 70% of serum levels, in contrast to amphotericin B for which cerebrospinal fluid levels are less than 5% of serum levels. The primary organ of excretion for flucytosine is the kidney; upwards of 90% of an oral dose can be recovered intact in the urine. Urine concentrations of the drug tend to be high. The elimination half-time of the drug is around 6 hours.

Toxicity. Flucytosine therapy is usually continued for several weeks to several months. Unlike amphotericin B, few patients are forced to discontinue medication due to toxic reactions. Nausea and diarrhea appear in roughly one-fourth of the patients treated with flucytosine. Blood dyscrasias and transient liver abnormalities have been reported. Since flucytosine is now frequently administered with amphotericin B, it may be difficult to distinguish which toxic reactions are caused by flucytosine.

The rationale for combining flucytosine and amphotericin B therapy for serious infections caused by fungi is twofold. First, the combination allows the dose of amphotericin B to be lowered somewhat, thereby reducing toxicity. Second, the development of resistance to flucytosine is minimized by combination chemotherapy. Full evaluation of the effectiveness of combined therapy has not been completed.

■ Rarely used drugs for systemic fungal infections

Amphotericin B and flucytosine are the drugs most appropriate for the vast majority of systemic fungal diseases. However, a few other drugs are used in rare instances. For example, *2-hydroxystilbamidine* is used to treat patients with blastomycosis. The drug is useful only for that disease. Patients with skin forms or noncavitary pulmonary forms of the disease benefit most from 2-hydroxystilbamidine therapy; more serious forms of blastomycosis require amphotericin B therapy (Table 47-1).

Clotrimazole and *miconazole* are compounds that, when applied topically, effectively control superficial fungal infections of various types (Table 47-2). In addition, these drugs have been used for systemic fungal infections. Current clinical data suggest clotrimazole to be toxic and relatively ineffective in the treatment of most serious fungal infections. Miconazole may be effective when administered intravenously to treat systemic *Candida, Cryptococcus,* and *Aspergillus* infections (Table 47-1).

TABLE 47-1. Summary of drugs used to treat systemic fungal infections

Generic name	Trade name	Drug class and mechanism of action	Dosage and administration	Clinical use	Principal toxic reactions
Amphotericin B	Fungizone	Polyene. Cell membrane disruption.	INTRAVENOUS: *Adults and children*—0.25 to 1 mg/kg infused at 0.1 mg/ml in 5% dextrose over 6 hr. Total drug course usually less than 4 Gm.	Disseminated, symptomatic fungal disease due to *Histoplasma, Blastomyces, Coccidioides, Cryptococcus, Aspergillus, Candida,* and others.	Initial headache, nausea, vomiting, and fever. Progressive nephrotoxicity, anemia, and renal electrolyte imbalance.
Flucytosine	Ancobon	Pyrimidine analog. Incorporated into defective nucleic acid.	ORAL: *Adults and children*—50 to 200 mg/kg daily in 4 doses. Lower drug doses are required when renal function is impaired.	Disseminated fungal infections due to sensitive *Candida* strains; combined with amphotericin B for cryptococcal meningitis.	Nausea and diarrhea are relatively common. Blood dyscrasias are less common and are usually mild.
2-Hydroxystilbamidine			INTRAVENOUS: *Adults*—225 mg in 200 ml of 5% dextrose or saline daily. Total drug course usually less than 8 Gm.	Blastomycosis of skin or lungs. Not for use in serious disseminated disease.	Hypotension and tachycardia during too rapid infusion. Nausea, vomiting, malaise, and headache are common. Dizziness, paresthesias, incontinence, and edema of face occur less commonly and usually clear rapidly.
Miconazole	Monistat-IV	Imidazole derivative. Disrupts fungal cell permeability.	INTRAVENOUS: *Adults and children over 1 yr*—25 to 30 mg/kg 2 or 3 times daily.	Systemic infections caused by *Candida, Cryptococcus,* and *Aspergillus.* Also used topically (see Table 47-2).	Thrombophlebitis, gastrointestinal distress, blood dyscrasias, and allergic reactions have been reported with intravenous use.

TABLE 47-2. Summary of drugs used to treat topical fungal infections

Generic name	**Trade name**	**Dosage and administration**	**Clinical use**	**Principal toxic reactions**	**Comments**
Acrisorcin	Akrinol	TOPICAL: *Adults and children*—cream (2 mg/Gm) applied twice daily.	Tinea versicolor only.	Blisters and skin irritation.	Do not use around eyes.
Amphotericin B	Fungizone	TOPICAL: *Adults and children*—3% cream, lotion, or ointment applied 2 to 4 times daily.	*Candida* infections of skin or mucous membranes.	Local tissue irritation.	Allergic reactions may rarely occur.
Candicidin	Candeptin Vanobid	INTRAVAGINAL: *Adults*—capsule, tablet, or ointment containing 3 mg drug twice daily.	Vaginal *Candida* infections only.	Irritation of vulvar area.	Male sexual partners should be treated for *Candida* to avoid reinfection.
Clioquinol or iodochlorhydroxyquin	Vioform	TOPICAL: *Adults and children*—3% cream, ointment, or powder applied several times daily.	Localized dermatophytoses.	Irritation of skin; usually mild but eyes must be avoided.	Clioquinol has both antifungal and antibacterial activity, aiding in therapy of mixed infections (nonprescription).
Clotrimazole	Gyne-Lotrimin Lotrimin Mycelex	TOPICAL: *Adults and children*—1% cream or solution applied twice daily. INTRAVAGINAL: *Adults*—Tablets or creams containing 100 mg inserted once daily.	Broad spectrum of antifungal activity.	Skin irritation, pruritus, urticaria. General irritation may be severe enough to cause drug to be discontinued.	Do not use around eyes.
Griseofulvin	Fulvicin Grifulvin Grisactin Gris-Peg	ORAL: *Adults*—500 mg microcrystalline form in single or divided daily dose. *Children*—10 mg/kg daily.	Tinea infections with the exception of tinea versicolor. Not for *Candida* infections.	Blood dyscrasias may rarely occur. Headache occurs early in treatment. Gastrointestinal disturbances, neuritis, allergies, and hepatotoxicity may occur.	Griseofulvin interferes with warfarin anticoagulant action. Barbiturates decrease griseofulvin activity.

Haloprogin	Halotex	TOPICAL: *Adults and children*—1% cream or solution applied twice daily.	Tinea and other superficial fungal infections.	Local tissue irritation or maceration.	Do not use around eyes.
Miconazole	Micatin Monistat	TOPICAL: *Adults and children*—2% cream or lotion applied twice daily. INTRAVAGINAL: *Adults*—2% cream once daily.	Dermatophytosis or *Candida* infections.	Local tissue irritation or maceration.	Use with care around the eyes.
Nystatin	Candex Mycostatin Nilstat O-V Statin	ORAL: *Adults and children*—0.5 to 1 million units 3 times daily. *Infants*—0.1 to 0.2 million units 4 times daily.	*Candida* infections of intestinal tract.	Nausea, vomiting, diarrhea.	Drug is not absorbed from intestinal tract.
		TOPICAL: *Adults and children*—ointments, creams, lotions (0.1 million units/Gm) applied twice daily.	*Candida* infections of skin.	Irritation of skin.	
		INTRAVAGINAL: *Adults*—tablets, 0.1 to 0.2 million units daily.	*Candida* infections of vagina.	Irritation is rare.	Relief of symptoms is rapid, but dosage should be continued for 2 wk or longer if necessary.
Tolnaftate	Aftate Tinactin	TOPICAL: *Adults and children*—1% cream, gel, solution, powder, or aerosol applied twice daily.	Tinea infections only. Not effective against *Candida*.	Rarely causes irritation or sensitization.	Avoid eyes. 2 to 3 wk of therapy is usually sufficient (nonprescription).
Undecylenic acid	Desenex Ting Undecylenic compound Unde-Jen	TOPICAL: *Adults and children*—ointment (5%, with 20% zinc undecylenate), powder (2%, with 20% zinc undecylenate), 10% solution, 2% soap applied twice daily.	Athlete's foot and ringworm in areas other than around nails or hairy areas.	Should not be allowed to contact eyes or mucous membranes.	Diabetics and others with impaired circulation should use only with physician's advice (nonprescription).
Calcium undecylenate	Caldesene Cruex	TOPICAL: *Adults and children*—10% powder applied as needed.	Tinea cruris (jock itch). Also used for diaper rash or other skin irritations of groin area.	Powder should not be inhaled or allowed to contact eyes or mucous membranes.	Diabetics and others with impaired circulation should use only with physician's advice (nonprescription).

■ DRUGS USED TO TREAT LOCALIZED OR TOPICAL FUNGAL INFECTIONS

In this section the drugs that are useful to treat fungal infections restricted to skin, mucous membranes, or gastrointestinal tract are considered. The properties of specific drugs are listed in Table 47-2. Most of these agents are used strictly locally, being applied at the site of infection. For example, *tolnaftate* is an effective agent for simple cases of tinea, but the effectiveness is limited by the accessibility of locally applied drug to the infective fungi. For this reason, tinea infections around nails and heavily keratinized skin are hard to eradicate.

Griseofulvin is an effective drug for the treatment of several types of dermatophytic infections. Griseofulvin is administered orally rather than used topically. For this reason, griseofulvin is especially useful for treating fungal infections of the scalp. The usefulness of this drug as an oral agent depends on the ability of griseofulvin to localize in the skin following oral absorption. Those skin cells containing high concentrations of griseofulvin are resistant to infection by dermatophytes. Ultimately, all infected cells will be lost through the natural sloughing off of skin cells and the disease will be cured. This process takes a considerable period of time and, accordingly, griseofulvin therapy may need to be continued for several weeks or several months, depending on the site and severity of the infection.

Nystatin is sometimes administered orally to treat intestinal fungal infections. This treatment may be considered topical, since nystatin is not absorbed orally and is retained in the intestinal tract. Nystatin is also used for treating vaginal infections, such as those caused by *Candida*. This treatment is also local, since the drug is administered intravaginally and is not significantly absorbed from that site. Nystatin is too toxic to be used for systemic infections.

Numerous over-the-counter preparations are available for treating fungal infections of the skin. Some of these preparations contain useful antifungal agents, whereas others are practically useless. The most effective preparations are identified in Table 47-2.

Antifungal agents are also available in combination with various antibacterial drugs. The rationale for these combinations is based on the fact that many infections diagnosed as fungal are, in fact, mixed bacterial and fungal infections. Full resolution of symptoms may therefore require treatment with an antibacterial and an antifungal agent. However, this therapy is best accomplished by using two separate preparations so that the most effective drugs for the patient's specific infection may be chosen. Moreover, dosage adjustment is easier with separate preparations.

■ PATIENT CARE IMPLICATIONS

Review the patient care implications section in Chapter 40.

Amphotericin B

1. Patients receiving amphotericin B via intravenous infusion will be hospitalized for 6 weeks or longer for the course of therapy.
2. Most patients will suffer some side effects while receiving amphotericin B. Common complaints include headache, fever, chills, nausea, anorexia, vomiting, and diarrhea. Infrequently seen side effects include hypertension or hypotension, coagulation defects, tinnitus, rash, and vertigo; anaphylactic reactions are rare. Treatment of side effects is symptomatic, and as it becomes clear what an individual patient's response will be, the anticipatory use of supportive therapy should proceed. Thus the patient may receive, in addition to the amphotericin B, antiemetics, antipyretics, antihistamines, or steroids.
3. Most patients will show some degree of renal damage; therefore appropriate studies (BUN, NPN, serum creatinine, creatinine clearance) should be done prior to therapy and at weekly intervals during therapy. In addition, serum electrolytes should be monitored twice a week, since hypokalemia is frequently observed. Symptoms of hypokalemia include muscle weakness, paresthesias, apathy, and, occasionally, abdominal distention.
4. Parenteral administration:
   a. See the manufacturer's literature for complete instructions about dilution. The final concentration should be less than 0.1 mg/ml.
   b. If an in-line intravenous filter is being used, the mean pore diameter should not be less than 1.0 μm.
   c. Thrombophlebitis often occurs; the addition of a small amount of heparin to the infusion may help. No other drugs should be added to the infusion. Avoid extravasation.
   d. The drug is light-sensitive so the medication must be protected from light during the infusion.
   e. Administer over 6 hours or longer. The use of an electronic infusion monitor may be appropriate.
   f. During infusions, monitor the temperature and vital signs. Fluid intake and output should be monitored during the course of therapy.
5. When amphotericin is used topically, there are virtually no side effects. The cream form may stain skin. A discoloration of fabrics from the cream or lotion can be removed with soap and water. Discoloration from the ointment on clothing can be removed with cleaning fluid.

■ THE NURSING PROCESS

■ Assessment

Fungal infections are relatively common and can occur in patients of any age. Examples of common fungal infections include thrush in the infant, athlete's foot, and vaginal monilial infections in the female. Serious systemic infections are possible with a variety of fungi and, although relatively uncommon, are life-threatening. Initially the patient should receive a thorough total assessment, with a focus on the specific subjective complaints or objective signs that indicate possible fungal infection. Parts of the history that may be important include recent exposure to possible new sources of infection, previous recent use of drugs which may alter the patient's immune response, and measures the patient has tried to this point for eradication of the problem. Obviously the depth of assessment will vary based on the nature of the problem as the patient presents it; the patient with a systemic infection could be obviously seriously ill and would thus need a different kind of assessment than an infant with the relatively common problem of oral thrush. Early diagnosis of fungal infections is enhanced by having a high degree of awareness; patients more likely to have fungal infections include those receiving cancer chemotherapy, immunotherapy, antibiotic therapy, or drugs that alter the normal pH of such areas as the vagina; patients receiving alimentation via peripheral or central venous catheters; and patients taking high doses of adrenocortical steroids.

■ Management

The management phase is often two-pronged. One aspect of the management phase is treatment with an appropriate drug for the fungal infection itself. The second aspect of care is removal of possible causative agents of the infection, including discontinuing drugs that may predispose the patient to fungal infections. For example, the adolescent female taking tetracycline for control of acne may need to have this drug discontinued at least temporarily to successfully treat vaginal monilial infections. During the management phase, the nurse needs to teach the patient about the drugs prescribed, about the infection itself, and about possible ways to limit the spread of the infection and to prevent its recurrence in the future. Treatment of systemic fungal infections is more serious. These patients often require long-term hospitalization with regular intravenous antifungal drug therapy. The nurse should monitor the vital signs and appropriate laboratory work to evaluate possible side effects. It may be appropriate, depending on the patient's response, to measure the fluid intake and output; to use additional drugs to control side effects such as headache, nausea, and vomiting; and to adjust meals and other patient activities to times in the day when the patient is better able to tolerate them. The use of an infusion monitoring device may be appropriate.

■ Evaluation

Therapy with antifungal agents should eradicate the infection. With the exception of the systemically used drugs, side effects are relatively uncommon. Before discharging a patient for self-management with an antifungal agent, the patient should be able to explain why the drug is being used, explain exactly how it should be used and under what circumstances, what to do if side effects should occur, and which side effects require notification of the physician. The patient should be able to explain any other measures suggested to provide relief of symptoms or treatment of the infection and what to do if symptoms do not begin to clear within 3 to 7 days. For further information, see the patient care implications section at the end of this chapter.

Flucytosine

1. Side effects of flucytosine include anorexia, nausea, vomiting, diarrhea, rash, headache, drowsiness, and vertigo. Side effects are seen less often with this drug than with amphotericin, although if both are being used concurrently, it may be difficult to decide which one is causing a specific side effect.
2. Blood work should be done at regular intervals to monitor for hematopoietic, renal, and hepatic changes that can occur. Most commonly, the drug produces neutropenia, eosinophilia, thrombocytopenia, and elevations of hepatic enzymes, BUN, and creatinine.
3. If nausea occurs, it may be reduced by giving the capsules a few at a time over a 15- to 20-minute period.

Miconazole

1. Side effects of intravenous therapy include phlebitis, pruritus, rash, anorexia, nausea, vomiting, diarrhea, and drowsiness. Nausea and vomiting may be reduced by giving an antiemetic or antihistamine before administering the drug, by not giving miconazole at mealtimes, and by reducing the rate of infusion.
2. Interaction with the coumarin anticoagulants results in enhancement of the anticoagulant effect; reduction in the dose of anticoagulant may be needed. Caution the patient to be alert for signs of bleeding and bruising.
3. For dilution, see the manufacturer's literature. The rate of infusion should be 30 to 60 minutes per dose.

Griseofulvin

1. Griseofulvin interferes with the activity of warfarin-type anticoagulants. It may be necessary to increase the dose of anticoagulants.
2. The drug may cause photosensitivity. Instruct patients to avoid prolonged exposure to the sun or ultraviolet light.

Nystatin

1. When nystatin is used to treat oral *Candida* infections, a drug suspension is used. The patient's mouth should be free of food particles when the suspension form is administered. Instruct the patient to place one half of the dose in each side of the mouth and to hold it as long as possible before swallowing.
2. The vaginal suppositories can also be used orally. Instruct the patient to suck on the tablet-like suppository to allow for prolonged contact in the mouth. The dose should not be chewed and swallowed.

Topical antifungal agents

1. Serious side effects with topical antifungal agents are rare but may occur. Instruct patients to report any local irritation (rash, burning, pruritus) or any systemic symptoms that occur.
2. Intravaginal medications should be used during pregnancy only when the physician considers it absolutely necessary.
3. Ascertain that women can accurately and correctly use the applicator supplied with intravaginal preparations. Use of the agent should continue during the menstrual period. Some women may find better treatment results if sanitary napkins are worn, not tampons. The routine use of douches is not recommended; consult the physician.

■ SUMMARY

Fungi are eucaryotic organisms and therefore offer little in the way of targets for selectively toxic agents. The polyene antifungal agents achieve some selective toxicity by interacting with fungal cell membranes more readily than with mammalian cell membranes. Other antifungal agents interfere with fungal metabolism in various ways.

Fungal diseases range from mild, self-limited pulmonary disease to serious systemic disease. Very few drugs are available for the treatment of systemic fungal infections. Amphotericin B is used to treat various systemic mycoses, but the drug is very toxic and successful therapy is difficult to achieve. The drug tends to bind to body tissues; nephrotoxicity, anemia, and electrolyte imbalances often occur during therapy.

Flucytosine is less toxic than amphotericin B but is frequently ineffective, since resistance to flucytosine can develop easily. Amphotericin B and flucytosine are sometimes used in combination. Combining the two drugs allows the dose of amphotericin B to be lowered, thereby lowering toxicity, and minimizes the development of resistance to flucytosine. Imidazole antifungal agents, including clotrimazole and miconazole, have also occasionally been used for the treatment of serious fungal infections.

Fungal infections localized to the skin are called dermatophytes. Since therapy can be applied topically in many cases, these infections may be treated with much more toxic agents than can systemic infections. An exception is the drug griseofulvin, which concentrates in the skin after oral administration and helps eliminate fungal infections of the skin.

■ STUDY QUESTIONS

1. Why are fungi resistant to drugs like penicillins and tetracyclines?
2. What animal species commonly spread fungal diseases to humans?
3. What types of infections are commonly caused by *Candida?*
4. What are dermatophytes?
5. What is the mechanism of action for the polyene antifungal agent amphotericin B?
6. By what route is amphotericin B employed?
7. What types of fungal infections are properly treated with amphotericin B?
8. How does the lipid solubility of amphotericin B influence its tissue distribution?
9. What are the characteristic toxic reactions associated with systemic use of amphotericin B?
10. What is the mechanism of action of flucytosine?
11. May flucytosine be employed as an oral agent?
12. What is the main route of excretion of flucytosine?
13. What toxic reactions occur with the use of flucytosine?
14. Why are flucytosine and amphotericin B sometimes combined for antifungal therapy?
15. For what purpose is the drug 2-hydroxystilbamidine prescribed?
16. May miconazole be employed for systemic fungal infections?
17. What is the mechanism of action of griseofulvin?
18. How is griseofulvin administered?
19. Is therapy with griseofulvin long or short term?
20. What types of fungal disease may be treated with the polyene nystatin?

■ SUGGESTED READINGS

Antifungal agents. In AMA drug evaluations, ed. 4, New York, 1980, John Wiley & Sons.

Heel, R.C., Brogden, R.N., Pakes, G.E., Speight, T.M., and Avery, G.S.: Miconazole: a preliminary review of its therapeutic efficacy in systemic fungal infections, Drugs **19:**7, 1980.

How to use intravenous antibiotics, Nurses' Drug Alert (special issue) **1:**89, June, 1977.

MacLeod, S.M., Ti, T.Y., Williams, R.B., Sellers, E.M.: Parenteral 5-flucytosine for candidiasis, Drug Intelligence and Clinical Pharmacy **13:**72, 1979.

Maddux, M.S., and Barriere, S.L.: A review of complications of amphotericin-B therapy: recommendations for prevention and management, Drug Intelligence and Clinical Pharmacy **14:**177, 1980.

Stranz, H.M.: Miconazole, Drug Intelligence and Clinical Pharmacy **14:**87, 1980.

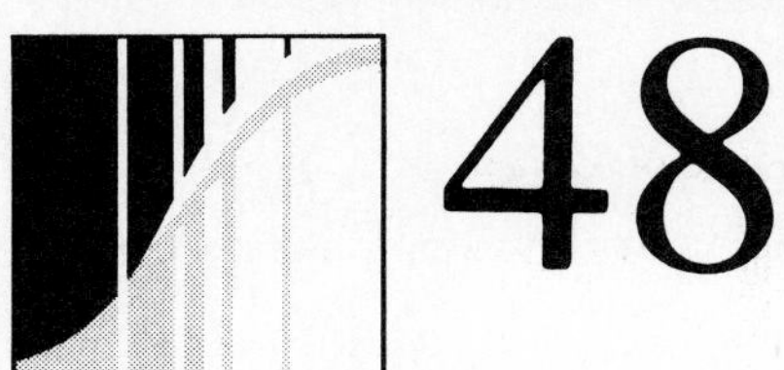

48 The treatment of viral diseases

Viral diseases are among the most common infections in humans, yet the prevention and treatment of these diseases has lagged far behind the ability to control bacterial infections. This chapter discusses the properties of viral diseases that make them difficult to prevent or treat and the mechanisms of action of antiviral drugs that have been developed.

■ NATURE OF VIRAL DISEASES

Viruses cause a wide variety of clinical disease, including some conditions that have only recently been recognized as viral in origin. Viral diseases may be classified as acute, chronic, or slow. Acute illnesses include the common cold, influenza, and various other respiratory tract infections. These illnesses frequently resolve very quickly and leave no latent infections or sequelae. Chronic infections are those in which the disease runs a protracted course with long periods of remission interspersed with reappearance of the disease. A classic example of this type of viral disease is herpes infection of the skin or conjunctiva in which active disease alternates with latent periods during which the virus remains dormant in nervous tissue. Slow virus infections are diseases that progress over a number of months or years, causing cumulative damage to body tissues and ultimately ending in death of the host. Diseases that are now thought to be slow virus diseases include multiple sclerosis, amyotrophic lateral sclerosis, Alzheimer-Pick disease, and various other degenerative diseases of the central nervous system.

Viral diseases may also be classified as local or generalized. Examples of local viral diseases include those that affect only the tissues of the respiratory tract. For these diseases, symptoms develop as the infection spreads from the original site to immediately adjacent cells. The severity of symptoms depends in part on how many host cells are affected.

Some viruses have the potential for more generalized invasion of tissues throughout the body. This spread may come about in several ways. Viruses such as rabies actually travel along the nervous tissue of humans and eventually invade the brain, causing the characteristic symptoms of rabies. Other viruses spread via the bloodstream; this mechanism is called *viremic spread*. The details of viremic spread are given in Table 48-1. The most important feature to recognize in this process is that clinical symptoms do not appear in most diseases spread in this manner until very late in the disease when the secondary viremia occurs. At this stage most viral infections are self-limiting and will resolve even without medical attention. However, certain viruses can attack the brain following the secondary viremia. An example is the polio virus, which causes relatively mild disease during the respiratory phase and secondary viremic stage but becomes life-threatening when it invades the central nervous system. Even with polioviruses, invasion of the central nervous system is a rare event and most infections end with the secondary viremia.

TABLE 48-1. Viremic spread in mammalian body

Site	Symptoms
PRIMARY SITE OF INFECTION (for example, the lung in pox, measles, mumps; the gastrointestinal tract in polio)	First wave of replication produces no symptoms.
BLOODSTREAM (viruses free or bound to blood cells)	Primary viremia produces no symptoms.
SECONDARY SITES OF INFECTION (for example, the liver, spleen, bone marrow, or lymphoid tissue)	Second wave of replication may produce mild symptoms for some viral diseases.
BLOODSTREAM (viruses free or bound to blood cells)	Secondary viremia may produce fever, rashes, and other symptoms whose severity depends on the number of viruses released.
CENTRAL NERVOUS SYSTEM (rarely involved)	Serious illness; specific symptoms are determined by the area of brain attacked.

TABLE 48-2. Vaccines useful in preventing viral diseases

Disease	Characteristics of vaccine	When administered
Poliomyelitis	Oral vaccine (trivalent) containing attenuated live polio virus mimics natural form of disease without risk of central nervous system involvement.	At 2, 4, 6 mo of age; boosters at 1½ and 6 yr.
Rubella (German measles)	Attenuated live rubella vaccine confers long-term resistance.	After 1 yr of age; especially important that females be immunized before puberty, since disease is most dangerous for fetuses in first trimester.
Measles (rubeola)	Attenuated live virus vaccine stimulates protective antibodies in 95% of children receiving it.	After 15 mo of age.
Mumps	Attenuated live virus vaccine stimulates protective antibodies in 95% of those receiving it.	After 1 yr of age.
Influenza	Inactivated viruses of types causing recent outbreaks. Differs from year to year.	During flu season to patients at high risk.
Smallpox	Success of vaccination is judged by response at vaccination site.	Given to persons traveling to countries recently experiencing outbreaks, or to contacts of victims.
Yellow fever	Live attenuated virus confers resistance on most persons receiving injection.	After 6 mo of age to persons traveling to areas of high exposure.
Rabies	Killed, fixed virus confers resistance to most patients exposed to infection.	Used after being bitten by rabid animal or animal suspected of being rabid.

The fact that symptoms appear late in most viral diseases has implications for chemotherapy of viral diseases: since symptoms occur after most of the virus particles have reproduced, therapy instituted at this stage of the disease can be expected to have limited effectiveness. This pattern is different from bacterial diseases where active bacterial reproduction accompanies the worst clinical symptoms. This relative delay in appearance of clinical symptoms in viral diseases is one of the most important reasons why drug therapy of viral diseases is difficult once the disease is established.

■ RESPONSE OF THE BODY TO VIRAL DISEASES

The external surface of viruses contains antigenic substances that promote the production of antibodies in humans. These humoral factors limit the spread of many types of viral disease and ultimately allow the body to eliminate the virus. Infected cells are also changed sufficiently in many viral diseases so that these cells are also eliminated. Many viral diseases are best controlled by inducing antibodies in healthy individuals prior to exposure to the viral disease. This prophylaxis is successful in the diseases listed in Table 48-2. Vaccines cannot be produced efficiently for many viral diseases, however. One example is rhinoviruses, which cause respiratory disease in humans. Among these viruses there are around 100 strains, each of which induces a specific antibody in humans; however, no antibody attacks more than one of the serotypes. Therefore successful immunization would require that an antibody be developed against each of the 100 pathogenic strains. Such a program is not feasible.

Influenza viruses illustrate another difficulty in immunizing against viral diseases. With influenza the antigenic properties shift every few years so that those persons who were immunized either naturally or artificially against the prevalent strain of the virus are unprotected when the new viral type arises. Therefore influenza immunizations are only effective for a specific viral strain and should not be expected to carry over when new strains appear. The most successful immunization programs are for those viral diseases where few pathogenic strains exist and where antigenic properties do not change. The vaccine for poliovirus fits these criteria. The oral vaccine is directed against the three major viral strains; these strains have not shifted in antigenic properties.

In addition to the traditional immune responses to viral infection, the body has another mechanism by which it limits the spread of viral diseases. This mechanism is the production of interferon. Interferons, released from virus-infected cells and T-type lymphocytes, alter the metabolism of uninfected cells to prevent the virus from attacking these new cells. This mechanism prevents the spread of the viral disease to new cells and allows the immune system to eliminate the viruses and infected cells. In theory interferons would be ideal antiviral agents to use where the natural defenses were insufficient. However, several properties of interferons have made them difficult to use in the clinic. First, interferons are host specific and not virus specific. This property means that interferons induce resistance to several types of viruses at once. This useful property is offset by the fact that the host specificity of interferons determines that only human interferon is effective in preventing viral disease in humans. The only interferon that has been acquired in sufficient quantities for testing has been from cultured leukocytes. Large-scale methods are not yet available for the production of interferon, and the material is therefore unavailable for clinical use. The second property of interferons that makes them less than ideal in the clinic is the fact that the resistance they confer is transient. Long-term protection does not develop as with antibody production. To overcome some of these problems, inducers of interferons have been tested. Although compounds have been developed that successfully induce interferons, the protection produced is again transient. Moreover, cells exposed to the inducers become refractory to further induction for a period of time, making it impossible to continuously maintain high interferon levels. For these reasons interferons remain an interesting class of substances whose clinical usefulness as routine antiviral agents is in doubt. Interferons may be useful in limited circumstances and research in this area continues.

■ SELECTIVE TOXICITY IN THE TREATMENT OF VIRAL DISEASES

Since viral reproduction is carried out mostly by host cell enzymes and ribosomes, targets for selective toxicity are difficult to identify. Virus reproduction can be divided into four steps (Table 48-3). Study of the details of each of these processes has revealed more potential for selective toxicity than was originally thought. It is now known that a few viral enzymes are involved in forming viral nucleic acid, for example. Viral enzymes or processes that occur only in virus-infected cells are likely points for attack with selectively toxic agents. Many agents have been tested as antiviral drugs, but only a few meet the test of effective action against virus-infected cells with low toxicity to uninfected host cells.

■ SPECIFIC ANTIVIRAL DRUGS (Table 48-4)

Amantadine

Amantadine has a narrow antiviral spectrum, being effective only against influenza type A. Moreover, clinical information suggests the drug is most effective at preventing the disease and has very limited ability to alter the course of the disease once symptoms have appeared. There is limited clinical evidence that if the drug is administered by a nebulizer so that it is breathed into the lungs, amantadine may help reduce the severity of the symptoms and the duration of influenza type A infections. At present, however, the drug is limited to prophylaxis in patients at great risk in influenza epidemics, that is, in elderly patients or others for whom influenza is likely to lead to life-threatening complications.

Routine administration of amantadine is by the oral route with most of the drug being excreted unchanged in the urine. The concentration of amantadine that reaches the epithelial surfaces of lung tissues is the determining factor in protecting against influenza A infections.

Toxic reactions to amantadine prophylaxis for viral diseases is ordinarily low, unless kidney failure is present and the drug accumulates in the bloodstream. Amantadine can cause amphetamine-like stimulation of the central nervous system, as well as lethargy, ataxia, slurred speech, and other symptoms. Because of these central nervous system effects, the drug should be used cautiously if at all in elderly patients with cerebral arteriosclerosis or in patients with a history of epilepsy.

Amantadine has been used to treat Parkinson's disease (Chapter 32). Since the doses used for this purpose are about twice those used for influenza prophylaxis, toxic reactions are more common.

Methisazone

Methisazone is one of a large group of chemically related substances that have been tested for antiviral

TABLE 48-3. Sequence of events in virus reproduction in mammalian cells

Step in reproduction	Biochemical events	Drugs that block process
1. Adsorption	Initial ionic, dissociable association become irreversible adsorption of virus to cell surface.	No clinically useful drugs block this process
2. Penetration and uncoating	Virus particles enter the cell and the outer coats dissolve, releasing the viral genetic material (either DNA or RNA).	Amantadine
3. Replication and transcription	All viruses synthesize new messenger RNA and, using host ribosomes, synthesize viral proteins.	Idoxyuridine (IUdR) Vidarabine (ara-A)
4. Assembly and release	Viral nucleic acids and proteins are assembled to form mature viruses, which are then released either by budding off from infected cell or by lysis of infected cell.	Methisazone

TABLE 48-4. Summary of drugs used to treat viral diseases

Generic name	Trade name	Dosage and administration	Clinical use	Principal toxic reactions
Amantadine	Symmetrel	ORAL: *Adults*—100 mg twice daily. *Children*—4.4 to 8.8 mg/kg, up to 150 mg daily.	Prophylaxis of influenza type A infections in high risk patients.	Central nervous system stimulation, ataxia, slurred speech, lethargy.
Methisazone	Marboran	ORAL: *Adults and children*—40 mg/kg daily or 200 mg/kg once, followed by 50 mg/kg every 6 hr for 2 days.	Prophylaxis of smallpox; treatment of vaccinia infections.	Interference with liver drug metabolizing systems.
Idoxuridine	Dendrid Herplex Liquifilm Stoxil	OPHTHALMIC: *Adults and children*—0.1% solution, 0.5% ointment used 5 times daily.	Topical use in the eye for herpes keratitis.	Local irritation and pitting defects in the cornea. Systemic toxicity is possible but rare by this route.
Vidarabine	Vira-A	OPHTHALMIC: *Adults and children*—3% ointment used 5 times daily. INTRAVENOUS: *Adults and children*—15 mg/kg daily by slow continuous infusion for 12 to 24 hr.	Topical use in the eye for herpes ketatitis. Herpes simplex encephalitis.	Local irritation, superficial punctate keratitis, allergy. Anorexia, nausea, vomiting, diarrhea, central nervous system disturbances, hepatotoxicity, blood dyscrasias.

activity. Methisazone (referred to in some literature as *N*-methylisatin-β-thiosemicarbazone) is the most active of this group, blocking replication of vaccinia virus, and various pox viruses including smallpox. Although other viruses are sensitive to the drug under laboratory conditions, methisazone is clinically useful only against vaccinia and pox viruses.

Methisazone is used clinically in two ways. The primary use in the past has been for prophylaxis in persons exposed to smallpox. Although the controlled trials with methisazone have shown variable degrees of protection against smallpox, the drug is still used in this way when a smallpox outbreak arises. However, many public health workers prefer to use vaccination of contacts as the primary mode of controlling the spread of smallpox. Smallpox has not existed in the United States since 1949 and has apparently been eliminated from India and Africa where the last cases of smallpox in the world were reported.

The second clinical use of methisazone is for treatment of vaccinia infections such as vaccinia eczema and vaccinia gangrenosa. These conditions involve progressive spread of viral infection from a primary skin site; vaccinia gangrenosa involves widespread destruction of tissues and leads to death. These conditions may arise following smallpox vaccination in patients lacking sufficient immune responses to halt the growth of the attenuated live virus in the vaccine. Methisazone has been used successfully in a few of these cases. Methisazone is not available in the United States but is used in England.

Methisazone is administered orally and is widely metabolized in the body. Little, if any, active drug appears in the urine of treated patients. Methisazone seems to be poorly absorbed from the gastrointestinal tract, and blood levels vary greatly among patients receiving the drug.

Methisazone may be cytotoxic and embryotoxic under laboratory conditions, but it is not known if these occur with clinical use of the drug. Methisazone does affect liver function, apparently interfering with the metabolism of a number of drugs including barbiturates and ethyl alcohol. Patients receiving methisazone may be overly sensitive to these drugs, as well as to other liver-metabolized agents.

Idoxuridine

Idoxuridine, also referred to as 5-iodo-2′-deoxyuridine or IUdR, is an analog of the thymidine normally found in DNA. Idoxuridine is incorporated into DNA in place of the normal thymidine, thereby preventing normal DNA replication and halting virus formation. Unfortunately, idoxuridine does not have a good therapeutic index and will harm rapidly growing normal host cells as well as virus-infected cells. For this reason, the use of idoxuridine is restricted to topical treatment of herpes simplex infections of the cornea, conjunctiva, and eyelids. These infections tend to recur, and idoxuridine does not prevent reappearance of the infection nor does it prevent scarring and resultant loss of sight in serious cases.

When used topically in the eye, little idoxuridine enters the systemic circulation. The drug can produce local reactions in the eye, the most serious being corneal defects. Idoxuridine may also interfere with corneal epithelial regeneration and healing. Systemic toxic reactions to idoxuridine include anorexia, nausea, stomatitis, vomiting, hair loss (alopecia), blood dyscrasias, and cholestatic jaundice. These toxic reactions preclude the safe use of this drug systemically. Idoxuridine does not enter the central nervous system in sufficient quantities to be useful in treating herpes encephalitis.

Vidarabine

Vidarabine, also referred to as *adenine arabinoside,* inhibits viral DNA synthesis in a variety of DNA viruses. Clinically, the drug is used primarily to treat herpes infections. For this use, vidarabine seems to be more selectively toxic to viral invaders than other antiviral drugs.

Vidarabine is used topically for eye infections caused by herpes in much the same way as idoxuridine. However, an important new use of vidarabine is in the treatment of herpetic encephalitis, a condition that kills up to 70% of its victims. Vidarabine, used intravenously, significantly reduces the mortality associated with this disease. Currently, vidarabine is the only agent recommended for use in herpes encephalitis.

Vidarabine is rapidly metabolized when administered parenterally, and the metabolites formed are less active than vidarabine itself. The drug is poorly absorbed orally or from intramuscular sites and is suitable only for intravenous use when systemic absorption of the drug is desired. Continuous infusions maintain blood levels of the active drug within a useful range.

■ Experimental antiviral agents

The success of agents such as vidarabine and an increased understanding of viral replication has spurred the search for even more effective antiviral agents. A few of these drugs have shown promise in clinical trials and may be released for more general use in the near future. *Trifluridine (Viroptic)* is being tested for use in herpes keratitis. *Ribavirin (Virazole)* is used in Latin America for prophylaxis of influenza B and may also be effective against herpes. *Acyclovir (Zovirax)* is perhaps the most promising of these agents, showing much greater antiherpetic activity than either idoxuridine or vidarabine. The clinical usefulness of these and other experimental drugs will depend on evaluations of short-term and long-term toxicity in human patient populations.

■ THE NURSING PROCESS

■ Assessment

Most patients who are diagnosed as having viral illnesses are treated symptomatically and not with an antiviral agent. Examples include patients who have the "flu," the common cold, influenza, and other kinds of viremias. Use of antiviral agents is limited to patients in whom supportive therapy has not been helpful or who have viruses known to be particularly virulent or frequently fatal. A total thorough patient assessment should be done in treating these patients. Emphasis should be placed on the subjective and objective complaints related to the virus, and data to be obtained would include appropriate laboratory work, cultures, and other studies that would be helpful in monitoring the progress of the disease.

■ Management

Even when antiviral agents are used, much of the care is supportive and symptomatic in nature. The nurse should monitor appropriate laboratory work, vital signs, and other objective data that will help chart the progress of the disease. If antiviral agents are being used, the nurse should monitor for the side effects known to occur with that drug. If it is anticipated that the patient will be receiving antiviral drug therapy after discharge, patient and family teaching should be done. If the virus is known to be a particularly virulent virus, patient isolation may be necessary during the hospitalization phase. For information about specific viruses, consult the infection control department, the local health department, or the Center For Disease Control in Atlanta, Georgia. Many of the serious viral illnesses should be reported to the health department, as they are used for epidemiological charting of viral spread; examples include polio and rabies. Finally, immunization of family members and health care team members should be done if appropriate for the specific virus being treated.

■ Evaluation

Success with antiviral agents is manifested by recovery from the virus being treated. Side effects with the most commonly used antiviral agents in the United States are relatively uncommon. Because new drugs and new dosage regimens are being used with the antiviral agents, it is important that health care personnel monitor these patients carefully for the appearance of signs and symptoms which may indicate possible side or toxic effects to the drugs. If patients are being discharged while taking these agents, before discharge they should be able to explain how to take the drug correctly, should know side effects that may occur, and should be able to describe situations that require notification of the physician.

■ PATIENT CARE IMPLICATIONS

Amantadine

See the patient care implications section in Chapter 32.

Vidarabine

1. The major side effects are anorexia, nausea, vomiting, diarrhea, malaise, and rash. Occasionally, central nervous system side effects occur, including tremor, dizziness, hallucinations, confusion, and ataxia.
2. The drug must be given via slow infusion. Rapid or bolus injections are to be avoided. See the manufacturer's literature for dilution instructions.

Other antiviral agents

Because many of these drugs are investigational or have not yet been released for use in the United States, check the information supplied by the manufacturer before administering these agents.

■ SUMMARY

Viral diseases are of three types: acute diseases that resolve quickly and leave no latent infections or sequelae; chronic infections in which the disease runs a protracted course with long periods of remission interspersed with reappearance of disease; and slow viral infections in which the disease progresses over a number of months or years, causing cumulative damage to body tissues and ultimately killing the host. Viral diseases may remain localized in the body in certain tissues or may spread by viremia. For most viral diseases the appearance of symptoms is late in the disease. This fact makes pharmacological treatment of viral diseases difficult.

The body produces antibodies against viruses. Immunization is therefore possible against some viral diseases. However, some viruses have too many virulent strains or change antigenic properties too often to allow efficient immunizations to be developed.

Interferons are part of the body's natural defense against viral disease, blocking the spread of viruses to uninfected cells. Only the interferon from humans is effective in humans, and limited amounts of this agent are available. In addition, disease resistance produced by interferons appears transient.

Selective toxicity against viral diseases is possible by attacking those viral enzymes that are involved in producing the viral genome in infected human cells. Agents that act in this way include idoxuridine and vidarabine. Idoxuridine is used only as a topical agent for herpetic infections of the eye, but vidarabine may also be used to treat herpetic encephalitis. Amantadine blocks the penetration and uncoating of the influenza A2 virus and is used in prophylaxis. Methisazone inhibits the assembly and release of smallpox and related viruses. This agent may be used prophylactically against smallpox or used to treat local vaccinia infections.

■ STUDY QUESTIONS

1. What are the differences between acute, chronic, and slow viral diseases?
2. What is viremic spread of viral disease?
3. What factors limit our ability to develop pharmacological agents to treat viral diseases?
4. Why is immunization not possible against all viral diseases?
5. What is interferon?
6. What are the drawbacks of interferon that make it less than ideal as an antiviral agent?
7. What is the mechanism of action of amantadine?
8. How is amantadine used in the therapy of viral diseases?
9. What side effects are associated with amantadine therapy?
10. What is the mechanism of action of methisazone?
11. How is methisazone used in the therapy of viral diseases?
12. What side effects are associated with the use of methisazone?
13. What is the mechanism of action of idoxuridine?
14. How is idoxuridine used in the therapy of viral disease?
15. What side effects are associated with the use of idoxuridine?
16. What is the mechanism of action of vidarabine?
17. How is vidarabine used in the therapy of viral disease?

■ SUGGESTED READINGS

Smith, R.A., Sidwell, R.W., and Robins, R.K.: Antiviral mechanisms of action, Annual Review of Pharmacology and Toxicology **20:** 259, 1980.

Whitley, R., Alford, C., Hess, F., and Buchanan, R.: Vidarabine: a preliminary review of its pharmacological properties and therapeutic use, Drugs **20:**267, 1980.

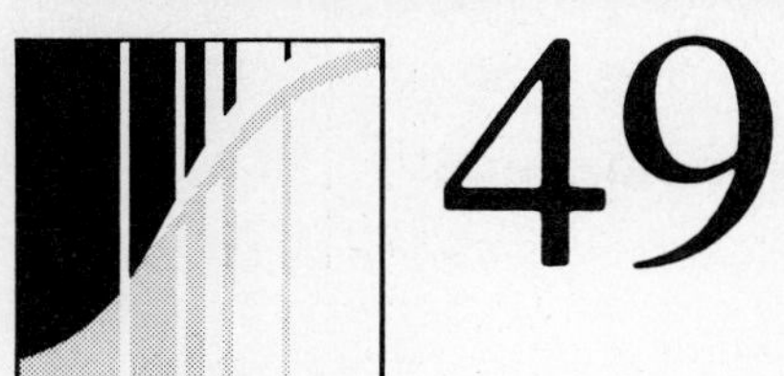

49 Drugs to treat protozoal and helminthic infestations

On a worldwide scale, chronic diseases caused by protozoal or helminthic infestations are the most commonly encountered afflictions of mankind. Although these diseases flourish primarily in tropical regions of the world, several are also encountered in North America. In this chapter the discussion centers on the treatment of diseases that occur in the continental United States. The first sections of this chapter relate individual drugs to specific diseases and explain the rationale for their use. The last section covers the pharmacological properties of the drugs.

■ THE TREATMENT OF DISEASES CAUSED BY PROTOZOANS

■ Amebic diseases

Entamoeba histolytica is a frequent pathogen of humans, commonly being passed from host to host by oral ingestion of fecally contaminated food or water. The organism is ingested as the cyst form. Cysts have thick walls and are resistant to dessication or to the action of stomach acids. Once in the intestine, the nonmotile cysts change to a motile, sexually active form called a *trophozoite*. Trophozoites produce the active disease as they reproduce and invade various tissues.

Amebic disease may be restricted to the intestinal lumen. However, trophozoites invade the intestinal lining in the course of the disease and may actually penetrate the intestinal wall and create abscesses in other tissues and organs. The liver and lung are most commonly affected in this way.

The choice of drug for treating amebic disease depends on the stage of the disease. For the acute colitis that occurs while the disease is limited to the intestinal tract, several drugs are available (Table 49-1). The best and safest of these drugs is metronidazole. Tetracyclines may be useful in combination with other agents. Tetracyclines may have mild antiamebic activity directly, but these broad spectrum antibacterial agents also alter the intestinal flora in such a way as to limit the growth of trophozoites.

Patients with organ abscesses receive metronidazole or a combination of emetine and chloroquine. These drugs not only attack trophozoites in the intestine, but by virtue of their distribution to other organs also attack liver and other soft organ sites of infestation.

■ Malaria

Malaria is caused when an infected mosquito injects a species of *Plasmodium* into the bloodstream of a person. Four species of *Plasmodium* produce human disease: *P. falciparum, P. vivax, P. ovale,* and *P. malariae*.

Plasmodia have complex life cycles. The form that enters the human bloodstream (sporozoites) travels immediately to the liver and may persist in the tissue for prolonged periods. Clinical malaria is produced when merozoites, the plasmodial form produced in liver cells, are released into the bloodstream. The merozoites attack red blood cells and ultimately cause them to rupture, thus producing the fever, chills, and sweating characteristic of the disease. A few gametocytes are also formed, which means that the patient at this stage of the disease can transmit the parasites to mosquitoes and thence to other human hosts. Only gametocytes cause a mosquito to become infectious and capable of transmitting the disease.

Therapy of malaria depends upon the stage of the disease and on which plasmodial species is involved. *P. falciparum* and *P. malariae* appear not to produce persistent tissue forms of the parasite. Therefore, therapy that destroys blood forms of the protozoan will be curative. With *P. vivax* and *P. ovale,* however, therapy must include a drug that destroys the persistent tissue forms of *Plasmodium*. A drug such as chloroquine is quite effective against blood forms (Table 49-2). Using chloroquine phosphate plus primaquine phosphate allows control of all four species of *Plasmodium*.

Chloroquine has been a mainstay in treating malaria for a number of years. Unfortunately, chloroquine-resistant malaria has now developed in several regions of the world. This type of disease should be treated with the combination of quinine, pyrimethamine, and sulfadiazine. Pyrimethamine and sulfadiazine are synergistic in activity and are given together for maximum benefit.

Several of the drugs used to treat malaria may also be used for prophylaxis. Chloroquine, hydroxychloro-

TABLE 49-1. Drugs used to treat amebic infestations (amebiasis)

Disease form	Drug used	Dosage and administration
Asymptomatic	Iodoquinol	ORAL: *Adults*—650 mg 3 times daily for 3 wk. *Children*—30 to 40 mg/kg divided in 3 doses daily for 3 wk.
	Diloxanide furoate	ORAL: *Adults*—500 mg 3 times daily for 10 days. *Children over 2 yr*—20 mg/kg daily in 3 divided doses for 10 days.
Intestinal symptoms only	Iodoquinol plus	As above.
	Tetracycline or	ORAL: *Adults*—250 to 500 mg 4 times daily for 2 wk. *Children*—10 mg/kg 4 times daily for 10 days.
	Emetine	INTRAMUSCULAR (deep), SUBCUTANEOUS: *Adults*—1 mg/kg up to 60 mg daily in single dose for 5 days. *Children*—same dosage but divided into 2 doses.
Abscesses in liver or other organs	Metronidazole	ORAL: *Adults*—750 mg 3 times daily for 10 days. *Children*—35 to 50 mg/kg divided into 3 doses daily for 10 days.
	Emetine plus	As above.
	Chloroquine phosphate	ORAL: *Adults*—1 Gm daily for 2 days, then 500 mg daily for 2 or 3 wk. *Children*—10 mg/kg up to 600 mg daily for 3 wk.

TABLE 49-2. Drugs used to treat malaria

Disease form	Drug used	Dosage and administration
Blood forms causing clinical symptoms.	Chloroquine phosphate	ORAL: *Adults*—600 mg initially; 300 mg at 6, 24, and 48 hr. *Children*—10 mg/kg initially; 5 mg/kg at 6, 24, and 48 hr.
	Chloroquine hydrochloride	INTRAMUSCULAR, INTRAVENOUS: *Adults*—3 mg/kg every 6 hr. *Children*—2 to 3 mg/kg repeated in 6 hr. Not for intravenous use in children under 7 yr.
	Hydroxychloroquine sulfate	ORAL: *Adults*—620 mg initially; 310 mg in 6 hr and again daily for 2 days. *Children*—10 mg/kg initially; 5 mg/kg in 6 hr and daily for 2 days.
	Amodiaquine hydrochloride	ORAL: *Adults*—600 mg initially; then 400 mg at 6, 24, and 48 hr. *Children*—10 mg/kg initially; then 5 mg/kg at 6, 24, and 48 hr.
	Quinine sulfate	ORAL: *Adults*—650 mg 3 times daily for 10 to 14 days. *Children*—25 mg/kg 3 times daily for 10 to 14 days.
	Quinine dihydrochloride	INTRAVENOUS: *Adults*—600 mg every 8 hr. *Children*—25 mg/kg divided into 2 1 hr infusions.
Persistent tissue forms of *Plasmodia (P. ovale, P. vivax)* or gametocytes	Primaquine phosphate	ORAL: *Adults*—15 mg for 14 days following therapy with one of the drugs listed above. *Children*—0.3 mg/kg for 14 days following therapy with one of the drugs listed above.
Chloroquine-resistant *P. falciparum*	Quinine sulfate or hydrochloride plus	As above.
	Pyrimethamine and	ORAL: *Adults and children*—50 mg daily for first 3 days.
	Sulfadiazine	ORAL: *Adults and children*—2 Gm daily for first 6 days.

TABLE 49-3. Drugs used to treat trichomoniasis, giardiasis, toxoplasmosis, and pneumocystosis

Disease form	Drug used	Dosage and administration
Trichomoniasis	Povidone-iodine	VAGINAL: *Adults*—10% gel applied nightly; 10% douche applied every morning. Therapy continues for 2 wk or longer.
	Metronidazole	ORAL: *Adults*—250 mg 3 times daily for 7 to 10 days.
Giardiasis	Quinacrine	ORAL: *Adults*—100 mg 3 times daily for 5 to 7 days. *Children*—7 mg/kg daily in 3 divided doses for 5 days. Daily dose should not exceed 300 mg in children.
	Metronidazole	ORAL: *Adults*—250 mg 3 times daily for 7 days.
Toxoplasmosis	Pyrimethamine plus	ORAL: *Adults*—50 to 100 mg for 1 or 2 wk, then 25 mg daily for up to 5 wk. *Children*—1 mg/kg daily in 2 doses for 2 to 4 days. Continue 0.5 mg/kg for 30 days.
	Sulfadiazine	ORAL: *Adults*—2 to 4 Gm for 1 or 2 wk, then 1 Gm every 4 to 6 hr for up to 5 wk. *Children*—150 mg/kg total divided in 4 to 6 daily doses after an initial dose equivalent to one-half the daily total.
Pneumocystosis	Trimethoprim with sulfamethoxazole	ORAL: *Adults*—20 mg/kg trimethoprim and 100 mg/kg sulfamethoxazole daily in 4 doses for 2 wk. *Children*—reduced doses are required.

quine, amodiaquine, and pyrimethamine are used at smaller doses than those normally used for therapy. Primaquine is used prophylactically at the same doses used for therapy.

■ Trichomoniasis

Vaginal infections caused by *Trichomonas vaginalis* occur commonly. The disease is marked by watery discharge from the vagina and signs of tissue irritation. *Trichomonas* may be unnoticed in the urinary tract and in the rectum, but these sites can serve as sources of infection.

Vaginal trichomoniasis may be treated with local agents applied as gels or douches (Table 49-3). Complete cure of the sites outside the vagina and of infections in the male urinary tract may require a systemic agent. Metronidazole is the drug of choice.

■ Giardiasis

Giardiasis is an intestinal infection caused by the protozoan *Giardia lamblia*. This disease, which is passed between human hosts by ingestion of fecally contaminated food, may be asymptomatic in many patients. For others, the disease may be much more severe, producing diarrhea, gastrointestinal distress, and malabsorption of food.

Quinacrine is the most commonly recommended drug for giardiasis in adults. Children should receive metronidazole. Many adults now also receive metronidazole (Table 49-3).

■ Toxoplasmosis

In the United States toxoplasmosis is primarily acquired from ingestion of the oocyte of *Toxoplasma gondii*. The most common source of infection is cat feces. In adult human beings the disease is usually mild and transitory, with symptoms resembling those of mild mononucleosis. Occasionally, the disease may involve the eyes or nervous system in adults.

The most dangerous form of toxoplasmosis is congenital, resulting from infection of a pregnant woman. Congenital toxoplasmosis is usually fatal, causing severe damage to eyes, brain, and other organs of the fetus. Because of the dangers this disease poses to unborn children, many obstetricians suggest that pregnant women avoid handling used cat litter and avoid any close contact with cats.

Pyrimethamine and sulfadiazine are employed in combination to treat this disease (Table 49-3).

■ Pneumocystosis

The parasite *Pneumocystis carinii* seldom causes disease in healthy human beings but may produce severe pulmonary disease in patients receiving immunosuppressive drugs. Young children are also susceptible. As many as half the patients who acquire this disease may die unless treated. Until recently, therapy of pneumocystosis was difficult, but today the fixed combination of trimethoprim and sulfamethoxazole (Bactrim, Septra [Chapter 45]) is successfully employed in many cases.

■ THE TREATMENT OF DISEASES CAUSED BY HELMINTHS

■ Ascariasis

Ascariasis, also called *roundworm infestation,* is produced by ingesting the eggs of *Ascaris lumbricoides*. This common disease is spread by fecally contaminated food and water. Larvae and adult worms migrate through lungs, liver, gallbladder, and other organs and may cause severe damage.

Ascaris infestations may be treated effectively with several agents, including mebendazole, pyrantel pamoate, and piperazine (Table 49-4).

■ Enterobiasis, or pinworm infestation

Pinworms are freely passed between individuals living in close proximity. Constant reinfection is the rule, since the eggs of these parasites are passed in great numbers and adhere to clothing, towels, and hands. The disease produced is usually mild and may be asymptomatic. However, patients may suffer pruritus ani and pruritus vulvae or more serious symptoms.

Since pinworms tend to stay within the intestinal tract, treatment of the disease is relatively simple. Mebendazole, pyrantel pamoate, and pyrvinium pamoate are all nearly 100% effective after a single dose. Piperazine is also effective, but therapy continues over a period of several days (Table 49-4).

■ Whipworm infestation

This intestinal infestation is usually asymptomatic, although large numbers of worms in small children may produce diarrhea, anemia, and cachexia. Whipworm infestations are easily and effectively treated with mebendazole or thiabendazole (Table 49-4).

■ Threadworm infestation

This disease, also called *strongyloidiasis,* is more serious than many infestations because the worms may reproduce in the human body. Larvae migrate from the wall of the intestine into systemic circulation and thence return to the intestine to mature and further increase the numbers of worms in the host. Malabsorption syndrome, diarrhea, and duodenal irritation may occur.

Most drugs used against worm infestations are ineffective against threadworms, since these worms live within the intestinal tissue. Thiabendazole is well-distributed to the tissues where this parasite lives and is effective in eliminating the infestation (Table 49-4).

■ Hookworm infestation

This disease, also called *uncinariasis,* is found in the southern United States. Although two species of worms may cause this disease, most infestations encountered in the United States are caused by *Necator*. Therefore, most patients may be treated with mebendazole or pyrantel pamoate.

Another type of hookworm from dogs and cats produces a cutaneous lesion called *creeping eruption,* or *cutaneous larva migrans*. Thiabendazole, either topically or orally, may be effective to kill the parasites and limit the allergic responses, which cause itching, burning, and skin damage (Table 49-4).

■ Trichinosis

This condition, also known as *pork roundworm infestation,* is much less common today than it once was. Ingested cysts from raw or improperly cooked meat develop into adult worms in the human intestine. Larvae are ultimately released into the circulation and enter muscle to form cysts. Patients suffer gastrointestinal upset, fever, muscle aches, and eosinophilia (accumulation of certain white cells in the blood).

Trichinosis can not yet be effectively treated. Most patients receive therapy designed to minimize symptoms rather than produce a cure, since most patients will survive the disease and carry the quiescent worms encysted in skeletal muscle for the rest of their lives. Thiabendazole has been used in selected cases to try to prevent the migration of the worms to the muscles (Table 49-4).

■ Tapeworm infestations

Tapeworms, or cestodes, of several types can infest humans. Beef, pork, fish, and dwarf tapeworms are all sensitive to niclosamide, a drug not yet marketed in the United States. Physicians may obtain the drug through the Parasitic Disease Drug Center of The Center for Disease Control. Quinacrine is also useful in treating tapeworm infestations (Table 49-4).

All detected infestations are treated even though the infestations are mostly asymptomatic. Pork tapeworm infestations may become serious if reflux of eggs from the intestine reach the stomach and hatch into larvae that invade tissues.

TABLE 49-4. Drugs used to treat infestations by helminths

Disease form	Drug used	Dosage and administration
Roundworms (ascariasis)	Pyrantel pamoate	ORAL: *Adults and children*—single dose of 11 mg/kg up to 1 Gm.
	Mebendazole	ORAL: *Adults and children*—100 mg twice daily for 3 days.
	Piperazine	ORAL: *Adults*—3.5 Gm in single dose for 2 days. *Children*—75 mg/kg up to 3.5 Gm once daily for 2 days.
Pinworms (enterobiasis)	Mebendazole	ORAL: *Adults and children*—100 mg single dose.
	Pyrantel pamoate	ORAL: *Adults and children*—single dose of 11 mg/kg up to 1 Gm.
	Pyrvinium pamoate	ORAL: *Adults and children*—single dose of 5 mg/kg.
	Piperazine	ORAL: *Adults and children*—65 mg/kg up to 2.5 Gm once daily for 1 wk.
Whipworms (trichuriasis)	Mebendazole	ORAL: *Adults and children*—100 mg daily for 3 days.
	Thiabendazole	ORAL: *Adults and children*—25 mg/kg up to 3 Gm twice daily for 1 or 2 days.
Threadworms (strongyloidiasis)	Thiabendazole	ORAL: *Adults and children*—25 mg/kg up to 3 Gm twice daily for 1 or 2 days.
Hookworms (uncinariasis)	Mebendazole	ORAL: *Adults and children*—100 mg twice daily for 3 days.
	Pyrantel pamoate	ORAL: *Adults and children*—11 mg/kg up to 1 Gm as single dose for 3 days.
	Thiabendazole	ORAL: *Adults and children*—25 mg/kg up to 3 Gm twice daily for 1 or 2 days.
Cutaneous larva migrans	Thiabendazole	ORAL: *Adults and children*—as for hookworms plus topical application of suspension (500 mg/5 ml) 4 times daily for 5 days.
Pork roundworms (trichinosis)	Thiabendazole	ORAL: *Adults and children*—25 mg/kg up to 3 Gm twice daily for 2 to 4 days.
Tapeworms (cestodiasis)	Niclosamide	ORAL: *Adults and children over 8 yr*—1 Gm; dose repeated 1 hr later. *Children 2 to 8 yr*—two 500 mg doses 1 hr apart. *Children under 2 yr*—two 250 mg doses 1 hr apart.

■ PHARMACOLOGICAL PROPERTIES OF SPECIFIC DRUGS

Amodiaquine, chloroquine, and hydroxychloroquine

Mechanism of action. Amodiaquine, chloroquine, and hydroxychloroquine are members of a drug family called *4-aminoquinolines*. This family of drugs has been the mainstay of antimalarial therapy worldwide since the late 1940's. All effective members of this family share the ability to bind tightly to DNA in its double-stranded form. The drugs are thought to *intercalate,* which is to slip into the groove between the two strands of DNA and bind to the bases and phosphate groups exposed within the groove. Binding of these drugs not only alters the physical properties of the DNA, but it also appears to inhibit the ability of the DNA to be replicated or transcribed. Therefore, cells whose DNA is affected by these drugs are incapable of cell division.

Absorption, distribution, and excretion. Amodiaquine, chloroquine, and hydroxychloroquine are all satisfactorily absorbed from the gastrointestinal tract. Chloroquine is available for intramuscular injection when oral dosage is impossible.

Drugs of the 4-aminoquinoline family are strongly concentrated in the liver, spleen, kidneys, and lung. More important to the therapeutic usefulness, the drugs are also concentrated in red blood cells. Infected red blood cells may concentrate the drug up to 1000-fold over the drug concentration in plasma.

The 4-aminoquinoline drugs may be metabolized in the liver by microsomal enzymes; some of the metabolites retain antiplasmodial activity. These drugs and metabolites are ultimately removed from the body by the kidney. Renal excretion of these drugs is enhanced by acidifying the urine, which converts the drug to a changed form that is not reabsorbed.

TABLE 49-5. Common reactions to antiparasitic drugs

Generic name	Trade name	Toxicity	References for uses and dosages
4-AMINOQUINOLINES			
Amodiaquine hydrochloride	Camoquin	Gastrointestinal distress is most common. Vision changes, central nervous system irritability, hemolysis can occur.	Malaria: treatment of clinical attacks or prophylaxis (Table 49-2).
Chloroquine	Aralen	As for amodiaquine.	Malaria: treatment of clinical attacks or prophylaxis (Table 49-2).
Dehydroemetine		As for emetine.	As for emetine.
Diloxanide furoate	Furamide	Flatulence is common. Other gastrointestinal symptoms are rare.	Amebiasis: eliminates cysts; eradicates carrier state (Table 49-1).
Emetine		Gastrointestinal irritation and cardiac toxicity are common.	Amebiasis: severe colitis with or without tissue abscesses (Table 49-1).
Hydroxychloroquine	Plaquenil sulfate	As for amodiaquine.	Malaria: treatment of clinical attacks or prophylaxis (Table 49-2).
Iodoquinol	Diiodohydroxyquin Yodoxin	Gastrointestinal upset and skin eruptions are most common. Blood levels of iodine may rise; optic neuritis may occur rarely.	Amebiasis: intestinal forms of disease (Table 49-1).
Mebendazole	Vermox	Abdominal discomfort may occur. Mebendazole is teratogenic in rats.	Roundworms, pinworms, whipworms, hookworms (Table 49-4).
Metronidazole	Flagyl	Gastrointestinal distress and pelvic discomfort may occur. Central nervous system effects are possible.	Amebiasis: intestinal or tissue abscesses (Table 49-1). Trichomoniasis, Giardiasis (Table 49-3).
Niclosamide	Yomesan	Mild gastrointestinal upset on day of therapy.	Tapeworms (Table 49-4).
Piperazine	Antepar Multifuge Citrate Vermizine	Gastrointestinal upset may occur. Skin rashes and transient neurological signs may be seen.	Roundworms, pinworms (Table 49-4).
Povidone-iodine		Tissue irritation may occur with topically applied drug.	Trichomoniasis (Table 49-3).
Primaquine		Gastrointestinal distress can occur. Hemolysis may occur, especially when G-6-PD deficiency exists.	Malaria: persistent tissue forms (Table 49-2).
Pyrantel pamoate	Antiminth	Mild gastrointestinal upset and transient changes in liver function occur. Headaches and dizziness are more rare.	Roundworms, pinworms, and hookworms (Table 49-4).
Pyrimethamine	Daraprim	Nausea and vomiting as well as blood dyscrasias occur, especially with higher doses.	Malaria: with quinine and sulfadiazine (Table 49-2). Toxoplasmosis: with sulfadiazine (Table 49-3).
Pyrvinium pamoate	Povan	Intestinal distress occurs in some patients. Bright red drug stains teeth, intestinal contents.	Pinworms (Table 49-4).
Quinine		Cinchonism is a dose-related sign of toxicity. Blood dyscrasias and pain on injection occur.	Malaria: with pyrimethamine and sulfadiazine (Table 49-2).

TABLE 49-5. Common reactions to antiparasitic drugs—cont'd

Generic name	Trade name	Toxicity	References for uses and dosages
Sulfadiazine		Gastrointestinal, allergic, and blood reactions are possible (see Chapter 45).	Malaria: with pyrimethamine and quinine (Table 49-2). Toxoplasmosis: with pyrimethamine (Table 49-3).
Sulfamethoxazole and trimethoprim	Bactrim Septra	Folic acid deficiency or sulfonamide toxicity may occur (see Chapter 45).	Pneumocystosis (Table 49-3).
Tetracycline		Gastrointestinal distress is common (see Chapter 43).	Amebiasis: with iodoquinol for intestinal forms (Table 49-1).
Thiabendazole	Mintezol	Gastrointestinal upset is common. Central nervous system effects and reduced liver function may be observed.	Threadworms, hookworms, cutaneous larva migrans, and trichinosis (Table 49-4).

Toxicity. Amodiaquine, chloroquine, and hydroxychloroquine are relatively safe drugs if care is taken to avoid overdose, prolonged use, or use in sensitive patients. Patients with glucose-6-phosphate deficiency are more likely than normal patients to suffer hemolysis when treated with these drugs. Children are also more sensitive to these agents than are adults. Patients with liver disease or retinal damage are also more at risk of severe toxic reactions.

At the doses commonly used in therapy, drugs of this family can produce nausea and other gastrointestinal symptoms (Table 49-5). These symptoms may be minimized by administering the drug with meals.

Visual changes may be observed with the 4-aminoquinolines. Blurred vision may signal reversible impairment of accommodation, but retinal or corneal changes are not reversible. Patients reporting misty vision, patchy vision, or foggy patches in the visual field may be developing serious eye damage. These complaints tend to arise in patients receiving the drugs for long periods.

Headache, dizziness, psychosis, and convulsions may be observed in patients treated with these drugs. In some patients, changes in heart function may be reported. Skin and blood changes may also occur.

The toxic reactions to 4-aminoquinolines are greatly increased when the drugs are used for prolonged periods, as for example when used for long-term malaria prophylaxis. When used in the routine short-term treatment regimens for malaria (Table 49-2), the drugs are better tolerated.

Diloxanide furoate

Mechanism of action. Diloxanide is an effective drug in eliminating *Entamoeba histolytica* from the intestine of persons mildly infected and passing cysts in their stools (Table 49-1). The drug has little effect against acute colitis produced by this parasite and no effect on tissue abscesses.

The biochemical basis for the ameba-destroying action of diloxanide is not known.

Absorption, distribution, and excretion. Diloxanide is administered orally and is well absorbed by that route. Nevertheless, diloxanide is useful alone only for intestinal amebiasis. Excretion of the drug is primarily by the kidney.

Toxicity. Diloxanide is relatively safe, producing few systemic side effects. Flatulence (intestinal gas) is the most frequently reported side effect. Other gastrointestinal disturbances such as nausea, diarrhea, and esophagitis may rarely be encountered.

Emetine and dehydroemetine

Mechanism of action. Emetine and dehydroemetine are alkaloids obtained from ipecac, a botanical used in the past as an emetic. Emetine has emetic properties when used orally but is now used primarily to treat amebiasis (Table 49-1). Dehydroemetine is similar to emetine and is marketed in Europe, but not the United States.

Emetine and dehydroemetine are thought to block protein synthesis in eukaryotes. Therefore, mammalian cells as well as the ameba may be sensitive.

Absorption, distribution, and excretion. Although emetine and dehydroemetine may be absorbed orally, the emetic and irritative properties of these drugs caused them to be poorly tolerated by that route. The drugs are more commonly given by intramuscular or subcutaneous injection. Intravenous injection is to be scrupulously avoided to prevent excessive toxicity to the heart. Emetine tends to accumulate in various tissues, including the liver, and is slowly released.

Toxicity. The heart is one site where accumulation of emetine occurs. Symptoms such as tachycardia (fast heart rate) and ECG changes signal that the drug should be discontinued to prevent further cardiac difficulty. Because of this potential for cardiac toxicity, every patient receiving emetine should be hospitalized and the nursing staff should carefully record pulse rates and blood pressure.

Emetine may also produce gastrointestinal irritation, even when administered parenterally. Muscle weakness and skin lesions may also occur. Dehydroemetine is similar to emetine in all respects. The claim that dehydroemetine is less toxic than emetine requires careful clinical evaluation.

Iodoquinol

Mechanism of action. Iodoquinol is an effective amebicidal agent (Table 49-1) whose action is thought to be related to the iodine content of the drug.

Absorption, distribution, and excretion. Iodoquinol is administered orally and is not significantly absorbed from the intestine. Iodine is increased in the bloodstream, however, suggesting that some drug is absorbed or that the iodine is absorbed following breakdown of the drug in the gut.

Toxicity. Iodoquinol is relatively nontoxic. Skin eruptions may occur. Nausea and other gastrointestinal symptoms have been reported.

Iodoquinol can affect the thyroid gland and increase blood iodine levels.

Prolonged high doses of iodoquinol may occasionally produce optic neuritis or atrophy and other signs of neuropathy.

Mebendazole

Mechanism of action. Mebendazole is an effective broad spectrum antihelminthic agent (Table 49-4). Mebendazole blocks glucose uptake in sensitive helminths. Since these organisms require externally supplied glucose to maintain energy levels, blockade of glucose absorption will ultimately destroy the worms.

Absorption, distribution, and excretion. Mebendazole is used orally for its action against intestinal helminths. Very little of the drug is absorbed into systemic circulation. The small amount of drug that enters the bloodstream is metabolized and excreted by the kidney.

Toxicity. Mebendazole produces few toxic reactions. A few reports of abdominal discomfort and diarrhea exist, but these symptoms may result from large masses of worms being expelled.

Mebendazole is teratogenic in rats but has not produced birth defects in dogs, sheep, or horses. It is difficult to predict the effects in humans. Therefore, some physicians limit the use of mebendazole, especially during pregnancy.

Metronidazole

Mechanism of action. Metronidazole attacks ameba at intestinal and other tissue sites (Table 49-1). The drug has also been used to treat trichomoniasis (Table 49-3). Metronidazole acts directly on sensitive organisms, but the exact mechanism for its lethal effects is unknown. Chemical relatives of metronidazole inhibit RNA synthesis; metronidazole may be effective by a similar mechanism.

Absorption, distribution, and excretion. Metronidazole is well absorbed following oral administration. The drug appears to be metabolized by various pathways. Both metabolites and the unchanged drug appear in urine. Some patients will observe a reddish brown discoloration of the urine while receiving metronidazole. This discoloration is caused by a colored metabolite of metronidazole. Patients should be reassured that the discoloration is harmless.

Toxicity. Metronidazole can produce gastrointestinal symptoms of various types. Some patients experience a sharp, metallic taste, as well as nausea, diarrhea, vomiting, epigastric pain, and abdominal cramping. While annoying, these symptoms rarely necessitate stopping the medication.

Metronidazole can rarely cause changes in function of the central nervous system. Dizziness, ataxia (incoordination affecting walking), numbness, and paresthesias may be seen. These symptoms may signal that metronidazole should be withdrawn.

Metronidazole may also produce discomfort in the pelvic organs. Patients describe a sense of pressure in that region. Dysuria, cystitis, and dryness of the vagina may be experienced.

Metronidazole causes an alarming reaction when ethyl alcohol is ingested. Patients experience intense flushing, nausea, headaches, and abdominal cramps. This reaction is similar to that experienced by patients taking both disulfiram and ethyl alcohol (Chapter 24).

Metronidazole may potentiate the action of warfarin. Patients receiving both drugs should be carefully observed for signs of bleeding.

Niclosamide

Mechanism of action. Niclosamide is an extremely effective drug against cestodes (tapeworms). These segmented flatworms are killed by a single dose of niclosamide, which blocks respiration and glucose uptake in the worms. The dead worm segments are frequently digested by proteolytic agents in the gut. For this reason, a cathartic may be given 1 or 2 hours after the drug to allow the dead but still intact worm parts to be identified in the feces. This purge is a therapeutic necessity when the tapeworm infestation is due to the pork tapeworm. With this organism, digestion of the dead worm segments releases living eggs, which can develop in humans and cause more serious, invasive disease. The purge removes the worm segments before they rupture and prevents this complication.

Absorption, distribution, and excretion. Niclosamide is not absorbed from the bowel and exerts all its actions within the lumen of the bowel.

Toxicity. Niclosamide is almost without toxicity. Systemic toxicity is not a problem, since the drug is not absorbed. Some patients have mild gastrointestinal symptoms on the day of therapy.

Piperazine

Mechanism of action. Piperazine is an effective agent for the treatment of ascaris and pinworm infestations (Table 49-4). The drug apparently blocks the action of the acetylcholine on the muscles of these parasites. As a result, the worms are paralyzed and are eliminated from the bowel by normal peristaltic flow. The worms eliminated are alive.

Absorption, distribution, and excretion. Piperazine is well absorbed following oral administration. A portion of the drug is metabolized to various inactive products. The kidney is the primary route for excretion. Patients with impaired renal or hepatic function may be more sensitive to piperazine than normal.

Toxicity. Piperazine produces few toxic effects at the doses routinely used to treat helminthic infestations. Gastrointestinal upset and occasional skin rashes have occurred. Transient neurological signs ranging from headache and dizziness to ataxia, paresthesias, or convulsions have been seen, but these more severe reactions are more common with overdoses. These more severe reactions also occur in patients with renal dysfunction, who tend to accumulate the drug.

Povidone-iodine

Mechanism of action. Povidone-iodine is a general antiseptic agent whose antiseptic effect is produced by the release of free iodine. The agent is widely used as a skin antiseptic for preparation before various medical procedures. In addition, povidone-iodine is used topically to treat *Trichomonas vaginalis* infections (Table 49-3).

Absorption, distribution, and excretion. Povidone-iodine is used topically in the vagina. Absorption of the drug is usually minimal, but some patients display a rise in iodine levels in the blood.

Toxicity. Povidone-iodine may prove irritating to tissues in some patients. Iodine toxicity is usually not a problem unless the patient is highly sensitive or is treated for extended periods.

Primaquine

Mechanism of action. Primaquine is a chemical relative of the 4-aminoquinoline family of antimalarial agents. Primaquine apparently has a different mechanism of action than those agents, but the exact mechanism by which primaquine kills certain forms of plasmodia remains unknown (Table 49-2).

Absorption, distribution, and excretion. Primaquine is well-absorbed following oral doses. Drug concentrations in the plasma peak within 6 hours of the dose, but the drug is extensively metabolized and rapidly cleared from the bloodstream.

Toxicity. Primaquine given at normal therapeutic doses produces little toxicity. Abdominal cramps and epigastric distress can occur, but these symptoms can usually be relieved by taking the drug with meals.

Primaquine may damage red blood cells. The drug blocks the production of an intracellular reducing agent, NADPH. In normal cells, this deficit is made up by glucose metabolism, and the cell continues to function normally. However, patients with reduced levels of glucose-6-phosphate dehydrogenase (G-6-PD) cannot utilize glucose rapidly enough to make up the deficit. The red blood cells in these patients accumulate oxidized products such as methemoglobin, which is not an efficient oxygen carrier. Cyanosis may result. Ultimately, these red blood cells may rupture. Hemolysis can be severe and is always a sign that drug dosage should be reduced or the drug terminated. One sign of hemolysis that may be seen easily is darkening of the urine.

Primaquine toxicity is more severe in the patients lacking G-6-PD. The lack of G-6-PD is genetically determined and exists in high proportions of certain populations such as Sardinians, Sephardic Jews, Greeks, and Iranians. Blacks are less prone to this deficiency than these groups, but have a higher incidence than the white population of the United States. Patients discovered to have these increased sensitivities to primaquine may be treated with reduced dosages of the drug.

Pyrantel pamoate

Mechanism of action. Pyrantel is a depolarizing neuromuscular blocking agent, similar in action to succinylcholine and decamethonium. Pyrantel causes spastic paralysis and gradual contraction of the muscle in worms (Table 49-4). The parasites are then eliminated from the body by normal peristalsis. Pyrantel is effective, when given in short courses, against a variety of worms. Purges are not necessary adjuncts to therapy with this drug. Piperazine may antagonize the action of pyrantel.

Absorption, distribution, and excretion. Pyrantel is not absorbed from the gastrointestinal tract to any great extent. What little drug is absorbed is excreted by the kidneys. Pyrantel produces its desired effects entirely within the lumen of the bowel.

Toxicity. Since pyrantel is not well absorbed following oral dosage, few systemic effects occur. Headache and dizziness may occur as a result of central nervous system effects of this drug. More commonly the drug causes mild gastrointestinal upset and transient changes in liver function tests.

Pyrimethamine

Mechanism of action. Pyrimethamine is an effective blocker of the enzyme dihydrofolate reductase in plasmodia. Pyrimethamine therefore blocks the formation of tetrahydrofolic acid (THFA), a cofactor required for several metabolic transformations. The enzyme blocked by pyrimethamine normally converts dihydrofolic acid (DHA) to THFA. The formation of DHA may be blocked by sulfonamides (Chapter 45). Combining pyrimethamine and a sulfonamide such as sulfadiazine is an example of synergistic effects being produced by drugs blocking sequential steps in a metabolic pathway. Another example is trimethoprim and sulfamethoxazole (Chapter 45).

Absorption, distribution, and excretion. Pyrimethamine is well absorbed following oral administration. The drug is metabolized and appears in the urine as metabolites. Pyrimethamine appears in the milk of nursing mothers.

Toxicity. Pyrimethamine, as it is normally used in treating chloroquine-resistant malaria, produces few side effects. In higher doses, such as those used to treat toxoplasmosis, the drug may impair host folic acid metabolism, leading to megaloblastic anemia and various other blood dyscrasias. Treatment with leucovorin (a folinic acid supplement) may be required. Large doses may also produce nausea and vomiting, which may be controlled partly by administering the drug with meals.

Pyrvinium pamoate

Mechanism of action. Pyrvinium inhibits energy metabolism in facultative anaerobic organisms such as the intestinal parasitic worms. The drug is most effective against pinworm infestations (Table 49-4), killing all the parasites in a large percent of cases following a single dose.

Absorption, distribution, and excretion. Pyrvinium is not absorbed from the gastrointestinal tract and is excreted in the feces. Since the drug is a cyanine dye, it colors the feces bright red.

Toxicity. Pyrvinium produces no dangerous toxicity. Older patients or patients receiving the drug in large doses or as the suspension may suffer intestinal distress, including emesis.

One of the most annoying aspects of pyrvinium is its bright red color and the fact that it can stain teeth and clothing. Patients should be cautioned not to chew the tablets. If emesis occurs, the vomitus may be red and capable of staining materials. The red color is not dangerous in any way but may make therapy less tolerable for the patient than therapy with other drugs might be.

Quinacrine

Mechanism of action. Quinacrine was first developed and used as an antimalarial agent but is now primarily used against tapeworms (Table 49-4). The drug acts on the attachment organ of the tapeworm and causes the head (or scolex) of the worm to release its hold on the intestinal wall and allows it to be eliminated.

Absorption, distribution, and excretion. Quinacrine is well absorbed from the gastrointestinal tract. However, when given orally the drug induces vomiting in many patients. To minimize this reaction, which usually prevents the dosage from being effective, quinacrine is frequently given by nasogastric tube so that the drug directly enters the duodenum. Residual materials in the bowel must be reduced for the drug to be maximally effective. Patients should receive a cathartic and cleansing enema before treatment. A purge after therapy allows the worm to be expelled before it can reattach.

Quinacrine is well distributed throughout the body and seems to bind strongly to tissues. Patients receiving quinacrine may notice a yellow discoloration of the skin. The reaction is not a sign of jaundice but simply illustrates the distribution of this yellow-colored drug to the skin.

Toxicity. Quinacrine causes few serious side effects when used in the short-term treatment courses required to eradicate tapeworms. Dizziness is occasionally noted as is toxic psychosis. Psoriasis may be exacerbated. Aplastic anemia has rarely been observed.

The most common reaction to quinacrine is nausea and vomiting.

Quinine

Mechanism of action. Quinine is a plant alkaloid with many actions on various tissues. The exact mechanism of the antimalarial action of quinine is unknown. Although quinine is the oldest antimalarial agent known and was once the mainstay of therapy, today its use is restricted to treating chloroquine-resistant *P. falciparum* (Table 49-2). Quinine should be combined with pyrimethamine and sulfadiazine for most effective action.

Absorption, distribution, and excretion. Quinine is rapidly absorbed following oral dosage. The drug is generally well distributed through the body, although it does not enter the cerebrospinal fluid to a significant degree.

Quinine is extensively metabolized and excreted in the urine. Excretion is enhanced in acidic urine.

■ THE NURSING PROCESS

■ Assessment

Because there are so many different kinds of protozoal and helminthic infections, patients may appear with a wide variety of symptoms and complaints. The nurse should perform a baseline total patient assessment, with a special emphasis on objective deviations from normal and subjective complaints by the patient. In addition, the patient history should include questions on such things as recent travel within the United States or to foreign countries, recent exposure to new food or water supplies, possible exposure through family members, school contacts, or business contacts who have had a similar illness recently, and any previous history of infection with protozoal or helminthic agents. Knowledge of local endemic health problems will be helpful in identifying some of these infestations. Before drug therapy is started, additional baseline data should be obtained for areas known to be affected by the medications to be prescribed. For example, since chloroquine and related drugs cause toxic reactions more commonly in patients with preexisting liver disease, baseline liver function tests should be obtained at the initiation of chloroquine therapy.

■ Management

Some of these infestations can be treated with very short courses of therapy; others require weeks to months of therapy. The nurse should monitor the overall patient condition, paying close attention to subjective and objective data related to the infection. Evaluation of objective data that could indicate side effects or toxic effects should be done at periodic intervals. During the start of the management phase the patient should be taught about the particular infestation, how it is transmitted, and how transmission can be prevented in the future. This process, of course, will be very individualized because of the wide variety of protozoal and helminthic infections that can occur. Evaluation of close family and social contacts may be appropriate to determine if these individuals have also contracted the particular disease. Referral to the local health department may be appropriate for assisting with this follow-up and for assistance in managing some of the various protozoal and helminthic infections. In addition, the health department will be interested in the epidemiological follow-up of some of these infestations for the purposes of general public health control.

■ Evaluation

The goal of therapy with these drugs is to rid the patient of the infestation. This is usually documented by a return to normal of abnormal smears and other laboratory tests and by a reduction of patient symptoms. The majority of drugs used for these infestations do not cause side effects except in rare instances. Before discharging the patient for self-medication the patient or family member should be able to explain why and how to take the drug, side effects that might occur, side effects that would necessitate notifying the physician, what symptoms would indicate unsuccessful treatment or reinfestation, and other measures that should be employed to assist in the eradication of the protozoan or helminth causing the problem. An example in this latter category might be abstaining from alcohol while taking metronidazole or the need to treat the sexual partner of a female for effective cure of trichomoniasis. For additional information, see the patient care implications section at the end of this chapter.

Toxicity. Quinine can produce an array of symptoms called *cinchonism* (quinine comes from cinchona bark). These symptoms include ringing in the ears, altered hearing acuity, headache, blurred vision, and diarrhea. At the doses used today, these symptoms are usually mild. If the dosage is increased or if the patient is hypersensitive, severe cinchonism can arise. Various blood dyscrasias may occur as well.

Quinine is irritating and causes severe pain on subcutaneous or intramuscular injections, which limits the use of these routes. Given intravenously, the drug can cause hypotension and circulatory failure.

Sulfadiazine

Sulfadiazine is a sulfonamide frequently used in combination with pyrimethamine for the treatment of chloroquine-resistant falciparum malaria (Table 49-2). For a full description of the properties of sulfadiazine, see the previous discussion of pyrimethamine in this chapter and Chapter 45.

Sulfamethoxazole and trimethoprim

Sulfamethoxazole and trimethoprim are used in combination to treat pneumocystosis (Table 49-3). For a full description of these drugs, see Chapter 45.

Tetracycline

Tetracycline is a broad spectrum antibacterial agent also used to amebic infestations (Table 49-1). For a full description of this agent, see Chapter 43.

Thiabendazole

Mechanism of action. Thiabendazole is an extremely potent and specific anthelminthic agent (Table 49-4). The exact mechanism of action of thiabendazole is unknown, but it is believed to attack a metabolic process essential in helminths but not found in humans.

Absorption, distribution, and excretion. Thiabendazole is well absorbed after oral administration, and peak blood levels may be expected within an hour of ingestion. Most of the drug is eliminated by hydroxylation and conjugation, these metabolites being the predominant forms of the drug excreted in the urine.

Very little unchanged drug appears in the feces.

Toxicity. Thiabendazole can cause a wide variety of transient, dose-related toxic reactions. The most common reactions are anorexia, nausea, vomiting, and dizziness. A few patients experience more severe gastrointestinal symptoms or central nervous system effects such as drowsiness, headache, or giddiness. Rarely, patients suffer tinnitus (ringing in the ears), abnormal sensations in the eyes, numbness, or metabolic derangements. Although these symptoms may incapacitate a patient, it is rare for the effect to persist beyond 48 hours and most subside much sooner.

Thiabendazole alters liver function in some patients. Therefore, patients with preexisting liver disease should be more carefully observed for progressive liver damage.

Patients frequently report a strong, unpleasant odor to their urine following thiabendazole therapy. The odor is reminiscent of that produced when asparagus is ingested. Patients may be reassured that this odor is harmless and caused by a metabolite of thiabendazole.

When thiabendazole is used to treat *Ascaris* infestations, migration of the worms may be triggered. Live *Ascaris* have appeared in the mouth and nose of patients receiving the drug.

■ PATIENT CARE IMPLICATIONS

General guidelines for patients receiving drugs to treat protozoal and helminthic infestations

1. Keep these and all medications out of the reach of children. Note that several of these drugs come in pleasant tasting chewable forms or liquids, and children may need special supervision in taking their medications and avoiding overdose.
2. Remind patients to keep all health care providers informed of all medications being taken.
3. Most of these drugs are not recommended for use during pregnancy unless the benefit outweighs the risks. Instruct patients to consult their physicians if questions arise.
4. Individuals contemplating international travel should be referred to the local health department for information regarding diseases that are endemic in areas which are to be visited. In addition, the booklet *Health Information for International Travel* is available from the U.S. Public Health Service, Center for Disease Control, Atlanta, Georgia. Raw fruits and vegetables, improperly cooked meats and food, and impure water can all be sources of parasitic infection, depending on the area to be visited.
5. Giardiasis is not common in the United States, although outbreaks have occurred. It is endemic in Russia, Mexico, Africa, and other countries and is usually transmitted from contaminated food, fruits, vegetables, and water.
6. Amebiasis is found in the United States where unsanitary conditions exist or where living conditions are crowded, as in institutions. Food handlers should always be instructed to wash their hands carefully to prevent possible spread of this disease. In areas where unsanitary conditions may exist, travelers should avoid eating raw fruit or vegetables or drinking the water.
7. Trichinosis can be prevented by cooking pork thoroughly. Smoking, drying, and salting are not reliable methods for killing trichinae.
8. Hookworms are easily transmitted in endemic areas because the larvae penetrate the skin. It is not possible to completely eradicate this infection, but instructing children and adults to avoid going barefoot outside will decrease the incidence.
9. Pinworms are difficult to eliminate because they are so easily transmitted. In the past patients were often instructed to boil their clothing and perform other overwhelming cleaning tasks. It is now thought that careful attention to hygiene is probably just as beneficial. Adults and children should be instructed to wash their hands before eating and after using the toilet. Underwear should be washed regularly. Fin-

gernails should be kept well-trimmed. Children's toys should be kept clean. To help children avoid scratching the perianal region, parents may find it helpful to wash the area several times a day. It is often necessary to treat the entire family for pinworms.

10. Roundworms are not so easily transmitted as pinworms, but hygiene, especially handwashing should be stressed.
11. In the case of worms, it is occasionally appropriate to make a public health referral. A referral may be necessary if a family is experiencing frequent reinfestations, where there is some question about the ability of the family to carry out hygiene activities, when there is concern about toilet or privy facilities, or when, in the assessment of the health care team, such a referral might be helpful.
12. To prevent toxoplasmosis, individuals should be instructed to avoid contact with cat feces. Pregnant women, in particular, should not empty the litter box. In addition, this disease is sometimes transmitted through food. Instruct patients to wash fruits and vegetables carefully and to cook meat thoroughly.
13. For malaria prevention, medication is often prescribed on a weekly basis, starting several weeks to a month before the individual is to go to the malaria infested area. Therapy is continued for 6 weeks to 3 months after leaving the infested area. Reinforce with patients the need to continue the drug for as long as prescribed and to find a way to remember to take the drug on a weekly basis.
14. For additional information about the treatment of and prevention of various parasitic infections, consult appropriate nursing and medical textbooks.

Individual drugs

Any drug not listed below is discussed fully in the text or is similar to others in its class.

4-aminoquinolines

1. Side effects are mild and usually reversible in antimalarial doses. In the high doses used to treat rheumatoid arthritis or lupus erythematosus, side effects are more common and may result in permanent damage. Of specific concern are retinopathy and other eye changes; patients receiving long-term therapy or high doses of these drugs should have regular ophthalmic examinations. Caution patients to report any visual changes.
2. Muscular weakness may develop with long-term therapy. Question patients carefully about subjective changes. Assess muscle strength and ankle and knee reflexes regularly.
3. Patients with a history of psoriasis may experience an exacerbation of their condition while taking these drugs.
4. Taking these medications with meals may reduce gastrointestinal irritation.
5. For suppression of malaria, patients should choose one day a week on which to take their medication.

Emetine and dehydroemetine

1. Toxicity with these drugs is cumulative and may result in degenerative changes in the heart, kidneys, liver, and other organs. Because of these changes and possible cardiac toxicity, patients should remain in bed during therapy and for several days afterward.
2. Monitor the pulse and blood pressure regularly during the course of therapy. If possible, the patient could be attached to a cardiac monitor for the course of therapy, or an electrocardiogram should be done at least every 2 days. Assess the patient's cardiovascular functioning at regular intervals during therapy, watching for precordial chest pain, dyspnea, tachycardia, arrhythmias, gallop rhythm, palpitations, and hypotension.
3. These drugs should be administered by deep subcutaneous or intramuscular injection; the intravenous route should be avoided.

Iodoquinol

1. This drug may interfere with thyroid function test, and this action may persist for up to 6 months after the drug is discontinued.
2. The relatively high concentration of iodine in this drug may cause certain side effects, including anal irritation and itching, skin changes, and discoloration of skin and nails. Instruct patients to report any unusual signs or symptoms.

Mebendazole

1. The tablet may be chewed, swallowed, or crushed and mixed with food.
2. Depending on the form of worm being treated, a single dose may be all that is necessary.

Metronidazole

1. The major side effects are discussed in the text.
2. Instruct patients to avoid the use of alcohol while taking this drug.
3. Caution patients that their urine may turn reddish brown during therapy.
4. Patients receiving oral anticoagulants may need a reduction in dose of anticoagulant while taking metronidazole. Caution patients to report any bleeding or excessive bruising.
5. If indicated, discuss with female patients the need to

treat sexual partners concomitantly if *Trichomonas* in the female seems resistant to treatment or if reinfection occurs.

Piperazine

1. It may be necessary to treat all members of a family.
2. Because the worms are excreted alive, parents should be cautioned to supervise bowel elimination of children carefully for several days after therapy. The worms may be safely flushed down the toilet.

Povidone-iodine

1. Patients should be questioned about possible allergy to iodine prior to use of this drug.
2. Review instructions for use carefully before sending the patient home. The gel comes with an applicator, and the usual dose is one applicator full at night followed by a povidone-iodine douch in the morning. It is important that women understand that therapy should continue even during the menstrual period. For information about douching, consult a fundamentals of nursing book.
3. Povidone-iodine preparations will not stain the skin and are not supposed to stain clothing or bed linens. Patients may wish to wear a sanitary napkin, however, to keep the medication off linens or clothing. Pads should be changed as needed or at least several times each day.

Primaquine

1. This drug should not be administered to patients who have recently received quinacrine as the incidence of side effects may be increased.
2. An acute intravascular hemolysis can occur in susceptible patients, especially dark-skinned individuals or blacks. Instruct patients to report any darkening or change in color of urine, which may represent hemoglobinuria.

Pyrantel pamoate

1. As indicated in the text, side effects are rare.
2. The drug may be mixed with fruit juice or milk.

Pyrimethamine

1. Check the dosage carefully. The dose for treatment of toxoplasmosis may be 10 to 20 times as high as the recommended antimalarial dose, and thus side effects are more common.
2. Taking the drug with meals may decrease gastrointestinal irritation and vomiting.
3. In usual antimalarial doses, side effects are rare, but with chronic use, folic acid deficiency may result. Symptoms of folic acid deficiency are macrocytic anemia, glossitis, diarrhea, and malabsorption.

Pyrvinium pamoate

1. This drug colors stools and vomitus red and will stain most materials.
2. Tablets should be swallowed without chewing to avoid staining the teeth. For patients who cannot swallow tablets, a suspension is available.

Quinacrine

1. Inform patients that the drug may cause urine and skin to turn yellow temporarily.
2. Patients with a history of psoriasis may experience an exacerbation of their disease while taking this drug.
3. For tapeworms, this procedure is often followed:
   a. Before receiving this drug, a cathartic and/or a cleansing enema will be ordered for patients. Some physicians will also request that patients receive a special diet for 24 to 48 hours prior to treatment.
   b. A saline cathartic should be given 1 to 2 hours after treatment. The worms passed will be stained yellow. The stool should be examined for the tapeworm scolex or head.

c. When given through a nasogastric tube directly into the duodenum, the dose should be diluted in 100 ml of warm water and administered via the tube. The dose should be followed by additional water to flush the tube. The cathartic can be given 30 minutes later via the tube; then the tube can be removed.
d. When given orally, the dose can be divided into 100 to 200 mg amounts and given at 10-minute intervals until the ordered dose is given. Sodium bicarbonate can be administered with each dose to help prevent nausea and vomiting.

4. For treatment of malaria or giardiasis, the dose should be taken after meals with a full glass of water, tea, or fruit juice.

Quinine

1. Observe the patient for signs of cinchonism (see text). Instruct the patient that the physician should be notified if any of these symptoms occur.
2. Intravenous doses of quinine dihydrochloride should be dissolved in 100 to 200 ml of Sterile Water or Normal Saline and administered over at least 30 minutes. Marked hypotension often accompanies this route of administration. Monitor the blood pressure. Administer only with the patient in a supine position. As soon as possible, the patient should be switched to oral medication.

Thiabendazole

1. Central nervous system effects occur frequently. Caution patients to avoid driving, operating machinery, or engaging in other hazardous activities requiring mental alertness until the effect of the drug can be evaluated.
2. Oral tablets should be chewed before swallowing and should be taken after meals. An oral suspension is also available.

■ SUMMARY

Parasitic diseases are caused by higher organisms against whom selective toxicity is sometimes difficult to achieve. The selection of an effective drug involves matching the tissue distribution of the drug with the sites of infestation of the parasite, as well as choosing an agent that possesses intrinsic activity against the parasite.

Amodiaquine, chloroquine, and hydroxychloroquine are 4-aminoquinoline derivatives that are widely used to treat malaria. These drugs tend to concentrate in red blood cells and in various organs including the liver and are most effective against the blood form of the disease. Toxicity is rare when the drugs are used for short-term treatment of malaria but more common when used for long-term prophylaxis.

Emetine and dehydroemetine are used to treat amebiasis either localized in the intestine or abscesses in lung and liver. These drugs are given by intramuscular or subcutaneous injection. Emetine accumulates in tissues and may cause cardiac toxicity. These drugs also cause gastrointestinal irritation.

Mebendazole is an effective broad spectrum antihelminthic agent that blocks glucose uptake in sensitive helminths. The drug is not absorbed from the intestinal tract and is therefore useful only for helminths within the intestine, including hookworms, roundworms, pinworms, and whipworms.

Metronidazole is used to treat amebiasis and trichomoniasis, an infestation of the genital tract in males and females. The drug is well absorbed from the intestine. Metronidazole produces gastrointestinal symptoms and central nervous system effects.

Piperazine blocks acetylcholine action on the muscles of *Ascaris* and pinworms, paralyzing the parasites and allowing them to be eliminated by normal peristaltic flow.

Primaquine is an antimalarial drug with a different mechanism of action than the 4-aminoquinolines. Primaquine normally causes little toxicity, but certain populations are sensitive to the hemolytic effects of this drug. Patients with reduced levels of glucose-6-phosphate dehydrogenase are more frequently found in black and Mediterranean populations and are most at risk of this reaction.

Pyrantel is a depolarizing neuromuscular blocking agent that paralyzes intestinal worms, which are then eliminated by peristalsis. The drug is not very efficiently absorbed from the intestinal tract.

Pyrimethamine blocks dihydrofolate reductase in plasmodia, an action similar to that of trimethoprim. Combining pyrimethamine with sulfadiazine gives synergistic effects against plasmodia. Used alone at high doses to treat toxoplasmosis, pyrimethamine may produce blood dyscrasias due to folic acid deficiency in the host.

Quinacrine is used to cause the attachment organ of the tapeworm to release from the intestinal wall. A subsequent purge eliminates the worm from the system. Quinacrine causes vomiting in many patients.

Thiabendazole is a potent antihelminthic agent well absorbed after oral administration. This drug may produce transient gastrointestinal and central nervous system symptoms. Thiabendazole is well distributed in body tissues and may trigger migration of live *Ascaris* from various sites.

■ STUDY QUESTIONS

1. What are the main sites of amebic infestation?
2. What are the two sites where plasmodia exist in the human body?
3. What is the site of trichomonas infections?
4. What type of disease is produced by *Giardia lamblia?*
5. What patients are most at risk from toxoplasmosis?
6. What type of patient is most likely to contract pneumocystosis?
7. Where may *Ascaris* worms locate in the body?
8. Why is threadworm infestation more serious than pinworm or whipworm infestation?
9. What is the fate of the pork roundworm in the human body?
10. What two forms of hookworm infestation occur?
11. What is the mechanism of action of the 4-aminoquinoline antimalarial drugs?
12. How does the tissue distribution of the 4-aminoquinolines increase the usefulness of the drugs in treating malaria?
13. What toxicity is associated with the 4-aminoquinolines?
14. What is the major use of diloxanide?
15. What is the major use of emetine?
16. What toxicity is associated with emetine?
17. What is the mechanism of action of iodoquinol?
18. What is the mechanism of action of mebendazole?
19. How does the tissue distribution of mebendazole affect its use?
20. What types of parasitic diseases are treated with metronidazole?
21. What toxicity is associated with the use of metronidazole?
22. Why should patients receiving metronidazole avoid ethyl alcohol?
23. What is the mechanism of action of niclosamide?
24. What is the tissue distribution of niclosamide administered orally?
25. What is the mechanism of action of piperazine?
26. What toxicity is associated with piperazine?
27. What type of parasitic infestation is povidone-iodine used to treat?
28. What difference exists between the action of primaquine and chloroquine?
29. What toxicity is associated with primaquine?
30. What is the mechanism of action of pyrantel pamoate?
31. Is pyrantel pamoate absorbed from the intestinal tract?
32. What is the mechanism of action of pyrimethamine?
33. What toxicity is associated with pyrimethamine?
34. What is the mechanism of action of pyrvinium pamoate?
35. What harmless side effect of pyrvinium pamoate may be most distressing to patients.
36. What is the mechanism of action of quinacrine?
37. What reaction is common with oral administration of quinacrine?
38. What is cinchonism?
39. What transient effects follow thiabendazole administration?

■ SUGGESTED READINGS

Beck, J.W., and Davies, J.E.: Medical parasitology, ed. 3, St. Louis, 1981, The C.V. Mosby Co.

Bossche, H. Van den: Chemotherapy of parasitic infections, Nature **273:**626, 1978.

Botero, D.: Chemotherapy of human intestinal parasitic diseases, Annual Review of Pharmacology and Toxicology **18:**1, 1978.

Dennerstein, G.: Effective treatment of vaginitis, Drugs **19:**146, 1980.

Kuntz, R.E.: Parasites of children in the United States, Pediatric Nursing **5:**12, Nov.-Dec., 1979.

Yoshikawa, T.T.: Antiparasitic drugs, American Family Physician **21**(3):132, 1980.

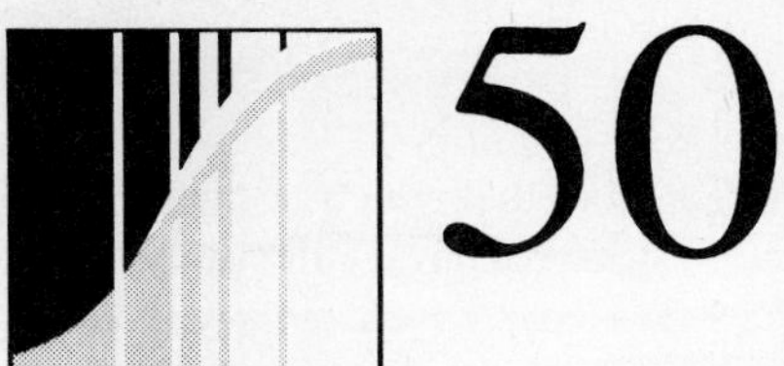

50 Drugs to treat neoplastic diseases

Neoplastic disease occurs when normal cells become transformed by chemicals, viruses, or unknown agents and thereby become resistant to normal controls that regulate cell division and other cellular processes. To understand the treatment regimens used in cancer chemotherapy, it is necessary to understand cell proliferation processes in normal and cancerous tissues. Therefore, in this chapter the cell cycle and the principle of selective toxicity as applied to neoplastic disease are discussed, as well as specific agents used in cancer therapy and the rationale behind certain successful therapeutic regimens.

■ THE CELL CYCLE

The cell cycle is the orderly sequence of events that occurs during the process of cell division, or reproduction. The cycle is usually divided into several segments, according to the processes which occur during that phase. The first event in the cycle is a rapid increase in RNA synthesis compared to the low level of RNA formation found in nonproliferating cells. RNA is formed from the sugar ribose and the purine and pyrimidine bases uracil, cytosine, adenine, and guanine. The phase during which RNA synthesis begins is called G_1 (Fig. 50-1).

The next phase in the cell cycle is the S phase, during which DNA synthesis occurs. DNA is the nucleic acid that forms the chromosomes and contains the genetic information for the cell. DNA is formed from the same components as RNA except that thymine is substituted for uracil and deoxyribose is substituted for ribose.

When DNA synthesis is complete, the cell contains twice the amount of DNA found in a nondividing cell. At this point, RNA and protein synthesis increase and the cell enters the G_2 phase. At the end of this phase, the cell contains enough material to form two complete cells, and mitosis begins.

In mitosis, the DNA condenses to form chromosomes. As mitosis begins, the cell has two copies of each chromosome. To separate these pairs so that one copy of each chromosome goes into each daughter cell, the cell forms microtubules, which are organized into the mitotic spindle. Without the mitotic spindle to pull the chromosomes into opposite ends of the cell, reproduction would halt. Once the chromosomes have been successfully segregated into two complete sets, the division process may be completed by closing the cell membrane to divide the mother cell into two daughter cells.

FIG. 50-1

The proliferative cycle of mammalian cells. In actively dividing cells, the metabolic processes required for cell division take place at different times during the cycle. DNA synthesis precedes messenger RNA and protein synthesis; these processes must be complete before mitosis, or cell division, can occur. Because of their metabolic differences, cells at different phases of this cycle have different sensitivities to many of the drugs used to control cancer.

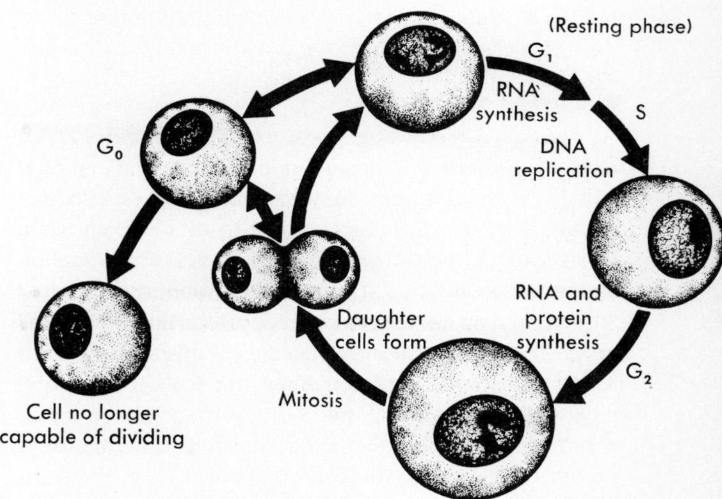

After cell division, a cell may either immediately re-enter the reproductive cycle or may become temporarily nonreproductive (G_0). In this nonreproductive phase, the cell does not carry out a large amount of nucleic acid or protein synthesis, although normal metabolic processes continue. A cell in the G_0 phase may become altered so that it is no longer capable of dividing or it may, after a variable time, return to the proliferation cycle and enter phase G_1 (Fig. 50-1).

Most normal tissues have very few cells actively reproducing at any one time. Most of the cells are either temporarily or permanently incapable of division. There are exceptions to this rule, however. For example, bone marrow is the site for formation of blood cells and as a result is constantly undergoing cell division. Lymphoid tissue is the site for formation of lymphocytes and monocytes and therefore has a high rate of cell division. The intestinal lining, testes, ovaries, and endometrium are all additional sites of relatively rapid cell division.

■ THE NATURE OF NEOPLASTIC DISEASE

■ Origin of cancer

Carcinogenesis is the process by which a normal cell is transformed into a cancerous cell. Although certain agents called *carcinogens* are known to induce this transformation, the exact mechanism producing this change is unknown. However, the outcome of this transformation is known. Cells that have been transformed gain the ability to proliferate indefinitely, as opposed to most normal cells that either do not proliferate or do so for a limited time. Cancer cells have an altered metabolism, which reflects this commitment to proliferation. DNA and RNA synthesis is increased, along with other metabolic processes necessary for growth and cell division.

■ Spread of cancer

Cancer cells also lose the normal property called *contact inhibition*. Contact inhibition prevents normal cells from dividing once they have begun to be crowded together, but cancer cells continue to divide even when the pressure of the surrounding cell mass is considerable. Uncontrolled proliferation and loss of contact inhibition explain in part how a cancer develops in the human body. In certain tissues as the cancer cell begins to proliferate in an uncontrolled manner, the cells form a solid mass and crowd surrounding normal tissue as the mass, or tumor, grows. In other tissues such as bone marrow, growth of the neoplastic cells is more diffuse, but ultimately normal marrow tissue is overwhelmed and crowded out by the cancerous tissues.

Cancer cells also possess the ability to *metastasize*. In this process cancer cells separate from the original mass and move directly or are transported by blood or lymph to distant sites in the body. There the cells lodge in healthy tissue and begin to divide, thus producing a metastasis (secondary tumor). Tumors have been produced in experimental animals with single cancer cells. This property of cancer cells is why cure of malignant neoplasms may require destruction of every cancer cell in the body.

■ Host responses to cancer

In theory one cancer cell left living after therapy is sufficient to cause recurrence of cancer in humans. This situation is quite different from that which occurs in antibacterial chemotherapy. With bacterial infections, therapy can be successful if the bacteria are simply stopped from growing long enough for the immune system to attack and eliminate the invaders. But with neoplastic disease, the immune system seems much less effective. One reason for this difference is that cancer cells are not easily recognized as foreign by the host immune system. Another factor which seems to lower the immune response to cancer is that as the tumors become massive, they produce a specific immune tolerance. Whatever the cause, for most cancers chemotherapy must proceed with little assistance from the host mechanism which so powerfully assists antibacterial agents. This factor helps explain why therapy of neoplastic diseases is so much less effective than therapy of bacterial infections.

■ Chemotherapy of cancer

Another difficulty in treating neoplastic diseases lies in the fact that the cancer cell offers fewer targets for selective toxicity than does a bacterial cell, for example. This similarity in structure and metabolic processes reminds us again that the cancer cell is derived from host cells. Luckily, some differences between normal and cancerous cells can be identified, but the differences are mostly quantitative rather than qualitative. The specific targets for selective toxicity are discussed with individual drug mechanisms.

Since cancer arises initially as a single, transformed cell, it is obvious that diagnosis cannot be expected until much later in the course of the disease. A single cell after 10 cycles of cell division could be expected to produce at most 1024 cells, a mass far too small to be noticed. By the time the tumor weighs about 1 Gm, it will have gone through about 30 division cycles. A 1 Gm tumor is roughly 1 cubic cm in volume or approximately the size of a small grape. In many locations within the body, a tumor this size may easily escape detection, yet in just 10 more cell divisions this tumor could exceed a mass of 1 kg (2.2 lb).

In fact most tumors do not grow nearly as rapidly as the theoretical example just cited, where it was assumed that every cell formed immediately re-entered the reproductive cycle. Certain cancers are rather slow growing and are described as having a low growth fraction. This description simply means that most of the tumor cells are temporarily or permanently incapable of division. Other tumors have a very fast growth rate with a high growth fraction.

■ Diseases called cancer

The lay public tends to think of cancer as a single disease, but in fact it is a large family of related diseases. Cancers may be categorized according to the tis-

TABLE 50-1. Tissue of origin for types of cancer

Cancer	Tissue of origin
Carcinoma	Epithelial cells (e.g., skin and mucous membranes of lung and gastrointestinal tract)
Leukemia	Blood-forming organ (e.g., bone marrow or lymphoid tissue)
Lymphoma	Lymphoid tissue
Melanoma	Pigmented skin cells
Myeloma	Bone marrow
Sarcoma	Connective tissue (e.g., bone, cartilage, and others)

TABLE 50-2. Selected neoplastic diseases

Disease	Characteristics
Burkitt's lymphoma	Rapidly growing tumor of lymphoid tissue; highly responsive to chemotherapy.
Choriocarcinoma (gestational trophoblastic tumors)	Rapidly growing tumor of embryonic cells; seeded in mother during abortion, childbirth, or following hydatidiform mole; highly responsive to chemotherapy.
Ewing's sarcoma	Rapidly growing tumor most frequently found in children; responsive to combination of surgery, radiation, and chemotherapy in early stages.
Hodgkin's disease	Tumor of the lymph nodes, spleen, and other lymphoid tissue; highly responsive to chemotherapy.
Lymphocytic leukemia	Cancer of lymphoid tissue causing leukocytes in blood to be lymphocytes or lymphoblasts; response to therapy is best in acute form of the disease.
Myelogenous leukemia	Cancer of myeloid tissue leading to excess granular polymorphonuclear leukocytes in blood; response to therapy not as good as in lymphocytic leukemia.
Wilms' tumor	Rapidly growing tumor of children; highly responsive to combination of surgery, radiation, and chemotherapy.

sue of origin (Table 50-1). Within these large categories, many subdivisions are possible. For example, leukemias can arise from any of the various cells within the bone marrow. Therefore myelogenous leukemias (arising from myeloid tissue in the marrow), lymphocytic leukemias (arising from cells forming lymphocytes), and other forms of the disease exist.

Some tumors give rise to very characteristic disease patterns. For example, Burkitt's lymphoma, Wilms' disease, Hodgkin's disease, and choriocarcinoma all tend to strike a certain age and sex of patient (Table 50-2).

■ SPECIFIC ANTINEOPLASTIC DRUGS

■ Agents that directly attack DNA

The genetic information necessary for cell reproduction resides in DNA. Although normal nucleated cells contain all the genetic information required to form new cells, this information is seldom expressed, since normal cells in most tissues rarely divide. For this reason, damage to the DNA of many normal cells will be undetectable, since the damage would only be revealed when the cell attempted to undergo division. This rationale explains the use of a large group of anticancer drugs called *alkylating agents*. These drugs form highly reactive compounds in the body, compounds that react with many chemicals including nucleic acids. The damage these chemicals do to DNA frequently makes the cell incapable of replication.

Alkylating agents may attack DNA in its double-stranded form, attaching various compounds to one strand or the other. Other agents may actually form cross-links, or chemical bonds between the strands. Since the strands must unwind and separate during replication, cross-linking effectively blocks replication. The specificity of agents that destroy nucleic acid is not great. All cells will suffer attack by these chemicals, although the action is lethal only when cells attempt division. Therefore, normal tissues with high growth fractions will be expected to show toxicity with these agents.

Because the alkylating agents chemically alter DNA, they are considered mutagenic and rarely may themselves induce cancers of various types.

The clinical properties of antineoplastic drugs that directly attack DNA are summarized in Table 50-3.

Mechlorethamine (nitrogen mustard)

Mechanism of action. Mechlorethamine is a potent alkylating agent that may attack DNA at one site or may cause cross-linking.

Mechlorethamine is especially useful in lymphomas but may also be useful in selected leukemias and solid tumors.

Absorption, distribution, and excretion. Mechlorethamine is so highly unstable that it must be administered intravenously immediately after the solution is pre-

TABLE 50-3. Clinical summary of anticancer drugs that directly attack DNA

Generic name	Trade name	Dosage and administration	Comments
Mechlorethamine or nitrogen mustard	Mustargen	INTRAVENOUS: *Adults*—0.4 mg/kg total dose in 1 or several doses. INTRACAVITARY: *Adults*—0.2 to 0.4 mg/kg.	Mechlorethamine is useful in treating Hodgkin's disease and other lymphomas. Mechlorethamine may be palliative for certain solid tumors and their pleural effusions. Bone marrow suppression is common, beginning soon after therapy and continuing to a nadir at 1 to 3 wk. Pain and severe tissue damage result if drug leaks from the intravenous line into surrounding tissue.
Melphalan	Alkeran	ORAL: *Adults*—0.15 mg/kg daily for 2 to 3 wk or 0.25 mg/kg daily for 4 days. After recovery of the bone marrow for 1 mo, 2 to 4 mg may be taken daily.	Melphalan is useful in treating multiple myeloma and may be helpful in certain tumors of the reproductive tract and malignant melanoma. Bone marrow suppression is an expected, dose-related reaction.
Chlorambucil	Leukeran	ORAL: *Adults and children*—0.1 to 0.2 mg/kg daily for 3 to 6 wk. Smaller doses may be used for maintenance therapy.	Chlorambucil is effective in treating lymphocytic leukemias and myelomas. Bone marrow suppression is the most commonly encountered side effect.
Cyclophosphamide	Cytoxan	ORAL: *Adults and children*—1 to 5 mg/kg daily. INTRAVENOUS: *Adults and children*—40 to 50 mg/kg total dose over 2 to 5 days for induction of remission. 3 to 5 mg/kg twice weekly for maintenance.	Cyclophosphamide is effective in treating lymphomas, lymphocytic leukemias, and myelomas. Hemorrhagic cystitis and bladder fibrosis may occur.
Busulfan	Myleran	ORAL: *Adults and children*—60 μg/kg daily or 1.8 mg/M² body surface area daily.	Busulfan may prolong survival in cases of chronic myelocytic leukemia. Toxicity is mainly observed in bone marrow or kidney (uric acid overload).
Thiotepa		INTRAVENOUS: *Adults*—0.2 mg/kg for 5 days every 4 wk. TOPICAL: *Adults*—60 mg in solution (sterile water) for application at tumor site.	Thiotepa is used in palliative therapy for certain carcinomas and rarely lymphomas. Bone marrow toxicity is dose related and delayed for several days or weeks after therapy is begun.
Carmustine	BiCNU	INTRAVENOUS: *Adults*—200 mg/M² as a single dose or divided into equal doses adminstered on successive days. Dose may be repeated no more frequently than every 6 wk.	Carmustine is used in palliative therapy of tumors of the central nervous system, certain myelomas, and lymphomas. Bone marrow suppression is delayed and may be severe. Carmustine penetrates the blood-brain barrier effectively. Gastrointestinal toxicity is characterized by transient nausea. Pain at injection site is common and severe if drug is infused too rapidly.
Lomustine	CeeNU	ORAL: *Adults*—130 mg/M² as a single dose. Repeated no more frequently than every 6 wk.	Lomustine is similar in use and properties to carmustine.

TABLE 50-3. Clinical summary of anticancer drugs that directly attack DNA—cont'd

Generic name	Trade name	Dosage and administration	Comments
Dacarbazine	DTIC-Dome	INTRAVENOUS: *Adults*—2 to 4.5 mg/kg for 10 days every mo or 250 mg/M² for 5 days every 21 days.	Dacarbazine is used to treat malignant melanoma and certain other solid tumors. Bone marrow suppression reaches its peak 10 to 15 days after therapy. Tolerance develops to the nausea and vomiting initially produced. Pain and tissue damage result if drug leaks from intravenous line into surrounding tissue.
Cisplatin	Platinol	INTRAVENOUS: *Adults*—100 mg/M² once every 4 wk, after heavy hydration to protect the kidneys.	Cisplatin is used to treat metastatic carcinoma and carcinomas of the ovary, bladder, and prostate gland. Renal damage may be severe and alter electrolyte balance in the patient. Myelosuppression, nausea and vomiting, ototoxicity, neurotoxicity, and anaphylactic reactions may occur.
Bleomycin	Blenoxane	INTRAMUSCULAR, INTRAVENOUS, SUBCUTANEOUS: *Adults*—0.25 to 0.50 units/kg weekly or twice weekly initially; decreasing to 1 unit daily or 5 units weekly for maintenance.	Bleomycin is used as palliative therapy for lymphomas, squamous cell carcinomas, testicular and ovarian carcinomas. Pulmonary toxicity, which may be fatal, occurs especially when the total dose exceeds 400 units. Skin reactions are common. Bleomycin does not produce bone marrow suppression.
Mitomycin	Mutamycin	INTRAVENOUS: *Adults*—20 mg/M² as a single dose or 2 mg/M² daily for 5 days separated by a 2-day interval. Neither schedule should be repeated more frequently than every 6 to 8 wk.	Mitomycin is useful in the treatment of gastrointestinal tumors. Bone marrow suppression is gradual and progressive. Gastrointestinal irritation, alopecia, and renal toxicity occur. Mitomycin produces local necrosis when it contacts skin or soft tissues.

pared. The drug is so highly reactive that it is destroyed within minutes of its injection into the bloodstream. No active drug appears in urine or is excreted by any other route.

Toxicity. Mechlorethamine is an extremely toxic agent with a very narrow margin of safety. Significant toxicity is to be expected in every treated patient.

Bone marrow suppression usually may be noted within a day of therapy and will progress to a nadir (lowest point) within 1 to 3 weeks. The platelet count may decrease sufficiently to cause bleeding gums and small subcutaneous hemorrhages. Recovery from the varied symptoms of bone marrow suppression may take several weeks. Nausea and vomiting are acute toxic reactions commonly encountered with mechlorethamine and are thought to be triggered by a central nervous system mechanism. A short-acting barbiturate and an antiemetic may be required to control this reaction.

Germinal tissue may be severely damaged by mechlorethamine. Males may suffer complete arrest of spermatogenesis. Females may suffer menstrual irregularities. Fetuses of treated mothers are damaged by mechlorethamine.

Mechlorethamine may induce malignancies of various kinds. The drug is also an immunosuppressant and predisposes the patient to infections.

Mechlorethamine is a potent vesicant (substance producing blistering). Patients and medical personnel must be rigorously protected from improper contact with the drug. Because of its instability, the drug must be dissolved immediately before use. The nurse or physician should wear surgical gloves for protection while the solution is being prepared and administered. Using a 10 ml sterile syringe, 10 ml of sterile water (or saline) should be injected into the vial. The vial should be shaken with the needle still in place and the appropriate amount of drug removed. This amount of the drug solution should be injected directly into a freely flowing intravenous line. This procedure avoids the danger of extravasation (leakage into tissues around the vein), which produces extreme pain and tissue destruction.

Melphalan (PAM, L-PAM, phenylalanine mustard)

Mechanism of action. Melphalan is a derivative of nitrogen mustard, which works very similarly to nitrogen mustard. Melphalan is therefore not specific for the cell cycle phase.

Some difference in mechanism must exist between melphalan and cyclophosphamide, another alkylating agent, since cross-resistance between these two drugs seems not to occur.

Absorption, distribution, and excretion. Melphalan is well absorbed orally and is usually given by that route. The drug persists in the blood longer than most alkylating agents, being detectable for up to 6 hours after a single dose.

Toxicity. Melphalan produces bone marrow suppression. Dosages are usually adjusted to produce mild leukopenia but no further damage. High doses can produce severe bone marrow depression and bleeding, as well as nausea and vomiting.

Chlorambucil

Mechanism of action. Chlorambucil is chemically related to mechlorethamine and is cytotoxic by the same mechanism. Chlorambucil is distinguished by being the slowest acting and the least toxic of the nitrogen mustard alkylating agents.

In addition to its cell cycle nonspecific cytotoxicity, chlorambucil displays a somewhat selective lympholytic action. This latter property makes chlorambucil an effective drug in treating chronic lymphocytic leukemia, Hodgkin's disease, lymphomas, and multiple myelomas.

Absorption, distribution, and excretion. Chlorambucil is administered orally. Large doses (20 mg or more) may produce nausea and vomiting, but more common doses are well tolerated and reliably absorbed. The drug is commonly given 2 hours after the evening meal or in the morning at least 1 hour before breakfast. The drug seems to be metabolized by the liver.

Toxicity. Chlorambucil commonly produces bone marrow suppression, although at normal doses the effects are usually mild and reversible.

Chlorambucil can produce central nervous system stimulation, gastrointestinal irritation, liver toxicity, and skin reactions at high doses, but these responses are not commonly seen with normal clinical doses.

Uric acid in the blood can reach dangerous levels following chlorambucil treatment. Patients should be observed for this reaction and treated appropriately to avoid severe renal damage.

Cyclophosphamide

Mechanism of action. Cyclophosphamide is a noncytotoxic form of nitrogen mustard that must be activated by liver microsomal enzymes. Several metabolites of cyclophosphamide are formed in the liver, and at least one of these metabolites is a potent alkylating agent with activity similar to nitrogen mustard. Since the drug as administered is not active, it does not possess the strong vesicant activity of other nitrogen mustards.

Cyclophosphamide seems especially effective against lymphoid or myeloid tissue proliferation. The drug is therefore useful to treat various lymphomas, myelomas, and lymphocytic leukemias.

Absorption, distribution, and excretion. Cyclophosphamide may be used either orally or parenterally, which is a distinct advantage over most alkylating agents. Absorption by the oral route is good, with the absorbed drug passing through portal circulation directly to the liver where the drug is activated.

The metabolites of cyclophosphamide are excreted primarily by the kidney. The plasma half-life of the drug and metabolites is 4 to 6 hours. The metabolites of cyclophosphamide are well distributed throughout the body and may enter the brain.

Toxicity. Cyclophosphamide produces all the expected side effects of nonspecific alkylating agents. Bone marrow suppression occurs and is frequently used to guide the physician in adjusting doses. In most patients the bone marrow begins to recover 7 to 10 days after the drug is discontinued.

Gastrointestinal toxicity with cyclophosphamide is common, usually consisting of nausea and vomiting although more severe reactions can occur.

Hair loss (alopecia) occurs with cyclophosphamide therapy much more commonly than with other drugs of this class. Most patients report regrowth of hair after therapy.

Immunosuppression is an expected side effect of cyclophosphamide. The drug has in fact been used directly for its immunosuppressive activity in rheumatoid arthritis and other nonneoplastic conditions.

Cyclophosphamide suppresses gonadal tissue, and the effects may be irreversible. Complete suppression of the menstrual cycles and of sperm formation have been reported.

Cyclophosphamide and its metabolites are excreted predominantly through the kidney. The accumulation of these cytotoxic compounds in the urinary bladder can produce a direct hemorrhagic cystitis. Patients should receive ample fluids while this drug is being used and should be encouraged to void frequently to reduce the damage to the bladder. Bladder fibrosis and carcinoma are somewhat increased in incidence in patients receiving long-term therapy with cyclophosphamide.

Several other drugs affect the metabolism and distribution of cyclophosphamide in the body. Allopurinol seems to prolong the plasma half-life of cyclophosphamide. Barbiturates induce the microsomal enzymes that activate cyclophosphamide, whereas corticosteroids and sex steroids may inhibit the enzymes and thereby lower the rate of formation of active metabolites of cyclophosphamide.

Busulfan

Mechanism of action. Busulfan is an alkylsulfonate capable of cross-linking DNA, as well as reacting with other substances. For reasons that are unclear, busulfan possesses a degree of selectivity which is unique among this class of drugs. Busulfan is a myelosuppressant at doses that do not significantly lower the levels of other blood cells, although platelets may be reduced. Because of this selectivity, busulfan is used in chronic myelocytic leukemia. The drug is not curative but prolongs life and improves its quality.

Absorption, distribution, and excretion. Busulfan is well absorbed orally and is used by this route in chronic intermittent therapy. The drug is highly reactive in blood and tissues and is rapidly converted in the body to a variety of breakdown products, which are excreted by the kidney and other routes.

Toxicity. Busulfan may produce leukopenia (lowered white blood cells), beginning usually after 7 to 10 days of therapy. Hemorrhage may ultimately result if the drug is not discontinued. With long-term therapy, many body systems may show signs of busulfan toxicity. The drug is especially dangerous in pregnant women, producing a very high percentage of fetal damage.

Busulfan may destroy large numbers of granulocytes during therapy. These dying cells release chemicals that may be converted to uric acid, excessively elevating the blood levels of uric acid. To avoid the toxicity produced by uric acid, allopurinol may be given during busulfan therapy.

Thiotepa (triethylenethiophosphoramide)

Mechanism of action. Thiotepa is the only member of the class of compounds called *ethylenimines* that remains useful as an anticancer drug. Thiotepa is a nonspecific alkylating agent.

Thiotepa is not curative but may alleviate the symptoms of certain carcinomas. Since the drug is so nonselective, attempts are often made to apply the drug directly to the tumor when possible. For example, bladder carcinoma may be treated by instilling the drug directly into the bladder. This type of therapy allows high doses to be achieved at the tumor site, with lower doses escaping into systemic circulation. Since toxicity is dose related, such a treatment regimen minimizes systemic toxicity.

Absorption, distribution, and excretion. Thiotepa is employed only by parenteral injection or topical application. Thiotepa is relatively nonirritating and can be administered rapidly through intravenous lines.

Impaired renal function may lower tolerance to thiotepa.

Toxicity. Thiotepa is primarily toxic to the bone marrow. Since the drug produces its effects slowly, care must be taken not to damage excessively the bone marrow by too high a dose in the early stages of therapy. White blood cell counts may be used as an index of toxicity.

Thiotepa may also produce nausea and anorexia.

Carmustine (BCNU) and lomustine (CCNU)

Mechanism of action. Carmustine is a rapidly acting alkylating agent affecting numerous enzymes as well as nucleic acids. The drug can cross-link the strands of DNA. Lomustine is chemically related to carmustine and, like that drug, not only alkylates DNA but has widespread metabolic effects as well. One advantage carmustine and lomustine have over many other alkylating agents is that both drugs penetrate the blood-brain barrier very well. They are therefore of primary use in controlling the symptoms produced by central nervous system tumors.

Absorption, distribution, and excretion. Carmustine is administered by intravenous infusion. The drug is very rapidly degraded so that only metabolites of the drug are detectable in blood or in tissues a few minutes after the dose is administered. The metabolites of carmustine are excreted by the kidney for several days following therapy. The suggestion has been made that the metabolites of carmustine are the active form of the drug.

Lomustine is used orally, being well absorbed by that route. Once absorbed, lomustine is metabolized and excreted similarly to carmustine.

Toxicity. Carmustine and lomustine cause a greatly delayed bone marrow suppression. Following a single dose of drug, bone marrow function may fall for an extended period, reaching its lowest point 4 to 6 weeks after therapy. For this reason, doses of these drugs must be given no more frequently than every 6 weeks or at more widely spaced intervals if the bone marrow does not promptly recover.

Nausea and vomiting are dose-related toxic reactions to carmustine and lomustine. Carmustine is highly irritating and may cause hyperpigmentation if it touches the skin. Pain during infusion of the drug is common. Patient discomfort can be reduced by slowing the rate of infusion of the drug and by properly diluting it before use.

Carmustine is a relatively unstable compound that decomposes in solution. The drug in the dry form in the unopened vial may also decompose at temperatures above 80° F (or 27° C). Only clear, colorless solutions freshly prepared (or stored for short periods in the cold) should be used.

Lomustine capsules are relatively stable when stored at room temperature in sealed containers.

Dacarbazine

Mechanism of action. Dacarbazine apparently acts as an alkylating agent after being activated in the liver. The drug may have other actions as well, but it clearly is cell cycle nonspecific.

Dacarbazine is used to treat malignant melanoma and occasionally other tumors.

Absorption, distribution, and excretion. Dacarbazine must be administered intravenously. The plasma half-life of the drug is about 30 minutes, and the drug appears to be concentrated in the liver.

Dacarbazine is secreted by the renal tubule, about half the drug dose being excreted by this route. The remaining half of the drug dose appears in the blood as a metabolite.

Toxicity. Dacarbazine causes delayed bone marrow toxicity (10 to 15 days after therapy). Many patients also report nausea and vomiting within a few hours following therapy. Tolerance to this symptom develops.

Dacarbazine can cause severe pain and tissue damage if allowed to escape from the vein into surrounding tissues.

Cisplatin (CPDD)

Mechanism of action. Cisplatin is an unusual, platinum-containing complex that apparently acts like an alkylating agent. Cisplatin causes cross-linking in DNA and is not cell cycle specific.

Cisplatin was first used to treat metastatic testicular tumors. Other genital and urinary tract tumors are now reported to respond to cisplatin. Clinical trials evaluating the usefulness of cisplatin in a variety of tumors are underway.

Absorption, distribution, and excretion. Cisplatin must be administered intravenously. The effects of a single dose of the drug last for weeks.

Toxicity. Cisplatin is a relatively toxic drug, which almost always causes severe nausea and vomiting. The drug is also toxic to the renal tubule and may cause serious damage with high doses or too frequent administration. Myelosuppression manifested by lowered leukocyte and platelet counts persists for 3 weeks or longer after a single injection of cisplatin.

Cisplatin causes hearing loss in the upper frequency ranges and ringing in the ears (tinnitus). Ototoxicity tends to progress with repeated doses.

Peripheral neuropathies may occur and may be irreversible. Loss of taste has also been reported.

Anaphylactoid reactions may occur when cisplatin is given to patients who have previously received the drug.

Bleomycin

Mechanism of action. Bleomycin is a complex mixture of glycopeptides derived from cultures of *Streptomyces*. The drug is therefore frequently referred to as an antibiotic (a compound produced by one life form with growth-inhibitory properties toward other life forms). Bleomycin directly attacks DNA, producing breaks in the strands. The drug may also inhibit enzymes that normally repair damaged DNA. Bleomycin apparently attacks cells at several stages of the cell cycle.

Bleomycin has been used against squamous cell carcinomas, lymphomas, and testicular carcinomas.

Absorption, distribution, and excretion. Bleomycin must be administered parenterally. Most tissues of the body rapidly inactivate bleomycin. Skin and lung are exceptions, and the drug tends to concentrate at those sites and there produce toxic reactions. Tumors tend not to inactivate bleomycin, so the drug is also concentrated there.

Toxicity. Bleomycin frequently produces skin and mucous membrane changes, as well as fever, chills, anorexia, and vomiting. Pulmonary reactions occur in 10% of treated patients and 1% may die. Lung toxicity begins as pneumonitis and progresses to pulmonary fibrosis. Anaphylaxis may also occur. Bleomycin does not suppress the bone marrow.

Mitomycin

Mechanism of action. Mitomycin is an antibiotic derived from cultures of *Streptomyces*. The drug is activated by enzymes in the human body so that it becomes capable of alkylating DNA. Like other alkylating agents, mitomycin is nonspecific for cell cycle.

Mitomycin seems most effective against tumors of the stomach, intestine, rectum, and pancreas, although the drug has been occasionally used against other tumors as well.

Absorption, distribution, and excretion. Mitomycin must be given intravenously, since the drug is not absorbed orally and is highly irritating to skin and muscle. The drug apparently enters several organs but not the brain.

Toxicity. Mitomycin produces severe and progressive myelosuppression. Leukopenia (lowered white blood cells) and thrombocytopenia (decreased platelets in the blood) persist for 4 weeks or longer after therapy. Mitomycin should not be readministered until platelet and white cell counts show the bone marrow to have recovered.

Mitomycin also frequently causes nausea and vomiting, skin rashes, and hair loss. A few patients may also suffer a type of kidney damage (glomerulosclerosis), liver toxicity, and lung damage.

Mitomycin causes local necrosis if allowed to escape into cutaneous tissues during intravenous injection.

Hexamethylmelamine

Hexamethylmelamine is an investigational agent chemically related to the alkylating agents. The drug may also have additional anticancer effects. Hexamethylmelamine shows typical toxicity, producing nausea and vomiting and blood dyscrasias due to bone marrow suppression. In addition, central nervous system effects have been observed, as well as peripheral neuropathy.

Hexamethylmelamine is one of the few drugs to show effects against bronchogenic carcinoma. In addition, the drug has been used to treat carcinoma of the cervix.

■ Agents that block DNA synthesis (S-phase inhibitors)

The uncontrolled proliferation of cancerous cells is frequently expressed as rapid cell division or as a high growth fraction. This property distinguishes cancers from most normal tissues, where a very low growth fraction is the rule. Since only those cells in the S phase of the cell cycle synthesize DNA, it is these cells that are most sensitive to agents which block the synthesis of DNA from purine and pyrimidines.

Drugs may block DNA synthesis in several ways. Some of the drugs in this section are specific enzyme inhibitors and prevent the action of an enzyme that is required for DNA synthesis. Other drugs that are chemically very similar to the natural purines and pyrimidines used to form DNA may actually be incorporated into DNA but make the DNA unstable and nonfunctional.

Obviously, a cell that is not forming DNA will not be damaged by a drug that inhibits DNA synthesis. For this reason, nonproliferating cells or cells in resting phase are relatively insensitive to the drugs discussed in this section. These drugs are referred to as *cycle-specific* or *phase-specific* drugs, since they affect primarily cells in S phase.

This property of phase specificity explains why these drugs must be given on a repeating schedule. In a single treatment, only the growing fraction of cells in the tumor will be affected. A recovery period with no drug given allows normal tissues with high growth fractions, such as bone marrow, to return to normal function. During this recovery period, many cells in the cancerous tissue will move from G_0 phase into the reproductive cycle. Other cells that were not in S phase during treatment will continue to proliferate and the tumor will continue to grow. Repeated widely spaced doses of the drug gives the maximal opportunity for the drug to catch the dividing cells in S phase when they will be sensitive.

Since the specificity of these drugs is only toward active DNA synthesis, many normal cells will be sensitive. At highest risk of toxicity are tissues with a high growth fraction. Bone marrow depression and suppression of lymphocyte formation are characteristic side effects of these drugs. Lowered lymphocyte formation reduces the ability of the patient to fight infection (immunosuppression), which may reduce the patient's chance for survival. Gastrointestinal mucosa also has a high growth fraction and is a target of serious toxic reactions to the drugs of this family.

The clinical properties of cycle-specific anticancer drugs are summarized in Table 50-4.

Cytarabine

Mechanism of action. Cytarabine is a chemical analog of cytidine, a normal component of DNA. Cytarabine resembles cytidine well enough to interfere with the function of the enzyme DNA polymerase, which inserts cytidine into DNA but which cannot insert cytarabine. Therefore, cytarabine slows or stops DNA synthesis.

Cytarabine is effective during the S phase of the cell cycle when DNA synthesis is occurring. Although cytarabine has been tested in other tumors, it is at present used almost exclusively in leukemias.

Absorption, distribution, and excretion. Cytarabine must be injected, either subcutaneously or intravenously. Subcutaneous injections are employed at present only to maintain remissions and are given once or twice a month.

Intravenous cytarabine may be given as a rapid bolus or as a slow continuous infusion. When the drug is given rapidly, higher doses may be tolerated, although nausea and vomiting are usually triggered. Infusion of the daily dose of the drug can take place over a 1-hour period or longer.

Cytarabine is rapidly inactivated by enzymes that deaminate the molecule. Blood and liver enzymes apparently contribute to this process. The drug persists in the bloodstream for only about 20 minutes, following a single rapid injection.

Cytarabine does not easily pass into the cerebro-

TABLE 50-4. Clinical summary of anticancer drugs that block DNA synthesis

Generic name	Trade name	Dosage and administration	Comments
Cytarabine, or Ara-C	Cytosar	INTRAVENOUS BOLUS: *Adults and children*—2 mg/kg daily for 10 days or until toxicity intervenes or remission occurs. INTRAVENOUS INFUSION: *Adults and children*—0.5 to 1 mg/kg daily for 10 days or until toxicity intervenes or remission occurs. SUBCUTANEOUS: *Adults and children*—1 mg/kg once or twice per wk.	Bone marrow suppression limits the use of this drug. Children tolerate higher doses than adults. Cytarabine is used to induce and maintain remission in leukemia patients.
Fluorouracil, or 5-FU	Adrucil	INTRAVENOUS: *Adults*—12 mg/kg for 4 days as initial therapy. Less frequent administration of the same dose is used for maintenance therapy when toxicity permits.	Fluorouracil is used as palliative therapy for solid tumors that are incurable by surgery or other means. Gastrointestinal and hematological toxicity limit the use of this drug. Irritation and ulceration may result when the drug escapes from the veins into surounding tissue.
	Efudex	TOPICAL: *Adults*—used as 1%, 2%, or 5% solution or cream.	Topical fluorouracil is used to treat multiple actinic (solar) keratoses. Local reactions include pain, dermatitis, swelling, and scarring.
Floxuridine	FUDR	INTRAARTERIAL: *Adults*—0.1 to 0.6 mg/kg over 24 hr.	Floxuridine is used as palliative therapy for solid tumors not treatable by other means. Toxicity as for fluorouracil.
Mercaptopurine	Purinethol	ORAL: *Adults and children over 5 yr*—2.5 mg/kg/day initially. May continue for weeks if toxicity does not supervene.	Mercaptopurine is used to produce remissions in leukemia, especially those of childhood. Hematological toxicity is delayed and may limit the use of this drug. Immunosuppression is a common side effect. Allopurinol inhibits the degradation of mercaptopurine, making lower doses of mercaptopurine necessary to avoid toxicity.
Thioguanine		ORAL: *Adults*—2 mg/kg daily initially. May continue for weeks if toxicity does not supervene.	Thioguanine is used as mercaptopurine. Delayed hematological toxicity occurs as with mercaptopurine. Allopurinol does not interfere with metabolism of thioguanine.
Methotrexate		ORAL: *Adults and children*—2.5 to 25 mg daily for various lengths of time, depending on the disease. INTRAMUSCULAR: *Adults and children*—15 to 30 mg daily for 5 days. INTRAVENOUS: *Adults and children*—0.4 mg/kg daily for 4 days of therapy or twice weekly to maintain remissions. INTRATHECAL: *Adults and children*—0.2 to 0.5 mg/kg up to 12 mg total. Administered every 2 to 5 days until response is noted.	Methotrexate is curative for choriocarcinoma. Methotrexate is used to maintain remissions in childhood lymphoblastic leukemia. Methotrexate is effective or palliative in certain lymphomas and solid tumors. Gastrointestinal toxicity frequently limits the use of this drug. Bone marrow depression commonly occurs. Immunosuppression may increase the susceptibility of the patient to infections.

TABLE 50-4. Clinical summary of anticancer drugs that block DNA synthesis—cont'd

Generic name	Trade name	Dosage and administration	Comments
Procarbazine hydrochloride	Matulane	ORAL: *Adults*—100 to 200 mg daily for the first wk; then 300 mg daily until bone marrow toxicity supervenes. On recovery of marrow, drug may be continued at 50 to 100 mg daily. *Children*—doses between 50 and 100 mg daily.	Procarbazine is used to palliate symptoms of Hodgkin's disease, lymphomas, and selected brain tumors. Bone marrow depression is frequently used to guide dosage adjustments. Gastrointestinal disturbances and neurological reactions occur. Unwanted drug interactions occur between procarbazine and sympathomimetics, tricyclic antidepressants, phenothiazines, tyramine, and ethyl alcohol.
Hydroxyurea	Hydrea	ORAL: *Adults*—doses range from 20 to 30 mg/kg daily up to 80 mg/kg every 3 days. *Children*—doses not established.	Hydroxyurea is used to treat melanoma, myelocytic leukemia, and carcinomas of various tissues. Bone marrow suppression occurs. Dosage of hydroxyurea may need to be reduced in elderly patients or in patients with renal impairment.

spinal fluid. If the drug is administered intrathecally, it may persist in the cerebrospinal fluid for several hours, since that fluid has a low level of the deaminating enzyme which inactivates cytarabine.

Toxicity. Cytarabine is a potent bone marrow suppressant, acting on that tissue by the same mechanism effective in cancer cells. Most treatment programs call for increasing the dose of cytarabine until the toxicity to the bone marrow becomes intolerable. Bone marrow depression is most profound roughly 5 to 7 days after the drug is stopped. Recovery of marrow function takes at least 2 weeks for most patients and longer for those receiving the drug for extended periods.

Cytarabine is also a potent immunosuppressant. The drug also causes significant gastrointestinal toxicity in many patients. Liver toxicity is reported in up to 7% of treated patients, but a clear relation of this toxicity to cytarabine has not been proven.

Fluorouracil and floxuridine

5-FU

Mechanism of action. Fluorouracil and floxuridine are synthetic pyrimidine bases, which may be converted in the body to an active agent (floxuridine monophosphate). This active form of fluorouracil resembles the pyrimidine that is directly incorporated into RNA or that is converted to the pyrimidine called *thymidylate*. Thymidylate is used exclusively for DNA synthesis. Fluorouracil and floxuridine disrupt these pathways in at least two ways. First, the activated drug may enter RNA, creating a defective form of that nucleic acid which does not support normal protein synthesis. Second and more importantly, thymidylate synthetase, the enzyme required to form thymidylate for DNA synthesis, is inhibited. With thymidylate synthetase blocked, DNA synthesis halts. Therefore, functionally both fluorouracil and floxuridine are S phase inhibitors. Both fluorouracil and floxuridine are used exclusively for solid tumors, and both must be considered palliative rather than curative.

Absorption, distribution, and excretion. Fluorouracil absorption by the oral route is erratic, and the drug is commonly given intravenously. For most patients, best results seem to be produced by giving loading doses intravenously for 5 consecutive days followed by lower doses administered once a week thereafter.

Fluorouracil is extensively metabolized by the liver and other tissues. Less than 15% of the drug dose appears as active drug in the urine. Fluorouracil is cleared from the bloodstream within 3 hours of an intravenous injection, but the effects of the drug persist much longer.

The route of administration of floxuridine determines its metabolic fate and its effectiveness. When floxuridine is given intravenously by rapid injection, the drug is broken down to fluorouracil and thence to the normal breakdown products of fluorouracil. If floxuridine is given slowly by intraarterial infusion, metabolism to fluorouracil is minimized and most of the drug is converted to floxuridine monophosphate, the metabolically active form. The intraarterial route requires a lower dose and yet is more effective than intravenous administration.

Toxicity. Both fluorouracil and floxuridine are highly toxic to the gastrointestinal tract. Inflammation of the membranes of the mouth and pharynx may be an early sign of such toxicity. Nausea, vomiting, and diarrhea almost always occur and if the drug is not discontinued, duodenal ulcers may occur and the bowel may perforate. Patients with preexisting poor nutritional status have a much greater risk with these drugs and are usually not considered candidates for therapy.

Blood dyscrasias also occur with fluorouracil and floxuridine and may cause termination of therapy. Leukopenia (reduced white blood cells) continues for 1 or 2 weeks after therapy is terminated. Various skin reactions and hair loss (alopecia) also occur but are not serious enough to cause the drug to be discontinued.

Mercaptopurine (6-mercaptopurine, 6-MP) and thioguanine (TG, 6-TG)

Mechanism of action. Mercaptopurine resembles both adenine and guanine and blocks several points in the synthesis of these nucleic acid precursors. Thioguanine blocks two reactions, which are also sensitive to mercaptopurine. As a result of the blockade of purine synthesis, DNA synthesis is blocked by either drug. Therefore, both mercaptopurine and thioguanine are S phase–specific inhibitors.

Absorption, distribution, and excretion. Mercaptopurine is well absorbed from the gastrointestinal tract following oral dosage. The drug is not directly irritating to the mucosal lining of the gastrointestinal tract.

Mercaptopurine has a half-life of about 90 minutes in the bloodstream. Part of the drug dose is excreted by the kidney but significant metabolic degradation also occurs. Mercaptopurine is used to produce remissions in leukemias, being most effective in acute lymphoblastic leukemias of childhood. The properties of thioguanine are similar to those of mercaptopurine.

Toxicity. Although bone marrow suppression may occur with mercaptopurine or thioguanine, it generally takes longer to develop than with most drugs of this class. Since bone marrow function continues to fall for several days after therapy is halted, the drug may need to be discontinued at the first sign of significant bone marrow toxicity.

Mercaptopurine is also an immunosuppressant. This action of the drug may reduce host immune defenses and contribute to increased risk of infection in the treated patient.

Mercaptopurine toxicity may be greatly increased by concomitant treatment of the patient with allopurinol. Allopurinol blocks uric acid synthesis and is frequently used to prevent toxic accumulation of that substance following extensive tumor cell destruction by chemotherapy. However, allopurinol is also an inhibitor of the metabolism of mercaptopurine. Therefore, when the drugs are combined, more mercaptopurine persists in the bloodstream and in tissues for longer periods, and greater toxicity results. Thioguanine metabolism is not affected by allopurinol (Table 50-4).

Methotrexate

Mechanism of action. Methotrexate is commonly described as a folic acid antagonist, since methotrexate prevents the conversion of the vitamin folic acid to its metabolically active form, tetrahydrofolate (THF). Without THF, cells are unable to carry out one carbon–transfer reactions, and normal metabolism is blocked at several points. One of these blockades prevents the formation of thymidylic acid, and another arrests adenine and guanine nucleotide synthesis in an early state. Without these precursors, DNA synthesis halts. Methotrexate is therefore specific for the S phase of the cell cycle.

Methotrexate is particularly effective in treating choriocarcinoma, an invasive tumor arising from disseminated fetal cells in new mothers. The drug is also used against a variety of other solid tumors. The most common current use for methotrexate is in maintaining remissions in various leukemias, especially acute lymphoblastic (stem-cell) leukemia of childhood.

Absorption, distribution, and excretion. Methotrexate may be administered by oral, intramuscular, intravenous, intraarterial, or intrathecal routes. For many patients, the oral route is satisfactory, since effective serum concentrations are reached within 1 hour. Parenteral administration results in a slightly faster absorption rate. The intrathecal route is required to treat leukemias that have penetrated the central nervous system. Methotrexate does not pass from the bloodstream into the cerebrospinal fluid in useful amounts.

Methotrexate is well distributed throughout the body and may accumulate to a degree in some tissues. Liver cells seem especially able to bind methotrexate for long periods. The drug also persists in the kidney. These tissue sites of drug accumulation normally account for a small fraction of the total dose of methotrexate. Most of the drug is excreted directly by the kidney. The human body apparently degrades methotrexate little, if at all, and the excreted drug is unchanged.

Toxicity. Methotrexate produces the classical signs of toxicity for drugs of this class. The rapidly dividing tissues of the gastrointestinal mucosal lining are severely damaged by the drug. Stomatitis (inflammation of the oral mucosa) and diarrhea are common signs of toxicity that call for discontinuation of the drug. If therapy continues in the face of these symptoms, severe gastrointestinal damage including perforation can result.

Bone marrow function is also compromised with methotrexate. The result, as with other drugs of this class, is leukopenia (lowered white cell count). Other blood changes may occur and may ultimately produce uncontrolled bleeding.

Methotrexate is an immunosuppressant and may damage the body's ability to fight infection.

The effectiveness and toxicity of methotrexate may be affected by a variety of other drugs. Salicylates (such as aspirin), sulfonamides, phenytoin, tetracycline, and chloramphenicol all tend to increase methotrexate toxicity by displacing methotrexate from plasma proteins. The increase in free plasma methotrexate frequently produces toxicity. Probenecid and other drugs excreted by renal tubular secretion may block the excretion of methotrexate and thereby increase toxicity of the drug.

Methotrexate uptake by cells may be affected by other drugs. The anticancer drugs vincristine and vinblastine apparently increase uptake, whereas penicillin, kanamycin, and bleomycin lower uptake.

Methotrexate produces its cytotoxic effects by blocking the conversion of folic acid to THF. It is therefore possible to prevent the action of the drug by supplying the body with THF. This fact has been exploited for treating methotrexate overdose. Certain tumors are now treated with massive doses of methotrexate. Under ordinary circumstances, these doses would destroy the bone marrow and be lethal. However, if the patient receives intravenous leucovorin (citrovorum factor), an agent containing THF and other folic acid forms, within an hour of the methotrexate dose, the bone marrow can be protected. This type of therapy is called *citrovorum,* or *leucovorin, rescue*.

Procarbazine hydrochloride

Mechanism of action. Procarbazine has multiple effects on cellular enzyme systems and nucleic acids. The drug apparently can cause oxidation of nucleic acids. In addition, nucleic acid synthesis is inhibited. Procarbazine is specific for the S phase of the cell cycle.

Procarbazine is useful in Hodgkin's disease and other lymphomas, as well as in brain tumors and bronchogenic carcinoma.

Absorption, distribution, and excretion. Procarbazine is well absorbed after oral administration. The drug rapidly equilibrates between plasma and cerebrospinal fluid, making the drug useful for treating brain tumors. Procarbazine is excreted primarily by the kidney. Excretion is rather slow, with less than half the drug being eliminated within 24 hours.

Toxicity. Procarbazine frequently produces bone marrow depression and gastrointestinal disturbance. Neurological signs may also appear. Procarbazine inhibits monoamine oxidase. Patients should therefore not receive both procarbazine and drugs that elevate biogenic amine levels (i.e., sympathomimetics, tricyclic antidepressants, phenothiazines, and tyramine-containing food). Ethyl alcohol can produce a disulfiram-like reaction.

Hydroxyurea

Mechanism of action. Hydroxyurea is an inhibitor of an enzyme that converts the ribonucleotide precursors of RNA to deoxyribonucleotides, which are used to form DNA. Hydroxyurea inhibition of the enzyme tends to block DNA synthesis. Hydroxyurea is specific for the S phase of the cell cycle.

Hydroxyurea has been used to treat melanoma, myelocytic leukemias, carcinoma of the ovary, and combined with radiation therapy to treat head and neck carcinoma.

Absorption, distribution, and excretion. Hydroxyurea is well absorbed when given orally. The drug is excreted by the kidney. Therefore patients with impaired renal function may be more sensitive to the drug than normal.

Toxicity. Hydroxyurea produces bone marrow suppression as the most common side effect. This reaction is reversible. Gastrointestinal disturbances, renal impairment, and skin reactions are reported less frequently.

■ Agents that block RNA or protein synthesis

The rapid proliferation of cancer cells can be inhibited by certain agents that block the formation of RNA or interfere with the use of RNA as a template for protein synthesis.

These agents are not highly specific for cancer cells but rather interfere with RNA and protein synthesis in any rapidly dividing tissue. The exception to this rule is asparaginase, a drug with some selectivity for cancer cells.

The clinical properties of these drugs are summarized in Table 50-5.

Asparaginase

Mechanism of action. Asparaginase is an enzyme that converts the amino acid asparagine to aspartic acid. The therapeutic effect of this agent arises because many types of cancer cells cannot form asparagine. Since the enzyme destroys circulating asparagine, those cells are starved for asparagine. Normal cells are spared, since they can form asparagine internally.

To be most effective, asparagine starvation should occur in the G_1 phase of the cell cycle. If asparagine levels are kept low during that period, the asparagine-dependent cancer cell will be unable to carry out protein synthesis and, ultimately, RNA and DNA synthesis will cease. If asparagine starvation occurs later in the cell cycle after many critical proteins and nucleic acids have been formed, the cell may not die.

Absorption, distribution, and excretion. Asparaginase is a protein and must therefore be administered by parenteral routes. The drug persists in the blood-

TABLE 50-5. Clinical summary of anticancer drugs that block RNA and protein synthesis

Generic name	Trade name	Dosage and administration	Comments
Asparaginase	Elspar	INTRAMUSCULAR: *Children*—6000 i.u./M^2 with doses administered every 3 days for one mo. INTRAVENOUS: *Adults and children*—200 i.u. (international units) daily for 28 days.	Asparaginase is used to induce remissions in acute lymphocytic leukemia in children. Allergy to asparaginase occurs frequently and may include anaphylaxis. Central nervous system depression or other signs of central nervous system effects may occur.
Dactinomycin	Cosmegen	INTRAVENOUS: *Adults*—0.5 mg daily for no more than 5 days in succession. Recovery period must be allowed between courses of drug. *Children*—0.015 mg/kg for 5 days.	Dactinomycin is useful to treat choriocarcinoma, Wilms' tumor, and various sarcomas. Bone marrow depression, gastrointestinal irritation, and skin reactions are common. Dactinomycin is extremely corrosive and must not be allowed to escape from the vein or to contact the skin during intravenous injection.
Doxorubicin	Adriamycin	INTRAVENOUS: *Adults*—60 to 75 mg/M^2 as a single injection repeated no more often than every 4 wk.	Doxorubicin is effective against leukemias, lymphomas, sarcomas, and various carcinomas. Bone marrow depression, gastrointestinal irritation, and alopecia are commonly encountered. Heart toxicity is encountered, especially when total doses approach 500 mg/M^2. Doxorubicin produces local necrosis when it contacts skin or soft tissues.
Mithramycin	Mithracin	INTRAVENOUS: *Adults*—0.025 to 0.030 mg/kg daily for 8 to 10 days. Therapy may be repeated monthly.	Mithramycin is useful for treating embryonal cell carcinoma and certain metastatic bone tumors associated with hypercalcemia. Mithramycin produces gastrointestinal, skin, liver, and kidney toxicity. Severe bleeding episodes may occur and progress after therapy. Mithramycin produces local necrosis when it contacts skin or soft tissues.

stream for extended periods and is apparently slowly degraded. The drug does not enter the cerebrospinal fluid in useful amounts and is not excreted in urine.

Toxicity. Asparaginase produces a wide range of toxic reactions. Since the drug is a protein, it is an effective antigen and may provoke severe allergic reactions in treated patients. Renal and kidney function may be impaired, and some patients suffer bleeding episodes, since the drug suppresses various clotting factors. Hyperglycemia has also been observed. Many patients show signs of central nervous system toxicity, including depression, lowered consciousness, coma, and others.

Asparaginase toxicity is increased by vincristine or prednisone. Nevertheless, these drugs are cautiously used together in certain combination treatment regimens.

Dactinomycin (actinomycin D)

Mechanism of action. Dactinomycin is an antibiotic derived from *Streptomyces*. The drug binds strongly to double-strand DNA and prevents the DNA from serving as a template for RNA synthesis. The cell, unable to form messenger RNA, is thus unable to synthesize proteins and complete cell division. Dactinomycin is cell cycle specific for G_1 and S phases.

Dactinomycin is useful in producing remission of choriocarcinoma (tumor of embryonic origin growing in the mother), Wilms' tumor (childhood renal tumor), and certain sarcomas.

Absorption, distribution, and excretion. Dactinomycin is not well absorbed from the gastrointestinal tract. The drug is also extremely corrosive to soft tissues and must therefore be given only by the intravenous route. Dactinomycin is rapidly cleared from the bloodstream, entering the liver and other tissues. The drug does not cross the blood-brain barrier in effective amounts. Excretion of dactinomycin is mainly into bile, with smaller amounts of unchanged drug also appearing in urine.

Toxicity. Dactinomycin is a very toxic drug, which must be administered with great care. The highly corrosive nature of the compound makes it imperative that intravenous injection be given properly, with no leakage of drug into tissues surrounding the vein. Such leakage, or extravasation, can cause extensive tissue damage.

Dactinomycin produces significant hematological changes, which can include aplastic anemia. These blood changes are most pronounced several days after therapy.

Gastrointestinal toxicity is severe with dactinomycin. Patients may experience extreme nausea and vomiting within hours of drug administration. Phenothiazine antiemetics may be required to control vomiting. Dactinomycin also irritates the lining of the entire gastrointestinal tract. Patients commonly report cheilitis (lip inflammation), dysphagia (difficulty in swallowing), ulcerative stomatitis (mouth sores), pharyngitis (inflammation of the pharynx), abdominal pain, and proctitis (anal inflammation).

Dactinomycin also severely damages hair follicles, causing hair loss (alopecia). The drug may cause reddening of the skin (erythema) and signs of inflammation, especially in an area also receiving irradiation.

Doxorubicin and daunorubicin

Mechanism of action. Doxorubicin and daunorubicin are antibiotics derived from cultures of *Streptomyces*. These drugs bind strongly to double-strand DNA and thus stop the formation of RNA. Cells are most markedly affected by these drugs during S and G_2 phases of the cell cycle.

Doxorubicin has a wide range of antitumor activity, including leukemias, lymphomas, sarcomas, genitourinary carcinomas, squamous cell carcinomas of the head and neck, and lung cancer. Daunorubicin has been used primarily for leukemias and neuroblastoma.

Absorption, distribution, and excretion. Doxorubicin is not well absorbed orally, is highly irritating to skin and soft tissues, and must therefore by given intravenously. The drug enters many tissues and organs, but it is the liver that metabolizes the drug rapidly and extensively. Most drug elimination occurs through the liver. Doxorubicin does not seem to enter the central nervous system.

Daunorubicin must also be administered intravenously.

Toxicity. Doxorubicin causes delayed leukopenia and other blood changes. Damage to bone marrow limits the amount of drug that may be used and the frequency of administration. Ordinarily, 21 days will be required for the marrow to recover.

Toxicity to the heart also limits the total amount of drug that can be administered. Total doses of more than 550 mg/M^2 may produce irreversible toxicity to the heart, including ECG changes and congestive heart failure. Preexisting heart disease, prior irradiation to the region of the heart, or prior use of the cardiotoxic drug cyclophosphamide all may greatly increase the likelihood for heart damage with doxorubicin.

Since doxorubicin is metabolized and eliminated by the liver, patients with impaired liver function may suffer drug accumulation and increased toxicity unless doses are appropriately reduced. Some metabolites of doxorubicin and daunorubicin appear in the urine of all treated patients and produce a harmless, red coloration of the urine. Doxorubicin can cause severe tissue necrosis if allowed to escape from the vein during drug administration. Damage to veins may occur if the same vein is used repeatedly.

Hair loss and gastrointestinal irritation commonly occur with doxorubicin.

Daunorubicin causes toxic reactions similar to those seen with doxorubicin.

Mithramycin

Mechanism of action. Mithramycin is an antibiotic derived from *Streptomyces*. The drug binds DNA, thereby preventing RNA synthesis. Mithramycin may be somewhat specific for the S phase of the cell cycle.

Mithramycin also blocks parathyroid hormone activity on osteoclasts, thereby lowering the release of calcium into the bloodstream. This ability to lower blood calcium levels may be useful in patients suffering hypercalcemia as a result of metastatic cancer of the bone.

Mithramycin is also used to treat embryonal cell carcinoma of the testes.

Absorption, distribution, and excretion. Mithramycin must be given intravenously, since oral absorption is poor and the drug damages skin and muscle tissues.

Toxicity. Mithramycin is a very toxic drug whose use must be limited to specific neoplasms where the beneficial results of therapy are known to outweigh the risks. Mithramycin produces a typical array of symptoms, including anorexia, nausea, vomiting, skin changes, liver damage, kidney damage, and lowered blood concentrations of calcium, potassium, and phosphorus.

Mithramycin also produces an unusual syndrome involving episodes of bleeding from various sites. Nosebleed (epistaxis) frequently signals the onset of this syndrome. The condition may stabilize after a few episodes or may progress to extensive hemorrhage, usually within the gastrointestinal tract, and death.

Mithramycin is irritating to skin and muscle tissues and causes tissue sloughing if allowed to leak from intravenous injection sites.

■ Agents that arrest mitosis

To segregate chromosomes, a dividing cell must form a mitotic spindle. The mitotic spindle is formed from microtubules. Microtubules normally function as part of the cytoplasmic transport systems in cells and are required for certain types of cell movement. The major component of microtubules is a protein called *tubulin*.

The structure of microtubules can be disrupted by certain substances that seem to bind to tubulin and cause it to be released from the microtubule. Breakdown of microtubular structure may not be lethal to a cell unless it is in the process of forming the mitotic spindle. Cells exposed at this stage of division are arrested at that point, and reproduction cannot proceed. Ultimately, these cells die. Substances that act in this way are frequently referred to as *mitotic poisons*.

The clinical properties of mitotic poisons used to treat cancer are summarized in Table 50-6.

Vincristine (VCR)

Mechanism of action. Vincristine crystallizes microtubular and spindle proteins, halting cell division in the midst of mitosis. Vincristine, which is a complex alkaloid obtained from the periwinkle plant, is cell cycle specific, since it is effective against cells in mitosis but not other phases.

Vincristine seems especially effective against lymphomas and lymphoblastic leukemias but is also used to treat various carcinomas and sarcomas as well.

Absorption, distribution, and excretion. Vincristine must be administered intravenously. The drug does not cross the blood-brain barrier well enough to combat central nervous system spread of leukemia but is distributed well to other tissues.

Vincristine is rapidly cleared from the bloodstream and is concentrated in the liver. The major route of excretion for this drug is via the bile, with less than 5% of the drug appearing in urine. Biliary obstruction or liver impairment can dangerously impede elimination of this drug.

Toxicity. Vincristine doses are usually limited by the peripheral neuropathy produced by the drug. Many symptoms of nerve dysfunction may be observed, but loss of the Achilles tendon reflex is taken as the first sign of neuropathy.

Vincristine is extremely irritating if it is allowed to escape from the vein into surrounding tissues during administration. Severe pain is produced and necrosis may develop in the exposed tissue.

Vincristine produces hair loss (alopecia) in approximately 20% of treated patients. Many patients complain of constipation and abdominal pain, but these symptoms can usually be relieved with enemas and laxatives.

Vincristine does not produce significant bone marrow depression.

Vinblastine (VLB)

Mechanism of action. Vinblastine, like the related vinca alkaloid vincristine, is a cell cycle specific inhibitor of cells in mitosis. The drug causes breakdown of microtubules and prevents formation of the mitotic spindle.

Vinblastine is used to treat various lymphomas and certain carcinomas.

Absorption, distribution, and excretion. Vinblastine must be administered intravenously. Like vincristine, vinblastine does not freely enter the central nervous system, is rapidly cleared from the blood, and is primarily excreted in bile.

Toxicity. Vinblastine produces neurological toxicity similar to that produced by vincristine. Mental depression and headache may accompany the signs of peripheral neuritis or other peripheral neurological disorders.

Vinblastine produces significant bone marrow suppression, primarily leukopenia (reduction of white cells). Leukopenia normally progresses to a low point 4 to 10 days after the dosage, but recovery usually occurs within 7 to 14 days.

Nausea and vomiting are frequently caused by vinblastine, but this reaction can frequently be controlled with antiemetic agents. Stomatitis, diarrhea, or constipation can also occur.

Vinblastine can cause phlebitis and cellulitis if the drug is allowed to leak into the tissues during intravenous administration.

Hair loss with vinblastine is common but often reverses even while the drug therapy is continued.

Podophyllotoxins (epipodophyllotoxin VM-26 and VP-16)

Mechanism of action. Podophyllotoxins are experimental anticancer drugs derived from compounds extracted from the root of the mandrake (or mayapple) plant. These compounds, like the vinca alkaloids, poison the mitotic spindle and destroy cells in mitosis.

Podophyllotoxins have been used in Europe to treat various lymphomas.

Absorption, distribution, and excretion. The pharmacokinetics of these agents is not yet thoroughly understood, but both drugs may be given intravenously. Epipodophyllotoxin VP-16 may be effective orally as well.

TABLE 50-6. Clinical summary of anticancer drugs that block mitosis

Generic name	Trade name	Dosage and administration	Comments
Vincristine, or VCR	Oncovin	INTRAVENOUS: *Adults*—1.4 mg/M² as a single dose. *Children*—2 mg/M² as a single dose.	Vincristine is effective in treating acute leukemia, lymphomas, various sarcomas, and Wilms' tumor. Hair loss (alopecia) and abdominal pain are not uncommon. Peripheral neuropathy is common and limits the drug dose. Vincristine causes local necrosis if allowed to seep around veins during intravenous injection.
Vinblastine, or VLB	Velban	INTRAVENOUS: *Adults*—0.15 to 0.2 mg/kg once weekly. Doses must start at 0.1 mg/kg and increase gradually. Final dose is limited by bone marrow toxicity.	Vinblastine is used in palliative treatment of various lymphomas and selected tumors of other tissues. Peripheral neuropathy and bone marrow suppression occur. Vinblastine causes local necrosis if allowed to seep around veins during intravenous injection.
Epipodophyllotoxin VM-26	Teniposide	INTRAVENOUS: *Adults*—100 mg/M² weekly. *Children*—dose has not been established.	Epipodophyllotoxin VM-26 is an investigational agent being tested against lymphomas and certain other tumors. Bone marrow suppression is the primary toxic reaction.
Epipodophyllotoxin VP-16	Etoposide	ORAL: *Adults*—100 mg/M² daily for 5 days. *Children*—dose has not been established. INTRAVENOUS: *Adults*—50 mg/M² daily for 5 days. *Children*—dose has not been established.	Epipodophyllotoxin VP-16 is an investigational agent being tested against leukemias and lymphomas. Bone marrow suppression is the primary toxic reaction.

Toxicity. Podophyllotoxins produce bone marrow suppression, anorexia, nausea, vomiting, and hair loss.

■ Tissue-specific agents

Most of the anticancer drugs discussed to this point are not tissue specific in their cytotoxic action. For example, although a drug like chlorambucil is clinically useful because it attacks lymphoid tissue, the drug also attacks other tissues, especially at higher doses.

A few drugs are effective anticancer agents because these drugs interact with specific receptors on or in certain cells. Most of the drugs in this category are derivatives of hormones and interact with those cells bearing specific receptors for the hormone. Glucocorticoids suppress lymphoid tissue because of the specific receptors in that tissue for glucocorticoids.

The sex steroids (androgens, estrogens, and progestins) are also used in cancer chemotherapy. These steroid hormones enter sensitive cells and, complexed with specific receptor proteins, are transported to the cell nucleus. Within the nucleus, these steroids alter RNA and protein synthesis, thereby changing the function of the cell. The use of these agents in cancer chemotherapy depends on a knowledge of the hormone dependence of certain tissues. For example, the prostate gland in males is dependent on androgens; without these hormones, the gland shrinks and loses function. Estrogens, hormones that produce feminization, antagonize the action of androgens on this tissue. Carcinoma of the prostate gland seems to retain a degree of this hormonal control, and tumor regression can frequently be produced by removing the source of internal androgens and supplying excess estrogens.

Similar results can be achieved with many breast carcinomas in females by treating with estrogens, antiestrogens, or androgens. To a certain extent, hormonal therapy of tumors of the reproductive tissues is empirical. However, the rationale behind all forms of this therapy is that (1) reproductive tissues proliferate in response to the proper balance of male and female hormones, and (2) tumors of reproductive tissues tend to retain a degree of dependence on hormones. Tumors in postmenopausal women respond to hormone therapy better than do those in premenopausal women.

The clinical properties of these tissue-specific anticancer drugs are summarized in Table 50-7.

TABLE 50-7. Clinical summary of drugs used to control cancer of specific tissues

Generic name	Trade name	Dosage and administration	Comments
ANDROGENS			
Dromostanolone propionate	Drolban	INTRAMUSCULAR: *Adults*—100 mg 3 times weekly for 8 to 12 wk.	Dromostanolone propionate palliates symptoms of selected carcinomas of the breast in postmenopausal women. Mild virilism may occur. Edema or hypercalcemia may require treatment with diuretics or other drugs.
Calusterone	Methosarb	ORAL: *Adults*—50 mg 4 times daily for 12 wk.	Calusterone palliates symptoms of selected carcinomas of the breast in postmenopausal women. Mild virilism may be seen in about one fourth of those patients treated. Edema or hypercalcemia may require treatment with diuretics or other drugs. Nausea and vomiting are observed in about 10% of treated patients.
Testolactone	Teslac	ORAL: *Adults*—250 mg 4 times daily for 12 wk. INTRAMUSCULAR: *Adults*—100 mg 3 times weekly for 12 wk.	Testolactone palliates symptoms of selected carcinomas of the breast in postmenopausal women. Pain and irritation at the injection site have been reported. Hypercalcemia may occur; appropriate therapy should be initiated.
ESTROGENS			
Estradiol	Progynon	SUBCUTANEOUS: *Adults*—25 mg pellet for subcutaneous implantation. Supplies estrogen for 3 wk.	Estradiol is used as palliative therapy for prostatic carcinoma. Increased risk of thromboembolitic disease occurs with estrogen therapy. Estrogens may cause edema, hypercalcemia, mood changes, breast tenderness, abdominal cramps, and increased pigmentation of breast areola.
Polyestradiol phosphate	Estradurin	INTRAMUSCULAR (DEEP): *Adults*—40 to 80 mg every 2 to 4 wk for at least 3 mo.	As for estradiol.
Diethylstilbestrol diphosphate	Stilphostrol	INTRAVENOUS: *Adults*—500 mg in 300 ml of saline or 5% dextrose on the first day; 1 Gm/300 ml diluent for subsequent 5 days or longer. Maintain with 250 to 500 mg IV once or twice weekly thereafter, or with oral dosage. ORAL: *Adults*—50 to 200 mg 3 times daily.	As for estradiol.

TABLE 50-7. Clinical summary of drugs used to control cancer of specific tissues—cont'd

Generic name	Trade name	Dosage and administration	Comments
ANTIESTROGENS			
Tamoxifen	Nolvadex	ORAL: *Adults*—10 or 20 mg twice daily.	Tamoxifen is used as palliative therapy for advanced carcinoma of the breast. Hot flashes, nausea, and vomiting occur in roughly one fourth of treated patients. Vaginal discharge, menstrual disturbances, and skin rashes may also occur.
PROGESTINS			
Megestrol acetate	Megace	ORAL: *Adults*—40 to 320 mg daily in divided doses for at least 2 mo for endometrial carcinoma; 160 mg daily, divided into 4 doses, for breast cancer.	Megestrol acetate is used as palliative therapy for advanced carcinoma of the breast or endometrium. Thromboembolitic disease and breast cancer may be increased in treated patients.
Medroxyprogesterone acetate	Depo-Provera	INTRAMUSCULAR: *Adults*—400 to 1000 mg in weekly injections.	Medroxyprogesterone acetate is used as palliative therapy for advanced carcinoma of the endometrium. Menstrual irregularities, breast tenderness, rashes, and thrombolitic disease have been reported.
GLUCOCORTICOIDS			
Prednisone	Deltasone Lisacort Meticorten Paracort Ropred Servisone Sterapred	ORAL: *Adults and children*—10 to 100 mg daily.	Prednisone is used to treat lymphoblastic leukemias and lymphomas. Long-term use of prednisone may produce Cushing's syndrome.
ADRENAL ANTAGONIST			
Mitotane	Lysodren	ORAL: *Adults*—6 to 15 mg/kg initially, daily in 3 or 4 doses. Daily dose may be increased gradually to 2 to 16 Gm.	Mitotane is used to control adrenal cortical carcinoma. Gastrointestinal disturbances are common. Central nervous system toxicity and skin reactions also occur in significant numbers of patients.

Androgens

Mechanism of action. Androgens can interact with certain reproductive tissues, altering RNA and protein synthesis. This action is independent of the cell cycle. For estrogen-dependent tissues, androgens frequently interfere with estrogen function. Androgens can therefore cause involution of these tissues. This action forms the basis for the use of androgen to control some forms of breast cancer in postmenopausal women. Results from this form of therapy usually do not become evident until after 8 weeks of treatment or longer.

Absorption, distribution, and excretion. Androgens are in general not well absorbed orally, although a few synthetic androgens are exceptions to this rule (Table 50-7). When given by injection, these oil-soluble substances are slowly absorbed from intramuscular sites.

Androgens are metabolized by the liver. Patients with impaired renal function may have difficulty in eliminating the amounts of androgen used therapeutically and may suffer excessive toxicity.

Toxicity. Androgens produce varying degrees of virilization, which in females is observed as an unwanted side effect. Increased libido, edema, hypercalcemia, nausea, and pain on injection occur occasionally with one or more of the androgens used in cancer chemotherapy. The androgens listed in Table 50-7 are used almost exclusively in cancer chemotherapy. Other androgens, used primarily in replacement therapy may occasionally be used to treat specific cancers. These drugs include fluoxymesterone, methyltestosterone, testosterone enanthate, and testosterone propionate (Chapter 38).

Estrogens

Mechanism of action. Estrogens can interact with certain reproductive tissues, altering RNA and protein synthesis. Ths action is independent of the cell cycle. For androgen-dependent tissues, estrogens frequently interfere with androgen function. Estrogens can therefore cause involution of these tissues. This action forms the basis for the use of estrogens to control prostatic carcinoma. A certain percentage of carcinomas of the breast also respond to exogenous estrogen therapy, especially in postmenopausal women.

Absorption, distribution, and excretion. Natural steroid estrogens are not absorbed orally, but several of the synthetic, nonsteroidal estrogens may be given successfully by this route. Estrogens are also available for subcutaneous implantation and intramuscular or intravenous injection.

Estrogens are metabolized by the liver. Patients with marked liver impairment may accumulate these compounds.

Toxicity. Estrogens increase the risks of thromboembolitic disease. Estrogens also increase salt and water retention, alter mood in some patients, decrease glucose tolerance, elevate calcium levels, produce nausea and vomiting, and cause breast tenderness and abdominal cramps. Of these reactions, thromboembolitic disease, hypercalcemia, and edema are the most threatening for cancer patients.

Of the many estrogen preparations available, three are recommended primarily for use in prostatic carcinoma (Table 50-7). Many of the estrogens discussed in Chapter 37 may also be used in palliative therapy for prostatic carcinoma or carcinoma of the female breast.

Tamoxifen

Mechanism of action. Tamoxifen is an antiestrogenic substance that seems to block estrogen binding at receptor sites in cells. This action of tamoxifen prevents estrogens from supporting the growth of estrogen-dependent cells. Tamoxifen is therefore most useful in palliating symptoms of breast carcinoma where estrogen dependence of the tumor has been established. Tamoxifen acts throughout the cell cycle.

Absorption, distribution, and excretion. Tamoxifen is administered orally. The drug is extensively metabolized. Tamoxifen and its metabolites enter the bloodstream rather slowly, with peak blood concentrations occurring 4 to 7 hours after an oral dose. However, the drug persists in the bloodstream for days as a result of its entry into enterohepatic circulation. Most of the drug is slowly eliminated from the body in the feces. The kidney contributes little to the excretion of this drug.

Toxicity. Tamoxifen may produce cancer and birth defects in animals. It is not known whether tamoxifen produces these effects in humans. Tamoxifen seems less toxic than the estrogens and androgens used for anticancer therapy. The drug may occasionally alter platelet or white cell counts, but the changes observed are mild and usually innocuous. The most frequent reactions to the drug are nausea, vomiting, and hot flashes. Fewer patients report vaginal bleeding or discharge or menstrual irregularities. These reactions do not usually require discontinuance of the drug.

Patients who are started on tamoxifen therapy sometimes report an increase in pain at the tumor site and within metastases in bone. Tumor metastases within soft tissue may actually temporarily increase in size and the surrounding tissue may become inflamed. This reaction, sometimes referred to as *disease flare,* may occur even when therapy is effective.

Progestins

Mechanism of action. Progestins normally function in the body to establish secretory function in the estrogen-primed endometrium. The use of progestins as antineoplastic agents has been limited primarily to using the drugs as palliative therapy for endometrial carcinoma.

Absorption, distribution, and excretion. Progestins are available in various forms suitable for oral or intramuscular administration. The drugs are metabolized primarily in the liver; derivatives of progestins appear in the urine.

Toxicity. Progestins usually produce few toxic reactions. Patients should be observed for signs of thromboembolitic disease or sudden changes in vision, which may be increased in treated patients. Fluid retention and disruption of normal menstrual cycles may also occur. Progestins that are injected may cause pain and tissue changes at the injection site.

Progestins in animals may increase the incidence of breast tumors.

Glucocorticoids: prednisone

Mechanism of action. Glucocorticoids are steroid hormones that regulate RNA and protein synthesis in various cells. This action is independent of cell cycle. Prednisone is the glucocorticoid most commonly used as an anticancer agent, although several of these agents are used for symptomatic relief. Prednisone is an effective anticancer agent because it attacks lymphoid tissue, causing regression of lymphatic tissue. Prednisone is therefore effective against lymphatic tumors and lymphoblastic leukemias, especially in children.

Absorption, distribution, and excretion. Prednisone is effectively absorbed orally and metabolized to the active form of the drug, prednisolone. Liver disease may impair this process and thus interfere with the effectiveness of prednisone.

Toxicity. Prednisone may produce all the well-known signs of glucocorticoid excess, if given long enough at high doses. These symptoms are outlined in Table 50-7 and also in Chapter 35.

Mitotane

Mechanism of action. Mitotane is a derivative of the insecticide DDT. Toxicity studies with the DDT family of insecticides showed specific effects on the adrenal cortex. Mitotane causes specific atrophy of the zona fasciculata and reticularis, the inner two layers of the adrenal cortex where the glucocorticoid cortisol is formed.

Mitotane is not cell cycle specific and is not a general cytotoxic agent. Because of its unusual tissue selectivity, the drug is used to treat adrenal cortical carcinoma.

Absorption, distribution, and excretion. Mitotane is satisfactorily absorbed when given orally. The drug is metabolized by the liver before excretion. If liver function is impaired, the drug may accumulate and toxic reactions increase.

Toxicity. Mitotane causes anorexia, nausea, and vomiting in nearly every treated patient. Nearly half of those treated experience lethargy or dizziness. Dermatitis occurs in 20% of people receiving mitotane. Less frequent but serious reactions include abnormalities of the eye, changes in blood pressure, and hemorrhagic cystitis.

Streptozotocin

Mechanism of action. Streptozotocin is a specific toxin for the beta (β) cells of the pancreatic islets. Other cells of the islets are relatively insensitive to the drug. For this reason, the drug is primarily used to treat insulin-secreting islet cell tumors of the pancreas. Other uses for streptozotocin are being explored.

Absorption, distribution, and excretion. Streptozotocin is relatively unstable and must be administered intravenously.

Toxicity. Streptozotocin can destroy beta cells. Therefore insulin production may cease. The drug is also toxic to the kidneys. Streptozotocin does not ordinarily affect blood-forming cells, so blood dyscrasias are rarely encountered.

■ COMBINATION CHEMOTHERAPY OF CANCER PATIENTS

Few of the anticancer drugs just discussed are used alone. Experience has demonstrated combinations of drugs to be much more effective than single agents. Several reasons for this increased success exist. First, combinations of drugs acting by different mechanisms are less likely to cause the development of drug resistance. Like microbial cells, cancer cells possess the ability to adapt and become drug resistant. This process occurs easily if only a single drug is used. If several are used, the cancer cell has greater difficulty in developing simultaneous resistance.

Second, drug combinations allow the physician to select agents that produce different patterns of toxicity and thereby reduce the damage directed at any one organ system. Most of the drugs discussed produce bone marrow suppression. Combining these drugs with drugs like bleomycin, vincristine, or prednisone, which do not damage the bone marrow, allows more anticancer effect to be achieved with no added damage to the bone marrow.

Finally, combining anticancer agents that act at different stages of the cell cycle allows for more tumor cells to be killed than would occur with the use of only one drug. For example, a drug like procarbazine is specific for the S phase of the cell cycle. Therefore tumor cells that pass into that phase while exposed to procarbazine will die, but cells in resting phase will survive. If an alkylating agent is added to the treatment regimen, we can expect a percentage of the cells that survive procarbazine treatment to be killed by the second drug. Adding a third drug with yet a different mechanism of action, such as vincristine, will further reduce the number of surviving cancer cells. Finally, if it is possible to add a tissue-specific drug to the regimen, even more anticancer effect may be gained. An established and effective treatment regimen such as has just been described exists for Hodgkin's disease. The regimen includes the alkylating agent mechlorethamine (Mustargen), the mitotic poison vincristine (Oncovin), the DNA synthesis inhibitor procarbazine (Matulane), and the lympholytic agent prednisone. This particular regimen is abbreviated MOPP. Many other established combination therapies exist for various types of cancer (Table 50-8).

■ Drugs used in supportive therapy of cancer patients

Cancer patients require many drugs during the course of their disease. The drugs previously discussed are designed to attack the cancer directly. In addition to these agents, cancer patients frequently require other drugs that relieve symptoms of the disease itself or ameliorate the side effects produced by the highly toxic antineoplastic drugs. A brief summary of drugs used in supportive therapy of cancer patients follows.

TABLE 50-8. Representative combination chemotherapeutic regimens

Regimen	Drugs included	Disease
ABVD	Doxorubicin (Adriamycin) Bleomycin (Blenoxane) Vinblastine (Velban) Dacarbazine (DTIC-Dome)	Hodgkin's disease
BACOP	Bleomycin (Blenoxane) Doxorubicin (Adriamycin) Cyclophosphamide (Cytoxan) Vincristine (Oncovin) Prednisone	Non-Hodgkin's lymphomas
CHOP	Cyclophosphamide (Cytoxan) Doxorubicin (Adriamycin) Vincristine (Oncovin) Prednisone	Non-Hodgkin's lymphomas
CMF	Cyclophosphamide (Cytoxan) Methotrexate Fluorouracil	Breast carcinoma
CVP	Cyclophosphamide (Cytoxan) Vincristine (Oncovin) Prednisone	Non-Hodgkin's lymphomas
MOPP	Mechlorethamine (Mustargen) Vincristine (Oncovin) Procarbazine hydrochloride (Matulane) Prednisone	Hodgkin's disease
POMP	Prednisone Vincristine (Oncovin) Methotrexate Mercaptopurine (Purinethol)	Acute lymphocytic leukemia

Allopurinol

Allopurinol may be included in treatment programs for cancer patients when large tumor masses are quickly destroyed by chemotherapy, releasing many breakdown products, including uric acid. Uric acid can severely damage kidney cells if it is allowed to increase unchecked. Allopurinol inhibits the formation of uric acid and therefore can prevent this complication. Allopurinol is also used in the treatment of gout.

Analgesics

The pain associated with advanced cancer can be severe. Therefore hospitals and all hospices specializing in care for the dying cancer patient have a policy of liberal use of narcotic analgesics. Frequent administration and high doses may be required to control pain. Addiction in this patient population is not a problem, and fear of addiction should not stand in the way of adequate control of pain in the terminal stages of the disease.

Antiemetics

Many of the drugs used to attack cancer cells also attack the gastrointestinal mucosa. Nausea and vomiting are therefore very commonly encountered as side effects of cancer chemotherapy. With some of the anticancer drugs, vomiting is so severe that it must be treated to prevent electrolyte imbalance. In other cases it is transient and less severe. Nevertheless, control of nausea and vomiting can greatly improve the patient's sense of well-being and aid in maintaining good nutritional status.

A variety of antiemetic agents are available (Chapter 11). The severe nausea and vomiting encountered in cancer patients receiving cytotoxic drugs frequently requires the strong antiemetic action of phenothiazines. Patients may also be sedated in an attempt to control nausea.

Isotopes

The use of radioactive isotopes is generally considered palliative therapy for certain results of cancer. These agents have their effect by virtue of the ionizing radiation they release. Sodium phosphate P 32 (^{32}P) enters forming DNA, so it tends to be concentrated where that process is highest. Clinically, the use of this drug is to attempt to control proliferation of blood cells in polycythemia vera or in myelocytic leukemia. Gold Au 198 (^{198}Au) is used to control ascites. Ascites occurs when tumor cells are widely disseminated in the abdominal cavity and large amounts of fluid accumulate. This condition differs from edema, since ascitic fluid is free within the abdominal cavity and not trapped in tissues. Pleural effusions may also be relieved by radioactive gold.

The use of ^{131}I, a radioactive isotope of iodine, to destroy overactive thyroid tissue was discussed in Chapter 35.

■ THE NURSING PROCESS

■ Assessment

Patients requiring chemotherapy for treatment of cancer may appear with a wide variety of symptoms; they may also be of any age. A complete and thorough total patient assessment should be done. Additional areas of focus should be based on the probable drugs that will be used for chemotherapy and their known side effects. Thus a detailed examination of the mouth might be done; the condition of the hair, skin, and nails recorded; and the height, weight, and vital signs should be recorded. A detailed history should be obtained, particularly if the patient has received chemotherapy previously. The patient's previous response to chemotherapy will be a guide to the nurse in anticipating response to a repeated dose of chemotherapeutic drugs. Certainly assessment should focus on any visible signs of cancer, and parameters should be outlined to measure the progress of the cancer and its response to chemotherapy. A variety of laboratory and other diagnostic studies may be obtained. Examples would include the hematocrit, hemoglobin, blood count, liver function studies, renal function studies, bone scans, liver scans, and other body scans. Depending on the specific type of cancer, there may be laboratory tests that can be used to monitor the cancer; an example might be alkaline phosphatase in the blood.

■ Management

Management of patients receiving chemotherapy may be very complex, particularly if multiple drugs are being used. Once the decision is made to use one or more agents, additional baseline data should be obtained as needed to identify normal function of certain organs known to be affected by the chemotherapy agents. The nurse should continue to monitor the vital signs, body weight, and the progress of anticipated side effects. For example, regular inspection of the mouth should be done if stomatitis is a frequent side effect of a drug. If alopecia is an anticipated side effect of the drug, the degree of hair loss should be noted. When a side effect is known to occur with regularity, preventive or prophylactic measures should be started as soon as possible. Thus oral rinses and gargles with products known to aid in stomatitis should be started as soon as the drug has been administered. Patients known to have serious bouts with nausea and vomiting in association with one or more agents should be treated prophylactically with antiemetics before the chemotherapeutic agents are given. Fluid intake and output should be monitored. Appropriate laboratory work should be monitored and nursing interventions developed in relation to the results of the laboratory work. Thus the person who is experiencing bone marrow depression should be put in a private room or other measures should be taken to reduce chances of infection. In some institutions, the policy is to put patients with bone marrow depression into protective isolation. Nursing personnel who have colds and other infections should not be permitted to care for individuals with bone marrow depression. If medications are being administered via constant infusion, an infusion control device should be used. Care should be taken to ensure that intravenous infusion lines are patent and that extravasation is avoided. Any new sign or symptom that develops should be thoroughly investigated. Any deviation from the patient's normal values should be noted and evaluated.

Continued.

■ **THE NURSING PROCESS—cont'd**

■ **Evaluation**

Ideally, chemotherapy drugs would eradicate cancer and allow the patient to lead a cancer-free life. Unfortunately, this rarely occurs. In most instances chemotherapy is used with the hope that in a small percentage of cases the cancer will be eradicated, but the goal of therapy for most patients is prolongation of life. An exception to this is adjuvant chemotherapy, which is administered to the patient who has had a surgical excision of the cancer but in whom there is a high chance that microscopic amounts of cancer remain behind. In a certain percentage of these patients the chemotherapy kills the few remaining cells, and these patients will be cured. There are only a few drugs that are used by the patient in the home situation for treatment of cancer. For the majority of patients, cancer chemotherapy is administered in the hospital or in the physician's office, since many of these drugs must be administered intravenously. Before discharging a patient with a medication to be taken in the home setting, the patient should be able to explain how to take the medication correctly, side effects that may occur, how to treat side effects, side effects that require notification of the physician, and any measures to be employed to prevent complications due to side effects. Much of the same information holds true even for the patient who receives chemotherapy in the physician's office. Because the nadir or most profound bone marrow suppression often occurs days to weeks after the drug is administered, it is important that the patient know when to anticipate the side effects and know what actions to take to deal with these side effects. Thus a patient who anticipates a period of bone marrow suppression should be cautioned to avoid exposure to children who often carry communicable diseases and to avoid crowds where infections are spread easily. Patients who have a good chance of developing thrombocytopenia should be cautioned to avoid activities that would cause excessive bruising and should be informed about restrictions that should be observed to prevent bruising or bleeding, such as limiting dental flossing or excessive brushing of teeth. Finally, all patients should be able to explain which situations require immediate notification of the physician. For additional specific guidelines, see the patient care implications section at the end of this chapter.

■ **PATIENT CARE IMPLICATIONS**

General guidelines for the administration of chemotherapy

1. Before a patient receives any antineoplastic agent, a full discussion about the side effects should be held with the patient and, if appropriate, the family. Unlike many medications that cause side effects only rarely, the majority of chemotherapy agents cause side effects regularly.
2. It is important to explain to the patient that it is the appearance and/or severity of side effects which serves as a gauge for the physician to know if the dose of medication is adequate.
3. The patient may not be interested in learning the cell cycle theory but may be interested in knowing on a simple level why various side effects occur. For example, stomatitis occurs in direct relation to the time that it takes normal mucosal cells of the mouth and of the gastrointestinal tract to go through their "life cycle." Thus if a dose of chemotherapy kills the normal cells at an early stage of development, then 5 to 10 days later, when those cells would be on the surface of the mouth, the mouth becomes sore and raw and stays that way until a new set of cells has a chance to develop and again line the mouth.
4. Although patients should be informed of the side effects of the medications they are to receive, an overemphasis on the side effects without a focus on the desired long-term benefit of the drug may cause patients to develop a fear of the medications. It is helpful to learn from patients before chemotherapy begins what the patient's expectations are related to drug therapy for cancer and what previous experiences the patient may have had with persons receiving chemotherapy.
5. Patients should be encouraged to return for follow-up blood tests and office visits. In time many pa-

tients will become very sophisticated in understandin their own body's response to the drugs being used and will know when to seek additional medical assistance. Patients should be helped to feel comfortable in calling the physician or nurse whenever a doubt or concern arises.

6. It is important for health care personnel to remember that each person's response to the diagnosis and treatment of cancer is different. Health care personnel who have or can develop an attitude of openmindedness, honesty, concern, and helpfulness may be the most helpful to the patients. Patients with a diagnosis of cancer often feel a great sense of isolation. Health care personnel who take the time to treat patients as people and take an interest in their personal lives will help the patient feel a little less isolated. The emotional care of the patient with cancer is beyond the scope and focus of this book. For additional information, consult the suggested readings at the end of the chapter or appropriate books and articles on the subject.
7. Fatigue is a common complaint of patients receiving chemotherapy. It may be due to the disease process, to anemia, to depression, to decreased food intake, or in some way to drugs.
8. Check ordered doses of medications carefully. Several chemotherapy drugs have similar names.
9. For information about dilution of intravenous doses, consult the manufacturer's instructions.
10. Although frequent and thorough patient assessment is important with patients receiving chemotherapy, monitoring laboratory results is also important, since changes in laboratory results may herald the onset of side effects before the clinical picture does. Although it is the physician's responsibility to monitor laboratory results, it is also a responsibility of all professional health care personnel caring for the patient.
11. Instruct the patient to keep all health care providers informed of all medications being taken. The patient should be instructed to limit the use of over-the-counter preparations, especially those containing aspirin, because of the potential for bleeding that exists with bone marrow suppression and high doses of aspirin.
12. Menstrual irregularities are common during chemotherapy. There may be temporary, and sometimes permanent, cessation of menses. The older the woman, the more likely that the cessation may be permanent. The patient should keep a record of menstruation while receiving chemotherapy. Any unusual or persistent bleeding or spotting should be reported to the physician, as should amenorrhea.
13. Antineoplastic drugs are not indicated for use during pregnancy. Women of childbearing age may wish to use birth control measures while receiving chemotherapy. A woman who becomes pregnant while receiving these drugs should report this immediately to the physician, as many of these drugs are mutagenic or teratogenic.
14. Chemotherapy may cause a reduction in the viability of sperm. Male patients who are to receive a drug that halts spermatogenesis may wish to arrange for deposit of sperm in a sperm bank before chemotherapy is started. This banked sperm would then be available for later use by the husband and wife. This is, of course, a decision for the couple to make. They should be advised, however, that this may be very expensive and of limited value.
15. Remind patients that these and all drugs should be kept out of the reach of children.
16. Mees' lines (ridges in the fingernails) may occur during chemotherapy and reflect the effect of the drugs on the dividing cells of the nails.
17. Some drugs used to treat cancer may also cause cancer. For most patients, the serious threat of the present cancer being treated makes the threat of a cancer in the future of relatively minor consequence. This later cancer may, however, be of significance to patients who achieve a cure with chemotherapy or in patients receiving adjuvant chemotherapy. Adjuvant therapy is given to patients who have had an apparently successful surgical removal of cancer, and it is given as a prophylactic therapy, usually for 1 or 2 years after the surgery. Patients receiving adjuvant chemotherapy should be informed of the possibility that chemotherapy received now might contribute to the development of cancer in the future.
18. For additional information about chemotherapy, drug protocols, protocols to deal with extravasation, oral gargles and mouthwashes, protein and other dietary supplements, patient teaching aids, and other cancer-related information, contact the chemotherapy department of your regional medical center; The American Cancer Society; the Office of Cancer Communications, National Cancer Institute, Bethesda, Md. 20205; local oncologists' offices; or current journals such as *Cancer Nursing*.
19. Elevation of the uric acid levels often accompanies the administration of chemotherapy to patients with leukemia or some lymphomas. This is due to the release of large quantities of breakdown products in these rapidly dividing forms of cancer. For this reason, chemotherapy given to these patients may be accompanied by routine orders for allopurinol. Monitor the uric acid levels. Keep the patient well hydrated (up to 3000 ml per day).

Patient care implications related to decreased white blood cell count (granulocytopenia)

1. Teach the patient to anticipate a period of greatest susceptibility to infection at a time 1 to 3 weeks after receiving a specific drug. During this time, patients should avoid contact with anyone with an infection, an infectious disease, a cold, bronchitis, and so on. Some patients may find it necessary to limit contact with young children or grandchildren during this time if the youngsters are having frequent colds or infections.
2. Review with each patient the anticipated nadir (point of greatest degree of bone marrow suppression or, stated differently, point of lowest blood count) for each drug being used.
3. Signs of infection include increased temperature (greater than 100° F or 38.3° C), malaise, altered level of consciousness, or development of new signs and symptoms: cough, sore throat, urinary frequency, or dysuria. If any of these appear or if the patient is in doubt, the physician should be notified to determine what treatment, if any, should be used.
4. Instruct the patient to report any wounds that are healing slowly.
5. If a patient is also receiving steroids, remember that the usual signs of infection may be masked. When symptoms do appear, the infection may be far advanced. Assess these patients frequently, carefully, and thoughtfully.
6. In the hospital, pay special attention to preventing the transmission of infection to patients receiving chemotherapy. Hands should be washed carefully between patients. Chemotherapy patients should not be assigned to multibed rooms in which any of the other patients has a known infection, whether pulmonary, urinary tract, wound, or otherwise. Many times it is necessary to assign chemotherapy patients to private rooms. In some instances the physician may choose to put the patient in protective isolation; other physicians feel that, although isolation has a sound theoretical base, it also forces the patient to have social isolation, which may be undesirable for the patient emotionally.
7. Avoid the use of rectal thermometers in these patients, since these may increase the chance of perirectal abscesses.

Patient care implications related to decreased platelet count (thrombocytopenia)

1. Caution the patient to report any sign of bleeding such as bleeding gums, nose bleeds (epistaxis), change of color of the urine that might indicate kidney or bladder bleeding, rectal bleeding, change of color of stools, excessive bruising, or the development of petechiae (minute hemorrhagic spots, pinpoint to pinhead size, seen on the skin). The development of petechiae in the lower extremities is often the first sign of thrombocytopenia the patient will notice.
2. Check stools for the presence of occult blood. It is only necessary to do this beginning about a week to 10 days after the drug is given, that is, a few days before the anticipated nadir of bone marrow suppression.
3. Instruct patients to avoid the use of a razor with a blade; an electric razor is preferred.
4. Avoid the use of intramuscular injections if the platelet count is low (below 60,000).
5. Avoid the use of dental floss if gums are bleeding or if the platelet count is below 10,000 to 15,000. Use a water-spraying oral care device only on the low setting. Brush the teeth with a soft bristle brush until the platelet count drops to 5000 to 10,000; then stop brushing. If the teeth are not being brushed, the mouth can be cleaned with a swab or 4 × 4 gauze pad wrapped around a tongue blade, using a mouthwash or other solution. Avoid the use of lemon-glycerin combinations as these are drying and may irritate the oral mucosa (Ostchega, 1980). See patient care implications for stomatitis also.
6. Instruct the patient to limit strenuous activity, based on the platelet count. The physician may have specific guidelines. One regimen from The American Cancer Society is listed below: for platelet counts greater than 100,000 up to 250,000, the patient may engage in tennis, jogging, basketball, and so on, but contact sports should be avoided; for platelet counts between 50,000 to 100,000, the patient may continue with moderate activity, including walking, swimming, and usual activities of daily living; when the platelet count falls below 50,000, the patient should only engage in mild activities such as walking, light housework, or yardwork. It may be necessary to clarify with each patient the specific activities that person engages in, as a general statement like "light yardwork" may be interpreted differently by each individual.
7. One of the most serious problems that can occur as the platelet count falls is intracranial bleeding; unfortunately, it is often fatal. Symptoms include headache, stiff neck, decreasing level of consciousness, pupillary inequality, and increasing blood pressure. If intracranial bleeding is suspected, the physician should be notified immediately. Many physicians will administer platelet transfusions to maintain the platelet level between 10,000 and 20,000 in an attempt to prevent this complication.

Patient care implications related to anemia

1. Anemia often accompanies chemotherapy and may be due to several factors, including bone marrow depression, anorexia and poor nutritional intake, and the cancer itself. Symptoms include malaise, easy fatigability, pale skin, and decreased hematocrit and hemoglobin levels.
2. Although iron preparations may be prescribed, they may have little effect until chemotherapy is concluded.
3. If anemia is a problem, diet counseling and teaching may be appropriate, although increasing the intake of iron-rich foods may not appeal to the patient if anorexia or nausea is a problem.
4. If anemia is severe, transfusions may be appropriate.
5. Fluoxymesterone (Halotestin) is sometimes prescribed for its androgenic properties.
6. Monitor the stools for the presence of occult blood. If the patient is bleeding, the anemia will be more severe.

Patient care implications related to diarrhea

1. If diarrhea occurs, instruct the patient to switch to a clear liquid diet. Oral fluid intake up to 2500 ml per day should be maintained. The patient should avoid food known to be irritating to the gastrointestinal tract. Common ones include fruit, fruit juices, spicy foods, raw vegetables, corn, and coffee.
2. If diarrhea persists longer than 1 or 2 days, the physician should be notified.
3. Teach the patient that diarrhea can lead to electrolyte imbalance. When possible, monitor serum electrolyte levels. Instruct the patient to consider using a commercially prepared electrolyte replacement solution (e.g., Gatorade) if the diarrhea persists, if the patient can afford the product, and if the physician approves. Rarely, in severe or protracted cases of diarrhea, the patient may have to be admitted to the hospital for intravenous replacement of fluids and electrolytes.
4. Instruct the patient to avoid the use of suppositories and rectal thermometers.
5. Showering or sitting in a tube of warm water a couple of times a day may decrease any anal irritation. Instruct the patient to wash the anal area after each loose bowel movement with soap and water and to dry the area carefully. Some patients may wish to wash the anal area with a prepackaged towelette such as those used to clean infants during diaper changes or with preparations such as Tucks or Wet Ones.
6. Diarrhea caused by chemotherapy may occur during the first 24 to 48 hours after the drug is administered or may occur in association with mucositis (stomatitis), which appears 5 to 10 days after therapy. The time of occurrence may be related to the individual drug and the individual patient response.
7. Refer to the discussion of diarrhea in Chapter 11.

Patient care implications related to constipation

1. Prevention of constipation is much easier than treatment. Individuals more prone to develop constipation are those whose activity level has decreased, those whose food intake has decreased in amount or in variety of foods (i.e., those who are anorexic or who have eliminated high fiber foods, fresh vegetables, etc.), those taking other medications that contribute to constipation, especially many narcotic analgesics, and those with severe anal stomatitis for whom defecating is very painful.
2. Advise the patient to keep a record of bowel movements. If the patient goes longer than 2 days without a bowel movement, consult the physician; the use of a stool softener may be appropriate.
3. In dietary counseling for constipation, advise the patient to increase and maintain the fluid intake at 2500 to 3000 ml per day. Patients should also increase the intake of foods known by that patient to be stimulants to the gastrointestinal tract. Examples of such foods include coffee, fruits and fruit juices, raw vegetables, and high fiber foods such as bran cereals.
4. Instruct the patient to consult the physician before using over-the-counter cathartics and enemas.
5. The actual treatment of constipation may vary with physician preference but most often begins with oral cathartics and stimulants, followed by enemas or manual disimpaction if necessary.
6. Refer to the discussion of constipation in Chapter 11.

Patient care implications related to stomatitis (mucositis)

1. Stomatitis can be both painful and unsightly. It may involve the mouth, anus, gastrointestinal tract (mucositis), and vagina. Since the turnover rate for mucosa cells of the gastrointestinal tract is about 5 to 10 days, mucositis/stomatitis can be expected to occur about 5 to 10 days after the chemotherapeutic agent is given and to last for about 5 to 10 days.
2. Before the first dose of chemotherapy is given, the mouth should be carefully inspected. If the teeth are carious or if there are other problems, the patient should be referred for dental care before the chemotherapy is begun. After chemotherapy is begun, the mouth of the hospitalized patient should be inspected carefully at least twice a day and the mouth of the outpatient on each return visit to the clinic.
3. If the patient experiences oral discomfort while eating, suggest switching to a diet more liquid in form,

including such things as ice cream or milk shakes. Some patients may decide to stop eating entirely until the stomatitis clears, but to prevent dehydration, fluid intake up to 2500 ml per day should continue.

4. Maintaining adequate nutritional intake can be a problem if stomatitis is severe. Suggest to the patient that homemade or commercially prepared food supplements that are high in calories and proteins be used. The physician may have some recipes available for homemade preparations or refer the patient to the nutritionist at the local health department. Many of these supplements can be frozen and eaten like ice cream and may be soothing to an irritated mouth.
5. Instruct patients to brush their teeth gently with a soft bristle brush. If bleeding from the gums is bad, the patient should forego brushing, using swabs instead to clean the mouth until healing has begun. Flossing should be avoided while stomatitis is at its worst. Water-spraying oral care devices should be used on a low setting only.
6. Oral fungal infections (thrush) often accompany stomatitis. To help avoid them, the patient should rinse the mouth or brush the teeth, if that is not too irritating after eating. If white patchy spots appear in the mouth, the patient should contact the physician, who may prescribe oral Mycostatin gargle or other treatment.
7. Instruct the patient to avoid foods that are irritating because of their consistency or spiciness (e.g., pizza, hard crusty bread).
8. Instruct the patient to avoid juices that cause a burning sensation.
9. Application of petrolatum (Vaseline) or a lip balm as needed to the lips will help decrease irritation due to sores and dry, cracking skin on the lips.
10. Instruct the patient to wear dentures and bridgework only when eating and to remove it at other times to decrease irritation to the mouth.
11. The use of a vaporizer at the bedside will help decrease irritation of mucous membranes, especially if the patient is mouth breathing.
12. The use of a local anesthetic gargle or mouthwash 10 minutes before eating may help some patients. Note, however, that the use of an anesthetic agent may decrease the swallowing reflex and contribute to aspiration. In addition, too frequent application of some anesthetic agents to denuded mucosa may result in increased incidence of systemic absorption and reaction to the agent.
13. Painting the oral cavity several times per day (up to every 4 hours) with substrate of milk of magnesia may help to prevent stomatitis. The substrate is obtained by allowing the milk of magnesia to settle out of solution. The liquid portion at the top of the dose or bottle is discarded, and the white, pasty portion remaining is painted over the inside of the mouth.
14. Regular use of specially prepared mouthwashes or gargles may also help prevent or lessen the stomatitis. There are a variety of "recipes" available (Ostchega, 1980); many include one or more of the following ingredients: peroxide, nystatin, tetracycline or other antibiotic, flavoring, and sterile water. Consult the physician, the hospital pharmacist, a regional medical center, and the American Cancer Society for additional formulas. These preparations should be used every 4 hours on a regular basis to be effective; use on an intermittent or "as needed" basis is apparently much less effective. Avoid the use of lemon-glycerin combinations, as they are irritating.
15. In children, stomatitis may develop more rapidly, occurring 2 to 3 days after chemotherapy.
16. For anal irritation, instruct the patient to avoid the use of rectal thermometers and suppositories. Soaking in a warm tub of water several times per day may be helpful. Clean the anal area well after each bowel movement. Some patients may find the use of a prepackaged towelette to clean the anal area after defecation to be helpful.
17. If the patient has severe anal stomatitis, the pain associated with defecation may cause the patient to avoid having bowel movements if possible, thus contributing to constipation. On the other hand, mucositis is severe enough in some patients to cause diarrhea.
18. For vaginal care, instruct the female to always wipe from front to back after a bowel movement. The vaginal-anal area should be kept clean and washed with soap and water; remind the patient to rinse off the soap well. Any vaginal discharge should be reported to the physician, as should a change in the color, odor, consistency, or amount of vaginal discharge. The patient should avoid douching or using tampons unless the physician has allowed it.
19. To decrease irritation during intercourse, the female may wish to use one of the commercially available lubricants designed for this purpose. She should not use hand lotion or other substances that are not designed for the more sensitive vaginal mucosa.
20. Some drugs alter the consistency and quantity of salivary production. Doxorubicin is such a drug. If dry mouth or thick saliva is a problem, there are now commercially prepared substitute saliva preparations available; an example is Xero-Lube.

Patient care implications related to alopecia

1. Inform patients about the possibility of hair loss before beginning chemotherapy. Some individuals may wish to invest in a wig resembling their own hair color and style before hair loss begins.
2. Patients who lose their hair require the emotional support of family members and health care personnel.
3. While less common, hair loss can occur from the pubic region, eyebrows, eyelashes, nose, and other body areas.
4. In most cases, attempts are made when feasible to prevent or reduce alopecia by using a head tourniquet or ice cap for the head. Both of these are used during infusion of the chemotherapeutic agent and for 15 to 30 minutes after infusion; the ice cap is applied 15 to 20 minutes before the infusion is begun. See the suggested readings for additional information. In patients with leukemia or lymphoma, or any cancer that may migrate to be found in the scalp, the use of a scalp tourniquet or ice pack should be avoided; check with the physician if in doubt.
5. Even when the tourniquet or ice pack is used, there will be varying degrees of alopecia with many drugs. In addition, there is no way to reduce alopecia from drugs given orally.
6. In most cases, hair will grow back after chemotherapy is finished, but patients on monthly or every 6 weeks doses will often continue to have little hair until the entire course of chemotherapy is completed. In other patients, hair will begin to grow back during the course of chemotherapy; this seems to be an individual response. Reassure patients that the resumption of hair growth does not mean the chemotherapy is no longer effective.
7. Usually, when the hair begins to return, it will be the same in color and texture as the hair that was lost. Sometimes, however, the hair that grows back is different in color and texture than the hair that was lost.
8. When hair loss is occurring, instruct the patient to wash the hair as little as possible and to brush and comb it gently. If all the hair has fallen out, a thin layer of baby oil applied to the scalp will help prevent dryness.
9. The scalp is very sensitive to sunlight and cold. The patient should be instructed to avoid direct exposure to the sun, either by keeping the head covered and/or applying a sun screen when outside. When the weather is cool, a hat should be worn.
10. Patients may be confused about hair loss due to radiation and to chemotherapy. With radiation therapy, hair loss usually occurs in the area irradiated; thus, alopecia usually only occurs with whole head radiation. With chemotherapy, the hair loss may occur anywhere on the body.

Patient care implications related to nausea and vomiting

1. Nausea and vomiting can be a difficult problem to treat. Each patient responds differently to drugs that cause nausea and vomiting and to regimens to treat nausea.
2. Medications ordered before or during administration of the chemotherapy should be given exactly as ordered, and the patient's response to the combination monitored.
3. For some patients, rescheduling the time of administration of chemotherapy in relation to meals or time of day may make a difference.
4. If vomiting is excessive, it may be necessary to hospitalize the patient to administer intravenous fluids and parenteral antiemetics.
5. Limiting the oral intake to clear fluids on the day of chemotherapy may help.
6. Keeping the environment clean and free of odors may help.
7. Instruct the patient to avoid spicy, fatty, or greasy foods.
8. Nausea and vomiting usually occurs within several hours of the chemotherapy dose and is usually self-limiting. In some patients it may be delayed and occur or recur 5 to 10 days after chemotherapy. This second bout of nausea and vomiting may be related to mucositis of the gastrointestinal tract.
9. The use of tetrahydrocannabinol (THC), the active ingredient in marijuana has been found to be helpful in some patients in preventing or decreasing nausea and vomiting. The use of this drug is still investigational. See the suggested readings for more information.

Patient care implications related to anorexia

1. Anorexia is a difficult problem to treat. It may be due to the underlying cancer or the treatment.
2. Foods with a strong smell or those that are hot in temperature sometimes seem to aggravate anorexia.
3. Small, frequent feedings that are attractively prepared and placed on the plate may be more appealing to the patient.
4. If the patient develops a craving for something, there is usually no reason the patient should not be encouraged to have as much as desired; the alternative is little or no oral intake.
5. Sometimes the activities required to prepare a meal

can so tire the patient that the appetite is diminished by the time the food is ready. If this is the case, suggest that the patient prepare foods ahead of time, on days the patient seems to have more energy, and to freeze them in individual portions that only need to be heated up. Another alternative is to have friends or family do the meal preparation for the patient.

6. Encourage the patient to keep snacks around and to nibble during the day or at bedtime. There should be high protein beverages or snacks available in the refrigerator. Examples include milk shakes, frozen yogurt, and ice cream. There are recipes available from dietitians, the American Cancer Society, and some oncologists' offices for high protein snacks or drinks that can be made at home. There are also available a variety of commercially prepared high protein supplements that the patient might find appealing, either as a drink or frozen and eaten as ice cream. Sometimes the best approach to a patient's anorexia is discovered after careful assessment and history taking.
7. In some patients and in some situations, the use of total parenteral nutrition may be helpful.

Patient care implications related to extravasation of chemotherapeutic agents

1. Extravasation of any chemotherapeutic medication is to be avoided, although several drugs are known to cause tissue necrosis and sloughing should extravasation occur. These agents include nitrogen mustard, vincristine, vinblastine, adriamycin, dactinomycin, mitomycin, mithramycin, carmustine, dacarbazine, daunorubicin, and streptozotocin.
2. In the ideal situation a fresh venipuncture should be done for the purpose of administering chemotherapy to ensure that the line is patent and in the vein. There are times, however, when an infusion in use needs to be used. If there is any doubt about the patency of the vein to be used, the chemotherapy drug should be withheld and a new infusion started.
3. Signs of extravasation would include any signs of intravenous infiltration: redness or swelling at the insertion site, decreased infusion rate, inability to get a blood return, pain, or resistance during the injection of medication.
4. Venipunctures done for the purpose of administering any of the drugs known to cause tissue necrosis following extravasation should be done in the forearm rather than the dorsum of the hand. Then, if extravasation occurs, the tissue necrosis in the forearm is not likely to be as severe as necrosis involving the tendons and muscles that control hand movement.
5. Patients receiving one of the aforementioned drugs should not be left unattended during the infusion.
6. If extravasation is thought to have occurred, discontinue the infusion immediately. There is not agreement about the next step to be followed, but many physicians recommend the intravenous or subcutaneous administration of corticosteroids (e.g., 40 mg Solu-Medrol via slow intravenous push), followed in some cases by topical steroids covered with an occlusive dressing. Most agree that heat should then be applied. Any remaining chemotherapy medication should be administered via another intravenous injection site. The physician should be notified that extravasation has occurred.
7. Medical orders for treatment of extravasation should be written at the time the chemotherapy is ordered. If standing orders exist, they should be readily available to and known by all persons who administer chemotherapy.
8. Because of the serious nature of this side effect of drug therapy, many hospitals and physicians' office limit the number of health care personnel who may administer intravenous chemotherapy.
9. Dacarbazine and carmustine can both cause pain during infusion that is unrelated to extravasation; slowing the rate of infusion may help.
10. Some chemotherapy agents are administered via direct intravenous infusion, that is, direct bolus. When administered this way, the drug should be prepared and drawn into the syringe; then a fresh sterile needle should be put onto the syringe before the venipuncture is performed. This prevents any medication that might be on the surface of the needle causing any irritation or necrosis at the venipuncture site.

Patient care implications for specific drugs

Mechlorethamine

1. See patient care implications for decreased platelet count, decreased white blood cell count, anemia, and nausea and vomiting. Rarely there may be alopecia, diarrhea, and stomatitis.
2. The drug is extremely caustic if it comes into contact with the preparer's hands (see text). If it does come in contact with the skin, flush with copious amounts of water for 15 minutes, followed by a flush with a 2% sodium thiosulfate solution. If the solution comes in contact with the eye, irrigate with copious amounts of normal saline, then see an ophthalmologist. To avoid these problems, the preparer should wear gloves and, ideally, goggles to shield the eyes. Review patient care implications for extravasation.
3. The drug must be administered immediately after re-

constitution. Length of administration should not exceed 5 minutes.

4. This drug is one of the most powerful emetics of the chemotherapy agents. Vomiting should be anticipated.

Melphalan

1. See the patient care implications for decreased white blood cell count, decreased platelet count, anemia, and nausea and vomiting.
2. Administering the dose at night before sleep may make the nausea more tolerable.
3. After reconstitution for intravenous use, this drug is stable only 20 minutes at room temperature; administer immediately.

Chlorambucil

1. See the patient care implications for decreased white blood cell count, decreased platelet count, and anemia. The drug has remarkably few side effects.
2. Bone marrow suppression may continue for up to 10 days after the last dose.

Cyclophosphamide

1. See the patient care implications for decreased white blood cell count, decreased platelet count, anemia, nausea and vomiting, and alopecia. The nadir for bone marrow suppression is 7 to 14 days.
2. For hemorrhagic cystitis, encourage the patient to increase the fluid intake, up to several liters per day. This will result in increased need for urination but will help dilute the drug as it passes through. In addition to drinking during the day, instruct the patient to drink a full glass of water at bedtime and, if the patient gets up to void during the night, to drink another full glass at that time. If given orally, it should be given in the morning so adequate hydration can continue all day. If given intravenously, increased hydration should continue for several days.
3. Cytoxan 25 and 50 mg tablets contain FD&C yellow number 5 (tartrazine), a coloring that may cause allergic-type responses in some individuals. Whereas overall incidence is rare, persons with aspirin hypersensitivity seem to be more susceptible.
4. The patient should be warned that skin and fingernails may darken during the course of therapy; this is temporary.

Busulfan

1. See the patient care implications for decreased white blood cell count, decreased platelet count, and anemia. Alopecia has been reported rarely.
2. Pulmonary reactions, including pulmonary fibrosis, can occur. The first symptom may be shortness of breath.

Thiotepa

See the patient care implications for decreased white blood cell count, decreased platelet count, anemia, nausea and vomiting, and anorexia.

Carmustine and lomustine

1. See the patient care implications for decreased white blood cell count, decreased platelet count, anemia, and nausea and vomiting. Alopecia and stomatitis have also been reported with lomustine. The nadir for bone marrow suppression may be as long as 4 to 6 weeks after therapy.
2. Carmustine often causes pain during infusion. Administer slowly and dilute well. Too rapid infusion may produce intensive flushing of the skin and suffusion of the conjunctiva; this side effect lasts about 4 hours. In addition, extravasation may cause tissue necrosis; see the patient care implications for extravasation.
3. Accidental contact with reconstituted carmustine may cause transient hyperpigmentation of the skin. Those preparing the drug should wear gloves.
4. Administering lomustine at night may decrease the incidence of nausea and vomiting. Administer lomustine on an empty stomach.

Dacarbazine

1. See the patient care implications for decreased white blood cell count, decreased platelet count, anemia, nausea and vomiting, diarrhea, and alopecia. The nadir for bone marrow suppression may be delayed 3 to 4 weeks.
2. Anaphylaxis can occur following administration of this drug. Epinephrine, corticosteroids, antihistamines, and oxygen should be readily available, as well as necessary equipment for possible resuscitation.
3. Rarely, photosensitivity has been reported. Caution patients to report any skin changes and to avoid exposure to the sun or to keep all parts of the body well covered when in the sun.
4. Extravasation of this drug during therapy may cause pain and tissue necrosis. See the patient care implications for extravasation.

Cisplatin

1. See the patient care implications for decreased white blood cell count, decreased platelet count, anemia, and nausea and vomiting. The nadir for bone marrow suppression is between 18 and 23 days.
2. Anaphylaxis can occur following administration of this drug. Epinephrine, corticosteroids, antihistamines, and oxygen should be readily available, as well as necessary equipment for possible resuscitation.

3. To prevent renal toxicity, this drug is usually given concomitantly with a high volume infusion of intravenous fluids, for example, 250 to 500 ml per hour for 4 hours. Some physicians also infuse mannitol during this time. It is important that the fluid infusion not be discontinued until completed, unless the patient's condition warrants it. Monitor the intake and output. Monitor the effects of the large fluid volume by assessing blood pressure and pulse, auscultating breath sounds, and monitoring cardiopulmonary status. Monitor the BUN and creatinine levels to assess renal function.
4. Assess the patient's hearing before each dose. Instruct the patient to report any ringing or noises in the ear or hearing loss. Hearing loss may be more severe in children. Ideally, audiometric testing should be done before the first dose is given, then on an annual or semiannual basis after that.
5. Needles or intravenous infusion sets having aluminum parts that might come in contact with the medications should not be used. If in doubt about the equipment being used, contact the manufacturer.
6. This drug causes severe nausea, which is often very difficult to control, even with high doses of antiemetics.
7. Peripheral neuropathy can occur. Symptoms of this would be numbness, tingling, or other unusual sensations in the extremities. Instruct the patient to report these symptoms if they occur.

Bleomycin

1. See the patient care implications for anorexia and nausea and vomiting. Stomatitis and alopecia have been reported rarely.
2. The pulmonary toxicity of bleomycin is difficult to detect. The first signs and symptoms may be fine rales and dyspnea; there may be changes on the chest x-ray film. This toxicity is usually dose related (in patients receiving more than 400 units total dose) and is more common in elderly persons.
3. An anaphylactic-type reaction can occur following administration of this drug. Epinephrine, corticosteroids, antihistamines, and oxygen should be readily available, as well as necessary equipment for possible resuscitation. This reaction seems to be more common in lymphoma patients, so it is suggested that these patients receive a test dose of 1 to 2 units, with the ordered dose withheld until the next day so the patient's response can be monitored.
4. Fever may occur as a side effect of this drug. It may appear within a day of receiving the dose, then disappear within 24 hours. In some patients the fever occurs or recurs, accompanied by flulike symptoms, 7 to 10 days after treatment. If the fever occurs, instruct the patient to take and record the temperature every 4 hours, maintain fluid intake (at least 2500 ml per day), and to take antipyretics as ordered. If the fever persists longer than 2 days or exceeds 100° F or 38.3° C, the physician should be notified. Often, the physician will elect to treat the patient with antibiotics, since it is difficult to tell initially if the fever is drug related or due to an infection in the patient.
5. Skin problems can occur with this drug, including rash, tenderness, swelling of the fingers, and vesicle formation over pressure points and the palms of the hands. Instruct the patient to report any skin changes.

Mitomycin

1. See the patient care implications for decreased white blood cell count, decreased platelet count, anemia, alopecia, nausea and vomiting, and stomatitis.
2. To monitor renal effects, assess serum creatinine and BUN levels regularly. Monitor the intake and output.
3. Fever may occur as a side effect of this drug. Instruct the patient to take the temperature at regular intervals if fever occurs, to maintain fluid intake (at least 2500 ml per day), and to take antipyretics as directed. If the fever persists longer than 2 days, or exceeds 100° F or 38.3° C, the physician should be notified. Because it is often difficult to differentiate a fever due to drug therapy versus one due to infection, the physician may elect to treat the patient with antibiotics.
4. The drug is harmful to tissues; see the patient care implications for extravasation.

Hexamethylmelamine

1. See the patient care implications for decreased white blood cell count, decreased platelet count, anemia, and nausea and vomiting. The nadir for bone marrow suppression may be delayed.
2. Visual hallucinations have been reported. Instruct the patient to report any visual changes.
3. Peripheral neuritis may be a problem. Symptoms include sensory loss and weakness in the hands and feet; there may be pain or discomfort. Some physicians may administer pyridoxine routinely to patients receiving hexamethylmelamine.

Cytarabine

1. See the patient care implications for decreased white blood cell count, decreased platelet count, anemia, stomatitis, diarrhea, and nausea and vomiting. Alopecia has been reported rarely. The nadir for bone marrow suppression is 5 to 7 days after the last dose.
2. Fever may occur as a side effect of this drug. Instruct the patient to take the temperature at regular intervals if fever occurs, to maintain fluid intake (at least 2500

ml per day), and to take antipyretics as directed. If the fever persists longer than 2 days, or exceeds 100° F or 38.3° C, the physician should be notified. Because it is often difficult to differentiate a fever due to drug therapy versus one due to infection, the physician may elect to treat the patient with antibiotics.

Fluorouracil and floxuridine

1. See the patient care implications for decreased white blood cell count, decreased platelet count, anemia, stomatitis, nausea and vomiting, diarrhea, and alopecia. The nadir for bone marrow suppression is usually 9 to 14 days after the last dose of drug.
2. Fluorouracil may be diluted and given as an infusion or as a bolus.
3. Some unusual side effects that can occur include darkening of the veins where infused, tearing (increased lacrimation), and cerebellar dysfunction manifested as gait abnormalities. Skin changes have also been reported, including photosensitivity. Instruct the patient to report any skin changes and to avoid prolonged direct exposure to the sun.

Mercaptopurine and thioguanine

See the patient care implications for decreased white blood cell count, decreased platelet count, anemia, nausea and vomiting, stomatitis (mucositis), and diarrhea.

Methotrexate

1. See the patient care implications for decreased white blood cell count, decreased platelet count, anemia, stomatitis, and diarrhea. Alopecia has been reported rarely.
2. There are a variety of medications that should not be taken with methotrexate, at least in the usual doses. Remind the patient to keep all health care personnel informed of all medications being taken.
3. This drug is sometimes prescribed for treatment for psoriasis. The epithelium of the patient with psoriasis is more rapidly dividing than normal skin and thus may respond to the drug therapy.
4. Patients taking vitamin preparations that contain folic acid may have an altered response to methotrexate. Encourage patients to discuss vitamin needs with the physician.
5. To monitor for renal toxicity, measure the fluid intake and output. Monitor the BUN and creatinine levels.
6. Prolonged use can result in liver toxicity. Monitor liver function tests. Assess the patient for development of jaundice.
7. Leucovorin rescue may be used with high dose methotrexate. The patient is kept well hydrated. The urine may be alkalinized to increase the solubility of the methotrexate; usually sodium bicarbonate is used. Monitor the fluid intake and output and renal function.
8. Skin rash may appear as a side effect. Some physicians feel this is a sign of toxicity and that it warrants discontinuing the drug. Instruct the patient to report any skin changes.

Procarbazine

1. See the patient care implications for decreased white blood cell count, decreased platelet count, anemia, and nausea and vomiting. Occasionally, constipation, diarrhea, or stomatitis has been reported.
2. The patient should be cautioned to avoid the use of alcohol while receiving procarbazine. Review with the patient the disulfiram (Antabuse) type reaction that may occur if alcohol is consumed (flushing, headache, nausea, hypertension).
3. Foods with a known high tyramine content should be avoided by the patient receiving procarbazine. A list of these foods is given in Table 26-5.

Hydroxyurea

1. See the patient care implications for decreased white blood cell count, decreased platelet count, and anemia. Occasionally constipation, diarrhea, alopecia, stomatitis, anorexia, and allergic dermatitis (rash) have been reported.
2. The capsules contain FD&C yellow number 5 coloring (tartrazine), which may cause allergic-type responses in some individuals. Although overall incidence is rare, persons with aspirin hypersensitivity seem to be more susceptible.
3. If the patient is unable to swallow capsules, the contents of the capsules may be emptied into a glass of water and taken immediately. There is some inert material within the capsule, so there may be some particulate matter that does not dissolve in the water; this is not harmful to the patient.

Asparaginase

1. See the patient care implications for nausea and vomiting; occasionally there is a decreased platelet count.
2. Monitor the urine and blood sugar concentrations regularly. Diabetics may find it necessary to increase insulin or oral hypoglycemic doses during therapy.
3. Because of the frequency of allergic responses, it is recommended that the patient be monitored closely during asparaginase administration. Epinephrine, corticosteroids, antihistamines, and oxygen should be readily available, as well as personnel, drugs, and equipment for resuscitation. The possibility of an allergic response should be anticipated with each dose.

4. Check the temperature every 4 hours during treatment as fatal hyperthermia has been reported.
5. Bleeding tendencies may occur as a side effect and may be due to decreased platelets and/or decreased clotting factors. Regardless of the cause, patients should be cautioned to report any bruising or bleeding, or development of petechiae.
6. Because of the high incidence of allergic reactions, it is recommended that each patient be skin tested prior to receiving the first dose of asparaginase. Directions for preparing the skin test solution and a possible desensitization schedule are included in the manufacturer's instructions. Note that a negative skin test does not completely rule out the possibility of an allergic response to the larger chemotherapy dose.
7. Pancreatitis can occur as a result of therapy. Signs and symptoms might include abdominal pain, enlarged pancreas (felt as an abdominal mass), tachycardia, jaundice, and elevation of serum amylase values.
8. When using more than one vial for a treatment, make certain that all vials used are from the same lot number. The lot number is printed on each vial.

Dactinomycin

1. See the patient care implications for decreased white blood cell count, decreased platelet count, anemia, nausea and vomiting, diarrhea, stomatitis, alopecia, and gastrointestinal irritations, probably due to mucositis. The nadir for bone marrow suppression is 7 to 10 days after the drug is given.
2. Extravasation should be avoided. See the patient care implications for extravasation.
3. Administer over 5 minutes for intravenous push. When given as intravenous drip, administer over 1 hour; protect intravenous bottle and infusion set from room light.

Doxorubicin

1. See the patient care implications for decreased white blood cell count, decreased platelet count, anemia, alopecia, and stomatitis (mucositis). The nadir for bone marrow suppression is 10 to 14 days after the dose is administered.
2. There is no agreement as to the best way to monitor for cardiac toxicity. Some physicians recommend monitoring the ECG for changes, and some feel the most predictive sign is persistent reductions in the QRS voltage. Other practitioners feel that echocardiography is the best tool. The toxicity is dose related. At a total dose of less than 400 mg per M^2, cardiac toxicity is rare; many physicians use 550 mg per M^2, total dose, as the highest possible dose that can be given safely. If there has been radiation to the heart, toxicity can occur at a lower dose than the values listed.
3. Inform patients that urine will be red during therapy and for 1 to 2 days after therapy; reassure them that this is not blood.
4. Skin contact with adriamycin may cause skin irritation. Individuals preparing the drug for administration should wear gloves. If contact with the skin occurs, the area should be rinsed well with water.
5. Extravasation should be avoided; see the patient care implications related to this problem.

Daunorubicin

1. See the patient care implications for doxorubicin.
2. The safe cumulative dose in relation to cardiac toxicity is less than or equal to 600 mg/M^2 for this drug.

Mithramycin

1. See the patient care implications for decreased white blood cell count, decreased platelet count, anemia, anorexia, and nausea and vomiting.
2. Because of the effect of this drug on calcium, potassium, and phosphorus, serum electrolyte levels should be monitored regularly.
3. In addition to monitoring platelets, the prothrombin time or bleeding time should be checked. Instruct the patient to report any bleeding or bruising. Often the first sign of bleeding difficulties with this drug is a severe nosebleed or hematemesis (vomiting of blood).
4. Observe the patient for possible renal failure. Monitor the fluid intake and output and regularly check the BUN and creatinine levels. The patient with a history of renal failure should receive only one half the usual dose.
5. This drug can also cause liver damage. Monitor the lactic dehydrogenase (LDH) level.
6. Extravasation should be avoided; see the patient care implications related to this problem.

Vincristine

1. See the patient care implications for alopecia and constipation. A drop in white blood cell count is rare unless the patient had a low count before therapy.
2. To monitor for peripheral neuropathy, check deep tendon reflexes, sensory loss, gait abnormalities. Instruct the patient to report any unusual sensations, tingling, or numbness of the feet or hands.
3. In addition to constipation, this drug can cause paralytic ileus, especially in children. Keep a record of the frequency of bowel movements. Auscultate for the presence of bowel sounds before each meal.
4. The routine use of a stool softener, starting before the vincristine is administered, is usually necessary.

5. An unusual side effect that can occur with this drug is jaw pain.
6. Orthostatic hypotension can occur after long-term use. Caution patients to move slowly from lying to sitting or standing positions. If, on changing positions quickly, the patient feels dizzy or lightheaded, the patient should sit or lie down.
7. Extravasation should be avoided; see the patient care implications related to this problem.

Vinblastine

1. See the patient care implications for decreased white blood cell count, decreased platelet count, anemia, nausea and vomiting, stomatitis, diarrhea, constipation, and alopecia. The nadir for bone marrow suppression is 4 to 10 days after the last dose.
2. Orthostatic hypotension can occur after long-term use. Caution patients to move slowly from lying to sitting or standing positions. If, on changing positions quickly, the patient feels dizzy or lightheaded, the patient should sit or lie down.
3. Jaw pain can occur as an unusual side effect of this drug.
4. Extravasation should be avoided; see the patient care implications related to this problem.

Epipodophyllotoxins: VM-26 and VP-16

1. See the patient care implications for decreased white blood cell count, decreased platelet count, anemia, nausea and vomiting, diarrhea, alopecia, and stomatitis.
2. Peripheral neuropathy has been reported with these two drugs. Instruct the patient to report any numbness, tingling, or other unusual sensations of the fingers, hands, or feet.
3. Orthostatic hypotension has been reported. Instruct the patient to move slowly from a lying to sitting or standing position. If the patient feels dizzy or lightheaded on arising, the patient should sit or lie down. In the hospital, it might be appropriate to monitor the blood pressure.
4. Blood pressure should be taken every 15 minutes during the administration of either of these drugs.
5. Anaphylaxis can occur with VP-16. Epinephrine, corticosteroids, antihistamines, and oxygen should be readily available, as well as personnel, drugs, and equipment for resuscitation.
6. Phlebitis can occur with VM-26 administration.

Androgens and estrogens

Patient care implications for these categories of drugs are discussed in Chapters 37 and 38.

Tamoxifen

1. See the patient care implications for nausea and vomiting.
2. Decreases in the platelet count of 50,000 to 100,000 have been reported, but this is rarely associated with bleeding problems.
3. Hypercalcemia may occur, but this is usually in patients with bone metastases. Signs and symptoms include thirst, polyuria, anorexia, nausea and vomiting, constipation, lethargy, and, eventually, coma. Instruct the patient to notify the physician if any of these symptoms occur.
4. Other side effects include hot flashes and abnormal uterine bleeding. Instruct the patient to report any vaginal bleeding or discharge.
5. Fluid retention may be a problem. Have the patient check weight at regular intervals. Monitor the blood pressure.
6. At high doses, there may be retinal changes, eventually leading to areas of blindness. Before beginning therapy, the patient should have a visual field examination done and an ophthalmological examination on a yearly basis.

Progestins

These drugs are discussed in detail in Chapter 37.

Glucocorticoids

These drugs are discussed in detail in Chapter 35.

Mitotane

1. See the patient care implications for anorexia and nausea and vomiting.
2. Treatment with mitotane may cause drowsiness and decreased mental alertness. Caution patients to avoid hazardous activities requiring mental alertness (e.g., driving, operating machinery) until the effects of the drug can be evaluated.
3. Monitor the blood pressure every 4 hours for hypertension. Orthostatic hypotension can also occur. Instruct the patient to move slowly from lying to sitting or standing positions. Symptoms of hypotension include dizziness, lightheadedness, and syncope. If the patient feels dizzy, the patient should sit or lie down.
4. Visual side effects include blurring of vision, diplopia, and lens opacities. Caution the patient to report any visual changes. Test for visual acuity on a regular basis.

Streptozotocin

1. See the patient care implications for nausea and vomiting, decreased white blood cell count, decreased platelet count, and anemia. The nadir is variable.

2. Monitor the blood and urine sugar levels, as hyperglycemia has been reported. Diabetics may find it necessary to increase the dose of insulin or oral hypoglycemic agents while receiving therapy.
3. Renal damage may be a problem. Monitor the fluid intake and output. Monitor the BUN, serum creatinine, and urinary protein levels.
4. Extravasation may cause tissue necrosis; see the patient care implications for extravasation.

■ SUMMARY

Selective toxicity against cancer cells has been difficult to achieve since few exploitable differences exist between normal cells and most cancer cells. The most successfully exploited difference has been the fact that most cancer cells proliferate, whereas the cells in most normal tissues do not.

One major class of antineoplastic agents directly attacks cell DNA, chemically altering it so that cell division becomes impossible. Within this group of drugs are alkylating agents such as mechlorethamine, chlorambucil, melphalan, cyclophosphamide, thiotepa, carmustine, lomustine, dacarbazine, and mitomycin; agents that cross-link DNA, such as busulfan and cisplatin; and bleomycin, which causes a breakdown of DNA structure. As a group, these drugs attack cells at any stage in the cell cycle. All these drugs are also toxic against one or more normal tissues that proliferate rapidly: bone marrow, gastrointestinal epithelium, and hair follicles.

A second group of antineoplastic agents blocks DNA synthesis. Therefore these drugs prevent the duplication of cell chromosomes and halt cell division. Only those cells actively forming DNA will be sensitive to these drugs. Therefore tissues with high growth fractions (high percentage of cells undergoing division) will be most sensitive. Cancers tend to have higher fractions than most normal tissues. Drugs of this class include agents that inhibit enzymes used in DNA synthesis, such as cytarabine, fluorouracil, floxuridine, mercaptopurine, thioguanine, procarbazine, and hydroxyurea; and agents that block folic acid formation such as methotrexate. As a group, these drugs are toxic toward one or more normal tissues with high growth fractions: gastrointestinal epithelium and bone marrow.

A third group of antineoplastic agents blocks RNA and/or protein synthesis. These drugs are most effective during the phases of the cell cycle when most RNA synthesis occurs. Agents in this class may bind to DNA and prevent RNA formation (dactinomycin, doxorubicin, daunorubicin, and mithramycin). Asparaginase specifically slows protein synthesis in cancer cells by starving them for asparagine, an amino acid required by cancer cells but which may be formed internally by normal cells. Drugs of this class produce toxicity against gastrointestinal epithelium, bone marrow, and hair follicles. In addition, several members of this class are toxic toward specific organs such as the heart (doxorubicin, daunorubicin) and kidney (asparaginase).

The fourth group of antineoplastic agents block mitosis by binding to tubulin and preventing the formation of the mitotic spindle. Drugs in this class include vincristine and vinblastine, as well as the experimental agents VM-26 and VP-16. All these agents except vincristine cause bone marrow suppression. In addition, nausea and vomiting and hair loss are common reactions to these agents.

A fifth group of agents are useful in cancer chemotherapy because they possess a degree of tissue specificity. Hormones may be used to alter the growth of cells that possess receptors for the hormone. Androgens, estrogens, antiestrogens, progestins, and glucocorticoids have been used in this way. In addition, certain cell-specific toxins have been used. Mitotane specifically destroys the cortisol-synthesizing layers of the adrenal cortex. Streptozotocin specifically destroys the B cells of the pancreas. These agents may therefore be effective against tumors arising in these specific tissues.

■ STUDY QUESTIONS

1. What are the phases of the cell cycle, and what events take place during each phase?
2. What is carcinogenesis?
3. What properties of cancer cells allow them to spread through the body?
4. How does the growth fraction of most normal tissues differ from that of most tumors?
5. On what property of cancer cells does most cancer chemotherapy depend?
6. What is the mechanism of action of alkylating agents used as anticancer medications?
7. What normal cells are especially vulnerable to attack by alkylating agents?
8. What type of toxicity is characteristically associated with the use of alkylating agents?
9. Which of the alkylating agents is not a strong vesicant as administered because the drug must be activated by liver microsomal enzymes?
10. Which of the drugs that directly damage the structure of DNA does *not* produce bone marrow suppression?
11. What is the mechanism of action of anticancer agents that block purine and pyrimidine formation or utilization?
12. Why are inhibitors of purine and pyrimidine formation or utilization considered phase-specific agents?
13. What type of toxicity is characteristic of drugs that inhibit DNA synthesis?
14. Which of the drugs that inhibit DNA synthesis are used exclusively against solid tumors?
15. Which useful anticancer drug inhibits DNA synthesis by preventing the conversion of folic acid to tetrahydrofolate (THF)?

16. What is the basis of the anticancer effect of drugs that block RNA or protein synthesis?
17. What toxicity is characteristic of anticancer drugs that inhibit RNA or protein synthesis?
18. What properties of asparaginase make it unique among anticancer drugs?
19. Which of the anticancer drugs that inhibit RNA formation have special toxicity toward the heart?
20. What is the basis of the anticancer effects of drugs that disrupt microtubule formation?
21. What toxicity is characteristic of mitotic poisons?
22. Which of the mitotic poisons is not associated with bone marrow suppression?
23. What is the basis for the anticancer effects of hormones such as androgens, estrogens, progestins, and glucocorticoids?
24. What is the mechanism of action of tamoxifen?
25. Mitotane is effective against what specific type of cancer?
26. What is the rationale behind combination chemotherapy in the treatment of cancer?
27. Why is allopurinol frequently used in cancer treatment programs?
28. What principle governs the use of analgesics in treating cancer patients?
29. Why are antiemetics frequently used as adjuncts to cancer chemotherapy?
30. What is the rationale for using isotopes such as ^{32}P or ^{198}Au in cancer treatment programs?

■ SUGGESTED READINGS

Accola, K.M., and Sommerfeld, D.P.: Helping people with cancer consider parenthood, American Journal of Nursing **79:**1580, Sept., 1979.

Akahoshi, M.: High-dose methotrexate with leucovorin rescue, Cancer Nursing **1:**319, 1978.

Andrysiak, T., Carroll, R.M., and Ungerleider, J.T.: Marijuana for the oncology patient, American Journal of Nursing **79:**1396, Aug., 1979.

Barlock, A.L., Howser, D.M., and Hubbard, S.M.: Nursing management of Adriamycin extravasation, American Journal of Nursing **79:**94, Jan., 1979.

Bender, R.A., Zwelling, L.A., Doroshow, J.H., Locker, G.Y., Hande, K.R., Murinson, D.S., Cohen, M., Myers, C.E., and Chabner, B.A.: Antineoplastic drugs: clinical pharmacology and therapeutic use, Drugs **16:**46, 1978.

Bingham, C.A.: The cell cycle and cancer chemotherapy, American Journal of Nursing **78:**1200, July, 1978.

Bochow, A.J.: Cancer immunotherapy: what promise does it hold? Nursing **6**(10):50, 1976.

Burns, N.: Cancer chemotherapy: a systemic approach, Nursing **8**(2): 56, 1978.

Carter, S.K.: The changing role of adjuvant chemotherapy, Drug Therapy **10**(6):111, 1980.

Carter, S.K.: Cancer chemotherapy: new developments and changing concepts, Drugs **20:**375, 1980.

Daeffler, R.: Oral hygiene measures for patients with cancer, Cancer Nursing, Part 1 **3**(5):347, 1980; part 2 **3**(6):427, 1980.

Davis, T.E., and Carbone, P.P.: Drug treatment of breast cancer, Drugs **16:**441, 1978.

DeMoss, C.J.: Giving intravenous chemotherapy at home, American Journal of Nursing **80:**2188, Dec., 1980.

Dustin, P.: Microtubules, Scientific American **243**(2):67, 1980.

Ellington, O.B.: Cis-platinum: a brief review of its use and nursing guidelines, Cancer Nursing **1**(5):403, 1978.

Ellison, N.M.: Unproven methods of cancer therapy, Drug Therapy **10**(7):73, 1980.

Gever, L.N.: Cisplatin. A breakthrough for the cancer patient. A nursing challenge for you, Nursing **10**(12):53, 1980.

Heel, R.C., Brogden, R.N., Speight, T.M., and Avery, G.S.: Tamoxifen: a review of its pharmacological properties and therapeutic use in the treatment of breast cancer, Drugs **16:**1, 1978.

Helping cancer patients—effectively, Horsham, Pa., 1978, Intermed Communications, Inc.

Hoffman, D.M.: Bleomycin: a review of its use and guidelines for administration, Cancer Nursing **1**(4):335, 1978.

Houde, R.W.: Nonnarcotic alternatives for controlling cancer pain, Drug Therapy **10**(8):59, 1980.

Houde, R.W.: The rational use of narcotic analgesics for controlling cancer pain, Drug Therapy **10**(7):63, 1980.

Kellogg, C.J., and Sullivan, B.P., editors: Current perspectives in oncologic nursing, vol. 2, St. Louis, 1978, The C.V. Mosby Co.

Kelsen, D.P., and Yagoda, A.: Toxic effects of antineoplastic agents, Drug Therapy **10**(3):63, 1980.

Kennedy, B.J.: The encouraging outlook for breast cancer patients, Drug Therapy **10**(5):63, 1980.

Krakoff, I.H.: Principles of cancer chemotherapy, Drug Therapy **10**(3):47, 1980.

Levine, M.E.: Cancer chemotherapy—a nursing model, Nursing Clinics of North America **13**(2):271, 1978.

Levitt, D.Z.: Cancer chemotherapy. Those dreaded side effects and what to do about them. Alkylating agents, RN **43:**56, June, 1980; Antibiotics, RN **43:**50, Sept., 1980; Nitrosoureas, vinca alkaloids, hormones, RN **43:**33, Dec., 1980.

Mackey, C., and Hopefl, A.W.: Keeping infections down when risks go up, Nursing **10**(6):69, 1980.

Maxwell, M.B.: Scalp tourniquets for chemotherapy-induced alopecia, American Journal of Nursing **80:**900, May, 1980.

Nicolson, G.L.: Cancer metastasis, Scientific American **240**(3):66, 1979.

Nirenberg, A.: High dose methotrexate, American Journal of Nursing **76:**1776, Nov., 1976.

O'Connor, A.B., editor: Nursing: the oncology patient. Contemporary Nursing Series, New York, 1980, American Journal of Nursing Co.

Ostchega, Y.: Preventing and treating cancer chemotherapy's oral complications, Nursing **10**(8):47, 1980.

Reich, S.D.: Daunorubicin: a brief review, Cancer Nursing **3**(6):465, 1980.

Satterwhite, B.E.: What to do when Adriamycin infiltrates, Nursing **10**(2):37, 1980.

Schwartz, M.K.: Breast cancer. Alternative therapy. Hormone receptor assay, American Journal of Nursing **77:**1445, Sept., 1977.

Scogna, D.M., and Smalley, R.V.: Chemotherapy-induced nausea and vomiting, American Journal of Nursing **79:**1562, Sept., 1979.

Stewart, C.: Current concepts of chemotherapy for brain tumors, Journal of Neurosurgical Nursing **12:**97, June, 1980.

Swartz, A.J.: Adriamycin: a review of its use and guidelines for administration, Cancer Nursing **1**(2):169, 1978.

Swartz, A.J.: Chemotherapy extravasation management. Part 1. Doxorubicin (adriamycin), Cancer Nursing **2**(5):405, 1979.

Van Scoy-Mosher, M.B.: Chemotherapy: a manual for patients and their families, Cancer Nursing **1**(3):234, 1978.

Welch, D., and Lewis, K.: Alopecia and chemotherapy, American Journal of Nursing **80:**903, May, 1980.

Willson, J.K.V., and Young, R.C.: Rising expectations for chemotherapy in gynecologic malignancies, Drug Therapy **10**(5):47, 1980.

Yagoda, A.: Chemotherapy of genitourinary tumors, Drug Therapy **10**(6):94, 1980.

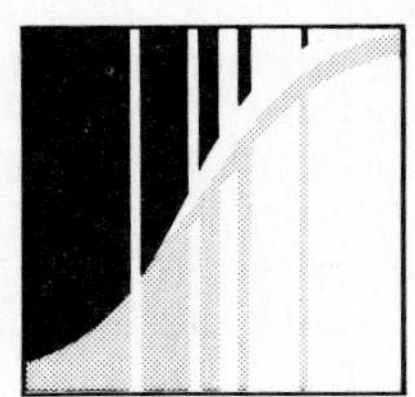

Index

C

F

J

K

L

M

O

P

S

T

W

X

Y

Z

Jim
Switzer
6365790

Pharmacological basis of nursing practice